Diseases of the Kidney

Diseases of the Kidney

SECOND EDITION

Editors

Maurice B. Strauss, M.D.
Professor of Medicine and Associate Dean,
Tufts University School of Medicine, Boston

Louis G. Welt, M.D.
Alumni Distinguished Professor and Chairman,
Department of Medicine, University of North Carolina
School of Medicine, Chapel Hill

By 59 Authors

Volume I

Little, Brown and Company
Boston

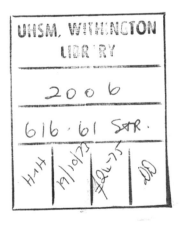

Contents

Volume I

v

Volume II

Contents

Preface to the Second Edition

In the preface to the first edition of *Diseases of the Kidney* (1963), reprinted in this edition, we commented on the impossibility of a single author's being able to embrace the entire area of renal disease, as a result of which a multiauthored text became obligatory. At that time it seemed entirely feasible to cover the consequences of renal failure and their management in a single chapter. The expansion of knowledge in the ensuing years has now made it necessary to subdivide this topic so that appropriate experts could discuss the general metabolic, hematopoietic, neurologic, and osseous consequences of renal insufficiency. The peculiarities of renal disease in children have made it advisable to add a separate chapter on pediatric nephrology for special consideration. We may well ask "Where will it all end?" and fervently hope that the development of unifying hypotheses in biology will bring order and simplification to the ever-increasing body of knowledge.

Other new chapters include those on atheroembolic renal disease, kidney transplantation, and the immunologic and genetic aspects of transplantation. Renal biopsy now deserves a separate chapter. One chapter has been eliminated; the use of an ileal conduit rather than a sigmoid bladder for urinary diversion has minimized the adverse effects often encountered with the latter procedure and rendered the topic one of historical rather than of current interest. We hope that future editions may see additional chapters eliminated for similar reasons.

With two exceptions, every chapter has been thoroughly revised, some by new authors. In the rapidly changing field of nephrology, only the areas involving the ultrastructure of the kidney and congenital malformations have remained relatively static. To the new authors, as well as to those who have so painstakingly revised their chapters, we can but repeat what we said in the preface to the first edition. This is their book, not ours, and the thanks of all those concerned with renal disease are due them for making this vast amount of learning available in these two volumes. Neither the binding nor the arms or chest of the reader would have withstood the weight of a single volume!

Numerous colleagues made important suggestions for the improvements embodied in this edition. We invite your suggestions for future editions.

Boston   M. B. S.
Chapel Hill   L. G. W.

Preface to the First Edition

The need for a critical and comprehensive clinical text dealing with diseases of the kidney has been manifest for many years. The growth of knowledge in this area in recent decades has been stupendous, and excellent monographs on one or another topic within the field have been published, but no single volume to which the student and clinician could turn for complete coverage has been available.

That this volume is multiauthored hardly requires comment. The day of Francis Bacon, when one man could embrace all human knowledge, is long past. Even if one author could encompass all of renal disease, the Herculean nature of the task would require so many years that the first chapter would be outdated long before the last was complete.

The editors have been most fortunate in obtaining the cooperation of a distinguished group of authorities who have labored long and assiduously in the compilation of this volume. We have thanked them individually and privately for their contributions. Now we wish to spread our appreciation on the written record. This is their book, not ours. The excellence of their individual chapters has made our editorial task light. We are profoundly grateful to them, and we know that both students of renal disease and those charged with the care of patients will share our gratitude that this vast amount of learning is now available in a single, if weighty, volume.

Finally we wish to express our appreciation to Miss Margaret F. Mutch, of Little, Brown and Company, who has succeeded in converting a multi-authored text into a cohesive whole without sacrificing the individual style of the separate contributors.

Boston	M. B. S.
Chapel Hill	L. G. W.

Contributing Authors

D. Bernard Amos, M.D.
James B. Duke Professor of Immunology and
Experimental Surgery, Duke University School
of Medicine, Durham, North Carolina
CHAPTER 43

Henry L. Barnett, M.D.
Professor and Chairman, Department of Pediatrics,
Albert Einstein College of Medicine of Yeshiva
University; Director of Pediatrics,
Bronx Municipal Hospital,
Bronx, New York
CHAPTER 42

Robert W. Berliner, M.D.
Deputy Director for Science, National Institutes
of Health, Bethesda, Maryland
CHAPTER 2

Lewis W. Bluemle, Jr., M.D.
President, State University of New York Upstate
College of Medicine; Attending Physician,
Upstate Medical Center, Syracuse
CHAPTER 10

William B. Blythe, M.D.
Professor, Department of Medicine,
University of North Carolina School of
Medicine; Attending Physician, North
Carolina Memorial Hospital,
Chapel Hill
CHAPTER 24

XV

Neal S. Bricker, M.D.
Professor and Chairman, Department of Medicine,
Albert Einstein College of Medicine
of Yeshiva University,
Bronx, New York
CHAPTER 27

Maurice B. Burg, M.D.
Head, Unit on Renal Transport, National
Institutes of Health, Bethesda, Maryland
CHAPTER 38

Norman W. Carter, M.D.
Associate Professor of Internal Medicine,
The University of Texas Southwestern
Medical School at Dallas
CHAPTER 6

Jacob Churg, M.D.
Professor of Pathology, Mount Sinai School of
Medicine of the City University of New York,
New York; Pathologist, Barnet Memorial
Hospital Center, Paterson, New Jersey
CHAPTER 22

O. Z. Dalgaard, M.D.
Medical Director, De Gamles By,
Copenhagen, Denmark
CHAPTER 35

Henry Dolger, M.D.
Clinical Professor of Medicine, Mount Sinai School
of Medicine of the City University of New York;
Attending Physician and Chief, Diabetes Clinic,
Mount Sinai Hospital, New York
CHAPTER 22

Chester M. Edelmann, Jr., M.D.
Professor of Pediatrics, Albert Einstein
College of Medicine of Yeshiva University;
Director of Pediatric Nephrology,
Bronx Municipal Hospital Center,
Bronx, New York
CHAPTER 42

R. H. Egdahl, M.D.
Chairman, Department of Surgery, Boston
University School of Medicine;
Surgeon-in-Chief, University
Hospital, Boston
CHAPTER 44

Franklin H. Epstein, M.D.
Director, Harvard Medical Services,
Boston City Hospital
CHAPTER 24

A. J. Erslev, M.D.
Cardeza Research Professor of Medicine and
Director, Cardeza Foundation for Hematologic
Research, Jefferson Medical College;
Attending Physician, Thomas Jefferson
University Hospital, Philadelphia
CHAPTER 7

Alfred J. Fish, M.D.
Assistant Professor of Pediatrics, University of
Minnesota School of Medicine, Minneapolis;
Established Investigator, American
Heart Association
CHAPTER 11

Lawrence R. Freedman, M.D.
Professor of Medicine, Yale University School of
Medicine, New Haven
CHAPTER 18

Robert A. Good, M.D.
American Legion Memorial Heart Research
Professor of Pediatrics and Microbiology,
University of Minnesota School of
Medicine, Minneapolis
CHAPTER 11

J. Hartwell Harrison, M.D.
Cutler Professor of Surgery, Harvard Medical
School; Chief of Urology, Peter Bent
Brigham Hospital, Boston
CHAPTER 41

A. McGehee Harvey, M.D.
Professor and Director, Department of Medicine,
The Johns Hopkins University School
of Medicine; Physician-in-Chief,
The Johns Hopkins Hospital,
Baltimore
CHAPTER 21

Joseph M. Hayman, Jr., M.D.
Dean Emeritus, Tufts University School
of Medicine, Boston
CHAPTER 39

R. H. Heptinstall, M.D.
Professor and Director, Department of Pathology,
The Johns Hopkins University School of
Medicine; Pathologist to The Johns
Hopkins Hospital, Baltimore
CHAPTERS 12, 14

Walter Hollander, Jr., M.D.
Associate Professor of Medicine, University of
North Carolina School of Medicine,
Chapel Hill
CHAPTER 25

Jerome P. Kassirer, M.D.
Associate Professor of Medicine, Tufts University
School of Medicine; Physician, Renal Department,
New England Medical Center Hospitals,
Boston
CHAPTERS 13, 28

Saulo Klahr, M.D.
Associate Professor of Medicine, Washington
University School of Medicine; Attending
Physician, Barnes Hospital, St. Louis;
Established Investigator,
American Heart Association
CHAPTER 27

Norman G. Levinsky, M.D.
Physician-in-Chief and Director, Evans
Department of Clinical Research,
University Hospital; Chairman of the
Division of Medicine, Boston University
School of Medicine, Boston
CHAPTER 3

Reginald William Luxton, M.D., F.R.C.P.
Honorary Lecturer in Medicine, University of
Manchester Faculty of Medicine; Consultant
Physician, Christie Hospital and Holt Radium
Institute, Manchester, England
CHAPTER 29

Carl B. Lyle, Jr., M.D.
Associate Professor of Medicine, University of
North Carolina School of Medicine;
Attending Physician, North Carolina
Memorial Hospital, Chapel Hill
CHAPTER 33

Edward M. Mahoney, M.D.
Associate in Surgery, Harvard Medical School;
Associate, Urologic Surgery, Peter Bent
Brigham Hospital, Boston
CHAPTER 41

J. A. Mannick, M.D.

Professor of Surgery, Boston University School
of Medicine; Visiting Surgeon,
University Hospital, Boston

CHAPTER 44

John P. Merrill, M.D.

Professor of Medicine, Harvard Medical School;
Director, Cardiorenal Section, Peter Bent
Brigham Hospital, Boston

CHAPTER 17

Alfred F. Michael, M.D.

Professor of Pediatrics, University of Minnesota
School of Medicine, Minneapolis

CHAPTER 11

Malcolm D. Milne, M.D.

Professor of Medicine, Westminster Hospital
Medical School, London, England

CHAPTER 30

Olle Olsson, M.D.

Professor and Chairman, Department of Diagnostic
Radiology, University of Lund; Medical Director,
University Hospital, Lund, Sweden

CHAPTER 4

Jack Orloff, M.D.

Chief, Laboratory of Kidney and Electrolyte
Metabolism, National Heart and Lung
Institute, National Institutes of Health,
Bethesda, Maryland

CHAPTER 38

Solomon Papper, M.D.

Professor of Medicine, University of Colorado
School of Medicine; Chairman, Department
of Medicine, General Rose Memorial
Hospital, Denver

CHAPTERS 19, 31

Gerald T. Perkoff, M.D.

Professor of Medicine, Preventive Medicine, and
Public Health and Director, Division of Health
Care Research, Washington University School
of Medicine; Associate Director, Private
Medical Service, Barnes Hospital,
St. Louis

CHAPTERS 34, 37

Floyd C. Rector, Jr., M.D.

Professor of Internal Medicine, The University of
Texas Southwestern Medical School
at Dallas

CHAPTER 6

Arnold S. Relman, M.D.

Frank Wister Thomas Professor of Medicine and
Chairman, Department of Medicine, University of
Pennsylvania School of Medicine; Chief of the
Medical Services, Hospital of the University
of Pennsylvania

CHAPTERS 3, 15

Johannes A. G. Rhodin, M.D., Ph.D.

Chairman and Professor, Department of Anatomy,
New York Medical College, New York

CHAPTER 1

George E. Schreiner, M.D., F.A.C.P.

Professor of Medicine, Georgetown University
School of Medicine; Director, Renal and Electrolyte
Division, Georgetown University Hospital,
Washington, D.C.

CHAPTERS 5, 16

William B. Schwartz, M.D.

Endicott Professor and Chairman, Department of
Medicine, Tufts University School of Medicine;
Physician-in-Chief, New England Medical
Center Hospitals, Boston

CHAPTER 13

Donald W. Seldin, M.D.

William Buchanan Professor of Medicine
and Chairman, Department of Medicine,
The University of Texas Southwestern
Medical School at Dallas; Chief of
Internal Medicine Service, Parkland
Memorial Hospital, Dallas

CHAPTER 6

S. S. Shapiro, M.D.

Associate Professor of Medicine, Cardeza
Foundation for Hematologic Research,
Jefferson Medical College; Assistant
Attending Physician in Medicine,
Thomas Jefferson University Hospital,
Philadelphia

CHAPTER 7

Ethan A. H. Sims, M.D.

Professor of Medicine and Director, Metabolic
Unit, Department of Medicine, University of
Vermont College of Medicine; Attending
Physician, Medical Center Hospital
of Vermont, Burlington

CHAPTER 32

William S. Sly, M.D.

Associate Professor of Pediatrics and Medicine,
Washington University School of Medicine;
Attending Physician and Director,
Division of Medical Genetics,
St. Louis Children's and Barnes
Hospitals, St. Louis

CHAPTER 34

Lloyd H. Smith, Jr., M.D.

Professor of Medicine, University of California
School of Medicine; Physician-in-Chief of
Medical Staff, University of California
Hospitals, San Francisco

CHAPTER 26

S. W. Stanbury, M.D., F.R.C.P.

Professor of Medicine, University of Manchester
Faculty of Medicine, England

CHAPTER 8

Maurice B. Strauss, M.D.

Professor of Medicine and Associate Dean,
Tufts University School of Medicine,
Boston

CHAPTER 36

Frank H. Tyler, M.D.

Professor of Medicine, University of Utah College
of Medicine; Physician, University Hospital,
Salt Lake City

CHAPTER 23

H. Richard Tyler, M.D.

Associate Clinical Professor of Neurology,
Harvard Medical School, Boston

CHAPTER 9

Carlos A. Vaamonde, M.D.

Associate Professor of Medicine, University
of Miami School of Medicine,
Coral Gables, Florida

CHAPTERS 19, 31

W. Gordon Walker, M.D.

Professor of Medicine, The Johns Hopkins
University School of Medicine; Physician,
The Johns Hopkins Hospital,
Baltimore

CHAPTER 21

Herman Wechsler, M.D.

Clinical Associate Professor of Urology, Albert
Einstein College of Medicine of Yeshiva
University; Attending Urologist, Veterans
Administration Hospital,
Bronx, New York

CHAPTER 40

Louis G. Welt, M.D.

Professor and Chairman, Department of
Internal Medicine, Yale University
School of Medicine, New Haven

CHAPTER 33

Hibbard E. Williams, M.D.

Associate Professor of Medicine, University of
California School of Medicine; Chief, Division of
Medical Genetics, University of California
Medical Center, San Francisco

CHAPTER 26

T. Franklin Williams, M.D.

Professor of Medicine, University of Rochester
School of Medicine and Dentistry; Medical
Director, Monroe Community Hospital,
Rochester, New York

CHAPTER 20

James W. Woods, M.D.

Professor, Department of Medicine, University of
North Carolina School of Medicine; Attending
Physician, North Carolina Memorial
Hospital, Chapel Hill

CHAPTER 20

John H. Yardley, M.D.
Associate Professor of Pathology, The Johns
Hopkins University School of Medicine;
Pathologist, The Johns Hopkins Hospital,
Baltimore
CHAPTER 21

Diseases of the Kidney

I

Structure of the Kidney

Johannes A. G. Rhodin

The *general architecture* of the mammalian kidney is well known and can be reviewed in any textbook of anatomy. Current concepts of the structure of the renal tissue, the histology of the nephron (Fig. 1-1) and some of the recent findings concerning its fine structure have been most knowledgeably compiled in the textbook of histology by Ham and Leeson [17]. Reviews of the normal ultrastructure have been presented by Mueller [27] on the glomerulus, and by Rhodin [35, 36] on the tubules. Electron microscopic studies of renal biopsies from the diseased kidney have been published by Farquhar [8, 9] and Bergstrand [3]. The histochemistry of the nephron has been reviewed by Wachstein [49] and Forster [11]. The article by Forster also deals with a variety of technics which have been used to clarify the structure and function of kidney cells, and is a most valuable source of condensed information for anyone interested in these aspects.

This chapter deals with the most recent findings related to the ultrastructure of the nephron. By presenting a series of low magnification electron micrographs, it is also intended to bridge the gap between light and electron microscopy in order to facilitate understanding of high magnification electron micrographs published in this book and elsewhere. The mouse kidney has been used almost exclusively in this series because of the convenience in obtaining specimens. However, there is basically little difference between the ultrastructure of the nephron in mouse kidney and in human kidney [4].

The tissue was prepared according to currently accepted technics for electron microscopy. The specimens were fixed in buffered osmium tetroxide and dehydrated in a graded series of alcohols. For low power surveys, the tissue blocks were embedded in methacrylates, and for detailed high power studies Epon was used as the embedding medium. All sections were cut with the LKB Ultrotome, and the electron microscopy was done with the Siemens Elmiskop I. The Epon sections were stained with lead hydroxide.

Glomerulus

The glomerulus is essentially a richly branched and interconnected capillary network (Fig. 1-2) which is indented at the

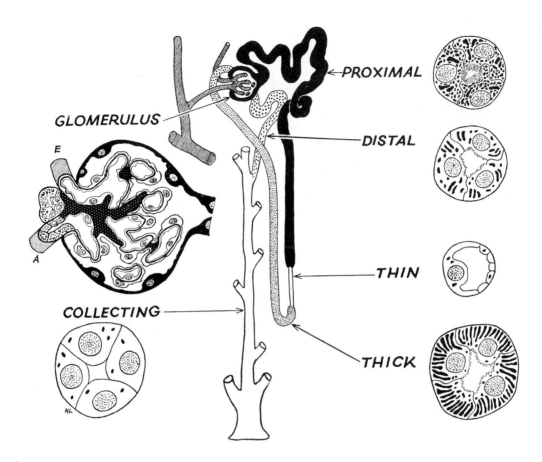

Figure 1-1. A simple diagram outlining the general histologic features of the mammalian nephron as studied in the mouse kidney. The afferent (A) and efferent (E) arterioles of the glomerulus split up and divide around the glomerular stalk (mesangium). The cross sections of the various segments of the tubule indicate roughly the size, distribution, and organization of the mitochondria based on electron microscopy.

beginning of the tubular duct. The word indentation, however, is used merely to explain the features of the glomerulus rather than to describe the actual process as it occurs during the development of the glomerulus. According to an earlier concept, the capillaries were thought to indent the Bowman's capsule by growing into the blind bulbous expansion at the beginning of the renal tubule. Recently, electron microscopic investigations [16, 17] have demonstrated that the glomerular capillaries develop in situ; i.e., a mass of mesenchymal cells differentiates into capillary endothelial cells. Only one cell type

seems to maintain its original mesenchymal structural and functional features [47]. This is the so-called mesangial cell (see below).

AFFERENT ARTERIOLE

The wall of the afferent arteriole is composed of endothelial cells, smooth muscle cells which form a distinct media, and a few pericytes investing the media with an incomplete cell layer (Fig. 1-3). At a distance of about 30 to 50 microns before the afferent arteriole enters the glomerulus at the vascular pole, the muscular cells of the media change their character of being purely muscle cells. Large,

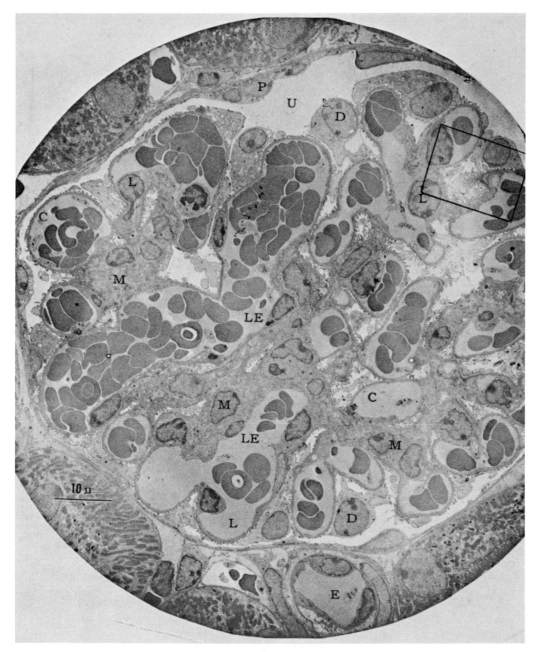

Figure 1-2. Survey of an entire renal corpuscle of the mouse kidney, surrounded by the capsule of Bowman. The glomerulus consists of richly branched capillaries (C) with intensely black-stained erythrocytes in their lumina. The two large capillaries (LE) represent the intraglomerular origin of the efferent arteriole (E) seen outside the renal corpuscle. The parietal layer of Bowman's capsule (P) consists of simple squamous cells, whereas the visceral layer is formed by podocytes (D) with numerous and elongated thin processes, the pedicels, which interdigitate and attach at the surface of the capillaries. Between the parietal and visceral layers is the urinary space of Bowman's capsule (U). The capillaries are lined with endothelial cells (L) which rest on a continuous basement membrane. Mesangial cells (M) are located in the centrolobular regions of the capillary tufts. The boxed-in area is enlarged in Figure 1-5, and the efferent arteriole (E) can be seen magnified in Figure 1-11. ×1500.

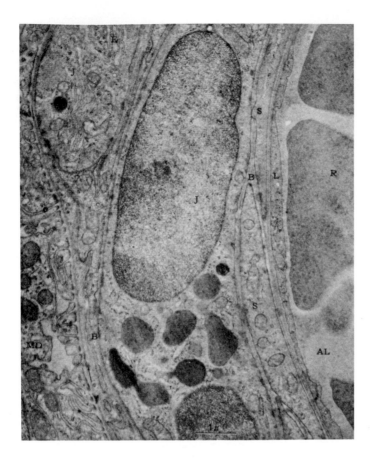

Figure 1-3. Detail of the wall of the afferent arteriole of the mouse glomerulus. The innermost layer next to the arteriolar lumen (AL) with red cells (R) is the thin endothelium (L). The main part of the vascular wall consists of ordinary smooth muscle cells (S) with delicate myofilaments and microvesicles as well as transformed muscle cells, the juxtaglomerular cells (J) with large secretory granules and sacs of rough-surfaced endoplasmic reticulum (E). Basement membranes (B) are interwoven within the arteriolar wall. Adjoining the juxtaglomerular cells is the basal part of some macula densa cells (MD) of the distal segment. The plasma membrane of the macula densa cells shows shallow infoldings. A distinct basement membrane (*arrows*), which is part of the continuous tubular basement membrane, separates the macula densa and the juxtaglomerular cells. ×11,000.

extremely electron-dense granules appear in the cytoplasm together with an increased amount of rough-surfaced endoplasmic reticulum [28]. The fine structure of the granules in these cells resembles that which characterizes secretory granules of glands elsewhere in the body. From a structural point of view, it is evident that the smooth muscle cell has been transformed into a secretory cell with a fair amount of endoplasmic reticulum with attached submicroscopic ribonucleoprotein (RNP) particles and numerous large granules of the secretory type. These cells have been called juxtaglomerular (JG) or epithelioid cells.

It has been suggested that the juxtaglomerular cells play a role in the production of the hormone renin [18]. If the large granules represent the structural precursor of renin,

their content cannot be discharged directly into the arteriolar lumen, because of the intervening endothelial lining. Supposedly, it reaches the bloodstream by diffusion, like other endocrine products. It has also been suggested that the granules of the juxtaglomerular cells may contain a hormone which regulates the amount of sodium in the bloodstream. When the sodium concentration is high, the juxtaglomerular cells become degranulated, whereas a reduced sodium concentration leads to an accumulation of granules in these cells.

GLOMERULAR CAPILLARIES

Just beyond the point at which it penetrates the parietal layer of Bowman's capsule, the afferent arteriole gives off several main capil-

Figure 1-4. Medium power election micrograph of capillaries in the mouse glomerulus. Epithelial cells (D) are located at the capillary surface in the urinary space of Bowman's capsule (U), which in turn is surrounded by the parietal layer of Bowman's capsule (P). Endothelial cells (L) line the inside of the capillaries with thin cytoplasmic sheaths. In the centrolobular region is evident a mesangial cell nucleus (Mn) with the mesangial cell cytoplasm (Mc) spreading out irregularly, and tying together at least seven capillary loops (C1–C7). *Arrows* point to strands of dense mesangial matrix. ×4000.

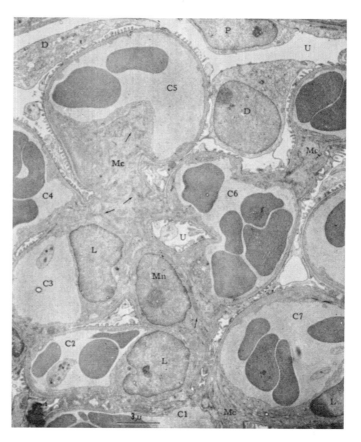

laries [14]. The capillary walls are composed of three layers (Fig. 1-4). The endothelial cells form the innermost layer and represent a direct continuation of the endothelium found in the afferent arteriole. A homogeneous, uninterrupted basement membrane establishes the middle component of the capillary wall, and the outside of the capillaries is covered by a layer of epithelial cells, which constitutes the visceral layer of Bowman's capsule (Fig. 1-5). A fourth component is also noted among the capillary loops. This is the mesangial cell, which also has been referred to as the intercapillary or intraluminal or deep endothelial cell [10, 19]. This cell is quite common in the avian glomerulus. It can easily be identified in the mouse and rat glomeruli but with less success in the normal human glomerulus. However, in the diseased human kidney it seems to be quite abundant.

Endothelium. The endothelium is formed by squamous endothelial cells which display a local protrusion into the capillary lumen in the vicinity of the nucleus (Fig. 1-5). The cytoplasm around the nucleus has a few mitochondria, a small Golgi apparatus, a varying number of RNP particles, and small vesicles of the type normally present in capillary endothelium elsewhere in the body. The attenuated portion of the endothelial cell, which is quite large, displays numerous round fenestrations with an average width of 600 angstroms (A). Each fenestra is bridged over by a thin diaphragm which measures 70A in thickness. A central knob-like structure is identified in the diaphragm (Fig. 1-6B).

Basement Membrane. The basement membrane forms a central continuous structure of the capillary wall (Fig. 1-5). It has an average thickness of about 800A in the mouse and is

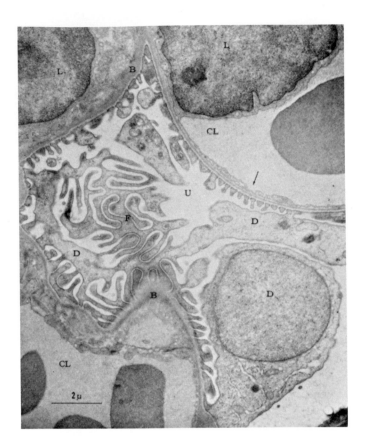

Figure 1-5. Detail of the elaborate interdigitation of epithelial (D) foot processes (F) as they attach at the capillary basement membrane (B). A perfectly perpendicular section of the capillary wall is seen at the *arrow* (compare with Figure 1-6) and a grazing section of a similar region occupies the left center of the picture. The endothelial cell (L) cytoplasm is spreading along the luminal part of the capillary wall. The capillary lumen (CL) shows a higher density than the urinary space (U). ×7000.

thicker in humans [4], in whom it averages 1200A. There is no consensus as to whether the basement membrane has a layered structure with a central dense zone and a less dense layer on either side. It has been suggested that this subdivision may be due to preparation artifacts, but it cannot be excluded that there is a true structural background to the layering. On the basis of observations made in tissue preparations which have been embedded in Epon, I favor the latter opinion. This embedding medium has proved to be most gentle to delicate cell components, and there is no reason to believe that the basement membrane of the glomerular capillaries is an exception. Whether the basement membrane is layered or not, it has been proposed that it is composed of short, delicate filaments arranged in an irregular meshwork similar to a filter paper. This is, however, an inconstant observation

and requires further investigation. All basement membranes of mammalian tissues are seen to have fine reticular filaments associated with the surface that faces the connective tissue space, but not attached at the surface which borders on a cell membrane. In the case of the glomerular capillaries, both sides of the basement membrane face cell membranes, and it should therefore not be expected that reticular filaments would be present.

Epithelium. The glomerular capillaries are covered by the visceral layer of Bowman's capsule. The layer is composed of epithelial cells that have developed from the inner layer of the metanephrogenic cells. The cells are of the cuboidal type, but shortly after birth they acquire a squamous shape as the capillaries grow, branch, and interconnect. The nucleus of the mature epithelial cell is surrounded by a fairly large amount of cytoplasm in which lie the

Figure 1-6. Detail of the glomerular capillary wall. A. The epithelial part of the glomerular capillary wall, with the urinary space of Bowman's capsule (U), the foot processes of the podocytes (F), and half of the basement membrane (M). B. The capillary part with the same basement membrane (M) as in A, and the thin endothelium (L) facing the capillary lumen (CL). The slit pores between the foot processes (F) are closed by a thin single membrane in which a central thickening can be distinguished (*arrows*). Note that the foot processes are completely surrounded by the triple-layered plasma membrane of the epithelial cells. The fenestrations of the endothelial cell (L) are closed by a diaphragm in which a central knob can be seen (*arrows*). A, ×75,000; B, ×70,000.

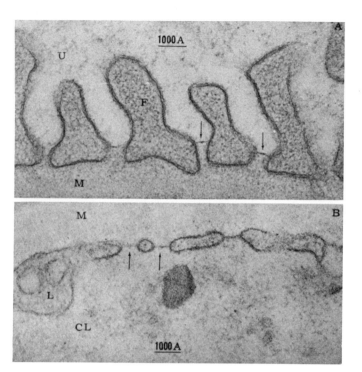

Golgi zone and the rough-surfaced endoplasmic reticulum. Several short mitochondria and a large number of vesicular components are found throughout the cytoplasm in addition to numerous RNP particles. Furthermore, the cytoplasm is traversed by fine filaments of varying length. This is particularly the case within the long cell processes, the podocytes, which extend over the capillaries. The podocytes in turn are subdivided into numerous small and narrow processes, the foot processes (or pedicels), which interdigitate with similar structures of the same cell and/or a neighboring epithelial cell (Fig. 1-5). The foot processes have a wide base which rests on the basement membrane and becomes narrower away from the basement membrane. The area between the foot processes, usually referred to as the slit pore, has an average width of about 400A although the claim has been made [15] that it can have a width of about 100A. This area is bridged by a membrane 70A thick, the so-called filtration slit membrane [50], in which

is found a filamentous central thickening or reinforcement (Fig. 1-6A).

Mesangium. Mesangium is a collective word for the dense arrangement of cells and branches of the capillary basement membrane that is located centrally in the capillary tufts (Fig. 1-4). The cells are also termed intercapillary [19] or deep endothelial cells [10]. They correspond to the cells which first were recognized by Zimmermann [53], who also suggested the name mesangial cells.

Structurally, the nucleus and the cytoplasm of the mesangial cell are almost identical with those of an endothelial cell, except in one respect. The mesangial cell cytoplasm displays a multitude of short and complicated processes which are surrounded by a material resembling basement membrane, the mesangial matrix [47]. The matrix consists of an amorphous substance which fills the irregular spaces between the mesangial cells and other structural elements such as capillary endothelial cells and the true capillary basement membrane. The

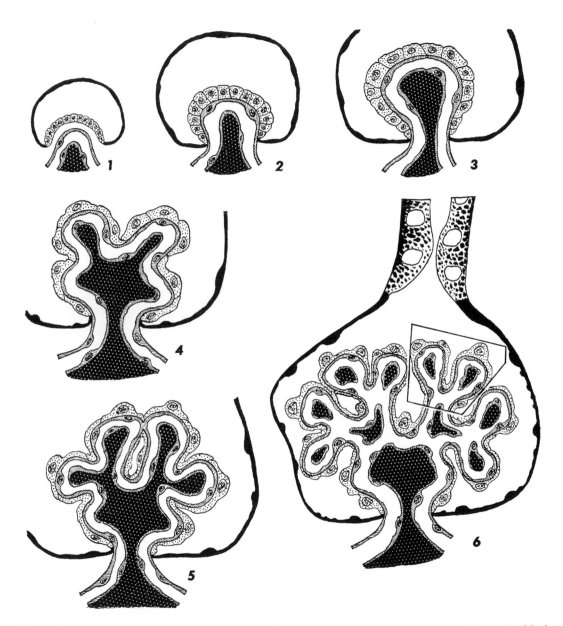

Figure 1-7. A series demonstrating the role and fate of the developing mesenchymal anlage cells (*dark-stippled*), the capillary endothelium (*crosshatched*), the inner layer of the metanephrogenic cells (*light-stippled*), and the parietal layer of Bowman's capsule (*solid black*). It is believed that the anlage cells give rise to the endothelial cells of the capillaries, which in turn gradually grow and branch (1–5). When the glomerulus reaches maturity, the development of anlage cells to capillary endothelium comes to an end, but the anlage cells are still present in the center of the capillary tufts, now termed mesangial cells (6). The boxed-in area is carried over to Figure 1-8 and there represented three-dimensionally. The interpretation of these developments is based on the electron microscopic investigations by Suzuki [47] and the light microscopic investigations by Lewis [20].

mesangial cell is in places incompletely enveloped by the mesangial matrix. The cytoplasmic processes, therefore, can be seen bordering directly on the capillary endothelial cell and in some instances, as pointed out by Yamada [50], even penetrate the endothelial cell to form so-called intracapillary colliculi. Because of the incomplete basement membrane, it is easy to mistake a mesangial cell for an endothelial cell, particularly since the cytoplasm in both cell types is so similar.

In 1933, Zimmermann [53] advanced the hypothesis that the mesangial cell represents a fibrocyte. Strong support for this idea is found in certain diseases in which reticular and collagen fibrils are laid down within the centrolobular region of the glomerular tufts. It is therefore likely that we are dealing with a connective tissue component located or trapped within the glomerular capillaries. This belief is strengthened even more when one considers the embryologic development of the mesangium as studied with electron microscopy (Fig. 1-7). According to Suzuki [47], an aggregation of cells, the so-called glomerular anlage cells, appears quite early between the primitive renal tubule and the inner layer of the metanephrogenic vesicle. The anlage cells are of mesenchymal origin. Blood channels form in the spaces between the anlage cells, and the cells flatten and become endothelial

cells. The glomerular anlage cells continue to proliferate and successively differentiate into endothelial cells, creating new blood cavities. This development of capillary ramifications [20] continues up to the period of glomerular maturity, when the differentiation of anlage cells to endothelial cells ceases and a definite change occurs in the structure of the anlage cells. The anlage cells now surround themselves with a basement membrane-like material, the mesangial matrix, and take up the role of supporting the blood cavities as intercapillary or mesangial cells.

In the mature glomerulus, the mesangial cell is to be regarded as a cell of mesenchymal origin which remains in its intercapillary location in a resting state (Fig. 1-8). Whenever there is a need for expansion of the capillary bed, the mesangial cells most probably are called upon to develop into endothelial cells and, therefore, be of great usefulness. However, less attractive abilities of the mesangial cell may be evoked, as under certain pathologic conditions [51], when the mesangial cell starts to lay down connective tissue elements such as an abundance of basement membranous material, or reticular or collagen fibrils, or when it starts to multiply and form a huge centrolobular mass of fibrocytic cells none of which easily can be said to be an endothelial or a mesangial type of cell.

Figure 1-8. A simplified three-dimensional presentation of small capillary tufts within the glomerulus of the mouse kidney. The cutaways are intended to demonstrate the means by which the mesangial or intercapillary cells (*dark-stippled*) are trapped in the center of the branching and interconnecting capillaries. The boxed-in area is carried over to Figure 1-9.

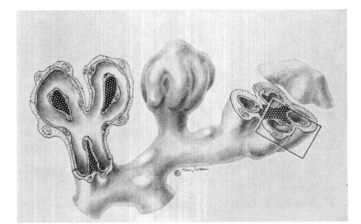

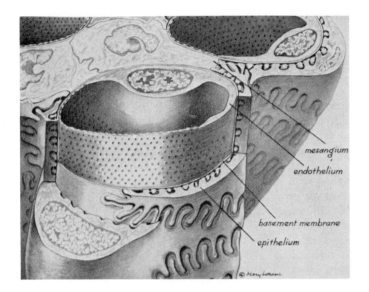

Figure 1-9. A three-dimensional representation of the fine structure and relationship between the mesangial cells and the basement membrane of the capillaries on the one hand, and between the capillary endothelium, the basement membrane, and the interdigitating epithelial cells on the other hand. The basement membrane can be incomplete as it borders on the mesangial (intercapillary) cells, although the diagram does not show this possibility. The fenestrations of the endothelium and the slits between the interdigitating foot processes of the epithelium are closed by a thin membrane, as indicated in Figure 1-10.

Functional Considerations Related to Filtration. The glomerular filtration membrane has three components: endothelium, basement membrane, and epithelium (Fig. 1-9). Until recently, it was considered that only one of these components, the basement membrane, represented a continuous, uninterrupted layer. The others were believed to have holes of two kinds: the endothelial pores were round, with an average diameter of about 600A, whereas the openings in the epithelial layer were elongated slits, with a minimum width of about 100A [13, 14, 31, 32, 34].

According to our current structural knowledge of the glomerular filtration membrane, the basement membrane is still to be regarded as a continuous layer in which no pores can be detected. Sitte [40] advanced the theory

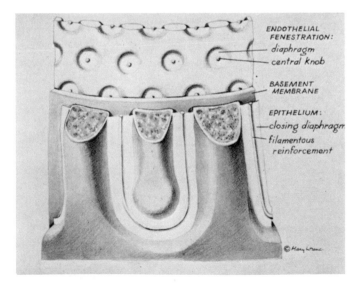

Figure 1-10. Detail of the glomerular capillary filtration membrane studied in the mouse kidney by electron microscopy of tissue fixed in buffered osmium tetroxide, embedded in Epon and stained with lead hydroxide. The thin part of the endothelium contains fenestrations which are closed by a thin diaphragm with a central knob-like structure. The basement membrane runs continuously as the central component. Three foot processes of the epithelial layer are shown. The spaces between the processes, the slit pores, are spanned by a thin membrane with a centrally located filamentous reinforcement. It is believed that in both epithelium and endothelium the closing membrane is derived from the plasma membrane of respective cells.

that the basement membrane could be compared to a filter paper composed of a feltwork of fibrils embedded in gel-like substance which consists mainly of mucopolysaccharides. As a result of the swelling that occurs in most kidney diseases which are accompanied by proteinuria, the filamentous components of the basement membrane would become separated and thus enable particles of a diameter larger than normal to penetrate the membrane. Sitte's theory of filaments has been neither confirmed nor disproved, and it is still justifiable to regard the basement membrane as one basic factor which helps to determine the size of the particles which may be allowed to escape from the capillary lumen into the urinary space of Bowman's capsule.

The facts that no discontinuities or holes exist in the capillary endothelium and that the slit pores of the epithelium are bridged by a diaphragm (Fig. 1-10) bring us back to theories about filtration mechanisms which existed before the alleged "pores" were discovered. Whatever leaves the capillary lumen must penetrate the plasma membrane of the endothelium, the basement membrane, and the plasma membrane of the epithelial cells. This fact has great functional significance, because now the endothelial cell as well as the epithelial cell determines the size of the molecules which will be filtered. This difficult task is not ultimately left to the structurally and functionally ill-defined basement membrane of the glomerular capillaries, as it would be if true holes existed in the endothelium as well as in the epithelium.

EFFERENT ARTERIOLE

The efferent arteriole has the structure of a typical arteriole with smooth muscle walls

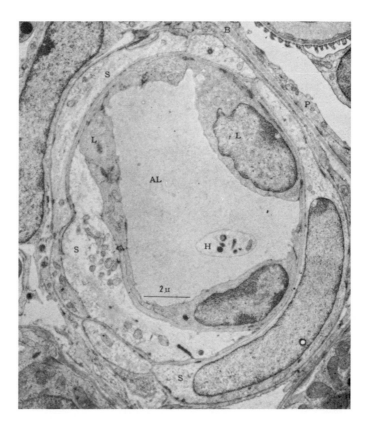

Figure 1-11. Cross section of the efferent arteriole of the mouse kidney glomerulus. The wall of the vessel is made up of smooth muscle cells (S) and an endothelial lining (L). No granulated cells can be identified in the wall of the efferent arteriole. In the lumen (AL) is seen a thrombocyte (H). The blood vessel borders on the capsule of the glomerulus with its basement membrane (B) and parietal cells (P). ×6000.

(Fig. 1-11). In the cortical nephrons, the diameter of the efferent arteriole is slightly less than that of the afferent arteriole.

The wall of the vessel has the usual composition of an endothelial layer, a media with one or several layers of smooth muscle cells, and an adventitia mostly characterized by occasional fibroblasts and an abundance of collagen fibers. As in blood vessels elsewhere in the body, the various layers of the efferent arteriolar wall are separated by basement membranes.

Granulated cells cannot be identified in the wall of the efferent arteriole. The smooth muscle cells show the typical features: abundant contractile elements, few and widely scattered ovoid mitochondria, a vestigial Golgi zone, and numerous vesicular inpocketings of the surface (plasma) membrane.

Peritubular Capillaries

The tubules are surrounded by an extensive network of freely anastomosing capillaries which usually are referred to as the peritubular capillaries. The capillaries are quite irregularly arranged in the cortex of the kidney. Each efferent arteriole decreases rather quickly in diameter after leaving a cortical glomerulus, and is transformed into the numerous peritubular capillaries which constitute the vascular bed of the cortex.

The capillaries are surrounded by a thin basement membrane which is closely applied at the basement membrane that envelops each tubule. The interstitial space is rather narrow and only occasionally can connective tissue elements like fibroblasts and collagen be identified within it. The capillary wall itself is extremely thin, most parts of it having a thickness of about 400A. The thin capillary wall displays an abundance of regularly dispersed fenestrations with an average width of 600A (Fig. 1-12). Each fenestra is bridged by a diaphragm 70A thick, in which a small central knob-like structure can be identified [37].

The fine peritubular capillaries of the kidney cortex eventually transform into venous capillaries which are drained by veins that gradually increase in diameter as they leave the cortex. From a functional point of view, the thinness of the walls of the peritubular capillaries and their close proximity to the base of the tubules seem to be of great importance. Because of the high rate of exchange between the tubular cells and the bloodstream, reabsorbed fluid and substances should be able to reach the peritubular capillaries as quickly as possible after they have undergone the proper processes within the tubule cells. As can be seen in Figure 1-12, the distance between the base of the tubule cells and the lumen of a peritubular capillary is only one-tenth of a micron, or even less.

The efferent arteriole of the juxtamedullary nephrons is slightly larger than the afferent arteriole of the same nephron. It soon achieves a direction toward the renal pelvis and continues as a single vessel into the renal pyramid, where it divides into a group of vessels, the arteriolae rectae or vasa recta. These arterioles develop retia mirabilia conjugata with two-directional flow. Longley and co-workers [21] studied them by electron microscopy in the rat and found that the vessels which direct the blood toward the papilla have an endothelium of medium thickness, whereas the arterioles which conduct the blood from the papilla back to the medulla have a very thin epithelium with a structure similar to that of the cortical peritubular capillaries. Such a rete mirabile seems to have functional importance in facilitating exchange between fluids flowing in opposing directions.

Tubules

It will be helpful to define the terms that will be employed in our discussion of the subdivision of the nephric tubule. Although different ways of subdividing the tubule have been used [33, 35, 36], it has become obvious

Figure 1-12. Thin peritubular capillary (C) in close apposition to two sections of proximal tubules (PT). The basement membrane of the tubules (B) is distinct, but that of the capillary is not visible as a structural entity in this micrograph. The capillary endothelium is provided with an abundance of fenestrations, all closed by a single membranous diaphragm in which can be seen a central point-like structure, the knob, when sectioned tangentially (*arrow*). The endothelial cell nucleus in the upper right-hand corner belongs to a neighboring capillary. ×14,000.

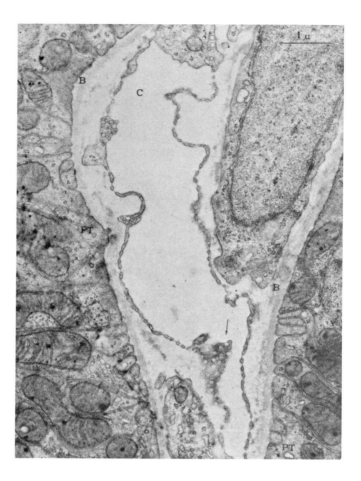

that the functional segments of the tubule which Smith [43] suggested represent an ideal subdivision also from a structural point of view.

The tubule distal to the glomerulus has the following segments, each of which can be further subdivided according to schemas proposed by various authors. Some of the synonyms are given.

Proximal segment
  Proximal convoluted tubule (proximal convolution; Hauptstück: pars contorta; H_1, H_2, H_3)
  Terminal part of proximal convolution (thick part of the straight descending limb of Henle's loop; Hauptstück: pars recta; H_4)
Thin segment (thin segment of Henle's loop; Überleitungsstück)
  Cortical nephrons: thin segment only

  Juxtamedullary nephrons:
    Descending thin segment
    Hairpin turn
    Ascending thin segment
Distal segment
  Thick ascending limb of Henle's loop (Mittelstück: pars recta)
  Macula densa
  Distal convoluted tubule (distal convolution; tubulus contortus II)
Collecting tubules
  Cortical collecting tubule (connecting tubule; arched collecting tubule)
  Collecting tubule
  Papillary duct (ducts of Bellini)

It should be remembered that this classification goes beyond the limits of the nephron proper, because the collecting tubules have a different developmental history than the rest of the tubules and do not belong to the nephron. Functionally, however, segments are important to consider, and it will be demonstrated below that the distal segment of the nephron and the collecting tubule have many structural features in common which seem to indicate that structurally and functionally the nephron includes more than its embryologic components.

BASEMENT MEMBRANE

The nephric and collecting tubules are enveloped by a continuous basement membrane throughout their length. It has an average thickness of about 800A (Fig. 1-13; see also Fig. 1-15). The membrane is connected with a similar structure that covers the parietal layer of Bowman's capsule. It is generally assumed that the homogeneous, structureless substance which forms the main component of all basement membranes is laid down by an interstitial process, probably mediated by certain connective tissue elements like fibroblasts which by enzymatic intracellular processes probably elaborate the precursors of the basement membranes. Since only few fibroblasts are present in the cortex of the mature kidney, it may be assumed that the formation of a basement membrane around the tubules either terminates when the nephron reaches its maturity, up to which time an abundance of fibroblasts are present, or is continued throughout life by action of the tubular cells. It seems likely that the formation of the basement membrane is completed by the time the nephron is ready to perform its full duty, and that the physicochemical properties are maintained by the limited number of fibroblasts

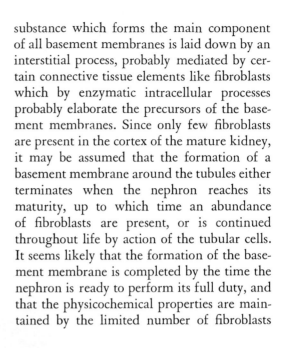

Figure 1-13. Low magnification electron micrograph of several cross-sectioned proximal tubules (PT) and one distal tubule (DT) surrounded by thin-walled capillaries. The numerous dense, spherical granules in the cells represent mitochondria. ×1300.

present in the interstitium. However, the fibroblasts appear to be present in a resting state, because they can be easily activated by pathologic processes that involve the connective tissue of the body.

It is doubtful that the basement membrane plays an active role in tubular function. The structure and function of a similar component present in the glomerular filtration membrane have been discussed above. The chief importance of the tubular basement membrane is that it forms an uninterrupted framework throughout the length of the nephron upon which the epithelium rests.

PROXIMAL SEGMENT

The proximal segment of the tubule has the widest diameter of all segments. It begins with a short part, termed the neck. In mammals this part does not show any peculiarities, but in certain frogs the cells are here provided with an abundance of long cilia.

The proximal segment, notably the convoluted part, has a tendency to collapse upon fixation for electron microscopy. Whether the lumen is open or closed in vivo has been a matter of controversy for some time. There seems to be no doubt at present that the lumen is open, provided the nephron is active and has steady filtration and reabsorption rates (Fig. 1-13). However, the moment the blood circulation is interrupted, as when small pieces of tissue are removed for electron microscopy, the filtration of urine ceases, and as a result the tubular urinary pressure falls rapidly, the tubular urine is resorbed, and the tubule collapses. On the other hand, if the nephrons are fixed with the blood circulating [32], it is possible to preserve the expanded tubule with an open lumen and thus presumably approximate the state in vivo as closely as it can be achieved.

The epithelium of the proximal segment is one cell-layer deep, and is composed of cuboidal or truncated pyramidal cells with coarsely granular cytoplasm and with large, basally placed, spherical nuclei. The cell boundaries, which are difficult to trace even in electron microscopy, are quite irregular and are interdigitated with the boundaries of adjacent cells. The interdigitation is less pronounced in the straight descending limb of Henle's loop, where the cell cytoplasm is less coarsely textured — which facilitates the tracing of the cell boundaries.

Luminal Cell Surface. Throughout the proximal segment, the cells are provided with an abundance of fine surface projections, the brush border, which by their multitude and free access to the urine of the tubular lumen highly increase the resorptive area of these cells. There are about 150 extensions per square micron, all covered by the plasma membrane (Fig. 1-14). Substances and fluid to be absorbed must be transferred across this membrane, actively or passively. It is well known that glucose is taken in by the cells of the proximal segment, probably mediated by the enzyme alkaline phosphatase, which shows its greatest concentration in the brush border zone of this segment [22, 49]. The exact localization of this enzyme is not quite clear, but with improved histochemical technics in electron microscopy it has been suggested that it is closely associated with the plasma membrane itself [25, 26].

The cell surface dips into shallow tubular invaginations between the bases of individual brush border extensions. These invaginations can become distended to vacuoles of varying size. It is believed that the vacuoles eventually become disconnected from the lumen and transported to deeper locations in the cell. The function of the invaginations and the vacuoles has been a mystery until recently. However, several independent investigations seem to indicate that these structures are a means by which the tubule cell can take in a substance, either as part of a normal metabolic process or as a defense mechanism. In capillaries [2] and the intestine [6, 30] similar surface structures are thought to be engaged in what has been called micropinocytosis or membrane flow.

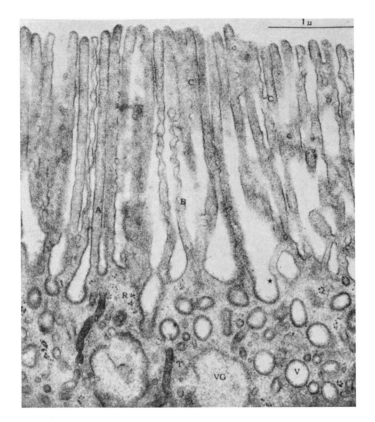

Figure 1-14. Detail of the brush border zone of the proximal tubule cell. The individual extensions show variation in shape and arrangement. Some are very straight, with inner longitudinal striations (A), others seem to be compressed and coiled (B), and in some instances two or more extensions seem to have fused (C). The invaginations (★) have a triple-layered wall with a central dense line, with a less dense zone on either side. It may be suggested that the invaginations can develop in two directions. They either collapse (T) or they become distended to vacuoles (V). In both cases, they seem to lose the outer surrounding dense line of their wall. The vacuoles eventually distend further and accumulate granular material inside (VG). This development of tubular invaginations of the surface membrane into vacuoles is called micropinocytosis or membrane flow. The submicroscopic ribonucleoprotein particles (R) of the cytoplasm are not found within the brush border extensions. ×23,000.

Large molecular proteins that cannot be absorbed through the surface membrane have been demonstrated to enter the invaginations of the tubular cells [23]. The content of the invagination and the vacuole seems to pass through several steps of transformation and condensation until it finally becomes a solid granule. Some of these granules seem to be discharged into the lumen of the tubule, probably as an end product. The vacuoles or granules correspond to structures with an easily demonstrable autofluorescence [41, 42].

Cell Organelles. The cell nucleus occupies a good portion of the cell near its base. The nuclear membrane has a triple-layered structure in which occasional constrictions can be seen, usually referred to as pores. It still has not been convincingly demonstrated that they represent open connections between the nu-

clear sap and the ground substance of the cytoplasm. Centrioles are rarely seen in cells of the proximal segment. A Golgi zone surrounds the luminal pole of the nucleus like a halo. The components of the Golgi apparatus, paired short membranes and small vesicles, most likely participate together with short pairs of rough-surfaced endoplasmic reticulum (membranes with attached ribonucleoprotein particles) in an intracellular fabrication of proteins to be used within the cells. In excretory cells, like the exocrine cells of the pancreas, the Golgi and the rough-surfaced endoplasmic reticulum elaborate the secretory granules.

The mitochondria are quite numerous in the convoluted part of the proximal segment but less so in the terminal straight part. They are mostly ovoid and located in the basal two-thirds of the cell. They have the usual fine

Figure 1-15. The basal part of a proximal tubule cell which borders on the basement membrane (B) is highly clefted by infoldings of the plasma membrane. Thus, the base of the cell is divided up into compartments, some of which house mitochondria (M) and vesicular structures of unknown origin. The mitochondria have a triple-layered outer capsule and a system of triple-layered inner membranes. The small, extremely dense areas are typical for kidney mitochondria but are of an unexplained nature. The thin capillary endothelium (L) is closely applied at the tubular basement membrane. ×22,000.

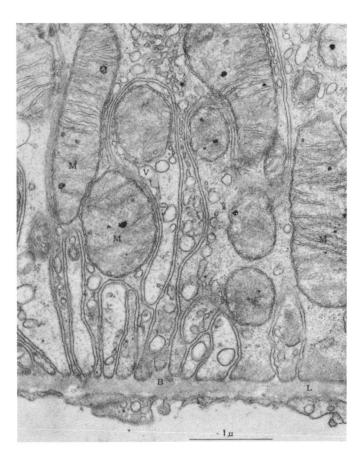

structural characteristics of this cell organelle (Fig. 1-15) and represent carriers of oxidative enzymes, mainly succinic dehydrogenase. It is not known whether mitochondria arise de novo in the cell, undergo division, or multiply by a budding mechanism. Structures were early analyzed in the cells of the proximal segment [33] which were thought to represent mitochondrial precursors. They have a single outside membrane and lack interior membranes, but their core has a density identical with that of the mitochondria. They were called microbodies, and since their discovery in kidney tubule cells, they have also been identified in liver cells. It is doubtful, however, that they really constitute mitochondrial precursors. It has recently been suggested that, in liver cells, they represent lysosomes [7], cytoplasmic particles which contain acid hydro-lytic enzymes which supposedly are involved in intracellular digestion. It may be assumed that the lysosomes participate in a cellular defense mechanism by dispersing both waste products derived from the breakdown of chemical compounds during the cell metabolism and materials taken into the cell via the tubular invaginations at the luminal cell surface.

Basal Cell Surface. The basal surface of the cells of the proximal segment is highly folded and the plasma membrane thrown into deep clefts which reach to varying depths. The infoldings are less numerous in the terminal part of the proximal segment. By the multitude of infoldings, the basal plasma membrane is brought into close proximity with the numerous mitochondria of these cells (Fig. 1-15).

The presence of a folded plasma membrane

was not discovered until electron microscopy was applied in morphologic research [33, 42]. The reason for this infolding and its functional interpretation are still not clear. It is usually found in cells noted for a high rate of fluid transport, such as those in the ducts of the salivary and lacrimal glands and in the choroid plexus. Intestinal cells do not show this feature, however.

The differentiation and development of the basal infoldings was studied in rats by Suzuki [46]. From this investigation it was concluded that the basal intussusceptions are formed by a reticular joining of original small vesicular inpocketings of the basal plasma membrane. Ruska et al. [38], upon using serial sectioning in electron microscopy, reconstructed the basal surface of these cells. They came to the conclusion that the base was highly clefted and digitated. Rhodin [33, 35, 36] suggested an even more complicated picture (Fig. 1-16) and proposed that not only was the base of the cell clefted and digitated, but also the lateral surfaces. The lateral clefts and ridges would then interdigitate with similar devices of a neighboring cell and some cell processes would even penetrate underneath and become intertwined with the basal clefts and ridges of that cell.

In view of Suzuki's investigations [46], it is doubtful that any description, simple or complicated, of the basal infoldings is of value in understanding the function of the basal plasma membrane infoldings. It seems quite likely that the plasma membrane is constantly moving, breaking up into vesicles, again joining to form membranes, and so forth. It is generally accepted that the membranes facilitate the transport of fluids across the tubule cell, but it seems less likely that a true mechanical pumping mechanism is involved [38].

A much more attractive solution to this problem is that advanced by Spater and co-workers [45], who were able convincingly to demonstrate ATPase activity within the membranes of the basal infoldings. Since the proximal tubule is engaged in active transfer of large quantities of solute and water, it may be assumed that the ATPase activity observed in the plasma membrane may be associated with either the type of membrane movement that Suzuki [46] observed or active transport of molecules across the membrane. This hypothesis, furthermore, is supported by the fact that the membranes with high ATPase activity are known to be in close contact with the ATP-synthesizing mitochondria by virtue of the extensive infolding.

THIN SEGMENT

Nephrons arising from glomeruli in the outer cortex turn in the cortex, and the thin segment is either extremely short or absent. In the juxtamedullary nephrons, the loop descends for a variable distance into the medulla, in some instances even to the papilla. In these deeper parts, the loop is composed of the thin segment. In man the shorter forms outnumber the longer ones by seven to one.

The thin segments which have been studied with electron microscopy were located in the medulla or papilla [31, 35, 36], and it is therefore not possible to predict anything about the fine structure of the short thin segment of the cortical nephrons. The transition between the columnar epithelium of the terminal part of the proximal segment and the flat squamous type of the thin segment is rather abrupt. At the same time the tubular diameter decreases considerably, and it is difficult to differentiate between capillaries and thin segments in cross sections of these structures in ordinary light microscopy. However, this difficulty is easily overcome in electron microscopy, where the capillaries display an even thinner cell wall than the thin segmental cells (Fig. 1-17). In addition, the plasma proteins present in the capillary lumen will be stained in most cases and give a noticeable density to the lumen of the capillaries.

The cytoplasm of the squamous cells of the thin segment is light. Only few and widely scattered small mitochondria are encountered

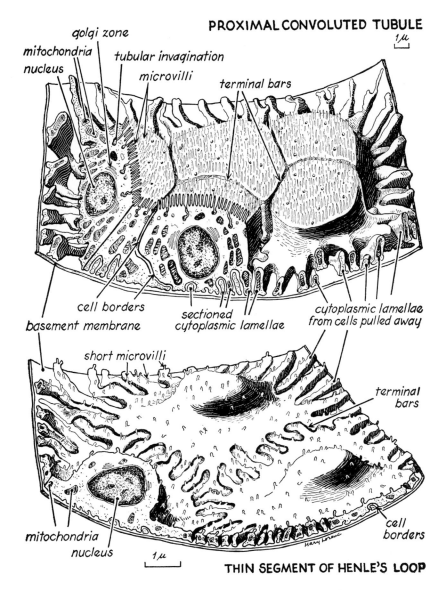

PROXIMAL CONVOLUTED TUBULE

golgi zone
mitochondria
nucleus
tubular invagination
microvilli
terminal bars
1μ

cell borders
basement membrane
sectioned cytoplasmic lamellae
cytoplasmic lamellae from cells pulled away

short microvilli
terminal bars
mitochondria
nucleus
1μ
cell borders

THIN SEGMENT OF HENLE'S LOOP

Figure 1-16. Three-dimensional reconstruction (not based on serial sections) of the basal and lateral interlocking mechanism of cells as analyzed in the proximal convoluted tubule and the thin segment of Henle's loop in the mouse kidney. (From Rhodin [36].)

in the cytoplasm, together with a vestigial Golgi zone and a scarcity of ribonucleoprotein particles (ribosomes). The luminal surface displays microvilli which are short and widely spread. They by no means represent a brush border structure of the abundance noted in the intestine or in the proximal segment of the nephron, but rather the type of surface specialization that characterizes the gallbladder or urinary bladder epithelium. Their resorptive capacity, therefore, is not considered to be extensive. The surface plasma membrane occasionally dips into the cell, forming small inpocketings. These structures are not

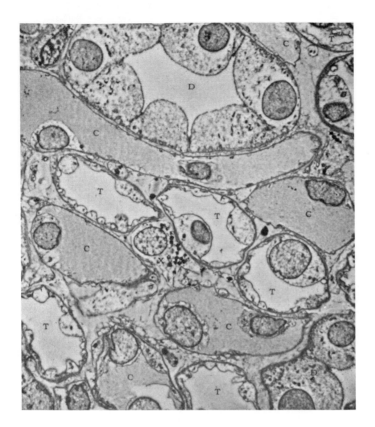

Figure 1-17. Survey of the papilla of the rat kidney showing mostly cross-sectioned collecting tubules (D), thin segments of Henle's loop (T), and capillaries (C). The cells of the collecting tubules are cuboidal, with few mitochondria, easily recognized cell boundaries, and tiny microvilli on the surface. The cells of the thin segments are squamous. They show in cross section a scalloped appearance due to narrow and elongated cell extensions which frequently interdigitate. The endothelium of the capillaries is extremely thin. The interstitial cell (X) is unidentified. ×1300.

nearly as frequent and elongated as the tubular invaginations of the proximal segment. They look more like the micropinocytosis vesicles of the capillary wall, but again occur less frequently.

The cells of the thin segment are shaped like starfish, with the cell nucleus located in the center and the cytoplasm extending as numerous arms (Fig. 1-16). The arm-like processes interdigitate with similar structures of neighboring cells. Near the luminal surface is seen a specialization of the plasma membrane, the so-called terminal bar. By means of this structure, which runs continuously along and within the plasma membrane of each cell, the cells and the arm-like processes of the cells are held together. It has been definitely established that some kind of cement substance exists in the intercellular space between the terminal bars, preventing substances

in the tubular lumen from using the intercellular space as a direct pathway to reach the peritubular capillaries. The basal surface is rather smooth in the thin segments encountered in the papilla (Fig. 1-18A), whereas in the medullary thin segments this surface is elaborately thrown into numerous narrow projections (Fig. 1-18B). It has not been possible to determine whether one or the other type of basal surface specialization is related to the descending or ascending parts of the thin segment.

The cells of the thin segment seem to offer little structural evidence that active transport may occur across their squamous epithelium. The amount of oxidative enzymes present is probably quite limited in view of the fact that so few mitochondria are encountered in the cells. The functional importance of the thin segment has recently been assumed to be re-

Figure 1-18. Two sections of the thin segment of Henle's loop as they appear deep in the papilla (1-18A) and in the medulla (1-18B). In the papilla, the luminal (TL) and the basal surfaces of the cells are rather smooth, whereas in the medulla these surfaces are elaborately thrown into numerous narrow projections. It has not been possible to determine whether one or the other structure is related to the descending or ascending parts of the thin segment. The cells of the thin segment are shaped like starfish. The arms of neighboring cells are interlocked and held together by terminal bars (*arrows*) near the luminal surface. The lumen and thin endothelium of the adjoining capillary (CL) are seen. A, ×17,000; B, ×13,000.

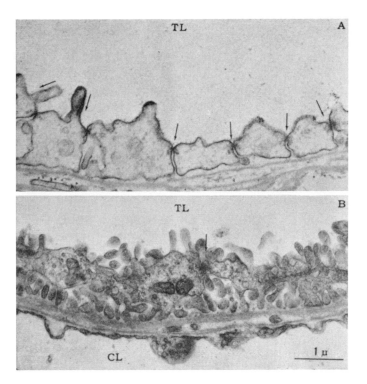

lated to the so-called countercurrent mechanism [48].

DISTAL SEGMENT

The cells of the distal segment are distinctly different from those present in the thin segment. However, they resemble in many ways the cells of the proximal segment, a fact which often makes it difficult for the student to tell them apart, especially in the diseased kidney. All cells of the distal segment are of the cuboidal type, with a coarsely granulated cytoplasm due to a heavy accumulation of mitochondria. The segment has the same average diameter as the proximal segment, but more often one sees a wide open lumen, even when the specimens have been fixed without the blood circulating. The nucleus is usually located in the apical part of the cell instead of at the base, as found in the proximal segment (Fig. 1-19).

Luminal Cell Surface. The cell bulges markedly into tubular lumen in the distal segment. This seems to be caused mainly by the nucleus but could also be due to the apical cell cytoplasm, which occupies a larger area than can be recorded in the proximal segment. The luminal cell surface is provided with numerous short microvilli. They are less abundant and coarser than the brush border extensions of the proximal segment. The microvilli are quite constant in size and number throughout the whole distal segment.

Only rarely are inpocketings of the plasma membrane identified in the distal segment. However, the entire apex of the cells is pervaded by a number of tiny vesicles which vary in number from cell to cell (Fig. 1-20). The vesicles are surrounded by a smooth single membrane with a slight granular condensation of the cytoplasm surrounding the vesicle. The vesicles may occasionally be seen to establish a contact with the surface plasma membrane and open up into the tubular lumen. Although the number of vesicles may vary from cell to cell within a local section of

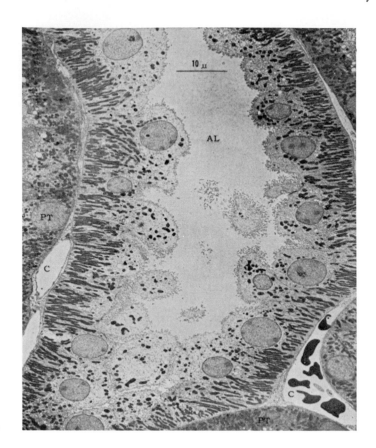

Figure 1-19. Low magnification electron micrograph of a longitudinally sectioned ascending thick limb of Henle's loop (AL) together with parts of proximal convolutions (PT) and capillaries (C). In the cells of the thick limb, the nuclei are located in the luminal half of the cell together with a few spherical mitochondria and an abundance of microvesicles. The cell surface displays a fair number of short microvilli. The basal half of the cell is occupied by long, rod-shaped mitochondria which are tightly packed. ×1300.

the distal segment, they are always found in the thick ascending limb of Henle's loop, in the macula densa cells, and in the distal convoluted tubule.

Because of their smooth-surfaced boundary toward the surrounding cytoplasm, they cannot be considered part of the rough-surfaced endoplasmic reticulum. Neither can they be looked upon as a structural variation of the tubular surface invaginations encountered in the proximal convoluted tubule, mainly because they so rarely are seen to establish an open connection with the lumen of the distal segment. Elsewhere in mammalian tissues, there seems to be at least one type of cell which is almost identical with the cell of the distal segment of the nephron in the number of vesicles the cytoplasm contains. This is the parietal cell of the gastric mucosa. Functionally, the parietal cell is supposedly engaged in the production of hydrochloric acid. If morphologic similarities reflect functional parallelism, one would be tempted to suggest that the vesicles in the cells of the distal segment represent a system engaged in elaborating hydrogen and hydroxyl ions, because it is commonly accepted that the acidification of the urine occurs in the distal segment.

Cell Organelles. Mitochondria are the most prominent cell organelle of the distal segment, but also the most variable structure within the various sections. They are long, rod-like and densely packed in the basal two-thirds of the cells in the thick ascending limb of Henle's loop (Fig. 1-21). They display a short, almost spherical shape in the apex of these cells (Fig. 1-20). As the distal segment is transformed into the distal convoluted tubule, the mitochondria become gradually less rod-like and less densely packed, until finally a state is

Figure 1-20. The luminal part of a cell located in the thick ascending limb of Henle's loop. The nucleus (N) is surrounded by a triple-layered membrane. The spherical mitochondria (M) show the typical fine structure of this cell organelle. Most characteristic is the abundance of smooth-surfaced vesicles (V), some of which are slightly flattened (F) and some in close proximity to the cell surface (*arrows*). Free RNP particles (R) are scattered throughout the cytoplasm. Short microvilli extend from the cell surface into the tubular lumen (AL). ×26,000.

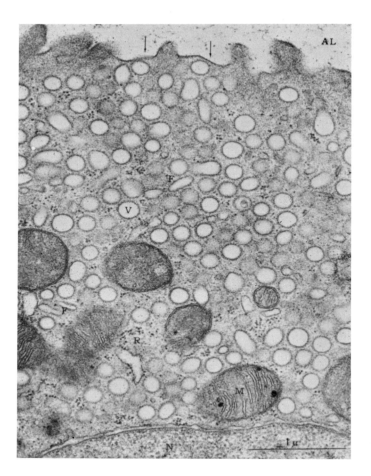

reached where a few spherical mitochondria are scattered throughout the cytoplasm.

The cytoplasm of the distal segment is denser than elsewhere in the nephron. This is partly caused by the numerous mitochondria, but also by the abundance of submicroscopic ribonucleoprotein particles (ribosomes). The ribosomes are mostly free, but occasionally they are seen attached to short, paired membranes, in which case the entire structural complex represents elements of rough-surfaced endoplasmic reticulum. The Golgi complex is small in these cells. Rarely are microbodies and and large, dense granules seen in the distal segment.

The abundance of mitochondria is an indication of the high enzymatic activity of these cells. The formation of ammonia requires a great deal of energy and so does the active transport of sodium chloride from the tubular lumen to the adjacent medullary interstitial fluid which allegedly takes place in the distal segment, possibly in connection with its role in a countercurrent multiplier system [48].

Basal Cell Surface. The basal surface of the cells of the distal segment shows clefts similar to those in the proximal segment. However, in the thick ascending limb of Henle's loop, the foldings of the basal plasma membrane are even more frequent and reach a level closer to the apex of these cells. The cytoplasm, therefore, is divided into narrow compartments. Most of these compartments house mitochondria, but some are too narrow for these cell organelles. Because of the large mitochondria, the extensive infoldings and

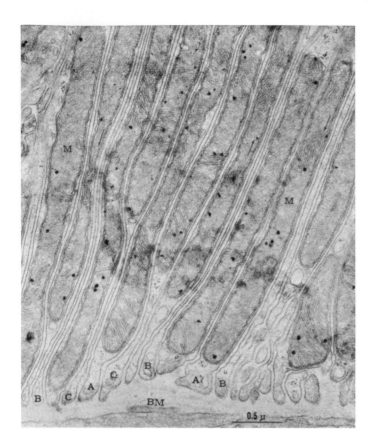

Figure 1-21. The basal part of a cell located in the thick ascending limb of Henle's loop. The basal plasma membrane is highly infolded, dividing the basal cell surface into narrow compartments. Most of these compartments (A) house mitochondria (M) but some (B) are too narrow for these cell organelles. Still others (C) are narrow toward the basement membrane (BM) and become wider some distance away from it. The mitochondria (M) are among the longest found in mammalian tissues. The inner triple-layered membranes are oriented mostly at an angle in relation to the long axis of the mitochondrion and in some instances (*arrows*) parallel to this axis. Notice the short distance between the infolded plasma membrane and the outer mitochondrion membrane. ×27,000.

narrow cytoplasmic compartments, the plasma membrane is brought into very intimate contact with the mitochondrial envelope (Fig. 1-21). This favors the interaction between the ATPase of the plasma membrane [45] and the ATP-synthesizing mitochondria discussed on page 18.

The base of the cells in the distal convoluted tubule is less extensively infolded, and where folds are recorded the cytoplasmic components are usually too short and narrow to permit large cell organelles like mitochondria to be located within them.

Macula Densa. A few words must be said about the macula densa. When the tubule returns to the glomerulus of its own origin after it has established its medullary loop of Henle, it makes a short tangential contact with the afferent arteriole just before this vessel enters the glomerular capsule. In the area of contact

the tubular epithelium adjacent to the arteriole is modified in such a way that the cells become narrow and the nuclei densely crowded together, giving rise to a characteristic feature known as the macula densa.

Because the cells are narrower in this region, and because of the prominence of the nuclei, the arrangement of deep basal infoldings of the plasma membrane and long rod-shaped mitochondria disappears temporarily. The mitochondria are few in number here and of a predominantly spherical shape; the basal infoldings are short and narrow (Fig. 1-3). It should be emphasized that the macula densa region of the distal segment is surrounded by a continuous basement membrane. This basement membrane borders on a similar structure which envelops the smooth muscle cells of the afferent arteriole whether these cells contain juxtaglomerular granules or not.

No functional explanation can be offered for the structural variation seen in the macula densa. Most likely the arrangement can be explained by the way this section of the distal segment develops embryologically.

COLLECTING TUBULES

The cells of the collecting tubules are mainly of the cuboidal type but they increase in height toward the ducts of Bellini, where a predominantly columnar type exists [39]. In general, the cells of the collecting tubules display a light cytoplasm with only few dense cell organelles (Fig. 1-22). However, a dark and coarsely granulated cell was early noticed to be mixed in with the light cells, particularly in the cortical collecting tubules [1]. This cell is usually described as being "intercalated." It is quite frequent in the cortical collecting tubules; gradually it becomes less frequent in the collecting tubules proper and disappears completely in the papillary ducts.

Luminal Cell Surface. Throughout the collecting tubule, the luminal cell surface is provided with quite short and coarse microvilli which are all covered by the plasma membrane. Tubular invaginations do not exist. As in the cells of the distal segment, the apical cytoplasm of the dark intercalated cell is interspersed with numerous vesicles. Neighboring light cells of the collecting tubules may have occasional vesicles, but not nearly to the same extent.

Cell Organelles. The submicroscopic ribonucleoprotein granules (ribosomes) are richly represented in the intercalated cells but are quite sparse in the other cells of the collecting tubules. Again, this reflects the rate of metabolic processes and turnover of proteins in these cells; it is certainly an indication that the

Figure 1-22. In the large collecting tubules, the ducts of Bellini (DB), the cells are of a columnar shape and stand out clearly against the squamous epithelium of the thin segment of Henle's loop (TS) and the very thin lining of the capillaries (C) of the papilla. The cells of the ducts of Bellini have a light cytoplasm with few mitochondria (M) and basally located lipid droplets (Li). Few and coarse protrusions characterize the luminal surface. The basal cell surface is relatively smooth but the lateral surfaces are highly irregular. The nucleus is located in the lower half of the cell. ×1300.

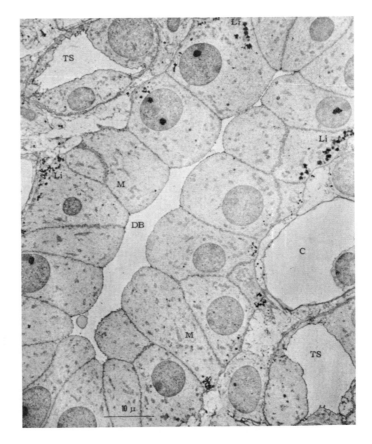

intercalated cells are more active than the light cells throughout the collecting tubule. The number of mitochondria is similarly greater in the intercalated cells than in the light cells. It was not demonstrated until the advent of electron microscopy that the majority of the granules of the intercalated cells represent mitochondria [5, 35]. Intensely dense granules with a great affinity to osmium tetroxide can be found in all cells of the collecting tubule. It was recently demonstrated [24] that these granules do not represent mitochondria although they have the same diameter. They have a highly ordered fine structure comparable to a crystalline lattice. Staining tests demonstrated that they contain acidic, unsaturated lipids, primarily phospholipids, and also some protein.

A different type of osmiophilic, electron-dense granule is located in the basal part of the cells in the larger collecting tubules and papillary ducts. Unlike mitochondria, the outlines of these organelles are irregular. The structure is similar to what is usually identified as a lipid granule in, for instance, the steroid-producing cells of the adrenal cortex [52]. The columnar cells of the papillary ducts have in addition a multitude of small, smooth-surfaced vesicles or short irregular tubules. These structures are not connected with the cell surface.

Basal Cell Surface. The basal cell surface is in most cases smooth or slightly infolded. Whenever infoldings are recorded, they seem to be small, narrow, and shallow. The lateral cell surfaces are irregular and characterized by slight indentations. Numerous desmosomes can be identified in an intercellular relationship.

Functional Considerations. Few functions have been assigned to the collecting tubules, mainly because of the simplicity of the epithelial cells. However, the most conspicuous cell type, the intercalated or dark cell, seems to offer a basis for the assumption that some processes related to the composition of the urine are located within the collecting tubules. It has been assumed [1, 5] that the dark and light cells of the cortical collecting tubules represent different functional states in a secretory process. This hypothesis is supported by other investigations [29], in which an increased number of intercalated cells and a decreased number of light cells were recorded after potassium depletion. The structural changes were associated with an electrolyte imbalance. Potassium depletion is also associated with droplet formation in the cells of the papillary ducts, probably as a result of disturbed sodium-potassium relationship within the papilla [44]. It is known [12] that the permeability of the cells of the collecting tubules may be influenced by the action of the antidiuretic hormone of the pituitary, which would result in a passive resorption of water, but structural evidence for this observation has not been provided.

Conclusion

A close and careful analysis of the ultrastructure of the mammalian nephron leaves the investigator with the notion that few cellular features are really unique along the nephron when reviewed in the light of similar investigations of cells elsewhere in the body. More impressive is the cellular pattern of arrangement within different segments of the nephron (Fig. 1-23). Each segment is characteristically organized with respect to luminal surface, mitochondrial arrangement, and differentiation of basal cell surface, which permits a functional interpretation compatible with the assumption that variation in structure or structural arrangement reflects a difference in function between the various segments. But in order to understand the meaning of the variation in ultrastructural arrangements within each segment, one has to compare a variety of vertebrate as well as invertebrate nephrons,

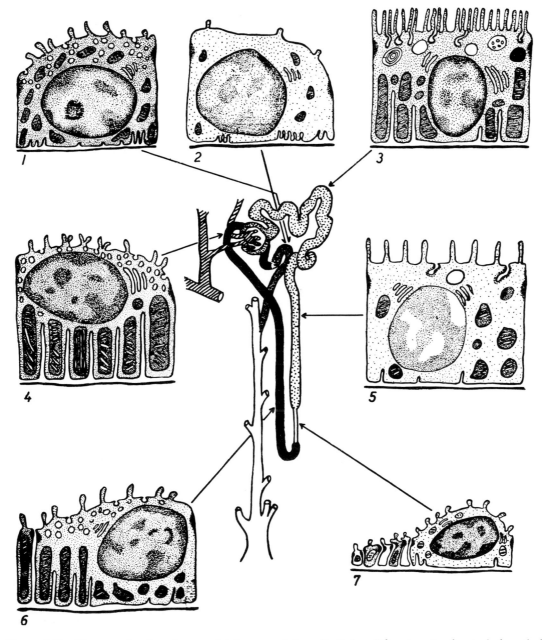

Figure 1-23. Diagram showing the essential features of the cells lining different parts of a typical cortical nephron in the mammalian kidney as seen with the electron microscope. (1) Distal convolution and collecting tubule, dark cell. (2) Distal convolution and collecting tubule, light cell. (3) Proximal convolution. (4) and (6) Thick ascending limb of Henle's loop. (5) Descending limb of Henle's loop. (7) Thin segment of Henle's loop. (From Rhodin [35].)

study the ultrastructure of the embryologic development, and last but not least, investigate the changes that will occur under various pathologic conditions. Using these studies as a basis, one might then be justified in drawing far-reaching conclusions related to the function of individual cells or sections of the mammalian nephron.

Acknowledgments

I am indebted to Mrs. Inger Terzakis and to Mr. Eugene Minner for their technical assistance and to Miss Marsha Rankin for making the photographic prints. I also gratefully acknowledge the artistic works by my wife, Mrs. Gunvor Rhodin (Fig. 1-23), and by Miss Mary Lorenc (Figs. 1-1, 1-7 through 1-10, 1-16), and I thank Mrs. Helen Stark for her valuable help during the preparation of the manuscript.

This investigation was supported in part by a research grant (A-2705) from the National Institutes of Health.

References

1. Andrejewitsch, A. T. Über das Epithel der Sammelröhren in der Säugerniere. Bern M.D. Thesis, 1919.

2. Bennett, H. S. The concepts of membrane flow and membrane vesiculation as mechanisms for active transport and ion pumping. *J. Biophys. Biochem. Cytol.* 2 (Suppl.): 99, 1956.

3. Bergstrand, A. Pathology: Kidney. In Clark, G. L. (Ed.), *Encyclopedia of Microscopy.* New York: Reinhold, 1961. P. 206.

4. Bergstrand, A., and Bucht, H. Anatomy of the glomerulus as observed in biopsy material from young and healthy human subjects. *Z. Zellforsch.* 48:51, 1958.

5. Clark, S. L., Jr. Cellular differentiation in the kidneys of newborn mice studied with the electron microscope. *J. Biophys. Biochem. Cytol.* 3:349, 1957.

6. Clark, S. L., Jr. The ingestion of proteins and colloidal materials by columnar absorptive cells of the small intestine in suckling rats and mice. *J. Biophys. Biochem. Cytol.* 5:41, 1959.

7. De Duve, C. Lysosomes, A New Group of Cytoplasmic Particles. In Hayashi, T. (Ed.), *Subcellular Particles.* New York: Ronald Press, 1959.

8. Farquhar, M. G. Review of normal and pathologic glomerular ultrastructure. *Proceedings of the Tenth Annual Conference on the Nephrotic Syndrome,* 1959.

9. Farquhar, M. G. Electron microscopy of renal biopsies. *Bull. N.Y. Acad. Med.* 36:419, 1960.

10. Farquhar, M. G., and Palade, G. E. Functional evidence for the existence of a third cell type in the renal glomerulus. *Abstracts of Papers Presented at the First Annual Meeting of the American Society for Cell Biology,* 1961.

11. Forster, R. P. Kidney Cells. In Brachet, J., and Mirsky, A. E. (Eds.), *The Cell,* Vol. 5. New York: Academic Press, 1961. Chap. 2.

12. Ginetsinsky, A. G., Sax, M. G., and Titova, L. K. The mechanism of the action of the antidiuretic hormone. *Nature* (London) 182:1218, 1958.

13. Hall, B. V. Studies on the normal glomerular structure by electron microscopy. *Proceedings of the Fifth Annual Conference on the Nephrotic Syndrome,* 1953.

14. Hall, B. V. Further studies of the normal structure of the renal glomerulus. *Proceedings of the Sixth Annual Conference on the Nephrotic Syndrome,* 1954.

15. Hall, B. V. The protoplasmic basis of glomerular filtration. *Amer. Heart J.* 54:1, 1957.

16. Hall, B. V., and Roth, L. E. Preliminary

studies on the development and differentiation of cells and structures of the renal corpuscle. *Proceedings of the Stockholm Conference on Electron Microscopy,* 1956.

17. Ham, A. W., and Leeson, T. S. *Histology.* Philadelphia: J. B. Lippincott, 1961.

18. Hartroft, P. M., and Newmark, L. N. Electron microscopy of renal juxtaglomerular cells. *Anat. Rec.* 139:185, 1961.

19. Latta, H., Maunsbach, A. B., and Madden, S. C. The centrolobular region of the renal glomerulus studied by electron microscopy. *J. Ultrastruct. Res.* 4:455, 1960.

20. Lewis, O. J. The vascular arrangement of the mammalian renal glomerulus as revealed by a study of its development. *J. Anat.* 92:433, 1958.

21. Longley. J. B., Banfield, W. G., and Brindley, D. C. Structure of the rete mirabile in the kidney of the rat as seen with electron microscope. *J. Biophys. Biochem. Cytol.* 7:103, 1960.

22. Longley, J. B., and Fisher, E. R. Alkaline phosphatase and the periodic acid-Schiff reaction in the proximal tubule of the vertebrate kidney. *Anat. Rec.* 120:1, 1954.

23. Miller, F. Hemoglobin absorption by the cells of the proximal convoluted tubule in mouse kidney. *J. Biophys. Biochem. Cytol.* 8:689, 1960.

24. Miller, F. Lipoprotein granules in the cortical collecting tubules of mouse kidney. *J. Biophys. Biochem. Cytol.* 9:157, 1961.

25. Mölbert, E., Duspiva, F., and v. Deimling, O. Die histochemische Lokalisation der Phosphatase in der Tubulusepithelzelle der Mäuseniere im elektronenmikroskopischen Bild. *Histochemie* 2:5, 1960.

26. Mölbert, E. R. G., Duspiva, F., and v. Deimling, O. H. The demonstration of alkaline phosphatase in the electron microscope. *J. Biophys. Biochem. Cytol.* 7:387, 1960.

27. Mueller, C. B. The structure of the renal glomerulus. *Amer. Heart J.* 55:304, 1958.

28. Oberling, C., and Hatt, P. Y. Étude de l'appareil juxtaglomérulaire du rat au microscope électronique. *Ann. Anat. Path.* (Paris) 5:441, 1960.

29. Oliver, J., MacDowell, M. C., Welt, L. G., Holliday, M. A., Hollander, W., Winters, R. W., Williams, T. F., and Segar, W. E. The renal lesions of electrolyte imbalance. I. The structural alterations in potassium depleted rats. *J. Exp. Med.* 106:563, 1957.

30. Palay, S. L., and Karlin, L. J. An electron microscopic study of the intestinal villus. II. The pathway of fat absorption. *J. Biophys. Biochem. Cytol.* 5:373, 1959.

31. Pease, D. C. The fine structure of the kidney seen by electron microscopy. *J. Histochem. Cytochem.* 3:295, 1955.

32. Pease, D. C. Electron microscopy of the vascular bed of the kidney cortex. *Anat. Rec.* 121:701, 1955.

33. Rhodin, J. Correlation of Ultrastructural Organization and Function in Normal and Experimentally Changed Proximal Convoluted Tubule Cells of the Mouse Kidney. Karolinska Institutets, Stockholm, Thesis, 1954.

34. Rhodin, J. Electron microscopy of the glomerular capillary wall. *Exp. Cell Res.* 8:572, 1955.

35. Rhodin, J. Anatomy of kidney tubules. *Int. Rev. Cytol.* 7:485, 1958.

36. Rhodin, J. Electron microscopy of the kidney. *Amer. J. Med.* 24:661, 1958.

37. Rhodin, J. The diaphragm of capillary endothelial fenestrations. *J. Ultrastruct. Res.* 6:171, 1962.

38. Ruska, H., Moore, D. H., and Weinstock, J. The base of the proximal convoluted tubule cells of the rat kidney. *J. Biophys. Biochem. Cytol.* 3:249, 1957.

39. Sakaguchi, H., and Suzuki, Y. Fine structure of renal tubule cells. *Keio J. Med.* 7:17, 1958.

40. Sitte, H. Veränderungen im Glomerulus der Rattenniere nach Fremdeeiweissgaben und hypothetische Erklärung der glomerulären Ultrafiltration. *Verh. Deutsch. Ges. Path.* 43. Tagung, 1959.

41. Sjöstrand, F. S. Über die Eigenfluoreszenz tierischer Gewebe mit besonderer Berücksichtigung der Säugetierniere. *Acta Anat.* (Basel) Suppl. 1, 1944.

42. Sjöstrand, F. S., and Rhodin, J. The ultrastructure of the proximal convoluted tubules

of the mouse kidney as revealed by high resolution electron microscopy. *Exp. Cell Res.* 4:426, 1953.

43. Smith, H. W. *Principles of Renal Physiology*. New York: Oxford University Press, 1956.

44. Spargo, B., Straus, F., and Fitch, F. Zonal renal papillary droplet change with potassium depletion. *Arch. Path.* (Chicago) 70: 599, 1960.

45. Spater, H. W., Novikoff, A. B., and Masek, B. Adenosinetriphosphatase activity in the cell membranes of kidney tubule cells. *J. Biophys. Biochem. Cytol.* 4:765, 1958.

46. Suzuki, Y. An electron microscopy of the renal differentiation. I. Proximal tubule cells. *J. Electron Micr.* (Tokyo) 6:52, 1958.

47. Suzuki, Y. An electron microscopy of the renal differentiation. II. Glomerulus. *Keio J. Med.* 8:129, 1959.

48. Ullrich, K. J., Kramer, K., and Boylan, J. W. Present knowledge of the countercurrent system in the mammalian kidney. *Progr. Cardiovasc. Dis.* 3:395, 1961.

49. Wachstein, M. Histochemical staining reactions of the normally functioning and abnormal kidney. *J. Histochem. Cytochem.* 3: 246, 1955.

50. Yamada, E. The fine structure of the renal glomerulus of the mouse. *J. Biophys. Biochem. Cytol.* 1:551, 1955.

51. Yamada, E. Collagen fibrils within the renal glomerulus. *J. Biophys. Biochem. Cytol.* 7:407, 1960.

52. Zelander, T. Ultrastructure of mouse adrenal cortex. *J. Ultrastruct. Res.* Suppl. 2, 1959.

53. Zimmermann, K. Z. Ueber den Bau des Glomerulus der Säugerniere. *Z. Mikr. Anat. Forsch.* 32:176, 1933.

2

Outline of Renal Physiology

Robert W. Berliner

The development of current concepts concerning the function of the kidney can be said to date from the studies of Bowman [18], who in 1842 first noted the continuity of the space within the glomerular capsule with the lumen of the conjoined tubule. The anatomic arrangement suggested that the glomerulus might be a filtering apparatus and led Bowman to propose that the glomerulus served to provide the water of the urine by filtration from the blood. However, he conceived that only water was derived from this process and that the water in turn served to convey distally the solutes secreted into the lumen by the tubule epithelium. (It is clear that at that time there was little understanding of the magnitude of osmotic forces, since to separate pure water from the plasma by filtration would require a hydrostatic pressure of approximately 6 atmospheres, almost 5 meters of mercury!)

Ludwig [92], at very nearly the same time and presumably independently, also reached the conclusion that the glomerulus was a filtering mechanism. He, however, proposed that all the urinary materials were derived from the filtration process. As the solution separated

by filtration in the glomerulus flowed down the tubules, it was concentrated by the reabsorption of water into the peritubular capillaries.

Heidenhain [63], in 1874, returned to a view closer to that of Bowman and initiated a controversy which lasted for many years. He noted that when the blood pressure was reduced to a level at which urine formation and, presumably, glomerular filtration ceased, certain dyes nevertheless accumulated in the tubule lumen. He also estimated that, to provide the urinary solutes, the volume of any glomerular filtrate would have to be extremely large relative to the volume of the excreted urine. He therefore placed the major burden of urinary excretion on the secretion of solute by the tubules.

In 1917, after reviewing the extensive literature on the subject, Cushny [32] attempted to bring some order out of the chaotic field by proposing what he called the "modern theory" of urine formation. He rejected entirely any secretion of materials from blood to urine, proposing that all the materials destined for excretion were contained in the glomerular filtrate. As this fluid flowed through the tubules, the lining epithelium was assumed to absorb from it a solution constant in composition and approaching in its makeup an ideal extracellular fluid. Cushny proposed that the "fluid reabsorbed is always the same, whatever the needs of the organism at the moment."

The extensive development of knowledge concerning the function of the kidney has shown that each of the above theories of renal function contains some elements which can be accepted as correct and others which can be definitely discarded. The glomerular filtrate is indeed an ultrafiltrate of plasma and does provide most of the materials which eventually appear in the urine. But the existence of processes by which materials can be transferred by the tubules directly from blood to urine has been established, as was first unequivocally shown by Marshall and Vickers [99]. The tubules do reabsorb much of the water and solute from the glomerular filtrate, but not in the form of an "idealized Locke solution," nor indeed as any "solution" at all; each component is reabsorbed by a more or less independent process, many of which are subject to modification in response to "the needs (or better, the physiologic state) of the organism at the moment."

Two technics in particular have been the basis of the rapid growth of understanding in renal physiology in the last 40 years.

1. The micropuncture technic, introduced by A. N. Richards [134] and his associates, provided a device for the collection and analysis of minute samples from identifiable locations within the nephron. The observations of Richards and his collaborators in the amphibian, and the subsequent work of Walker and his colleagues [169] in mammals, have provided the framework for interpretation of the large amount of data obtained by more indirect means. The current revival of this technic in a number of laboratories is providing the major impetus for progress in the field.

2. The clearance technic for measuring glomerular filtration, and hence the reabsorption and secretion of a wide variety of substances, was introduced largely through the leadership of Rehberg [130] and Homer Smith [152]. It has provided the means for evaluating the renal mechanisms involved in the excretion of many materials in intact, unanesthetized animals and in man under conditions that at least approach the normal.

General Nature of the Process of Urine Formation

Although the two kidneys of man are composed of some two million individual nephrons, it is frequently convenient to consider these collectively and speak of the kidney as if it constituted a single large nephron composed of *the* glomerulus, *the* proximal convoluted tubule, etc. This is a useful oversimplification which, for many purposes, is an adequate model. However, it is clear that the nephrons are not all identical, and the heterogeneity of structure and of function becomes important when certain activities of the kidney are to be interpreted. Moreover, although for many purposes each nephron can be considered an autonomous unit operating independently of all the others, it is essential to take account of their interdependence in certain functions, particularly that responsible for the formation of concentrated urine.

The process of urine formation is initiated by the separation, across the walls of the glomerular capillary loops, of an ultrafiltrate of plasma. Driven by the net filtration pressure, the glomerular filtrate flows through the tubules. Through the activities of the epithelium lining the tubules, the composition of the fluid is drastically modified. Many of the constituents of the filtrate are removed from the tubule lumen and returned to the peritubular capillaries to be retained in the body. Certain constituents (e.g., glucose, amino acids) are reabsorbed more or less completely under normal conditions, appearing in the urine in appreciable amounts only under unusual circumstances. Other filtrable components of the plasma (e.g., urea) are reabsorbed to only a limited extent and a major fraction of that filtered is, under normal conditions, excreted in the urine. Still others are reabsorbed to a variable extent, which is often determined by hormonal regulation. Water is perhaps the most important example of this class of substances. Finally, other components of the urine are removed from the blood by the cells of the tubule epithelium and secreted directly into the tubule lumen for excretion in the urine. Thus three major processes are involved in urine formation: (1) glomerular filtration, (2) tubular reabsorption, and (3) tubular secretion. These three processes and their integration are considered in the following pages.

Glomerular Filtration

The filtering function of the glomerular tuft was inferred by Bowman [18] and Ludwig [92] in 1842. Although in the intervening years this view had frequently been cast into doubt, it finally received virtually universal acceptance as a result of the work of A. N. Richards and his associates in the 1920's and 1930's (see Richards [134] for summary). The composition of fluid collected from the glomerular capsule of amphibians (frogs and the mud puppy *Necturus*) was determined in considerable detail and was found to be, with respect to an extensive list of constituents, that predicted for an ultrafiltrate of plasma. Each of the components measured was, within the limits of accuracy of the methods employed, present at the same concentration in the glomerular fluid as in the plasma water of blood obtained at the same time. In mammals, not only are the structures much smaller but the glomeruli are rarely directly available for puncture on the surface of the kidney. These technical problems delayed extension of the

observations to the mammal, but the results subsequently obtained by Walker et al. [169] were fully in accord with the results in the amphibians. In addition, it was shown by Hayman [62] that the hydrostatic pressure in the glomerular capillaries is great enough to supply the driving force for separation of the glomerular filtrate from the colloids of plasma.

The rate of glomerular filtration can be related to a series of forces favoring and opposing the filtration process and to the area and permeability of the membranes across which the filtration occurs. Thus, as in other capillaries, the main driving force is the hydrostatic pressure in the glomerular capillaries (Pb), and the filtration is opposed by the hydrostatic pressure in the glomerular capsule (Pc) and by the osmotic pressure attributable to the plasma proteins (πb). The rate of glomerular filtration may be related to these variables by the equation

$$(1) \qquad \text{GFR} = \text{Kp}([\text{Pb} - \text{Pc}] - \pi \text{b})$$

where Kp describes the filtration permeability of the glomerular capillaries and is a function of both the area and the porosity of the glomerular capillary surface.

The glomerular capillaries differ from capillaries elsewhere in the body in several respects. They are interposed between two arterioles, the afferent and efferent glomerular vessels; the hydrostatic pressure in the capillary lumen is maintained at a higher level, and they appear to have an appreciably higher permeability. Pappenheimer et al. [115] have estimated that the permeability of glomerular capillaries is roughly 100 times greater than that of capillaries in the cat hind limb (largely muscle capillaries). The difference is presumably largely in the fraction of the total capillary surface occupied by pores rather than in the average pore dimensions. It is probably the capillary basement membrane which is penetrated by the pores through which filtration occurs, and the basement membrane which supplies the major resistance to filtration.

The approximate dimensions of the glomerular capillary pores can be inferred from the dimensions of molecules which are or are not filtered. Albumin, a somewhat elongated molecule of molecular weight (MW) about 70,000, normally penetrates the glomerular membrane very little if at all. Hemoglobin (MW 68,000) with almost the same molecular weight but a more spherical configuration is estimated to be present in glomerular filtrate at a concentration about 5 per cent of its concentration in plasma (after the latter concentration has been corrected for the binding of hemoglobin to other larger proteins of plasma) [83]. It is clear that the size of the pores of the glomerular membrane cannot differ greatly from that of these molecules.

The permeability of the glomerular membrane to polysaccharides is of some interest not only for the information it may yield on pore size but because one polysaccharide, inulin, has played a major role in the study of renal function. Inulin is a polymer of fructose. It is usually assigned a molecular weight of 5200, but it is probably polydisperse — that is, the molecules vary in size, some being larger, some smaller, than the mean. It is a highly elongated molecule and has a lower diffusibility and penetrates membranes less readily than would be expected for a substance of its molecular weight. Nevertheless, it passes the glomerular membrane quite readily, and the concentration of inulin in glomerular filtrate is the same as that in plasma water [64]. Dextrans have also been used in the investigation of renal function. These polymers of glucose vary in molecular weight from a few thousand to several hundred thousand. Those with molecular weights approximating that of inulin appear to be completely filtrable across the glomerular capillary membrane. As the molecular weight increases, their penetration is progressively restricted, and in the study of Wallenius [170] no dextrans of molecular weight in excess of 55,000 appeared in the urine.

Although no definitive figure can be assigned to the capillary membrane pore dimensions and the figure derived depends to some extent on the theoretical treatment applied, the available data are compatible with the presence of pores approximately 100 angstroms (A) in diameter.

REGULATION OF GLOMERULAR
FILTRATION RATE

In considering the physiologic regulation of glomerular filtration rate, it is apparent from equation (1) that changes may result from modification of any of four variables: (1) glomerular permeability; (2) capillary blood pressure; (3) intracapsular hydrostatic pressure; and (4) colloid osmotic pressure.

1. *Glomerular permeability.* Although the specific permeability of the glomerular capillaries (i.e., the permeability per unit area) is ordinarily considered to remain constant under normal conditions, K_p of equation (1) cannot be considered a permeability constant, because it may vary with the area of the capillary bed exposed to filtration. How great a fraction of the total capillary bed contributes to glomerular filtration at any one time is a question that has evoked differences of opinion. The area available for filtration depends upon the number of functioning glomeruli and the number of capillaries in each glomerulus contributing to the process. It has at various times been proposed that the regulation of glomerular filtration is effected largely through changes in the proportion of functioning glomeruli. Physiologic data from some lower vertebrates are quite in accord with this view [47, 135]. However, in mammals the weight of evidence strongly favors the view that all the glomeruli are continuously active under normal conditions and that variations in glomerular filtration depend on changes in the volume of filtrate per glomerulus rather than in the number of glomeruli contributing to the process [27, 147, 162]. (The physiologic data on which these conclusions are based do

not bear on the possibility of variation in the number of capillary loops per glomerulus open at any time.)

2. *Capillary blood pressure.* The major variable in determining the rate of glomerular filtration is the intracapillary hydrostatic pressure. The latter in turn depends upon the aortic pressure and the resistances of the glomerular arterioles. Constriction of the afferent arteriole tends to lower the glomerular capillary pressure; dilatation of the afferent arteriole causes the glomerular capillary pressure to approach that in the aorta. Conversely, constriction of the efferent arteriole tends to raise the glomerular capillary pressure and filtration rate, dilatation to lower them. The degree of constriction of these arterioles is presumably under neural control; indeed, this is probably the only physiologic role of the renal nerves. Nevertheless the kidney, even when totally separated from nervous control, shows a capacity to maintain a reasonably constant blood flow and filtration rate despite wide changes in renal artery pressure [37]. This phenomenon, which has been designated *autoregulation,* has been the subject of considerable study [68, 172]. Although opinions as to its origin differ, it probably results from myogenic adjustments of arteriolar tone to variations in distending pressure [163].

It should be noted that it is the pressure in the glomerular capillaries, not the flow through them, that is the determinant of glomerular filtration rate. The flow becomes a limiting factor only to the extent that filtration of a large fraction of the plasma flowing through the glomerular capillaries raises the concentration of the plasma proteins and thus their osmotic effect opposing filtration. Because of the dependence on pressure rather than flow, there is no obligatory relationship between cardiac output and glomerular filtration rate. As long as arterial pressure is maintained, a low cardiac output is compatible with a normal rate of filtration except insofar as afferent arteriolar constriction is a part of the

vasoconstrictor response involved in the maintenance of arterial pressure in the face of the decreased cardiac output.

3. *Intracapsular hydrostatic pressure.* Variations in the pressure in the glomerular capsule probably contribute little to the regulation of glomerular filtration under normal physiologic circumstances.* The level of intracapsular pressure becomes important, however, when it is increased by resistance to the outflow of urine from the tubules. In massive solute diuresis the pressure required to drive the increased flow through the tubules may well contribute to the decrease in glomerular filtration rate which is frequently observed. Total obstruction of the ureter reduces glomerular filtration to very low levels, presumably through the very high intracapsular pressure it produces.

4. *Colloid osmotic pressure.* The osmotic effect of the plasma proteins is roughly equivalent to a hydrostatic pressure of 25 to 30 mm. Hg opposing the filtration of fluid from the glomerular capillaries. Consequently, when hydrostatic pressure in the glomerular capillaries falls to the level of 25 to 30 mm. Hg, glomerular filtration ceases. Because the concentration of the plasma proteins is relatively stable under physiologic conditions, it is probably not an important variable in regulating the rate of glomerular filtration.

MEASUREMENT OF GLOMERULAR FILTRATION

The measurement of glomerular filtration plays a central role in the evaluation of renal

* However, note should be taken of the view proposed by Bojesen [17], and strongly supported by Leyssac [88], that intracapsular hydrostatic pressure is a major determinant of filtration rate. Since (1) this pressure is in part determined by the resistance to flow through the tubule, (2) the resistance is related to the rate at which flow diminishes along the nephron as a result of reabsorption of fluid, and (3) the rate of reabsorption of fluid is determined largely by the rate of reabsorption of sodium salts (see page 59), it would follow that glomerular filtration rate varies with sodium reabsorption rather than the reverse as is generally held!

function. The difference between the rate at which a substance is filtered at the glomeruli and the rate at which it is excreted in the urine is equal to the rate at which it is reabsorbed from or secreted into the urine by the activity of the renal tubules. The rate at which the substance is filtered is given by the product of the rate of glomerular filtration and the concentration of the substance in the water of plasma (with correction, if necessary, for binding to plasma protein and for Donnan effects in the case of electrolytes). The rate of excretion may be determined as the product of the volume flow of urine and the concentration in that urine of the particular substance in question. The difference between the rates of filtration and excretion yields a quantitative estimate of the net activity of the tubules in adding the substance to or subtracting it from the urine. Thus, determination of the rate of glomerular filtration is important not only as an evaluation of the initial step in the formation of urine but also as an essential for the quantitative assessment of the processes of reabsorption and secretion by the tubules.

The measurement is based upon the excretion of some substance which can be neither reabsorbed nor secreted by the tubules. In the steady state the rate of excretion of such a substance must be equal to the rate at which it is filtered at the glomeruli. Thus:

$$(2) \quad U_x V = GFR\, P_x \ \textit{or}\ GFR = \frac{U_x V}{P_x}$$

where U_x is the concentration of substance X in the urine, V is the volume flow of urine (usually in milliliters per minute), GFR is the rate of glomerular filtration, and P_x is the concentration of X in the plasma (assuming X to be freely filtrable at the glomeruli).

It is now generally accepted that inulin fulfills the necessary criteria to serve as the reference substance in the measurement of glomerular filtration rate. This starch-like polymer of fructose is derived from dahlia tu-

bers and appears to be suitable for the measurement of glomerular filtration rate in all vertebrates, including man.

The expression $U_x V/P_x$ denotes a quantity which is generally referred to as the clearance of X and abbreviated as C_x. It is equal to the volume of plasma required to supply substance X at the rate at which the latter is excreted in the urine. It is thus a measure of the efficiency of the kidney in excreting the substance in question; the higher the clearance, the more effectively the material is removed from the plasma by the activity of the kidney. In other words, the term *clearance* may be considered as designating that volume of plasma which yields its entire content for renal excretion and is thus "cleared" of the substance in question. Some confusion has arisen from this interpretation of the term clearance because the volume is often a virtual rather than a real one. Thus the same value of the clearance is obtained if 100 ml. of plasma yield all of their content for excretion, 200 ml. of plasma half of their content, or 400 ml. one-fourth of their content.

The clearance of inulin or some other substance handled in like manner by the renal tubules is equal to the rate of glomerular filtration. Comparison of the clearance of some other substance with that of inulin can be used to investigate the effects of the tubules on the excretion of the other substance. If its clearance is greater than that of inulin, it is secreted by the tubules; if the clearance is lower, it is reabsorbed. Thus, the rate at which a substance X is filtered is given as the product of the inulin clearance (C_{IN}) and the concentration of X free in the plasma water.

$$\text{Filtered X} \quad = C_{IN} P_x$$

$$\text{Excreted X} \quad = U_x V$$

$$\text{and (3)} \quad C_{IN} P_x + T_x = U_x V$$

where T_x is equal to the rate at which X is transported by the tubules into (sign positive) or out of (sign negative) the urine.

If equation (3) is divided through by P_x we obtain

$$(4) \qquad C_{IN} + \frac{T_x}{P_x} = \frac{U_x V}{P_x} = C_x$$

From inspection of equation (4) it can be seen that if the value of T_x is limited, the clearance of X will approach the clearance of inulin as the concentration of X in the plasma is increased, since as P_x approaches infinity the term T_x/P_x approaches zero. This type of behavior is typical of many of the substances transported by the renal tubules.

RATE OF GLOMERULAR FILTRATION IN MAN

The average-size, well-hydrated man has a glomerular filtration rate of a little more than 125 ml. per minute. If fluids have been withheld for 12 to 18 hours, the level of glomerular filtration is likely to be somewhat lower, but in man, as opposed to many other mammalian species, the rate of glomerular filtration is remarkably constant. To make it possible to compare function in individuals of varying physical stature it is customary to normalize all measurements of renal function by "correcting" them to the standard normal body surface area of 1.73 square meters. Even after such normalization, women have rates of glomerular filtration averaging some 10 per cent lower than those of men [155].

A consideration of the magnitude of the process of glomerular filtration gives a picture of the rather impressive magnitude of the reabsorptive processes carried out by the tubules. An average-size man forms some 180 liters of glomerular filtrate each day; of this, all but a liter or two is reabsorbed by the tubules. Since the average-size man has a total body water of some 45 liters, all the body water is filtered on the average of four times a day; similarly the extracellular fluid passes through the glomeruli some fifteen times per day and the plasma volume more than twice each hour. The daily glomerular filtrate contains more than a kilogram of sodium chloride, less than 1 per cent of which is excreted in the urine. It is apparent from the very large amounts filtered and reabsorbed each day that only a small percentage change in these quantities could result in very considerable changes in the rate of excretion.

OTHER MEASURES OF GLOMERULAR FILTRATION

Except for inulin, no substance has yet been found which can be considered to yield a reliable measure of the rate of glomerular filtration in man. Because of technical difficulties in the determination of inulin concentrations, many attempts have been made to find a substitute which would simplify the analytic procedure. Some of these have been moderately successful in yielding methods for approximating the filtration rate and following the direction and rough magnitude of large changes. None of the substitutes can be considered useful for the quantitative assessment of the contributions of reabsorption and secretion to the excretion of some other substance.

The most commonly used substance for approximating glomerular filtration in man is creatinine. The endogenous creatinine clearance on the average is fairly close to the inulin clearance [21]. This is the result of compensating factors; creatinine is secreted by the renal tubules in man [145], so that the clearance of creatinine itself is actually higher than the inulin clearance. However, the plasma contains other substances that give the color reaction by which creatinine concentrations are measured; since these creatinine-like materials of plasma do not appear in the urine, their presence lowers the apparent creatinine clearance. The creatinine clearance, particularly in the presence of renal disease, may vary widely from the inulin clearance and in either direction [101]. Endogenous creatinine clearances in man should be interpreted with considerable caution.

On the other hand, creatinine appears to be excreted by certain mammals (e.g., cat and rabbit) and by amphibians by a mechanism which does not involve secretion or reabsorption [47, 50, 73, 74, 136, 146]. In these species, the clearance of exogenous creatinine is the same as that of inulin and can be substituted for it. Creatinine is secreted by the tubules in the rat [46].

Vitamin B_{12} labeled with radioactive cobalt has been found to have a clearance that gives a reasonably close approximation of the rate of glomerular filtration. Binding of vitamin B_{12} to plasma protein markedly reduces the clearance when the vitamin is present in physiologic amounts, but the binding capacity of the protein can be saturated by the administration of a relatively large dose of nonradioactive vitamin B_{12} [110].

Other substances that have been used to approximate glomerular filtration in man are certain hexitols (particularly mannitol) and allantoin; the mannitol clearance is fairly uniformly some 10 per cent lower than the inulin clearance [5].

Tubular Reabsorption

The magnitude and importance of tubular reabsorption are indicated by a comparison of the volume and composition of glomerular filtrate with the volume and composition of urine. The tubular reabsorptive processes are divided into two groups: passive and active.

PASSIVE REABSORPTION

It is clear that the volume flowing through the renal tubules is markedly reduced by the processes of reabsorption. If, in the course of this reabsorption, some substance is reabsorbed less rapidly than water, its concentration in the remaining fluid rises. Conditions favorable to the diffusion of such a substance from lumen to interstitial fluid and blood are thus created, and if the tubule epithelium is permeable to the substance it will escape from the lumen at a rate determined by this permeability and the concentration gradient from lumen to peritubular fluid. Such a process is designated passive reabsorption. The common example of a substance subject to this type of reabsorption is urea, the excretion of which will be considered in more detail later.

In general, the transport of materials across membranes is considered passive when it can be attributed to easily defined physical forces: gradients of concentration, gradients of electrical potential in the case of charged particles, and frictional forces due to the flow of solvent through channels through the membrane [165]. (In biologic systems it is usual to discount the possible existence of temperature gradients, which could also cause passive movement.) The significance of such defined forces is that they make it unnecessary to assume that metabolic energy is required to move the substance in question at a greater rate or in a direction other than that in which it would move spontaneously. It is not, however, justifiable to interpret passive movement as indicating that the entire system in which it occurs is independent of metabolic energy. The energy is required to produce the movement of other substances, which in turn produce the osmotic, concentration, or electrical gradients that can cause the movement of the passively transported material. The importance of distinguishing lies in the fact that when it can be shown that the movement of a substance is passive there is no need to seek a specific chemical process involved in its transport or to look for the mechanism by which metabolic energy is specifically channeled into the process. In the case of the passive movement of urea out of the tubule, it will be shown that the metabolic energy is required to effect the movement of sodium out of the tubules; this creates an osmotic gradient which causes the (passive) movement of water out of the lumen. As a result, the urea concentration is increased and it may diffuse from the lumen in a process of passive reabsorption.

ACTIVE REABSORPTION

The reabsorption of many substances from the renal tubules cannot be explained as the consequence of concentration gradients. In some instances very marked concentration gradients *opposing* the movement of the substance may be established in the process of reabsorption. Such processes fall in the category of active transport and are designated by the term *active reabsorption*. The classic example of active reabsorption is the process by which glucose is removed from the tubular fluid. A consideration of the process of glucose reabsorption will illustrate many of the features of this type of mechanism.

REABSORPTION OF GLUCOSE

Glucose is normally present in the plasma, and, since it is completely filtrable, must also be present in the glomerular filtrate (as, indeed, micropuncture study [134] has shown it to be). Under normal conditions, however, glucose is absent from the urine except for negligible traces. Clearly, then, glucose is reabsorbed by the tubules, against the gradient established by its removal which lowers the concentration in the tubule lumen to virtually zero. Since glucose bears no electrical charge, its reabsorption requires an active transport process.

If the concentration of glucose in the plasma is increased progressively, it is found that the urine remains free of glucose until the concentration in the plasma reaches a critical value. Glucose then appears in the urine. As the plasma concentration is increased further, the amount in the urine increases in proportion to the increment in plasma glucose. These relationships may be examined in detail by the measurement of the arterial* plasma glucose

concentration, the inulin clearance (glomerular filtration rate), and the rate of excretion of glucose. It is found that as the plasma glucose concentration is increased, the rate of reabsorption initially remains equal to the rate at which glucose is filtered and none appears in the urine. At a certain point, however, reabsorption fails to increase further, and with additional increases in the amount filtered the excess is excreted in the urine [150]. These relationships are illustrated in Figure 2-1.

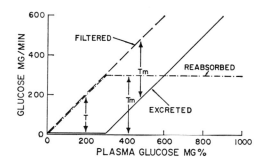

Figure 2-1. Relationship of filtration and reabsorption to excretion of glucose. (Glomerular filtration rate assumed constant at 100 ml. per minute, glucose Tm 300 mg. per minute.)

The relationship between the several variables may be expressed by the equation

$$(5) \qquad U_G V = C_{IN} P_G - T_G$$

where T_G is the rate of reabsorption of glucose from the tubule and the subscripts G and IN refer to glucose and inulin, respectively.

T_G increases progressively, remaining equal to the filtered glucose until it reaches a limiting value. With further increases in the filtered load ($C_{IN} P_G$) there is no further change in T_G and the limiting value of glucose reabsorption is designated as Tm_G or the transport maximum for glucose [150].

---

* For many substances it is sufficient and convenient to measure venous plasma concentrations. However, it is arterial plasma that is filtered in the glomeruli, and the venous plasma concentration is the same as the arterial only when the arterial concentration is stable with time and when the substance in question cannot be produced in or metabolized by the peripheral tissues. The latter condition is not fulfilled for glucose.

Such limiting transport rates are characteristic of many active processes. They are generally interpreted as indicating the involvement of a "carrier" in the transport process [149]. The concept of carrier-mediated transport depends upon the assumption that the transported substance combines reversibly with some component of the transporting membrane. This membrane component or carrier is then assumed to rotate or diffuse to the other surface of the membrane,* carrying with it the substance being transported. The substance may then dissociate from the carrier on the far side of the membrane. Such carrier-mediated transport may occur in the direction of the concentration gradient, as appears to be the case for glucose entry into the human red blood cell [84]. In this case the movement is passive, even though carrier-mediated, and no source of energy other than the concentration gradient is required. In the renal tubule, however, the transport is against the concentration gradient, and without some chemical energy to drive the movement of glucose the spontaneous movement would be in the other direction.

One may visualize the reactions involved as represented by the equation

$$\overset{(1)}{A_1 + B} \rightleftharpoons \overset{(2)}{AB} \rightarrow A_t + B$$

where A_1 represents the glucose in the tubule lumen, B the carrier, AB the glucose-carrier complex in the membrane, and A_t the glucose liberated on the other side of the membrane. Since the concentration of A_t becomes greater than that of A_1 — as a result of the falling concentration in the lumen — some means of forcing the reaction to the right is required. This might be achieved by driving the dissociation of AB to A_t and B, or possibly some change in

the carrier might occur in reaction (2) requiring the carrier to be regenerated at the luminal surface before it is able again to combine with A.

When the transport reaction is saturated, e.g., glucose is being transported at a rate equal to Tm_G, all of the carrier is considered to be tied up in the combined form. Under these circumstances the rate of transport will be determined by the concentration of total carrier and the rate constant for the dissociation of the glucose-carrier complex. While one might suppose that the available energy for driving the transport process might become rate-limiting, there is no evidence that this is the case, and the renal tubules are able to carry out simultaneously a wide variety of transport processes without evidence of mutual interference.

Although the existence of carriers is fairly widely accepted and the concept is a very useful one in explaining a number of phenomena related to membrane transport, it is important to recognize their hypothetical nature. No carrier has yet been isolated or even identified. The presumed interaction of carrier and transported substance is analogous to the interaction of an enzyme and its substrate and, in fact, the reactions above are formally identical with those which form the basis of the Michaelis-Menten equation for the kinetic analysis of enzymatic reactions. Transport reactions also share with enzymatic reactions the property of being inhibited either competitively or noncompetitively. The transport of glucose is rather specifically inhibited by the glycoside, phlorizin. Adequate doses of the latter compound may completely abolish the reabsorption of glucose, so that the clearance of glucose becomes equal to that of inulin. Several other monosaccharides also appear to be transported by the same mechanism by which glucose is reabsorbed, although in these other cases the reabsorption is far less efficient [50]. These various saccharides are mutually competitive for transport, and their reabsorption is inhibited by phlorizin.

---

* The membrane here need not include the full thickness of the cell concerned, e.g., the tubule epithelial cell; it may be the cell membrane itself, in the case of the renal tubule either the membrane facing the tubule lumen or the membrane at the basal aspect of the cell.

Micropuncture studies in both amphibians and mammals have shown that glucose is reabsorbed in the proximal convoluted tubule [134, 169]. The concentration of glucose normally drops quite rapidly, so that most of the glucose has disappeared about halfway down the proximal tubule. In animals given phlorizin, glucose becomes concentrated in the proximal tubule as a result of the reabsorption of water without glucose, and its concentration pattern becomes that of substances excreted by filtration only.

In normal man of "standard" size (1.73 square meters of body surface area) the capacity to reabsorb glucose (Tm_G) averages 375 mg. per minute; in women, approximately 300 mg. per minute [154]. If this figure is considered in relation to the normal rate of glomerular filtration of about 125 ml. per minute, it may be calculated that glucose reabsorptive capacity should become saturated when the plasma glucose concentration is 3 mg. per milliliter or 300 mg. per 100 ml. In accordance with the idealized relationship illustrated in

Figure 2-1, one should then expect to find no glucose in the urine until the plasma glucose concentration exceeded 300 mg. per 100 ml., and at this point glucose reabsorption should become maximal and equal to Tm_G and show no further increase at higher plasma glucose concentrations. In practice this is clearly not the case. It is common experience that in the presence of hyperglycemia, glucose may be expected to appear in the urine at considerably lower plasma concentrations.

The actual relationship between filtered and excreted glucose observed by Smith [154] and his associates is shown in Figure 2-2. It may be seen from this figure that glucose begins to appear in the urine (T falls below load) when the load (the amount of glucose filtered) is only some 70 per cent of the capacity to reabsorb glucose. Furthermore, the full capacity to reabsorb glucose is not utilized until the amount filtered is some 50 per cent greater than the reabsorptive capacity. The real relationship between filtration and reabsorption differs from the idealized one considered ear-

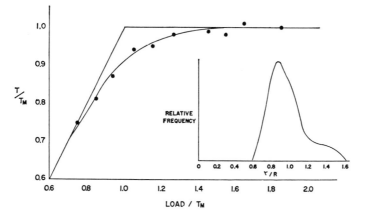

Figure 2-2. Titration of the capacity to reabsorb glucose. Based on average data from 10 normal individuals. The ordinate (T/Tm) is the ratio of glucose reabsorbed at a particular value of filtered glucose to the maximum capacity to reabsorb glucose in the same individual. It is thus the fractional saturation of glucose reabsorptive capacity. The abscissa (load/Tm) is the amount of glucose available for reabsorption, again related to the capacity of the individual to reabsorb glucose. The frequency distribution curve shows the proportion of nephrons having various ratios (r) of filtration rate to reabsorptive capacity as related to the average of this ratio (R) for the two kidneys as a unit. The data are those of Smith, Goldring, Chasis, Ranges, and Bradley (*J. Mt. Sinai Hosp.* 10:59, 1943).

lier because, in arriving at the idealized relationship, two implicit assumptions have been made. While satisfactory for first approximations, these assumptions cannot be considered entirely in conformity with the true situation. The two assumptions are: (1) as the plasma glucose is increased, all the filtered glucose in each nephron is *completely* reabsorbed right up to the point at which the transport capacity is fully saturated; and (2) all the nephrons of the two kidneys are identical — or, at least, the ratio of glomerular filtration rate to glucose reabsorptive capacity is identical in all.

Assumption (1) can be analyzed in terms of what is believed to be the first step in the transport process, the reversible combination of glucose with carrier $(A_1 + B \rightleftharpoons AB)$. The mass action expression corresponding to this reaction can be written as

$$\frac{[A_1]\,[B]}{[AB]} = K$$

From this it can be seen that there must always be a finite concentration of A_1 (residual unreabsorbed glucose) and a finite concentration of B (unutilized carrier transport capacity). However, if the dissociation constant for the complex is very small, the values of $[A_1]$ and $[B]$ can both be very small simultaneously, which would yield a situation *close* to that required by assumption (1). If K is not very small, then $[A_1]$, the concentration of unresorbed substrate, can be very small only when there is an appreciable excess of B, unused transport capacity; conversely, B can be very small (i.e., the transport capacity saturated) only when there is a considerable excess of residual, unreabsorbed substrate. It has been shown that in the case of glucose (but this is probably not true of a number of other substances reabsorbed by the tubules) the value of K must, indeed, be very small and that most of the departure of the titration curve of glucose reabsorption (Fig. 2-2) from the idealized version (Fig. 2-1) is related to the unrealistic nature of assumption (2) [24].

It is apparent a priori not only that nephrons are not all identical but that they cannot be expected to have the same balance of glomerular filtration rate against glucose reabsorptive capacity. Thus there must be some heterogeneity of the ratio of filtration rate to reabsorptive capacity, referred to as glomerulo-tubular balance. Those nephrons with a high ratio of filtration rate to glucose reabsorptive capacity will become saturated when the plasma glucose concentration is too low to saturate the average nephron. Such nephrons account for the appearance of glucose in the urine when the total amount of glucose filtered is too low to saturate the reabsorptive capacity of all the nephrons if the filtered glucose were distributed among the nephrons in proportion to their capacity to reabsorb. Conversely, those nephrons with low ratios of filtration rate to reabsorptive capacity will not become saturated until the plasma glucose concentration is considerably higher than is required to effect saturation of the average nephron. Smith [154] and his associates have calculated the distribution of ratios of filtration rate to glucose reabsorptive capacity in normal man. The results, included in Figure 2-2, indicate that the ratio varies from about 40 per cent below to 60 per cent above that for the average of the two kidneys taken as a unit.

OTHER SUBSTANCES ACTIVELY REABSORBED BY THE TUBULES

Glucose reabsorption has been treated in detail as the most typical and best studied of a number of active reabsorptive processes. Except for the reabsorption of strong monovalent electrolytes and water, which will be considered separately, all the active reabsorptive processes of the kidney that have been studied have proved to be located in the proximal convoluted tubule. Most of these processes share the general features of glucose reabsorption.

Amino Acids. Although amino acids are normally present in the plasma they are, except for traces, absent from the urine and must therefore be reabsorbed by the tubules. Several distinct transport mechanisms have been recognized, each apparently responsible for the reabsorption of a group of generally structurally related amino acids [15, 119]. The basic amino acids arginine, lysine, and histidine appear to be reabsorbed by a common mechanism. Raising the concentration of one of these amino acids depresses the reabsorption of the others. A limited capacity to reabsorb arginine and lysine has been demonstrated, but in the case of histidine no evidence of saturation of the transport mechanism has been obtained at the highest concentrations attained experimentally. Leucine and isoleucine are reabsorbed by another process, which they share and for which they compete. Glycine, proline, and hydroxyproline have been reported to compete for another transport process [144], and there is some evidence that creatine may be reabsorbed by the same mechanism as glycine [118].

Phosphate. Phosphate is reabsorbed by an active process in the proximal convoluted tubule [97, 121]. The mechanism is subject to saturation and is probably inhibited by parathyroid hormone although the latter point is disputed [60, 65, 70]. There is some evidence that acidosis increases the excretion of phosphate by increasing the "splay" of the titration curve, i.e., the extent of its departure from the idealized form (Fig. 2-1) [140]. There have been repeated poorly documented reports that phosphate is secreted into as well as reabsorbed from the renal tubules, but there is no convincing evidence for the existence of a phosphate secretory process in the dog or in man.

Sulfate. Sulfate is reabsorbed by a process which is rather unusual in that it becomes saturated at plasma sulfate concentrations only slightly in excess of normal [90]. Thiosulfate is reabsorbed in the dog by the same mechanism responsible for sulfate reabsorption, and these two divalent anions compete for the transport capacity [6].

Urate. Urate is reabsorbed by a process that is unique in its susceptibility to inhibition by a wide variety of agents, some of which are secreted by rather than reabsorbed by the tubules. The capacity to reabsorb is far greater than that required to reabsorb the filtered urate under any conditions which might be encountered in the ordinary course of events in the normal individual [10]. Nevertheless, urate is normally excreted at an appreciable rate, an amount equal to some 5 to 10 per cent of the filtered urate appearing in the urine. Increasing evidence supports the suggestion that the excretion may be attributable, not to residual filtered and unreabsorbed urate, but to urate deposited in the tubule lumen by a separate secretory process [58].

Tubular Secretion

The term tubular secretion is used to designate processes by which substances are removed from the peritubular capillary blood and transported into the tubule lumen. This phenomenon is also sometimes called tubular excretion. Consideration in this section is limited to the processes by which organic electrolytes are transferred into the urine. These appear to be confined to the proximal tubule. The processes by which potassium, hydrogen, and ammonium ion enter the urine will be considered separately.

The first clear demonstration of tubular secretion was provided by Marshall and Vickers [99] in studies with phenol red. It was shown that as much as 75 per cent of the phenol red brought to the kidney in the plasma might be excreted in the urine; however, because of the binding of phenol red to plasma protein, only about 25 per cent of the plasma dye was filtrable and available for excretion by glomerular filtration. Since the amount excreted was greater than that which could be provided by the filtration of any fraction of the perfusing plasma, tubular secretion must be involved in the process.

A large number of substances are now recognized as secreted by the renal tubules. Excluding the strong monovalent cations (K^+, H^+, NH_4^+) these fall into two groups, organic anions and organic cations. Within each group there is a wide variation in the structure of the secreted materials, but for members of each group the transport mechanism appears to be identical. Thus among the organic anions transported are sulfonic acids, such as phenol red and a number of structurally related substances: carboxylic acids, such as para-aminohippurate (PAH), iodopyracet (Diodrast), penicillin, and a number of the iodinated urographic contrast media;* glucuronides, ethereal sulfates, and the sulfonamide structure represented by chlorothiazide and acetazolamide (see Taggart [160] for review). In those instances in which it has been examined there is mutual competition among these substances for transport, and a single highly nonspecific process seems to be involved. It is noteworthy that among the substrates none is a normal constituent of the body fluids, and the biologic role of this phylogenetically widely distributed transport system is not known. It may be involved primarily in the rapid excretion of conjugation products of foreign substances that enter the body.

The organic cations appear to be secreted by a separate and functionally independent transport system (see Peters [116] for review). This, too, has a very low specificity, the excreted substances including quaternary ammonium ions (e.g., tetraethyl ammonium), tertiary amines (e.g., N-methyl-nicotinamide, tolazoline), and secondary amines (e.g., mecamylamine).

* The iodine is important to their radiologic density, but not to their transport.

Despite the reversal of the direction of transport, the mechanisms involved in tubular secretion resemble in many respects those involved in active tubular reabsorption. When relatively small amounts of material are presented to it, the transport mechanism is able to reduce the substrate concentration virtually to zero, moving the transported material against what may be very steep concentration gradients. As the amount presented for transport increases, the amount secreted increases only up to a point. The mechanism becomes saturated, and a maximum rate of transfer is achieved which does not increase with further increases in load.

The substance most frequently used for study of this type of mechanism is para-aminohippuric acid† and the excretion of PAH illustrates some of the features of these processes. When PAH is administered in such a way that the concentration in plasma is held constant at rather low levels (generally 2 mg. per 100 ml. or less), the concentration in renal venous plasma is generally only some 10 per cent of that in arterial or peripheral venous plasma — i.e., some 85 to 90 per cent of the PAH brought to the kidney by the plasma is removed during its passage through the kidney (see Smith [156] for summary). Since at least some of the blood flowing through the renal vessels must perfuse structures (e.g., capsule, connective tissue, possibly medulla) which do not transport PAH, there is reason to believe that an even greater fraction of PAH is removed from that plasma which actually comes in contact with the transporting tissue.‡ It is generally believed that extrac-

† The hippurates as a group are rapidly secreted by the renal tubular secretory mechanism for organic anions; the amino group is important only in that it facilitates chemical determination in blood and urine.

‡ It is currently popular to equate the nonextracted fraction of the renal plasma flow with that volume of renal plasma flow that perfuses the medulla, on the assumption that renal cortical plasma is completely freed of PAH, but that PAH is not extracted by medullary segments [117, 132]. It is questionable that renal medullary plasma flow can even be approximated in this way, and

tion is virtually complete in the latter case. Accepting this assumption, it is apparent that the plasma perfusing functioning tissue is completely cleared of PAH and that its clearance is therefore equal to the plasma flow to such tissue. This is the basis of the use of the clearance of PAH and other similarly handled substances for the estimation of effective renal plasma and blood flow; this application is considered in more detail below.

If the excretion of PAH is studied as a function of plasma PAH concentration, a relationship such as that illustrated in Figure 2-3

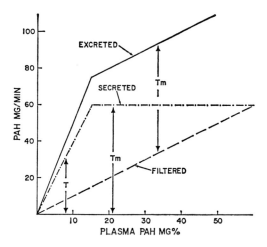

Figure 2-3. Relationship between plasma PAH and PAH excretion, assuming renal plasma flow of 500 ml. per minute, glomerular filtration rate of 100 ml. per minute, and Tm_{PAH} 60 mg. per minute.

is found. In evaluating this relationship it is necessary to take into account the PAH filtered at the glomeruli, subtracting the amount filtered from the total excreted to estimate the amount reaching the urine as a result of the secretory process. The amount filtered is determined by the simultaneous estimation of glomerular filtration rate (inulin clearance)

and is equal to the product of filtration rate and plasma PAH concentration when the latter has been corrected for a small amount of binding to plasma albumin. The amount filtered is represented by the dashed line in Figure 2-3. The difference between the rate of excretion and the rate of filtration is the rate of tubular secretion:

$$U_{PAH}V = C_{IN}P_{PAH}f + T_{PAH}$$

where f is the fraction of the plasma PAH not bound to plasma protein.

It is seen that the rate of excretion exceeds that attributable to filtration throughout and that the rate of secretion increases in direct proportion to plasma concentration so long as the plasma concentration remains low. When the latter exceeds a critical value, the rate of secretion no longer increases, further increments in excretion being due solely to the increased amounts in the glomerular filtrate. The secretory mechanism is saturated and the rate of secretion is designated as Tm_{PAH}.

In actual practice, the observed relationship departs, as in the case of reabsorption, from the idealized intersection of two straight lines. Thus the extraction of PAH from the perfusing blood falls below the maximal value found at low plasma concentrations before the secretory mechanism is saturated, and conversely the secretory mechanism does not become saturated until the amount delivered to it is considerably in excess of its capacity to transport [154]. This splay in the PAH titration curve is analogous to that observed with glucose and has a similar basis: (1) the dissociation of substrate-carrier complex; and (2) heterogeneity of the nephron population. In this case it is not, of course, the heterogeneity of glomerulo-tubular balance which is pertinent, but the dispersion of perfusion with plasma to transport capacity.

There is a large group of organic anions and another of organic cations that are rapidly secreted by the same mechanisms under consideration here, but which, because of the high

---

the calculation frequently yields preposterously high values of medullary perfusion (i.e., when total renal plasma flow is high and extraction is low).

lipid solubility of their undissociated forms, are able to escape from the tubule lumen by diffusion in more distal portions of the nephron [173]. Thus the amount of such substances excreted may fall far below the amount secreted and may often be even less than the amount filtered. Included in this group of weak acids that are secreted but subsequently escape the lumen by nonionic diffusion (see page 77) are several that had originally been considered specific inhibitors of transport not themselves subject to transport. These substances (e.g., probenecid, phenylbutazone) are now recognized to be competitive inhibitors which, however, appear in the urine in small amounts because in their undissociated acid forms they readily penetrate the lining epithelium of the tubules [174]. The usefulness of PAH and Diodrast as measures of secretion (and plasma flow) derives not only from their rapid transport but from their low solubility in lipid, which prevents their passive penetration of cells.

UTILIZATION OF TUBULAR SECRETION FOR
MEASUREMENT OF RENAL BLOOD FLOW

As indicated above, several substances are removed virtually completely from the plasma that perfuses the kidney. This characteristic has rendered them particularly useful for the estimation of renal plasma and blood flow. Diodrast and PAH have been most often used for this purpose, the latter particularly because of the ease with which it may be chemically detected, the former because it was the first substance found to suit the purpose and more recently because of the ease with which it may be labeled with radioactive iodine (^{131}I) and its concentration measured from its radioactivity. The application to measurement of blood flow may be developed using Diodrast as an example.

The Fick principle holds that if the rate of removal of a substance from the blood during its passage through an organ is known and the concentration of the substance in the blood entering and leaving the organ can be determined, then the flow can be determined since

$$\text{Flow} = \frac{\text{Removal rate}}{\text{A–V concentration difference}}$$

This equation can be applied to the measurement of renal plasma flow with Diodrast if all the Diodrast removed from the blood appears in the urine. Then the excretion rate may, in the steady state, be taken as the removal rate. It is also important that all the Diodrast removed from the blood during passage through the kidney be removed from the plasma and that the red cells contribute none of the excreted Diodrast.* One may then say that

$$\text{RPF} = \frac{U_D V}{P_D{}^A - P_D{}^{RV}}$$

where RPF is renal plasma flow, $U_D V$ the rate of Diodrast excretion, and $P_D{}^A$ and $P_D{}^{RV}$ the concentrations of Diodrast in arterial and renal venous plasma, respectively.

All the terms in the right-hand member of this equation are determinable. However, the collection of renal venous blood is considerably more difficult than the collection of either urine or arterial blood, and even the latter can be replaced by peripheral venous blood since, when the plasma Diodrast concentration is stable, peripheral venous and arterial Diodrast concentrations are identical. Taking into account the fact that Diodrast is extracted virtually completely from the plasma during its passage through the kidney, i.e., that $P_D{}^{RV}$ is close to zero when $P_D{}^A$ is low, we may write as a first approximation

$$\text{ERPF} = \frac{U_D V}{P_D} = C_D$$

---

* Certain organic bases have clearances even higher than that of Diodrast or PAH because the red cells contribute to that which appears in the urine [111, 143].

or the effective renal plasma flow is equal to the Diodrast clearance at low plasma Diodrast concentrations. (As the plasma Diodrast concentration is increased, the extraction of Diodrast from the perfusing plasma is less complete and the Diodrast clearance is no longer an adequate approximation of the renal plasma flow.)

From the effective renal plasma flow and the hematocrit, the effective renal blood flow (ERBF) can be calculated:

$$ERBF = \frac{ERPF}{1 - Hct}$$

It is noteworthy that the application of the Diodrast clearance to measurement of renal plasma flow was introduced by Homer Smith [152] and his associates before the technic of venous catheterization made possible the collection of renal venous blood. Their deduction was based on the very large value of the Diodrast clearance (over 600 ml. per minute), which made it seem improbable that the renal plasma flow could be much higher. It should also be noted that if renal venous plasma is collected and analyzed, PAH, Diodrast, etc., have no unique value for the measurement of plasma flow. Then any substance excreted in the urine and not produced or stored in or metabolized by the kidney could be used. Under these conditions the advantage in the use of Diodrast, etc., is only that a high extraction ratio minimizes experimental error.

RENAL BLOOD FLOW IN MAN

The application of the clearance of PAH and Diodrast to the estimation of renal plasma flow has made possible the measurement of this physiologic function in the relatively intact and undisturbed individual. (In fact, methods have been devised which, though of limited usefulness, make unnecessary even the collection of urine [43].) Consequently, considerable information has been obtained concerning the renal blood flow under various physiologic stresses and in disease [153].

The very large renal plasma flow in normal man has already been mentioned. The average normal blood flow of some 1200 ml. per minute indicates that roughly one-quarter of the cardiac output perfuses the kidneys under basal conditions. This "renal fraction" of the cardiac output is, of course, subject to variation with the physiologic or pathologic state of the individual.

The value of the renal plasma flow is also used for calculation of another significant variable, the extent to which fluid is lost from the plasma as it passes through the glomerular capillaries. Since virtually all the renal plasma flow must pass through the glomerular capillaries, the glomerular filtrate is derived more or less evenly from all the perfusing plasma, and the ratio of the rate of glomerular filtration to the renal plasma flow, or *filtration fraction,* is a measure of the fluid loss from the plasma and the extent to which the plasma proteins are concentrated in the process. In normal man the filtration fraction averages about 0.2.

Although the rate of glomerular filtration in man is a relatively stable function, the renal blood flow is subject to wide and frequently rapid fluctuations. Variations in renal blood flow result largely from changes in renal vascular resistance which are mediated chiefly, but not entirely, via the renal nerves. In fact, although the question of a nervous control of renal tubular transport has been the subject of inconclusive debate, there is good reason to hold to the view that the only significant role of the renal nerves is in the regulation of vascular tone, and hence blood flow.

Renal blood flow is reduced by exercise, by fright, by norepinephrine, by stimulation of certain areas in the central nervous system, and, in general, by anything that tends to reduce systemic blood pressure. When the systemic pressure is decreased, the reduction of renal blood flow is generally far greater than can be explained by the reduction in pressure alone and is attributable to increases in renal vascular resistance. These increases reflect the fact that the renal vasculature takes part in the generalized vasoconstriction in response to a reduction in arterial pressure. Renal blood flow may be markedly reduced when the drop in blood pressure is minimal. Renal blood flow is also reduced by most of the drugs that reduce blood pressure. In this instance, the reduction in flow is usually considerably smaller than when equivalent hypotension is due to hemorrhage, etc., because the vasoconstriction is usually inhibited by the drug.

A marked increase in renal blood flow is a striking and characteristic feature of the response to pyrogen. The renal hyperemia, however, is independent of the febrile response itself since it occurs even when the temperature rise is prevented by the prior administration of antipyretic drugs.

With all of the cited changes of renal blood flow, changes in glomerular filtration rate are generally comparatively slight and may, in fact, be absent. Thus the filtration fraction usually varies inversely with the renal blood flow.

Reabsorption and Excretion of Water

One of the most striking and important features of mammalian renal function is the capacity to produce urine differing very markedly in total solute concentration from the plasma from which it is derived. It is through the production of urine considerably more concentrated or dilute than the body fluids that the concentration of those fluids is, under normal conditions, maintained within very narrow limits despite wide fluctuations in the intake and extrarenal loss of water. When the body fluids are diluted by an excess of water, the urine becomes dilute and the excess is rapidly excreted; conversely, when because of excessive intake of solute or loss of water the concentration of the body fluids

rises above normal, the urine becomes highly concentrated so that solute is lost in excess of water, the water retained tending to return the body fluids to a normal solute concentration.

It is desirable, before considering the processes involved in these events, to review the concept of osmotic pressure and define the units in which it is measured. If two solutions of differing solute concentration are separated by a membrane permeable to the solvent (water in all cases pertinent here) but not to the solute, water will move from the solution which has the lower solute concentration into that which has the higher concentration. The net movement is based on the fact that the presence of solute reduces the activity of the water and the water moves from the place where its activity is high to that in which it is low. (For most purposes activity may be considered very closely related to concentration.) The water movement will continue until the solutions on both sides of the membrane have attained the same concentration or, if the water movement is opposed by the application of a hydrostatic pressure to the more concentrated side, until the hydrostatic pressure just balances the concentration difference. This hydrostatic pressure is then said to be equal to the osmotic pressure difference between the two solutions. The osmotic pressure of a solution is that pressure which would be required to prevent the entry of water into it if it were separated from pure water by an ideal semipermeable membrane.* It is common usage to speak of the osmotic pressure of solutions even though osmotic pressure is virtually never measured. However, several other properties of solutions vary in exact proportion to the osmotic pressure and these are more easily measured — e.g., depression of the freezing point, decrease of the vapor pressure. In fact, even the use of the term osmotic pressure is a

---

* An ideal semipermeable membrane is one that is freely permeable to the solvent but totally impermeable to the solute.

rather loose application since in physiology it is usually expressed in units of concentration rather than pressure (see below).

The osmotic pressure, freezing point depression, vapor pressure lowering, etc., are what are referred to as the colligative properties of a solution. These properties depend upon the ratio of solute particles to solvent particles and ideally are independent of the nature of the solute. Thus, ideally the freezing point is depressed to the same extent by a millimol of albumin (MW 70,000) as by a millimol of urea (MW 60), and, because it is dissociated into two particles, a millimol of sodium chloride (MW 58) will depress the freezing point by twice as much as a millimol of urea. One mol of an ideal, undissociated solute dissolved in a kilogram of distilled water yields a solution with a freezing point of $-1.86°$C. Such a solution is defined as an *osmolal* solution and contains one *osmol* per kilogram of water.* Since most physiologic solutions are more dilute than this, it is useful to avoid decimals and speak of *milliosmols* and *microosmols,* a milliosmol being one thousandth of an osmol and a microosmol one thousandth of a milliosmol. The milliosmolality of a solution is defined as its freezing point depression divided by 0.00186. Normal plasma is about 285 milliosmolal (abbreviated 285 mOsm).

Under most normal circumstances the urine flow is relatively low and the urine has an osmotic concentration considerably in excess of the plasma. If under these conditions an individual drinks a moderately large volume of water (e.g., 1000 to 1500 ml.), it is found that the urine produced remains more or less unchanged in composition for a period of some 15 to 20 minutes. Urine flow then begins to increase more or less rapidly and is likely to reach a maximum level some 40 to 60 minutes after the ingestion of the water. Although the exact level attained may be rather variable, it

* Note that the units are per unit weight of solvent, *not* per unit volume of solution.

is generally of the order of 10 to 15 per cent of the rate of glomerular filtration. Flow remains high until most of the ingested water has been excreted, urine flow then falling rapidly to the control level. The high rate of flow may be sustained, however, if a positive water balance is maintained by continuing intake.

A more detailed analysis of the events which take place during such a water diuresis reveals the following significant features. Before the onset of the increasing urine flow there is a slight but definite fall in the osmotic pressure of blood indicating its dilution by the ingested water. The change in flow is almost entirely a change in the rate of excretion of water; there is virtually no change in the excretion of solute, so that the urinary solute concentration (osmotic pressure) varies inversely with the flow. If the rate of glomerular filtration is measured, it is found to change only slightly if at all; the change in water excretion is thus attributable almost entirely to a change in the extent to which water is reabsorbed from the tubules. If at the height of the diuresis the positive balance is increased by ingestion of additional water, the rate of urine flow is not appreciably changed. If, at any time in the course of the diuresis, vasopressin, the antidiuretic hormone (ADH) of the pituitary, is administered, there is an abrupt drop in urine flow to or close to control levels, and the osmotic pressure of the urine promptly rises above that of the blood.

The basis of these features of water diuresis becomes clear from a consideration of the renal mechanisms involved and their extrarenal regulation. The concentration of the urine is normally continuously controlled by the secretion of antidiuretic hormone from the posterior lobe of the pituitary. This hormone has been identified in man and most mammals that have been studied as the octapeptide arginine vasopressin [42]. (In the pig, the arginine is replaced by lysine.) The hormone is believed to be formed by the cells of the hypothalamic supraoptic nuclei and to migrate via the supraoptico-hypophyseal tracts to the posterior lobe of the pituitary gland, where it is stored and released into the blood in response to stimuli believed to be mediated over the same neural pathways.

A number of vesicular cells in the supraoptic nuclei have been tentatively identified as the *osmoreceptors* [168]. These, as other cells, are presumed to behave as tiny osmometers, taking up water and swelling when the osmotic pressure of their environment is diminished and giving up water and shrinking when the solute concentration of the extracellular fluid rises. Shrinkage of the osmoreceptors, indicative of an increased osmotic pressure, is the stimulus leading to release of ADH, which in turn is carried to the kidney, where it effects conservation of water. Conversely, swelling of the osmoreceptors results from an excess of water over solute, and signals an interruption of ADH release; as the circulating ADH disappears, the urine becomes dilute and the excess of water is rapidly excreted.

The current views of the hypothalamic control of ADH secretion outlined above are based heavily on the work of Verney [168], who showed that hypertonic solutions injected into the internal carotid artery of the dog evoked prompt antidiuresis whereas similar amounts injected peripherally were without significant effect. An amount of sodium chloride calculated to increase the osmotic pressure of the carotid blood by about 2 per cent was an effective stimulus to ADH release. Injection of the osmotically equivalent amount of urea, however, was virtually without effect, presumably because urea penetrates cell membranes relatively easily and rapidly. When the urea concentration is raised in their environment, the osmoreceptors presumably take up urea rather than lose water.* Since they do not

shrink, there is no stimulus for ADH release. It is necessary, therefore, to distinguish between the total osmotic pressure and the *effective osmotic pressure* of the body fluids. The total osmotic pressure is that due to all the solutes and is that which would theoretically be found if it were measured with an ideal semipermeable membrane. However, cell membranes are not ideal semipermeable membranes, and the osmotic pressure effective in regulating ADH release is that due to solutes which penetrate cell membranes slowly or not at all. It does, then, include that due to electrolytes and many of the organic constituents of extracellular fluid but excludes substances such as urea, alcohol, etc., which are distributed rapidly and more or less uniformly in body water.

Dilution and concentration of the urine are normally regulated so as to maintain the osmotic pressure of the body fluids within a narrow normal range. However, there are a number of nonosmotic stimuli which can cause the release of antidiuretic hormone and which can therefore lead to the production of concentrated urine even when body fluids are abnormally dilute. Among such stimuli appear to be a diminished circulating blood volume, fear, trauma, and a number of drugs [161].

The results of micropuncture studies are largely responsible for our knowledge of the location and nature of the processes which effect the conversion of the isotonic glomerular filtrate to a urine differing widely in osmotic pressure from the fluid from which it is originally derived. All but a few of the micropuncture studies that have been carried out in mammals have been done in rodents, particularly the rat. However, additional studies have been done in dogs [4, 30] and in the Rhesus monkey [3] and although the re-

---

* In theory, at least, and probably in reality, there is a transient loss of water when the urea concentration of the surroundings is raised. However, the initial rate of water loss, even before any urea has entered the osmore- ceptors, would be lower than when an equivalent concentration of nonpenetrating solute is added. These phenomena can be more clearly demonstrated with red blood cells [53].

sults differ in certain respects from those in the rat, these differences are outweighed by the general similarity. The glomerular filtrate has been shown to have the same osmotic pressure* as the plasma from which it is derived [3, 30, 46, 169]. As the fluid passes down the proximal tubule, the volume flow is rapidly reduced by reabsorption. In the rat and dog only the first 60 per cent of the proximal tubule is available on the surface of the kidney; up to 85 per cent of the proximal tubule can be punctured in the monkey since the surface tubules represent cortical nephrons that have short straight segments. The findings indicate that some 60 to 80 per cent of the glomerular filtrate is reabsorbed in the proximal tubule of hydropenic animals. This reabsorption occurs without change in the osmotic pressure of the remaining fluid *whether the final urine is to be dilute or concentrated* [56, 169, 180]. Thus this portion of the reabsorption of glomerular filtrate, which has been termed *isosmotic reabsorption,* plays no role in osmoregulation and has been designated *obligatory reabsorption* by Smith [152] to indicate that it goes on irrespective of the state of water balance and to distinguish it from the *facultative reabsorption* in the distal nephron, which

---

* Actually there must be a very small difference, owing to the virtual absence of protein from the glomerular filtrate, but the contribution of protein to the osmotic pressure of plasma is so small as to be within the limits of error of the micro methods used for determining the osmotic pressure of micropuncture samples. It is important to distinguish between the total osmotic pressure, with which we are concerned in dealing with the formation of dilute and concentrated urine and which is due to all the solutes in solution, and the osmotic pressure due to the plasma proteins or oncotic pressure of plasma. The latter plays an important role in regulating the distribution of fluid across capillary membranes, because these membranes are highly permeable to all the smaller solutes. However, the tubule lining epithelium does not have this high permeability to smaller solutes, and all solutes are therefore more or less equivalent in this respect. In this context, then, the plasma proteins make a negligible contribution to osmotic pressure because of their very low molal concentration. The concentration of plasma proteins is of the order of 2 mOsm (equivalent to an osmotic pressure of about 25 mm. Hg), whereas the total concentration is 285 mOsm (equivalent to roughly 6 atmospheres).

is subject to regulation in accord with the osmotic pressure of the body fluids.†

The reabsorption of water in the proximal tubule is entirely a passive process and secondary to the active removal of solute, particularly sodium salts, by the tubule epithelium. As solute is removed from the tubule lumen and transferred to the surrounding interstitium, the osmotic pressure of the urine tends to fall below that of the surroundings. The small osmotic gradient presumably created causes water to move from the more dilute lumen to the peritubular interstitium through the cells lining the proximal tubule, which has a demonstrably high permeability to water [176].

The events that occur in the loop of Henle have been studied somewhat more sketchily because of the limited accessibility of the medullary structures for micropuncture. However, the tips of the longest loops are accessible in certain desert rodents which have elongated renal papillae [56], and procedures have been devised for exposing most of the rat papilla [137]; additional information is available from perfusion studies of the rat papilla in vitro [103, 104]. Data from such preparations taken with observations on the composition of fluid emerging into the distal tubule [56, 180] and with the results of analysis of slices of renal medulla [86, 164] yield a fairly reliable picture of events in the loop of Henle. The descending limb of the loop retains the high permeability to water that characterizes the proximal tubule. The high concentration of salt, which characterizes the interstitial space of the medulla through which the loop courses (see below), requires, if the fluid is to retain the osmotic pressure of the surroundings, that there be a further reduction in the volume of fluid as it flows through the descending limb

---

† The volume reabsorbed in the proximal tubule does not vary in relationship to the osmolality of body fluids, but recent studies indicate that the fraction of the glomerular filtrate reabsorbed in the proximal tubule does vary markedly in response to changes in the volume of extracellular fluid [39, 79].

or that sodium chloride diffuse into the lumen. Fluid collected from loops at the tip of the papilla in desert rodents indicates that both processes probably occur [36a, 54].

There is an abrupt change in the permeability characteristics of the lining epithelium just before the turn of the loop. The high permeability to water is replaced by a low one, and the continued outward transport of salt dilutes the remaining fluid so that the fluid in the ascending limb has an osmolality appreciably lower than that in the descending limb at the same level [71]. This fluid emerges into the distal tubule with an osmotic pressure less than that of plasma by 50 per cent or more. This dilution occurs whether the final urine is to be dilute or concentrated [54, 180].

The fluid entering the distal convoluted tubule is always dilute. When the final urine is also less concentrated than the plasma, the urine remains hypotonic during its passage through the remainder of the nephron. This is made possible by the low permeability to water of the distal tubule and collecting duct in the absence of ADH. This low permeability serves to insulate the lumen contents from their surroundings and to prevent dissipation of the osmotic gradient. At the same time the continued abstraction of salt by the tubular transport mechanisms enhances the dilution, reducing the osmotic pressure to levels which may be only one-fifth to one-tenth that of plasma.

Antidiuretic hormone has been shown in a number of biologic systems to have the specific property of increasing the permeability of certain membranes to the osmotic movement of water [75, 93, 139]. Its role in inducing the production of hypertonic urine is adequately explained by the property of increasing the permeability to water of the lining epithelium of certain parts of the distal nephron. In the rat, in the presence of ADH the fluid arriving in the distal tubule loses its excess of water, and its osmotic concentration approaches that

of the surrounding interstitial fluid in the latter portion of the distal tubule, despite the continuing abstraction of sodium salts. Thus the fluid regains isotonicity before it enters the collecting system [56, 180]. Note, however, that the urine does not become hypertonic to plasma in the distal tubule; the final loss of water which leads to the production of a solute concentration in excess of that of plasma occurs in the collecting system. Recent work has shown that, in the dog and monkey, the permeability to water of the distal convoluted tubule is unaffected by ADH [3, 4]. The first segment affected by the hormone in these species appears to be the cortical collecting tubule, and it is apparently in the latter structure that isotonicity is regained before the fluid enters the medullary collecting ducts.

The mechanism by which urine is rendered more concentrated than plasma has long been one of the more challenging problems in renal physiology, and the apparent elucidation of at least its essential features in line with a mechanism proposed by Wirz, Hargitay, and Kuhn [181] has been one of the major developments of recent years. It had previously been necessary to assume that the final removal of water leading to the production of hypertonic urine was the result of active transport of water which moved water from its region of low activity in the concentrated urine to a region of higher water activity (lower osmotic pressure) in the surrounding interstitium and blood. No such process has been clearly shown to exist anywhere in nature, and the problems in proposing an adequate model for such a mechanism are many. The type of mechanism suggested for some of the solute transport, in which substrate combines molecule by molecule with a carrier, presents great stoichiometric problems since the number of water molecules in plasma is 150 to 200 times that of all other particles combined. Moreover, the "osmotic diffusion pump" taken up by many as at least a step in the right direction was shown to be thermodynamically incapable of carrying out the necessary transfer [22, 48].

The mechanism proposed by Wirz, Hargitay, and Kuhn and, in its essential features, now generally accepted eliminates any consideration of active water transport and derives its driving force from the transport of sodium salts which, of course, is well known to occur not only in the kidney but in virtually every living cell. Furthermore, it depends upon the unique architecture of the kidney, to which no functional significance had previously been attributed. Phylogenetically the development of the loop of Henle had long been known to be highly correlated with the capacity to produce hypertonic urine [25], yet the evidence pointed clearly to the collecting system as the site at which the final water removal occurred [125, 157]. The proposed mechanism provided a reconciliation of this apparent conflict, showing how the loop provides the driving force for removing water from the collecting system.

In its essentials the mechanism for forming concentrated urine is quite simple and straightforward. The details, involving countercurrent exchangers and countercurrent multipliers, are more complex and their consideration may be momentarily deferred so as not to obscure the uncomplicated outline of the mechanism which relates closely to the anatomic organization of the kidney into cortex and medulla. The glomeruli and the convoluted tubules are cortical structures; the loops of Henle and the collecting ducts are limited to the medulla. Thus the latter structures are not only in intimate anatomic relationship to each other, but are isolated from the many transport processes that occur in the cortex. The blood supply to the medulla is also unique in that no large vessels enter this region; the vasa recta which supply the medulla are derived from the efferent arterioles of the juxtamedullary glomeruli. They

flow down into the medulla and then loop back into the cortex before being gathered into venules. The loop-like arrangement becomes important in consideration of countercurrent systems.

As was noted above, the fluid that flows through the loops of Henle becomes diluted before it reenters the cortex in the distal tubule. The salt removed from the loop to produce this dilution is transferred to the interstitial space of the medulla and raises the osmotic pressure of the interstitial fluid and blood to an extent determined by the amount of salt transferred and the volume of the effective blood flow. Having given up a major fraction of its salt content in the loop of Henle, the fluid in the lumen reenters the cortex, where, in the distal tubule and cortical collecting tubule and in the presence of ADH, the excess of water is dissipated. This loss of water occurs in a region which is spatially separated from the medulla and one in which, because of the high blood flow in the renal cortex, the excess of water produces very little change in osmotic pressure of the cortical interstitium and blood. Having regained isotonicity with blood and having been greatly reduced in volume as it flows through the distal tubule, the fluid now reenters the medulla in the collecting ducts. Because of the salt deposited in medullary interstitium by the loops, the collecting ducts are surrounded by a medium of high osmotic pressure. The high permeability of the collecting ducts in the presence of ADH permits the escape of water from the urine until the latter attains the same high osmotic pressure as the surroundings. Because the volume flow through the loops of Henle is several times that in the collecting ducts, a relatively small change in osmotic pressure of the loop contents may produce a very much greater osmotic pressure change in the urine.

Before considering the nature and role of countercurrent mechanisms in these processes it is appropriate to digress to point out that the production of dilute urine requires only a loss of the permeability to water in the distal tubule and collecting system. All the other processes may remain more or less unchanged, and there is evidence that the medullary interstitium is considerably more concentrated than the blood even in water diuresis [19, 54]. However, in the absence of ADH, insulated from the surroundings by the poorly permeable tubule lining, the urine flows through distal tubule and collecting duct, probably losing small amounts of water in the process, but not enough under most conditions to lose its markedly hypotonic character.

As was noted above, the extent to which a certain amount of salt deposited in the medulla will raise the osmotic pressure of interstitial fluid and blood is inversely related to the effective blood flow. In this sense the flow of blood competes with the collecting duct urine for the osmotic effects of the salt from the loops of Henle because the osmotic pressure of the blood must be raised to the same high level as that of the urine. In the cortex,

for example, the flow of blood is about ten times the highest flow of tubular fluid, and a given amount of salt added in this area would be very ineffective in raising the osmotic pressure of the tubule fluid. The best available estimates indicate that the blood flow is very much lower in the medulla than in the cortex, being of the order of 0.2 ml. per minute per gram of tissue in the medulla and about 4 ml. per gram per minute in the cortex [77]. Furthermore, the effective medullary blood flow is lower than the actual flow because it is in the form of a countercurrent exchanger [14].

The principle of the countercurrent exchanger has been known and used in engineering for many years. Its involvement in biologic systems has been pointed out particularly by Scholander [142]. The principle is illustrated in Figure 2-4. In A, we imagine a pipe through which water flows at a rate of 10 ml. per minute. The pipe is insulated from its surroundings except as it passes through a heat source. The latter is arranged so as to supply 100 calories per minute to the water as

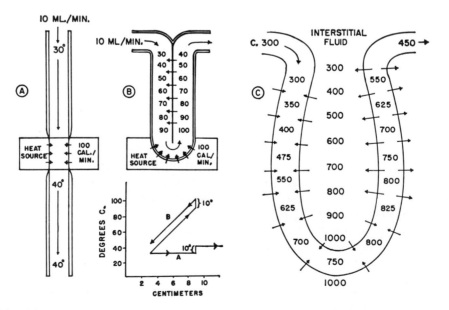

Figure 2-4. Principle of the countercurrent exchanger. (Berliner, Levinsky, Davidson, and Eden, *Amer. J. Med.* 24:730, 1958.)

it flows through. Each 10 ml. of water therefore absorbs 100 calories and its temperature is raised by 10°C. If the temperature of the inflow is 30°, that of the outflow will then be 40° and the profile of the temperature along the apparatus will be as illustrated by curve A of the graph.

If the pipe is made to double back upon itself with no insulation between the inflowing and outflowing limbs, the situation is drastically changed. When the heat source is first turned on, the water entering at 30° is heated to 40°, but as it emerges from the heat source into the outflowing limb it encounters water entering at 30°. It therefore gives up some of its heat to the inflow and has its temperature reduced below 40°. But the inflowing water has its temperature raised above 30°, e.g., to 35°. Since the temperature rises 10° in the heat source no matter what the entering temperature, such water will leave at a temperature of 45°. This process will continue until a steady state is reached when all of the heat is carried away by the water leaving the system at the end of the outflow pipe. The latter will then have a temperature of 40°, but the temperature along the remainder of the system will be higher, perhaps as illustrated in B and indicated by curve B of the graph.

The model is brought closer to the situation with blood flow in the renal medulla if we consider the flow as intended to cool the heat source. Then we see that the effective flow is much greater in A with through flow, since it keeps the temperature at about 35°, than it is in B with countercurrent exchanging flow, since the temperature now rises to about 95°. Although the model is set up for heat exchange, it is equally applicable to movements of solute, particularly since the laws of diffusion are formally identical with those for heat movement. It is not necessary that inflowing and outflowing limbs be in direct contact as in B. They need only tend to equilibrate with the same medium, e.g., interstitial fluid. The only requirements are that the latter be relatively unstirred and that the distance for diffusion between limbs of the exchanger (capillary loops) be small relative to the distance for diffusion along the full length of the system.

On this basis, it may be seen that the effective flow for removal of solute from the medulla may be appreciably lower than the actual blood flow. Data are not available to assign a quantitative factor to the diminution attributable to the countercurrent exchanger, but it has been amply shown to exist [80, 94]. Furthermore, no single factor can be assumed to exist, since it will vary for each substance involved; flow is more effectively reduced the more diffusible the substance. It seems likely that one of the more important consequences of the countercurrent exchanger arrangement of the renal medullary blood flow is the trapping of urea in the medulla, which is considered further below. Finally it should be noted that although the countercurrent exchanger has a lower effective than actual flow, it has an exaggerated response to *changes* in flow. The concentration achieved by a given addition to a countercurrent exchanger is inversely related to the *square* of the flow rather than to the flow itself as in an ordinary through-flowing system [14].

The capillary loops constitute the countercurrent exchanger, a passive system which reduces the effective blood flow in the renal medulla. The loops of Henle, however, are believed to form a countercurrent multiplier, a system of an entirely different nature. Such systems, first elucidated by Kuhn [59], constitute a mechanism whereby the capacity to produce small concentration differences can be exploited so as to yield a greatly enhanced concentration at one end of the system. The principle of such a system is illustrated in Figure 2-5.

Imagine a tube consisting of two compartments separated by a membrane as represented by the dashed line in A. The system may be filled by inflow at the left end of the upper chamber, fluid passing through the loop

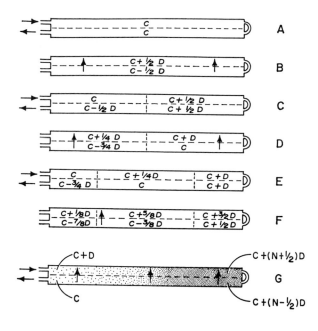

Figure 2-5. Principle of the countercurrent multiplier.

at the right-hand end into the lower chamber and out at the left-hand end of the lower compartment. In A the chamber is filled throughout with fluid of concentration C. Suppose that the membrane has the property of transporting solute from the lower compartment to the upper. The capacity to carry out this transport is, however, limited so that the membrane is able to create a difference of concentration between the two sides equal to but not exceeding D. Such a limitation is not uncommon in biologic systems; it might be interpreted as being due to a limited capacity to transfer solute actively from the lower to the upper side of the membrane. At the same time the membrane may be considered to have a certain passive permeability to the solute, so that as a concentration gradient is established across the membrane there is net diffusion from the upper to the lower side. When the gradient is sufficient to produce a net diffusion equal to the maximum rate of active transport, net movement of solute will stop. In B, the membrane has been permitted to carry out this transport to the limit of its capacity. Assuming, for simplicity, equal volumes for the two compartments, further transport ceases when the

concentration in one compartment is reduced to $C - \frac{1}{2} D$ and that in the other raised to $C + \frac{1}{2} D$. The latter represents the most concentrated solution which can be produced in such a single step.

In panel C, the factor of flow is introduced; fresh solution is introduced into the left-hand half of the upper chamber. The solution of concentration $C + \frac{1}{2} D$ which formerly occupied the upper compartment fills the right-hand half of both compartments, and half of that which formerly occupied the lower compartment has been displaced from the system. The concentration difference across the membrane is now smaller than its limiting value at all points along the membrane. Transfer is therefore resumed until, as in panel D, the concentration gradient again reaches its maximum value.

Fresh solution is again introduced as in panel E so as to fill the left-hand one-fourth of the upper compartment, displacing the other elements of solution accordingly around the counterflowing system. Accomplishment of the transport capacity of the membrane yields the situation shown in panel F.

Note that in this small number of discontinuous steps it has been possible to produce a solution of concentration C + ¾ D, or one increased in concentration by three times the increment which could be achieved by the membrane itself. The small "single effect" (½ D) has been multiplied by the counter-current flow. In practice, of course, flow is continuous and a situation such as that shown in panel G results, the contents of the entire system becoming more concentrated as we move from left to right, with only a small concentration gradient from top to bottom; the solution becomes progressively concentrated as it flows from left to right and correspondingly (and a trifle more) diluted as it returns from right to left.

In considering the application of this principle to the loop of Henle it is assumed that the capacity to produce a concentration difference between lumen and interstitium is, in some fashion, limited. It might, for example, be impossible to transfer sodium from a concentration of 50 mEq. per liter inside to one of, say, 500 to 600 mEq. per liter in the interstitium. If, however, the concentration in the lumen has first been increased to a value close to that in the interstitium, the transfer might easily be accomplished. It is uncertain to what extent the initial increase in the loop of Henle is accomplished by the passive entry of sodium chloride into the lumen and to what extent by loss of water from the descending limb to the hypertonic interstitium. In either case the concentration of sodium salts in the lumen approaches that in the surroundings. As sodium salts are transferred out of the water-impermeable ascending limb, diluting that which remains, the fluid is at the same time flowing upward away from the tip of the papilla, where the interstitial concentrations are highest, to the more superficial regions of the medulla, where interstitial concentrations are lower. The transport, therefore, need never occur against a steep concentration gradient.

The foregoing description of the concentrating and diluting mechanisms has dealt only with the extremes of concentration and dilution. There are, of course, many intermediate states due to the presence of less than maximally effective amounts of ADH, and the concentration and flow of urine may be found to be anywhere within the range of its extremes. In man the most dilute urines are of the order of 30 mOsm although concentrations below 50 to 60 mOsm are not often observed. Inability to produce maximally dilute urine may result not only from the presence of ADH but also from failure of sufficient amounts of sodium salts to reach the segment of the tubule in which the urine is diluted, as when glomerular filtration is depressed or in certain states associated with intense sodium retention [9, 114].

On the other hand, the maximum concentration that can be achieved in man is 1200 to 1500 mOsm (a rather poor showing compared with certain other mammals — e.g., dog, 2500 mOsm; rat, 3200 mOsm; kangaroo rat, 5000 mOsm). The capacity to produce maximally concentrated urine is impaired in a number of pathologic and physiologic states.

One physiologic variable that determines the ability to produce maximally dilute and concentrated urine is the rate of solute excretion. The extremes of hypotonicity and hypertonicity can be achieved only when solute excretion is relatively small. The basis for the limitation can be deduced from the mechanisms described above, but is more easily understood in terms of the analysis and terminology introduced by Homer Smith and his associates [156], which have found wide currency in renal physiology. This analysis views the volume of urine excreted per minute as consisting of one fraction required to excrete the solute of the urine in solution isotonic with plasma (the osmolal clearance, C_{OSM}) and the excess of water (the free water clearance, C_{H_2O}).

$$V = C_{OSM} + C_{H_2O}$$

The osmolal clearance is determined by dividing the rate of solute excretion by the osmolality of plasma, the rate of solute excretion being estimated (with certain inescapable inaccuracies because of the different dimensions) as the product of flow and urine osmolality. Thus,

$$C_{OSM} = \frac{U_{OSM}V}{P_{OSM}}$$

When the urine is dilute, flow exceeds C_{OSM} by an amount, designated the free water clearance, which is that amount of water which would have to be removed from one minute's flow of urine to leave the remainder isotonic with plasma. In terms of the mechanism by which the dilution is produced, it may be seen that the free water clearance is the osmotic equivalent of the salt removed in the dilution process, provided it is assumed that no water has escaped from the tubule beyond that point at which the dilution process begins. While the latter assumption is not entirely correct, it is clear that C_{H2O} cannot exceed this hypothetical value; and to the extent that there is a limit on the capacity of loop, distal tubule, and collecting system to transport salt out of the urine, the free water clearance can never be greater than the osmotic equivalent of this limited capacity (although it may be smaller because of subsequent water losses). This limitation accounts for the fact that as solute excretion increases, dilute urine becomes less hypotonic — under these conditions C_{OSM}, the isotonic fraction of the urine, increases, while the solute-free fraction C_{H2O} remains relatively constant. This may be seen from combination and rearrangement of the equations above to yield

$$U_{OSM} = P_{OSM}\left(1 - \frac{C_{H2O}}{V}\right)$$

This indicates that as V increases without an equivalent increase in C_{H2O}, U_{OSM} approaches P_{OSM}.

On the other hand, when the urine is hypertonic, C_{H2O} assumes a negative value, the amount of water which must be *added* to the urine to render it isotonic with plasma. This "negative free water clearance" has been designated as T^C_{H2O}, where for hypertonic urines

$$V = C_{OSM} - T^C_{H2O}$$

If it is assumed that the urine entering the collecting system is isotonic and that water but no solute is lost from the collecting ducts where the concentration of urine occurs, then T^C_{H2O} would represent this water loss. Since there is solute loss from the urine during its traversal of the collecting system [66] and since the urine may be hypotonic when it enters the collecting system, the measured value of T^C_{H2O} is always less than the true loss of water from the collecting ducts. However, there is an inherent limitation on the loss of water from the collecting ducts. The driving force for this loss of water is provided by the salt transported in excess of water out of the loops of Henle. T^C_{H2O} cannot be greater than the osmotic equivalent of the excess salt transported by the loop and therefore approaches a maximum value as flow increases. Thus, in analogy to the equation for dilute urine,

$$U_{OSM} = P_{OSM}\left(1 + \frac{T^C_{H2O}}{V}\right)$$

and as solute excretion increases without an equivalent increase in T^C_{H2O}, the urine concentration approaches that of plasma.*

Important as the capacity to produce hypertonic urine may be in facilitating the maintenance of normal osmotic pressure of the body fluids in the face of restricted water intake, loss of this capacity is by no means the

---

* In practice it has been found that if very high rates of solute excretion are produced, particularly when there is some impairment of the concentrating mechanism, the urine may become hypotonic to plasma despite maximal ADH activity [85, 113]. This may reflect the entry of a dilute urine into the collecting system as the result of failure to regain isotonicity in the collecting tubules.

handicap entailed by the total absence of ADH. Quantitatively, the most important effect of ADH is to prevent the excretion of a dilute urine; the production of one more concentrated than plasma is a less important adaptation. This is reflected by the ordinarily observed values of C_{H2O} and T^C_{H2O}. In moderate water diuresis C_{H2O} may easily reach 10 to 15 ml. per minute, while under most conditions T^C_{H2O} is of the order of 1 ml. per minute, reaching maximum values of about 5 ml. per minute only with very high rates of solute excretion. Thus the water saved in not excreting a dilute urine is many times greater than that saved in rendering it maximally concentrated.

Reabsorption and Excretion of Sodium and Chloride

The active process by which sodium salts are reabsorbed in the renal tubules exceeds in magnitude by a considerable margin any other energy-requiring function of the kidney. Several studies have indicated that so long as filtration is maintained the oxygen consumption of the kidney is directly related to the rate of reabsorption of sodium from the tubules [76, 81]; the energy requirement for all the other transport processes is so much smaller that the effects of loading with such substances as glucose and PAH cannot be detected in the oxygen consumption [23, 31].

The distribution of sodium reabsorption along the nephron has been referred to in connection with the reabsorption of water. Although complete quantitative data are not available, it is clear that a very large fraction of the filtered sodium is reabsorbed in the proximal tubule. This fraction, probably in the range of 60 to 80 per cent under most conditions, may vary outside of this range with expansion and contraction of the volume of extracellular fluid. Under ordinary conditions the concentration of sodium in the tu-

bule lumen remains virtually the same as that in the plasma as proximal tubular reabsorption goes on. This is an automatic consequence of two factors: (1) by the rapid escape of water along the small osmotic gradient presumably established by removal of sodium, the lumen fluid retains an osmotic pressure virtually the same as that of plasma; and (2) sodium salts constitute the bulk of the total solute of the glomerular filtrate and much of the other solute is, under normal conditions, reabsorbed as fast as or faster than the sodium. Since sodium reabsorption does not usually occur against a gradient of chemical concentration and since recent work suggests that there is no electrical potential gradient across the wall of the proximal convoluted tubule [49], the criteria for active transport of sodium are not met under ordinary conditions. This has even led to the proposal that the movement of sodium might be a passive process. However, the results obtained when a considerable amount of poorly reabsorbed solute is present in the glomerular filtrate indicate that the transport is indeed active. For example, during the infusion of mannitol the concentration of sodium in the lumen falls appreciably below that in plasma [54, 177]. The decline occurs because mannitol is very poorly reabsorbed from the tubule lumen; hence, as sodium is reabsorbed, the mannitol constitutes an increasing fraction of the remaining solute and the sodium concentration decreases.

It is, however, a fact of some importance that the proximal tubule does not appear to be able to reduce the sodium concentration in the lumen below a limiting value. This value appears to be about 75 per cent of the concentration in the plasma, and when this limiting gradient is reached there is no further reabsorption of sodium [178, 179]. The basis of this limitation probably lies in a relatively high passive permeability of the proximal tubule to sodium. The concentration gradient between plasma and lumen is probably sufficient to drive the diffusion of sodium into the lumen at a rate equal to the capacity of the tubules actively to transport it out.

The nature of the process by which chloride leaves the lumen of the proximal tubule is somewhat uncertain at the present time. It is reported that the chloride concentration cannot be reduced below that in the plasma, a finding that would be compatible with an entirely passive process; additional confirmation of this finding is needed. However, the rates of movement of chloride, both into and out of the proximal tubule (as measured with isotopes), are higher than would be expected for free diffusion alone, suggesting the involvement of exchange diffusion [7, 51]. In addition, there are observations that suggest active chloride reabsorption in the distal tubule [127].

Reabsorption of sodium in the distal tubule (and collecting system) differs in several important respects from that in the proximal tubule. There appears to be no limit to the reduction of sodium concentration, which, from the fact that the urine can be virtually sodium-free, clearly may fall to negligibly small levels. Furthermore, since there is a large gradient of electrical potential (45 to 120 millivolts, lumen negative [49, 95, 127, 158]), the electrochemical gradient opposing sodium transport is even greater than is suggested by concentration alone. The greater ability of the distal tubule to produce sodium gradients probably is due to a lower passive permeability rather than to any fundamental difference in the sodium transport mechanism itself. The latter possibility cannot, however, be excluded.

In addition, in the distal system, not all the sodium reabsorbed is accompanied by an equivalent amount of anion. A part of the sodium removal occurs by a process of cation exchange in which the sodium removed is replaced in the tubule fluid by other cations (potassium, hydrogen). The processes involved are considered in relation to potassium excretion and the regulation of acid-base balance.

The nature of the mechanism by which sodium is reabsorbed in the kidney is by no means clear. Sodium is transported by virtually every cell in the body, by means which are almost equally unclear, but it is a reasonable working assumption that transport by the renal tubular cell is an adaptation for transcellular ion movement of that process by which most body cells extrude sodium from their interiors.

The chloride concentration may also be reduced to very low levels in the distal portions of the nephron. Although this reduction of the chloride concentration is favored by the electrical gradient, lumen being negative to interstitial fluid by 60 to 100 mv or more, recent observations indicate that this is not sufficient to balance the concentration gradient, and suggest that chloride is also removed from the lumen by an active process [127].

REGULATION OF SODIUM EXCRETION

A number of factors are known to modify the excretion of sodium; there are almost certainly other influences which remain to be identified. The development of an adequate quantitative description of the way in which these influences are integrated to determine the rate of sodium excretion remains a major problem.

Because the sodium salts constitute all but a very small fraction of the solute of extracellular fluid, the sodium concentration varies with the osmotic pressure of plasma. Since the osmotic pressure is regulated by the excretion and retention of water, it follows that the concentration of sodium in the plasma is regulated through the control of water excretion and not by modulation of sodium excretion. It also follows that the amount of sodium in the extracellular fluid need bear no relation to its sodium concentration; the latter reflects osmotic pressure. Since the osmotic pressure is maintained within a rather narrow range, the amount of sodium in the extracellular fluid, and hence in the body, is related much more closely to the extracellular fluid volume. It would be anticipated, therefore, that sodium excretion should be modulated in relation to the volume of extracellular fluid, and this appears to be the case, although in what fashion this regulation is achieved remains rather uncertain. The rate of sodium excretion is, of course, determined by the balance between filtration and reabsorption, but each of these is varied and regulated in a way which cannot yet be subjected to detailed analysis.

Rate of Filtration of Sodium. The filtration of sodium is varied largely by changes in the rate of formation of glomerular filtrate. This is a consequence of the fact that the plasma sodium concentration is generally maintained within a narrow range by the processes that regulate osmotic pressure.

Under most physiologic conditions, all but a very small fraction of the filtered sodium is reabsorbed by the renal tubules. The excretion of sodium by a normal person on a moderate sodium intake averages between 0.5 and 1 per cent of the amount filtered. It is therefore clear that if the amount filtered were to increase by 1 per cent and all of the increment were to escape reabsorption, the amount excreted would double or triple. While it is plain that under such conditions reabsorption does not remain constant and the increment of the filtered load is not excreted, these considerations point up the potential sensitivity of sodium excretion to small changes in glomerular filtration rate. They also emphasize the problem of evaluating the contribution of changes in glomerular filtration to changes in excretion since few measurements of glomerular filtration can be considered to have potential errors of less than several per cent.

However, as mentioned above, the reabsorption of sodium does not remain constant in the face of changes in filtered load, and in this respect it differs from the reabsorption of such substances as glucose, amino acids, etc. When glomerular filtration increases, sodium reabsorption increases, and vice versa. However, because the changes in filtration and reabsorption are concordant but not proportional, the change in sodium excretion is relatively much greater than the change in filtration. Thus acute changes in glomerular filtration are frequently accompanied by very large changes in sodium excretion. If such changes are maintained, however, compensatory modification of reabsorption generally returns sodium excretion toward normal levels.

These characteristics of the filtration and excretion of sodium are clearly illustrated by the illuminating experiments of Mueller and his associates [107], who implanted clamps on one renal artery in dogs and collected the urine separately from each kidney. They found that a very slight constriction of the artery might give a very significant decrease in sodium excretion by the kidney even though the reduction of glomerular filtration might be too small to be clearly detected. When constriction of the artery was sufficient to reduce glomerular filtration by a small but definitely detectable amount, there was a very marked reduction of sodium excretion. Such a kidney might excrete only 10 to 20 per cent of the daily sodium intake, balance being maintained by increased excretion by the other undisturbed kidney. This situation could continue for long periods. Apparently so long as the normal kidney was present, balance could be maintained and there was no stimulus to induce those compensatory changes in reabsorption which ordinarily return sodium excretion toward normal in the face of a sustained reduction of glomerular filtration rate. However, if the normal kidney was removed, placing the full load for maintaining sodium excretion on the clamped kidney, operation of these compensatory factors yielded a marked increase in sodium excretion, and sodium balance was restored despite the clamp.

Adrenocortical Steroids. The steroids secreted by the adrenal cortex exert one of the best-known influences on sodium reabsorption by the renal tubules. The property of increasing the reabsorption of sodium is shared by a large number of the natural steroids and some of their synthetic congeners. It is probable, although not established with certainty, that all exert their effects through a common mechanism and thus that these effects, so far as they are limited to electrolyte transport, are qualitatively identical. However, the steroids differ not only in the intensity of their effects, but in the relationship between their ability to enhance sodium transport and their capacity to produce those effects generally designated as glucocorticoid effects.

The biochemical nature of the influence of adrenal steroids on sodium transport is completely unknown. In the renal tubule they appear to enhance sodium reabsorption in all of its forms — that is, reabsorption along with chloride as well as by exchange for potassium and hydrogen ions. There is some evidence that their effect is exerted primarily in the distal portions of the nephron, but this conclusion should not be accepted without some reservation. It is important to recognize that the effect of steroids on sodium transport is to moderate fine adjustments. Although in the absence of adrenal steroids a somewhat larger fraction of the filtered sodium is excreted, the actual fraction is so small that a moderately increased intake is sufficient to maintain balance.

Just as prolonged reduction of glomerular filtration is not associated with continued reduction of sodium excretion, continued secretion (or administration) of salt-retaining steroids does not yield sustained retention of sodium. The early retention of salt is followed by restoration of sodium balance essentially to normal.* Although increases in glomerular fil-

tration rate may play some role in this "escape" phenomenon [2], it is probable that the major role is played by as yet poorly defined factors that are the major regulators of sodium reabsorption (see below); these influences are sometimes lumped together in the (optimistic) designation "third factor."

Aldosterone is recognized as the hormone by which most adrenocortical influences on renal sodium transport are mediated [151]. Although the mechanisms by which aldosterone secretion is controlled have not yet been established with certainty, the evidence strongly indicates that the renin-angiotensin system plays an important role.

Additional Influences on Sodium Reabsorption by the Tubules. A number of studies over the last few years have shown that when isotonic saline solutions are infused there is a marked increase in the excretion of sodium and chloride and that this increased excretion is not prevented by reduction of glomerular filtration rate or the administration of maximally effective doses of mineralocorticoids [16, 38, 87, 129]. It has been shown that the expansion of extracellular fluid volume is accompanied by a marked depression of reabsorption in the proximal tubule; in fact, the additional sodium that escapes reabsorption in the proximal tubule is greater than the amount excreted in the urine, indicating that there is actually an increase in the amount reabsorbed in more distal segments of the nephron [39, 79]. However, the depressed reabsorption in the proximal tubule is not the entire explanation of the increased salt excretion since it is possible to produce similar depression of proximal reabsorption with only a minor increase in the amount excreted [69].

The nature of the processes by which this inhibition of sodium reabsorption is produced remains obscure. One popular view is that the inhibition is produced by the secretion of an as yet unidentified hormone. Several attempts to

* There is usually a continuing loss of potassium which in all probability is replaced by additional retained sodium, but the amounts of sodium involved are likely to be too small to detect easily by balance methods.

reproduce the diuresis by the transfer of blood from saline-infused animals to hydropenic recipients or to perfuse the blood of the saline-infused animal through an isolated kidney have yielded equivocal results [38, 72, 89], some of which have been interpreted as positive but which are not entirely convincing.

Another view holds that the relevant changes are largely hemodynamic. This view derives from observations that indicate that manipulations that might be thought to increase the hydrostatic pressure or decrease the protein oncotic pressure in peritubular capillaries increase sodium excretion while interventions that decrease peritubular capillary pressure or increase oncotic pressure decrease the rate of sodium excretion [44, 100]. While it is easy to see that such changes in pressure would probably vary renal extravascular volume, it is not so readily apparent how these volume changes would influence active transport out of the tubules.

Osmotic Diuresis. When the glomerular filtrate contains appreciable concentrations of solute that cannot be reabsorbed by the renal tubules, the sodium concentration of proximal tubule contents must fall as proximal reabsorption progresses. Since the gradient against which sodium can be transported is limited, sodium reabsorption is impaired and large amounts of sodium appear in the urine. This phenomenon is known as osmotic diuresis [106, 175]. It has frequently been produced, in physiologic studies of renal function, by the administration of mannitol or urea. It has a spontaneous counterpart in marked glycosuria secondary to hyperglycemia of whatever origin.

Inhibition of Sodium Reabsorption. Enhancement of the excretion of sodium is frequently a desirable therapeutic measure and most of the useful diuretics owe their activity to the ability to inhibit the reabsorption of sodium. Although the various groups of diuretics probably differ in the mechanisms by which their effects are produced, the mercurial diuretics, chlorothiazide and its congeners, the carbonic anhydrase inhibitors and, presumably, the xanthine diuretics owe their effects to a capacity to interfere with one or another step in the process of sodium reabsorption.

Excretion of Potassium

Potassium is one of the few normal constituents of the body fluids that are both reabsorbed and secreted [8, 85]. The rate of excretion of potassium under normal conditions is about 15 per cent of the rate at which potassium is filtered by the glomeruli. On the other hand, when large amounts of potassium are administered or when acidification of the urine is inhibited, the excretion of potassium may be more than twice that which could be due to filtration alone. Although the amount excreted is usually well below the amount filtered, there is a considerable body of evidence that indicates that the potassium that is excreted, even at low rates of excretion, is derived in large part from the secretory process [5].

The concentration of potassium in the proximal tubule lumen remains close to that in plasma so that the fraction of the filtered potassium reabsorbed in the proximal tubule is very close to the fraction of the filtered volume that is reabsorbed, 60 to 80 per cent [3, 4]. Although the observations that have been made are insufficient to warrant a definite statement, it appears that the reabsorption of potassium in the proximal tubule is a passive process probably driven by the small concentration gradient that must be established by the reduction of volume. The fraction of the filtered potassium reabsorbed in the proximal tubule depends only on the fraction of the glomerular filtrate reabsorbed and is not related to the state of potassium balance. Thus, in the change from potassium depletion, in which the amount of potassium excreted may be only 1 or 2 per cent of the amount filtered, to potassium loading or during carbonic anhydrase inhibition, when the potassium excreted may be considerably in excess of the amount filtered, the concentration of potassium in proximal tubule fluid remains equal to that in plasma, and the fraction reabsorbed remains relatively constant [4, 171]. The adjustments that regulate potassium excretion are entirely the function of more distal nephron segments.

The concentration of potassium in samples obtained from the loop of Henle has been found to be quite high (of the order of four times that of plasma) [71, 98]. It is probable that this represents passive inward movement (in the descending limb) of potassium that has been reabsorbed from the collecting ducts. The potassium that enters the loop probably leaks out again from the ascending limb, although this is not established. In any case the fluid that reaches early segments of the distal convoluted tubule regularly has a concentration of potassium appreciably below that in plasma, a fact that indicates the presence of an active reabsorptive process, the more so since reabsorption is opposed by an electrical gradient of 45 to 65 mv, lumen negative [95].

As fluid passes down the distal tubule, both the concentration and the content of potassium increase owing to entry of potassium. The increase may be minimal to absent during potassium depletion, moderate in normal hydropenia, and marked during potassium loading [3, 4, 95]. The net entry of potassium is always down the electrochemical gradient since the electrical potential is large enough to provide opposing chemical concentration gradients greater than any that have yet been observed. In fact, it has been shown that the concentration in the distal tubule is kept below the equilibrium concentration by an active reabsorptive process [95]. It thus appears that the accumulation of potassium (secretion) in the distal tubule is driven by the electrical forces which in turn are presumably the consequence of the active reabsorption of sodium. In this sense potassium secretion is an ex-

change for sodium, though not on an ion-for-ion basis.

The amount of potassium present at the end of the distal convoluted tubule has been found to be adequate to explain the largest amounts excreted in the urine. Thus net addition does not seem to occur in the collecting system. However, the amount of potassium in the urine is frequently much less than that which leaves the distal tubule indicating reabsorption of potassium in the collecting system [3, 95, 166].

REGULATION OF POTASSIUM EXCRETION

Potassium Concentration in Cells. The variation of potassium excretion with depletion and loading has been referred to above. Under many circumstances the rate of excretion is poorly related to the potassium concentration in plasma. It is, on the other hand, well correlated to what may be inferred to be the potassium concentration of cells, particularly the cells of the renal tubules. The plasma concentration is related to excretion only to the extent that the concentrations in cells and plasma are in turn related. Since potassium is predominantly an intracellular ion, such a relationship is well adapted to maintaining a normal potassium content of the body. The effect of cell potassium concentration is probably exerted through modification of the active reabsorptive process in distal segments.

Delivery of Sodium to Distal Sites. Since reabsorption of sodium provides the electrical driving force for potassium to enter the lumen, and since this driving force is opposed by the active reabsorption of potassium, exhaustion of the sodium from the lumen presumably causes a drop in electrical potential and permits the reabsorptive process to operate unopposed; thus potassium may virtually disappear from the lumen [166]. This series of events is presumed to occur in the collecting system when sodium excretion is minimal. Thus when sodium excretion is very low, potassium excretion is also likely to be low, and increased delivery of sodium to distal segments increases potassium excretion.

Factors Modifying Hydrogen Ion Excretion. The secretion of hydrogen and potassium ions has been found to vary inversely under a wide variety of conditions [12, 13]. The exact mechanism by which high potassium suppresses hydrogen secretion, and vice versa, is not certain. It may be related to an inverse relationship of the concentration in cells [126].

Regulation of Acid-Base Balance

The products of intake and metabolism include a number of potential sources of acid. The sulfur of the sulfur-containing amino acids (cysteine, methionine) is oxidized to sulfuric acid, and the phosphorus of protein and phospholipid is converted to phosphoric acid. In addition, if ammonium chloride is ingested, the ammonium ion is converted to urea in the liver, leaving a residue of hydrochloric acid. When calcium chloride is taken by mouth, a large part of the calcium may be converted to insoluble calcium soaps and excreted in the stool, while hydrochloric acid is absorbed. Organic acids may be produced in excess of the capacity to metabolize them further, as in starvation or diabetic ketosis.

Since none of these can exist in the body fluids as the free, undissociated acid, they must react with the buffers of the body. Because bicarbonate is present in high concentration and because the anhydride, CO_2, is volatile, most of the buffering occurs by reaction of the acid with bicarbonate to yield the corresponding sodium salt and carbonic acid. The carbonic acid then decomposes to water and CO_2, the latter being excreted in the lungs.

$$(1) \quad H^+A^- + Na^+HCO_3^- \rightleftharpoons Na^+A^- + H_2CO_3$$
$$\Updownarrow$$
$$H_2O + CO_2$$

The net result is the replacement, in the extracellular fluid, of one equivalent of bicarbonate by one equivalent of the anion of the strong acid. The anion is eventually excreted by the kidneys. If it were to be excreted along with the sodium ion by which it is balanced in the extracellular fluid, the net result would be the disappearance from the extracellular fluid of one mol of sodium bicarbonate for each mol of acid formed or ingested. In the face of the continuing excess of acid radicles derived from intake and metabolism, the bicarbonate of body fluids would be quite rapidly exhausted.

The bicarbonate and buffer capacity of the extracellular fluid can be restored only if the sodium bicarbonate can in some way be regenerated. This could be accomplished if it were possible to excrete the metabolic acid in un-ionized form in the urine, in essence by reversal of reaction (1) above:

$$(2) \quad H_2O + CO_2$$
$$\Updownarrow$$
$$H_2CO_3 + Na^+A^- \rightarrow$$
$$Na^+HCO_3^- \text{ (to blood)} + HA \text{ (to urine)}$$

To the extent that the kidney is able to form urine more acid than blood, and to the extent that certain weak acids are less ionized at the pH of urine than at the pH of blood, the kidney can carry out the net process represented by the series of reactions indicated in (2).* The kidney is capable of producing urine considerably more acid (pH as low as 4.0) than the blood (pH 7.4), and there are a number of acids appreciably less ionized at pH 4.0 or 5.0 (the latter more often representing the maximum acidity achieved) than at pH 7.4. The most important of these is phosphate (pK 6.8 for the second ionization, i.e., $HPO_4^{--} + H^+ \rightleftharpoons H_2PO_4^-$). Others that fit the category are creatinine, pKa 5.0 (for the reaction

---

* While the overall effect is accomplished, this is not to be interpreted as meaning that the steps involved are those represented.

$Cr + H^+ \rightleftharpoons CrH^+$) and β-hydroxybutyric acid, pK 4.7.* The amount of bicarbonate regenerated in the excretion of these un-ionized acids is equal to the amount of alkali required to titrate this acid back to the pH of plasma and is called the *titratable acid* of the urine. It is clear that the titratable acid that can be excreted is limited to some fraction of the number of mols of suitably weak acid excreted in the urine. Furthermore it is clear that, to the extent these acids originally enter the body fluids as the free acid, the bicarbonate regenerated in excreting them as titratable acid in the urine never can make up for the loss of bicarbonate initially incurred. The mechanism is merely one for minimizing these losses. There must, then, be some mechanism for making up the remainder.

The existence of such a mechanism becomes even clearer when hydrochloric and sulfuric acids are considered. These are strong acids and completely ionized at all pH's. At a pH of 4.0 the concentration of such an acid is only 0.1 mEq. per liter. The anions of these acids must therefore always be balanced in both blood and urine by an equivalent amount of cation.

The excretion of such anions in the urine without the expenditure of the cations of blood is made possible by the substitution of a metabolically produced cation, the ammonium ion, for sodium in the urine. The processes involved in this substitution can be summarized by the reactions:

(1) $RNH_2 + H_2O \rightarrow NH_3 + ROH$

(ROH may be oxidized to CO_2 and H_2O.)

(2) $NH_3 + Na^+A^- + H_2CO_3 \rightarrow$
$$NH_4^+A^- \text{ (to urine)}$$
$$+ Na^+HCO_3^- \text{ (to blood)}$$

Although neither of these reactions should be literally interpreted as indicative of those occurring in ammonia formation and excretion, they do describe the overall processes involved.

Thus the recovery of bicarbonate temporarily displaced by the access of acid to body fluids is effected by two mechanisms: (1) the excretion of acid urine containing a part of the suitably weak acids in un-ionized form, and (2) the substitution of ammonium ion for sodium ion in the excretion of the anions of strong acids. The disposal of alkali is more directly accomplished. Alkali added to the body fluids is directly converted to bicarbonate by reaction with CO_2:

$$B^+OH^- + CO_2 \rightarrow B^+HCO_3^-$$

Thus it may be excreted as the bicarbonate with only the expenditure of metabolically derived CO_2.

This summary of the elements of acid-base balance will serve as an introduction to a consideration of the renal mechanisms that effect the excretion of acid and alkali and their integration to achieve the regulation of the acid-base balance of body fluids.

Three processes are important in determining the amount of acid or alkali excreted: (1) glomerular filtration, particularly as it determines the amount of bicarbonate salts delivered to the tubules; (2) the processes by which bicarbonate is reabsorbed and the urine rendered acid; (3) the synthesis of ammonia by the renal tubules.

The glomerular filtrate contains bicarbonate at a concentration very close to that in plasma water.† As the filtrate flows through the proximal tubule, the concentration of bicarbonate is considerably reduced by the activity of the reabsorptive processes, and the pH

---

* The pK of an acid is the pH at which it exists half as the un-ionized acid and half in the dissociated form as defined by the equation $pH = pK + \log [A^-]/[HA]$. At pH's above the pK, the un-ionized acid predominates; at pH's above the pK the dissociated form is in excess.

† As a consequence of the Donnan equilibrium, filtrable anions are present in glomerular filtrate at a concentration some 5 per cent higher than in the plasma water, while the concentration of filtrable cations, including hydrogen ion, is some 5 per cent lower than in plasma water.

Table 2-1. Renal Regulation of Acid-Base Balance

Process	Initially in Lumen	Secreted	Reabsorbed	Remains in Lumen	Further Reactions
Bicarbonate reabsorption	$Na^+HCO_3^-$	H^+	Na^+	H_2CO_3	$\leftrightarrows CO_2 \uparrow + H_2O$
Formation of titratable acid	Na^+A^-	H^+	Na^+	HA	
Formation of ammonium ion	Na^+Cl^-	H^+	Na^+	H^+Cl^-	$H^+ + NH_3 \leftrightarrows NH_4^+$

of the proximal tubule fluid is reduced by 0.5 to 1.0 pH unit [3, 30, 52, 55]. Since these changes are accompanied by a large reduction in volume, all but a small fraction of the filtered bicarbonate is ordinarily reabsorbed in the proximal tubule. Most of the remaining bicarbonate is usually removed from the urine in the distal tubule and collecting system, where the extremes of urinary acidity may be attained.

The changes in pH that occur as bicarbonate is removed from the urine depend upon the relative rates of loss of bicarbonate and water. If water removal proceeds more rapidly than that of bicarbonate, the bicarbonate concentration rises, and vice versa. Changes in bicarbonate concentration are accompanied by concordant changes in pH because carbonic acid concentration tends to remain proportional to the carbon dioxide tension (pCO_2), which in turn remains close to that of blood. These relationships are expressed in the Henderson-Hasselbalch equation

$$pH = 6.10 + \log \frac{[HCO_3^-]}{[H_2CO_3] + [\text{dissolved } CO_2]}$$

Since $[\text{dissolved } CO_2] = \alpha pCO_2$, where α is a solubility constant, and since, when the reaction $CO_2 + H_2O \rightleftharpoons H_2CO_3$ is at equilibrium, $[H_2CO_3] = \text{constant} \times [CO_2]$, the denominator of the above equation, may be expressed as a constant multiplied by the pCO_2 of the tubular fluid, and the pCO_2 of tubular

fluid may be assumed to remain close to that of blood. To the extent that these approximations are correct, the pH will be a linear function of the log of the bicarbonate concentration. One consequence of these considerations is the conclusion that the formation of alkaline urine with a pH higher than that of blood requires no specific mechanism, but only that the fraction of the filtered water reabsorbed be greater than the reabsorbed fraction of the filtered bicarbonate.

MECHANISM OF BICARBONATE
REABSORPTION AND URINE ACIDIFICATION

Largely as a result of the work of Pitts [120] and his associates, it is generally accepted that the urine is acidified by the secretion of hydrogen ion and that this secretion occurs by an exchange of hydrogen ions for sodium ions. This single process can* provide the driving reaction for all the renal tubular activities which go into the renal regulation of acid-base balance, as indicated in Table 2-1.

The nature of the process by which hydrogen ion is made available and secreted in exchange for sodium remains unknown. The original proposal of Pitts and Alexander [122] (Fig. 2-6) that the hydrogen is derived from carbonic acid is undoubtedly a considerable oversimplification of the actual steps involved, but it remains a good description of the overall process since it indicates the initial and final

* Although it has not been shown that this process is alone responsible, the assumption is retained in the absence of evidence to the contrary.

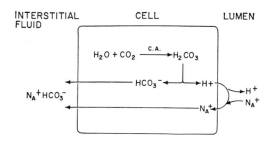

Figure 2-6. Mechanism for acidifying the urine deriving hydrogen ion from splitting of carbonic acid as proposed by Pitts and Alexander.

products. No matter what intermediate steps are assumed, the sodium ion reabsorbed is returned to the blood along with bicarbonate ion. The proposal provides a role for carbonic anhydrase, which has been shown to be essential for the normal acidification of the urine. On the other hand, it does not provide for the participation of metabolic energy in the secretory process, nor is it clear how hydrogen and bicarbonate ions could be directly separated. To take account of these deficiencies, but still leaving the mechanism unspecified, a process resembling that proposed by Davies [35] for gastric acid secretion may be suggested (Fig. 2-7). Here hydrogen and hydroxyl ions are generated from water in spatially separated loci: the hydrogen ion is secreted in exchange for sodium; the hydroxyl ion reacts with carbonic acid to yield bicarbonate ion. Note that

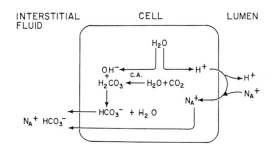

Figure 2-7. Acidification of urine deriving hydrogen ion indirectly from water by generation of H+ and OH− in spatially separated loci.

the initial materials, CO_2 and H_2O, and the final products, secreted hydrogen ion and sodium bicarbonate returned to the blood, are the same as in the earlier proposal. The role of carbonic anhydrase is slightly different — in this case, to maintain the level of carbonic acid necessary for keeping down the concentration of hydroxyl ion.

Whatever may be the nature of the hydrogen ion secretory process, it is clear that its net result is the return of one equivalent of sodium bicarbonate for each equivalent of hydrogen ion delivered to the lumen. This is independent of the fate of the hydrogen ion after it has been extruded into the lumen. Although bicarbonate reabsorption, formation of titratable acid, and formation of ammonium ion are, for clarity, treated as separate processes, all three occur simultaneolsy and utilize the same hydrogen ion secretion. The distribution of secreted hydrogen ion among the three processes is dependent entirely upon the composition of the fluid into which it is secreted. The hydrogen ion is distributed in conformity with the requirement that all the buffers of any fluid must simultaneously be at equilibrium at the same pH. Thus,

$$pH = pK_{H2CO3} + \log \frac{[HCO_3^-]}{[CO_2]}$$

$$= pK_{buffer\ A} + \log \frac{[A^-]}{[HA]}$$

$$= pK_{buffer\ B} + \log \frac{[B]}{[BH^+]}, \text{etc.}$$

In general, hydrogen ion will combine with buffers present in highest concentration and to an extent that increases as the pH of the fluid approaches the pK of the buffer. However, in the proximal tubule, although bicarbonate *is* present in far higher concentration than other buffers, these considerations are dwarfed by the fact that only in the case of bicarbonate can addition of acid fail to lower the pH. A fall in pH will not occur if volume reduction keeps pace with bicarbonate conversion to CO_2 via carbonic acid. The loss of the CO_2 tends to keep the denominator of the Henderson-Hasselbalch equation constant. For any other buffer the ratio is not appreciably affected by volume changes and therefore pH changes are independent of volume changes. Thus the effect of bicarbonate on pH change predominates until bicarbonate concentration has been much reduced. Other buffers receive hydrogen ion in the proximal tubule only to the extent that bicarbonate *concentration* falls and pH is reduced. In the distal tubule, as the concentration of other buffer rises and the bicarbonate approaches exhaustion, the hydrogen ion is increasingly diverted to the formation of titratable acid and ammonium ion.

In considering the contribution of renal mechanisms to regulation of acid-base balance it is frequently useful to calculate net acid excretion as the sum of titratable acid and ammonium ion excreted minus any bicarbonate which may have escaped into the urine. Since the excreted titratable acid and ammonium ion are the equivalent of the bicarbonate regenerated by the renal tubules and returned to the body, the calculation has meaning relative to the maintenance of the "alkali reserve" of the body. However, it should not be considered a measure of the activity of the renal tubules in acidifying the urine. Under most conditions the hydrogen ion secreted by the tubules is in large part expended in bicarbonate reabsorption. Thus, even a relatively limited capacity for hydrogen ion secretion can produce large amounts of titratable acid if the bicarbonate requiring reabsorption is sufficiently reduced in amount — i.e., if the plasma bicarbonate concentration is low. On the other hand, since bicarbonate reabsorption merely returns to the body fluids bicarbonate that was temporarily lost in the glomerular filtrate, its function is primarily conservative, and despite the magnitude of this operation it does not appear in the balance sheet when only the final urine is examined.

EXCRETION OF AMMONIA

As mentioned above, the excretion of ammonia, like the excretion of titratable acid, represents regeneration of bicarbonate for the body fluids. Under most conditions it is quantitatively the more important. The site of formation and the precursors of the urinary ammonia were the subject of debate for many years. Nash and Benedict [109] showed that the amount of ammonia leaving the kidney in renal venous blood exceeded that delivered in the arterial blood and thus established that the urinary ammonia is formed in the kidney. Van Slyke and his associates [167] demonstrated that most of the urinary ammonia could be accounted for by the disappearance of the amide nitrogen of glutamine. Ammonia is also produced by the deamination of several amino acids (e.g., glycine, alanine, aspartic acid, leucine) [91].

The fact that ammonia excretion varies with urine pH is best interpreted as being due to the entry of ammonia into the urine by diffusion from the cells in which it is produced and its accumulation in the urine by combination with hydrogen ion to form ammonium ion [112, 120]. The nature of these processes can be understood from a consideration of the permeability characteristics of cell membranes and the behavior and solubility characteristics of weak electrolytes.

Most cell membranes have the characteristics of thin layers of lipid permeated by aqueous pores. The aqueous pores seem generally to have very small dimensions and to occupy only a very small fraction of the cell surface area. Since substances which are highly soluble in lipid can pass through the membrane by dissolving in the lipid, such materials can easily penetrate the entire cell surface, while those that are soluble in water but not in lipid must enter and leave the cells through the water-filled pores. Consequently, the passage of lipid-soluble materials is many times more rapid than that of lipid-insoluble, water-soluble substances. Among such water-soluble substances are most ions; they would be expected to penetrate cell membranes relatively slowly. On the other hand, many weak acids and bases are highly soluble in lipid *in their un-ionized form*. The ammonium ion (NH_4^+) is highly soluble in water and would be expected to penetrate cell membranes relatively poorly. The un-ionized free ammonia (NH_3) is highly lipid-soluble and diffuses readily through cell membranes.

Now suppose that we have two solutions of differing pH separated by a lipid membrane of the type just described. To one of these solutions, ammonia is added. Since the ammonia readily penetrates the membrane, it will immediately begin to diffuse across into the other solution and will continue to do so until the concentration of ammonia is the same in both solutions. However, in each solution ammonia will also react with hydrogen ion to yield ammonium ion:

$$NH_3 + H^+ \rightleftharpoons NH_4^+$$

and this reaction will in each solution be continuously at the equilibrium dictated by the dissociation constant of this reaction:

$$pH = pKaNH_4 + \log \frac{[NH_3]}{[NH_4^+]}$$

$$(pKaNH_4^+ = 8.9)$$

If it is assumed that the permeability of the membrane to NH_4^+ is so small as to be negligible relative to the permeability to NH_3, then equilibrium in the total system will be reached when two conditions are satisfied: when $[NH_3]$ is the same in both solutions, and when the dissociation equilibrium is satisfied in each solution.* When these conditions

have been achieved, the above equation may be rewritten:

$$pH = pKa + \log [NH_3] - \log [NH_4^+]$$
$$= \text{constant} - \log [NH_4^+]$$

Since in blood, cells, and urine $[NH_3]$ is rarely more than one-tenth of $[NH_4^+]$ and more often less than one one-hundredth, the concentration of total ammonia ($NH_3 + NH_4^+$) reflects almost entirely the concentration of ammonium ion, and the total ammonia concentration will also change approximately tenfold for each unit change in pH.

This model may be considered to represent the renal mechanism involved in the entry of ammonia into the urine and its accumulation there if one phase is taken to be the contents of the cells in which ammonia is produced and the other phase the fluid in the tubule lumen. The pH of the ammonia-producing cells and their ammonia concentration may, as a first approximation, be considered to be held constant. The concentration achieved in the tubule lumen will then increase tenfold for each decrease of one unit in the pH of the lumen fluid.†

Because several of the assumptions involved in the foregoing model are at best approximations, ammonia excretion does not vary with urine pH precisely as required by the model. The rate of excretion of ammonia rather than its concentration in the urine is generally closely related to the urine pH, especially when the urine pH is low, and a change of 2.0 to 2.5 pH units is usually required to produce a tenfold increase in ammonia excretion [112].

Ammonia has been found to accumulate in tubule fluid beginning in the proximal tubule in the rat [29, 52a, 61]. The extent of accumulation can be considered to reflect the degree

---

* As NH_3 diffuses through the membrane and reacts with H^+, the pH of the solution tends to rise. It must be assumed that the pH difference between the two solutions is maintained by continuous addition of hydrogen ion as necessary.

†A similar equilibrium must be assumed to exist between blood and cells, but because the pH of urine is generally considerably lower than the pH of blood, most of the ammonia will enter the urine rather than the blood.

to which fluid in the lumen becomes acid, since there is evidence to suggest that all the fluids of the renal cortex attain approximately the same concentration of free ammonia, i.e., a more or less uniform pNH_3 [36].

A unique feature of ammonia excretion is its adaptation to meet the requirements for maintenance of acid-base balance. If some acidifying salt (NH_4Cl, $CaCl_2$) is administered, there is an immediate fall in urine pH and a corresponding increase in ammonia excretion. However, without further change in urine pH, or even with a return of pH toward control values, the excretion of ammonia gradually increases over a period of three to five days, at the end of which it may be several times greater at any given urine pH than it was before the acidifying regimen was instituted [120, 128, 138]. The mechanism of this adaptation is uncertain, but it appears to involve changes in the enzymatic processes by which ammonia is produced [34] and is presumably accompanied by an increase of the ammonia concentration of the secreting cells.

In the rat it has been amply shown that this adaptation is well correlated with an increase in glutaminase activity in the kidney, but such changes in glutaminase apparently do not occur in the dog [128]. Since ammonia excretion in man varies with urine pH in a manner similar to that observed in the dog but different from that in the rat, there is reason to suspect that the changes observed in the rat probably do not occur in man.

The nature of the immediate stimulus which leads to adaptation is also unclear. It does not appear to be extracellular acidosis since, on prolonged administration of acid, ammonia excretion may continue at a high level even though the plasma bicarbonate has returned to essentially normal levels [67].

QUANTITATIVE ASPECTS OF

URINE ACIDIFICATION

Factors Related to Filtered Load. As with nearly all renal excretory processes, the acidifi-cation of the urine depends upon the balance between glomerular filtration and tubular transport processes. The component of the glomerular filtrate most pertinent to urinary acidification is its bicarbonate concentration. For reasons which remain unexplained, the capacity of the renal tubules to reabsorb bicarbonate appears to vary with the rate of glomerular filtration [124].* The capacity to reabsorb, however, is not related to the plasma bicarbonate concentration. Consequently the plasma bicarbonate concentration is a much more important determinant of bicarbonate excretion and urine acidification than is the rate of glomerular filtration. For these reasons, and to facilitate the quantitative description of the processes involved and to render them, to some extent, orderly and predictable, it is customary to factor the filtration, reabsorption, and excretion of bicarbonate by the rate of glomerular filtration and to present these processes in units of amount per unit volume of glomerular filtration — e.g., milliequivalents per liter or per 100 ml. of glomerular filtrate.

When the plasma bicarbonate concentration is low, the urine is highly acid and essentially free of bicarbonate, all of the filtered bicarbonate being reabsorbed by the tubules. As the plasma bicarbonate is progressively increased, the urine remains virtually bicarbonate-free until the concentration in plasma approaches 27 to 28 mEq. per liter [123].† Small but rapidly increasing amounts of bicarbonate then appear in the urine. Further increases in plasma bicarbonate concentration are not accompanied by increases in bicarbonate reabsorption, which remains stable at about 28 mEq. per liter of glomerular filtrate and the

* Such behavior would be easily explained if the change in glomerular filtration were due to changes in the number of functioning nephrons, but data relative to other tubular processes indicate that in mammals under most conditions all the nephrons are continuously active.

† The figures quoted are for man. In the dog, frank bicarbonate excretion begins at 23 to 25 mEq. per liter in the plasma.

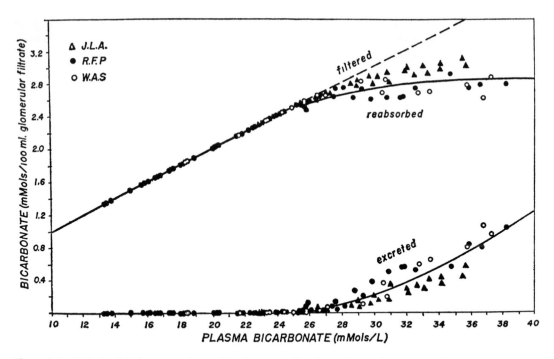

Figure 2-8. Relationship between plasma bicarbonate and reabsorption and excretion of bicarbonate in man. (Pitts, Ayer, and Schiess, *J. Clin. Invest.* 28:35, 1949.)

excess of the filtered bicarbonate is excreted in the urine.* These characteristics are illustrated by the data of Pitts and associates [123] in Figure 2-8. Thus the plasma bicarbonate concentration tends to become stabilized at about 28 mEq. per liter. As the plasma bicarbonate concentration falls below this level, the urine becomes acid, titratable acid and ammonia are excreted, and the bicarbonate thus regenerated tends to return the plasma bicarbonate concentration to the equilibrium level of approximately 28 mEq. per liter. When plasma bicarbonate rises above this level, the excess is rapidly excreted in the urine.

To the extent that the secretion of hydrogen ion is expended in bicarbonate reabsorp-

tion, little is available to appear as titratable acid and ammonia. Thus, as the plasma bicarbonate concentration approaches 28 mEq. per liter and the urine pH rises toward that of plasma, titratable acid and ammonia tend to disappear from the urine even though very little bicarbonate may be excreted.† When the bicarbonate concentration in the plasma is lower, the filtered bicarbonate is exhausted higher in the nephron and increasing amounts of secreted hydrogen ion are converted to titratable acid and ammonium ion. Under these conditions the limits of acidity may be reached and all the available ammonia trapped

* The maximum rate of bicarbonate reabsorption is sometimes referred to as a Tm. It should be noted, however, that it differs from the usual Tm in being an amount per unit of glomerular filtrate and thus has the dimensions of concentration rather than amount per unit time.

† Under certain abnormal conditions (e.g., hyperaldosteronism) ammonia may be excreted in rather large amounts although the urine is alkaline [41]. The most probable basis for this is an increase in the ammonia-forming processes with a high concentration of ammonia in the tubule cells. The urine pH is probably high *because* of its high ammonia concentration rather than in spite of it. Diffusion of ammonia into the urine is the equivalent of titration with alkali.

in the urine before the capacity to secrete hydrogen ion is fully utilized. Consequently, the capacity to secrete hydrogen ion is not subject to evaluation when the urine is acid; furthermore, hydrogen ion secretion, paradoxically, is usually greatest when the urine is alkaline. However, reduction of the urine pH to low levels is a manifestation of another capacity of the renal tubules — that of producing a normal maximum gradient of pH between blood and urine. The capacity to secrete hydrogen ion may, under some conditions, vary independently of the capacity to establish gradients of pH [133].

Factors Modifying Hydrogen Ion Secretion. The foregoing discussion has been based on renal tubular behavior under normal conditions with respect to several variables that affect renal tubular acid secretion. The effect of changes in these variables may be considered individually.

CARBON DIOXIDE TENSION. When the carbon dioxide tension is increased (respiratory acidosis), the plasma bicarbonate concentration rises and remains at a higher level. The initial increase in bicarbonate concentration is in large part due to titration of the buffers of blood by CO_2 (carbonic acid). However, maintenance of the increased level requires a change in renal activity since otherwise the excess of bicarbonate above the normal value would be rapidly excreted in the urine. It can be shown that there is, in fact, an increase in renal tubular capacity for bicarbonate reabsorption and that, as the increased level of pCO_2 is maintained for prolonged periods, there is a further increase in this capacity [20, 40, 131, 159]. Although the nature of the latter adaptive change remains obscure, the initial change in hydrogen ion secretion is readily interpreted in terms of the assumption that the rate of secretion is directly related to the hydrogen ion concentration of cells. In view of the high permeability of cells to CO_2, it is a reasonable assumption that the CO_2 tension and consequently the hydrogen ion concen-

tration of cells vary promptly and concordantly with the CO_2 tension of the blood.*

The effects of reduction of CO_2 tension (respiratory alkalosis) are the opposite of those described above, although no prolonged experiments have been performed to determine whether or not there is any adaptation analogous to that with prolonged respiratory acidosis.

POTASSIUM METABOLISM. The administration of potassium salts to normal persons depresses acid secretion, and the urine may become alkaline in spite of a low plasma bicarbonate concentration. The mechanism by which this effect is produced is not entirely clear. It may reflect an inverse relation of the concentration of potassium and hydrogen ions in the secreting cells [13]. Potassium depletion has been recognized for some time as being associated with a sustained increase in plasma bicarbonate concentration [33]. However, it has been shown that chloride depletion is also a concomitant of this alkalosis [1]. It is not entirely clear whether the increased hydrogen ion secretion, which maintains the high plasma bicarbonate concentration, is a consequence of the chloride deficit alone [1] or whether the depletion of potassium also is a factor in increasing urinary acidification [78].

CARBONIC ANHYDRASE. As already indicated, carbonic anhydrase is essential for the normal operation of the acidifying mechanism. When the enzyme is inhibited there is a marked reduction in the capacity to secrete hydrogen ion [13, 122]. However, when the plasma bicarbonate concentration is sufficiently reduced, even this reduced capacity may yield a normally acid urine. The enzyme activity is almost certainly rate-limiting only when it is drastically reduced by inhibitors. Under other conditions, other factors set the limit on hydrogen ion secretion. There is no convincing evidence that the carbonic anhydrase activity

* On the other hand, there is little evidence to suggest that the bicarbonate concentration of cells is closely related to that of extracellular fluid.

is adaptively modified in the face of acid loads.

ADRENAL STEROIDS. The secretion of hydrogen ion appears to participate in the enhancement of sodium reabsorption produced by the "mineralocorticoids."

Excretion of Urea

Urea is the major end product, in mammals, of the metabolism of nitrogen-containing substances. The mechanism by which it is excreted is of particular interest not only for this reason but because urea excretion is so often considered a clinical index of renal function and because the excretion of urea has certain unique features.

The reabsorption of urea from the renal tubules has long been regarded as the prototype of a passive reabsorptive process. Certainly, most of the features of urea excretion in man and in the dog can be readily interpreted in the framework of such a hypothesis. However, note should be taken of the view that urea excretion is, at least to some extent, a "regulated" process, an interpretation somewhat better supported by evidence in the ruminant (camel, sheep) than it is in most other mammals [108, 141]. The evidence that such regulation occurs in man or in the dog is not sufficiently convincing to warrant modification of the following description based on the assumption of passive processes only.

Most cell membranes have a high permeability to urea. It is therefore to be expected that as water is reabsorbed from the glomerular filtrate, thus tending to concentrate the urea that remains, the urea tends to diffuse out of the tubule lumen. More remarkable, in view of this generally high permeability, are the very considerable extent to which urea can be concentrated in the urine and the large fraction of the filtered urea which may be excreted in the urine. Two factors may be considered responsible:

1. Some portions of the renal tubule have an unusually low permeability to urea, particularly in the absence of antidiuretic hormone. This low permeability is not too surprising in view of the uniquely low permeability to water of some of these same segments.

2. Urea escaping from the nephron in the collecting ducts is accumulated in the interstitial fluid of the medulla because of the low effective blood flow in this region. Thus the concentration gradient from lumen to interstitium is considerably lower than that represented by the concentrations in urine and blood and the tendency for escape of urea by diffusion is correspondingly reduced.

Since the tendency to raise the concentration of urea in the tubule is proportional to the fraction of the filtered water reabsorbed, the reabsorption of urea is dependent upon the reabsorption of water and varies with the urine flow. In water diuresis in man as in the dog (Fig. 2-9), some 60 to 70 per cent of the filtered urea is excreted in the urine; i.e., the urea clearance is 60 to 70 per cent of the rate of glomerular filtration [147]. If the urine flow is increased beyond that attainable by water diuresis by the superimposition of an osmotic diuresis (e.g., with mannitol or sodium sulfate), the fraction of the filtered urea appearing in the urine is further increased. Extrapolation of the resulting curve suggests that no urea would be reabsorbed if no water were reabsorbed [148]. Conversely, in the absence of osmotic diuresis, as the urine flow falls in antidiuresis the excreted fraction of the filtered urea falls progressively and may be only 10 to 20 per cent at very low flows.

The change from the low urea clearance of antidiuresis to the value attained in water diuresis reflects changes in the reabsorption of urea in the more distal segments of the nephron, since the changes in water reabsorption that occur in the transition from water diuresis to antidiuresis are in large part limited to the distal nephron and collecting system. The

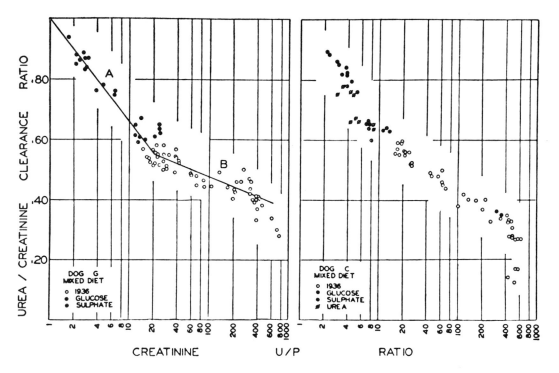

Figure 2-9. Fraction of filtered urea excreted (urea/creatinine clearance ratio) as a function of water re-absorption (creatinine U/P). (Shannon, *Amer. J. Physiol.* 122:782, 1938.)

distal convoluted tubule has been shown to have a relatively low permeability to urea in the rat, even in the presence of antidiuretic hormone [26], and in the rabbit, the cortical collecting tubules have a low permeability to urea even when the water permeability has been markedly increased by antidiuretic hormone [57]. However, the permeability of the rat medullary collecting ducts to urea is markedly enhanced by vasopressin [104]. The effects of vasopressin in the distal region are of two sorts, both of which can be considered to increase urea reabsorption: (1) the increased permeability to water increases water reabsorption, raising the urea concentration in the remaining fluid and increasing the concentration gradient driving the outward movement of urea; and (2) the permeability to urea is itself increased, largely in the medullary portion of the collecting system.

The fraction of the filtered urea that is un-affected by water diuresis is presumably largely reabsorbed in the proximal tubule, and it is this fraction that is depressed by osmotic diuresis, which is known to interfere with proximal water reabsorption. The observed gross behavior thus fits with the micropuncture findings that some 30 to 40 per cent of the filtered urea is ordinarily reabsorbed in the proximal tubule in the presence or absence of antidiuretic hormone [28, 82]. In water diuresis the remaining urea is excreted almost quantitatively in the urine. In the presence of antidiuretic hormone the mechanism becomes considerably more complicated. The permeability of the collecting duct to urea is increased. However, as urea escapes from the collecting ducts, it tends to accumulate in the medullary interstitial fluid and to reenter the tubules by diffusion into the descending limb of the loop of Henle [54]. Thus a fraction of the urea is recirculated through the distal portion of the nephron and the amount of urea leaving the medulla in the loop of Henle to enter the distal tubules is considerably greater than that which enters the medulla from the proximal tubules. The recirculation of urea through the distal portions of the nephron in antidiuresis and the absence of this recirculation in water diuresis* should not lead to the misconception that there is less urea loss in antidiuresis; the losses of urea are considerably greater under the latter condition since only a fraction of the escaping urea is recirculated.

The accumulation of urea in the interstitium of the medulla has particular significance for the formation of concentrated urine. This accumulation may be considered to result from the low absolute blood flow in this region and from the countercurrent exchanger arrangement of this flow. The removal of urea in the blood is largely prevented by its diffusion into the blood entering the medulla with a low urea concentration. In fact, the results of micropuncture study in the rat suggest that the major fraction of the urea that escapes from the collecting ducts leaves the medulla by reentering the tubule in the descending limb of the loop of Henle and only a small fraction is carried away in the blood. Thus, by a small net loss from the collecting ducts a very high concentration of urea can be maintained in the medullary interstitium. This concentration in the interstitium can be shown to approach the very high concentration of urea in the bladder and collecting duct urine [85, 164]. Consequently, the urinary urea is balanced osmotically to a very considerable extent by urea in the fluid surrounding the collecting ducts, and the sodium chloride of the interstitial fluid, which initiates the concentrating process, can balance, for the most part, the urinary solutes other than urea. Thus

urine can be rendered considerably more concentrated when urea is a major fraction of the excreted solute than when it is not; and, in effect, urea can be excreted in water already largely obligated for the excretion of other solutes. Thus the addition of urea to the urinary solute creates an exception to the rule (see page 57) that as solute excretion increases, urine concentration falls; when urea appears in the urine (in moderate amounts), concentration rises despite the increased total solute excretion [45, 85].

The frequent use of the urea clearance as a clinical index of renal function warrants brief further comment. Because the concentration of urea in red blood cell water is the same as that in plasma water, the concentration of urea in whole blood is very close to that in the plasma (being some 15 per cent lower since about this fraction of whole blood is red blood cell solids). It is therefore common to use whole blood rather than plasma for the clinical determination of urea clearances; the value thus derived is nearly the same. To take account of the variation of urea clearance with urine flow it is usual to divide urea clearances into two classes. When urine flow is in excess of 2 ml. per minute, the clearance of urea tends to approach that in water diuresis — some 60 per cent of the rate of glomerular filtration — and is relatively unaffected by further increases in flow. Under these conditions, the clearance of urea is calculated in the usual fashion (UV/B) except for the substitution of the concentration in whole blood (B) for that in plasma (P). The value obtained is called the *maximal urea clearance* and can be considered to be roughly 60 per cent of the glomerular filtration rate. When the urine flow is lower, it has been found empirically that the use of the formula $U\sqrt{V}/B$ yields a value which does not vary much with the urine flow. This value, which is called the *standard urea clearance,* is an empirical one not indicative of any physical process, and

---

* The recirculation of urea in antidiuresis is established on the basis of micropuncture studies in the rat [54]. Its absence in water diuresis is assumed.

averages somewhat less than half the rate of glomerular filtration [102].

The blood urea concentration itself is sometimes used as an index of renal function but must be interpreted with caution since it not only varies inversely with the rate of glomerular filtration, but is also directly proportional to the rate of urea formation in the body and is markedly affected by any unusual level of urinary flow.

Nonionic Diffusion

The phenomenon known as nonionic diffusion has been referred to in several previous sections and the physicochemical principles that underlie it have been considered in connection with the excretion of ammonia. These principles may be summarized as follows:

1. Cell membranes generally have the characteristics of a layer of lipid perforated by minute aqueous pores which occupy only a very small fraction of the surface area.

2. Lipid-soluble materials can pass through the entire cell surface, while water-soluble substances are limited to passage through the pores (or by specific transport mechanisms); lipid-soluble particles, therefore, penetrate much more readily.

3. Many organic acids and bases in their un-ionized state are highly lipid-soluble; their ions generally are virtually insoluble in lipid. Since the rate at which a substance penetrates a membrane depends on the concentration of the penetrating substance, the rate of penetration by weak organic acids and bases increases as the un-ionized fraction increases.

Thus, if the tubule lumen contains such a weak acid or base at a given concentration, the rate at which the weak electrolyte diffuses out of the lumen will depend upon the pH of the fluid in the lumen. Bases will diffuse out more rapidly as the pH of the fluid increases, since the ionization of weak bases decreases as the pH increases. Conversely, weak acids will escape from the lumen more readily as the pH of the fluid diminishes, since a fall in pH suppresses the ionization of weak acids. Typically, then, the urinary excretion of weak bases increases as the urine is acidified, and the urinary excretion of weak acids increases as the urine becomes alkaline. This is not, however, uniformly the case, because even the un-ionized weak electrolyte may have too low a solubility in lipid to penetrate the lining membranes with any facility; PAH and Diodrast are examples of this type of weak acid.

It happens that many of the weak acids and bases that tend to escape from the tubule lumen by nonionic diffusion are also subject to secretion in the proximal tubule by one or the other of the two active transport mechanisms responsible for the secretion of organic anions and cations into the tubule.* These substances are thus presumably delivered in large amounts into the proximal tubule lumen and subsequently escape back to the blood at rates dependent upon the pH of the fluid and the lipid solubility of their un-ionized forms. The frequency with which active secretion in the proximal tubule is associated with passive reabsorption by nonionic diffusion has considerably complicated the study of the secretory process — a clearance well below glomerular filtration rate cannot be considered to exclude rapid and active secretion.

---

* Although nonionic diffusion is discussed here as governing the rate of escape of weak acids and bases from the urine, it can be involved primarily in their accumulation in the urine, as appears to be the case in ammonia excretion. In such instances the un-ionized species enters the urine and may or may not be trapped, depending upon the extent to which it is converted to the ionized form in the latter phase. It is at least theoretically possible that under proper conditions of urine volume and pH the clearance of such substances might exceed the rate of glomerular filtration even though there is no active transport of the substance. However, in most instances in which the latter considerations have been thought to apply, developments have shown that the process involves initial active secretion and passive reabsorption by nonionic diffusion (e.g., salicylate, quinine, Atabrine) [116, 173].

References

1. Atkins, E. L., and Schwartz, W. B. Factors governing correction of the alkalosis associated with potassium deficiency; the critical role of chloride in the recovery process. *J. Clin. Invest.* 41:218, 1962.

2. August, J. T., and Nelson, D. H. Adjustment to aldosterone or desoxycorticosterone acetate induced sodium retention in patients with Addison's disease. *J. Clin. Invest.* 38:1964, 1959.

3. Bennett, C. M., Brenner, B. M., and Berliner, R. W. Micropuncture study of nephron function in the rhesus monkey. *J. Clin. Invest.* 47:203, 1968.

4. Bennett, C. M., Clapp, J. R., and Berliner, R. W. Micropuncture study of the proximal and distal tubule in the dog. *Amer. J. Physiol.* 213:1254, 1967.

5. Berger, E. Y., Farber, S. J., and Earle, D. P., Jr. Renal excretion of mannitol. *Proc. Soc. Exp. Biol. Med.* 66:62, 1947.

6. Berglund, F., Helander, C-G., and Howe, R. B. Inorganic sulfate and thiosulfate: Transport and competition in renal tubules of the dog. *Amer. J. Physiol.* 198:586, 1960.

7. Berliner, R. W. Membrane transport. *Rev. Mod. Phys.* 31:342, 1959.

8. Berliner, R. W. Renal mechanisms for potassium excretion. *Harvey Lect.* 55:141, 1961.

9. Berliner, R. W., and Davidson, D. G. Production of hypertonic urine in the absence of pituitary antidiuretic hormone. *J. Clin. Invest.* 36:1416, 1957.

10. Berliner, R. W., Hilton, J. G., Yü, T. F., and Kennedy, T. J., Jr. The renal mechanism for urate excretion in man. *J. Clin. Invest.* 29:396, 1950.

11. Berliner, R. W., and Kennedy, T. J., Jr. Renal tubular secretion of potassium in the normal dog. *Proc. Soc. Exp. Biol. Med.* 67:542, 1948.

12. Berliner, R. W., Kennedy, T. J., Jr., and Hilton, J. G. Renal mechanisms for excretion of potassium. *Amer. J. Physiol.* 162:348, 1950.

13. Berliner, R. W., Kennedy, T. J., Jr., and Orloff, J. Relationship between acidification of the urine and potassium metabolism. Effect of carbonic anhydrase inhibition on potassium excretion. *Amer. J. Med.* 11:274, 1951.

14. Berliner, R. W., Levinsky, N. G., Davidson, D. G., and Eden, M. Dilution and concentration of the urine and the action of antidiuretic hormone. *Amer. J. Med.* 24:730, 1958.

15. Beyer, K. H., Wright, L. D., Skeggs, H. R., Russo, H. F., and Shaner, G. A. Renal clearance of essential amino acids: Their competition for reabsorption by the renal tubules. *Amer. J. Physiol.* 151:202, 1947.

16. Blythe, W. B., and Welt, L. G. Dissociation between filtered load of sodium and its rate of excretion in the urine. *J. Clin. Invest.* 42:1491, 1963.

17. Bojesen, E. The renal mechanism of "dilution diuresis" and salt excretion in dogs. *Acta Physiol. Scand.* 32:129, 1954.

18. Bowman, W. On the structure and use of the malpighian bodies of the kidney, with observations on the circulation through that gland. *Phil. Trans. Roy. Soc.* (London) 132:57, 1842. Reprinted with Bowman's biography and bibliography in *Medical Classics* 5:258, 1940.

19. Bray, G. Freezing point depression of rat kidney slices during water diuresis and antidiuresis. *Amer. J. Physiol.* 199:915, 1960.

20. Brazeau, P., and Gilman, A. Effect of plasma CO_2 tension on renal tubular reabsorption of bicarbonate. *Amer. J. Physiol.* 175:33, 1953.

21. Brod, J., and Sirota, J. H. The renal clearance of endogenous "creatinine" in man. *J. Clin. Invest.* 27:645, 1948.

22. Brodsky, W. A., Rehm, W. S., Dennis, W. H., and Miller, D. G. Thermodynamic analysis of the intracellular osmotic gradient hypothesis of active water transport. *Science* 121:302, 1955.

23. Bucht, H., Werko, L., and Josephson, B. The oxygen consumption of the human kidney during heavy tubular excretory work. *Scand. J. Clin. Lab. Invest.* 1:277, 1949.

24. Burgen, A. S. V. A theoretical treatment

of glucose reabsorption in the kidney. *Canad. J. Biochem. Physiol.* 34:466, 1956.

25. Burgess, W. W., Harvey, A. M., and Marshall, E. K., Jr. The site of the antidiuretic action of pituitary extract. *J. Pharmacol. Exp. Ther.* 49:237, 1933.

26. Capek, K., Fuchs, G., Rumrich, G., and Ullrich, K. J. Harnstoffpermeabilitat der corticalen Tubulusabschnitte von Ratten in Antidiurese und Wasserdiurese. *Pflueger. Arch.* 290:237, 1966.

27. Chasis, H., and Smith, H. W. The excretion of urea in normal man and in subjects with glomerulonephritis. *J. Clin. Invest.* 17:347, 1938.

28. Clapp, J. R. Urea reabsorption by the proximal tubule of the dog. *Proc. Soc. Exp. Biol. Med.* 120:521, 1965.

29. Clapp, J. R., Owen, E. E., and Robinson, R. R. Contribution of the proximal tubule to urinary ammonia excretion by the dog. *Amer. J. Physiol.* 209:269, 1965.

30. Clapp, J. R., Watson, J. F., and Berliner, R. W. Osmolality, bicarbonate concentration, and water reabsorption in proximal tubule of the dog nephron. *Amer. J. Physiol.* 205:273, 1963.

31. Clark, J. K., and Barker, H. G. Effect of work on renal oxygen utilization. *Fed. Proc.* 8:26, 1949.

32. Cushny, A. R. *The Secretion of the Urine.* London: Longmans, Green, 1917.

33. Darrow, D. C., Schwartz, R., Iannucci, J. F., and Coville, F. The relation of serum bicarbonate concentration to muscle composition. *J. Clin. Invest.* 27:198, 1948.

34. Davies, B. M. A., and Yudkin, J. Studies in biochemical adaptation. The origin of urinary ammonia as indicated by the effect of chronic acidosis and alkalosis on some renal enzymes in the rat. *Biochem. J.* 52:407, 1952.

35. Davies, R. E. Hydrochloric acid production by isolated gastric mucosa. *Biochem. J.* 42:609, 1948.

36. Denis, G., Preuss, H., and Pitts, R. The P_{NH_3} of renal tubular cells. *J. Clin. Invest.* 43:571, 1964.

36a. de Rouffignac, C., and Morel, F. Net solute addition, the major concentrating

factor in descending limb of Psammomys kidneys. *Proc. Twenty-fourth Intern. Congr. Physiol. Sci.* 1968. P. 376.

37. de Wardener, H. E., and Miles, B. E. The effect of haemorrhage on the circulatory autoregulation of the dog's kidney perfused in situ. *Clin. Sci.* 11:267, 1952.

38. de Wardener, H. E., Mills, I. H., Clapham, W. F., and Hayter, C. J. Studies on the efferent mechanism of the sodium diuresis which follows the administration of intravenous saline in the dog. *Clin. Sci.* 21:249, 1961.

39. Dirks, J. H., Cirksena, W. J., and Berliner, R. W. The effect of saline infusion on sodium reabsorption by the proximal tubule of the dog. *J. Clin. Invest.* 44:1160, 1965.

40. Dorman, P. J., Sullivan, W. J., and Pitts, R. F. The renal response to acute respiratory acidosis. *J. Clin. Invest.* 33:82, 1954.

41. Dustan, H. P., Corcoran, A. C., and Page, I. H. Renal function in primary aldosteronism. *J. Clin. Invest.* 35:1357, 1956.

42. Du Vigneaud, V. Hormones of the posterior pituitary gland: Oxytocin and vasopressin. *Harvey Lect.* 50:1, 1956.

43. Earle, D. P., Jr., and Berliner, R. W. A simplified clinical procedure for measurement of glomerular filtration rate and renal plasma flow. *Proc. Soc. Exp. Biol. Med.* 62:262, 1946.

44. Earley, L. E., and Friedler, R. M. The effects of combined renal vasodilatation and pressor agents on renal hemodynamics and the tubular reabsorption of sodium. *J. Clin. Invest.* 45:542, 1966.

45. Epstein, F. H., Kleeman, C. R., Pursel, S., and Hendrikx, A. The effect of feeding protein and urea on the renal concentrating process. *J. Clin. Invest.* 36:635, 1957.

46. Fingl, E. Tubular excretion of creatinine in the rat. *Amer. J. Physiol.* 169:357, 1952.

47. Forster, R. P. The use of inulin and creatinine as glomerular filtrate measuring substances in the frog. *J. Cell. Comp. Physiol.* 12:213, 1938.

48. Frank, J., and Mayer, J. E. An osmotic diffusion pump. *Arch. Biochem.* 14:297, 1947.

49. Fromter, E., and Hegel, U. Transtubulare

Potentialdifferenzen an proximalen und distalen Tubuli der Rattenniere. *Pflueger. Arch.* 291:107, 1966.

50. Gammeltoft, A., and Kjerulf-Jensen, K. The mechanism of renal excretion of fructose and galactose in rabbit, cat, dog, and man (with special reference to the phosphorylation theory). *Acta Physiol. Scand.* 6:368, 1943.

51. Giebisch, G. Measurements of electrical potentials and ion fluxes on single renal tubules. *Circulation* 21:879, 1960.

52. Giebisch, G., Windhager, E. E., and Pitts, R. F. Mechanism of Urinary Acidification. In Quinn, E. L., and Kass, E. H. (Eds.), *Biology of Pyelonephritis* (Henry Ford Hospital International Symposium). Boston: Little, Brown, 1960. Chap. 19.

52a. Glabman, S., Klose, R. M., and Giebisch, G. Micropuncture study of ammonia excretion in the rat. *Amer. J. Physiol.* 205:127, 1963.

53. Goldstein, D. A., and Solomon, A. K. Determination of equivalent pore radius for human red cells by osmotic pressure measurement. *J. Gen. Physiol.* 44:1, 1960.

54. Gottschalk, C. W. Micropuncture studies of tubular function in the mammalian kidney. Fifth Bowditch Lecture. *Physiologist* 4:35, 1961.

55. Gottschalk, C. W., Lassiter, W. E., and Mylle, M. Localization of urine acidification in the mammalian kidney. *Amer. J. Physiol.* 198:581, 1960.

56. Gottschalk, C. W., and Mylle, M. Micropuncture study of the mammalian urinary concentrating mechanism: Evidence for the countercurrent hypothesis. *Amer. J. Physiol.* 196:927, 1959.

57. Grantham, J. J., and Burg, M. B. Effect of vasopressin and cyclic AMP on permeability of isolated collecting tubules. *Amer. J. Physiol.* 211:255, 1966.

58. Gutman, A. B., Yü, T. F., and Berger, L. Tubular secretion of urate in man. *J. Clin. Invest.* 38:1778, 1959.

59. Hargitay, B., and Kuhn, W. Das Multiplikationsprinzip als Grundlage der Harnkonzentrierung in der Niere. *Z. Elektrochem. Angew. Physik. Chem.* 55:539, 1951.

60. Harrison, H. E., and Harrison, H. C. The renal excretion of inorganic phosphate in relation to the action of vitamin D and parathyroid hormone. *J. Clin. Invest.* 20:47, 1941.

61. Hayes, C. P., Jr., Mayson, J. S., Owen, E. E., and Robinson, R. R. A micropuncture evaluation of renal ammonia excretion in the rat. *Amer. J. Physiol.* 207:77, 1964.

62. Hayman, J. M. Estimations of afferent arteriole and glomerular capillary pressures in the frog kidney. *Amer. J. Physiol.* 79:389, 1927.

63. Heidenhain, R. Versuche über den Vorgang der Harnabsonderung. *Arch. Ges. Physiol.* 9:1, 1874.

64. Hendrix, J. P., Westfall, B. B., and Richards, A. N. Quantitative studies of the composition of glomerular urine: XIV. The glomerular excretion of inulin in frogs and *Necturi. J. Biol. Chem.* 116:735, 1937.

65. Hiatt, H. H., and Thompson, D. D. The effects of parathyroid extract on renal function in man. *J. Clin. Invest.* 36:557, 1957.

66. Hilger, H. H., Klumper, J. D., and Ullrich, K. J. Wasserrückresorption und Ionentransport durch die Sammelröhrzellen der Säugetierniere. *Pflueger. Arch.* 267:218, 1958.

67. Hilton, J. G. Potentiation of diuretic action of mercuhydrin by ammonium chloride. *J. Clin. Invest.* 30:1105, 1951.

68. Hinshaw, L. B., Day, S. B., and Carlson, C. H. Tissue pressure as a causal factor in the autoregulation of blood in the isolated perfused kidney. *Amer. J. Physiol.* 197:309, 1959.

69. Howards, S. S., Davis, B. B., Knox, F. G., Wright, F. S., and Berliner, R. W. Depression of fractional sodium reabsorption by the proximal tubule of the dog without sodium diuresis. *J. Clin. Invest.* 47:1561, 1968.

70. Jahan, I., and Pitts, R. F. Effect of parathyroid on renal tubular reabsorption of phosphate and calcium. *Amer. J. Physiol.* 155:42, 1948.

71. Jamison, R. L., Bennett, C. M., and Berliner, R. W. Countercurrent multiplica-

tion by the thin loops of Henle. *Amer. J. Physiol.* 212:357, 1967.

72. Johnston, C. I., and Davis, J. O. Evidence from cross circulation studies for a humoral mechanism in the natriuresis of saline loading. *Proc. Soc. Exp. Biol. Med.* 121:1058, 1966.

73. Kaplan, B. J., and Smith, H. W. Excretion of inulin, creatinine, xylose, and urea in normal rabbits. *Amer. J. Physiol.* 113:354, 1935.

74. Kennedy, T. J., Jr., Hilton, J. G., and Berliner, R. W. Comparison of inulin and creatinine clearance in the normal dog. *Amer. J. Physiol.* 171:164, 1952.

75. Koefoed-Johnsen, V., and Ussing, H. H. The contributions of diffusion and flow to the passage of D_2O through living membranes. Effect of neurohypophyseal hormone on isolated anuran skin. *Acta Physiol. Scand.* 28:60, 1953.

76. Kramer, K., and Deetjen, P. Beziehungen des O_2-Verbrauchs der Niere zu Durchblutung und Glomerulusfiltrat bei Änderung des arteriellen Druckes. *Pflueger. Arch.* 271:782, 1960.

77. Kramer, K., Thurau, K., and Deetjen, P. Hämodynamik des Nierenmarks. I. Mitteilung. Capillare Passagezeit, Blutvolumen, Durchblutung, Gewebshämatokrit und O_2-Verbrauch des Nierenmarks in situ. *Pflueger. Arch.* 270:251, 1960.

78. Kunau, R. T., Jr., Frick, A., Rector, F. C., Jr., and Seldin, D. W. Micropuncture study of the proximal tubular factors responsible for the maintenance of alkalosis during potassium deficiency in the rat. *Clin. Sci.* 34:223, 1968.

79. Landwehr, D. M., Klose, R. M., and Giebisch, G. Renal tubular sodium and water reabsorption in the isotonic sodium chloride-loaded rat. *Amer. J. Physiol.* 212:1327, 1967.

80. Lassen, N. A., and Longley, J. B. Countercurrent exchange in vessels of renal medulla. *Proc. Soc. Exp. Biol. Med.* 106:743, 1961.

81. Lassen, N. A., Munck, O., and Thaysen, J. H. Oxygen consumption and sodium reabsorption in the kidney. *Acta Physiol. Scand.* 51:371, 1961.

82. Lassiter, W. E., Gottschalk, C. W., and Mylle, M. Micropuncture study of net transtubular movement of water and urea in nondiuretic mammalian kidney. *Amer. J. Physiol.* 200:1139, 1961.

83. Lathem, W. The renal excretion of hemoglobin: Regulatory mechanisms and the differential excretion of free and protein-bound hemoglobin. *J. Clin. Invest.* 38:652, 1959.

84. LeFevre, P. G. Sugar transport in the red blood cell: Structure-activity relationships in substrates and antagonists. *Pharmacol. Rev.* 13:39, 1961.

85. Levinsky, N. G., and Berliner, R. W. The role of urea in the urine concentrating mechanism. *J. Clin. Invest.* 38:741, 1959.

86. Levinsky, N. G., Davidson, D. G., and Berliner, R. W. Effects of reduced glomerular filtration on urine concentration in the presence of antidiuretic hormone. *J. Clin. Invest.* 38:730, 1959.

87. Levinsky, N. G., and Lalone, R. C. The mechanism of sodium diuresis after saline infusion in the dog. *J. Clin. Invest.* 42:1261, 1963.

88. Leyssac, P. P. The regulation of proximal tubular reabsorption in the mammalian kidney. *Acta Physiol. Scand.* 70 (Suppl.): 291, 1966.

89. Lichardus, B., and Pearce, J. W. Evidence for a humoral natriuretic factor released by blood volume expansion. *Nature* (London) 209:407, 1966.

90. Lotspeich, W. D. Renal tubular reabsorption of inorganic sulfate in the normal dog. *Amer. J. Physiol.* 151:311, 1947.

91. Lotspeich, W. D., and Pitts, R. F. The role of amino acids in the renal tubular secretion of ammonia. *J. Biol. Chem.* 168:611, 1947.

92. Ludwig, E. *Beiträge zur Lehre vom Mechanismus der Harnsecretion.* Marburg: N. G. Elwert, 1843.

93. Maffly, R. H., Hays, R. M., Lamdin, E., and Leaf, A. The effect of neurohypophyseal hormones on the permeability of the toad bladder to urea. *J. Clin. Invest.* 39:630, 1960.

94. Maganzini, H. C., and Lilienfield, L.

Demonstration of countercurrent diffusion exchange in the vasa recta of the renal medulla. *Proc. Soc. Exp. Biol. Med.* 107:872, 1961.

95. Malnic, G., Klose, R. M., and Giebisch, G. Micropuncture study of distal tubular potassium and sodium transport in rat nephron. *Amer. J. Physiol.* 211:529, 1966.

96. Malnic, G., Klose, R. M., and Giebisch, G. Microperfusion study of distal tubular potassium and sodium transfer in rat kidney. *Amer. J. Physiol.* 211:548, 1966.

97. Malvin, R. L., Wilde, W. S., and Sullivan, L. P. Localization of nephron transport by stop-flow analysis. *Amer. J. Physiol.* 194: 135, 1958.

98. Marsh, D. J., and Solomon, S. Analysis of electrolyte movement in thin Henle's loops of hamster papilla. *Amer. J. Physiol.* 208: 1119, 1965.

99. Marshall, E. K., Jr., and Vickers, J. L. The mechanism of the elimination of phenolsulphonephthalein by the kidney — a proof of secretion by the convoluted tubules. *Bull. Johns Hopkins Hosp.* 34:1, 1923.

100. Martino, J. A., and Earley, L. E. Demonstration of a role of physical factors as determinants of the natriuretic response to volume expansion. *J. Clin. Invest.* 46:1963, 1967.

101. Miller, B. F., Leaf, A., Mamby, A. R., and Miller, Z. Validity of the endogenous creatinine clearance as a measure of glomerular filtration rate in the diseased human kidney. *J. Clin. Invest.* 31:309, 1952.

102. Möller, E., McIntosh, J. F., and Van Slyke, D. D. Studies of urea excretion: II. Relationship between urine volume and the rate of urea excretion by normal adults. *J. Clin. Invest.* 6:427, 1929.

103. Morgan, T., and Berliner, R. W. Permeability of the loop of Henle, vasa recta, and collecting duct to water, urea, and sodium. *Amer. J. Physiol.* 215:108, 1968.

104. Morgan, T., Sakai, F., and Berliner, R. W. In vitro permeability of medullary collecting ducts to water and urea. *Amer. J. Physiol.* 214:574, 1968.

105. Mudge, G. H., Foulks, J., and Gilman, A.

The renal excretion of potassium. *Proc. Soc. Exp. Biol. Med.* 76:545, 1948.

106. Mudge, G. H., Foulks, J., and Gilman, A. Effect of urea diuresis on renal excretion of electrolytes. *Amer. J. Physiol.* 158:218, 1949.

107. Mueller, C. B., Surtshin, A., Carlin, M. R., and White, H. L. Glomerular and tubular influences on sodium and water excretion. *Amer. J. Physiol.* 165:411, 1951.

108. Murdaugh, H. V., Jr., Schmidt-Nielsen, B., Doyle, E. M., and O'Dell, R. Renal tubular regulation of urea excretion in man. *J. Appl. Physiol.* 13:263, 1958.

109. Nash, T. P., and Benedict, S. R. The ammonia content of the blood and its bearing on the mechanism of acid neutralization in the animal organism. *J. Biol. Chem.* 48:463, 1921.

110. Nelp, W. B., Wagner, H. N., Jr., and Reba, R. C. Renal excretion of vitamin B_{12} and its use in measurement of glomerular filtration rate in man. *J. Lab. Clin. Med.* 63:480, 1964.

111. Orloff, J., Aronow, L., and Berliner, R. W. The transport of priscoline by the renal tubules. *J. Pharmacol. Exp. Ther.* 109:214, 1953.

112. Orloff, J., and Berliner, R. W. The mechanism of the excretion of ammonia in the dog. *J. Clin. Invest.* 35:223, 1956.

113. Orloff, J., Wagner, H. N., Jr., and Davidson, D. G. The effect of variations in solute excretion and vasopressin dosage on the excretion of water in the dog. *J. Clin. Invest.* 37:458, 1958.

114. Orloff, J., Walser, M., Kennedy, T. J., Jr., and Bartter, F. C. Hyponatremia. *Circulation* 19:284, 1959.

115. Pappenheimer, J. R., Renkin, E. M., and Borrero, L. M. Filtration, diffusion and molecular sieving through peripheral capillary membranes. A contribution to the pore theory of capillary permeability. *Amer. J. Physiol.* 167:13, 1951.

116. Peters, L. Renal tubular excretion of organic bases. *Pharmacol. Rev.* 12:1, 1960.

117. Pilkington, L. A., Binder, R., de Haas, J. C. M., and Pitts, R. F. Intrarenal distribution of blood flow. *Amer. J. Physiol.* 208:1107, 1965.

118. Pitts, R. F.   A renal reabsorptive mechanism in the dog common to glycin and creatine. *Amer. J. Physiol.* 140:156, 1943.

119. Pitts, R. F.   A comparison of the renal reabsorptive processes for several amino acids. *Amer. J. Physiol.* 140:535, 1944.

120. Pitts, R. F.   Renal excretion of acid. *Fed. Proc.* 7:418, 1948.

121. Pitts, R. F., and Alexander, R. S.   The renal reabsorptive mechanism for inorganic phosphate in normal and acidotic dogs. *Amer. J. Physiol.* 142:648, 1944.

122. Pitts, R. F., and Alexander, R. S.   The nature of the renal tubular mechanism for acidifying the urine. *Amer. J. Physiol.* 144:239, 1945.

123. Pitts, R. F., Ayer, J. L., and Schiess, W. A.   The renal regulation of acid-base balance in man: III. The reabsorption and excretion of bicarbonate. *J. Clin. Invest.* 28:35, 1949.

124. Pitts, R. F., and Lotspeich, W. D.   Bicarbonate and the renal regulation of acid-base balance. *Amer. J. Physiol.* 147:138, 1946.

125. Rapaport, S., Brodsky, W. A., West, C. D., and Mackler, B.   Urinary flow and excretion of solutes during osmotic diuresis in hydropenic man. *Amer. J. Physiol.* 156:433, 1949.

126. Rector, F. C., Jr., Bloomer, H. A., and Seldin, D. W.   Effect of potassium deficiency on the reabsorption of bicarbonate in the proximal tubule of the rat kidney. *J. Clin. Invest.* 43:1976, 1964.

127. Rector, F. C., Jr., and Clapp, J. R.   Evidence for active chloride reabsorption in the distal renal tubule of the rat. *J. Clin. Invest.* 41:101, 1962.

128. Rector, F. C., Jr., and Orloff, J.   The effect of the administration of sodium bicarbonate and ammonium chloride on the excretion and production of ammonia. The absence of alterations in the activity of renal ammonia-producing enzymes in the dog. *J. Clin. Invest.* 38:366, 1959.

129. Rector, F. C., Jr., Van Giesen, G., Kiil, F., and Seldin, D. W.   Influence of expansion of extracellular volume on tubular reabsorption of sodium independent of changes in glomerular filtration rate and aldosterone activity. *J. Clin. Invest.* 43:341, 1964.

130. Rehberg, P. B.   Studies on kidney function: I. The rate of filtration and reabsorption in the human kidney. *Biochem. J.* 20:30, 1926.

131. Relman, A. S., Etsten, B., and Schwartz, W. B.   The regulation of renal bicarbonate reabsorption by plasma carbon dioxide tension. *J. Clin. Invest.* 32:972, 1953.

132. Reubi, F.   Objections à la théorie de la séparation intrarénale des hématies et du plasma (Pappenheimer). *Helv. Med. Acta* 25:516, 1958.

133. Reynolds, T. B.   Observations on the pathogenesis of renal tubular acidosis. *Amer. J. Med.* 25:503, 1958.

134. Richards, A. N.   Processes of urine formation. Croonian Lecture. *Proc. Roy. Soc. [Biol.]* 126:398, 1939.

135. Richards, A. N., and Schmidt, C. F.   A description of the glomerular circulation in the frog's kidney and observations concerning the action of adrenalin and various other substances upon it. *Amer. J. Physiol.* 71:178, 1924.

136. Richards, A. N., Westfall, B. B., and Bott, P. A.   Inulin and creatinine clearances in dogs, with notes on some late effects of uranium poisoning. *J. Biol. Chem.* 116:749, 1936.

137. Sakai, F., Jamison, R. L., and Berliner, R. W.   A method for exposing the rat renal medulla in vivo: Micropuncture of the collecting duct. *Amer. J. Physiol.* 209:663, 1965.

138. Sartorius, O. W., Roemmelt, J. C., and Pitts, R. F.   The renal regulation of acid-base balance in man: IV. The nature of the renal compensations in ammonium chloride acidosis. *J. Clin. Invest.* 28:423, 1949.

139. Sawyer, W. H., and Schisgall, R. M.   Increased permeability of the frog bladder to water in response to dehydration and neurohypophyseal extracts. *Amer. J. Physiol.* 187:312, 1956.

140. Schiess, W. A., Ayer, J. L., Lotspeich, W. D., and Pitts, R. F.   The renal regulation of acid-base balance in man: II. Factors affecting the excretion of titratable acid by

the normal human subject. *J. Clin. Invest.* 27:57, 1948.

141. Schmidt-Nielsen, B., Schmidt-Nielsen, K., Houpt, T. R., and Jarnum, S. A. Urea excretion in the camel. *Amer. J. Physiol.* 188:477, 1957.

142. Scholander, P. F. The wonderful net. *Sci. Amer.* 196:96, 1957.

143. Scribner, B. H., Crawford, M. A., and Dempster, W. J. Urinary excretion by nonionic diffusion. *Amer. J. Physiol.* 196:1135, 1959.

144. Scriver, C. R., Schafer, I. A., and Efron, M. L. Evidence for a renal tubular amino acid transport system common to glycine, l-proline and hydroxy-l-proline. *J. Clin. Invest.* 40:1080, 1961.

145. Shannon, J. A. The renal excretion of creatinine in man. *J. Clin. Invest.* 14:403, 1935.

146. Shannon, J. A. The excretion of inulin and creatinine at low urine flows by the normal dog. *Amer. J. Physiol.* 114:362, 1936.

147. Shannon, J. A. Glomerular filtration and urea excretion in relation to urine flow in the dog. *Amer. J. Physiol.* 117:206, 1936.

148. Shannon, J. A. The renal reabsorption and excretion of urea under conditions of extreme diuresis. *Amer. J. Physiol.* 123:182, 1938.

149. Shannon, J. A. Renal tubular excretion. *Physiol. Rev.* 19:63, 1939.

150. Shannon, J. A., and Fisher, S. The renal tubular reabsorption of glucose in the normal dog. *Amer. J. Physiol.* 122:765, 1938.

151. Simpson, S. A., Tait, J. F., Wettstein, A., Neher, R., von Euw, J., and Reichstein, T. Isolierung eines neuen kristallisierten Hormons aus Nebennieren mit besonders höher Wirksamkeit auf den Mineralstoffwechsel. *Experientia* 9:333, 1953.

152. Smith, H. W. *The Physiology of the Kidney.* New York: Oxford University Press, 1937.

153. Smith, H. W. The physiology of the renal circulation. *Harvey Lect.* 35:166, 1941.

154. Smith, H. W. *Lectures on the Kidney.* Lawrence (Kan.): University Extension Division, University of Kansas, 1943.

155. Smith, H. W. *The Kidney. Structure and Function in Health and Disease.* New York: Oxford University Press, 1951. Pp. 544–545.

156. Idem. P. 161.

157. Smith, H. W. Renal excretion of sodium and water. *Fed. Proc.* 11:701, 1952.

158. Solomon, S. Transtubular potential differences of rat kidney. *J. Cell. Comp. Physiol.* 49:351, 1957.

159. Sullivan, W. J., and Dorman, P. J. The renal response to chronic respiratory acidosis. *J. Clin. Invest.* 34:268, 1955.

160. Taggart, J. V. Mechanisms of renal tubular transport. *Amer. J. Med.* 24:774, 1958.

161. Theobald, G. W., and Verney, E. B. The inhibition of water diuresis by afferent nerve stimuli after complete denervation of the kidney. *J. Physiol.* 83:341, 1935.

162. Thompson, D. D., Barrett, M. J., and Pitts, R. F. Significance of glomerular perfusion in relation to variability of filtration rate. *Amer. J. Physiol.* 167:546, 1951.

163. Thurau, K., and Kramer, K. Weitere Untersuchungen zur myogenen Natur der Autoregulation des Nierenkreislaufes. Aufhebung der Autoregulation durch muskulotrope Substanzen und druckpassives Verhalten des Glomerulusfiltrates. *Pflueger. Arch.* 269:77, 1959.

164. Ullrich, K. J., and Jarausch, K. H. Untersuchungen zum Problem der Harnkonzentrierung und Harnverdünnung. Über die Verteilung von Elektrolyten (Na, K, Ca, Mg, Cl, anorganischem Phosphat), Harnstoff, Aminosäuren und exogenem Kreatinin in Rinde und Mark der Hundeniere bei verschiedenen Diuresezuständen. *Pflueger. Arch.* 262:537, 1956.

165. Ussing, H. H. The distinction by means of tracers between active transport and diffusion. *Acta Physiol. Scand.* 19:43, 1949.

166. Vander, A. J. Potassium secretion and reabsorption in distal nephron. *Amer. J. Physiol.* 201:505, 1961.

167. Van Slyke, D. D., Phillips, R. A., Hamilton, P. B., Archibald, R. M., Futcher, P. H., and Hiller, A. Glutamine as source material of urinary ammonia. *J. Biol. Chem.* 150:481, 1943.

168. Verney, E. B.   Antidiuretic hormone and the factors which determine its release. *Proc. Roy. Soc.* [*Biol.*] 135:25, 1947.

169. Walker, A. M., Bott, P. A., Oliver, J., and MacDowell, M. C.   The collection and analysis of fluid from single nephrons of the mammalian kidney. *Amer. J. Physiol.* 134:580, 1941.

170. Wallenius, G.   *Renal Clearance of Dextran as a Measure of Glomerular Permeability.* Uppsala: Almqvist & Wiksells Boktryckeri AB, 1954.

171. Watson, J. F., Clapp, J. R., and Berliner, R. W.   Micropuncture study of potassium concentration in proximal tubule of dog, rat, and *Necturus. J. Clin. Invest.* 43:595, 1964.

172. Waugh, W. H., and Shanks, R. G.   Cause of genuine autoregulation of the renal circulation. *Circ. Res.* 8:871, 1960.

173. Weiner, I. M., Garlid, K. D., Romeo, J. A., and Mudge, G. H.   Effects of tubular secretion and reabsorption on titration curves of tubular transport. *Amer. J. Physiol.* 200: 393, 1961.

174. Weiner, I. M., Washington, J. A., II, and Mudge, G. H.   On the mechanism of action of probenecid on renal tubular secretion. *Bull. Johns Hopkins Hosp.* 106:333, 1960.

175. Wesson, L. G., Jr., Anslow, W. P., Jr., and Smith, H. W.   The excretion of strong electrolytes. *Bull. N. Y. Acad. Med.* 24:586, 1948.

176. Whittembury, G., Oken, D. E., Windhager, E. E., and Solomon, A. K.   Single proximal tubules of *Necturus* kidney: IV. Dependence of H_2O movement on osmotic gradients. *Amer. J. Physiol.* 197:1121, 1959.

177. Windhager, E. E., and Giebisch, G.   Micropuncture study of renal tubular transfer of sodium chloride in the rat. *Amer. J. Physiol.* 200:581, 1961.

178. Windhager, E. E., and Giebisch, G.   Comparison of short-circuit current and net water movement in single perfused proximal tubules of rat kidneys. *Nature* (London) 191:1205, 1961.

179. Windhager, E., Whittembury, G., Oken, D. E., Schatzmann, H. J., and Solomon, A. K.   Single proximal tubules of the *Necturus* kidney: III. Dependence of H_2O movement on NaCl concentration. *Amer. J. Physiol.* 197:313, 1959.

180. Wirz, H.   Der osmotische Druck in den corticalen Tubuli der Rattenniere. *Helv. Physiol. Pharmacol. Acta* 14:353, 1956.

181. Wirz, H., Hargitay, B., and Kuhn, W.   Lokalisation des Konzentrierungsprozesses in der Niere durch direkte Kryoskopie. *Helv. Physiol. Pharmacol. Acta* 9:196, 1951.

3

Clinical Examination of Renal Function

Arnold S. Relman and Norman G. Levinsky

I t is the purpose of this chapter to discuss a number of relatively simple laboratory studies which are useful in evaluating the patient suspected of renal disease. The tests to be described include the determination of the *urine protein* content, examination of the *urine sediment,* and the commonly applied *clinical measurements of renal function.* All are readily available to the clinician and nearly all can be performed with only the simplest laboratory facilities. Examination of the urine sediment and determination of the presence of proteinuria are of the utmost value in the recognition and differential diagnosis of renal disease, while the clinical function tests discussed are often of great help in evaluating the severity and progression of kidney disease. The technics considered are but a small fraction of the available laboratory aids. Renal radiography and angiography are discussed in Chapter 4, and renal biopsy in Chapter 5; split function tests, etc., are considered in other chapters as they seem pertinent.

Proteinuria

Although the occurrence of protein in urine had been discovered more than a century before, it was Richard Bright [37] who first noted the relationship between proteinuria and diseases of the kidney. Despite the continuous interest of innumerable investigators in this subject since that time, many key questions remain unsettled. Thus, while it is widely agreed that increased proteinuria is an important sign of renal disease, there is still considerable uncertainty about the anatomic and physiologic changes in the kidney responsible for proteinuria. This is in no small part due to the lack of adequate information about the normal handling of plasma proteins by the human kidney. Nevertheless, much important and practical information about the nature and extent of renal disease may be gained from measurements of protein, and the qualitative and quantitative analysis of urine for protein remains one of the most valuable tests of renal integrity available to the physician.

In this section only a brief review of normal and abnormal proteinuria will be presented. The subject has been reviewed in a recently published monograph, to which the reader interested in further details is referred [165].

DEFINITION

Protein excretion is abnormal when the total daily excretion exceeds 150 mg. — that is, when the average rate of excretion exceeds 10 or 11 micrograms per minute. Although there is usually a small amount of protein in the normal urine, the term *proteinuria* generally refers only to rates in excess of normal, and this convention is used throughout this chapter. For any given rate of protein excretion, the concentration of protein in a single voided sample of urine will vary inversely with urine flow. However, even at low flow rates, the concentration of protein in normal urine does not exceed 10 to 20 mg. per 100 ml. Thus, the occurrence of a higher concentration in any specimen of urine implies the existence of proteinuria. It should be clearly understood, however, that at relatively high rates of urine flow (which usually mean a dilute urine) proteinuria may occur with concentrations well below 20 mg. per 100 ml. — so low, in fact, as to be undetectable by routine methods. Therefore, a negative qualitative test for protein on a dilute sample of urine does not exclude proteinuria.

METHODS

Only brief mention will be made of the various technics for measuring urinary protein. Details are to be found in any of the standard references on clinical laboratory methods [9, 62, 153]. Reliable and accurate quantitative determinations of total protein in urine can be obtained by application of the classic nitrogen method of Kjeldahl or with the biuret reaction. In urine specimens containing relatively little protein it may be necessary to precipitate the protein or to concentrate it by dialysis or ultrafiltration prior to analysis with the above technics. Very low concentrations of albumin can be accurately measured by a radioimmunoassay method [126], but neither this nor the quantitative chemical procedure is suitable for routine office or clinic use.

For routine use, a number of more practical semiquantitative procedures are available. One type depends on the precipitation of protein by heat and acetic acid, nitric acid, or sulfosalicylic acid. In our opinion, the most satisfactory of these is the heat and acetic acid method. The precipitation methods are usually sensitive to protein concentrations of 5 to 10 mg. per 100 ml. or sometimes even lower, but they are not very precise or specific and give false-positive reactions to nonprotein substances in the urine such as radiopaque materials and tolbutamide [62, 89, 137, 160, 213]. The other type of procedure, perhaps the one most commonly used at present, is based upon a color-producing reaction between albumin and paper strips or tablets impregnated with the dye tetrabromphenol blue [89, 137]. This method is fairly specific for albumin. It does not, for example, register the presence of abnormal globulin chains in the urine. However, it is slightly less sensitive than the heat and acetic acid method and cannot be relied upon to detect albumin concentrations of less than 15 to 20 mg. per 100 ml. [89, 137, 213].

In routine clinical practice the total concentration of protein in a single voided specimen is reported in terms of milligrams per 100 ml. of urine or, more frequently, simply as zero to 4 plus. As already mentioned, it is possible for an abnormally increased rate of protein excretion to be concealed by a high urine flow which results in a protein concentration too low to be detected by the conventional methods. For this reason, it is always well to determine the specific gravity of the urine as a rough index of urine flow when evaluating tests for protein. More meaningful information about proteinuria may be obtained by carrying out determinations of the total 24-hour excretion of protein. The turbidity of an aliquot of a pooled 24-hour specimen after addition of sulfosalicylic acid can be quantitatively expressed in terms of protein concentration by comparison with known standards [132, 150]. Another simple and widely employed method requires only the precipitation of protein in an aliquot of the pooled 24-hour urine specimen with the use of Tsuchiya's phosphotungstic acid reagent or of Esbach's picric acid–citric acid reagent [150, 239]. The quantity of protein is then estimated from the volume of the precipitate formed after centrifugation or sedimentation in specially calibrated tubes. There is evidence suggesting that the turbidometric method is the more reliable [150].

PROTEINS OF NORMAL URINE

It has long been known that normal urine contains small quantities of protein [181]. Estimates of the total amount have varied with the methods employed, but most workers agree that the upper limit is between 100 and 150 mg. per day, with a mean value in the range of 40 to 80 mg. per day [32, 59, 167, 172, 216, 272]. Considering that the average normal daily volume of urine is approximately 1000 to 1500 ml., this implies that the average concentration of protein in random normal specimens would be of the order of 2 to 8 mg. per 100 ml. Precise chemical measurements of protein concentrations as low as this are difficult, but estimates of "apparent protein" concentration, based on surface activity, have yielded similar figures [107, 259]. By electrophoretic fractionation it has been shown [32, 167, 216, 273] that two-thirds to three-quarters of the normal urine protein has the mobility of plasma globulin; the remainder, the mobility of plasma albumin. The major part of the globulin migrates in alkaline buffers to the alpha globulin zone. A large number of discrete plasma proteins have been identified in normal urine. With the application of immunochemical technics it has been possible to demonstrate that at least 18 proteins in the urine are antigenically similar to their counterparts in the plasma [24, 25, 103, 195, 225, 274]. Ultracentrifugal measurements of molecular weight indicate probable identity of the urine and plasma albumin [274]. On the other hand, the urine globulin fractions appear to be much smaller molecules than those proteins comprising the major part of the plasma globulins [88, 225, 274], and may be metabolic precursors or derivatives of the latter. Of interest is the fact that some of these globulins, antigenically related to serum gamma globulin, resemble Bence Jones protein in their macroscopic behavior on heating [253], and probably represent light-chain proteins [76, 254].

Among the plasma fractions *not* detectable in normal urine or present only in traces are α_2-lipoproteins and β-lipoproteins and the β_2-macroglobulin [24, 103, 195, 225]. These molecules may be unable to pass through the glomerular filter because of their relatively large effective diameters. On the other hand, there are apparently several fractions in urine either not found in plasma or present in undetectably small concentrations. Most prominent among these is the high-molecular-weight mucoprotein described by Tamm and Horsfall [257] which migrates as an alpha globulin at pH 8.6 and is normally excreted at a rate of approximately 25 mg. per day per 1.73 square meters of body-surface area [168]. This substance, sometimes called "uromucoid," is apparently formed in the cells of the loop of Henle and the distal convolutions and collecting ducts [204], and it is the major protein constituent of urinary casts [169]. In addition to the Tamm-Horsfall mucoprotein, there are about a dozen discrete antigenic components, probably of protein nature, which appear to arise from the lower urinary tract, including the semen and the prostatic and urethral secretions [104, 195].

MECHANISM OF PROTEINURIA

As described in Chapter 2, micropuncture data show that the glomerulus is normally an effective barrier to the passage of most plasma protein molecules from plasma into the glomerular filtrate [68, 270]. The normal glomerulus ordinarily restrains the passage of molecules the size of serum albumin and larger, but allows excretion of smaller-sized proteins [19] or dextrans [271]. This could be explained by assuming the presence of pores of suitable size in the filtering membrane. However, electron microscopy fails to reveal any such pores [108]; and observations on the penetration of ferritin molecules through the glomerular basement membrane suggest a more random type of movement than would be expected through fixed pores [84]. This question remains to be settled.

The extent to which small quantities of plasma proteins normally may penetrate the glomerular filter remains conjectural. Early analyses of rat and guinea pig glomerular and proximal tubular fluid failed to reveal protein in 25 of 41 specimens collected by micropuncture [270], but the best method of microanalysis then available was incapable of detecting protein in a concentration less than 30 mg. per 100 ml. Other studies in the dog, using an immunochemical technic capable of detecting concentrations of 2 mg. per 100 ml. or higher, have demonstrated no protein in 18 of 38 samples from the proximal tubule, but albumin concentrations of 2 to 8 mg. per 100 ml. in most of the others [68]. The positive samples in both of these studies may have been due to changes in glomerular permeability caused by the stress of the experimental procedures, but it is also possible that normal glomerular filtrate always contains small amounts of protein, sometimes too low in concentration to be detected by the technics available. If the concentration were normally only 1 mg. per 100 ml. of filtrate in man, the total quantity of protein filtered per day would still be several times greater than the daily normal excretion of plasma protein, thus implying reabsorption of protein by normal tubules. However, until more data are available, this question must be regarded as unsettled.

Direct evidence of tubular reabsorption of protein in man is lacking. Physiologic studies of the effects of albumin infusions in proteinuric patients [105, 109, 163] provide suggestive but not conclusive support, as does the development of "hyaline droplets" in the proximal tubular cells of such patients [188]. In other species, however, the evidence for tubular reabsorption of protein is stronger. In the rat, there is a large body of physiologic, morphologic, and histochemical data to suggest that plasma proteins are normally filtered through the glomerulus and subsequently removed by active processes in tubular cells [189, 190, 210, 235]. Other studies suggest that protein penetrating the normal glomerular basement membrane of the rat may also be removed from the filtrate by the epithelial cells of the glomerular tuft itself [82]. In the proteinuric dog, stop-flow experiments appear to demonstrate tubular reabsorption of protein [13]. In addition, in both normal and proteinuric dogs the stop-flow procedure seems to provoke addition of protein to the urine from some distal tubular site [13].

To explain the occurrence of proteinuria in renal disease, therefore, one might reasonably propose at least three discrete, though not mutually exclusive, mechanisms: (1) increased glomerular filtration of proteins; (2) decreased removal of filtered protein; and (3) addition of protein to the urine from renal tubular cells or possibly from renal lymphatics. This problem remains unsettled at present, but it is fair to say that the weight of available evidence strongly favors the conclusion that gross proteinuria in man always is the result, at least in part, of increased glomerular filtration of protein. Some of the most salient facts implicating increased filtration of protein are the following:

1. In almost all situations associated with increased proteinuria there is anatomic evidence, although sometimes only ultramicroscopic [83, 247], of glomerular involvement; by contrast, in many disorders characterized by physiologic or anatomic evidence of severe tubular damage, proteinuria may be minimal or absent.

2. The relative clearance rates of some of the serum proteins in the nephrotic syndrome appear to be roughly inversely proportional to the effective molecular diameter of each protein [109, 248]. Furthermore, the electrophoretic distribution and the average molecular weights of the proteins separated from normal and nephrotic sera by ultrafiltration through a semipermeable nitrocellulose membrane closely resemble those of nephrotic urine [224]. These observations strongly suggest that proteinuria in the nephrotic syndrome results from the molecular "sieving" action of an abnormally permeable glomerular filter. A similar conclusion would also seem to follow from the fact that the dextran molecules excreted when proteinuric patients are infused with dextran mixtures of varying molecular weight are considerably larger than those excreted by normal subjects given similar infusions [271].

3. Following the infusion of human albumin into nephrotic patients, proteinuria may far exceed the estimated maximal rate of filtration of protein in normal subjects. The minimum concentration of albumin in the glomerular filtrate of such patients, calculated from the rate of excretion of albumin and the glomerular filtration rate, may be increased several times over the estimated upper limit for the normal filtrate [55].

With the exception of a few noteworthy situations to be discussed later, the increased urine protein appears to consist largely of an albumin fraction chemically and immunologically indistinguishable from that found in normal plasma [97, 224]. Furthermore, infusion of plasma from proteinuric patients into normal subjects does not produce proteinuria [115]. From these considerations it follows that if there is increased glomerular filtration of protein, it is mainly caused by increased permeability of the normal glomerular barrier, rather than by the presence in the plasma of abnormal proteins which might be more filtrable than normal proteins.

These considerations do not, however, rule out coexistent defects in tubular reabsorption of filtered protein or even the addition of plasma protein to the tubular fluid through lymphatics or damaged cells.

FRACTIONATION OF URINE PROTEINS
IN RENAL DISEASES

With the use of relatively crude chemical technics for fractionation, it was established many years ago that most of the protein excreted in the urine in the common disorders causing marked proteinuria had the characteristics of serum albumin [26]. However, it was not until immunologic and electrophoretic methods were applied that detailed and reliable information on the fractionation of urine proteins became available. It is now generally agreed that an albumin fraction, apparently identical with that in serum, constitutes some 60 to 90 per cent of the total urinary protein in the majority of the diseases associated with significant proteinuria [38, 98, 156, 224, 242, 281]. Much smaller quantities of each of the four major plasma globulin electrophoretic fractions are excreted. There have also been identified in urine small amounts of a lipoprotein which appears to be electrophoretically and immunologically similar to the β-lipoprotein in plasma. However, there is evidence to suggest that those plasma globulins which are excreted may represent fractions of relatively low molecular weight [224]. This is generally the case in the nephrotic syndrome, acute and chronic glomerulonephritis, intercapillary glomerulosclerosis, malignant nephrosclerosis, secondary amyloid disease of the kidney, lupus erythematosus and scleroderma of the kidney, severe congestive heart failure, and most of the so-called "functional" and "benign" proteinurias [59, 184, 243].

In contrast to the relatively high proportion of albumin to globulin in the disorders just noted, there are a few diseases in which the excretion of globulins usually exceeds that of albumin. Most patients with *multiple myeloma* have proteinuria, and, unless amyloid disease of the kidney is superimposed, globulins are predominant and sometimes may represent the only proteins to be found in the urine [112, 191, 192, 261, 286]. Heavy albuminuria in a patient with multiple myeloma usually means that glomerular permeability is increased due to amyloid infiltration, but even in such cases, large amounts of globulin are also present.

In most patients with myeloma, the urine globulin consists, at least in part, of so-called Bence Jones proteins, which are abnormal light-chain proteins of low molecular weight (approximately 22,500 or 45,000). These proteins are structurally and antigenically identical with the light chains of the IgG or IgA myeloma proteins that are found in the plasma [76, 112, 254]. In addition, some patients have intact IgG or IgA myeloma protein in their urine [112].

As first described by Henry Bence Jones over 100 years ago [20], the low-molecular-weight light-chain myeloma protein in urine has a thermal characteristic quite different from that of ordinary urine proteins: it coagulates on heating from 45° to 55°C. and redissolves partially or wholly on boiling. This simple heating test is often useful in the initial clinical diagnosis of plasma cell myeloma, but it is not wholly reliable. The test is positive in only 50 to 60 per cent of patients. This is partly because, as noted above, some patients excrete little or no abnormal protein in their urine. However, even when electrophoresis of the urine discloses the presence of myeloma proteins, a positive "Bence Jones test" may not be elicited; this is probably explained by the effects of varying urine pH on the thermal behavior of the different types of myeloma protein [207].

The other group of renal diseases in which globulinuria apparently may equal or exceed albuminuria includes some patients with pyelonephritis [31, 262] as well as patients with a variety of inherited or acquired disorders of tubular transport [45, 61, 111]. In the Fanconi syndrome, for example, the urine may contain increased quantities of low-molecular-weight proteins with electrophoretic and immunologic properties similar to those of plasma globulins. These proteins are cleared at rates inversely proportional to their molecular size, and may be found even in the absence of significant albuminuria, thereby suggesting that impaired tubular reabsorption may be at fault [111].

The *relative clearance rates* of various plasma proteins have been of considerable interest, ever since it was first suggested that this information might give some idea of the selective permeability of the glomerular filter [109]. In general, it has been found that the clearance of plasma proteins is inversely proportional to their effective molecular diameter [109, 248]. Loss of "selectivity" of the glomerulus seems to reflect the severity of the lesion. Thus, in nephrotic patients with significant glomerular lesions the ratio of the clearance of large protein molecules (e.g., IgG or alpha-2 macroglobulin) to that of smaller molecules (e.g., transferrin or albumin) is relatively higher than in proteinuric patients with minimal glomerular lesions [46, 123]. Furthermore, it has been claimed that a high degree of "selectivity" (i.e., a relatively lower permeability to large molecules) correlates well with a good prognosis and response to therapy [46, 123], but it seems likely that this correlation simply reflects the fact that the glomerulus becomes more permeable to high-molecular-weight plasma proteins with any type of advanced renal damage [159, 161].

QUANTITATIVE ASPECTS OF PROTEINURIA

Some renal diseases characteristically have little or no effect on protein excretion, and others increase proteinuria only moderately. In some varieties of disease, however, the urine has a grossly increased protein content, with the daily excretion rising to 20 to 30 gm. or more. It is usually greater during the day than at night, and is often increased during periods of activity and upright posture or during febrile illnesses [26]. Even in healthy subjects protein excretion is often much increased in the upright position. In the nephrotic syndrome, proteinuria may be increased by a high protein intake [26, 197]. Wide variations in protein excretion may occur with treatment or in association with spontaneous changes in the stage and severity of the underlying renal lesion. Such variations are in most instances presumably caused by changes in glomerular permeability or tubular transport of protein, but there is evidence that the level of plasma albumin and the rate of glomerular filtration also affect protein excretion [26]. Thus, a reduction in the excretion of protein may mean improvement in the underlying renal lesion, but alternatively may reflect progressing hypoalbuminemia or increasing destruction of glomerular units. Sometimes, when proteinuria is relatively minimal, it may repeatedly disappear and then reappear either spontaneously or as the result of transient disorders not necessarily related to the underlying renal disease. Intermittent proteinuria is often seen as a stage of either the development or the healing of renal disease [63]. In general, however, once a constant proteinuria has become established as the result of renal disease,

it will not completely disappear unless the underlying disorder heals.

The following generalizations may be of some diagnostic help in interpreting the significance of proteinuria:

1. *Continuous proteinuria* is more apt to be caused by renal disease than by physiologic or functional conditions. Even in the absence of any obvious clinical or laboratory evidence of renal damage, persistent proteinuria should be considered presumptive evidence of renal disease.

2. *Heavy proteinuria* (more than 4 gm. daily) is usually caused by renal diseases that grossly increase glomerular permeability. These include acute and chronic glomerulonephritis, so-called pure or lipoid nephrosis, intercapillary glomerulosclerosis, amyloid disease, malignant nephrosclerosis, systemic lupus erythematosus, and severe venous congestion of the kidney such as may be caused by renal vein thrombosis, severe congestive heart failure, or constrictive pericarditis.

3. *Minimal or moderate continuous proteinuria* (0.5 to 4.0 gm. per day) may also be a manifestation of any of the disorders listed above. In addition, this is the characteristic finding in latent or inactive chronic glomerulonephritis and in many patients with nephrosclerosis or pyelonephritis with hypertension.

4. *Intermittent or minimal proteinuria* (less than 0.5 gm. per day) is found frequently in chronic pyelonephritis, renal tubular disorders, polycystic disease of the kidneys, and benign nephrosclerosis. This pattern is often caused by latent glomerulonephritis or healing acute glomerulonephritis. The so-called benign varieties of proteinuria are usually intermittent.

5. Renal diseases often occurring in the *absence of proteinuria* include: acute and chronic pyelonephritis, obstructive nephropathy, nephrolithiasis, the nephropathies of hypercalcemia and potassium depletion, tumors of the kidney, and congenital malformations.

POSTURAL AND "FUNCTIONAL"
PROTEINURIA

Just as the absence of proteinuria does not rule out renal disease, so its presence does not inevitably imply an organic renal lesion. It is common, in fact, for *intermittent* and relatively mild proteinuria to be found in occasional urine specimens of apparently healthy individuals under certain conditions (described briefly below).

Postural Proteinuria. In approximately 3 to 5 per cent of healthy adolescents and young adults, mild proteinuria occurs during the day and disappears during the nocturnal period of recumbency [67, 154]. It is very likely that posture is the most important factor in producing this pattern of proteinuria, because in such patients proteinuria can be induced simply by the assumption of the erect position. However, there is evidence that the rate of protein excretion is increased, in comparison with controls, even in the recumbent position, suggesting that the effect of posture may be superimposed upon some underlying abnormality [218]. An exaggerated lordotic position will induce proteinuria in a substantial percentage of healthy young subjects; Bull [43] demonstrated this effect in 77 per cent of a group of healthy boys aged 14 to 16 and in 36 per cent of a group of healthy medical students aged 20 to 30. Postural proteinuria is maximal in erect lordosis but can be induced in some subjects in recumbent lordosis as well. Following the assumption of a recumbent or erect kyphotic position, proteinuria usually disappears, but only after an interval sufficient to allow washout of urinary "dead space" [243].

Individual urine specimens may have protein concentrations as high as 1000 mg. per 100 ml., but in the majority of instances the concentration is much less. Total daily excretion of protein is usually less than 1 gm. Electrophoretic fractionation reveals a preponderance of albumin and a relative proportion of albumin to the major globulin fractions which approximates that of normal serum [154, 243]. There may also be an increase in the output of all formed elements in the urine, including red and white blood cells, epithelial cells, and hyaline and granular casts [43, 228]. As already noted, the erect posture may also increase the rate of protein excretion in patients with established renal disease and preexisting proteinuria. In such patients the acute effect of the passive erect position is apparently variable, although protein concentration always increases [129, 143]. Orthostasis may decrease protein excretion in patients with relatively severe renal disease and low glomerular filtration rates [143], but it usually increases proteinuria in those with milder disease [129].

The explanation of the effect of posture on protein excretion is still somewhat uncertain. The role of renal venous congestion has been emphasized by some studies [43, 275], but it seems likely that reductions in plasma flow and filtration rate are also important. Lordotic or passively erect posture usually produces renal vasoconstriction as well as venous congestion, and a number of workers have suggested that the vasoconstriction may be the critical factor [106, 129]. A similar mechanism has been proposed for a variety of other physiologic stimuli which are known to cause proteinuria (see *"Functional" Proteinuria*). Supporting this hypothesis is the interesting observation that proteinuria in the passively erect position does not occur if peripheral pooling of venous blood is prevented by the application of external pressure [106]. However, the relative significance of renal ischemia, venous congestion, and other possible factors remains to be settled. Although the electrophoretic pattern of the urine proteins in orthostasis resembles that of lymph proteins and of the urine proteins in chyluria [154], there is no direct evidence to support the hypothesis [154] that the erect posture results in the addition of protein to the urine from renal lymphatics. To the contrary, studies with labeled proteins suggest instead that there is a direct transfer of plasma protein to urine [243].

"Functional" Proteinuria. By this term is meant the proteinuria which is caused by *exercise* [8, 49, 59, 122, 184, 278], *fever* [276], *exposure to heat or cold* [54, 229], and by *emotional stress* associated with increased sympathetic nervous activity [250]. The proteinuria commonly occurring in *congestive heart failure* [209] probably also belongs in this group. It is well established that such conditions may induce proteinuria in previously nonproteinuric subjects without renal disease, or increase protein excretion in those with pre-existing proteinuria. The urinary protein excreted after exercise has variously been reported to consist mainly of albumin [184] or globulin [59], but other evidence indicates the predominance of albumin, as well as the presence of many of the medium- and low-molecular-weight serum globulins. Little is known in detail about the mechanisms responsible for these "functional" proteinurias, but they are all characterized by relatively marked renal vasoconstriction, and it is widely believed that a change in the circulation may be the important underlying factor here, as in postural proteinuria. Of interest in this connection is the fact that infusions of epinephrine and norepinephrine, which regularly produce renal vasoconstriction, increase proteinuria in subjects with renal disease [131] and may induce proteinuria in normal subjects [131, 260].

There has been increased interest in the effect of *athletic exertion* on the excretion of protein and formed elements in the urine. Numerous reports [8, 49, 59, 93, 136, 184, 229, 260, 278] have indicated that proteinuria, as well as cylindruria and hematuria, is frequently induced by such activities in healthy young men, and usually disappears soon thereafter. In one study, for example, it was found that 100 per cent of long-distance runners and 70 to 80 per cent of all other college athletes had proteinuria immediately after competitive play; 50 to 80 per cent also showed microscopic hematuria and cylindruria [8]. Proteinuria appears to be related to the intensity and duration of the physical exertion [260, 278] and tends to decrease with training [260]. It is not restricted to sports in which body contact, and hence direct trauma to the kidney, might be important [136]. It may continue during the 24-hour period following exercise [59], but how much longer postexercise proteinuria will continue in the resting subject is not known. Severe muscular exertion, particularly when involving untrained muscle groups, may occasionally result in hemoglobinuria [12, 96, 120, 249] (a condition sometimes referred to as "March hemoglobinuria") and even myoglobinuria [120].

Clinical Significance of Postural and "Functional" Proteinuria. It is obvious that if proteinuria occurs in the majority of apparently healthy young people with the assumption of an exaggerated lordotic position [43] and after violent exercise [8], this phenomenon cannot be considered indicative of renal disease. Nevertheless, proteinuria should not be dismissed simply because it is first discovered in subjects shortly after exercise; failure of the protein excretion to disappear within a few days must be considered suspicious of renal disease. What is not so clear, however, is the significance of "postural" proteinuria, which, as already described, occurs in apparently healthy subjects under the much less extreme stimulus of simply being up and about while carrying on normal, quiet activities. This latter type of proteinuria is a frequent source of concern to patients and constitutes a perplexing dilemma for the physician. There can be no doubt that intermittent proteinuria of this type may occur in certain vascular or interstitial diseases of the kidney and may also be seen in the healing or latent stages of glomerulonephritis [63, 128, 129]. Although sometimes the evidence of the underlying disease is clear, many such cases may not be recognized at first because casual examination of the urine sediment and the usual clinical tests of renal function may be normal.

Renal biopsies in asymptomatic and otherwise normal young patients with orthostatic or intermittent proteinuria have revealed nonspecific focal or diffuse glomerular, interstitial, or vascular lesions in more than half the cases [180, 183, 219, 220]. Despite this fact, there is an old and widely held opinion that postural or intermittent proteinuria, in the absence of other evidences of systemic or renal disease, has a generally benign prognosis [4, 67, 85, 280]. Life insurance actuarial data [124] tend to support this view, for they indicate that people with minimal degrees of intermittent proteinuria and normal blood pressure do not have a significantly increased mortality rate. A retrospective study of the long-term mortality of young men found to have asymptomatic proteinuria in college comes to similar conclusions [148]. On the other hand, prospective follow-up studies of young patients with orthostatic proteinuria have reported the development of persistent proteinuria or definite abnormalities in the urine sediment within 5 to 8 years in a significant number [130, 145], suggesting the possibility that some of these patients may be going on to progressive renal disease. It is clear, however, that most patients with intermittent proteinuria as an isolated finding do *not* have an active renal disease. Even those with renal lesions on biopsy seem to have a good short-term prognosis. Large numbers of carefully studied patients will have to be followed over long periods of time before the natural history of postural and intermittent proteinuria can be finally elucidated.

ASYMPTOMATIC PERSISTENT PROTEINURIA

The clinical significance of persistent proteinuria is probably different from that of the postural or intermittent variety. Even in the absence of any of the usual clinical or laboratory evidences of renal functional impairment, the finding of increased protein in *all* urine specimens obtained over a period of time under various conditions usually means the existence of some type of renal disease, however minimal this may be. Biopsy studies of patients with persistent proteinuria as an apparently isolated finding have revealed significant lesions in the majority, most commonly glomerulonephritis or interstitial nephritis [199, 200, 203].

Many patients with asymptomatic persistent proteinuria may remain in good health for years without evidence of change [11]. However, there is no doubt that there is a significantly increased incidence of progressive renal disease among this group and their long-term mortality is increased [148]. The limited actuarial experience of life insurance companies in this regard suggests that the more severe the proteinuria the more likely the renal disease will progress. Thus, a constant "trace" of protein (10 to 50 mg. per 100 ml.) has so far been found to have little or no effect on overall mortality, whereas persistent proteinuria of "moderate" degree (51 to 100 mg. per 100 ml.) increases the mortality rate even in patients with normal blood pressure [124]. It is also claimed that the coexistence of microscopic hematuria is another factor that worsens the prognosis of persistent proteinuria [11].

Urine Sediment

The microscopic examination of the formed elements in the urinary sediment is an indispensable part of any clinical evaluation of the kidney. Although it provides no information about renal function, it does constitute the most valuable single test of the anatomic integrity of the kidneys that is readily available to the clinician. Furthermore, it not only provides reliable evidence of the existence of renal disease but also frequently affords accurate clues to the nature and extent of the lesion.

In this section a brief description will be

given of those formed elements in the sediment that may have significance in the diagnosis of renal disease. Some of the practical aspects of the examination of urine sediment will also be considered. A more detailed consideration of this subject is to be found in Lippman's monograph [153].

FORMED ELEMENTS OF THE SEDIMENT
AND THEIR ORIGINS

Cells. The cells in the urine sediment arise either by desquamation from the lining of the urinary tract or by entrance of cellular elements of the blood into the urinary tract. In females additional desquamated epithelial elements from the mucosal surfaces of the vulva and vagina are usually present unless the specimen has been obtained by catheterization of the bladder. The epithelial cells to be found in urine include those forming the tubular walls of the nephron as well as cells from the transitional and squamous epithelium of the renal pelvis, ureters, bladder, and urethra [221]. In normal urine these elements are presumably sloughed off in small numbers as the result of normal wear and tear, but degenerative, inflammatory, or neoplastic changes may result in increased shedding of cells. Inclusion-bearing epithelial cells may occur in certain viral infections [28] but are not specific for such conditions, because they are also common in normal urine and in urine from patients with a variety of systemic disorders as well as local inflammatory and neoplastic conditions of the urinary tract [171].

In renal disease of all types, tubular epithelium degenerates and cells may slough off into the urine in increased numbers. This process is particularly striking in severe acute glomerulonephritis or pyelonephritis, malignant nephrosclerosis, the diuretic phase of acute tubular necrosis, and in most disorders characterized by profuse proteinuria. When heavy proteinuria is present, tubular epithelial cells are especially prone to undergo fatty degeneration; the coarse fatty droplets in their cytoplasms are anisotropic and have a typical "Maltese cross" appearance under polarized light [57, 215, 285]. Anisotropic particles are also found free in the urine sediment. There is evidence that the free anisotropic lipid particles, as well as the material that appears in cells and urinary casts, consist mainly of cholesterol esters [57, 285]. However, it is not clear whether this material is derived from the tubular ingestion (athrocytosis) and subsequent cellular metabolism of filtered lipoproteins [285], or whether the urinary lipid simply represents the desquamation of material from cells that are undergoing spontaneous fatty degeneration [57]. The direct excretion of unreabsorbed plasma lipoproteins, which apparently may leak through diseased glomeruli in small amounts [27, 233], is probably responsible for the presence of dissolved lipids in the urine of nephrotic patients [41, 285], but it is of interest that the excretion of cholesterol is the same in nephrotic as in other types of patients, and bears no direct relation to the degree of proteinuria [57]. Tubular epithelial cells swollen with fat are called oval fat bodies and, when they are found in large numbers, are characteristic of the nephrotic syndrome. However, occasional oval fat bodies may be seen in a great variety of clinical conditions [208]; in general, the number of oval fat bodies in the sediment is proportional to the degree of proteinuria [186].

Leukocytes and erythrocytes are found in normal urine in small numbers. It is not at all clear how and where they enter the normal urine, nor is it even certain that they come from the kidney. That these blood cells do not come simply from minute hemorrhages into the urine is suggested by the fact that the ratio of erythrocytes to white blood cells in the urine is much lower than it is in blood. In renal disease, increased numbers of red blood cells and leukocytes may be added to the urine from the kidney. Increased numbers of red and white cells may also be derived from any part of the urinary passages below the kidney. Only when these elements are seen in casts can it be stated with confidence that they derive from the kidney itself.

Some years ago there was a revival of interest in the possible diagnostic significance of the appearance and staining properties of the polymorphonuclear leukocytes in the urine. It has been suggested that leukocytes arising from infections in the kidney characteristically tend to be pale and swollen and to show Brownian movement in their cytoplasm [252]. With a gentian violet and safranin stain these cells appear pale blue in contrast to the red or deep violet stain of other leukocytes [252]. However, it seems probable that the appearance of these so-called glitter cells or granular motility cells is caused by the hypotonicity of the urine and possibly by other changes in urine composition [23]. Thus, although "glitter cells" are very commonly found in dilute urine specimens from patients with pyelonephritis [23, 214, 252], they are not specific for this disease and may also be observed in hypotonic urines in cases of lower urinary tract infection [23, 214].

Casts. Casts [234] are more or less cylindrical masses of agglutinated material which are formed usually in the distal parts of the nephron and are then later washed out into the urine. The width of a cast is determined by the dimensions of the conduit in which it is formed, the broadest casts presumably coming from the collecting tubules and the ducts of Bellini. The presence of many broad casts in the sediment suggests widespread stasis of urine and cessation of excretion in large segments of the kidney. It is probably for this reason that, as pointed out by Addis [2], these broad casts are characteristically found in advanced renal disease. They are sometimes referred to as *renal failure casts.*

Two processes acting alone or in concert seem to be responsible for the formation of casts: (1) agglutination of masses of cells in the tubular lumina; and (2) intratubular precipitation or gelling of protein present in tubular fluid. This latter process is favored by increased acidity and by relatively low flow and increased urine concentration in the distal nephron. Normally, there are not enough epithelial cells, red blood cells or leukocytes in the tubular lumina to form cellular casts, and in the distal parts of the nephron where the urine is normally concentrated and acidified there is usually not enough protein to provide more than an occasional cast. *Cylindruria* (excretion of increased numbers of casts) therefore usually means either increased proteinuria or renal excretion of cells, or both. For any given degree of proteinuria the formation and excretion of casts, particularly of the hyaline varieties (see below), will presumably be affected by the rate of flow in the distal portions of the nephron and by the pH of the urine in those areas.

Current evidence indicates that the protein matrix material in hyaline and granular casts is largely, if not entirely, composed of the Tamm-Horsfall mucoprotein [169]. This material is apparently secreted by the cells lining the distal parts of the nephron [204], and it appears in increased quantities in the urine of patients with various types of proteinuria [168]. It has an isoelectric point at pH 4.8 and is readily precipitated by a low urine pH and by increased electrolyte concentrations [170], thus apparently explaining the effects of the acidity and concentration of the urine on the formation of urinary casts. Similarly, the ready solubility of Tamm-Horsfall mucoprotein at high pH explains why casts disappear so rapidly in alkaline urines.

Many classifications of casts have been proposed, some of which have been unnecessarily elaborate. In the absence of detailed information about the genesis and physicochemical structure of the various types of casts, it would seem sufficient for most purposes to use a simple descriptive classification such as the following:

Cellular casts and their derivatives
    Leukocyte casts
    Red blood cell casts
    Epithelial cell casts
    Mixed cellular casts
    Degenerating cellular casts
Granular casts
Waxy casts
Fatty casts
Hyaline casts and their derivatives
    Pure hyaline casts
    Hyaline casts with cellular inclusions
    Hyaline casts with granular or fatty debris
    Pigmented hyaline casts

Leukocyte casts (Fig. 3-1) are usually easily recognized as cylindrical plugs of tightly packed leukocytes [125, 211]. Sometimes they are well preserved, their nuclei and cell boundaries clearly discernible. Often, however, the cells are degenerating, and no details are visible. It is not always possible to distinguish such casts from degenerating epithelial casts or from casts containing mixtures of epithelial

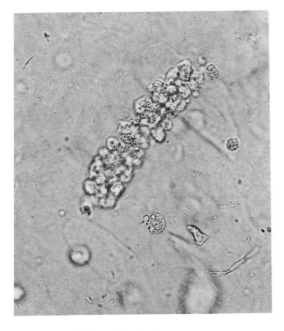

Figure 3-1. Leukocyte cast.

cells and white cells, or even red cells. Leukocyte casts also need to be distinguished from clumps of white cells, which may at times be packed by centrifugal force into cylindrical forms. Casts usually have harder, sharper outlines than such clumps, and the cells composing them tend to be more tightly packed, with less distinct margins.

Red blood cell casts usually have the characteristic rusty or reddish-brown hue of hemoglobin, which distinguishes them from all other cellular casts. Sometimes, however, much of this color may be washed out of the cells, which may appear simply as "ghosts." The distinctive, uniformly spherical outlines of the erythrocytes may be discernible in the casts, but often the cells are deteriorated beyond recognition and may be fused into a granular mass of cellular debris. Such casts, if they retain their color, are referred to as *blood casts.* Erythrocytes are often mixed with epithelial cells or white cells in the form of *mixed cellular casts.*

Epithelial cell casts are clearly identifiable as such only when the cell outlines are preserved well enough to make possible their distinction from leukocytes. Epithelial cells in casts in general are larger than leukocytes and show more fatty and hyaline degeneration of their cytoplasm.

Degenerating cellular casts (Fig. 3-2). The cellular elements in casts are usually degenerated to some extent even in freshly voided urine. Epithelial cells may undergo fatty or hyaline changes before they slough off into casts, but it is generally believed that degenerative changes more often occur after cells have been formed into casts. Badly degenerated leukocyte and epithelial casts may be indistinguishable as to cell type, while the characteristic tint of hemoglobin may be the only clue that a degenerated cast contains red blood cells. Prior to such deterioration it is often possible to recognize that casts contain at least a few epithelial cells because they tend

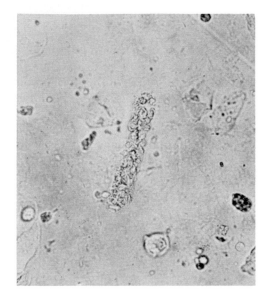

Figure 3-2. Degenerating cellular cast, probably composed of leukocytes and renal epithelial cells.

to disintegrate into larger, more refractile and more irregular particles than do leukocytes.

Granular casts are composed of homogeneous, presumably proteinaceous, material which may have a finely stippled or a more coarsely granular texture (Fig. 3-3). They are colorless, but often have a sharp outline and may at times be dense enough to look rather black against a light background. Following Addis [4], most contemporary textbooks consider that granular casts represent a further stage of degeneration in the life history of the cellular cast. Evidence for this is indirect, mainly the fact that types of casts intermediate between cellular and granular may be identified. However, this explanation does not easily account for the showers of apparently freshly formed granular casts which can be abruptly produced in normal subjects by orthostasis or exercise.

Waxy casts (Fig. 3-4) are usually relatively broad. They consist of a colorless, waxy-looking homogeneous material which seems structureless under ordinary light microscopy and has a hard, refractile outline. Addis and his school believe that these casts represent the ultimate stage in the degeneration of cellular casts [4], and in support of this hypothesis point to the occurrence of what seem to be in-

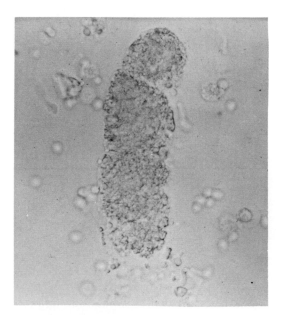

Figure 3-3. Broad, coarsely granular cast.

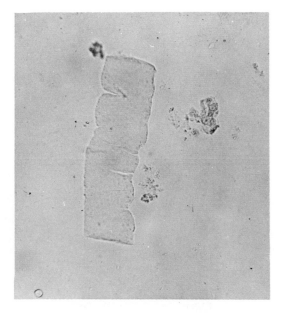

Figure 3-4. Broad waxy cast.

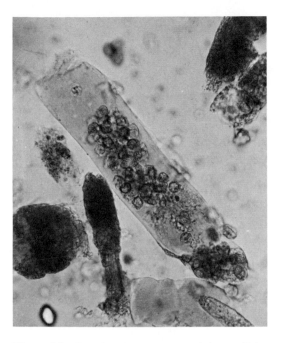

Figure 3-5. Broad waxy cast containing cellular and granular material, possibly an example of an intermediate form. Several coarsely granular casts are also shown at the top right and bottom left.

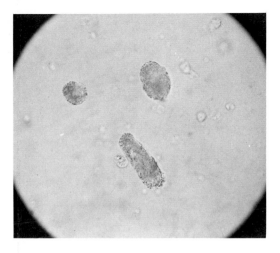

Figure 3-6. Two oval fat bodies (*top*) and a narrow fatty cast (*bottom*).

termediate types of casts, partly granular or cellular and partly waxy (Fig. 3-5).

Fatty casts are coarsely granular casts, the granules of which are apparently composed chiefly of lipoidal material. These casts are usually narrow and rather short. When viewed under white light with the low power objective, they often appear black. Closer examination under higher power reveals that they contain coarse, refractile granules or droplets. These casts characteristically take any stain for fat such as Sudan III, and exhibit anisotropism under polarized light. They are usually seen together with oval fat bodies (Fig. 3-6).

Hyaline casts appear to represent the results of the precipitation of pure protein, and they are characteristically clear, structureless, and colorless cylinders with an optical density barely greater than that of the usual background. They have faint outlines and are seen best when the substage light is reduced. They are usually relatively narrow and often very elongated, sometimes ending in a tapering, thread-like tail. The latter type of hyaline cast is referred to as a *cylindroid* (Fig. 3-7). Hyaline casts may include within their protein matrix a few cells or small amounts of coarsely or finely granular material. Sometimes, when the urine contains a pigment such as hemoglobin, myoglobin, or bile pigment, hyaline casts stained with the characteristic color of these pigments will be excreted in the urine. Hyaline casts, unlike the cellular, granular, or waxy varieties, readily dissolve in dilute saline solutions and are usually not found in very hypotonic urine specimens. They also differ from waxy casts in being very susceptible to variation in pH, rarely occurring in urines of relatively marked alkalinity.

QUALITATIVE EXAMINATION OF THE
URINE SEDIMENT

For most clinical purposes it suffices to examine the centrifuged sediment of the urine in a qualitative or only semiquantitative manner, with the purpose of ascertaining only the types and relative numbers of formed elements. For this examination to be of value,

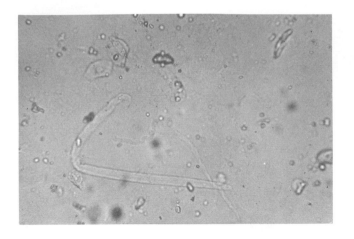

Figure 3-7. Elongated hyaline cast with a tapering tail, sometimes called a cylindroid.

however, it is essential that it be performed with care and that proper attention be paid to a number of relatively simple technical points enumerated below.

The urine specimen must be freshly voided and as concentrated as possible. There is rarely any need to obtain specimens by catheter if the patient is able to void. In male patients urine specimens suitable for examination of the sediment as well as for quantitative bacterial culture (see Chapter 18) can be obtained simply by collecting the second half of the voiding in a sterile container. This is usually also true in females, but it is necessary to cleanse the external genitalia thoroughly prior to voiding. Proper attention to this will usually avoid significant contamination of the urine with vaginal secretions and other extraneous debris.

Approximately 15 ml. of urine should be centrifuged in a tapered centrifuge tube at 3000 rpm for 5 minutes. If there is no visible sediment at the bottom of the tube, an attempt should be made further to concentrate any sediment. This is most easily done by allowing the freshly voided urine to stand in a beaker for 30 minutes before pipetting off 15 ml. for centrifugation from the bottom of the beaker. After centrifugation, the sediment should be identified; then the supernatant urine is gently decanted without disturbing the sediment. When the sediment is abundant, it can be resuspended in a small amount of supernatant urine in order to avoid too dense a mass. On the other hand, if the sediment is scanty, it may consist entirely of a very small speck of material confined to the tip of the tube and it is important that this not be overlooked or poured off with the supernate. Such sediments should be directly pipetted onto a slide without prior dilution or mixing.

Systematic examination of an entire drop of fresh, unstained sediment prepared as described above will usually reveal all elements of diagnostic significance. Although many types of special stains have been suggested to help in the identification of various cells or casts [125, 153, 221, 234], we are of the opinion that they do not ordinarily contribute enough to justify their routine use. For special investigations, however, or for cytologic studies in endocrinology or cancer diagnosis, staining technics may be important. We have found that ordinary bright-field microscopy suffices for most routine examinations of the sediment, but it is essential that the substage diaphragm be stopped down to allow for adequate contrast, particularly of hyaline casts. Others have advocated the use of phase-contrast microscopy, which is said to facilitate the recognition of all formed elements [40].

The most important practical point to be

made about the examination of the sediment is that it should be done by the physician interested in the patient and should not be delegated to anyone else. It is undoubtedly a practical necessity that laboratory technicians be assigned the responsibility of doing routine urinalyses. When a patient is suspected of renal disease, however, it becomes imperative that the sediment be examined carefully and competently by a physician in the light of the entire clinical picture. Dock [69] makes this observation: "It is as essential for the renal specialist to look at sediments obtained under standard conditions as for the heart specialist to do his own auscultation." While endorsing this opinion warmly, we would add that this obligation should be laid upon *all* physicians dealing with renal problems, not just the "specialist." There can be no doubt that casual or inexperienced examination of the sediment is commonly responsible for failure to recognize the existence of renal disease and to identify it with precision.

QUANTITATIVE EXAMINATION OF THE
URINE SEDIMENT

Technics for the measurement of the rates of excretion of the formed elements were first developed by Addis and his collaborators and subsequently applied by them to the study of the natural history of glomerulonephritis. The details of these technics can be read elsewhere [4, 153]. In essence they depend upon the collection of a carefully timed specimen of urine collected over a period of 8 to 12 hours. A specified aliquot of this volume is then centrifuged, and the sediment resuspended in 0.5 ml. of urine. A drop of this suspension is transferred with a pipette to the chamber of a standard hemocytometer. Under appropriate microscopic magnification the total number of casts, red cells, white blood cells, and epithelial cells in a given area is counted. (Addis believed that it was difficult and often impossible to distinguish between the latter two cell types with this technic.) Ap-

plying appropriate factors to these counts, the total number of each type of formed element excreted per day can be calculated. Recently, two modifications of the "Addis count" method have been suggested which permit the quantitative determination of cellular elements in urine specimens collected over shorter periods [118, 221].

These methods possess the obvious advantage of being quantitative. Quantitation of the sediment may be of value in studying the natural history of certain renal diseases or in recognizing relatively minor degrees of pathologic hematuria or pyuria. However, such counts require the collection of timed urine specimens, no mean feat in everyday clinical practice. They also are a technically more demanding procedure than the simple qualitative examination and, even when carried out with great care, are subject to considerable methodologic error. Furthermore, Addis counts are not ideal for distinguishing between types of casts and cells, because these elements may have begun to disintegrate before the examination can be completed. Finally, although there is some difference of opinion about this, most authorities agree that *qualitative* information about the sediment is more useful than *quantitative* data in the recognition of renal disease. For these reasons Addis counts, although sometimes employed in clinical investigation, have not generally replaced the simple qualitative technics for examination of the urine sediment.

NORMAL SEDIMENT

Red Blood Cells. With the Addis technic, up to approximately 1,000,000 red blood cells may be excreted in the 24-hour urine of the healthy adult while at normal quiet activity [3, 100]; the mean excretion rate is approximately 150,000 to 300,000 cells per day [3, 100]. In children from 4 to 12 years of age the maximum normal rate was found to be approximately 250,000 red cells per day [158]. With another counting technic that utilizes shorter collections and differential staining of the sediment [205], it has been reported that the mean rate of excretion is 38,500 cells per hour in adult males and 28,800 cells per hour in females.

With the usual qualitative technic of examination it is normal to see occasional erythrocytes in the sediment. Normal limits are difficult to define because of many variables in the technic, but it should not be considered abnormal to find as many as one or possibly two red blood cells in every high power field. In support of this clinical impression is the observation that 600,000 red cells added to 300 ml. of clear urine will give about two red cells per high power field when this specimen is handled in the usual manner [140]. Most normal urines show fewer cells than this; thus, in 6000 consecutive male and female specimens examined by one insurance company, 94 per cent had no more than one red cell per high power field and 78 per cent apparently had "none" [282]. This per cent may be greatly increased by vigorous exercise, lordotic posture, and by bodily trauma to the region of the kidneys. Microscopic hematuria is also increased during the febrile phases of acute febrile diseases without necessarily implying any serious disease of the kidney or urinary tract [100].

White Blood Cells and Epithelial Cells. With the Addis method, up to approximately 2,000,000 leukocytes and nonsquamous epithelial cells per day may be excreted by the normal adult male [3, 100]; the mean rate of excretion is approximately 600,000 to 1,000,000 cells per day [3, 100]. In children from 4 to 12 years of age the excretion rates are about the same, with the rate for girls (uncatheterized) slightly higher than that for boys [158]. As with red cells, this number may be increased by exercise [217] or febrile illness [100]. Using a modification of the Addis technic on shorter-timed urine specimens, a mean rate of 66,000 cells per hour was found for males and females, with extremes of 18,000 and 196,000

[118]. In young children the normal rates are much lower, and they increase with age until the adult rate is reached at about age 8 to 10 [119]. When differential stains are employed to separate renal tubular cells from leukocytes, and longer collection periods are used, it is found that the mean rate of excretion of tubular cells is 78,200 per hour for adult males and 68,000 per hour for adult females. The mean rate of leukocyte excretion is 28,700 per hour in males and 107,800 per hour in females, but these results are for clean-voided specimens, and it is not known whether the large difference between the sexes would persist with catheter specimens [205]. In general, the excretion of leukocytes tends to be more variable than that of renal tubular cells.

On qualitative examination most normal men will be found to have a "rare" to "occasional" leukocyte or nonsquamous epithelial cell. (As noted previously, it is often difficult to distinguish between these, and most observers report them together.) Of 5000 consecutive urine specimens from males examined for life insurance purposes, 89 per cent had no more than two leukocytes or nonsquamous epithelial cells per high power field [217]. Of 1000 consecutive urine specimens obtained without catheter from females, 69 per cent had two or fewer cells per high power field, and 76 per cent had five or fewer [217]. Since directly voided urine from women is not infrequently contaminated with vulval or vaginal secretions, it is sometimes difficult to interpret increased leukocyte counts in such specimens. Special care in obtaining clean-voided specimens will usually obviate this difficulty. In noncatheterized specimens from postpubertal females, it is also common to find large numbers of squamous epithelial cells caused mainly by contamination by vaginal secretions. Squamous cells also originate from the anterior urethra. Such cells, although a nuisance to the observer interested in renal disease, can sometimes provide valuable endocrinologic information, for their number and appearance in suitably stained smears reflect estrogenic activity [48, 240], and they vary with the phases of the menstrual cycle [266].

Casts. Normal subjects may excrete up to 5000 or 10,000 casts per 24 hours [3, 100]; children excrete approximately the same number [158]. Thus, it is not unusual to find an occasional cast, perhaps one every 10 or 20 high power fields, in perfectly healthy subjects. These casts are almost always of the narrow hyaline or cylindroid varieties, with a rare finely granular type. Exercise, fever, posture, trauma, and other "functional" disturbances which may produce proteinuria in normal subjects can also induce cylindruria [8, 43, 100, 136, 217]. With these types of stress, granular and even cellular casts may appear. Except for such circumstances, however, the occurrence of even an occasional granular or cellular cast should be viewed with suspicion.

URINE SEDIMENT IN RENAL DISEASE

Descriptions of the characteristic findings in the urinary sediment in the major types of renal disease will be found in the chapters devoted to these subjects. This topic is also discussed in detail in Lippman's monograph [153]. Some important generalizations may be presented here:

1. Marked *hematuria* is found in such a large variety of renal and extrarenal disorders that it is of little diagnostic value unless accompanied by *red blood cell casts* or mixed cellular casts stained with hemoglobin. These casts, however few, are almost invariably found in the presence of acute or subacute inflammatory lesions of the glomeruli such as occur in active glomerulonephritis, diffuse angiitis, and lupus erythematosus or periarteritis. They are also occasionally found in malignant nephrosclerosis and acute tubular necrosis and are common following violent exercise or renal trauma (including needle or surgical biopsies of the kidney). In the absence of trauma or violent exercise the finding of red blood cell casts or mixed red cell and epithelial cell casts

may be considered strongly suggestive of some type of active vascular or inflammatory process in the glomerulus.

2. *Leukocytes,* when slightly increased in number, may be seen in almost any renal disease, but when found in profusion or in clumps, they usually indicate infection somewhere in the urinary tract. However, markedly increased pyuria is not infrequently seen in cases of acute exudative glomerulonephritis. It has recently been suggested that the leukocyte excretion in response to intravenous injection of bacterial pyrogen may be helpful in the diagnosis of chronic pyelonephritis [121, 196]. Control rates of cell excretion may be normal or increased, but injection of pyrogen usually causes a marked rise to over 400,000 cells per hour [121].

The only convincing sign of the renal origin of leukocytes is their presence in casts. As already noted, "glitter cells" are not specifically of renal origin and cannot be considered diagnostic of pyelonephritis, although they do occur frequently in this disease. On the other hand, casts consisting wholly or largely of leukocytes, or leukocytes mixed with epithelial cells, are an important sign of pyelonephritis although they are not specific for this disorder [211]. *White blood cell casts,* and more commonly mixed cellular casts containing leukocytes, are also seen frequently in exudative varieties of acute and subacute glomerulonephritis and sometimes in disseminated lupus erythematosus and periarteritis. However, when white cell casts occur in a sediment which does not contain many other types of casts, a strong presumptive diagnosis of pyelonephritis can be made. Sometimes they may be the only evidence of pyelonephritis when all other clinical and laboratory findings suggest merely a lower urinary tract infection [211]. Not infrequently an occasional white blood cell cast will betray the presence of pyelonephritis in the absence of bacteriuria or a significant degree of pyuria.

3. *Hemoglobin casts* and *bile-stained casts*

may be found in acute tubular necrosis and "hepatorenal syndrome," respectively, but they are not pathognomonic of these conditions, because they may occur in any situation where the serum concentration and renal excretion of these pigments are elevated.

4. Droplets of *fatty debris,* cellular or granular *casts showing fatty degeneration* and *oval fat bodies* are characteristic of renal disorders producing heavy proteinuria. Such elements when found in profusion are the hallmark of the nephrotic syndrome, irrespective of the nature of the lesion producing it. Occasionally, however, urine from a nephrotic patient may contain only hyaline casts and renal cells which show little or no fatty change; conversely, occasional fatty cells and casts may be found in a variety of renal diseases in the absence of the nephrotic syndrome.

5. The excretion of large numbers of relatively well-preserved, free *renal epithelial cells and casts containing such cells* is a sign of an active degenerative process involving the tubules. This may occur, of course, as part of glomerulonephritis, in which case there will also be many other casts of the hyaline and granular varieties as well as red blood cells and possibly red blood cell casts. In acute tubular necrosis, and occasionally in cases of necrotizing papillitis, plaques of renal epithelial cells, representing necrotic fragments of tubular walls, may be found in the urine. Active pyelonephritis may also cause a particularly striking excess of epithelial cells and epithelial cell casts.

6. *Renal failure casts* in large numbers usually indicate the presence of renal insufficiency, and in general have an ominous significance [2]. It should be noted, however, that such casts may occur in the diuretic phase of acute tubular necrosis and following recovery from the oliguric phase of a severe attack of acute glomerulonephritis.

Clinical Tests of Renal Function

Tests of kidney function are useful in clinical medicine chiefly as means for evaluating the severity of renal disease and following its progress. Abnormalities of renal function may be discovered by clinical laboratory tests well before symptoms have developed; hence, these tests may sometimes have diagnostic significance. However, for the early recognition and differential diagnosis of kidney disease one must rely mainly on other types of evidence, some of which have been discussed in previous

Table 3-1. Renal Function Tests

Function	Specific Tests	Clinical Tests
Glomerular filtration	Inulin clearance	Creatinine clearance Urea clearance Plasma creatinine Plasma urea
Renal plasma flow	PAH clearance Diodrast clearance	PSP excretion
Proximal tubular transport	Tm glucose (reabsorptive) Tm_{PAH} or Tm Diodrast (secretory)	PSP excretion
Distal tubular transport	Concentration and dilution $T^C_{H_2O}$, C_{H_2O} Maximal and minimal U/P osmolality	Concentration and dilution Maximal and minimal specific gravity

sections of this chapter. Using more sophisticated laboratory studies of renal physiology, it has been possible to recognize patterns of functional changes more or less characteristic of certain types of kidney disease [33, 74, 75], but even this type of information is rarely of value in differential diagnosis. With the relatively blunt tools ordinarily used in clinical medicine for the evaluation of renal function, the data obtained are even less likely to have diagnostic significance.

In discharging its urinary function the kidney performs an enormous number of complexly interrelated steps, and in theory one might wish to evaluate any or all of these functional processes in order to determine the effect of a given disease process on the kidney. In the second column of Table 3-1 are shown some of the reasonably specific and selective tests of discrete aspects of renal function which are available in the laboratory. None of the clinical tests listed in the last column of this table is quite so clearly related to a single discrete functional mechanism. The clearance of urea and creatinine or their plasma levels, while in general related primarily to the glomerular filtration rate, are also determined in part by tubular processes. Conversely, the excretion of PSP is largely a proximal* tubular function, but the clinical PSP test is also a function of the renal plasma flow. The ability to concentrate and dilute the urine is intrinsically a distal* tubular function, but the tubular mechanisms are often considerably modified by changes in glomerular filtration. Although none of the common clinical tests of kidney function is specific, taken together and backed by a considerable amount of empiric information they usually provide an adequate overall view of kidney function in clinical renal disease.

A number of additional clinical tests have

* *Proximal* is used here to mean the proximal convolution; *distal* refers to any part of the nephron beyond this, including the loop of Henle, the distal convolution, and the collecting tubules.

been employed for the evaluation of special physiologic functions of the kidney, such as sodium conservation, response to parathormone, or the regulation of acid-base balance, and these are sometimes useful in certain clinical situations. Description of these other procedures will be omitted, however, in favor of discussion of the three types of clinical tests shown in Table 3-1, which are used widely and have greater clinical importance.

CLINICAL MEASUREMENTS OF THE
GLOMERULAR FILTRATION RATE

There is no technic by which the glomerular filtration rate (GFR) can be measured directly. All available methods depend on estimations of the rate at which substances excreted by glomerular filtration are cleared from the plasma. If the clearance of a material is to be an accurate index of GFR, it must be filtered freely at the glomerulus and neither rcabsorbed nor secreted by the renal tubule. As described in Chapter 2, an impressive body of evidence demonstrates that inulin, a fructose polymer, fulfills these criteria in a wide variety of species including man. Hence, the inulin clearance is an accurate index of GFR in normal man. It is uncertain, however, whether the inulin clearance is an exact measurement of GFR in the presence of renal disease. It is conceivable that inulin diffuses back across damaged tubules [17] or that it is not freely filtered through diseased glomeruli [244]. On the other hand, to the extent that the "intact nephron hypothesis" is correct and only normal nephrons continue to function, the inulin clearance should be a valid index of GFR even in advanced renal disease [36]. The inulin clearance is the standard of reference for all other methods of estimating GFR. Hence, until the validity of the inulin clearance in the diseased kidney can be determined by independent means, there is some uncertainty with regard to all methods when renal disease is present.

The inulin clearance is too demanding for

routine clinical purposes principally because inulin must be infused intravenously at a constant rate. The clearance of radioactive vitamin B_{12} has been proposed as an alternative. When plasma binding sites have been saturated with nonlabeled vitamin B_{12}, the clearance of the radioactive vitamin is approximately equal to that of inulin [34, 185]. The vitamin B_{12} method does not circumvent the need for a continuous intravenous infusion. With the advent of automated methods for inulin analysis, the analytic technics for radioactive vitamin B_{12} and inulin are now comparably simple. However, the correlation between vitamin B_{12} and inulin clearances is not always exact [162]. Hence, the vitamin B_{12} clearance would seem inferior to the inulin clearance for investigative or clinical purposes. Various technics involving simple intravenous injections of inulin or vitamin B_{12} have been proposed from time to time, but the accuracy of clearance calculations based on a falling plasma level is debatable [244]. These methods seem to have no advantages over the still simpler technics which depend on reference substances normally present in blood. The measurement of GFR for clinical purposes would be greatly simplified if the clearance of some substance normally present in plasma were equal to that of inulin. No such material has been found. However, the clearances of creatinine and urea can serve as convenient clinical approximations of the filtration rate.

Creatinine Clearance. If creatinine is infused into man to raise the normally low plasma creatinine levels and minimize analytic error, the exogenous creatinine clearance so determined is regularly from 10 to 40 per cent greater than the clearance of inulin [42, 60, 237, 238]. As the plasma level of creatinine is raised from 10 mg. to 100 mg. per 100 ml., the creatinine-to-inulin clearance ratio falls from 1.4 to 1.1 [237, 238]. At any of these plasma levels the administration of phlorizin [237] or Diodrast [238] abruptly lowers the creati-

nine-to-inulin clearance ratio toward 1.0. This behavior is characteristic of substances excreted in part by the secretory activity of the tubules and indicates beyond reasonable doubt that tubular secretion of creatinine can occur. In patients with elevated plasma creatinine levels due to chronic renal failure, creatinine clearance exceeds the inulin clearance by 10 to 100 per cent [21, 70, 164, 177].

However, the mode of excretion of creatinine at normal endogenous plasma levels has not been determined; in spite of a vast number of clinical and experimental observations, the existence of creatinine secretion at endogenous plasma levels is still very much a matter for debate. Part, at least, of the difficulty in settling this problem results from the nonspecificity of the classic Folin picrate method for determination of creatinine. The apparent plasma levels of creatinine determined by this method are some 10 to 40 per cent higher than those determined by more specific methods involving the use either of a creatinine-destroying bacterial enzyme [175] or of selective creatinine adsorbents [110, 114]. However, it has never been established that even these latter methods are completely specific, and hence it is not certain that they measure all the creatinine in plasma and creatinine alone [113, 144, 193]. The nature of the so-called "noncreatinine chromogens" which give a color with the picrate reagents has never been fully elucidated, but whatever their chemical nature, they apparently are not excreted into the urine to any significant degree [110, 114, 175, 193]. In other words, the clearance of these materials is vanishingly low. Since the picrate reaction measures both creatinine itself and these various nonspecific chromogens, it follows that the overall clearance of chromogenic substance should be lower than the exogenous true creatinine clearance. This is in fact the case, and in nearly all the published observations the total chromogen-to-inulin clearance ratio approximates 1.0 [39, 114, 251]. This of course is an average figure, and individual correlations of endogenous total chromogen clearance and inulin clearance are relatively poor. It should in any case be clear that the apparent correspondence of the two clearances may be fortuitous and may occur because the numerator of the fraction UV/P is proportionately increased approximately as much by the secretion of true creatinine as the denominator is increased by virtue of its complement of non-creatinine chromogen.

From these considerations one would expect that the endogenous true creatinine clearance should, like the exogenous creatinine clearance, give evidence of tubular secretory activity and exceed the inulin clearance by a considerable margin. Such indeed is the case in several series of observations of normal subjects. However, in many apparently equally careful investigations the endogenous true creatinine clearance is on the average equal to the inulin to clearance [78, 114, 164]. Other studies have demonstrated that the endogenous true creatinine clearance is regularly less than the exogenous clearance determined immediately thereafter in the same subjects [176]. No adequate explanation for these observations has been offered; it is possible that creatinine secretion is minimal at normal plasma levels, but is enhanced at increased concentrations. In any case, the endogenous creatinine clearance in man cannot be safely used as an exact measure of the filtration rate [21]. It has been shown, for example, that cortisone may depress the creatinine-to-inulin clearance ratio [44], presumably by suppressing tubular secretion of creatinine at endogenous plasma levels. Conversely, there is suggestive evidence in man that creatinine may sometimes be reabsorbed by the renal tubules, since in infants [164] and in some patients with congestive cardiac failure [15, 177] the true endogenous creatinine clearance is *less* than the inulin clearance. (In dogs there is reasonably definitive evidence that creatinine is reabsorbed somewhere in the urinary

tract at very low urine flows [139, 146].) It has also been suggested that creatinine secretion is increased in patients with heavy proteinuria [21], but this is uncertain [34]. The creatinine clearance is thus not an exact measure of the glomerular filtration rate in man, but it is nevertheless a valuable clinical tool in following the progress of renal disease.

An extensive study of simultaneous inulin and creatinine clearances in normal subjects and patients with renal failure [230] suggests that the creatinine-to-inulin clearance ratio increases progressively as the inulin clearance decreases. When the inulin clearance was about 80 ml. per minute, the creatinine clearance was within 15 to 25 per cent of the inulin clearance. With increasing renal failure, the clearance ratio appeared to increase progressively, so that the mean creatinine clearance exceeded the inulin clearance by as much as 50 to 80 per cent at inulin clearances of 30 ml. per minute or less. This discrepancy is important in clinical investigations, but the creatinine clearance is adequate for most practical purposes even in advanced renal failure. For example, in advanced azotemia, the creatinine clearance may be 15 ml. per minute when the true glomerular filtration rate is 10 ml. per minute. Although the fractional error is large, the absolute error of 5 ml. per minute is insignificant for most clinical purposes. The creatinine clearance is very convenient in clinical use because excretion of creatinine is independent of the rate of urine flow [236], except perhaps at flows of much less than 0.5 ml. per minute [53]. Moreover, the plasma creatinine level is relatively stable, usually varying no more than 10 per cent of its average value in a 24-hour period [6, 241]. These facts permit the creatinine clearance to be measured over long periods, such as 24 hours, which minimizes collection errors and obviates the need of special procedures for hydration of the patient. Furthermore, the 24-hour clearance may perhaps derive some special clinical significance from the fact that it represents an estimate of the filtration rate integrated through the total range of the patient's daily activities.

The technic for the measurement of the 24-hour creatinine clearance is quite simple. It is usually most convenient for the patient to void and discard when he arises on a given morning; thereafter, he can collect all urine up to and including the urine which he passes at the corresponding time on the following morning. A single blood specimen is obtained at any convenient time during or close to the 24-hour period. The analytic procedures for urine and plasma creatinine are relatively simple, but an analytic error of at least 10 per cent in the determination of endogenous plasma creatinine is to be expected even in the best clinical laboratories [9]. The exact normal values for 24-hour creatinine clearance depend somewhat on the particular analytic methods chosen. In general the range of true creatinine clearance for men is approximately 140 to 200 liters per day (97 to 140 ml. per minute) and for women 120 to 180 liters per day (85 to 125 ml. per minute) [78]. The fall in the average clearance of total creatinine chromogen with progressing renal disease is usually caused by true creatinine [175, 177, 222]. Since the clearance of creatinine itself is much higher than that of the noncreatinine chromogens, the total chromogen clearance will not fall in proportion to the fall in glomerular filtration rate [177]. The true creatinine clearance may therefore be a somewhat more satisfactory means of following the functional progress of renal disease than the total chromogen clearance, but the difference is of little practical significance.

Urea Clearance. The urea clearance is of considerable historic interest since it was in their studies of urea excretion that Van Slyke and his co-workers first coined the word "clearance" [14, 179]. In addition, a large body of clinical information about urea clearance in man is available, and it is still widely used as a function test. Therefore, the principles underlying the urea clearance are presented here, although in our opinion the urea clearance is a much less satisfactory test of renal function than the creatinine clearance.

Urea is freely filtered at the glomerulus, but a variable proportion of the filtered load of urea is reabsorbed by the renal tubules, presumably as a passive consequence of the urea concentration gradient established by water reabsorption (see Chapter 2). Physiologic studies indicate that the fraction of the filtered urea which is reabsorbed is an inverse function of the rate of urine flow (or, more precisely, of the U/P ratio for inulin) over the entire range of urine flow rates in man [52]. However, Van Slyke and his associates [14, 179] found that at flow rates ranging from 2 ml. per minute to those found in maximal water diuresis, the urea clearance can be considered, for clinical purposes, to be roughly constant. In other words, at flow rates greater than 2 ml. per minute the rate of excretion of urea is proportional to the plasma urea concentration. Van Slyke called 2 ml. per minute the "augmentation limit" and named the urea clearance obtained at flows of 2 ml. per minute or more the "maximum clearance." At flows of less than 2 ml. per minute, Van Slyke and his associates found that the clearance of urea is roughly proportional to the square root of the rate of urine flow. In order to permit comparison of clearances obtained at varying flows of less than the augmentation limit, Van Slyke "corrected" the observed urea clearance to a "standard clearance" of 1 ml. per minute by the formula $U\sqrt{V}/B$. The normal values obtained by Van Slyke and his associates were 75 ml. per minute for the maximum clearance and 54 ml. per minute for the standard clearance of urea. As would be expected from the approximate nature of the flow correction, the maximum clearance was found by Van Slyke and later workers to be a more accurate and reproducible measurement than the standard clearance. An extensive series of simultaneous measurements of urea and inulin clearances in normal subjects and in patients with renal failure has shown that the mean urea-to-inulin clearance ratio is relatively stable at about 0.60 to 0.65 when the inulin clearance exceeds 30 ml. per minute, but it is increased to a mean of about 0.75 at lower rates of glomerular filtration [231].

To measure the maximum clearance of urea the subject should be instructed to drink several glasses of fluid prior to the performance of the test, thus ensuring a high rate of urine flow. Two accurately timed periods, each approximately one hour in length, are obtained to provide a check against collection errors caused by inaccurate timing or incomplete emptying of the bladder. A single blood specimen is obtained at about the midpoint of the test for determination of blood urea values. Since the blood urea varies considerably during the course of a day and since urea excretion is markedly dependent on the rate of urine flow, urea clearance tests must be carried out over relatively short time intervals. The analytic methods for urea are relatively simple and accurate [9].

Comparison of the Creatinine and Urea Clearances. While one can obtain useful and approximately equivalent information by the performance of either the urea or the creatinine clearance, as a practical clinical matter the 24-hour creatinine clearance is much the superior test. The errors caused by inaccurate timing of collection periods and incomplete emptying of the bladder are proportionately much more important over the short intervals of time required by the urea clearance test. These factors in most clinics more than balance the slightly greater analytic precision of the urea method and the occasional difficulty in obtaining complete 24-hour urine collections for creatinine. Moreover, the urine flow rates required for accurate maximal urea clearance measurements are sometimes difficult to obtain, particularly in patients with advanced renal disease. Attempts at rapid hydration in such patients are occasionally dangerous be-

cause they may lead to acute water intoxication. For these practical reasons, the urea clearance is a less satisfactory means than the creatinine clearance for following the functional history of renal disease in a given individual. As already noted, there may be a tendency for the creatinine-to-inulin clearance ratio to increase with increasing renal failure [230]. The urea-to-inulin clearance ratio also increases as GFR falls, presumably because of the increasing osmotic diuresis per nephron, which retards urea reabsorption [52, 155, 231]. Therefore, changes in either clearance may tend to underestimate the magnitude of decreases in GFR as chronic renal failure progresses.

*Plasma Creatinine and Blood or Plasma Urea.** Much more commonly used by clinicians to follow the functional changes in renal disease than either clearance measurement are the levels of creatinine and urea in the blood. Tacit in such use is the assumption that these concentrations are inversely related to the clearance of the respective substances. Since the clearance of a substance is given by the equation

$$\text{Clearance} = \frac{\text{Excretion rate}}{\text{Plasma concentration}}$$

it follows that the clearance and the plasma level of a reference material will have a precisely inverse relation only when the excretion of the material is constant. This relation between the clearance and plasma levels of urea and creatinine is illustrated in Figure 3-8. The figure is based on a constant urea nitrogen excretion of 11.5 gm. and a creatinine excretion of 1.2 gm. per day, which would be

---

* Since the concentrations of urea in the water of plasma and red cells are the same, plasma and whole blood concentrations may, for practical purposes, be considered equivalent. Actually, the whole blood urea is roughly 10 per cent lower than the concentration in plasma, because of the relatively low water content of red cells [198]. The blood urea concentration is usually expressed in terms of blood urea nitrogen (BUN), which constitutes approximately half of the weight of urea.

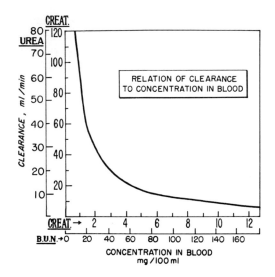

Figure 3-8. Relation of clearance of urea or creatinine to the concentration of these substances in blood, assuming a constant urea nitrogen excretion of 11.5 gm. per day (8 mg. per minute) and a creatinine excretion of 1.2 gm. per day (0.84 mg. per minute).

average values for a 70-kg. man ingesting 80 gm. of protein daily. To the mathematically minded, it should be obvious that if excretion is constant, the equation relating clearance and plasma level describes a rectangular hyperbola. Such a curve means that the absolute rate of rise in plasma level progressively increases as the clearance falls. For example, as can be seen from the figure, a 50 per cent reduction in urea clearance from 80 to 40 ml. per minute increases the BUN by about 10 mg. per 100 ml. (from 10 to 20). By contrast, a similar percentage reduction in clearance from 10 to 5 ml. per minute raises the BUN by 80 mg. per 100 ml. (from 80 to 160).

In the steady state the rate of excretion of metabolic end products like creatinine and urea must equal the rate of production. Therefore, if changes in plasma creatinine or urea are to reflect changes in clearance alone, rates of production must also be constant. For creatinine, this is very nearly the case. The daily excretion in a given individual varies only

within 10 to 15 per cent of the mean value over long periods of time [71, 86, 236, 262, 268]. The rate of excretion seems to be a function of muscle mass [86, 236], since nearly all of the creatinine excreted in the urine derives from the creatine of muscle [198]. It is presumably because of the greater muscular development of the male that the rate of creatinine excretion tends to be higher in a man than in a woman of equivalent total body-surface area or weight. The normal range for creatinine excretion in males is about 1000 to 2000 mg. (20 to 26 mg. per kilogram) per 24 hours; in females about 800 to 1500 mg. (14 to 22 mg. per kilogram) per 24 hours [198]. Even with the largest variation in preformed creatinine that is likely to occur, as, for example, when the amount of cooked meat protein is increased from 0.5 to 1.5 gm. per kilogram of body weight per day, creatinine excretion in the urine increases by only 10 per cent [18].

On the other hand, since urea is the chief end product of nitrogen metabolism in man, the production and excretion of urea depend on the many factors which affect nitrogen metabolism. These include the protein intake of the diet, caloric balance, the function of the liver and certain endocrine glands, and the accelerated degradation of endogenous protein associated with trauma, infection, and fever, and the breakdown of blood in tissues or the gastrointestinal tract [198]. Inasmuch as the plasma level of urea depends on the relation of urea production to urea excretion, it will change with alterations in any of these factors. This is illustrated in Figure 3-9, which shows the extreme changes in blood urea which can result from changes in protein intake in the diet without any significant change in urea clearance. Thus, with different dietary protein intakes, a family of curves can be obtained similar to that in Figure 3-8. At any given protein intake, and with all other factors affecting urea production held constant, the inverse relation between clearance and blood level can be expected. On the other hand, since

Figure 3-9. Marked variations in blood urea without significant changes in urea clearance, produced by alterations of protein consumption in a patient with renal disease. (From Goldring, W. [100]; reproduced by permission.)

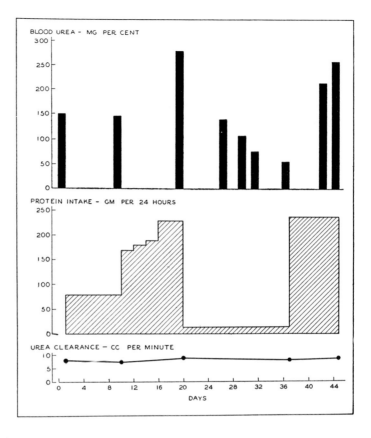

creatinine excretion is largely independent of diet, a single curve is sufficient to describe the relation of plasma creatinine to creatinine clearance in any one subject, regardless of diet.

One can safely assume that a doubling of the plasma creatinine at any absolute level of plasma creatinine represents approximately a 50 per cent fall in the creatinine clearance [71, 79, 230]. However, a similar change in blood urea concentration may reflect only a doubling of urea production caused by increased protein consumption or some other cause of accelerated nitrogen turnover. Late in the course of renal disease creatinine excretion may decrease somewhat [79, 99, 251, 265], presumably because of decreased muscle mass due to malnutrition. Under these circumstances the relation between plasma creatinine and creatinine clearance in a given individual will be altered. Creatinine clearance will de-

crease without proportionate rise in plasma creatinine. Other causes of reduction in muscle mass may have similar effects, in that plasma creatinine will be lower than expected from a given clearance. These exceptions aside, serial measurements of plasma creatinine afford a satisfactory means of following the functional progress of patients with renal disease and of making some reasonably quantitative inferences about the change in glomerular filtration rate. Because of the many factors that may cause gross changes in urea production, changes in blood urea concentration provide a less reliable guide to the urea clearance. As noted previously, the urea clearance, and possibly also the creatinine clearance, may tend to increase in proportion to the glomerular filtration rate (inulin clearance) in advanced renal failure. The plasma levels of urea and creatinine may therefore rise less rapidly than would be predicted from the fall in filtration rate.

The plasma concentration of urea or creatinine in normal individuals is the result of two independent factors, production and clearance, which may vary greatly among different subjects. Hence the range of "normal" values is rather wide.* Plasma urea nitrogens of 8 to 22 mg. per 100 ml. and plasma true creatinines of 0.4 to 1.2 mg. per 100 ml. are within the accepted normal range.† This relatively wide normal range may prevent recognition of early changes in renal function [71, 101, 230, 265]. For the detection of early functional impairment a clearance measurement is often necessary.

It is sometimes stated that the plasma levels of urea or creatinine do not increase significantly until their clearance falls below 50 per cent of normal. Such statements confuse the significance of the range of values in groups of normal subjects with that of changes within this range in any one individual. It should be obvious from the foregoing discussion that in any given individual, other things being equal, the clearances of urea or creatinine and their respective plasma levels have a mathematically exact inverse relation *throughout* their range. If a normal creatinine clearance of 200 liters per day is halved, for example, or if an already reduced creatinine clearance of 100 liters per day is halved, the plasma creatinine

will in each case be doubled. In the first instance, the normal plasma creatinine of perhaps 0.5 mg. per 100 ml. will increase only to 1 mg. per 100 ml., a value still within the accepted "normal" range. In the latter case, however, the plasma creatinine will rise from 1 to 2 mg. per 100 ml., which is ordinarily considered abnormal. Unless serial observations have been made, or the creatinine clearance measured, it would be difficult to recognize the plasma value of 1 mg. per 100 ml. as abnormal *for the particular individual*.

In Figure 3-10 the inverse relation between clearance and blood urea concentration is illustrated by data from patients with a wide range of normal and abnormal clearances. In this figure, logarithmic scales are used, which show equal percentage changes as equal distances along the axes. Hence the rectangular hyperbola of Figure 3-8 is converted to a straight line. Plotted in this manner, it is obvious that plasma urea rises continuously and at the same proportionate rate over the entire range of urea clearance.

Nonprotein Nitrogen (NPN). The nonprotein nitrogen of the plasma is the sum of all the nitrogenous materials not precipitated by the usual protein precipitants. Detailed analysis indicates that when the plasma NPN is normal (15 to 35 mg. per 100 ml.), roughly half of the nitrogen derives from the plasma urea and the rest from a mixture of nitrogenous compounds of which the principal known members are amino acids (3 to 5 mg. of nitrogen per 100 ml.), uric acid, and creatinine [198]. The NPN has been used as a substitute for the direct determination of blood urea nitrogen concentrations because at one time analytic methods for urea were rather difficult. Analysis for urea nitrogen by the urease method is now as simple and accurate as the Kjeldahl analysis for NPN, and there is no further reason for the use of NPN measurements as an indicator of renal function. The mechanisms for excretion of urea, amino acids, creatinine, uric acid, and the other materials which make up the NPN are all

---

* The dependence of plasma concentration on the relation of production to clearance and not on either factor alone is well illustrated by the fact that women tend to have somewhat lower plasma creatinine concentrations than men even though their glomerular filtration rates are also somewhat lower. This is because their rates of production of creatinine are proportionately still lower, so that clearance in relation to production is higher in women than in men.

† Such limits cannot be taken too literally, for they vary according to the methods used and the "normal" population chosen for study. In our laboratory the mean plasma (or serum) urea nitrogen levels in 32 normal subjects was 15.2 mg. ± 3.7 (S.D.) per 100 ml. with no difference between the sexes. In 16 normal men the mean plasma creatinine was 0.83 mg. ± 0.20 per 100 ml. and in 16 women 0.69 mg. ± 0.12 per 100 ml. This difference was significant at the 5 per cent level [10].

Figure 3-10. Relation between blood urea and urea clearance, plotted logarithmically to show that they are inversely related over the entire range of normal and abnormal clearance values. Each point represents a measurement on one patient. (From Goldring, W. [100]; reproduced by permission.)

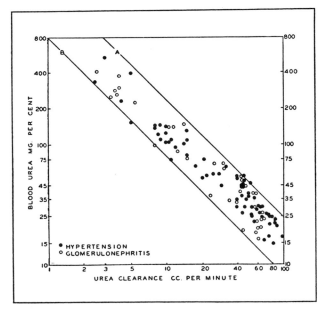

different, so that changes in plasma NPN reflect changing filtration rates only very approximately. As renal disease progresses, plasma amino acids do not change significantly; plasma creatinine and uric acid concentrations increase somewhat, but nearly all of the rise in NPN is caused by the increasing concentrations of urea in the blood [198]. Thus, in one series of observations [182], when the NPN was less than 30 mg. per 100 ml., urea accounted for 55 per cent of the total NPN; with NPN's in the range of 31 to 60 mg. per 100 ml., it accounted for 65 per cent; and with NPN's over 61 mg. per 100 ml., 75 per cent of the NPN was contributed by urea. Because of the variable relations of changes in the various components of the NPN to changing renal function, the NPN should be discarded in favor of measurements of plasma creatinine or urea.

Tests of Concentrating and Diluting Function

Although measurements of urine specific gravity have been made at least since the time of Richard Bright [37], the systematic clinical use of concentration tests as measures of renal tubular function was apparently first undertaken by Volhard [269] and has subsequently been emphasized and given impetus in this country by Addis [5] and Fishberg [85]. Considering that the tubules perform many different transport and metabolic functions, that many of these are localized to certain parts of the nephron, and that disease can affect these separate functions and anatomic sites to different degrees, it should be obvious that no single test can adequately measure the total anatomic and functional integrity of the tubules. Nevertheless, tests of the concentrating and diluting functions have firmly established themselves as the most convenient and widely used clinical estimates of tubular function.

As described in Chapter 2, the concentrating and diluting operations of the kidney take place in the distal portions of the nephron. To function normally, they require active tubular transport of sodium as well as the ability of the tubules to vary their permeability to water in response to the action of the antidiuretic hormone. The anatomic integrity of the medulla is also important, for it is here that the tubular and vascular loops play their special roles as countercurrent multipliers and countercurrent exchangers, respectively, in the complex process of urine concentration. These distal tubular mechanisms, however, are modified by a number of other renal and extrarenal factors that may thereby affect concentration or dilution. If the glomerular filtration rate is decreased, maximal urine concentration may be reduced even if tubular function is intact [147, 149]. On the other hand, a reduced filtration rate, or a reduced amount of sodium and water reaching the distal tubules, may impair diluting ability. Furthermore, maximal urine concentration is an inverse function of the rate of total solute excretion, provided that the rate of urea excretion is at least that produced by the usual diet.

As discussed in Chapter 2, the concentrating function of the kidney can be described both in terms of the maximal urine-plasma concentration gradient which can be achieved and in terms of the maximal amount of "free" water which is conserved ($T^C_{H_2O}$). Similarly, the diluting function can be measured by the minimal urine-plasma concentration gradient and by the maximal content of "free" water excreted (C_{H_2O}). Maximal and minimal osmolality can be attained only at the lowest rates of solute excretion; $T^C_{H_2O}$ and C_{H_2O} are greatest when solute excretion is high. The maximal osmolality of urine from dehydrated normal subjects is usually 800 to 1400 mOsm per kilogram of water [29, 87, 152, 174, 283]; the minimal osmolality during water diuresis is 40 to 80 mOsm per kilogram of water [232]. $T^C_{H_2O}$ is about 5 ml. per minute per 1.73 square meters in normal subjects [29, 283]. Systematic data on C_{H_2O} over a wide range of solute excretion are not available. At relatively high rates of solute excretion induced by diet [133] or by prehydration [138], C_{H_2O} is approximately 8 to 20 ml. per minute per 1.73 square meters. Measurements of $T^C_{H_2O}$ and C_{H_2O} are too complicated for routine use, and in clinical

practice it is customary to test only maximal and minimal urine concentrations. It should be noted, however, that these two types of tests measure different aspects of the renal concentrating and diluting function. For this reason, it is theoretically possible for changes in maximal and minimal U/P gradients to be dissociated from changes in free water clearances. This may be illustrated in early sickle cell disease, where $T^C_{H_2O}$ may be fairly well preserved despite reduced maximal concentration [212].

OSMOLALITY AND SPECIFIC GRAVITY

Because of the simplicity and ready availability of the hydrometer, specific gravity rather than osmolality is commonly used as a clinical measure of urine concentration. When a freezing-point depression apparatus is available, measurements of osmolality are easy, rapid, and quite precise. Such measurements of urine concentration are to be preferred over any other because the physiology of the concentrating process is best described in terms of the number of solute particles per unit of solvent. This is precisely the quantity defined by the osmolality. The specific gravity of urine depends on both the *number* and the *nature* of the particles in solution whereas, as just defined, the osmolality depends only on the number of dissolved particles and is independent of the nature of each particle. Thus, relatively large, dense molecules like sugar, protein, and the dyes used for intravenous pyelography raise the specific gravity of the urine proportionately much more than its osmolality. The reverse is true of relatively small molecules like urea [92].

Figure 3-11 shows the relation between specific gravity and osmolality for a large number of urine specimens of widely differing concentration and composition. It is clear that relatively large differences in osmolality among various urines may not be reflected in their specific gravity because of variations in the exact nature of the urine solutes. Fur-

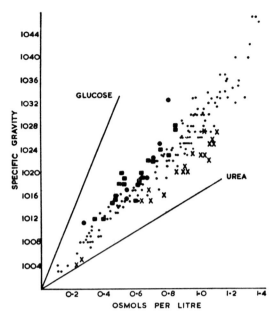

Figure 3-11. Relation between osmolality and specific gravity of urine. Different urines are shown as follows: no sugar or protein (•); 3+ sugar (•); 3+ protein (■); after 25 gm. of urea by mouth (×). The lines show the relation of specific gravity to osmolality for pure glucose and urea solutions. (From Miles, B. E., Paton, A., and de Wardener, H. E. [174]; reproduced by permission.)

thermore, the measurement of specific gravity with a hydrometer, though simple, is technically crude in comparison with the precision with which osmolality can be determined. Obviously, maximal specific gravity can serve only as an approximate measure of concentrating function. In spite of these limitations, much useful clinical information about the concentrating function can be obtained from measurements of maximal urine specific gravity. The technical limitations of urinometry can be minimized by attention to detail. Glassware should be clean and free of detergent which may alter surface tension and hence apparent specific gravity; each new hydrometer should be calibrated in distilled water, and measurements should be made at the temperature at which the instrument has been calibrated (commonly 15° or 20°C.).

FACTORS AFFECTING MAXIMAL CONCENTRATING ABILITY

Most clinical tests of concentrating function depend on measurements of maximal urine specific gravity in suitably dehydrated subjects. It has already been explained that total *solute excretion* as well as urea excretion may affect maximal concentration. Since both of these rates are normally dependent in large part on diet, one might expect that careful attention to prior diet might be necessary for proper interpretation of concentration tests. In clinical practice, however, it is sufficient to collect urines after the customary overnight fast in dehydrated patients who have previously eaten a normal diet.* Rigorous diet control prior to the test, such as the special three-day diets proposed by Lashmet and Newburgh [141], seems to add little value to the specific gravity measurements. However, some attention should be paid to an adequate *protein intake* prior to the test, since maximal urine concentration is reduced by a protein-deficient diet [81]. It should also be borne in mind that, irrespective of diet, high rates of solute excretion which might diminish maximal concentration can occur in a variety of clinical conditions — for example, in patients with glucosuria or in those undergoing diuresis of edema fluid.

In clinical testing, maximal urine concentration is usually arbitrarily defined as that obtained after a specified period of dehydration. It should be understood, however, that in many normal subjects urine osmolality may continue to increase slightly as the *period of dehydration* is prolonged. In Figure 3-12 are plotted some data of Miles et al. [174] showing that at least 22 hours of dehydration are required for normal subjects to achieve 90 per cent or more of the final "maximum" concen-

* This statement does not apply to infants. On ordinary diets they are unable to concentrate as well as adults, but it has been shown that the addition of urea or protein to their diet and sufficient prior restriction of fluid overcome this deficiency [77].

tration after 30 hours of dehydration. Hence, in tests employing substantially shorter periods of dehydration occasional patients with normal renal function may be expected to excrete urine significantly less concentrated than the true maximum which they can achieve.

To avoid the inconvenience of prolonged dehydration, long-acting *vasopressin* preparations may be used as an alternative stimulus to urine concentration. In this case, fluid intake need not be restricted. However, the urine concentrations achieved after dehydration are normally somewhat greater (100 to 300 mOsm per kilogram of water) than those obtained when vasopressin is given without fluid restriction [174]. There is apparently little or no difference between dehydration and exogenous vasopressin in patients with reduced concentrating ability [64, 174].

The difference in normal subjects between the effects of dehydration and exogenous vasopressin on urine concentration suggests that water restriction increases urine concentration not only by promoting the secretion of antidiuretic hormone but by some other mechanisms as well. Evidence to this effect also comes from studies of patients with compulsive polydipsia and of normal subjects who drink large volumes of fluid in experimental studies. After several days of excessive fluid intake, subjects with normal renal function may have gross defects in urine-concentrating ability during subsequent dehydration [66, 80]. Obviously, in ordinary clinical work concentration tests cannot be accepted as reliable indicators of tubular function if *prior fluid intake* has been abnormally large.

TEST PROCEDURES

Many specific procedures for testing urine-concentrating ability have been described, each differing from the others largely in terms of such factors as the length of dehydration and the emphasis placed on control of previous diet [5, 85, 141]. In the light of the various factors discussed above, the following pro-

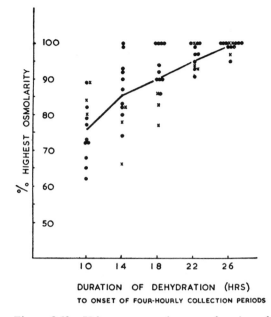

Figure 3-12. Urine concentration as a function of length of dehydration in a group of normal subjects. The osmolality is given as a percentage of the highest osmolality attained by each subject during 30 hours of dehydration. (From Miles, B. E., Paton, A., and de Wardener, H. E. [174]; reproduced by permission.)

cedure can be recommended. If a random urine specific gravity is 1.023 or more, concentrating function may be considered intact within the limits of clinical testing and no further studies need be done. If the specific gravity is less than 1.023, the subject is instructed to take no more fluids after breakfast on a given day and to void and discard after awakening the following morning. The specific gravity of the next voided specimen is determined.

NORMAL RESULTS AND INTERPRETATION OF CONCENTRATION TESTS

Normal subjects taking an average diet and drinking ordinary volumes of fluid prior to the above test should be able to concentrate their urines to a specific gravity of 1.026 or more [5, 151]. Although the maximal specific gravity tends to fall slightly with increasing age, subjects up to the age of 65 should still be able to reach this maximum. Even patients in their nineties can concentrate to 1.023 [151]. In view of the minimal control, in tests of this general type, of the various physiologic factors affecting urine concentration, it is obvious that so-called normal standards should not be interpreted too rigidly. For example, Storey [255] found that 10 to 25 per cent of a large group of subjects carefully selected for the absence of impaired renal function were unable to reach the standard maximal specific gravity even after repeated retesting. Like any other factor in the evaluation of a patient with possible renal disease, the concentration test must be interpreted in the light of the total clinical picture.

Certain technical points already alluded to are worth reemphasis. Tests should not be done when drugs or medications that unpredictably elevate specific gravity out of proportion to osmolality (e.g., the dyes used for intravenous pyelography) are likely to be in the urine. The temperature of the urine at the time of measurement should be that at which the urinometer has been calibrated; for each 3°C. above or below this temperature, 0.001 should be added to or subtracted from the observed value. If proteinuria is present, 0.003 should be subtracted from the observed reading for each 10 gm. of protein per liter [141]. When for any reason a solute diuresis is present, the concentration test cannot be interpreted as a measure of tubular function and should not be performed. A correction factor of 0.003 or 0.004 for each 10 gm. of glucose per liter of urine is sometimes employed. However, marked glucosuria represents a solute diuresis and under these circumstances the concentration test is invalid for the reasons already discussed. In the presence of the solute diuresis regularly associated with azotemia, the test is worthless as an independent measure of renal function. Furthermore, dehydration may involve some risk to the patient.

Fluid restriction can be avoided by giving the patient 5 units of vasopressin [64, 174] in oil and collecting urine specimens at any time in the next 24 hours.* Fluids and food may be taken ad lib. during this time. Normal values for this procedure have not been firmly established, but urine specific gravity over 1.020 is adequate clinical evidence of normal concentrating function since, as already noted, in normal subjects urine concentration after vasopressin tends to be somewhat lower than after prolonged dehydration. Vasopressin should not be administered to patients with possible coronary artery disease because it is a coronary vasoconstrictor. The special use of vasopressin and dehydration tests in differentiating diabetes insipidus and allied conditions has been reviewed by de Wardener [65].

DILUTION TESTS

Dilution of the urine, like concentration, is a tubular function and theoretically can be used as a measure of tubular functional integrity. While both are intrinsically distal tubular functions, they are neither anatomically nor functionally precisely coextensive. Moreover, antidiuretic hormone is required for maximal concentration of the urine but not for dilution. It is therefore possible for concentration and dilution of the urine to be affected more or less independently in the course of a pathologic process. In addition to the obvious case of the various forms of diabetes insipidus, defects in concentration with preservation of diluting ability may occur in potassium depletion, sickle cell disease, and possibly in pyelonephritis [212] and hyperparathyroidism [56]. Diluting ability may be grossly defective and concentrating ability relatively less affected in adrenal insufficiency, hepatic disease, and cardiac failure. In these latter situations extratubular factors such as the ab-

* The vasopressin tannate usually sediments at the bottom of the ampule as a brownish discoloration. It must be thoroughly suspended before use, by shaking and warming in the hand.

sence of adrenal steroids, depressed glomerular filtration rates, or abnormal release and metabolism of antidiuretic hormone are presumably involved.

In practice, dilution tests are much less useful than tests of concentrating ability, because nonspecific factors such as emotion or nausea may interfere with a water diuresis in otherwise normal subjects. A number of protocols for clinical dilution tests have been described [85, 255]. The patient may be given a liter of plain or suitably flavored water to drink in a 30-minute period and urine collected at intervals over the next three hours. In normal subjects the specific gravity of one sample should be less than 1.003. In addition, most normal subjects will excrete more than half of the ingested volume in three hours, although this criterion is particularly variable. Since decreases in filtration rate or the presence of a solute diuresis may prevent the excretion of urines of minimum specific gravity even when tubular function is normal, and since large water loads may lead to water intoxication in patients with reduced glomerular filtration rates, dilution tests are neither useful nor safe in subjects with frank azotemia.

CONCENTRATION AND DILUTION TESTS
IN RENAL DISEASE

The results of tests of concentrating and diluting ability show a fairly characteristic pattern during the course of chronic progressive renal failure [8, 35, 135]. In the early stages of the disease process, before clinical testing shows any significant decrease in glomerular filtration, concentrating function may sometimes be significantly impaired. As the filtration rate falls from three-quarters to one-quarter of normal, maximum urine specific gravity progresses more or less regularly toward 1.010 and diluting capacity becomes progressively limited [135]. It is sometimes stated that concentrating ability is regularly decreased before diluting ability in the course

of chronic renal disease. That such dissociation may occur in some cases has already been indicated. However, some of the apparent preservation of diluting function is undoubtedly merely a technical and conceptual artifact. Conceptually, a 50 per cent fall in maximal osmolality from 1400 to 700 mOsm per kilogram of water is more impressive than a proportionate rise in minimal osmolality from 50 to 100. Moreover, the insensitivity of specific gravity measurements is such that the fall in maximal osmolality might be reflected by an easily measurable decrease of specific gravity from 1.028 to 1.019, whereas the increase in minimal osmolality would perhaps be associated with a rise in specific gravity of from 1.001 to 1.002, still well within "normal limits." By the time that the filtration rate has reached 20 per cent of normal, urine specific gravity has usually become fixed at around 1.010, the specific gravity of the glomerular filtrate. Obviously, as further decreases in filtration rate occur, no additional changes in urine specific gravity can be expected. Hence, it is apparent that the concentration test is much more suitable as a means for detecting functional changes in early renal disease than it is for following the functional progress of chronic renal failure.

The pathophysiology responsible for this pattern of decreasing concentrating and diluting ability in chronic renal disease is not fully understood. Two kinds of factors are thought to be important. On the one hand, it is obvious that specific damage to the sites involved in the concentrating and diluting operations would interfere with their normal function. Hence, when the nature of the pathologic process is such as to damage the loops of Henle, the distal convoluted tubules, or the collecting ducts, or to disrupt the circulation or architecture of the renal medulla, one may reasonably expect relatively early and severe impairment of the concentrating function of the kidney. Such damage probably accounts for the early loss of concentrating ability which is fairly common in pyelonephritis [212]. On the other hand, it has become evident [35, 198, 256] that one mechanism known to depress concentrating capacity is common to all forms of chronic renal failure — namely, the presence of a relative solute diuresis. Since, as renal failure proceeds, the normal load of solute must be excreted by a progressively decreasing number of nephrons, each nephron unit must undergo an osmotic diuresis of increasing intensity. Even in the absence of disproportionate tubular damage, progressive reduction of the number of relatively normal nephrons might of itself be sufficient to account for the gradual development of restricted concentrating and diluting capacity, because of the well-known effects of a solute diuresis on these functions (see Chapter 2). Available data suggest that a relative solute diuresis may well be sufficient to account for the diluting defect [135] but is not the entire explanation for the concentrating defect in chronic renal disease [16, 72, 73, 135].

Occasionally, vasopressin-resistant hyposthenuria, rather than isothenuria, may characterize certain patients with renal damage due to obstruction [22, 223, 279], hypercalcemia [223, 284], amyloidosis [47], sarcoidosis [194], and potassium depletion [227]. Recent reports indicate that patients with a variety of common types of advanced renal disease, including pyelonephritis and glomerulonephritis, not infrequently respond to exogenous vasopressin and dehydration with the excretion of slightly hypotonic urine [116, 134, 258]. The excretion of urine hypotonic to plasma in spite of the presence of adequate amounts of antidiuretic hormone sometimes occurs during extreme osmotic diuresis. An increase in the solute load per nephron may therefore explain the hyposthenuria in patients with advanced azotemia. However, in other patients a decrease in the intrinsic permeability of the distal tubules or a decrease in tubular response to antidiuretic hormone would seem to be a more likely explanation.

Phenolsulfonphthalein Excretion

In 1923 Marshall and Vickers [166] showed that phenolsulfonphthalein (PSP) was excreted into the urine much faster than it could be supplied by any likely rate of glomerular filtration, and thereby provided the first unequivocal demonstration of tubular secretion in the mammalian kidney. It was, however, on the purely empiric grounds that PSP is excreted very rapidly that Rowntree and Gheraghty [226] had suggested some dozen years earlier that PSP excretion could be a useful clinical test of tubular function. The value of the test was greatly enhanced when Chapman [50, 51] suggested that PSP excretion be measured separately in fractional urine specimens rather than in terms of total two-hour excretion as described by Rowntree and Gheraghty.

PSP is remarkably nontoxic; in a review of the English-language literature we were unable to find a single reported instance of a toxic effect attributed to PSP administration. The analytic methods for PSP are so simple that they can easily be performed without the assistance of a clinical laboratory. PSP is not metabolized, and the greater part of an administered dose is rapidly excreted via the kidneys. For all these reasons, measurement of the rate of PSP excretion has become a popular and useful empiric test of renal function.

MECHANISM OF EXCRETION OF PSP

Physiologic studies have indicated that at the plasma levels of PSP attained in the course of the clinical test, PSP excretion is ordinarily a measure not of tubular excretory capacity, as originally assumed, but of the renal plasma flow. Tubular capacity to excrete PSP does not become saturated until the plasma level reaches 1 mg. per 100 ml. [102]. With the usual 6 mg. clinical dose, plasma PSP is probably no more than one-fifth of this value. Hence, in the normal subject the limiting factor in PSP excretion is the rate of delivery to the tubules via the renal plasma flow, not tubular excretory capacity. Only when tubular transport mechanisms are grossly reduced without a comparable fall in plasma flow does the rate of PSP excretion become to any great extent a function of tubular excretory capacity.

At the plasma concentrations to be expected in the clinical test, more than 80 per cent of the PSP in the blood is bound to albumin [102] and therefore only about 4 per cent of the PSP which reaches the kidney can be excreted by glomerular filtration.* The rest passes into the peritubular circulation, from which it is removed by the cells of the proximal convolutions. Since competitive inhibition in the excretion of PSP, para-aminohippurate (PAH), Diodrast, penicillin, and a number of other substances has been demonstrated [245, 246], it is assumed that they are secreted into the urine via a common transport mechanism. PAH is almost completely (92 per cent) removed in one circulation through the kidney, and the clearance of PAH is therefore a measure of renal plasma flow (see Chapter 2). However, only 50 to 60 per cent of the PSP which reaches the kidney is extracted in one circulation [244, 246]; hence, the clearance of PSP is only an approximate index of plasma flow to the kidney.

In the clinical test a single intravenous dose of PSP is given. Since, at the plasma levels achieved, tubular transport capacity for PSP is not saturated, the rate of excretion of PSP is proportional to its concentration in the plasma. Hence, the absolute rate of removal is fastest just after PSP is given, and it decreases rapidly thereafter. If sufficient time is allowed for repeated recirculations, even the kidney with markedly diminished plasma flow may finally excrete a relatively normal

amount of PSP. Therefore, the rate of excretion during the first few minutes after PSP is given is the most sensitive indicator of the decreased renal circulation.

In two hours, 60 to 85 per cent of a 6 mg. dose of PSP is excreted by the kidneys. The final disposition of the remaining PSP has not been studied in man. When 3 mg. of PSP is given, 85 to 98 per cent is excreted into the urine in four hours [58]. In dogs, part of a subcutaneous dose of PSP is excreted into the bile initially, but it is later apparently reabsorbed in the intestinal tract, since little or no PSP appears in the feces [1]. Patients with liver disease may excrete an unusually high proportion of a 6 mg. dose of PSP in two hours, suggesting impaired excretion into the bile [277]. While there is no direct evidence on this point, it would seem to be a reasonable inference from these various observations that part of the clinical 6 mg. dose of PSP in man is initially excreted into the bile, but that this is later reabsorbed and excreted by the kidneys, so that final urinary excretion is nearly complete.

THE PSP TEST AND ITS INTERPRETATION

The details of the test as ordinarily done are as follows: The patient drinks two or three glasses of water 30 minutes before the PSP is to be given. Exactly 1 ml. of PSP solution containing 6 mg. of PSP is rapidly given intravenously and the exact time noted. It is essential that this dose be measured very accurately with a 1 ml. syringe since interpretation of the result of the test is wholly dependent on the exact amount of PSP administered. For the same reason, it is important to look for any evidence of extravasation of the dye into the tissues. Urine specimens are obtained precisely 15, 30, 60, and 120 minutes after the dye is given. The patient should not void just before the PSP is administered, since he may then find it difficult to void again in 15 minutes. Supplementary fluid intake during the test may be necessary to facilitate

---

* The glomerular filtration rate is about 20 per cent of the renal plasma flow and only the fraction of the PSP in plasma not bound to albumin is filtrable; hence, 0.20 times 0.20, or about 4 per cent, of the total PSP reaching the kidney is filtered.

voiding. An aliquot of each urine specimen is diluted appropriately and alkalinized to develop maximum red color, which is then compared with appropriate standards, either visually or by the use of a colorimeter. Bromsulphalein (BSP) gives a similar color and therefore BSP and PSP tests should not be done on the same day. If blood or bile is present in the urine in large amounts, it may be necessary to precipitate them from the urine prior to color development since they interfere with the reading [9]. The normal values for fractional PSP excretion are shown in Table 3-2 [51].

Table 3-2. Excretion of PSP by Normal Subjects

Time (minutes)	Excretion of PSP (per cent)		
	Minimum	Maximum	Average
15	28	51	35
30	13	24	17
60	9	17	12
120	3	10	6
Total for 2 hr.	63	84	70

This test should be interpreted as a rough measure of renal plasma flow, as already discussed. There is evidence that PSP excretion is correlated linearly with renal plasma flow (PAH clearance) in man, but PSP excretion at any given plasma flow may vary over a wide range [95, 173]. The 15-minute excretion is by far the most significant value, because even a damaged kidney may remove normal amounts of PSP from the plasma in the number of circulations through the kidney afforded by the two-hour interval. Thus, in their original paper Rowntree and Geraghty [226] showed that removal of half the normal kidney mass experimentally did not alter two-hour PSP excretion. This has been confirmed in the clinical studies of Van Slyke et al. [267], who found that two-hour PSP excretion was nor-

mal in half of their patients whose urea clearances were in the range of 40 to 60 per cent of normal, and in one-fourth of patients whose clearances were 20 to 40 per cent of normal. The increased sensitivity of the fractional test is illustrated in the data of Chapman [51], who found that about one-third of his patients with renal disease excreted abnormally low amounts of PSP in 15 minutes but normal amounts in two hours.

A variation of the PSP test which has recently been described [94, 95] avoids errors due to problems in collecting adequate urine specimens. In this procedure, a plasma PSP index is calculated from the rate of decrease of PSP in plasma 15 to 35 minutes after injection of 1 mg. of PSP per kilogram of body weight intravenously. A single venipuncture suffices for PSP injection and blood sampling, since an in-dwelling venous catheter is used. This test correlates very closely with the 15-minute PSP excretion. The advantage of the plasma PSP index is that urine collections are not required, which eliminates errors due to such factors as antidiuresis and incomplete voiding. The principal disadvantage is the somewhat greater amount of analytic work required.

The PSP test, like tests of concentrating ability, is primarily useful for the detection of functional damage early in the course of renal disease. PSP excretion may be decreased before clinical tests demonstrate a significant fall in glomerular filtration rate [51]. When renal disease has progressed to the point of azotemia, PSP excretion will almost uniformly be decreased [51, 90], and the rapid hydration required for the test may be uncomfortable or even dangerous. Hence, it is not recommended in the presence of azotemia. Since the PSP test correlates best with renal blood flow, excretion may be diminished even when intrinsic kidney function is normal if renal blood flow is decreased by extrarenal factors such as oligemia or severe congestive heart failure [157, 178]. The 15-minute PSP excretion may also be reduced in the last trimester of pregnancy [90, 91], even if the urine is obtained via catheter. However, the two-hour excretion is usually normal. Transplacental circulation of PSP and the effects of upper urinary tract dilatation have been invoked to account for this phenomenon.

Technical or physiologic considerations unrelated to renal function may sometimes result in abnormal patterns of excretion in the fractional test. Greater excretion in a later specimen than in the 15-minute urine suggests either incomplete emptying of the bladder or subcutaneous extravasation and later slow release of the administered PSP. If two-hour total excretion is more than 85 per cent, it is likely either that an overdose of PSP was given or that hepatic excretion of the dye has been reduced by liver disease [277]. Excretion in the first 15 minutes is not affected by liver disease [277].

PSP AS A TEST FOR BLADDER RESIDUAL

Cotran and Kass [58] have suggested an ingenious use for PSP as a measure of bladder residual without the need for catheterization. The patient voids (this urine is discarded) and then 3 mg. of PSP is given intravenously. Three hours later the patient voids and drinks a glass of water. After another hour he urinates again. Since renal excretion of PSP normally is essentially complete within three hours, it can be assumed that all the dye in the second specimen is present because of incomplete bladder emptying during the first voiding. The bladder residual (V_R) can then be calculated from a knowledge of the concentrations of PSP in the two specimens (C_1 and C_2) and the volume of the second specimen (V_2):

$$V_R = \frac{C_2 V_2}{C_1 - C_2}$$

Direct comparison of this method with catheterization gave satisfactory checks.

This test is not applicable in patients with

reduced renal PSP excretion, in whom the assumption that all the PSP has been excreted in three hours may not be correct. For this reason, Cotran and Kass suggest that the test be considered invalid when the two urine specimens contain less than 85 per cent of the administered PSP. Also implicit in the procedure is the assumption that the residual volume after each of the two voidings is the same. Since results from this procedure are in good agreement with those obtained by catheterization, this assumption is in most cases apparently sufficiently valid for clinical purposes.

Correlation of Clinical Function Tests

By the use of specific physiologic technics, such as the clearance of inulin, PAH clearance, and PAH Tm, it has been found that certain functional patterns are in a general way characteristic of many of the more common types of renal disease [33, 74, 75]. For example, in the early phases of nephrosclerosis caused by benign hypertension, renal plasma flow tends to be decreased out of proportion to the reduction in filtration rate and tubular transport capacity for PAH. In acute glomerulonephritis, the glomerular filtration rate is commonly reduced out of proportion to the variable falls in renal plasma flow and tubular transport functions which may occur; this relative predominance of glomerular involvement tends to persist into the chronic stage of glomerulonephritis even after plasma flow and tubular transport functions begin to decline. In pyelonephritis, disproportionate depression of the transport function of the tubules is common. However, it should be noted that even with the relatively specific physiologic tests, there are many individual exceptions to these general functional patterns, and such studies have very limited diagnostic value.

It has been emphasized that the clinical

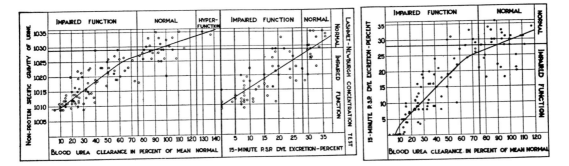

Figure 3-13. Correlation of clinical renal function tests in patients with chronic glomerulonephritis. Urea clearance, concentrating ability, and PSP excretion in each patient were measured on the same day. (From Freyberg, R. H. [90]; reproduced by permission.)

tests are relatively crude and correlate only imperfectly with the specific functional capacities of the kidney. It is therefore not surprising that the patterns described above are somewhat difficult to discern from the relative changes in the clinical function tests. Data correlating the clinical clearance tests with concentrating ability and fractional PSP excretion are rather scarce. In Figure 3-13 are shown the observations of Freyberg [90] in a group of patients with chronic glomerulonephritis. The predominance of glomerular impairment so often evident from more specific tests is not apparent from the data in Figure 3-13, which on the whole show a proportionate decrease in the three clinical function tests. In occasional cases in which the urea clearance is normal, however, PSP excretion or concentrating ability may be reduced, and less commonly, the reverse situation is seen. Similarly, the observations of Van Slyke and his collaborators [267] show that an early and persistent depression of concentrating ability out of proportion to the changing urea clearance often occurs in acute glomerulonephritis; this observation is somewhat unexpected from the specific functional pattern noted above.

To summarize, clinical tests of renal function are useful, first, in the recognition and evaluation of acute or early chronic renal disease and, second, as a quantitative index of the progress of established disease. They are not likely to be of much use in differential diagnosis. In acute and early chronic disease, each of the clinical tests may at times give evidence of functional damage when the results of the other tests are normal (see Figure 3-13). Hence, creatinine clearance, concentrating ability, and PSP excretion should all be measured in the initial workup of patients with early renal disease, and serial measurements of any or all may be helpful in evaluating the progress of the disorder. With rare exceptions, when azotemia supervenes, PSP and concentration tests change more or less in proportion to the decreasing filtration rate. When glomerular filtration is greatly reduced maximum specific gravity becomes fixed near 1.010 and can no longer reflect changes in glomerular filtration rate. PSP excretion is already minimal and changes in excretion become too small to be evaluated. Serial measurements of the filtration rate are therefore the only suitable method of following chronic azotemic renal disease. The reasons for considering measurements of creatinine clearance and plasma creatinine as the best means to this end have already been discussed in detail.

References

1. Abel, J. J., and Rowntree, L. G. On the pharmacological action of some phthaleins and their derivatives, with especial reference to their behavior as purgatives. I. *J. Pharmacol. Exp. Ther.* 1:231, 1909.

2. Addis, T. Renal failure casts. *J.A.M.A.* 84:1013, 1925.

3. Addis, T. The number of formed elements in the urinary sediment of normal individuals. *J. Clin. Invest.* 2:409, 1926.

4. Addis, T. *Glomerular Nephritis.* New York: Macmillan, 1948.

5. Addis, T., and Shevky, M. C. A test of the capacity of the kidney to produce a urine of high specific gravity. *Arch. Intern. Med.* 30:558, 1922.

6. Addis, T., Barrett, E., Poo, L. J., Ureen, H. J., and Lippman, R. W. The relation between protein consumption and diurnal variations of the endogenous creatinine clearance in normal individuals. *J. Clin. Invest.* 30:206, 1951.

7. Alving, A. S., and Van Slyke, D. D. The significance of concentration and dilution tests in Bright's disease. *J. Clin. Invest.* 13:969, 1934.

8. Alyea, E. P., and Parish, H. H., Jr. Renal response to exercise: Urinary findings. *J.A.M.A.* 167:807, 1958.

9. Annino, J. S. *Clinical Chemistry: Principles and Procedures* (3d ed.). Boston: Little, Brown, 1964.

10. Annino, J. S., and Relman, A. S. The effect of eating on some of the clinically important chemical constituents of the blood. *Amer. J. Clin. Path.* 31:155, 1959.

11. Antoine, B., Symvoulidis, A., and Dardenne, M. La stabilité évolutive des états de proteinurie permanente isolée. *Nephron* 6:526, 1969.

12. Arnett, J. H., and Gardner, K. D., Jr. Urinary abnormalities from over-use of muscles. *Amer. J. Med. Sci.* 241:55, 1961.

13. Aukland, K. Stop flow analysis of renal protein excretion in the dog. *Scand. J. Clin. Lab. Invest.* 12:300, 1960.

14. Austin, J. H., Stillman, E., and Van Slyke, D. D. Factors governing the excretion rate of urea. *J. Biol. Chem.* 46:91, 1921.

15. Baldwin, D. S., Sirota, J. H., and Villarreal, H. Diurnal variations of renal function in congestive heart failure. *Proc. Soc. Exp. Biol. Med.* 74:578, 1950.

16. Baldwin, D. S., Berman, H. J., Heinemann, H. O., and Smith, H. W. The elaboration of osmotically concentrated urine in renal disease. *J. Clin. Invest.* 34:800, 1955.

17. Bank, N., Mutz, B. F., and Aynedian, H. S. The role of "leakage" of tubular fluid in anuria due to mercury poisoning. *J. Clin. Invest.* 46:695, 1967.

18. Barrett, E., and Addis, T. The serum creatinine concentration of normal individuals. *J. Clin. Invest.* 26:875, 1947.

19. Bayliss, L. E., Kerridge, P. M. T., and Russell, D. S. The excretion of protein by the mammalian kidney. *J. Physiol.* (London) 77:386, 1933.

20. Bence Jones, H. On a new substance occurring in the urine of a patient with mollities ossium. *Phil. Trans. Roy. Soc. London* 138:55, 1848.

21. Berlyne, G. M., Varley, H., Nilwarangkur, S., and Hoerni, M. Endogenous creatinine clearance and glomerular filtration rate. *Lancet* 2:874, 1964.

22. Berlyne, G. M. Distal tubular function in chronic hydronephrosis. *Quart. J. Med.* 30:339, 1961.

23. Berman, L. B., Schreiner, G. E., and Feys, J. O. Observations on the glitter-cell phenomenon. *New Eng. J. Med.* 255:989, 1956.

24. Berggärd, I. Studies on the plasma proteins in normal human urine. *Clin. Chim. Acta* 6:413, 1961.

25. Berggärd, I., Cleve, H., and Bearn, A. G. The excretion of five plasma proteins previously unidentified in normal human urine. *Clin. Chim. Acta* 10:1, 1964.

26. Bing, J. Studies on proteinuria. *Acta Med. Scand.* Suppl. 76, 1936.

27. Blainey, J. D., Brewer, D. B., Hardwicke, J., and Soothill, J. F. The nephrotic syndrome. *Quart. J. Med.* 29:235, 1960.

28. Bolande, R. P. Inclusion-bearing cells in

the urine in certain viral infections. *Pediatrics* 24:7, 1959.

29. Boyarsky, S., and Smith, H. W. Renal concentrating operation at low urine flows. *J. Urol.* 78:511, 1957.

30. Boyce, W. H., and King, J. S., Jr. Total nondialyzable solids (TNDS) in human urine: IV. Electrophoretic properties of RS-1 subfraction. *J. Clin. Invest.* 38:1525, 1959.

31. Boyce, W. H., and King, J. S., Jr. Total Nondialyzable Solids in Human Urine: IV. Pyelonephritis of Bacterial Origin. In Quinn, E. L., and Kass, E. H. (Eds.), *Biology of Pyelonephritis.* (Henry Ford Hospital International Symposium.) Boston: Little, Brown, 1960. P. 551.

32. Boyce, W. H., Garvey, F. K., and Norfleet, C. M., Jr. Proteins and other biocolloids of urine in health and in calculous disease: I. Electrophoretic studies at pH 4.5 and 8.6 of those components soluble in molar sodium chloride. *J. Clin. Invest.* 33:1287, 1954.

33. Bradley, S. E., Bradley, G. P., Tyson, C. J., Curry, J. J., and Blake, W. D. Renal function in renal diseases. *Amer. J. Med.* 9:766, 1950.

34. Breckenridge, A., and Metcalfe-Gilson, A. Methods of measuring glomerular-filtration rate. *Lancet* 2:265, 1965.

35. Bricker, N. S., Morrin, P. A. F., and Kime, S. W., Jr. The pathologic physiology of chronic Bright's disease. *Amer. J. Med.* 28:77, 1960.

36. Bricker, N. S., Klahr, S., Lubowitz, H., and Rieselbach, R. E. Renal function in chronic renal disease. *Medicine* (Balt.) 44:263, 1965.

37. Bright, R. *Reports of Medical Cases.* London: Longmans, Rees, Orme, Brown and Green, 1827.

38. Broch, O. J., and Brodwall, E. Urinary proteins in renal diseases. *Acta Med. Scand.* 160:353, 1958.

39. Brod, J., and Sirota, J. H. The renal clearance of endogenous "creatinine" in man. *J. Clin. Invest.* 27:645, 1948.

40. Brody, L., Webster, M. C., and Kark, R. M. Identification of urinary sediment with

41. Bruger, M. Cholesteroluria in Bright's disease. *Amer. J. Clin. Path.* 5:504, 1935.

42. Bucht, H. On the tubular excretion of thiosulphate and creatinine under the influence of caronamide. *Scand. J. Clin. Lab. Invest.* 1:270, 1949.

43. Bull, G. M. Postural proteinuria. *Clin. Sci.* 7:77, 1948.

44. Burnett, C. H. The Actions of ACTH and Cortisone on Renal Function in Man. In *Transactions of the Second Conference on Renal Function.* New York: Josiah Macy, Jr. Foundation, 1950. P. 106.

45. Butler, E. A., and Flynn, F. V. The proteinuria of renal tubular disorders. *Lancet* 2:978, 1958.

46. Cameron, J. S., and Blandford, G. The simple assessment of selectivity in heavy proteinuria. *Lancet* 2:242, 1966.

47. Carone, F. A., and Epstein, F. H. Nephrogenic diabetes insipidus caused by amyloid disease: Evidence in man of role of collecting ducts in concentrating urine. *Amer. J. Med.* 29:539, 1960.

48. Castellanos, H., and Sturgis, S. H. Cytology of human urinary sediment: Diagnostic value of the non-nucleated cell. *J. Clin. Endocr.* 18:1369, 1958.

49. Castenfors, J., Mossfeldt, F., and Piscator, M. Effect of prolonged heavy exercise on renal function and urinary protein excretion. *Acta Physiol. Scand.* 70:194, 1967.

50. Chapman, E. M. Further experience with the fractional 'phthalein test. *New Eng. J. Med.* 214:16, 1936.

51. Chapman, E. M., and Halstead, J. A. The fractional phenolsulphonephthalein test in Bright's disease. *Amer. J. Med. Sci.* 186:223, 1933.

52. Chasis, H., and Smith, H. W. The excretion of urea in normal man and in subjects with glomerulonephritis. *J. Clin. Invest.* 17:347, 1938.

53. Chesley, L. C. Renal excretion at low urine volumes and the mechanism of oliguria. *J. Clin. Invest.* 17:591, 1938.

54. Chesley, L. C., Markowitz, I., and Wetchler, B. B. Proteinuria following momen-

tary vascular constriction. *J. Clin. Invest.* 18:51, 1939.

55. Chinard, F. P., Lauson, H. D., Eder, H. A., Greif, R. L., and Hiller, A. A study of the mechanism of proteinuria in patients with the nephrotic syndrome. *J. Clin. Invest.* 33: 621, 1954.

56. Cohen, S. I., Fitzgerald, M. G., Fourman, P., Griffiths, W. J., and de Wardener, H. E. Polyuria in hyperparathyroidism. *Quart. J. Med.* 26:423, 1957.

57. Comings, D. E. Anisotropic lipids and urinary cholesterol excretion. *J.A.M.A.* 183: 128, 1963.

58. Cotran, R. S., and Kass, E. H. Determination of the volume of residual urine in the bladder without catheterization. *New Eng. J. Med.* 259:337, 1958.

59. Coye, R. D., and Rosandich, R. R. Proteinuria during the 24-hour period following exercise. *J. Appl. Physiol.* 15:592, 1960.

60. Crawford, B. Depression of the exogenous creatinine/inulin or thiosulfate clearance ratios in man by Diodrast and p-aminohippuric acid. *J. Clin. Invest.* 27:171, 1948.

61. Creeth, J. M., Kekwick, R. A., Flynn, F. V., Harris, H., and Robson, E. B. An ultracentrifuge study of urine proteins with particular reference to the proteinuria of renal tubular disorders. *Clin. Chim. Acta* 8:406, 1963.

62. Davidson, I., and Henry, J. B. H. (Eds.). *Todd-Stanford Clinical Diagnosis by Laboratory Methods* (14th ed.). Philadelphia: W. B. Saunders, 1969.

63. Derow, H. A. The diagnostic value of serial measurements of albuminuria in ambulatory patients. *New Eng. J. Med.* 277: 827, 1942.

64. de Wardener, H. E. Vasopressin tannate in oil and the urine concentration test. *Lancet* 2:1037, 1956.

65. de Wardener, H. E. Polyuria. *J. Chronic Dis.* 11:199, 1960.

66. de Wardener, H. E., and Herxheimer, A. W. The effect of a high water intake on the kidney's ability to concentrate the urine in man. *J. Physiol.* (London) 139:42, 1957.

67. Diehl, H. S., and McKinley, C. A. Albu-

minuria in Young Men. In Berglund, H., and Medes, G. (Eds.), *The Kidney in Health and Disease.* Philadelphia: Lea & Febiger, 1935. Chap. 28.

68. Dirks, J. H., Clapp, J. R., and Berliner, R. W. The protein concentration in the proximal tubule of the dog. *J. Clin. Invest.* 43:916, 1964.

69. Dock, W. Proteinuria and the associated renal changes. *New Eng. J. Med.* 227: 633, 1942.

70. Dodge, W. F., Travis, L. B., and Daeschner, C. W. Comparison of endogenous creatinine clearance with inulin clearance. *Amer. J. Dis. Child.* 113:683, 1967.

71. Doolan, P. D., Alpen, E. L., and Theil, G. B. A clinical appraisal of the plasma concentration and endogenous clearance of creatinine. *Amer. J. Med.* 32:65, 1962.

72. Dorhout Mees, E. J. Role of osmotic diuresis in impairment in concentrating ability in renal disease. *Brit. Med. J.* 1:1156, 1959.

73. Dorhout Mees, E. J. Relation between maximal urine concentration, maximal water reabsorption capacity, and mannitol clearance in patients with renal disease. *Brit. Med. J.* 1:1159, 1959.

74. Dustan, H. P., and Corcoran, A. C. Functional interpretation of renal tests. *Med. Clin. N. Amer.* 39:947, 1955.

75. Earle, D. P., Jr. Renal function tests in the diagnosis of glomerular and tubular disease. *Bull. N.Y. Acad. Med.* 26:47, 1950.

76. Edelman, G. M., and Gally, J. A. The nature of Bence Jones proteins. *J. Exp. Med.* 116:207, 1962.

77. Edelmann, C. M., Jr., Barnett, H. L., and Troupkou, V. Renal concentrating mechanisms in newborn infants. *J. Clin. Invest.* 39:1062, 1960.

78. Edwards, K. D. G., and Whyte, H. M. Plasma creatinine level and creatinine clearance as tests of renal function. *Aust. Ann. Med.* 8:218, 1959.

79. Enger, E., and Blegen, E. M. The relationship between endogenous creatinine clearance and serum creatinine in renal failure. *Scand. J. Clin. Lab. Invest.* 16:273, 1964.

80. Epstein, F. H., Kleeman, C. R., and Hendrikx, A. The influence of bodily hydration on the renal concentrating process. *J. Clin. Invest.* 36:629, 1957.

81. Epstein, F. H., Kleeman, C. R., Pursel, S., and Hendrikx, A. The effect of feeding protein and urea on the renal concentrating process. *J. Clin. Invest.* 36:635, 1957.

82. Farquhar, M. C., and Palade, G. E. Segregation of ferritin in glomerular protein absorption droplets. *J. Biophys. Biochem. Cytol.* 7:297, 1960.

83. Farquhar, M. C., Vernier, R. L., and Good, R. A. An electron microscope study of the glomerulus in nephrosis, glomerulonephritis, and lupus erythematosus. *J. Exp. Med.* 106:649, 1957.

84. Farquhar, M. C., Wissig, S. L., and Palade, G. E. Glomerular permeability: I. Ferritin transfer across the normal glomerular capillary wall. *J. Exp. Med.* 113:47, 1961.

85. Fishberg, A. M. *Hypertension and Nephritis* (5th ed.). Philadelphia: Lea & Febiger, 1954.

86. Folin, O. Laws governing the chemical composition of urine. *Amer. J. Physiol.* 13:66, 1905.

87. Frank, M. N., Dreifus, L. S., Rarick, F., and Bellet, S. Urinary osmolar concentration in the hydropenic state as a measure of renal tubular function: A test for early renal impairment: Preliminary report. *Amer. J. Med. Sci.* 233:121, 1957.

88. Franklin, E. C. Physicochemical and immunologic studies of gamma globulins of normal human urine. *J. Clin. Invest.* 38:2159, 1959.

89. Free, A. H., Rupe, C. O., and Metzler, I. Studies with a new colorimetric test for proteinuria. *Clin. Chem.* 3:716, 1957.

90. Freyberg, R. H. The choice and interpretation of tests of renal efficiency. *J.A.M.A.* 105:1575, 1935.

91. Freyberg, R. H., Gillard, J. L., and Ganesbauer, F. A comparison of different methods for measuring renal function during pregnancy. *Amer. J. Obstet. Gynec.* 31:511, 1936.

92. Galambos, J. T., Herndon, E. G., Jr., and Reynolds, G. H. Specific-gravity determinations fact or fancy? *New Eng. J. Med.* 270:506, 1964.

93. Gardner, K. D., Jr. "Athletic pseudonephritis." Alteration of urine sediment by athletic competition. *J.A.M.A.* 161:1613, 1956.

94. Gault, M. H. The plasma phenolsulfonphthalein index (PSPI) of renal function: I. Theoretical consideration and investigative studies. *Canad. Med. Ass. J.* 94:61, 1966.

95. Gault, M. H., Kinsella, T. D., Gonda, A., and Ferguson, G. A. The plasma phenolsulfonphthalein index (PSPI) of renal function: II. Correlation with other parameters of renal function and indications for use. *Canad. Med. Ass. J.* 94:68, 1966.

96. Gilligan, D. R., and Blumgart, H. L. March hemoglobinuria: Studies of clinical characteristics, blood metabolism and mechanism, with observations on three new cases, and a review of the literature. *Medicine* (Balt.) 20:341, 1941.

97. Gitlin, D., and Janeway, C. A. An immunochemical study of the albumins of serum, urine, ascitic fluid and edema fluid in the nephrotic syndrome. *J. Clin. Invest.* 31:223, 1952.

98. Glass, R. H., Risinger, C., Wide, L., and Gemzell, C. A. Urinary albumin/total protein ratio in toxemia of pregnancy. *Amer. J. Obstet. Gynec.* 86:241, 1963.

99. Goldman, R. Creatinine excretion in renal failure. *Proc. Soc. Exp. Biol. Med.* 85:446, 1954.

100. Goldring, W. Studies of the kidney in acute infection: III. Observations with the urine sediment count (Addis) and the urea clearance test in lobar pneumonia. *J. Clin. Invest.* 10:355, 1931.

101. Goldring, W. Clinical application of current tests of renal function. *J.A.M.A.* 153:1245, 1953.

102. Goldring, W., Clarke, R. W., and Smith, H. W. The phenol red clearance in normal man. *J. Clin. Invest.* 15:221, 1936.

103. Grant, G. H. The proteins of normal urine. *J. Clin. Path.* 10:360, 1957.

104. Grant, G. H. The proteins of normal

urine: II. From the urinary tract. *J. Clin. Path.* 12:510, 1959.

105. Gregoire, F., Malmendier, C., and Lambert, P. P.   The mechanism of proteinuria, and a study of the effects of hormonal therapy in the nephrotic syndrome. *Amer. J. Med.* 25:516, 1958.

106. Greiner, T., and Henry, J. P.   Mechanism of postural proteinuria. *J.A.M.A.* 157:1373, 1955.

107. Gunton, R., and Burton, A. C.   On the concentration of protein in samples of normal urine measured by its surface activity. *J. Clin. Invest.* 26:892, 1947.

108. Hall, V.   The protoplasmic basis of glomerular ultrafiltration. *Amer. Heart J.* 54:1, 1957.

109. Hardwicke, J., and Squire, J. R.   The relationship between plasma albumin concentration and protein excretion in patients with proteinuria. *Clin. Sci.* 14:509, 1955.

110. Hare, R. S.   Endogenous creatinine in serum and urine. *Proc. Soc. Exp. Biol. Med.* 74:148, 1950.

111. Harrison, J. F., and Blarney, J. D.   Low molecular weight proteinuria in chronic renal disease. *Clin. Sci.* 33:381, 1967.

112. Harrison, J. F., Blarney, J. D., Hardwicke, J., Rowe, D. S., and Soothill, J. F.   Proteinuria in multiple myeloma. *Clin. Sci.* 31:95, 1966.

113. Haugen, H. N.   The determination of endogenous "creatinine" in plasma and urine. *Scand. J. Clin. Lab. Invest.* 5:48, 1953.

114. Haugen, H. N., and Glegen, E. M.   The true endogenous creatinine clearance. *Scand. J. Clin. Lab. Invest.* 5:67, 1953.

115. Hayman, J. M., Jr., and Bender, J. A.   Nephritic albuminuria. *Arch. Intern. Med.* 51:447, 1933.

116. Holliday, M. A., Egan, T. J., Morris, C. R., Jarrah, A. S., and Harrah, J. L.   Pitressin-resistant hyposthenuria in chronic renal disease. *Amer. J. Med.* 42:378, 1967.

117. Hopper, J., Jr.   Creatinine clearance: A simple way of measuring kidney function. *Bull. Univ. California Med. Center* 2:315, 1951.

118. Houghton, B. J., and Pears, M. A.   Cell excretion in normal urine. *Brit. Med. J.* 1:622, 1957.

119. Houston, I. B.   Urinary white cell excretion in childhood. *Arch. Dis. Child.* 40:313, 1965.

120. Howenstine, J. A.   Exertion-induced myoglobinuria and hemoglobinuria. *J.A.M.A.* 173:493, 1960.

121. Hutt, M. S. R., Chalmers, J. A., MacDonald, J. S., and de Wardener, H. E.   Pyelonephritis: Observations on the relation between various diagnostic procedures. *Lancet* 1:351, 1961.

122. Javitt, N. B., and Miller, A. T., Jr.   Mechanism of exercise proteinuria. *J. Appl. Physiol.* 4:834, 1952.

123. Joachim, G. R., Cameron, J. S., Schwartz, M., and Becker, E. L.   Selectivity of protein excretion in patients with the nephrotic syndrome. *J. Clin. Invest.* 43:2332, 1964.

124. Joint Committee on Mortality. *1951 Impairment Study.* Chicago: Society of Actuaries, 1954.

125. Kaye, M.   A peroxidase-staining procedure for the identification of polymorphonuclear leukocytes and leukocyte casts in the urinary sediment. *New Eng. J. Med.* 258:1301, 1958.

126. Keen, H., and Chlouverakis, C.   An immunoassay method for urinary albumin at low concentrations. *Lancet* 2:913, 1963.

127. King, J. S., Jr., Little, J. M., Boyce, W. H., and Artom, C.   Total nondialyzable solids (TNDS) in human urine: III. A method for subfractionation of RS-1 solids. *J. Clin. Invest.* 38:1520, 1959.

128. King, S. E.   Patterns of protein excretion by the kidneys. *Ann. Intern. Med.* 42:296, 1955.

129. King, S. E.   Postural adjustments and protein excretion by the kidney in renal disease. *Ann. Intern. Med.* 46:360, 1957.

130. King, S. E.   Albuminuria (proteinuria) in renal diseases: II. Preliminary observations on the clinical course of patients with orthostatic albuminuria. *New York J. Med.* 59:825, 1959.

131. King, S. E., and Baldwin, D. S.   Production of renal ischemia and proteinuria in

man by the adrenal medullary hormone. *Amer. J. Med.* 20:217, 1956.

132. Kingsbury, F. B., Clark, C. P., Williams, G., and Post, A. L. The rapid determination of albumin in urine. *J. Lab. Clin. Med.* 11:981, 1926.

133. Kleeman, C. R., Epstein, F. H., and White, C. The effect of variations in solute excretion and glomerular filtration on water diuresis. *J. Clin. Invest.* 35:749, 1956.

134. Kleeman, C. R., Hewitt, W. L., and Guze, L. B. Pyelonephritis. *Medicine* (Balt.) 39: 3, 1960.

135. Kleeman, C. R., Adams, D. A., and Maxwell, M. H. An evaluation of maximal water diuresis in chronic renal disease: I. Normal solute intake. *J. Lab. Clin. Med.* 58:169, 1961.

136. Kleiman, A. H. Athlete's kidney. *J. Urol.* 83:321, 1960.

137. Knights, E. M., Jr., and Jablokow, V. A one-drop method for detection of albuminuria. *J.A.M.A.* 165:1277, 1957.

138. Ladd, M. Renal excretion of sodium and water in man as affected by prehydration, saline infusion, Pitressin and Thiomerin. *J. Appl. Physiol.* 4:602, 1952.

139. Ladd, M., Liddle, L., and Gagnon, J. A. Renal excretion of inulin, creatinine and ferrocyanide at normal and reduced clearance levels in the dog. *Amer. J. Physiol.* 184:505, 1956.

140. Larcom, R. C., Jr., and Carter, G. H. Erythrocytes in urinary sediment: Identification and normal limits. *J. Lab. Clin. Med.* 33:875, 1948.

141. Lashmet, F. H., and Newburgh, L. H. An improved concentration test of renal function. *J.A.M.A.* 99:1396, 1932.

142. Lathem, W. Renal circulatory dynamics and urinary protein excretion during infusions of *l*-norepinephrine and *l*-epinephrine in patients with renal disease. *J. Clin. Invest.* 35:1277, 1956.

143. Lathem, W., Roof, B. S., Nickel, J. F., and Bradley, S. E. Urinary protein excretion and renal hemodynamic adjustments during orthostasis in patients with acute and chronic renal disease. *J. Clin. Invest.* 33: 1457, 1954.

144. Lauson, H. D. Sources of error in plasma creatinine determination. *J. Appl. Physiol.* 4:227, 1951.

145. Lecocq, F. R., McPhaul, J. J., and Robinson, R. R. Fixed and reproducible orthostatic proteinuria: V. Results of a 5-year follow-up evaluation. *Ann. Intern. Med.* 64: 557, 1966.

146. Levinsky, N. G., and Berliner, R. W. Changes in composition of the urine in ureter and bladder at low urine flow. *Amer. J. Physiol.* 196:549, 1959.

147. Levinsky, N. G., Davidson, D. G., and Berliner, R. W. Effects of reduced glomerular filtration on urine concentration in the presence of antidiuretic hormone. *J. Clin. Invest.* 38:730, 1959.

148. Levitt, J. E. The prognostic significance of proteinuria in young college students. *Ann. Intern. Med.* 66:685, 1967.

149. Levitt, M. F., Levy, M. S., and Polimeros, D. The effect of a fall in filtration rate on solute and water excretion in hydropenic man. *J. Clin. Invest.* 38:463, 1959.

150. Lewis, B., and Richards, P. Measurement of urinary protein. *Lancet* 1:1141, 1961.

151. Lewis, W. H., Jr., and Alving, A. S. Changes with age in the renal function in adult men. *Amer. J. Physiol.* 123:500, 1938.

152. Lindeman, R. D., van Buren, H. C., and Raisz, L. G. Osmolar renal concentrating ability in healthy young men and hospitalized patients without renal disease. *New Eng. J. Med.* 262:1306, 1960.

153. Lippman, R. W. *Urine and the Urinary Sediment* (2d ed.). Springfield, Ill.: Charles C Thomas, 1957.

154. Löwgren, E. Studies on benign proteinuria with special reference to the renal lymphatic system. *Acta Med. Scand.* Suppl. 300, 1955.

155. Lubowitz, H., Slatapolsky, E., Shankel, S., Rieselbach, R. E., and Bricker, N. S. Glomerular filtration rate: Determination in patients with chronic renal disease. *J.A.M.A.* 199:252, 1967.

156. Luetscher, J. A., Jr. Electrophoretic analysis of plasma and urinary proteins. *J. Clin. Invest.* 19:313, 1940.

157. Lundsgaard, C., and Møller, E. Investiga-

tions into the value of the phenolsulphon-phthalein test in renal and circulatory diseases. *Acta Med. Scand.* 63:242, 1925.

158. Lyttle, J. D. The Addis sediment count in normal children. *J. Clin. Invest.* 12:87, 1933.

159. MacLean, P. R., and Robson, J. S. Unselective proteinuria in acute ischaemic renal failure. *Clin. Sci.* 30:91, 1966.

160. Magath, T. B. Minimal Albuminuria and Tests for Albumin in the Urine. In Berglund, H., and Medes, G. (Eds.), *The Kidney in Health and Disease*. Philadelphia: Lea & Febiger, 1935. Chap. 27.

161. Maiorca, R., Scarpioni, L., Cambi, V., Carrara, G. C., and Dall'aglio, P. Urinary protein clearances in chronic renal diseases with and without uremia. *Clin. Chim. Acta* 16:253, 1967.

162. Malamos, B., Dontas, A. S., Koutras, D. A., Marketos, S., Sfontouris, J., and Papanicolaou, N. The determination of glomerular filtration rate in clinical practice. *Lancet* 1:943, 1966.

163. Malmendier, C., DeKoster, J. P., and Lambert, P. P. Effects of an increase in plasma volume on glomerular permeability to albumin in proteinuric patients. *Clin. Sci.* 19: 605, 1960.

164. Mandel, E. E., Jones, F. L., Willis, M. J., and Cargill, W. H. Renal excretion of creatinine and inulin in man. *J. Lab. Clin. Med.* 42:621, 1953.

165. Manuel, U., Revillard, J. P., and Betuel, H. (Eds.), *Proteins in Normal and Pathological Urine*. Baltimore: University Park Press, 1970.

166. Marshall, E. K., Jr., and Vickers, J. L. The mechanism of the elimination of phenolsulphonphthalein by the kidney; a proof of secretion by the convoluted tubules. *Bull. Johns Hopkins Hosp.* 34:1, 1923.

167. McGarry, E., Sehon, A. H., and Rose, B. The isolation and characterization of the proteins in the urine of normal subjects. *J. Clin. Invest.* 34:832, 1955.

168. McKenzie, J. K., Patel, R., and McQueen, E. G. The excretion rate of Tamm-Horsfall urinary mucoprotein in normals and in patients with renal disease. *Aust. Ann. Med.* 13:32, 1964.

169. McQueen, E. G. The composition of urinary casts. *Lancet* 1:397, 1966.

170. McQueen, E. G., and Engel, G. B. Factors determining the aggregation of urinary mucoprotein. *J. Clin. Path.* 19:392, 1966.

171. Melamed, M. R., and Wolinska, W. H. On the significance of intracytoplasmic inclusions in the urinary sediment. *Amer. J. Path.* 38:711, 1961.

172. Melo, E. H. L., Manani, I., Martirani, I., and Cintra, A. B. V. Protein, hexose, and hexosamine in the nondialyzable fraction of the filtered urine in normal young men. *J. Lab. Clin. Med.* 54:739, 1959.

173. Mertz, D. P., and Sarre, H. Über dur diagnostischen Wert semiquantitative Nierenfunktiosproben: II. Korrelation Zwischen Phenolrottest und PAH-Clearance. *Klin. Wschr.* 40:692, 1962.

174. Miles, B. E., Paton, A., and de Wardener, H. E. Maximum urine concentration. *Brit. Med. J.* 2:901, 1954.

175. Miller, B. F., and Dubos, R. Determination by a specific enzymatic method of the creatinine content of blood and urine from normal and nephritic individuals. *J. Biol. Chem.* 121:457, 1937.

176. Miller, B. F., and Winkler, A. W. The renal excretion of endogenous creatinine in man. *J. Clin. Invest.* 17:31, 1938.

177. Miller, B. F., Leaf, A., Mamby, A. R., and Miller, Z. Validity of the endogenous creatinine clearance as a measure of glomerular filtration rate in the diseased human kidney. *J. Clin. Invest.* 31:309, 1952.

178. Møller, E., and Lundsgaard, C. Continued investigations into the excretion of phenolsulphonphthalein by the kidneys. *Acta Med. Scand.* 63:268, 1925.

179. Møller, E., McIntosh, J. F., and Van Slyke, D.D. Studies of urea excretion: II. *J. Clin. Invest.* 6:427, 1929.

180. Morel-Maroger, A. L., Leroux-Robert, C., Amiel, C., and Richet, G. Étude histologique de 33 cas de proteinurie isolée. *Nephron* 4:13, 1967.

181. Mörner, K. A. H. Untersuchungen über

die Proteinstoffe und die Eiweissfällenden Substanzen des normalen Menschenharns. *Skand. Arch. Physiol.* 6:332, 1895.

182. Mosenthal, H. O., and Miller, A. The relation of the non-protein nitrogen to the urea nitrogen of the blood. *J. Urol.* 1:75, 1917.

183. Muth, R. G. Asymptomatic mild intermittent proteinuria. *Arch. Intern. Med.* (Chicago) 115:569, 1965.

184. Nedbal, J., and Seliger, V. Electrophoretic analysis of exercise proteinuria. *J. Appl. Physiol.* 13:244, 1958.

185. Nelp, W. B., Wagner, H. N., Jr., and Reba, R. C. Renal excretion of B_{12} and its use in measurement of glomerular filtration rate in man. *J. Lab. Clin. Med.* 63:480, 1964.

186. Neumann, M., West, M., and Zimmerman, H. J. The relationship between proteinuria and fatty elements in the urine sediment. *Amer. J. Med. Sci.* 241:617, 1961.

187. Oliver, J. New directions in renal morphology: A method, its results and its future. *Harvey Lect.* 40:102, 1944.

188. Oliver, J., and MacDowell, M. Cellular mechanisms of protein metabolism in the nephron: VII. The characteristics and significance of the protein absorption droplets (hyaline droplets) in epidemic hemorrhagic fever and other renal diseases. *J. Exp. Med.* 107:731, 1958.

189. Oliver, J., MacDowell, M., and Lee, Y. C. Cellular mechanisms of protein metabolism in the nephron: I. The structural aspects of proteinuria; tubular absorption, droplet formation, and the disposal of protein. *J. Exp. Med.* 99:589, 1954.

190. Oliver, J., Moses, M. J., MacDowell, M., and Lee, Y. C. Cellular mechanisms of protein metabolism in the nephron: II. The histochemical characteristics of protein absorption droplets. *J. Exp. Med.* 99:605, 1954.

191. Osserman, E. F. Plasma cell myeloma: II. Clinical aspects. *New Eng. J. Med.* 261: 952, 1006, 1959.

192. Osserman, E. F., and Lawlor, D. Immunoelectrophoretic characterization of the serum and urinary proteins in plasma cell myeloma and Waldenström's macroglobulinemia. *Ann. N.Y. Acad. Sci.* 94: 93, 1961.

193. Owen, J. A., Iggo, B., Scandrett, F. J., and Stewart, C. P. The determination of creatinine in plasma or serum, and in urine; a critical examination. *Biochem. J.* 58:426, 1954.

194. Panitz, F., and Shinaberger, J. H. Nephrogenic diabetes insipidus due to sarcoidosis without hypercalcemia. *Ann. Intern. Med.* 62:113, 1965.

195. Patte, J.-C., Baldassaire, G., and Loret, J. Étude immunoélectrophorétique des protéinuries normales et pathologiques. *Rev. Franç. Étud. Clin. Biol.* 3:960, 1958.

196. Pears, M. A., and Houghton, B. J. Response of infected urinary tract to bacterial pyrogens. *Lancet* 2:1167, 1959.

197. Persike, E. C., and Addis, T. Food protein consumption in glomerulonephritis. *Arch. Intern. Med.* 81:612, 1948.

198. Peters, J. P., and Van Slyke, D. D. *Quantitative Clinical Chemistry.* Vol. 1: *Interpretations.* Baltimore: Williams & Wilkins, 1946.

199. Phillippi, P. J., Robinson, R. R., and Langelier, P. R. Percutaneous renal biopsy. *Arch. Intern. Med.* (Chicago) 108:139, 1961.

200. Phillippi, P. J., Reynolds, J., Yamauchi, H., and Beering, S. C. Persistent proteinuria in asymptomatic individuals: Renal biopsy studies on 50 patients. *Milit. Med.* 131: 1311, 1966.

201. Platt, R. Structural and functional adaptation in renal failure. *Brit. Med. J.* 1:1313, 1952.

202. Poirier, K. P., and Jackson, G. G. Characteristics of leukocytes in the urine sediment in pyelonephritis: Correlation with renal biopsies. *Amer. J. Med.* 23:579, 1957.

203. Pollak, V. E., Pirani, C. L., Muehrcke, R. C., and Kark, R. M. Asymptomatic persistent proteinuria; studies by renal biopsies. *Guy Hosp. Rep.* 107:353, 1958.

204. Pollak, V. E., and Arbel, C. The distribution of Tamm-Horsfall mucoprotein (uromucoid) in the human nephron. *Nephron* 6:667, 1969.

205. Prescott, L. F.   The normal urinary excretion rates of renal tubular cells, leucocytes and red blood cells. *Clin. Sci.* 31:425, 1966.

206. Putnam, F. W.   Plasma cell myeloma and macroglobulinemia: I. Physicochemical, immunochemical and isotopic turnover studies of the abnormal serum and urinary proteins. *New Eng. J. Med.* 261:902, 1959.

207. Putnam, F. W., Easley, C. W., Lynn, L. T., Ritchie, A. E., and Phelps, R. A.   Heat precipitation of Bence Jones proteins: I. Optimum conditions. *Arch. Biochem.* 83: 115, 1959.

208. Quinn, J. R., and Zimmerman, H. J.   Significance of oval fat bodies in urinary sediment. *Amer. J. Clin. Path.* 24:787, 1954.

209. Race, G. A., Scheifley, C. H., and Edwards, J. E.   Albuminuria in congestive heart failure. *Circulation* 13:329, 1956.

210. Rather, L. J.   Filtration, resorption, and excretion of protein by the kidney. *Medicine* (Balt.) 31:357, 1952.

211. Relman, A. S.   Some Clinical Aspects of Chronic Pyelonephritis. In Quinn, E. L., and Kass, E. H. (Eds.), *Biology of Pyelonephritis*. (Henry Ford Hospital International Symposium.) Boston: Little, Brown, 1960. P. 355.

212. Relman, A. S., and Levinsky, N. G.   Kidney disease: Acquired tubular disorders. *Ann. Rev. Med.* 12:93, 1961.

213. Rennie, I. D. B., and Keen, H.   Evaluation of clinical methods for detecting proteinuria. *Lancet* 2:489, 1967.

214. Reubi, F., Goodgold, A., and Schmid, A.   La présence de cellules de Sternheimer-Malbin dans le sédiment urinaire, est-elle liée à l'existence d'une pyélonéphrite? *Helv. Med. Acta* 20:392, 1953.

215. Rifkin, H., Parker, J. G., Polin, E. B., Berkman, J. I., Spiro, D.   Diabetic glomerulosclerosis: Clinical and pathologic observations with special reference to doubly refractile fatty cells and casts in the urine. *Medicine* (Balt.) 27:429, 1948.

216. Rigas, O. A., and Heller, C. G.   The amount and nature of urinary proteins in normal human subjects. *J. Clin. Invest.* 30: 853, 1951.

217. Roberts, A. M.   Some effects of exercise on the urinary sediment. *J. Clin. Invest.* 14: 31, 1935.

218. Robinson, R. R., and Glenn, W. G.   Fixed and reproducible orthostatic proteinuria: IV. Urinary albumin excretion by healthy human subjects in the recumbent and upright postures. *J. Lab. Clin. Med.* 64:717, 1964.

219. Robinson, R. R., Glover, S. N., Phillippi, P. J., Lecocq, F. R., and Langelier, P. R.   Fixed and reproducible orthostatic proteinuria: I. Light microscopic studies of the kidney. *Amer. J. Path.* 39:291, 1961.

220. Robinson, R. R., Ashworth, C. T., Glover, S. N., Phillippi, P. J., Lecocq, F. R., and Langelier, P. R.   Fixed and reproducible orthostatic proteinuria: II. Electron microscopy of renal biopsy specimens from five cases. *Amer. J. Path.* 39:405, 1961.

221. Rofe, P.   The cells of normal human urine. *J. Clin. Path.* 8:25, 1955.

222. Roscoe, M. H.   Plasma chromogen and the endogenous creatinine clearance. *J. Clin. Path.* 11:173, 1958.

223. Roussak, N. J., and Oleesky, S.   Water-losing nephritis: Syndrome simulating diabetes insipidus. *Quart. J. Med.* 23:147, 1954.

224. Rowe, D. S.   The molecular weights of the proteins of normal and nephrotic sera and nephrotic urine, and a comparison of selective ultrafiltrates of serum proteins with urine proteins. *Biochem. J.* 67:435, 1957.

225. Rowe, D. S., and Soothill, J. F.   Serum proteins in normal urine. *Clin. Sci.* 21:75, 1961.

226. Rowntree, L. G., and Geraghty, J. T.   An experimental and clinical study of the functional activity of the kidneys by means of phenolsulphonephthalein. *J. Pharmacol. Exp. Ther.* 1:579, 1910.

227. Rubini, M. E.   Water excretion in potassium-deficient man. *J. Clin. Invest.* 40: 2215, 1961.

228. Rytand, D. A.   The renal lesion in orthostatic albuminuria. *Arch. Intern. Med.* 59: 848, 1937.

229. Sargent, F., II, and Johnson, R. E.   The effects of diet on renal function in healthy men. *Amer. J. Clin. Nutr.* 4:466, 1956.

230. Schirmeister, J., Willmann, H., Kiefer, H., and Hallauer, W. Für und wieder die Brauchbarkeit der endogen Kreatininclearance in der funktionellen Nierendiagnostik. *Deutsch. Med. Wschr.* 89:1640, 1964.

231. Schirmeister, J., Lotzen, H., and Willmann, H. Symposium über aktuelle Fragen der klinischen Nephrologic, Freiburg. Stuttgart: Thieme-Verlag, 1966.

232. Schoen, E. J. Minimum urine total solute concentration in response to water loading in normal men. *J. Appl. Physiol.* 10:267, 1957.

233. Schradl, W., Böhle, E., and Becker, G. Über die Ausscheidung von Lipoprotein in Urin bei der songenannten Albuminurien. *Deutsch. Arch. Klin. Med.* 202:415, 1955–56.

234. Schreiner, G. E. The identification and clinical significance of casts. *A.M.A. Arch. Intern. Med.* 99:356, 1957.

235. Sellers, A. L. The mechanism and significance of protein excretion by the normal kidney. *A.M.A. Arch. Intern. Med.* 98:801, 1956.

236. Shaffer, P. The excretion of kreatinin and kreatin in health and disease. *Amer. J. Physiol.* 23:1, 1908.

237. Shannon, J. A. The renal excretion of creatinine in man. *J. Clin. Invest.* 14:403, 1935.

238. Shannon, J. A., and Ranges, H. A. On the renal tubular excretion of creatinine in normal man. *J. Clin. Invest.* 20:169, 1941.

239. Shevky, M. C., and Stafford, D. D. A clinical method for the estimation of protein in urine and other body fluids. *Arch. Intern. Med.* 32:222, 1923.

240. Silver, H. K. Cytology of urinary sediment in childhood. *Pediatrics* 26:255, 1960.

241. Sirota, J. H., Baldwin, D. S., and Villarreal, H. Diurnal variations of renal function in man. *J. Clin. Invest.* 29:187, 1950.

242. Slater, R. J., and Kunkel, H. G. Filter paper electrophoresis with special reference to urinary proteins. *J. Lab. Clin. Med.* 41:619, 1953.

243. Slater, R. J., O'Doherty, N. J., and De-Wolfe, M. S. Studies on human proteinuria: I. The mechanism of postural proteinuria. *Pediatrics* 26:190, 1960.

244. Smith, H. W. *The Kidney: Structure and Function in Health and Disease.* New York: Oxford University Press, 1951.

245. Smith, H. W. *Principles of Renal Physiology.* New York: Oxford University Press, 1956.

246. Smith, H. W., Goldring, W., and Chasis, H. The measurement of the tubular excretory mass, effective blood flow and filtration rate in the normal human kidney. *J. Clin. Invest.* 17:263, 1938.

247. Spiro, D. The structural basis of proteinuria in man. *Amer. J. Path.* 35:47, 1959.

248. Squire, J. R. The nephrotic syndrome. *Advances Intern. Med.* 7:201, 1955.

249. Stahl, W. C. March hemoglobinuria. *J.A.M.A.* 164:1458, 1957.

250. Starr, I., Jr. The production of albuminuria by renal vasoconstriction in animals and in man. *J. Exp. Med.* 43:31, 1926.

251. Steinitz, K., and Türkand, H. The determination of the glomerular filtration by the endogenous creatinine clearance. *J. Clin. Invest.* 19:285, 1940.

252. Sternheimer, R., and Malbin, B. Clinical recognition of pyelonephritis, with a new stain for urinary sediments. *Amer. J. Med.* 11:312, 1951.

253. Stevenson, G. T. Detection in normal urine of protein resembling Bence Jones protein. *J. Clin. Invest.* 39:1192, 1960.

254. Stevenson, G. T. Further studies of the gamma-related proteins of normal urine. *J. Clin. Invest.* 41:1190, 1962.

255. Storey, W. E. Variations in urinary dilution and concentration among healthy males under simple standard conditions. *Ann. Intern. Med.* 34:737, 1951.

256. Strauss, M. B. *Body Water in Man.* Boston: Little, Brown, 1957.

257. Tamm, I., and Horsfall, P. L., Jr. A mucoprotein derived from human urine which reacts with influenza, mumps, and Newcastle disease viruses. *J. Exp. Med.* 95:71, 1952.

258. Tannen, R. L., Regal, E. M., Dunn, M. J., and Schrier, R. W. Vasopressin-resistant

hyposthenuria in advanced chronic renal disease. *New Eng. J. Med.* 280:1135, 1969.

259. Tarnoky, A. L. "Apparent protein" in human urine: Some surface film measurements. *Biochem. J.* 49:205, 1951.

260. Taylor, A. Some characteristics of exercise proteinuria. *Clin. Sci.* 19:209, 1960.

261. Ten Thije, O. J. Urinary and serum proteins in myelomatosis. *Acta Med. Scand.* 153:253, 1956.

262. Tidstrøm, B. Urinary protein in glomerulonephritis and pyelonephritis. *Acta Med. Scand.* 174:385, 1963.

263. Tidstrøm, B. Quantitative determination of protein in normal urine. *Scand. J. Clin. Lab. Invest.* 15:167, 1963.

264. Tidstrøm, B. Urinary protein in normal human subjects. *Scand. J. Clin. Lab. Invest.* 15:259, 1963.

265. Tobias, G. J., McLaughlin, R. F., Jr., and Hopper, J., Jr. Endogenous creatinine clearance: A valuable clinical test of glomerular filtration and a prognostic guide in chronic renal disease. *New Eng. J. Med.* 266:317, 1962.

266. Tyler, D. E. Urinalysis and urine cytology correlated with the menstrual cycle and age. *Amer. J. Obstet. Gynec.* 90:147, 1964.

267. Van Slyke, D. D., McIntosh, J. F., Møller, E., Hannon, R. R., and Johnston, C. Studies of urea excretion. *J. Clin. Invest.* 8:357, 1930.

268. Vestergaard, P., and Leverett, R. Constancy of urinary creatinine excretion. *J. Lab. Clin. Med.* 51:211, 1958.

269. Volhard, F. Über die funktionelle Unterscheidung der Schrumpfnieren. *Verh. Deutsch. Kongr. Inn. Med.* 27:735, 1910.

270. Walker, A. M., Bott, P. A., Oliver, J., and MacDowell, M. C. The collection and analysis of fluid from single nephrons of the mammalian kidney. *Amer. J. Physiol.* 134:580, 1941.

271. Wallenius, G. Renal clearance of dextran as a measure of glomerular permeability. *Acta Soc. Med. Upsal.* Suppl. 4:1, 1954.

272. Wang, C., and Wu, H. A method for the determination of protein in normal urine with some observations. *Chin. J. Physiol.* 12:371, 1937.

273. Webb, T., Rose, B., and Sehon, A. H. Biocolloids in normal human urine: I. Amount and electrophoretic characteristics. *Canad. J. Biochem. Physiol.* 36:1159, 1958.

274. Webb, T., Rose, B., and Sehon, A. H. Biocolloids in normal human urine: II. Physicochemical and immunochemical characteristics. *Canad. J. Biochem. Physiol.* 36:1167, 1958.

275. Wegria, R., Capeci, N. E., Blumenthal, M. R., Kornfeld, P., Hays, D. R., Elias, R. A., and Hilton, J. G. The pathogenesis of proteinuria in the acutely congested kidney. *J. Clin. Invest.* 34:737, 1955.

276. Welty, J. W. Febrile albuminuria. *Amer. J. Med. Sci.* 194:70, 1937.

277. Wernze, H., and Becker, G. Zur Frage der renalen und hepatischen Phenolrot-Ausscheidung bei chronischen Leberkrankungen. *Klin. Wschr.* 39:963, 1962.

278. White, H. L., and Rolf, D. Effects of exercise and of some other influences on the renal circulation in man. *Amer. J. Physiol.* 152:505, 1948.

279. Winberg, J. Renal function in water-losing syndrome due to lower urinary tract obstruction before and after treatment. *Acta Paediat.* 48:149, 1960.

280. Wolman, I. J. The incidence, causes and intermittency of proteinuria in young men. *Amer. J. Med. Sci.* 210:86, 1945.

281. Wolvius, D., and Verschure, J. C. M. The diagnostic value of the protein excretion pattern in various types of proteinuria. *J. Clin. Path.* 10:80, 1957.

282. Wright, W. T. Cell counts in urine. *A.M.A. Arch. Intern. Med.* 103:76, 1959.

283. Zak, G. A., Brun, C., and Smith, H. W. The mechanism of formation of osmotically concentrated urine during the antidiuretic state. *J. Clin. Invest.* 33:1064, 1954.

284. Zeffren, J. L., and Heinemann, H. O. Reversible defect in renal concentrating mechanism in patients with hypercalcemia. *Amer. J. Med.* 33:54, 1962.

285. Zimmer, J. G., Dewey, R., Waterhouse, C., and Terry, R. The origin and nature of anisotropic urinary lipids in the nephrotic syndrome. *Ann. Intern. Med.* 54:205, 1961.

286. Zinneman, H. H., Glenchur, H., and Gleason, D. F. The significance of urine electrophoresis in patients with multiple myeloma. *Arch. Intern. Med.* (Chicago) 106: 172, 1960.

4

Renal Radiography

Olle Olsson

Diagnostic roentgenology plays an important role in the diagnosis and treatment of diseases of the kidney and urinary pathways. One reason is that the roentgen diagnostic methods are well adapted to both the morphology and the physiology of the urinary tract. No other part or organ of the body can be approached roentgenologically by such a variety of suitable methods.

Formerly it was the circumscript, so-called surgical renal diseases that attracted most roentgen diagnostic interest. In recent years, however, interest has been focused also on the generalized so-called nonsurgical renal diseases. These two groups are united by a generalized disease, pyelonephritis, which per se or as a complication of surgical renal disease is very common. Particularly, the advent of suitable antibiotics and the development of the artificial kidney have resulted in an increase of the therapeutic contributions and thereby of the demands for diagnosis of generalized kidney disease.

This chapter outlines the various methods available for roentgen examination of renal diseases and indicates the information they can yield. It also includes a description of the roentgenographic features of various renal diseases.

Examination Principles

Diagnostic radiology yields information on anatomic, pathologic, and physiologic conditions. Cumulative experience, technical advances, and clinical research have given diagnostic radiology a value of its own. It should therefore not be regarded or used simply as a supplement to the clinical investigation.

The examination should consist of a detailed study of normal and pathologic conditions using all necessary variations of the different technics. The examination results in a series of films demonstrating as unequivocally as possible the pertinent pathologic and physiologic findings. To take a film or a standardized set of films and study these films has nothing to do with serious diagnostic radiology. The examination should be complete. If a roentgen examination is performed only halfheartedly, or if it is interrupted simply because preliminary findings happen to fit in with a preconceived opinion, or if technically poor examinations are accepted, the examination may result in a serious misdiagnosis.

Estimation of Renal Parenchymal Mass

In many instances of renal disease, especially chronic generalized disease of the renal parenchyma, the estimation of actual renal parenchymal mass is important.

At roentgen examination the size of each kidney can be seen, and thus a rough estimation of parenchymal mass can be made. In the presence of renal or perirenal edema, the fat capsule surrounding the kidney may be infiltrated with edema fluid to such an extent as to erase the radiation absorption difference between fat and renal tissue. This has been the case in several patients with acute renal failure. Reduction of the edema by therapeutic means will make possible the delineation of the kidneys.

The size of the kidney is a very crude basis for estimating parenchymal mass. Edema within the kidney will increase kidney size. A somewhat diminished kidney in an acute edematous stage will thus be normal in size or even be larger than normal.

The size as a measure of parenchymal mass has another important source of error. The kidney may be more or less excavated by a pathologic process. The kidney may have normal or greater-than-normal dimensions, but the sinus part of the kidney may be more or less widened and the parenchyma reduced to a thin layer. This is very often seen in dilation of the kidney pelvis caused by different factors. In fibrolipomatosis in the renal sinus, specific functioning parenchyma is replaced by unspecific fibromatous or lipomatous tissue. Although kidney size is normal, the amount of renal parenchyma may, in such cases, be markedly reduced.

In amyloidosis, for instance, specific functioning parenchyma may be markedly reduced, although kidney size and shape are

normal. Tumor tissue sometimes may have the same effect as have leukemic infiltrates.

In order to study more reliably the amount of parenchyma, it has been proposed to measure the calyx-surface distance at urography or pyelography. This is a crude and often unreliable method, since the calyces are not at right angles to the usual plane of recording.

Plain radiography, eventually with tomography, can give a good impression of kidney size, including the size of the sinus. Urography and pyelography can add information by adding the width of renal pelvis and the extension of calyces if proper projections are used.

The best information on the amount of renal parenchyma is provided by the use of renal angiography. In the arterial phase the width of the arteries mirrors the amount of functioning parenchyma. In a urographically silent kidney with long-standing stasis, it may not be evident whether either the stasis had been permanent or intermittent or the loss of function is permanent or temporary. Angiography will solve the problem. If the caliber of the renal artery is normal or only slightly reduced, the functional capacity of the kidney will be restored after the release of the obstacle. If, on the other hand, the caliber is markedly reduced, the functional capacity is definitely lost.

In the nephrographic phase angiography demonstrates the amount of renal parenchyma, and general or localized reduction can be appreciated. Densitomographic study of the angiograms in the nephrographic phase with Bolin's [12] method adds very detailed information regarding functional parenchyma (see page 154).

Hypertensive Disease

In hypertensive disease a renal cause is common, calling for examination of the kidneys. The changes to be looked for are primary-parenchymal or primary-vascular. The first-mentioned group includes generalized renal parenchymal disease of different kinds, most commonly pyelonephritis (the reader is referred to the respective chapters).

Among vascular changes responsible for hypertensive disease of renal origin, renal artery stenosis is the most common. This may be arteriosclerotic, traumatic, or of the fibromuscular hyperplasia type. The stenosis may be of every degree from slight to complete. It is usually short, and a poststenotic dilation of the artery is often seen. It may be localized at the origin of the renal artery, in which case the sclerotic plaque of the artery is often seen to involve the aortic wall adjacent to the mouth of the renal artery. It may be localized far out in the main artery or in one or more branches. The stenotic lesion may be unilateral or bilateral. In multiple arteries it may affect one or all of the arteries. In multiplicity the stenotic process may vary in degree in the different localizations.

In complete or severe stenosis a collateral circulation is often seen, originating from capsular, suprarenal, and lumbar arteries.

In an angiographic study indicated by hypertensive disease, it is often rational to perform an aortic study in proper projections to demonstrate the first part of the renal artery. This means that two slightly oblique views are needed, one with the patient turned to the right, one to the left. This aortic study will demonstrate stenosis unilaterally or bilaterally in one of two or more renal arteries to one kidney, collateral circulation, and changes in the aortic wall.

In moderate to severe stenosis it may be helpful in the same sitting to replace the aortic catheter with a thin, selective catheter that can be passed through the stenotic segment to measure the pressure gradient across the stenosis. A stenotic process without a pressure gradient can be supposed not to have any pathogenetic significance regarding the hypertensive state.

In order to select cases for angiography, several methods have been proposed. The simplest one is a plain film study of differences in kidney size, on the both sides. A difference in length of 1 cm. between the two kidneys is supposed to be suggestive of arterial stenosis.

A stenotic lesion of a renal artery will reduce production of urine and slow down the flow through tubules. The first-mentioned factor will cause delay in the demonstration of contrast urine in the parenchyma and the kidney pelvis. This delay may be noticeable in comparison of the two sides in a series of films taken in fairly rapid sequence after injection of the contrast medium. The other factor will cause a production of more highly concentrated urine from the stenotic side, which in a late phase of the examination is discernible as a difference in concentration between the two kidneys.

The modification of urography to the socalled washout urography [4] consists of forcibly inducing diuresis by performing urography with urea and saline solution and of checking washout time from the kidney pelvis of the contrast urine. The diminished production of urine from the kidney with the stenotic artery will increase washout time.

In phlebography, washout time of the contrast medium from the renal vein is increased on the stenotic side because of diminished flow and back pressure. Winding collaterals may cause characteristic impressions in the kidney pelvis and the ureter in urography or pyelography.

PREPARATION OF THE PATIENT FOR
ROENTGEN EXAMINATION

To secure the best possible result of an examination the patient must be properly prepared. For plain radiography of the urinary tract and for pyelography and urography the gastrointestinal tract should be empty if possible. This can be achieved by the taking of a laxative the day before the examination, with an enema the evening before or the morning of the examination day, and maintaining a fasting state on the examination day. Every department usually has its own detailed prescription for preparation.

It is very important to get rid of intestinal gas. Most gas consists of swallowed air. To diminish the amount of air passing into the intestine, the patient should, when possible, be up and about.

Many clinicians recommend strict fluid restriction many hours before urography. This is important if diiodized contrast media are to be used, but not if the examination is performed with triiodized contrast medium. An enema can be given before the examination despite water absorption from the intestine. In the presence of large amounts of intestinal gas and fecal contents in the colon, a tannic acid enema may be given immediately before the examination; the tannic acid content causes intestinal contraction and therefore often has a very good immediate effect. In younger patients with large amounts of intestinal gas a subcutaneous injection of vasopression (Postacton) helps to clear the bowel of gas. For angiography premedication in the form of a sedative may be suitable, for example, with atropine or barbiturate or both.

Acute examinations can be made without preparation.

An important part of the preparation of a patient and one often neglected is the giving of proper information as to why an examination has to be made and what type of procedure the patient may expect. During the examination it is valuable whenever possible to keep the patient continuously informed as to different parts of the procedure, not least in order to secure the patient's full cooperation.

RADIATION PROTECTION

A few simple rules fulfill requirements for radiation protection in urologic diagnostic radiology. Every examination should have a good indication. The preparation of the patient, the planning of the examination, the performance of it, and the equipment used should make it possible to extract the desired information using the smallest possible amount of radiation and making reexamination unnecessary.

Gonad regions should, whenever possible, be covered with lead rubber when in primary beam. This beam should always be carefully collimated. Fluoroscopy should be restricted to a minimum.

Examination Methods

All roentgen examinations of the kidneys and urinary pathways are based on the simplest form of examination, plain radiography. This basic method must precede all other examination methods, such as pyelography, urography, and angiography. Additional technics supplementing these methods are tomography and zonography and, in strictly selected cases, retroperitoneal pneumography. Technically satisfactory results can be expected only if the patient is properly prepared for the examination.

PLAIN RADIOGRAPHY

The density of the kidney is approximately the same as that of the surrounding tissues, from which it can be distinguished, however, because of its fatty capsule. If the capsule is thin, as it always is in infancy and in old age as well as in very lean persons, it may be difficult to outline the kidney. Definition may be improved by the use of oblique views. Such projections are always necessary to demonstrate whether a calcification projected over the kidney is situated inside or outside.

The normal range of variation of the shape of the kidney is wide. This may be due to true anatomic differences, but also to the angle of projection. For example, if a kidney is displaced caudally along the psoas muscle, its lower pole will be directed ventrally and the object-film distance will be increased. This re-

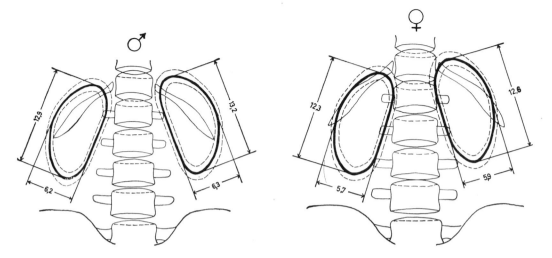

Figure 4-1. Graphic representation of normal variation of kidney size. (From Moëll, H. [33].)

sults in a radiographic enlargement of that pole, which then appears plump.

The surface of the kidney is usually smooth. In the medial part the hilus is often demonstrable.

The kidneys vary considerably in size. Figure 4-1 illustrates this normal variation in adults. The size does not vary appreciably with body build (stature, body weight, area of body surface, etc.).

The position of the kidneys varies within a fairly wide range. They are usually related to the twelfth rib. The right kidney is usually somewhat lower than the left. In one-third of all persons, both kidneys are situated at the same level, and rarely the left is lower than the right (Fig. 4-2). The kidneys are relatively lower in children than in adults, assuming their definite position at the age of 5 to 10 years.

The position of the kidneys in relation to the midline (distance and angle) is apparent from Figure 4-3. In males both kidneys are situated more laterally than in females, and the angle between the longitudinal axis of the kidney and the midline is greater.

The kidneys have a certain range of mobil-

ity in the craniocaudal direction. This is limited by the vascular pedicle, by the attachment of the kidney to the suprarenal gland and by connective tissue running from the renal fascia through the fatty capsule to unite with the fibrous capsule of the kidney. Nevertheless the range of movement is about 3 cm., somewhat less on the right side than on the left. On deep respiration, however, excursions up to 10 cm. can be recorded. The mobility in the ventrodorsal and the mediolateral directions is small.

TOMOGRAPHY AND ZONOGRAPHY

Tomography or zonography may be useful to outline the kidneys completely if it is impossible, for instance, to get rid of intestinal gas overlying the kidney, or to demonstrate thin calcifications or the amount of fat in the sinus in fibrolipomatosis. In connection with angiography, tomography may be useful in the nephrographic phase to demonstrate or exclude pathologic density in circumscribed areas. Retroperitoneal pneumography is facilitated by the use of tomography.

Tomography is performed preferably as multilayer examination and with circular

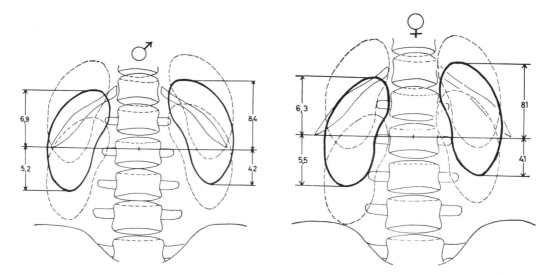

Figure 4-2. Distance upward and downward from middle of vertebra L_{11} of poles of normal adult kidneys in plain roentgenograms. Dashed lines indicate ±2 s. Figures are in centimeters. (From Moëll, H. [33].)

movement, whereas zonography is useful especially in combination with urography when contrast excretion is poor or the bowel content disturbing.

RETROPERITONEAL PNEUMOGRAPHY

If the fatty capsule of the kidney is thin, and also if the adrenal glands are to be studied, retroperitoneal pneumography may be indi-

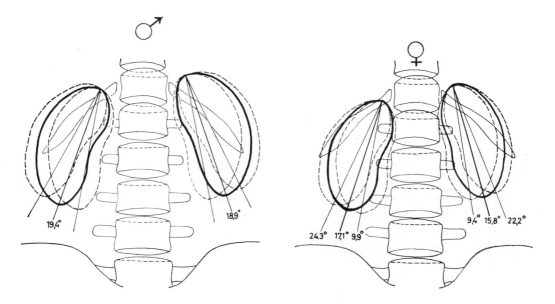

Figure 4-3. Angle between length of kidneys and midline. Dashed lines indicate ±2 s. (From Moëll, H. [33].)

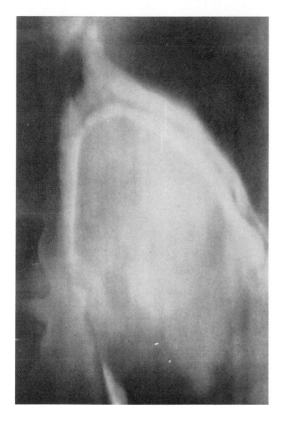

Figure 4-4. Retroperitoneal pneumography and body section radiography showing left kidney and suprarenal and renal fascia.

cated. The best method is that of Ruiz Rivas, in which gas is injected into the retrorectal space. The pelvic connective tissue continues directly upward in the retroperitoneum, and since the renal fascia surrounds the kidney and is open caudally, the gas can enter the fascia, surround the kidney and suprarenal gland, and find its way into the interstices in the connective tissue between these two organs (Fig. 4-4). The connective tissue within the renal fascia may be abundant, particularly on the dorsal part of the kidney. When gas fills this tissue, the kidney may be very mobile.

The gas used for retroperitoneal pneumography should preferably be carbon dioxide, which is rapidly absorbed and readily soluble in the blood.

Technic. The coccyx is identified and puncture is done with an ordinary lumbar puncture needle, which is introduced immediately adjacent to this bone. The tip of the needle is directed medially and cranially and toward the sacrum. Penetration of the rectal mucosa is avoided by palpation with a finger in the rectum. From 1.0 to 1.5 liters of gas is injected with the patient in the knee-elbow position or lying on his side, with the side of greater diagnostic interest uppermost. This technic of examination has few indications. Large series have been published, demonstrating that it has often been employed with inadequate indications.

Risks. In a survey by Ransom et al. (1956) including over 9000 retroperitoneal pneumographies by the presacral route, 24 patients had died and 33 had suffered severe nonfatal reactions. The frequency of fatalities was equal whether air or oxygen had been used. Therefore carbon dioxide should be used, which is twenty times more soluble in blood than is oxygen. If large amounts of gas enter the vascular system, the patient should be placed on the left side as soon as the reaction occurs, because in this posture no air trap arises in the left ventricular outflow tract.

PYELOGRAPHY

In pyelography a contrast medium is injected directly into the renal pelvis (i.e., antegrade pyelography) or via catheter into the ureter (i.e., retrograde pyelography). In antegrade pyelography the contrast medium is injected via a pyelostomy or after percutaneous puncture of the kidney pelvis. In retrograde pyelography the tip of the catheter should be placed in the upper part of the ureter. The position of the catheter must be checked before starting the injection of the contrast medium. Reflux of contrast medium from the bladder can also be utilized for pyelography.

Pyelography should be performed under fluoroscopic control, preferably with an image intensifier (with or without television). This is the only way to secure a suitable degree of filling. Incomplete filling means incomplete examination. Overdistention may cause reflux, which in addition to certain risks makes study of morphologic detail impossible.

The kidney consists of 14 papillae: 4 in the cranial part, 4 in the caudal part, and 6 in the intermediate part. In the cranial part, but also in the caudal part, the papillae may fuse with one another when the kidney "rolls in" to assume its definitive form, and then the number of papillae will be smaller. The cranial part is the part above the primary bifurcation angle of the renal pelvis. In a double kidney the upper of the two kidneys represents this cranial part.

The papillae are arranged in a dorsal row and a ventral row, but because of a displacement in the mediolateral direction the dorsal row lies more medially (more frequently on the left side) than the ventral, or vice versa. In the former case the hilus faces ventrally; in the latter, dorsally. These very characteristic anatomic variations are usually readily demonstrable in pyelography. Their existence often makes assessment of the amount of kidney parenchyma by measurements from a calyx to the kidney surface in ventrodorsal urograms misleading.

Owing to this position of the papillae, the calyces also are positioned in different planes. Therefore *it is necessary to examine the patient at various angles in order to be able to study all the papillae and calyces at suitable projections*. Sometimes it is necessary to turn the patient over in prone position to obtain a filling of ventrally directed calyces.

The contrast medium is heavy, and its physical density is higher than that of urine and blood; therefore, it first and preferably fills the lower parts of a fluid-filled space. Failure to give proper attention to this *layer formation* invites diagnostic errors.

Nomenclature. The shape of the renal pelvis, particularly its width as well as the shape of the pelviureteric junction, varies widely. I have found the nomenclature which is given in Figure 4-5 suitable. A renal pelvis that is not dilated will sometimes show filling defects along its border or as transverse bands. These defects are due to the edge of the renal parenchyma at the sinus and to vessels, usually the arteries.

The motility of the renal pelvis and the ureters can be studied by cineradiography with an image intensifier.

UROGRAPHY

In urography a filling of the renal pelvis is obtained by excretion of contrast urine after injection of contrast medium, usually intravenously. The molecule of the contrast medium contains two or three iodine atoms bound to a pyridine or benzene ring, and a carboxyl group is incorporated to make the medium water-soluble. The best media have a low toxicity and are excreted in high concentration in the urine. The excretion occurs partly by ultrafiltration in the glomeruli and partly by excretion from the tubular epithelium, the amount excreted by either route varying with the medium. The amount filtered is directly proportional to the concentration of the contrast medium in the plasma. A high concentration of contrast medium not bound to the plasma protein will therefore result in high ultrafiltration, which, however, is accompanied by an increase in diuresis. The increased excretion is thus balanced by the increased volume of urine, so that the concentration of the contrast medium in the urine is unchanged. Dehydration of the patient promotes a greater reabsorption of water with increase in the concentration as a result, well observable when diiodine contrast media are used.

The concentration of the contrast medium excreted by the tubules is proportional to the blood concentration if this is low, but since the tubular excretion has a maximum rate which is easily reached with the ordinary doses used for urography, the concentration

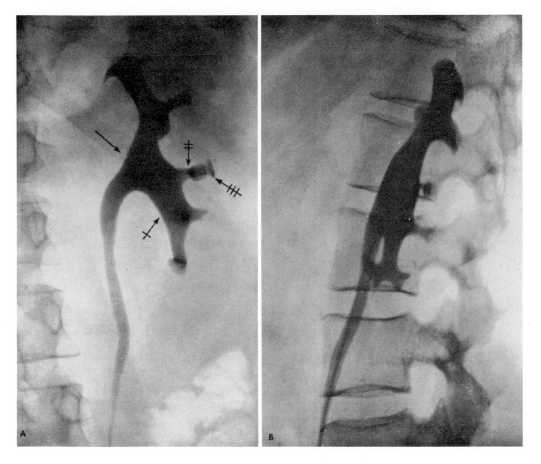

Figure 4-5. Pyelography, frontal and lateral view. Note, in lateral view, position of kidney with cranial part dorsalmost. Nomenclature: → confluence; ─╀→ branch; ─╫→ stem of calyx; ─╫╫→ calyx.

will not increase further with larger doses. The wide variation in the width of the renal pelvis from case to case and in the same patient under different examination conditions gives the contrast-filled renal pelvis varying density in the film. The film in addition poorly reveals small variations in density. These facts are fundamental for judging the excretion of contrast medium in the urine. It is therefore to be hoped that the literature will no longer be encumbered with reports of "100 cases of urography for evaluation of a new contrast medium." Such papers reflect the shortcomings of the author rather than the qualities of the contrast medium.

The excretion is dependent mainly on the secretory pressure in the kidney (in reality the blood pressure) and the intrapelvic pressure. When no excretion can be seen, these two basic factors must be borne in mind. Lack of excretion may be due to fall in blood pressure. Unilateral absence of excretion need not be a manifestation of injury to the renal parenchyma; it may indicate that the intrapelvic pressure in urinary stasis exceeds the secretory pressure. Relief of the intrapelvic pressure may result in resumption of secretion.

Since the excretion is dependent on so many factors and the functional reserve ca-

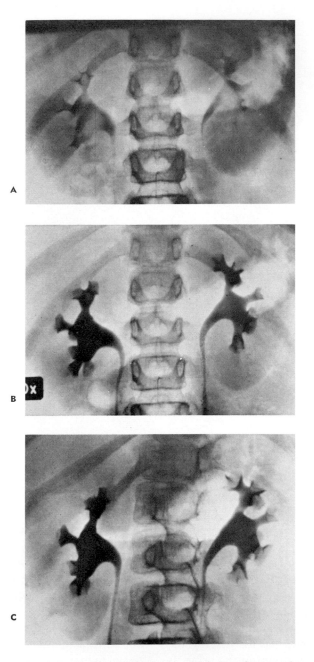

Figure 4-6. Urography. Plain films showing kidneys of normal size, shape, and position. No calcifications. A. 3 minutes after injection of 20 ml. of contrast medium; ordinary excretion of contrast urine on both sides. B. 7 minutes after application of ureteric compression; this was applied after the film in A had been studied. C. Oblique view during ureteric compression. B and C demonstrate normal morphology. The oblique view makes it possible to distinguish between ventral and dorsal calyces and to study each calyx separately. D. Film immediately after removal of ureteric compression; ureters and bladder filled.

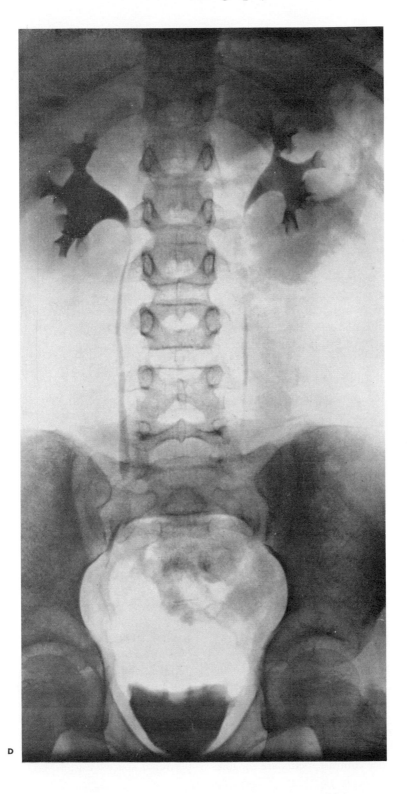

D

pacity of a kidney is high, caution should be exercised in assessing renal function from the urogram. One must recollect that renal function may be severely impaired before any substantial reduction in concentration of the contrast urine is demonstrable.

Morphologic Examination by Urography. If excretion is good, a filling may be obtained of the entire renal pelvis by using ureteric compression, and then the pelvis and ureter will be demonstrated by urography just as well as by pyelography. Compression should be applied over each ureter separately and the pressure should be increased gradually and in intimate cooperation with the patient (Fig. 4-6). The ureteric compression should not be applied until excretion of contrast medium has been seen on preliminary films.

Intravenous injection of great amounts of contrast medium or of blood-diluting fluid together with the contrast medium (infusion urography) will cause better filling of the kidney pelvis than conventional examination without compression. Large comparative series demonstrate that urography with compression generally gives better filling with better possibilities of studying details in the kidney-pelvis morphology. In patients who have difficulties in tolerating ureteric compression, or in cases where this is contraindicated, infusion urography may be used instead.

The most important point in urography is that the technic should be modified according to circumstances in the given case and from one stage of the examination to another according to the findings. *Any examination performed according to a rigidly standardized procedure is a poor examination.*

Tolerance to Contrast Media. Injection of 20 ml. of contrast medium is usually sufficient for urography, but further doses of the same size may be injected during the examination if the contrast density is not satisfactory or if the ureteric compression has to be adjusted.

One must always consider the possibility of side reactions since contrast media are capable of causing local or general reactions. With the best media available, damage to the kidneys through the urographic procedure is rare. Even in patients with severely impaired renal function, infusion urography can be performed. In many of these patients, however, excretion of the contrast medium will be so poor that only limited information can be gained through the procedure.

Hypersensitive reactions can occur. They are usually mild, with sneezing or a few urticaria rashes. They may take a serious turn in exceptional instances, with laryngeal edema or shock. The injection of the contrast medium may cause decrease in blood pressure, with fainting. Injection of a suitable drug counteracts this effect. Therefore emergency remedies must be easily within reach in the examination room.

To prevent reactions to the contract medium, preliminary tests have been recommended, preferably provocation tests with the injection of 1 to 2 ml. intravenously or intracutaneously. This test dose should be given, when possible, the day before the examination. However, the result of the test dose and the reaction to the definitive injection dose do not always agree, just as some patients who fail to react positively to the test dose may experience reactions to the dose used for the examination.

BACKFLOW

If the capacity of the renal pelvis is exceeded and the pressure in it rises, backflow of the contents of the renal pelvis may occur in the renal parenchyma, in the tubules, or interstitially. Usually, however, a sinus reflux occurs by rupture of the fornix calyx at one or more papillae, and then the contrast medium flows out into the sinus. The reflux may be limited to a small sinus extravasate near a papilla, a so-called fornix reflux, but it may increase and then the extravasate spreads in the sinus and may escape through the hilus into the perirenal space (Fig. 4-7). The contrast me-

Figure 4-7. Fornix-sinus reflux in urography. A. All calyces well filled. B. At border of calyx in middle of kidney a small extravasation is seen adjacent to calyceal border. C. Extravasate has spread around calyx and around stems of nearby calyces.

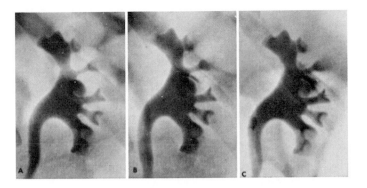

dium may flow along the edge of the fornix into lymphatics, with pyelolymphatic reflux as a result. It may also flow along the vascular channels branching from the sinus toward the parenchyma and there dissect the veins, which readily rupture and permit the entry of contrast medium, with pyelovenous backflow as a result. The term pyelovenous backflow is often erroneously used to cover all these types.

Backflow is a common complication of retrograde pyelography, especially if the examination is performed without fluoroscopy or pressure control (Fig. 4-8). It may also occur during urography after prolonged ureteric compression, usually as a small fornix-sinus reflux, but other types may also develop, particularly pyelolymphatic reflux [38].

The reflux is mainly an artifact and its frequency varies with the technic applied. One

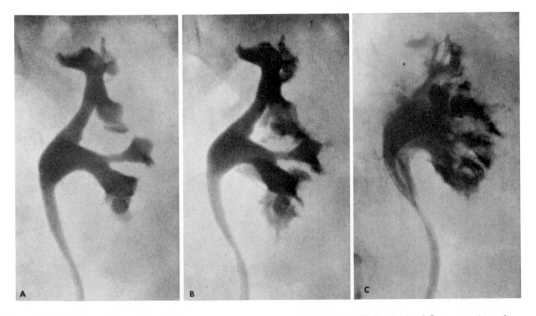

Figure 4-8. Pyelography without fluoroscopy or pressure control. A. Small fornix backflows at edge of upper calyces. B. Backflows from most calyces. Extravasates spread around branches of kidney pelvis. C. Extravasate has spread through hilus and around upper part of ureter. Contrast-filled thin lymph vessels are seen medial to confluence and ureter.

type, however, the reflux seen in acute renal colic, may be part of a pathophysiologic combination. In such cases contrast medium may occasionally be seen to spread in an early stage of the examination from the sinus out through the hilus and down along the ureter on the painful side. This extravasation of contrast medium is diffusely outlined and fades off toward the sides, and is fairly rapidly absorbed. The rate at which the reflux occurs shows that the contrast urine follows a reflux route already paved by the urine. Such backflow is probably the cause of the retroperitoneal edema, the tenderness, and the elevation of the erythrocyte sedimentation rate sometimes found in renal colic.

Reflux into a tumor or around a cyst sometimes occurs.

Tubular backflow is seen as a diffusely outlined increase in contrast at the site of one or more renal papillae. It is observed during pyelography and is then a true reflux, but it is not uncommon in urography and should then be conceived as a sign of slight stasis in association with ureteric compression. In interstitial reflux, which occurs only in association with pyelography, streaks of contrast medium are seen to extend up into the renal parenchyma, sometimes out to the capsule, over a varying portion of the kidney.

The fornix-sinus reflux often shows a diffusely outlined accumulation of contrast medium adjacent to the fornical edge. When this reflux increases, it spreads along the neck of the calyx and then the wall of the calyx is seen as a filling defect between the contrast urine in the calyx and that in the sinus. In pyelolymphatic backflow, contrast-filled fine lymphatics are seen running medially and usually swinging off in the caudal direction at the spine. Pyelovenous backflow is seldom observable; if seen, it is very transitory.

Pyelograms with severe backflow are of little diagnostic value. A small reflux may appear as a papillary ulceration. It can be diagnosed as a reflux if compression is maintained and

films are taken at intervals of a few minutes. In such films the contrast extravasate will be seen to change in size and assume the characteristic spread of the sinus reflux. If this is not decisive, the examination must be repeated a few days later since the path of the reflux soon closes.

In pyelography, backflow may result in intravenous "injection" of contrast medium and the excretion of contrast urine by the other kidney. If, for instance, pyelography is done instead of urography in renal insufficiency, the examination must be performed most carefully to avoid such an injection of the contrast medium into the bloodstream via a backflow.

Much clinical importance has been attached to the backflow phenomenon. It has been regarded as the cause of shock-like fall in blood pressure, spread of infection in the kidney and from the kidney to other parts of the body, and spread of metastases from renal tumors. Though the risks possibly are exaggerated, care should be taken to perform the examination in such a way as to minimize the risk of backflow. This means that the use of pyelography should be limited, and that, when indicated, it should be done under fluoroscopic control. Urography should be done in an individualized and not in a standardized way.

RENAL ANGIOGRAPHY

Most types of renal disease affect the vasculature. Therefore the importance of angiography in the study of many renal diseases is rapidly growing. Transplantation surgery stresses demands on this specific examination method.

Renal angiography* may be performed by direct puncture of the lumbar aorta, but should preferably be done by catheterization after percutaneous puncture of the femoral artery. As in all types of angiography, selectivity should be the goal — i.e., the renal artery

* For more detailed description of renal angiography, see Olsson [39].

should be catheterized. The tolerance of the kidneys to the contrast medium to be used is important. Histologic and physiologic studies have shown that the kidneys tolerate certain triiodide contrast media — e.g., sodium diatrizoate (Hypaque) and natrium amidotrizoas meglumin amidotrizoas (Urografin) — well. On selective catheterization of one of the renal arteries a dose of 4 to 5 ml. of 60 per cent Urografin may be used. The medium should be injected during diastole, because then the dose will be diluted least and give optimal filling. In the films, taken preferably with an automatic cassette or film changer, all the angiographic phases should be well represented.

The contrast medium should be injected into the aorta only if there is reason to suspect that the kidneys have multiple arteries (double kidney, malrotation, fusion, hydronephrosis) and when both renal arteries are to be compared with one another. We then inject 30 ml. of 60 per cent Urografin.

The catheter for selective angiography must have a hole in the tip and not side holes because through side holes a continuous flow of blood can come from the outer end of the catheter, although the tip of the catheter

blocks an arterial branch. If a catheter with only an end hole blocks the artery, this is easily noted through the fact that no blood flows from the outer end of the catheter. A catheter with side holes will allow blood flow even if the catheter blocks the renal artery.

The catheter should not be so wide that it could plug a renal artery. This is specifically important if the renal artery is thin or if a supplementary artery has been catheterized.

The tip should be advanced only a short distance in the renal artery; otherwise it may be passed into a branch, usually the dorsal artery. The dose injected into that part will then be too large and the resulting angiogram incomplete or misleading [25].

Thorough knowledge of the vascular anatomy of the kidney is necessary for interpretation of the angiogram (Fig. 4-9) [7]. The kidney has a ventral artery and a dorsal artery running ventrally and dorsally, respectively, to the renal pelvis. Usually the ventral artery feeds the ventral part of the middle and the ventral pyramids in the inferior part, but also the dorsal pyramids in the lower pole. The dorsal artery feeds the dorsal middle part, the dorsal part of the upper pole, and sometimes the ventral part of the upper pole. The vascu-

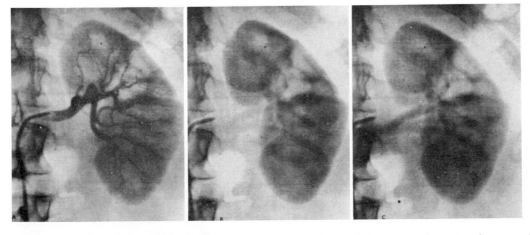

Figure 4-9. Renal angiography. Normal case. Selective examination. Radiopaque catheter put into mouth of left renal artery. A. Arteriographic phase. Dorsal arterial branch most medial in hilus. B. Nephrographic phase. C. Phlebographic phase.

larization of the poles varies considerably. The supply to the inferior pole is most important because of the now common partial resection for stone. This part is usually fed by one artery. In 60 per cent of our cases the ventral artery supplied the whole inferior pole, in 20 per cent the dorsal artery fed the dorsal part, and in the remaining 20 per cent the supply of the dorsal part was divided between the ventral and dorsal arteries.

Owing to the tilted position of the kidney and the characteristic appearance of the dorsal and ventral branches of the renal artery, a single projection is often sufficient to chart the course and field of supply of the branches, but sometimes an oblique view is helpful.

The arteriographic phase is followed, after a few seconds, by the nephrographic phase, which is initially due to a very slight vascular phase but mainly to accumulation of the contrast medium in the tubular epithelium of the cortex and in the urine inside the tubules. This phase offers good possibilities of examining the shape and surface of the kidneys as well as the anatomy of the hilus, the relationship between the cortex and the medulla, and the extent of any destruction of the parenchyma. *While urography and pyelography demonstrate changes in the renal parenchyma indirectly, largely by their effect on the shape of the renal pelvis, these parenchymal changes are seen directly in the nephrogram.*

The nephrographic phase is followed by the phlebographic phase, in which the renal veins appear. These veins can also be studied by renal phlebography, usually after injection of contrast medium via a catheter passed selectively into the renal vein, preferably with introduction of the catheter from the femoral vein through percutaneous puncture. Injection of epinephrine into the renal artery immediately prior to the injection of contrast medium into the renal vein will result in a complete retrograde phlebogram with filling as far back as to the stellate veins [36].

Renal angiography has been used for mor-

phologic studies so far, but important modifications in the technic make possible important physiologic conclusions. Bolin [12] has designed a densitometric method for estimation of renal function in which variations in contrast density of the kidney during angiography will allow estimation of renal cortical blood flow, tubular cell mass, and filtration. The study of these physiologic parameters can be made at the same examination as the study of morphology.

Olin and Redman [35] have constructed a cineradiographic flowmeter based on the spillover of contrast medium from the renal artery into the aorta during injection for renal angiography. Through this method the renal blood flow can be studied and easily compared with flow data obtained by means of other technics [5].

The technics mentioned are still in an early stage of development. Pharmacoangiography of different kinds will also refine renal angiographic studies.

Renal angiography requires careful consideration of a wide variety of details in a well-elaborated technic. If properly performed it can yield valuable information with only slight risks. Judging from the literature, however, the technic applied in renal angiography is often poor and, among other things, ignores the tolerance of the kidneys to contrast media.

In renal angiography selectivity means adherence to some basic roentgen diagnostic principles: superimposition can be avoided, the correct projections can be chosen, and the dose of contrast medium can be kept low. In addition, the timing can be chosen exactly and the filling be the best possible.

The examination method called nephrotomography may have certain indications. Selective renal angiography, however, gives far better possibilities for studying the kidney.

RADIATION HAZARDS

In all radiologic departments a careful watch should be held to prevent undue exposure of the staff and the patients to radiation. All members of the staff should be well acquainted with the risks of irradiation, and the examination room and the examination technic should be such as to guarantee full protection against radiation. *In urologic diagnostic roentgenology the reproductive organs are often included in the beam; therefore, strict observance of all rules and regulations of radiation protection is necessary.* Simple arrangements such as lead shielding of the testes and ovaries can reduce the exposure to radiation considerably, particularly in males, but also in females.

It cannot be stressed enough that control of radiation should always be uppermost in the minds of all persons working in a department of radiology.

The foregoing brief survey of the examination technic and the normal roentgen anatomy represents an introduction to the diagnostic radiology of renal diseases. The most common diseases will now be discussed with special reference to the characteristic roentgen features of each.

Anomalies

Anomalies of the kidneys and the upper urinary tract constitute a major part of all malformations. The anomalies discovered on roentgen examination are: changes in size, shape, position, and number of kidneys, demonstrable in plain roentgenograms; malformations including abnormal number and shape of the renal pelvis, seen in urography or pyelography; and vascular anomalies detectable by angiography. These anomalies are sometimes combined with extrarenal anomalies.

In *malrotation* (see Fig. 4-13), which is in reality inhibited rotation, one or both of the kidneys are often situated lower down than is usual, with the renal pelvis facing anteriorly and the dorsal calyces medially. Malrotation is often a characteristic feature of fused or ectopic kidneys.

The *fusion* is usually caudal, i.e., the caudal renal poles are united by a connective tissue bridge or a parenchymal bridge (Fig. 4-10), the latter readily demonstrable in the nephrographic phase of angiography. Ectopies are usually caudal (Fig. 4-11), sometimes cranial or crossed (Fig. 4-12). In a caudally ectopic kidney the renal artery springs from a low segment of the aorta or from the iliac artery, while in ptosis the renal artery springs from the usual site. Malrotated and fused kidneys often have multiple arteries [44].

Most common is double renal pelvis, which is of diagnostic significance in incontinence because the cranial pelvis is often drained by a ureter with an ectopic orifice or with a ureterocele. It should be remembered that a stone in one ureter of a double kidney can cause stasis in only one part of the kidney. In many other respects, the presence of a double kidney is of diagnostic importance. Double kidneys often have two renal arteries.

Blind ureter, which may be short or long, may be regarded as an incomplete development of a double kidney.

Anomalies of the calyces, microcalyces, calyx border evaginations, etc., are common. Some of the changes described as anomalies — e.g., many so-called pyelogenous cysts — are definitely pathologic changes, such as old papillary necroses or communicating renal cysts.

Hypoplasia is a not uncommon disorder consisting of a small kidney with irregular, dilated calyces. The changes may involve an entire kidney, part of a kidney, or only one part of a double kidney. Definite distinction between developmental anomaly of the kidney or part of it and shrinkage through pyelonephritis is often impossible. Undoubtedly many of the changes described as hypoplasia are manifestations of pyelonephritis and vascular changes.

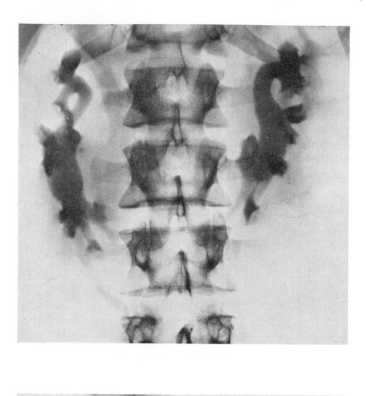

Figure 4-10. Horseshoe kidney fused caudally. Urography. Kidney pelves and ureters swing medially. Some calyces directed medially.

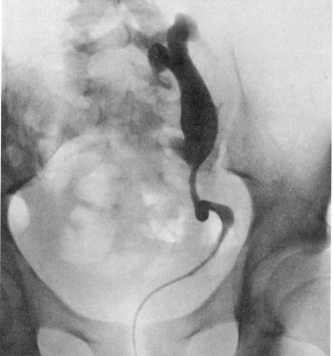

Figure 4-11. Caudal ectopy. Pyelography.

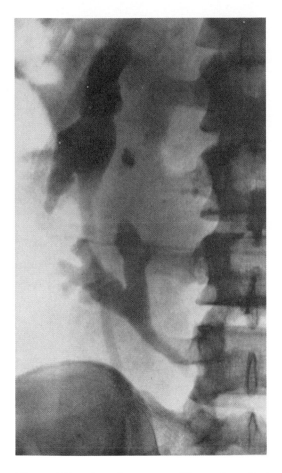

Figure 4-12. Crossed ectopy. Urography. Both kidneys fused on the right side, "left" kidney caudal to right. Ureter swings over to left.

VASCULAR ANOMALIES

Multiple renal arteries represent the most common vascular abnormality. We have found multiple arteries in 23.8 per cent of a large series. After exclusion of cases of hydronephrosis, the frequency was 20.6 per cent. About half of the supplementary arteries arose at a distance up to 19 mm. from the main renal artery. Then the frequency of multiple arteries decreased with increasing distance from the main artery. After a distance of 80 mm., however, the frequency again began to increase. The distribution of supplementary arteries in our material showed a preponderance of arteries to the lower pole segment, which was supplied by more than 70 per cent of the multiple arteries. In double kidney, malrotation (Fig. 4-13), fusion, and hydronephrosis, multiple arteries are common.

On selective angiography special attention must be given to the possibility of multiple arteries. Therefore the pattern of the arteries must be checked and the nephrogram studied for any defects. If the catheter for selective angiography is passed into a small supplementary artery and the entire dose of contrast medium is deposited there, the result will be a high concentration of the medium in a small portion of the kidney. If the tip of the catheter lies in the main renal artery but a supplementary artery is present, branches to a portion of the kidney will be missing in the arteriogram and a corresponding defect will be seen in the nephrogram. Unless the possibility of a supplementary artery is borne in mind, an erroneous diagnosis may result.

RETROCAVAL URETER

Retrocaval ureter (e.g., anteureteric caval vein) is a vascular anomaly intruding upon the ureter. Owing to disturbance in the embryologic development of the inferior caval vein, this vein runs anterior to the ureter and obstructs drainage of the renal pelvis and the upper part of the ureter, which then shows a severe kink. Combined pyelography and cavography will demonstrate this anomaly clearly.

Stone

Practically all concrements in the kidneys and ureters contain apatite and triple phosphate, and the calcium content is so high that even small stones can usually be demonstrated by plain radiography. The group of less radiopaque stones, such as uric acid calculi,

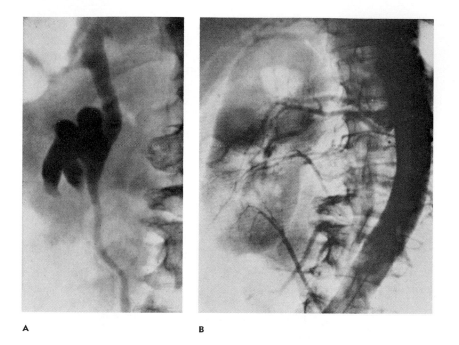

A   B

Figure 4-13. Malrotation. A. Urography. Caudal calyces point medially. B. Renal angiography of same patient. Hilus directed anteriorly. Three arteries supply the kidney.

represents a very low percentage of all urinary tract stones. In cystinuria the concrements are less opaque, but they can usually be demonstrated in plain films.

Stones are prone to appear in certain conditions such as metabolic disorders with an elevated concentration of oxalic acid, uric acid, and cystine, and often in familial metabolic disorders. Certain diseases such as hyperparathyroidism and sarcoidosis favor stone formation, and nephrocalcinosis may occur (Fig. 4-14). In vitamin A deficiency, myeloma, and leukemia, stones are common. Stone formation may also be favored by certain types of treatment which produce increased precipitation of calcium in the urine, such as vitamin D in too large a dose, parathormone or AT 10, mandelic acid, etc. Acetazoleamide may also induce stone formation. So-called recumbency stones may occur in patients who have been bedridden for a long time.

It is important to ascertain whether a calcification seen is actually situated in the kidney. This can be readily decided by taking films in different projections, so-called oblique views. Once this point has been clarified and the calcification has been found to be lodged in the kidney, the next point to decide — usually by urography — is whether the calcification is situated inside the renal pelvis and is thus a stone, or whether it is situated outside the pelvis, i.e., in the renal parenchyma, in which case it is a parenchymal calcification.

The shape of the stone often suggests the existence or nature of renal anomalies or pathologic processes. It may thus, for instance, correspond to a separated papilla (see Fig. 4-39). Multiple stones may have the appearance characteristic of medullary sponge kidney (see Fig. 4-31). The position of the stone may show that it is situated in a cavity near the surface of the kidney, or it may have the shape of one of the pelves in a double kidney, etc.

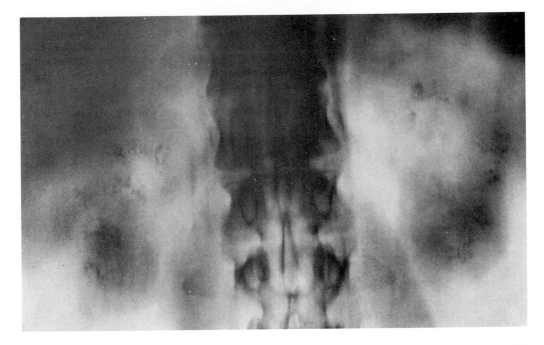

Figure 4-14. Body section radiography of both kidneys showing nephrocalcinosis in hyperparathyroidism.

Concrements may change rapidly in position as well as in size and shape. Differences in the shape of a stone are often simply due to differences in projection. An irregularly shaped concrement may rotate, with change in shape and size in the roentgenogram as a result, but a change in size may also be a true change due to rapid calcification of the organic matrix, with increase in the size of the stone. Decrease in the size of a stone may be due to fragmentation and passage of some of the fragments. If check roentgenography fails to show a previously demonstrable stone, the explanation usually is passage of the stone, but it might also be migration of the stone to that part of the ureter projected over the pelvic bones. If a stone situated in the ureter is no longer demonstrable on check roentgenography, it is usually because the stone has passed, but it should be borne in mind that stones may be displaced in the cranial direction right up into the renal pelvis, especially if dilatation of the ureter is present.

Roentgen examination may give a clue to the understanding of the formation of stone. Thus, small stones are sometimes seen to form at the fornix calyces (Fig. 4-15), but stone is more frequently seen in an organic matrix, such as a detached papilla.

Urography often shows signs of contraction or shrinkage around the stone in the renal pelvis, and sometimes the mucosa is high and irregular. When such changes are seen, malignant metaplasia may be suspected.

It is important to ascertain whether the stone impairs renal function, particularly by obstructing drainage of the renal pelvis or part of it. Urography is a good examination method for this purpose. Even if the renal pelvis is full of large stones, excretion usually is demonstrable unless there is severe renal stasis (Figs. 4-16, 4-17). If a stone is impacted in the stem or a branch of a calyx and produces stasis, excretion from that part of the kidney will be impaired. If the stone is impacted at the pelviureteric junction or in the

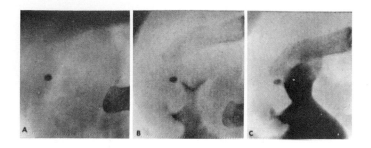

Figure 4-15. Stone at calyx edge. A. Plain film. B. Urography before application of ureteric compression. C. During compression.

ureter, urography may show complete absence of excretion.

If no contrast medium is excreted, the reason may be that obstruction of the drainage has raised the intrapelvic pressure above the secretory pressure of the kidney. It might be, on the other hand, that prolonged stasis has produced atrophy of the kidney. This can be checked by renal angiography because, in the presence of potential renal function, the renal artery is of ordinary width or only slightly narrowed, while in renal atrophy it is appreciably narrower than normal. If the caliber of the artery has decreased to at least half that on the other side, renal function cannot recover even after removal of the obstruction.

In *acute renal colic,* urography is an indispensable examination method. The examina-

tion should be done as quickly as possible, i.e., during the attack. If the pain is due to renal colic, urography will show one or more signs of stasis: the kidney is enlarged, excretion of contrast urine is delayed, the renal pelvis is dilated, an uninterrupted filling of the ureter is obtained down to the site of the stone, and emptying of the renal pelvis is retarded. Severe stasis stops excretion of contrast urine but causes an accumulation of contrast medium in the entire renal parenchyma. If the pain is due to a process outside the urinary pathways, it will not cause stasis. If the pain is on the right side, differential diagnosis of appendicitis versus renal colic can be difficult clinically. Then urography is a rapid and reliable method. Acute appendicitis never produces stasis of the urinary pathways; renal

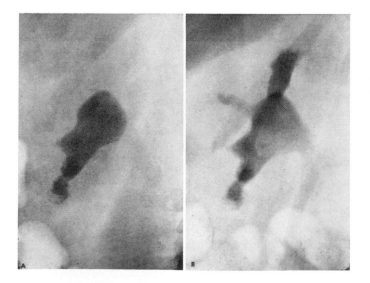

Figure 4-16. Large staghorn calculus filling confluence and inferior branch of kidney pelvis. A. Plain film. B. Urography showing fairly good excretion of contrast medium. No distention of calyces.

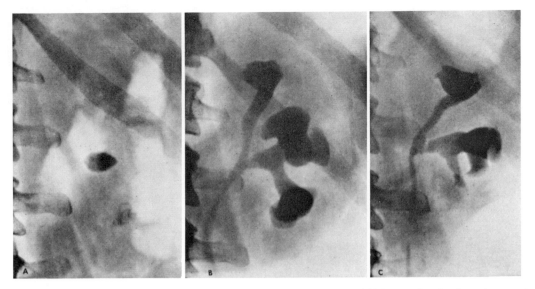

Figure 4-17. Kidney stones. A. Plain film showing stone in hilar part of kidney and collection of stones in caudal pole. B. Urography with ureteric compression. Stone at confluence of branches from middle and caudal part of kidney. Stones in caudal pole lodged in lowermost calyces. C. Urography after removal of stones and caudal polar nephrectomy.

colic, on the other hand, always does, provided the examination is done *during* the attack of pain.

When the pain of renal colic has abated, the signs of stasis decrease or disappear. Within a few hours of the cessation of pain, only 80 per cent of all cases will show roentgenographic signs of stasis, and after one day only 50 per cent.

The fact that the pain proves to be due to renal colic does not necessarily imply that it is due to concrement. If no stone is demonstrable, roentgenologically or clinically, the possibility that the pain is due to a blood clot, for example, must be considered. Then the examination should be repeated after about one week, following ordinary preparation of the patient and with the application of ureteric compression for examination of the anatomy of the renal pelvis. Renal tuberculosis and renal tumor, for example, may cause hemorrhage, and subsequent clot formation may cause renal colic. Such a lesion is detected by urography at the check examination.

It is pertinent to comment here on the term *reflex anuria* in renal colic. My experience in experimental investigations and in the examination of more than a thousand patients in the acute stage of renal colic has convinced me that this term may be deleted in discussions of this disease. If no excretion of contrast medium is demonstrable on either side in acute renal colic, obstruction is bilateral or secretion pressure of the kidneys is low because of shock.

If a ureteric stone is the cause of renal colic, the question arises whether or not the stone may be expected to pass spontaneously. On analysis of our very large material it was found that small stones, with a roentgenographic width of less than 4 mm., in the lower half of the ureter will usually pass spontaneously. Medium-sized stones, 4 to 6 mm., in the lower half of the ureter will pass spontaneously in about half of the cases. Large stones, more than 6 mm., in the lower half of the ureter only occasionally pass spontaneously.

If expectant treatment is decided upon, renal function should be regularly evaluated. This is best done with urography.

Tumor

Benign renal tumors are less common than malignant tumors — renal carcinoma in adults and embryoma in infants.

The appearance of renal carcinoma in plain roentgenography varies widely with the size, mode of growth, and site of the tumor. There may be a generalized enlargement of the kidney with or without preservation of shape, or part of the kidney may show a protuberance. A well-defined pathologic process will have a sharp outline, but if the growth infiltrates contiguous tissue, the outline will be diffuse. Small tumors situated deep in the renal parenchyma cannot be demonstrated by plain roentgenography.

Some tumors contain calcifications. A localization of the calcifications in the center of an expanding lesion means that the lesion is a tumor, and not a cyst (Fig. 4-18). Both tumors and cysts can give rise to thin peripheral calcifications.

Pyelography and urography may show the renal pelvis, and possibly the upper part of the ureter, to be deformed by the tumor, particularly if it is central and large, but to a lesser degree if it is situated in the periphery or if it is small. The deformation varies widely from case to case with the size of the tumor, its position, shape, and mode of growth, and also with the primary anatomic form of the renal pelvis. The deformation is to a large extent dependent on the fixation of the kidney. An infiltrative growth may encroach upon the pelvic wall, which then becomes stiff and irregular, and the tumor may protrude into the renal pelvis. A large tumor may severely impair the excretion of contrast urine in urography. Those parts of the skeleton included in

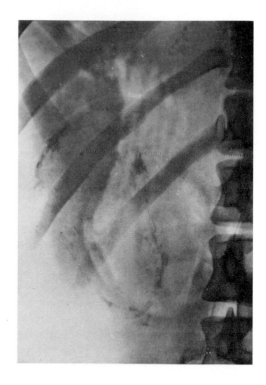

Figure 4-18. Intrarenal irregular calcifications in renal carcinoma. Calcifications are localized peripherally and centrally.

roentgenograms of the kidney should always be studied for possible metastases.

If a space-occupying process is rounded and shows no signs of infiltration or metastases, plain roentgenography, pyelography, or urography will not indicate whether or not the tumor is malignant. The first question is to decide whether the change is due to a solid tumor or to a simple cyst. Renal angiography will nearly always give the answer (Fig. 4-19). This method in addition can give the diagnosis where other methods have failed, as in the case of a patient with a small but nevertheless clinically important tumor.

With good timing of the exposures so that they cover the end of the arterial phase and the beginning of the nephrographic phase, angiography will show pathologic vessels, usually with several arteriovenous fistulas, in

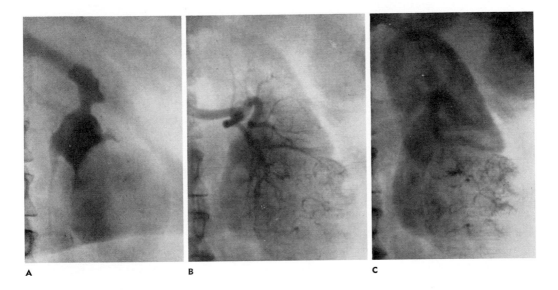

A   B   C

Figure 4-19.   Renal carcinoma. A. Urography: marked displacement of lowermost calyces around spherical well-defined expansive growth with even surface. Differential diagnosis of well-defined renal carcinoma versus simple cyst not possible in plain radiography and urography. B and C. Renal angiography. B. Arterial phase. Arteries to lower pole of kidney displaced. Multiple pathologic arteries. C. Nephrographic phase. Tumor well-defined against normal kidney parenchyma. Thus, renal angiography allows a definite diagnosis of renal carcinoma.

at least 90 per cent of all cases. The rare avascular or poorly vascularized tumors are ill-defined against the normal renal parenchyma.

Cysts, on the other hand, contain no vessels at all and show a sharp border against the renal parenchyma, which is best demonstrated in tangential projections against the pit in the parenchyma caused by the cyst. Vessels are seldom, if ever, seen in that part of the cyst wall protruding outside the kidney.

Renal angiography should be done selectively; otherwise, superimposition of irrelevant vessels will diminish the possibility of definitive interpretation. Folin [19], in a large series of angiographically examined renal carcinomas and cysts, demonstrated the high reliability of angiography in the diagnosis and differential diagnosis of these processes.

The nature of an expansive process may also be studied by percutaneous puncture (see Fig. 4-22). There is, however, an understandable antipathy to puncture of a malignant tumor. Puncture of a cyst yields clear fluid. Contrast medium should be injected into the cyst and the examination done in such a way as to make sure that the inner wall of the cyst filled with contrast medium is smooth, that it contains only fluid, and that its outline coincides exactly with that of the process seen in the plain roentgenogram and pyelogram. Careful attention should be given to these features, because renal tumors often necrotize and undergo a varying degree of cystic degeneration, sometimes probably complete.

Renal angiography also provides a possibility of detecting metastases in lymph nodes near the kidney as well as local recurrences after nephrectomy for renal carcinoma. In carotid or vertebral angiography the appearance of cerebral metastases from a renal tumor is in many cases the same as that in renal angiography of the primary tumor.

Experience has shown that in the presence of a large space-occupying lesion and absence of excretion of contrast urine during urography, hydronephrosis or pyonephrosis should always be borne in mind. For differential diagnosis of hydronephrosis from renal tumor, angiography is the method of choice.

Renal carcinoma may also occur in infancy, though the most common malignant renal tumor in this stage of life is embryoma. This tumor may develop even during intrauterine life and may be of familial occurrence. It metastasizes to the lungs and liver but, in contrast to sympathicoblastoma, not to the skeleton.

The roentgen findings, including angiographic findings, are principally the same as in renal carcinoma (described above). In the differential diagnosis it must be distinguished from simple cyst, multicystic unilateral kidney disease, and hydronephrosis.

Tumors of the renal pelvis and ureter are polypous and papillomatous, and often malignant — usually transitional cell papillary carcinoma or, less often, squamous cell carcinoma. They are diagnosed by pyelography or urography, during which procedure care must be taken to secure a suitable density of contrast in the renal pelvis (Figs. 4-20, 4-21). The papilloma causes filling defects and then resembles a stone or blood clot. Cancer of the

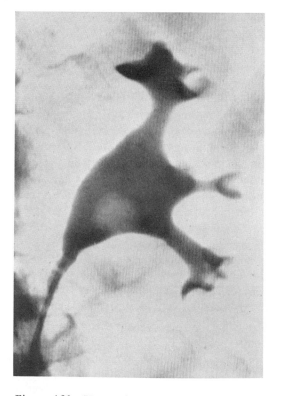

Figure 4-20. Urography showing small polypous carcinoma in confluence of kidney pelvis. (Always remember stone and blood clot as possibilities in the differential diagnosis.)

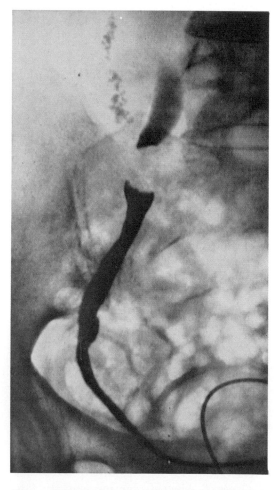

Figure 4-21. Pyelography showing papillomatous ureteric carcinoma causing slight distention of ureter.

renal pelvis can infiltrate the renal pelvic wall along a wide front and also encroach upon the renal parenchyma, in which case it may be difficult to distinguish from a primary renal carcinoma. Angiography is excellent for diagnosis of renal pelvis tumors that have caused hydronephrosis [7]. In these cases angiography is characterized by a combination of signs of renal atrophy and pathologic vessels. The preoperative diagnosis of renal pelvis carcinoma as the cause of a hydronephrosis in which nephrectomy is indicated is important for the planning of the operation. In carcinoma-hydronephrosis total ureterectomy should also be included in the operative procedure.

Ureteric papillomas may be very elongated but nevertheless produce only slight or no stasis. Carcinoma of the ureter causes an irregular narrowing of varying length, eventually with severe dilatation proximal thereto.

One must remember that tumors of the renal pelvis and ureter are often multiple. The examination must therefore include the renal pelvis, ureter, and urinary bladder.

Renal Cyst

Among cystic formations, in the kidney, roentgenologically the simple cyst is of greatest interest. Its differentiation from renal carcinoma is described in the preceding section.

The simple cyst may be small and may communicate with the renal pelvis. It may, however, be very large and even extend across the midline. Sometimes two or more simple cysts may occur in the same kidney, and cyst formation may be bilateral. As a rule, the cysts grow slowly or cease to grow after they have assumed a certain size. A cyst may also rupture spontaneously and collapse.

Cysts are more or less deep-seated in the renal parenchyma, in which they produce a cavity which gives a characteristic appearance, especially when viewed tangentially, in the nephrographic phase. Capsular cysts are situated outside the parenchyma, as is the peripelvic lymphatic cyst.

The diagnosis and differential diagnosis were described in the previous section (Fig.

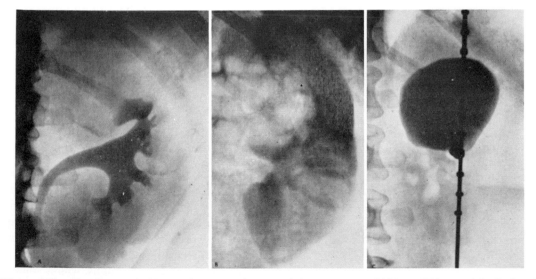

Figure 4-22. Simple cyst. A. Urography: expansive growth in upper part of kidney. Kidney pelvis displaced downward and cranial calyces flattened. Differential diagnosis of renal carcinoma versus simple cyst not possible. B. Renal angiography, nephrographic phase: characteristic filling defect caused by cyst. C. Percutaneous puncture of cyst (clear fluid) and filling with contrast medium. Cyst has even inner surface and corresponds exactly to filling defect seen in nephrogram.

4-22). It is often stated in the literature that cysts and well-defined renal carcinoma can be distinguished from one another because the contents of the cysts in plain roentgenograms are less radiopaque than the cancer tissue. This difference in density is exceptional and is therefore of no importance from the point of view of differential diagnosis.

At plain roentgenography a well-defined round or oval space-occupying lesion is seen. The outline is smooth. Only if two or more cysts are situated adjacent to one another is it irregular. Calcifications are rare. They may occasionally be seen in a minor part of the cyst capsule. Very rarely is this capsule completely calcified. In such cases tumor should be suspected.

As a rule, the excretion of contrast urine will be good. Only if the cyst is very large will it impair renal function. Deformation of the renal pelvis varies with the size and position of the cyst. Cysts situated in the periphery, even large ones, produce only slight deformation of the renal pelvis, e.g., a slight flattening of a calyx, which is demonstrable in suitable projection. At angiography tangential views of the lesion should be secured for the demonstration of the characteristic outline of the cyst. Only small, deep-seated cysts in the renal parenchyma are likely to escape detection and need tomography in the nephrographic phase for their demonstration. In this connection, once more the importance of selective angiography should be stressed. The possibility of multiple arteries should be kept in mind. So-called nephrotomography may be useful but is less dependable than selective angiography.

The multilocular cyst is, as was pointed out, significant in the differential diagnosis of embryoma.

Hydatid cysts are of less importance despite the increasing international travel and trade of today, which increase the possibilities of infestation. These cysts are much more common in the liver than in the kidneys. They often have an irregularly calcified capsule.

Polycystic disease is a bilateral, congenital, hereditary disease (see Chap. 35). Both kidneys contain a number of cysts varying widely in size and spread.

The kidneys may be only slightly enlarged or they may fill the major part of the abdomen (Fig. 4-23). Single or multiple cysts may show peripheral calcifications, which may be of irregular shape because the cysts influence one another's shape. Urography will show multifocal, moderate to grotesque deformation. In advanced cases renal function is impaired and the contrast medium is only of low to moderate concentration, though as a rule it is sufficiently opaque to reveal the changes. The roentgenographic appearance of the kidney on one side may differ widely from that on the other.

Only in exceptional cases is angiography indicated, and then to assess the amount of functioning renal parenchyma for judging the prognosis. The angiographic findings are usually characteristic: the arteries are thin and stretched, and in the nephrographic phase multiple, closely crowded, filling defects of varying size can be seen, due to innumerable cysts in the cortex.

Tuberculosis

Treatment of renal tuberculosis has undergone radical changes during the last few years. The roentgen diagnostic methods have been modified accordingly. When nephrectomy was the rule in the treatment of unilateral renal tuberculosis, the purpose of roentgen examination was to demonstrate the tuberculous parenchymal focus in communication with the renal pelvis, and pyelography was a suitable method. With conservative therapy, however, possibly in combination with selective surgery, urography and angiography have become

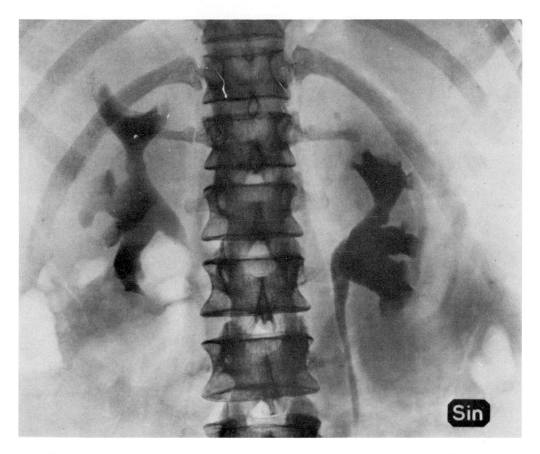

Figure 4-23.   Polycystic kidneys. Plain radiography showed both kidneys enlarged and with bulging surface. Urography. Good contrast excretion. On right side, several calyces are flattened and moderately displaced by a multicentric expansive lesion. On left side, lowermost calyces slightly flattened. Increased distance between periphery of calyces and kidney surface.

more important. On repeated check examination, urography places a much less severe strain on the patient than pyelography. If partial nephrectomy is planned, knowledge of the extent of the process within the renal parenchyma as well as of the vascular anatomy is valuable, and such information can be obtained from angiography.

Renal tuberculosis usually is a slow process, particularly since the advent of tuberculostatics. The earliest demonstrable change consists of caseation of one or more papillae. The process may involve the entire renal parenchyma; necrotic masses may undergo calcification; new-formed tissue may shrink, particularly in the renal pelvis, the ureter, and the urinary bladder. This last course (accentuated by tuberculostatics) explains the wide variability of the roentgenologic appearance of the disease.

In early cases *plain roentgenography* will show no changes. If the disease is extensive, the kidney may show a generalized increase in size or local bulges. The tuberculous contracted kidney may appear as a kidney considerably reduced in size.

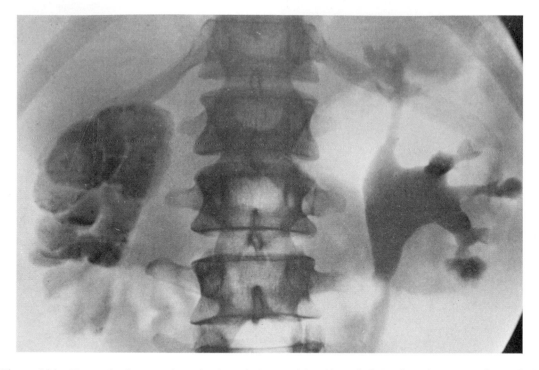

Figure 4-24. Urography in case of renal tuberculosis. On right side, calcified tuberculous pyonephrotic kidney — so-called putty kidney. On left side, small ulcerations in most papillae conflowing in upper part of kidney.

Calcifications in the renal parenchyma are common and usually of irregular shape. They may be small and they may involve the entire kidney, with so-called putty kidney as a result (Fig. 4-24). Judging from our experience, calcifications occur in about half of the cases, often in patients reporting no symptoms whatsoever from the urinary tract. Most of our patients were examined because of epididymitis. This implies that even an extensive lesion may progress asymptomatically. The ureter, also, may calcify, and sometimes, though rarely, the bladder.

If the pathologic process is of limited or moderate extent, *urography* will show only a slight or no decrease in the density of the contrast medium. An advanced process may be manifested by poor density or absence of excretion of contrast medium. Thus, small changes may give favorable examination conditions. Large processes, on the other hand, can be demonstrated even if excretion is poor. If properly performed, urography will demonstrate even the earliest changes, and pyelography will seldom be necessary.

The earliest change is ulceration of a papilla, seen as a contrast filling of a usually irregularly outlined cavity in the periphery of the papilla, or more centrally with a fistula into the renal pelvis (Fig. 4-25). Destruction of renal parenchyma may be extensive, and then a contrast filling will be obtained of large, irregularly outlined cavities that may displace the calyces. Stricture of the originally narrow parts such as the stems of the calyces, the pelviureteric junction, and the ureteric orifice is common. As in all types of tuberculosis, shrinkage is marked and produces considerable deformation of the renal pelvis, sometimes with obstruction of drainage and dilatation, which

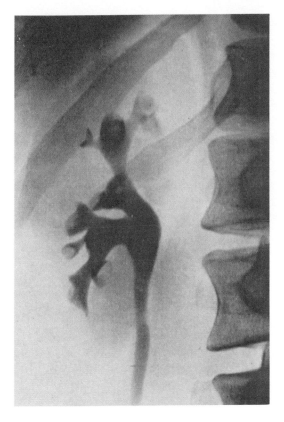

Figure 4-25. Renal tuberculosis. Solitary papillary ulceration. Contrast medium fills irregular cavity in connection with uppermost calyx.

accelerates the destruction of parenchyma still more. The irregular shrinkage may cause a pursing of parts of the renal pelvis. This is a very characteristic change of renal tuberculosis.

Early cases of renal tuberculosis must be differentiated from anomalies of the calyx and from fornix reflux (see earlier discussion). A very important differential diagnosis is papillary necrosis in pyelonephritis.

The urinary bladder shows local irregular mucosal thickening, usually near the orifice of the ureter draining the diseased kidney. The changes may progress and result in a small, contracted bladder. Urethrocystography will reveal irregular abscesses situated in the prostatic gland and communicating with the

lumen in the urethra. Strictures may develop in the urethra, which, in constrast to what is seen in gonorrhea, are located in its posterior part.

Renal angiography will demonstrate the vascular anatomy and displacement of intra-renal arterial branches. Endarteritic vascular changes are often demonstrable. The nephrographic phase, however, is the most important, because it yields valuable information on the extension as well as the exact position of the tuberculous process within the kidney parenchyma, which is of importance in the planning of selective surgery. It should be remembered that, broadly speaking, pyelography yields only indirect information on the size and shape of the process, i.e., its effect on the shape of the renal pelvis. Angiography, on the other hand, gives direct information because it demonstrates the lesion directly in the renal parenchyma.

Conservative treatment requires repeated check examination, which should preferably be done with plain radiography and urography. During such treatment a minor or major part of the renal pelvis is liable to be shut off by strictures of a branch or neck of a calyx. Such occlusion is suggestive of healing, but behind the stricture the process in the parenchyma may progress and spread, with further destruction of the parenchyma. This must be borne in mind in the evaluation of therapy, just as it must be recollected that even untreated tuberculosis of the kidneys and urinary tract may show such cicatrization.

Urinary Tract Dilatation

Dilatation of the urinary pathways, unilateral or bilateral, complete or partial, moderate or severe, is common and plays a prominent role in urologic diagnostic roentgenology. It may be a readily explainable and more or less important component of some disease of known pathogenesis, or it may dominate the

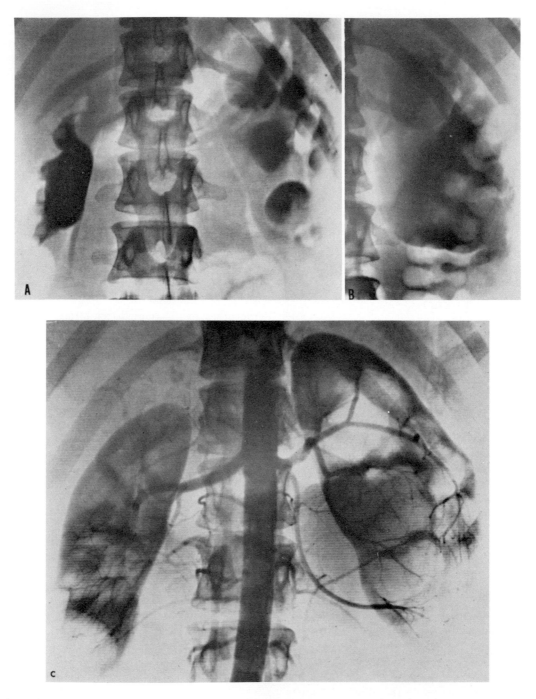

Figure 4-26. Hydronephrosis due to obstruction at pelviureteric junction. A. Urography showing marked dilatation of calyces. B. Prone position filling of ventrally situated dilated confluence part of kidney pelvis. C and D. Renal angiography shows polar artery to lower pole of left kidney displaced in a medially convex curve corresponding to medial border of dilated pelvis. D. Nephrographic phase shows dilated renal sinus. E and F. Check urography: dilatation of kidney pelvis has diminished considerably.

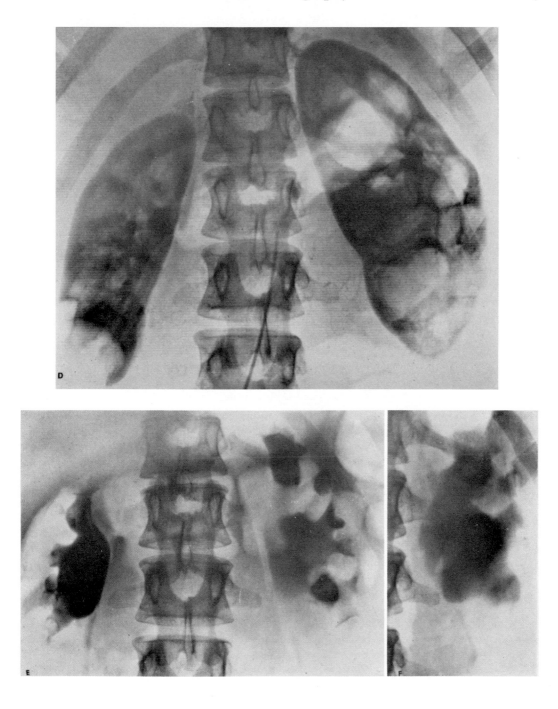

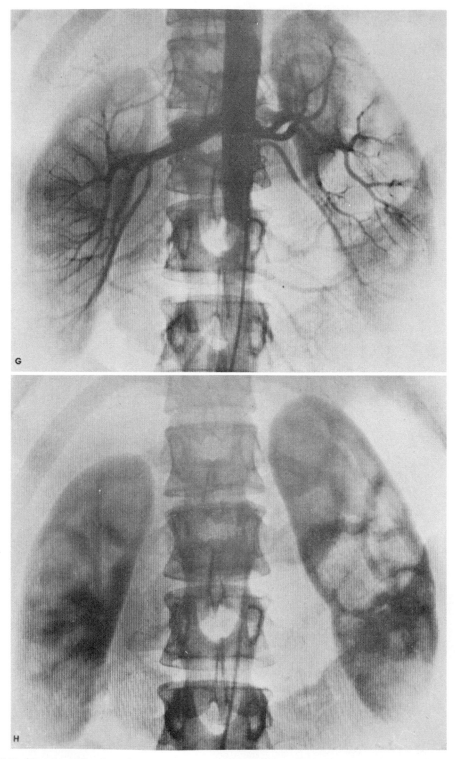

Figure 4-26 (Continued).   G and H. Angiography. Postoperative check after transposition of displaced vessel. The vessel runs a straight course. Kidney size close to normal.

pathologic picture to such an extent as to be regarded as a disease *sui generis*.

Roentgen examination of dilatation of the urinary tract has numerous facets. Only certain fundamental facts are dwelt on here. The tactics of examination may be best exemplified in the investigation of the obstructed pelviureteric junction.

It is widely believed that pyelography is the method of choice in the examination of dilatation of the renal pelvis, because it offers possibilities of studying the anatomy at the pelviureteric junction, particularly in patients with high intrapelvic pressure. Pyelography with retrograde injection of fluid into a dilated renal pelvis with obstructed drainage, however, is attended by the risk of infection of an organ in a state of retention and by the risk of converting a decompensated organ into an uncompensated one. I consider that it is important to study the effect of the dilatation on renal function; hence I believe that urography combined with angiography is preferable in the examination of hydronephrosis.

A markedly dilated renal pelvis in *plain roentgenography* will show up as a large, soft tissue mass at the site of the kidney. In moderate dilatation the dilated renal pelvis may appear as a medially well-defined soft tissue mass at the hilus. The excretion of contrast urine is usually good in cases of moderate dilatation. In the beginning of the examination, when the patient is in the supine position, contrast urine will fill only the most dorsal, i.e., cranial, calyces, after which the other calyces and the confluence will be filled, but slowly. Since the pelviureteric junction is uppermost when the patient is on his back, this will be filled last. Instead of waiting for this part to be filled, which may sometimes take a long time, one may turn the patient over into prone position. The pelviureteric junction will then be lowermost and will be filled immediately with contrast medium, which usually overflows into the ureter.

If the intrapelvic pressure is increased, excretion will be delayed or absent. In intermittent hydronephrosis the roentgenographic appearance may be normal during remissions, but during exacerbations the renal pelvis will be severely dilated and excretion impaired.

In *angiography* the nephrogram will demonstrate any dilatation of the renal sinus and reveal the extent of parenchymal atrophy. The arterial phase will make it possible (see page 154) to judge the potential function of the kidney. Finally, angiography enables evaluation of the vascular anatomy, particularly the presence of multiple arteries and their significance.

Urography and angiography in combination thus yield invaluable information for judging a given case and deciding upon the form of therapy (Fig. 4-26).

The narrowing of the pelviureteric junction is due to intrinsic stenosis, extraureteral adhesions, and vascular anomalies either separately or in combination. Roentgen examination offers good possibilities of assessing which of these factors is responsible. Judging from our experience, bilateral changes are nearly always due to intrinsic stenosis. Stenosis or adhesions (or both) are sometimes seen in patients with vascular anomalies. In less than half of our operated cases with multiple vessels it was the vascular anomaly alone that was responsible for the dilatation of the renal pelvis. In all the cases in which the dilatation was due to a supplementary artery the latter ran ventral to the renal pelvis and regularly arose within 40 mm. of the origin of the main renal artery from the aorta. The supplementary artery runs in a caudolateral direction to the lower pole of the kidney and is displaced in a curve with the convexity facing caudally. If angiography is followed immediately by urography with the patient in the same position, it is possible to trace the urogram onto the angiogram and thereby form a good opinion of the relation of the supplementary vessel to the renal pelvis and to the cranial part of the ureter. It should be observed that not only supplementary arteries but also anomalous veins can cause obstruction.

Angiography is also useful for assessing the results of surgical transposition of a supplementary artery and, as mentioned previously, to distinguish between the type of hydronephrosis described and hydronephrosis caused by renal pelvic carcinoma.

DILATATION OF THE URINARY
TRACT DURING PREGNANCY

A special and important form of urinary tract dilatation is that occurring in almost all women during pregnancy. It is more common on the right side and involves the renal pelvis and the ureter down to the level of the iliac artery. It is sometimes very marked. As a rule, it disappears after delivery, but in some women a slight dilatation persists throughout the rest of life. If pregnancy is complicated by pyelonephritis, persistent dilatation may be marked.

URINARY TRACT DILATATION IN INFANCY

The large majority of urologic diseases in children are due to stasis and infection. Suffice it here to stress that it is important that the roentgen examination in these cases should always include examination of the urethra and bladder. Urethrocystography should be done to check the possibility of urethral valves, for example. During this procedure it is often possible to secure retrograde filling of the urinary tract by holding the child upside down. Dilatation of the bladder and urinary tract in children is often due to voiding difficulties combined with insufficiency and reflux through the ureteral orifice. Unilateral dilatation due to obstruction of flow from the bladder may be produced when only one of the ureteral orifices is incompetent. The diagnosis of incompetency of a ureteric orifice, dilatation of the ureter and the kidney pelvis and of papillary changes suggestive of pyelonephritis is made through retrograde filling obtained during voiding cystography.

MISCELLANEOUS TYPES OF
URINARY TRACT DILATATION

Dilatation of the urinary pathways occurs in a wide variety of diseases, such as hyperplasia of the prostatic gland, stone, periureteral fibrosis, ureteric tumors, and certain genital tumors. In some diseases the dilatation may be local. Thus a tuberculous stricture of a branch of a corresponding part of the renal pelvis, or a stone impacted in the stem of a calyx may cause hydrocalycosis.

Dilatation is of special interest in patients with a double kidney, particularly when only one of the renal pelves is dilated. It is nearly always the cranial renal pelvis that is dilated, and the dilatation is often due to a ureterocele or ectopic opening of a ureter. If urography shows excretion of contrast urine in both pelves of a double kidney, the diagnosis is, of course, easy. As a rule, however, stasis has existed so long in the cranial renal pelvis that the excretion of contrast urine is impaired. In some cases plain radiography and urography will show a space-occupying lesion in the upper part of the kidney, and then the possibility of dilatation of a double kidney should be considered. Renal angiography may be useful and will show a very narrow border of renal parenchyma around the dilated pelvis.

Trauma

Injury to the trunk is common, especially with the increasing number of motorcar accidents. It sometimes results in injury to a kidney or ureter. The severity of the lesion varies widely — from small ruptures of the capsule to complete crushing of the kidney. The trauma as such, but also rapid deceleration, can also cause tearing of the kidney stalk. Tearing of the artery then is the most serious lesion in the acute stage; tearing of the ureter is more serious in the long run. Roentgen examination can reveal the extent of the lesion, and should be performed in such a way as to demonstrate the passage in the ureter.

Plain radiography will show that the kidney, or part of it, is ill-defined. The kidney may be displaced or enlarged, but the enlargement may be only apparent and due to ventral displacement of the kidney by a hematoma. Increased density of the retroperitoneal space with loss of the normal soft tissue anatomy owing to hematoma is characteristic, and fractures of ribs or of transverse processes near the kidney are common. The formation of a hematoma is an important factor. A small injury with a large hematoma can give the impression that the injury is much more severe than it is in reality.

Renal function and the passage of urine through the ureter is best studied with urography. Pyelography is rarely necessary. It is indicated only if passage through the ureter cannot be judged because of delayed secretion of contrast urine. In urography as well as in pyelography, contrast medium from the renal pelvis may be seen to enter the renal parenchyma (Fig. 4-27). The renal pelvis may be deformed. Such deformation can be due to a perirenal hematoma or to a blood clot in the renal pelvis. The hematoma compresses and deforms the renal pelvis, and therefore the extent of the damage cannot be estimated exactly in all cases from the results of the examination of the patient in the acute stage. Reexamination one or two weeks later usually shows rapid regression of the hematoma. If a small rupture is detected by the passage of contrast medium from the renal pelvis into the parenchyma, check radiography some days later will as a rule show that the lesion is closed and that there is no longer any escape of contrast medium.

The basis for the diagnosis can be widened by renal angiography, which shows the extent and type of the damage and will indicate whether there is a rupture or whether it is only a question of a perirenal hematoma and to what extent the rupture or hematoma is

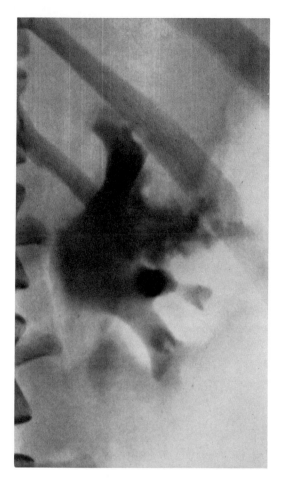

Figure 4-27. Kidney rupture. Trauma against back; hematuria. Acute stage. Urography without ureteric compression. From calyx at middle of kidney extravasation of contrast medium occurs into kidney parenchyma and out into renal sinus.

responsible for the changes. In later stages angiography may show atrophy of parts of the kidney owing to lacerations of blood vessels and displacement of kidney fragments with or without adequate blood supply.

The end results depend mainly on the extent of the injury. Ruptures are said to have excellent healing tendency. Check examination with urography or pyelography will as a rule show normal conditions or only scar formation with consequent slight deformation of the renal pelvis. In the majority of the healed cases, as angiographic studies show, no real rupture existed, but a large hematoma, which caused the changes and which was rapidly resorbed. On the other hand, angiography as a check examination of a real rupture years after may show considerable changes although only slight changes were demonstrated with urography or pyelography. Sometimes, however, renal function may be impaired and the renal pelvis deformed. Occasionally cysts or concrements are seen.

Perirenal hematomas sometimes undergo cystic degeneration or calcification.

The kidney and ureter may also be damaged by the introduction of a catheter. Such injuries are of roentgen diagnostic interest because they produce characteristic changes which are readily explainable by technical mishaps, e.g., subcapsular deposition of contrast medium on passage of the catheter through the renal pelvis in under the renal capsule.

Renal Carbuncle, Abscess, Perinephritis

Local inflammatory processes in the kidney may be due to a renal carbuncle or a renal abscess. The carbuncle is a tumor-like multilocular process consisting of multiple abscesses with a marked reactive tissue zone. The abscess is unilocular and may be solitary or multiple. At roentgen examination the changes in the kidney resemble a space-occupying process, and the differential diagnosis of these fairly rare lesions is largely the same as that of tumors and cysts.

These inflammatory processes in the kidney can break through the renal capsule or infect perirenal tissue via the lymphatics and cause perinephritis. Such perinephritis may also be secondary to an inflammatory process adjacent to the kidney, such as osteomyelitis, or it may be hematogenous. It may also be due to violence, with penetrating wound.

In perinephritis, plain radiography will show severe edema around the kidney. The latter is often enlarged or appears to be enlarged when the patient is examined in the supine position. The abscess usually tends to be thicker posteriorly and therefore lifts the kidney, with the result that the object-film distance will be increased with projection enlargement. A local bulge of the kidney may indicate a local inflammatory process. The kidney is displaced, usually laterally and distally. Gas may be seen in the abscess, sometimes as small bubbles.

The skeletal parts near the kidney should be studied for signs of osteitis.

The changes vary with the extent of the pathologic process, its age, and severity.

Contracture of the muscles in the flank and scoliosis, with the concavity facing the injured side, are often seen. It should be observed that scoliosis, permanent or temporary, may prevent the edge of the psoas muscle from appearing in the usual way. This should not be misconceived as a sign of retroperitoneal edema.

Plain radiography may show a generalized or local meteorism, and the intestine or stomach may then be seen displaced. If the pathologic process is on the left side, for instance, the descending colon may be displaced outward and be narrowed, and examination of the colon will show that the mucosa is edematous (Fig. 4-28). Perforation to the intestine as well as to the skin may sometimes occur. Fistulography may then be useful.

The diaphragm is often high on the affected side, and its excursions are limited. In the basal parts of the lung on that side, lamellar atelectases are common. Fluid in the corresponding pleural cavity is also common. The examination for fluid should be performed with the patient in the lateral decubitus position and with the beam horizontal. Only in this way is it possible to demonstrate small quantities of fluid.

In some patients with perinephritic abscess, urography and pyelography will show no

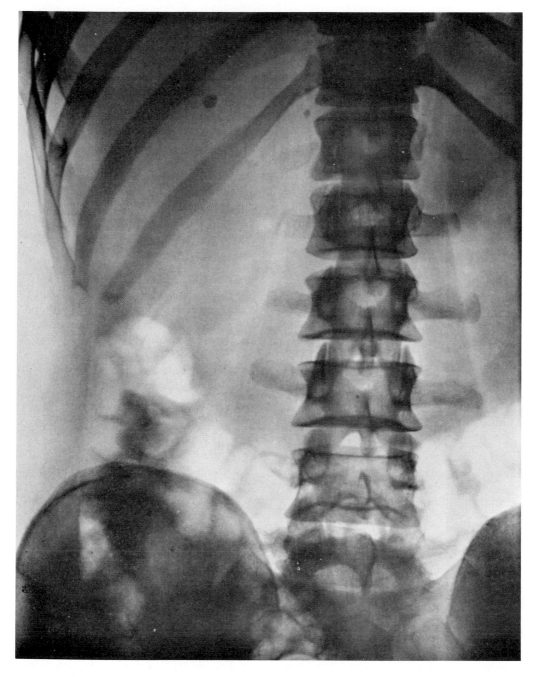

Figure 4-28. **Perinephritis.** Right kidney enlarged, partly with blurred outline. Retroperitoneal edema with blurring of anatomy in retroperitoneal space. Edge of psoas muscle cannot be seen on the right side. It is sharply outlined on the left.

change in the shape of the renal pelvis, while in other patients the extrarenal process may compress and markedly deform it. A proper examination technic, particularly views from suitable angles, will enable distinction between an extrarenal and an intrarenal process. The type of deformation varies with the site of the abscess, and the severity with its size.

Calcifications may occur in old abscesses.

The roentgen diagnosis of perinephritic abscess is sometimes difficult because the patients are often very ill and because clinical symptoms of the abscess are often not characteristic or are masked by other symptoms. The various roentgen abnormalities are not specific but, taken together, they allow a roentgen diagnosis of perinephritic abscess with a high degree of certainty.

Primary Vascular Changes

The foregoing discussion of the angiographic appearance of various renal diseases included a description of more or less characteristic secondary vascular changes occurring, for example, in renal tumor and tuberculosis, etc. Primary vascular changes as a cause of certain diseases, particularly in some cases of hypertension, are of great diagnostic importance. The most common is arteriosclerosis. Plain radiography will sometimes show calcifications in the vessel walls, usually intimal calcifications, but sometimes characteristic medial calcifications. They are localized to the main trunk, but they may also occur in intrarenal arterial branches. Tortuous, rigid vessels can also cause marked impressions in the wall of the renal pelvis, which are demonstrable by urography and pyelography. Angiography will show tortuosity of vessels, varying caliber or even complete obliteration, but also fairly local changes in the form of narrowings of varying length around the entire circumference of the vessel or part of it, with or without poststenotic widening (Fig.

4-29). The arteriosclerotic changes may cause only a short narrowing, such as contraction at the site of departure of the renal artery from the aorta. More extensive changes may be part of generalized arteriosclerosis with advanced changes in the aorta and both renal arteries. Collateral circulation from the aorta to the kidney bypassing the stenotic segment is often seen. Check radiography at various intervals will sometimes show rapid progression of the changes. Fibromuscular hyperplasia affects the renal artery, causing single or multiple narrowings, often with marked beading of one or both arteries.

Aneurysms in the renal arteries are well known (Fig. 4-30), since they can sometimes be seen as characteristic calcifications, rings 1 to 3 cm. in diameter, and often with a small defect corresponding to the neck of the aneurysm. The calcifications are usually situated outside but close to the kidney, but sometimes they are seen within the kidney. By no means do all aneurysms calcify. Uncalcified aneurysms demonstrated by renal angiography produce the same signs as aneurysms elsewhere, i.e., a more or less spherical or a fusiform widening of the vessel. The latter type is frequently seen as a poststenotic widening distal to a narrowing. Aneurysms are often bilateral.

Arteriovenous aneurysms are rare, but are readily diagnosed angiographically. They produce the same radiologic signs in the kidney as they do in the cerebrum, for example. Arteriovenous fistulas, for instance, caused by needle biopsy can also be well demonstrated by angiography.

Emboli in the renal artery may be diagnosed in the acute stage of the disease by angiography, which will show total occlusion of the renal artery, or one or more branches peripherally. Plain radiography will usually show a slight enlargement of the kidney, and urography demonstrates absence of excretion of contrast urine, while pyelography will show a renal pelvis of ordinary outline. Check

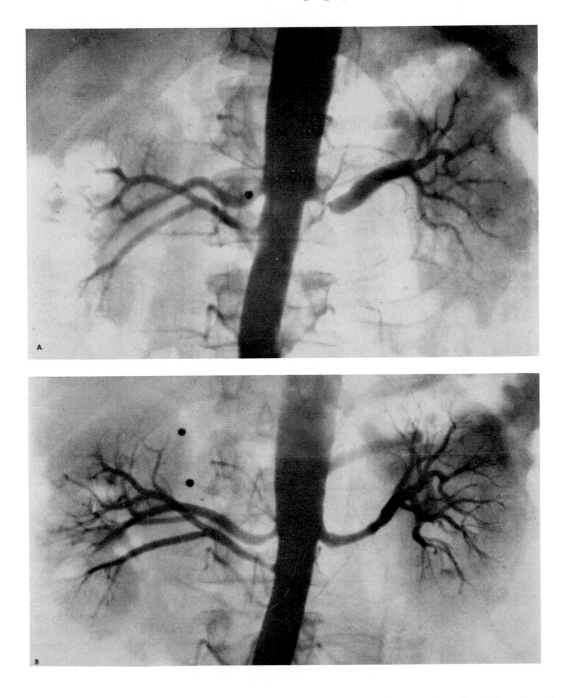

Figure 4-29. Aortic renal angiography. A. Marked stenosis in intrarenal arterial branch. Wide collateral arteries via the renal pelvic arteries, a common collateral pathway. B. After reparative surgery on the left side, slight fibromuscular changes in left renal artery.

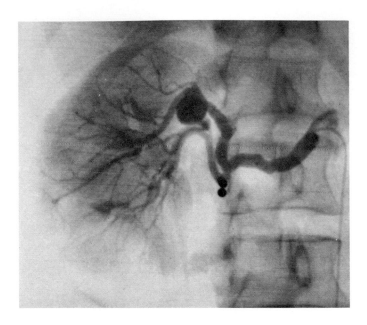

Figure 4-30. Arterial aneurysm and arteriosclerosis. Selective renal angiography shows marked arteriosclerotic changes in main renal artery and in ventral branch in which a saccular aneurysm, 1 cm. in diameter, is seen at entrance of artery into sinus. (Selective angiography contralateral side: no aneurysm.)

examinations after the acute stage has passed will show that the kidney gradually decreases markedly in size, with corresponding reduction in the size of the renal pelvis. In renal infarction a small or large, single or multiple indentation may be seen in the surface of the kidney. At angiography in the acute stage an ill-defined avascular area is seen. In later stages this area diminishes in size and is well defined. Old infarctions and pyelonephritic scars have the same appearance angiographically.

Renal vein thrombosis may develop in the same way as thrombosis elsewhere. If the onset is acute, examination may show an enlargement of the kidney and perirenal edema, while urography will show absence of excretion of contrast urine. Toward the end of the acute stage, cavography may reveal thrombosis manifested by filling defects or a filling of collateral veins. Varicosities of venous trunks forming the renal vein can cause hematuria and can sometimes be seen at urography as irregularly shaped filling defects in the kidney pelvis. Their nature can be demonstrated by retrograde phlebography.

Medullary Sponge Kidney

Medullary sponge kidney consists of a malformation of the pyramids with a widening of the collecting tubules in one, several, or all pyramids in one or both kidneys. The changes may be part of a disease complex, for instance, with cystic disease of the liver. The changes are most readily demonstrated by urography, at which a filling will be obtained of the wide excretory ducts in the frequently hypertrophic papillae (Figs. 4-31, 4-32). Medullary sponge kidney can often be demonstrated even by plain radiography, because concrements of characteristic appearance form in the diseased papillae. The concrements are usually small, often numerous, and localized to the papilla or papillae involved. The change is important for differential diagnosis in papillary ulceration and papillary necrosis, e.g., tuberculosis, pyelonephritis.

Gas in the Urinary Pathways

A more or less complete filling of the renal pelvis with gas — a spontaneous gas pyelo-

Figure 4-31. Sponge kidney. A. Plain film showing multiple small stones corresponding to hypertrophic papilla in cranial kidney pole. B. Urography showing widened, stone-containing ducts in hypertrophic papillae in uppermost part of kidney.

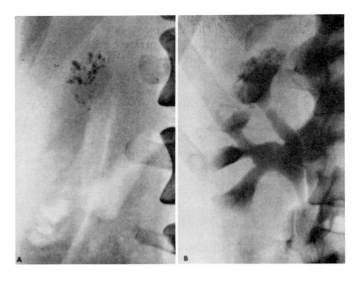

gram, so to speak — can be seen in the presence of fistulization between the urinary tract and a gas-containing organ (Fig. 4-33) such as the digestive tract. Such fistulas may be surgical, as in ureterosigmoidostomy, or they may be spontaneous, caused by perforation of

concrement from the renal pelvis or ureter to the intestine.

Gas can also form in the urinary tract in the presence of gas-producing bacteria with an inflammatory renal lesion. In urine from diabetic patients, for example, fermentation can

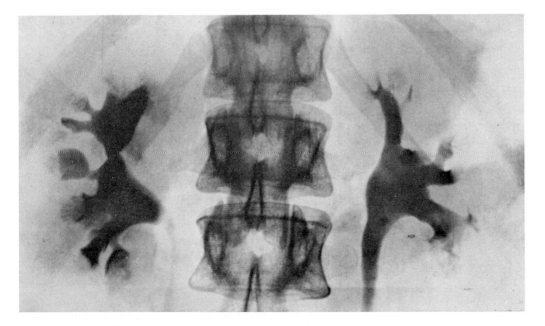

Figure 4-32. Sponge kidneys with dilated papillary ducts bilaterally and slight papillary hypertrophy on the right side.

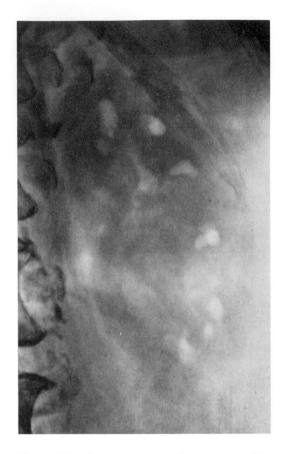

Figure 4-33. Spontaneous gas formation in kidney in diabetic patient with papillary necrosis. Gas fills cavities of shed papillae.

take place with the formation of carbon dioxide.

Gas may be produced in the wall of the urinary tract, and bullae can be formed which may rupture, with the content of gas escaping into the lumen of the bladder or kidney pelvis, as in emphysematous or phlegmonous cystitis.

Generalized Renal Disease

This group includes particularly pyelonephritis, glomerulonephritis, and tubular nephritis — renal diseases which, though of great surgical interest, represent the major part of urologic diseases usually falling within the field of the specialty often called nephrology. They are common causes of acute and chronic renal insufficiency, and in this respect have a common roentgen diagnostic basis.

In a discussion of generalized renal disease it should be borne in mind that the differential diagnosis, as a rule, is made clinically and is sometimes very uncertain, and that at least in the case of pyelonephritis the renal disease is often seen in association with some other pathologic process with its own roentgen diagnostic characteristics.

ACUTE RENAL FAILURE

Acute renal failure is a life-threatening condition. In the examination of patients with this disease the first step is to decide whether the acute failure is due to a lesion preventing the production of urine or to obstructed drainage. In the latter case, provisional or permanent passage of the urine can be secured by surgical intervention. In the former, the situation requires measures to prevent the formation of urinary toxic products, or to remove them. The primary purpose of the roentgen examination is thus to decide whether the renal failure is due to changes in the renal parenchyma such as generalized parenchymatous changes, toxic damage, tumor, etc., or to obstructed drainage by stone, tumor, edema after radiotherapy, periureteritis obliterans, etc. A tumor arising in the colon, for example, or the bladder, or in the female genital organs can occlude both ureters. Attention should therefore be given to the size of the kidneys and the width of the renal pelves. Dilatation, as mentioned, can often be demonstrated in plain roentgenograms. Stone in the kidneys or in the ureters is, as a rule, readily recognized in plain roentgenograms. It must be realized, however, that the general condition of the patient, meteorism, retroperitoneal edema, etc., often prevent adequate examination. Hence only positive findings are of value.

Roentgen examination in the acute stage

can yield valuable information regarding the severity of edema, which may be of significance in the pathophysiology of acute renal failure. Plain radiography offers good possibilities of estimating the degree of retroperitoneal edema. In the presence of marked edema the opacity of the retroperitoneal space is increased and all tissues have the same roentgenographic density with disappearance of the fatty layers. If edema is less marked, it is possible to recognize the kidney and the border of the psoas muscle, for example, though they are seen less clearly than is normal. On regression of the edema the anatomy of the soft tissues in the retroperitoneal space will gradually reappear. Edema is often accompanied by a varying degree of meteorism, and ascites is often demonstrable.

Highly important is the detection of pulmonary edema. Extensive life-threatening renal lung edema may produce hardly any respiratory trouble or clinical symptoms or signs, yet roentgen examination may reveal widespread changes (Figs. 4-34, 4-35). Roentgenologically the uremic lung edema is characteristic. The air content of the lungs is decreased centrally, while the peripheral parts have good air content. This applies to each lobe separately. The changes may be strictly localized to the center of the lungs or spread a varying distance toward the periphery of the individual lung lobes. In characteristic pulmonary edema the most peripheral part of the lungs is always free; i.e., the alveoli contain a normal amount of air.

Various theories have been offered to explain this characteristic localization of the changes. In experimental and clinical investigations (Boijsen and Lunderquist, 1963) it was found that the localization of the edema corresponds to the branching of the bronchial arteries. There is reason to assume that toxic injury to the vessels, with impairment of their permeability, particularly in the region supplied by the bronchial artery, may be the basic factor and that fluid retention is secondary.

Clinically and therapeutically, however, the fluid retention is important. The term *fluid lung* stresses this fact.

Uremic lung edema can vary in extent and degree. If the toxic effect is controlled or the fluid balance made favorable, it can disappear rapidly and completely but may recur repeatedly with exacerbation of the underlying condition. In association with lung edema or as an independent symptom of edema, fluid is often found in the pleural cavities. Small amounts of fluid can be demonstrated only by examination of the patient in the lateral position with the beam horizontal.

Roentgenologically, physiologically, and clinically, renal lung edema differs from cardiac edema. The latter is mainly peripheral, involving the alveoli and often running a dramatic clinical course. Since many generalized renal diseases affect the circulation by their toxic effect on the heart or by secondary hypertension, uremic lung edema and cardiac lung edema are not infrequently associated with one another. In addition to vascular stasis, bronchial retention of mucus, small atelectases, and small or widespread bronchial pneumonia may be superimposed on the renal pulmonary edema or may mimic edematous changes.

GLOMERULONEPHRITIS

The primary purpose of roentgen examination (as a rule, plain radiography only) is to make possible the estimation of the size of the kidney and thereby the stage of the disease, and to follow its further course. In acute glomerulonephritis the kidneys are moderately enlarged and after a certain time decrease to normal size, which they maintain. In some cases the disease may persist in a subacute form for a very long period with usually moderate and bilateral renal enlargement. In some cases the acute stage is rapidly followed by the stage of contraction. The kidneys then become smaller than normal — sometimes very small — and may be irregular in outline.

Knowledge of the stage of the disease is

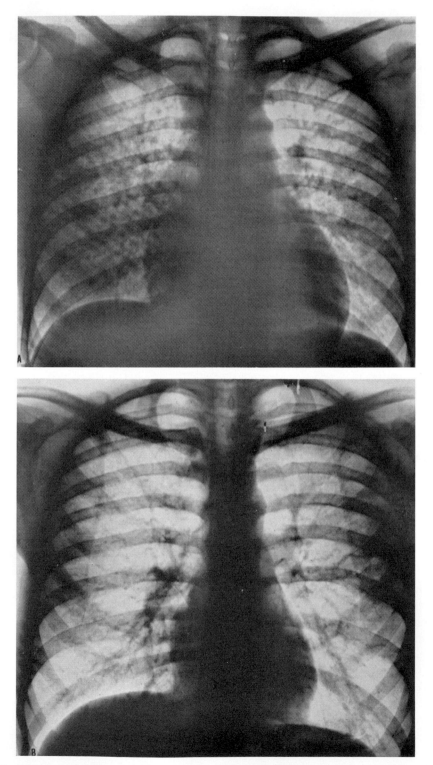

Figure 4-34. Uremic pulmonary edema. Subacute glomerulonephritis in anuric state. A. Bilateral wide-spread changes. B. After dialysis, changes have completely disappeared. C. Recurrence of changes. D. After new treatment, complete disappearance of edema. All examinations made at bedside.

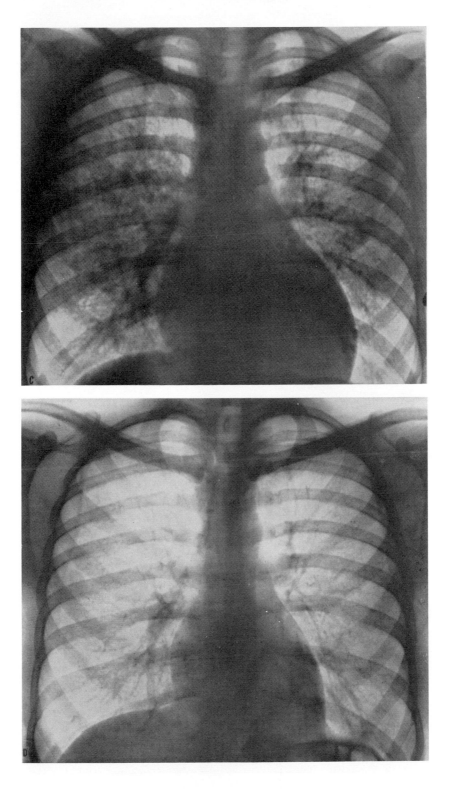

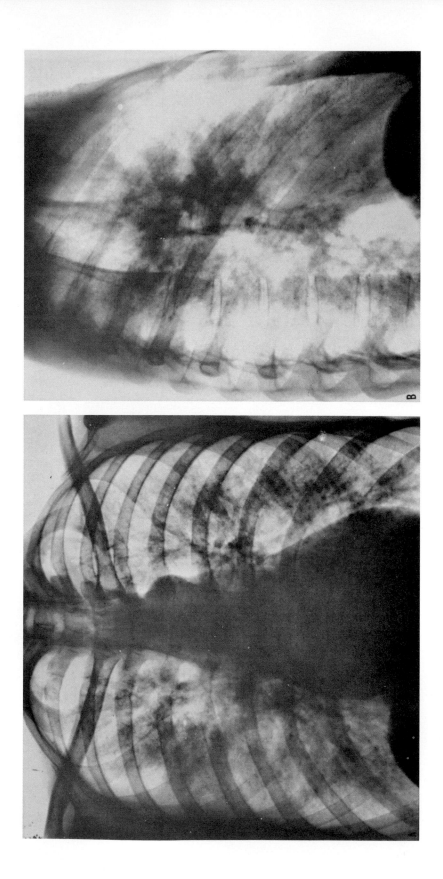

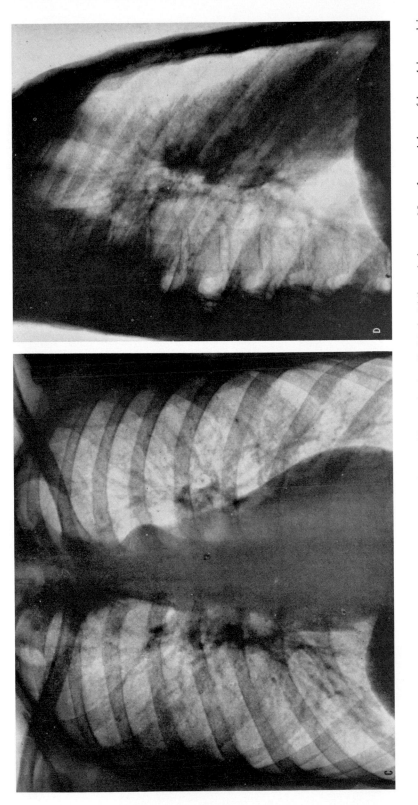

Figure 4-35. Uremic pulmonary edema in acute glomerulonephritis with anuria. A & B. Marked bilateral changes. Note free periphery of lung lobes and in lateral view the typical central localization of the changes. C & D. After dialysis, changes have completely disappeared three days later.

important in the examination of patients with oliguria or anuria. If the kidneys are very small, they represent advanced chronic glomerulonephritis and the prognosis is poor. The cause of the uremia, however, may be glomerulonephritis in the acute stage, in which instance the kidneys are enlarged.

TUBULAR NEPHRITIS (ACUTE TUBULAR NECROSIS)

This disease is referred to in the literature by a wide variety of names. Burn nephritis, crush syndrome, traumatic anuria, and lower nephron nephrosis are all used to describe it. The acute form is usually called acute renal failure. What was said concerning acute renal failure holds for acute tubular necrosis, which may be regarded as part of the renal failure group of disorders (Fig. 4-36).

In the acute stage the kidneys show fairly marked general enlargement. They can be defined in more than half the cases despite retroperitoneal edema, but in some cases they cannot be outlined until the edema has regressed. In the course of two or three weeks the kidneys decrease in size, which usually becomes normal again after some weeks [33].

Clinically, the disease is divided into the anuric or oliguric stage, which is defined as the period during which the daily urinary

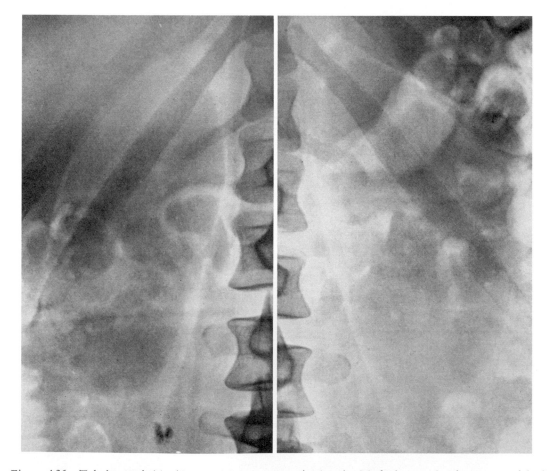

Figure 4-36. Tubular nephritis (due to delirium tremens). Anuria. Marked general enlargement of both kidneys. Three weeks later kidneys returned to normal size.

volume is 400 ml. or less; the diuretic stage, defined as beginning when the daily urinary volume exceeds 400 ml. and with still reduced renal function; and finally the late diuretic stage, when kidney function gradually improves, and in most cases becomes normal (Fig. 4-37). Broadly speaking, the first stage

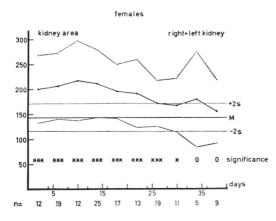

Figure 4-37. The area of both kidneys in acute renal failure in 66 cases. The straight lines represent the mean value and the standard deviation in 100 cases with "healthy" kidneys. (From Moëll, H. [33].)

may be regarded as that period during which the kidneys are markedly enlarged; the second stage, as that in which they begin to decrease in size; and the third, as that in which they have returned to ordinary size.

Because of the wide normal variation of the size of the kidneys, moderate renal enlargement may be difficult to ascertain in the beginning, particularly in males, unless roentgenograms from some previous examination are available.

In some cases the process progresses with shrinkage of the kidneys as a result. Characteristic of this course is renal cortical necrosis.

Gross bilateral cortical necrosis occurs most frequently in association with concealed accidental hemorrhage. The disease thus starts as ordinary tubular nephritis, but the oliguric stage is very long, particularly if the patient

is treated with the artificial kidney (Fig. 4-38). After about two months, irregular calcifications of low density usually occur in the cortex and gradually increase in opacity. At the same time the kidneys decrease markedly in size, and their surface becomes irregular.

Pyelonephritis and Papillary Necrosis

In pyelonephritis the interest for a long time was focused on the kidney pelvis (pyelitis). The disease, however, has been found to have its main and important changes in the renal parenchyma itself. This change in knowledge has caused a change in attitude toward the disease, not the least in the radiologic diagnosis of the disease. From observations mainly of the shape of the renal pelvis and its mucosa, the roentgenologist broadened his interest to include a close scrutiny of the boundary between pelvis and parenchyma, the calyces and the papillae, and now focuses his attention on the size and shape of the kidney and on a close study of the parenchyma with a variety of methods. The roentgen appearance of pyelonephritis varies widely with the extent, severity, and age of the process. In addition, the roentgen findings are influenced by coexistent diseases secondary to pyelonephritis or primary to it. Thus, dilatation of the urinary pathways and stone are common.

It is apparent from the literature that surveys of the roentgen findings described as characteristic of pyelonephritis are often based on clinical grounds and are not founded on pathoanatomic verification. In addition, the examination technic used for the demonstration of the changes is not always adequate.

In the differential diagnosis of acute abdominal conditions acute pyelonephritis must be distinguished from renal stone with renal colic. Regarding the examination in the acute stage of the disease, we have found that at urography during an attack of acute pyelonephritis with pain, usually the excretion of

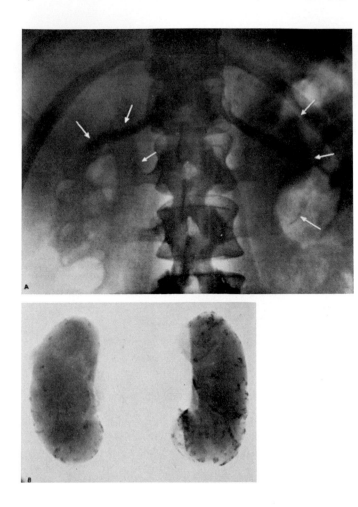

Figure 4-38. Bilateral cortical necrosis in woman 27 years of age. Proteinuria during pregnancy. Vaginal cesarean section performed because of suspected separation of the placenta. Prolonged drop in blood pressure. Marked oliguria. The patient lived under treatment for 119 days with continual shrinkage of the kidneys, in which calcifications appeared. A. Plain film. Small kidneys with peripheral calcifications (*arrows*). B. Roentgenogram of autopsy specimens.

contrast urine is not delayed, and the density and drainage are normal. However, sometimes excretion may be delayed. The contrast density may be somewhat low and drainage slow because of slight stasis caused by inflammatory edema of the ureteric mucosa.

In early cases of chronic pyelonephritis at plain radiography no signs of a pathologic process are seen. If the changes are more extensive, examination of the kidney during an acute exacerbation may show enlargement on one or both sides, but usually the two kidneys differ in size. Advanced changes cause contraction with reduction in the size of the kidney, which then has an irregular surface. Single scar formations cause marked indentation in the kidney surface. The change may be unilateral and involve mainly one part of the kidney. A slight thickening of the fat capsule is often the only discernible sign of a slight shrinkage. In contrast to other types of generalized kidney disease, differences between the two kidneys are characteristic of pyelonephritis. Scattered small calcifications may sometimes be seen in the kidney. In papillary necrosis (see below) one or more concrements may be seen in the renal pelvis or ureter and bladder, and they are often of characteristic papillary shape (Fig. 4-39).

If the changes are less advanced, urography will show ordinary contrast density and normal excretion of contrast urine. It is striking that in very advanced cases without acute symptoms the density of the contrast urine may be fairly good. It may, however, also vary widely from slightly decreased density to almost no excretion of contrast urine at all.

If the excretion is good, the morphology of the kidney can be examined by urography; otherwise pyelography must be performed. The renal pelvis is abnormally plastic and readily impressed by the border of the renal parenchyma in the sinus and by normal vessels, usually arteries, and then most commonly the dorsal artery. The impressions vary in degree and appearance and are usually best seen

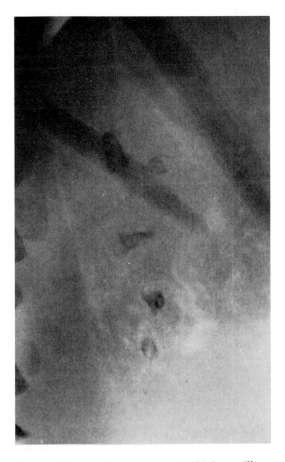

Figure 4-39. Papillary necrosis. Multiple papillary-shaped stones — calcified shed papillae — in left kidney.

in the cranial part of the confluence. Sometimes the renal pelvis is slightly dilated, as the ureter may be, down to the level where it crosses the iliac artery. The calyces are slightly widened and the fornices are rounded.

Papillary necrosis is combined with pyelonephritis, and accordingly papillary changes are common in pyelonephritis. The early stages of papillary necrosis demonstrate contrast medium penetrating more or less regularly into zones of demarcation in a papilla or at the base of the corresponding pyramid. One or more papillae may be affected, and often the changes are bilateral. In later stages one or more papillae detach and result in filling defects in the renal pelvis (Fig. 4-40). Corresponding cavities occur in the papillae and pyramids, in early stages irregular, later well defined and most easily seen in the cranial poles. The detached tissue is apt to calcify and cause stone formation. Shed papillae lodged in the kidney pelvis may thus continuously increase in calcium content and thereby give the impression of increasing in size and number. Loosened papillae, calcified or uncalcified, may pass, or they may be stuck in the ureter, causing renal colic.

In acute pyelonephritis the renal pelvis may show mucosal changes with edema displacing the stems of the calyces or entire branches. Sometimes severe shrinkage is seen in the renal pelvis. In chronic processes granular or cystic pyelitis, demonstrable as crowded filling defects, may occur. Sometimes the cicatricious contraction of the renal pelvis results in narrowing or complete occlusion of a calyx or a branch. On destruction of parenchyma and local scar formation the calyces at the sites of the scars may be widened and extend out to the periphery of the kidney (Fig. 4-41).

Pyelonephritis secondary to renal stone or hydronephrosis may result in almost complete parenchymal atrophy, with a nonfunctioning kidney consisting entirely of a hydro-pyonephrotic sac.

The angiographic characteristics of pyelo-

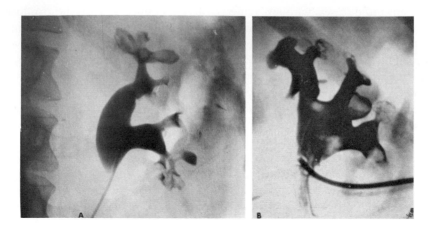

Figure 4-40. Papillary necrosis. Pyelography via pyelostomy made because of obstruction of ureter by shed papillae. Around several calyces bands of contrast medium are seen penetrating into necrotic zones at base of papillae. Shed papilla appearing as filling defects in pyelogram in B.

nephritis are less widely known. In our experience angiography can demonstrate the degree of vascular atrophy accompanying parenchymal destruction and widening of the distal intrarenal branches which can be seen stretching more laterally than in the unaffected kidney. The nephrographic phase will show the amount of surviving renal parenchyma. The degree of atrophy of the cortex can be assessed, besides which the examination offers good possibilities of judging cicatrization in the kidney with generalized unevenness of its surface or more localized deep scars. A local florid process can be demonstrated by the finding of an area of increased vascularization. Angiography is important because with this method of examination the significant part of the kidney involved by the pathologic process can be studied. Thus in patients with a unilateral process urographically, angiography may demonstrate bilateral changes. In a patient with localized changes at urography, angiography may demonstrate generalized changes in addition.

The destruction of the parenchyma may sometimes be mainly centrally in the kidney, in which case there may be no decrease in overall size. Instead the sinus widens and is filled by a lipofibromatous tissue. The change is called fibrolipomatosis renis or replacement lipomatosis. This may be extensive and become a source of error to be borne in mind in the evaluation of the amount of renal parenchyma as judged by the size of the kidney. Fibrolipomatosis is very common, usually in moderate degree. It may be generalized or more or less local. The change is readily demonstrated by tomography, preferably with circular motion, and by angiography, particularly in the nephrographic phase. Local, marked fibrolipomatosis may give rise to suspicion of tumor. At angiography this suspicion can be eliminated and the true nature of the process be definitely established.

Compensatory Renal Hypertrophy

If one of the kidneys is missing, as in aplasia, or if function is poor, as in severe hypoplasia, or if one of the kidneys has been removed or has ceased to function owing to such conditions as stasis, infection, or degeneration, the other kidney will, as a rule, increase in size. This so-

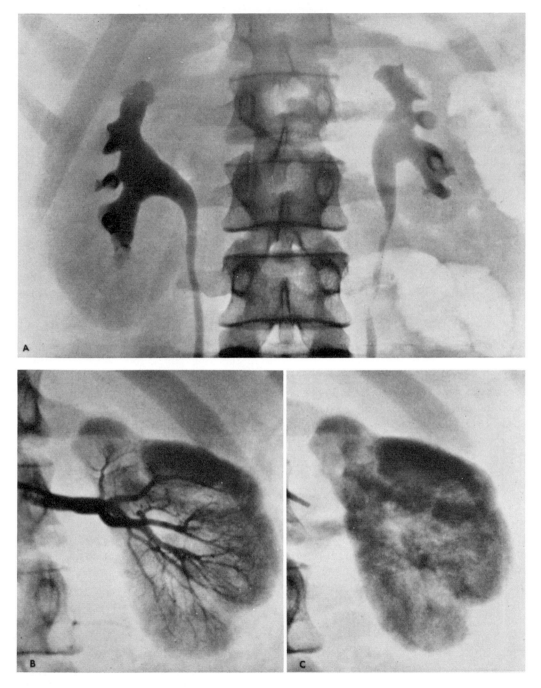

Figure 4-41. Pyelonephritis. A. Urography: right kidney normal; left kidney small. Distal calyces deformed and distance of calyceal edge to kidney surface diminished. B & C. Selective renal angiography: slight arterial atrophy. Large scars laterally in inferior, and medially in superior pole of kidney. Marked reduction in width of cortex in both poles.

called compensatory hypertrophy is due to growth in size of different parts of the nephron, whereas the number of nephrons does not increase. Plain roentgenography will show the increase in size of the kidney. It is less marked in older persons. The increase usually is rapid, but continuous increase for two to three years has been noted. Urography often shows the width of the renal pelvis to be slightly increased and angiography shows that the renal artery is somewhat wider than normal. The process usually involves the whole kidney, but local hypertrophy may be seen in parts of the kidney where other parts of the kidney are atrophic or destroyed by, for instance, pyelonephritis.

Extrarenal Manifestations of Renal Disease

In connection with roentgen examination of the kidneys, changes in other organs or tissues may be seen which are caused by, or are concomitant with, a renal lesion. In renal carcinoma, for instance, metastases may be present or suspected, indicating examination of the lungs, skeleton, liver, or brain. In angiographic studies of cerebral tumor, for instance, the vascularity of the tumor may be characteristic enough to make obvious the diagnosis of a metastasis from a renal carcinoma, and direct attention to the kidneys. On the other hand, tumors primary in other organs sometimes may metastasize to the kidney, as can leukemia, eosinophilic granuloma, etc.

In renal stone, skeletal changes, i.e., osteitis fibrosa, may be present, indicating hyperparathyroidism. Production of stone or nephrocalcinosis is a common feature in several general disorders producing hypercalcemia or hyperphosphatemia. Sarcoidosis is often combined with renal stone, and stone production is seen in decalcifying tumors such as carcinoma and myelomatosis. Uric acid calculi may be seen in leukemia, for example, and osteo-

myelosclerosis. Neurologic disorders, cerebral or medullary, may affect urine drainage, and long bed rest for any disease may be responsible for stone production.

Gout, myeloma, or systemic lupus erythematosus may have radiologically uncharacteristic renal involvement. Renal tuberculosis is often only one manifestation of primary tuberculosis, concomitant lesions being seen in the skeleton, lungs, or abdomen. Nonspecific infectious lesions may have several foci, one, for instance, in the kidney as a localized abscess or as more generalized inflammatory changes.

In chronic renal disease, so-called renal osteodystrophy, characteristically localized changes may be presented. The changes in this disease may consist of osteoporosis with, for instance, disappearance of the lamina dura of the teeth and local decalcification with superficial destruction in the metaphyseal parts of the long bones, most characteristically at the medial part of the proximal end of the tibia. The changes may affect any part of the skeleton including fingers and toes. Sometimes metastatic calcifications such as peritendinitis calcarea are seen. Changes of this type may be very marked in patients under chronic dialysis, with decalcification of the skeleton and calcium deposits close to several joints.

Anomalies are sometimes combined, one localization being the kidney. In polycystic disease, cysts may also be present in the liver. Tuberous sclerosis, in addition to characteristic cerebral calcifications, may have renal changes.

Lesions adjacent to the kidney may affect the kidney. Suprarenal tumors and other retroperitoneal tumors may displace, or even infiltrate, the kidney.

Renal disease in a uremic stage may cause gastrointestinal symptoms which, to begin with, may attract clinical attention completely. Roentgen examination of the stomach and bowel in uremic patients usually demonstrates mucosal edema and disturbances of motility.

Lung changes are common in uremic patients and are described separately. In connection with lung and pleural changes, pericarditis may also be present.

This incomplete review will only bring to the reader's attention the necessity in many instances of widening the diagnostic interest outside the urinary tract in patients with urinary symptoms and also, in certain diseases, of paying interest to conditions in the kidneys and the urinary tract, even without direct symptoms from this area.

References

1. Abrams, H. The response of neoplastic renal vessels to epinephrine in man. *Radiology* 82:217, 1964.
2. Abrams, H., Baum, S., and Stamey, T. Renal venous washout time in renovascular hypertension. *Radiology* 83:597, 1964.
3. Abrams, H., Boijsen, E., and Borgström, K.-E. Effect of epinephrine on the renal circulation. *Radiology* 79:911, 1962.
4. Amplatz, K. Assessment of curable renovascular hypertension by radiographic technics. *Radiology* 83:816, 1964.
5. Bodforss, B., Muth, T., and Olin, T. Renal function test with radioactive Diodrast in dogs. *Acta Radiol. [Diagn.]* (Stockholm) 2:433, 1964.
6. Bodforss, B., Muth, T., and Olin, T. Renal function judged with radioactive Diodrast after selective renal angiography in dogs. *Acta Radiol. [Diagn.]* (Stockholm) 2:449, 1964.
7. Boijsen, E. Angiographic studies of the anatomy of single and multiple renal arteries. *Acta Radiol.* (Stockholm) Suppl. 183, 1959.
8. Boijsen, E., and Folin, J. Angiography in carcinoma of the renal pelvis. *Acta Radiol.* (Stockholm) 56:81, 1961.
9. Boijsen, E., and Folin, J. Angiography in the diagnosis of renal carcinoma. *Radiologe* 1:173, 1961.
10. Boijsen, E., and Köhler, R. Renal artery aneurysms. *Acta Radiol. [Diagn.]* (Stockholm) 1:1077, 1963.
11. Boijsen, E., and Köhler, R. Renal arteriovenous fistulae. *Acta Radiol.* (Stockholm) 57:433, 1962.
12. Bolin, H. Contrast medium in kidney during angiography: A densitometric method for estimation of renal function. *Acta Radiol.* (Stockholm) Suppl. 257, 1966.
13. Borgström, K.-E., Ising, U., Linder, E., and Lunderquist, A. Experimental pulmonary edema. *Acta Radiol.* (Stockholm) 54:97, 1960.
14. Cronqvist, S. Renal osteonephropathy. *Acta Radiol.* (Stockholm) 55:17, 1961.
15. Edholm, P., and Seldinger, S. Percutaneous catheterization of the renal artery. *Acta Radiol.* (Stockholm) 45:15, 1956.
16. Elkin, M., Meng, C.-H., and de Paredes, R. Correlation of intravenous urography and renal angiography in kidney injury. *Radiology* 86:496, 1966.
17. Ekström, T., Engfeldt, B., Lagergren, C., and Lindvall, N. *Medullary Sponge Kidney.* Stockholm: Almquist & Wiksell, 1959.
18. Fish, G. Large solitary serous cysts of the kidney. *J.A.M.A.* 112:514, 1939.
19. Folin, J. Angiography in renal tumours: Its value in diagnosis and differential diagnosis as a complement to conventional methods. *Acta Radiol.* (Stockholm) Suppl. 267, 1967.
20. Folin, J. Complications of percutaneous femoral catheterisation for renal angiography. *Radiologe* 8:190, 1968.
21. Idbohrn, H. Renal angiography in experimental hydronephrosis. *Acta Radiol.* (Stockholm) Suppl. 136, 1956.
22. Johnsson, S. A contribution to the diagnostics of nephromata. *Acta Radiol.* (Stockholm) Suppl. 60, 1946.
23. Kincaid, O. *Renal Angiography.* Chicago: Year Book, 1966.
24. Kjellberg, S., Ericsson, N., and Rudhe, U. *The Lower Urinary Tract in Childhood.* Chicago: Year Book, 1957.

25. Köhler, R. Incomplete angiogram in selective renal angiography. *Acta Radiol. [Diagn.]* (Stockholm) 1:1011, 1963.

26. Lagergren, C. Biophysical investigations of urinary calculi. *Acta Radiol.* (Stockholm) Suppl. 133, 1956.

27. Lindblom, K. Diagnostic kidney puncture in cysts and tumors. *Amer. J. Roentgen.* 68:209, 1952.

28. Lindblom, K. Percutaneous puncture of renal cysts and tumors. *Acta Radiol.* (Stockholm) 27:66, 1946.

29. Lindvall, N. Renal papillary necrosis: A roentgenographic study of 155 cases. *Acta Radiol.* (Stockholm) Suppl. 192, 1960.

30. Lindvall, N. Roentgenologic diagnosis of medullary sponge kidney. *Acta Radiol. [Diagn.]* (Stockholm) 51:193, 1959.

31. Moëll, H. Size of normal kidneys. *Acta Radiol.* (Stockholm) 46:640, 1956.

32. Moëll, H. Gross bilateral renal cortical necrosis during long periods of oliguria-anuria. *Acta Radiol.* (Stockholm) 48:355, 1957.

33. Moëll, H. Kidney size and its deviation from normal in acute renal failure. *Acta Radiol.* (Stockholm) Suppl. 206, 1961.

34. Ödmann, P. Percutaneous selective angiography of the main branches of the aorta. *Acta Radiol.* (Stockholm) 45:1, 1956.

35. Olin, T., and Redman, H. Spillover flowmeter. *Acta Radiol. [Diagn.]* (Stockholm) 4:217, 1966.

36. Olin, T., and Reuter, S. A pharmaco-angiographic method for improving nephrophlebography. *Radiology* 85:1036, 1965.

37. Olsson, O. Die Urographie bei der Nierentuberkulose. *Acta Radiol.* (Stockholm) Suppl. 47, 1943.

38. Olsson, O. Studies on backflow in excre-tion urography. *Acta Radiol.* (Stockholm) Suppl. 70, 1948.

39. Olsson, O. Renal Angiography. In Abrams, H. (Ed.), *Angiography.* Boston: Little, Brown, 1961.

40. Olsson, O. Renal Angiography in Pyelonephritis. In Viamonte, M., and Parks, R. (Eds.), *Progress in Angiography.* Springfield, Ill.: Thomas, 1964.

41. Olsson, O., Alwall, N., and Lunderquist, A. Studies on electrolyte-fluid retention: I. Uremic lung-fluid lung? On pathogenesis and therapy. A preliminary report. *Acta Med. Scand.* 56, 1953.

42. Olsson, O., and Lunderquist, A. Angiography in renal trauma. *Acta Radiol. [Diagn.]* (Stockholm) 1:1, 1963.

43. Olsson, O., and Weiland, P.-O. Renal fibrolipomatosis. *Acta Radiol. [Diagn.]* (Stockholm) 1:1061, 1963.

44. Olsson, O., and Wholey, M. Vascular abnormalities in gross anomalies of kidneys. *Acta Radiol. [Diagn.]* (Stockholm) 2:420, 1964.

45. Sandegard, E. Prognosis of stone in the ureter. *Acta Chir. Scand.* Suppl. 219, 1956.

46. dos Santos, R., Lamas, A., and Caldas, J. Arteriografia da aorta e dos vasos abdominais. *Med. Contemp.* 47:93, 1929.

47. Steinert, R. Renal tuberculosis and roentgenologic examination. *Acta Radiol.* (Stockholm) Suppl. 53, 1943.

48. Vogeler, E., and Herbst, R. *Angiographie der Nieren.* Stuttgart: Thieme, 1958.

49. Widén, T. Renal angiography during and after unilateral ureteric occlusion. *Acta Radiol.* (Stockholm) Suppl. 162, 1958.

50. Wulff, H. Die Zuverlässigkeit der Röntgendiagnostik — besonders hinsichtlich des Wertes der Urographie — und die Prognose bei Nieren- und Harnleitersteinen. *Acta Radiol.* (Stockholm) Suppl. 32, 1936.

5

Renal Biopsy

George E. Schreiner

The introduction of percutaneous renal biopsy has contributed in a major way to our understanding of renal disease. The general use of the renal biopsy procedure is a recent event. It is not clear why it lagged behind similar developments in the technics of liver, bone marrow, and even splenic biopsy. In retrospect, the delay was probably based more on emotional than on rational grounds. To many the mere idea of introducing a needle into a pulsatile, mobile kidney through which flows one-fifth or more of the cardiac output remains a somewhat frightening idea. Actually, the kidney has many unique features which make biopsy both feasible and relatively safe. Unlike the liver, for example, the kidney is retroperitoneal, it is a paired organ, it lies almost subcutaneously behind a thin-roofed anatomic triangle, it is enclosed in a tight fascial compartment which aids hemostasis from the biopsy puncture, and its fine anatomy affords usually easy verification of a satisfactory specimen, because of the arcuate vessels which demarcate the cortical zone. These can be seen, often with the naked eye, and, indeed, with a hand lens even glomeruli can be counted. Location of the kidney is a relatively simple x-ray procedure which, even in the obese individual, may be rendered more precise by the administration of a radiopaque dye excreted by the renal parenchyma, and the taking of a simple x-ray film during the nephrogram phase.

Brun and Raaschou [3] credited Jungmann (1924) [13] as the first to carry out surgical renal biopsy. The reports of Castleman and Smithwick [4], Heptinstall [11], and Saltz et al. [39] wrought widespread recognition of the value of kidney biopsies which they had obtained during the course of a sympathectomy, and which they used to study the renal aspects of hypertension and the relationships of hypertension in nephrosclerosis.

Alwall [1] attempted percutaneous renal biopsy in 1944 (reported in 1952), but apparently abandoned the technic because of a single fatality. Perez Ara [34] reported biopsy experience in 1950, but the modern biopsy era really began with the report of Iversen and Brun [12], and the technic spread rapidly by means of direct demonstrations given by Brun in nephrology centers in many countries throughout the world. Early biopsy series were reported in this country before 1960 from the laboratories of Parrish (1953 to 1957) [30, 31, 32], A. J. Merrill (1954 to 1957) [24, 25, 26], Kark [17, 18], Jackson [20], Good (1956 to 1958) [16, 47], Schreiner (1957) [42], Kellow et al. [19], and others. Some idea of the rapid acceptance of the technic is indicated from the result of a questionnaire circulated by Welt in June, 1967, in which 21 nephrology centers reported that in the previous five years 8081 biopsies had been performed in these centers. There were 6699 done on patients above and 1382 below the age of 14. From our own information on smaller centers that have performed a fewer number of biopsies, we would estimate that in excess of 20,000 percutaneous renal biopsies have now been performed in the United States since the introduction of the technic.

Technical Considerations

X-RAY ANATOMY

In the average adult the long diameter of the renal shadow usually measures between 11 and 14 cm., with a width of 6 to 8 cm.; this corresponds to an average weight of 120 to 180 gm. of kidney substance. Simon [44] examined the data concerning renal size from 100 consecutive autopsies and found that the ratio of kidney length to the height of the second lumbar vertebra is 3.7 ± 0.37 and that the statistical range of normal values is 3.0 to 4.4. The ratio of renal length to the height of the second lumbar vertebra and its disk is 3.4 ± 0.27 (range, 2.6 to 3.6), and unlike kidney weight, kidney length does not decrease with age. The kidney is enclosed in a dense fat pad which may, in some persons, have a radiographic opacity resembling that of the kidney parenchyma. The hilus of the kidney is usually opposite the second lumbar vertebra. Usually the right kidney is lower by the breadth of one lumbar vertebra. Arteriographic technics and clinical experience with renal biopsy emphasize the fact that the kidney may move as

much as 3 cm. on deep inspiration. The lower pole of the kidney is usually chosen for biopsy because latex perfusion studies indicate that this area contains the smallest number of large vessels and is the least vascular portion of the renal parenchyma. This is most fortunate since in its posterior aspect the lower pole of the kidney falls usually within a natural anatomic triangle formed by the lateral border of the sacrospinalis muscle, the inferior border of the last rib, and the upper border of the quadratus lumborum muscle. At this point the kidney is almost subcutaneous.

LOCALIZATION OF THE KIDNEY

Localization of the kidney is usually carried out by means of x-ray technics. The simplest method is a plain film of the abdomen performed after the gastrointestinal tract has been cleansed. Most operators prefer intravenous pyelograms, if obtainable. Recent widespread use of intravenous drip pyelography is capable of increasing the density of the renal shadow in most persons, even those with moderate functional impairment. The optimum time for the taking of the nephrogram may be delayed in azotemic subjects with a blood urea nitrogen (BUN) in excess of 60 mg. per 100 ml. Berlyne [2] has employed ultrasonics for locating the kidney, but this technic has not been widely applied. Other technics which have been used are localization with isotopes [35, 45] and direct fluoroscopic visualization [23, 27]. With the use of an image intensifier or television monitoring, even greater precision has been obtained [7, 9, 10, 16]. In general, the direct methods have been more widely employed by pediatricians who are performing biopsies on children. The Welt questionnaire indicated that 6393 percutaneous biopsies were done by the direct technic, and 1398 employed image-intensification fluoroscopy.

Figure 5-1 shows the anatomic relationships of the midspinal line, the lowest rib, and the proposed biopsy site in the lower pole of the

Figure 5-1. Dots outline the lower and lateral borders of the left kidney. Dashed lines indicate the midspinal line and the lowest rib. *X* marks the proposed biopsy site in the left lower pole.

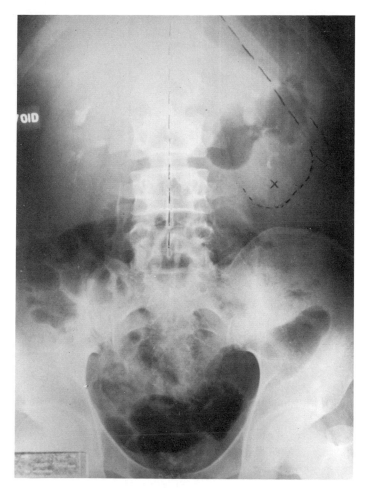

left kidney. Figure 5-2 indicates the biopsy site in relationship to major anatomic markings.

VARIATIONS IN POSITION AND
TYPE OF NEEDLE EMPLOYED

Perez Ara [34] first used the lateral and later the prone position, and aspirated the biopsy specimen through an ordinary cannula and a syringe or a special "nephro biotome." Iversen and Brun [12] employed both the sitting and the lateral position, using the Iversen-Roholm cannula with a 1.5 mm. bore. DiGaddo et al. [5] and Fiaschi et al. [8] used perirenal air insufflation and roentgenography in the prone position and a Vim-Sil-

verman cannula, the respiratory motions serving as a guide to localization. In 1953 Payet et al. [33] reported on 55 aspiration biopsies in the prone position, a sandbag being placed under the abdomen.

The literature does not adequately reflect the role of personal demonstrations in the rapid spread and improvement of the percutaneous biopsy technic among experienced nephrologists. For example, it was Parrish who familiarized himself with the technique through the writings of Brun, then gave a demonstration at the University of Illinois that was witnessed by Kark and Kellow. Arthur Merrill and his colleagues graciously supervised my first human biopsy, after I had

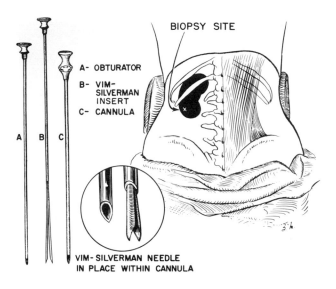

BIOPSY SITE

A- OBTURATOR

B- VIM-
SILVERMAN
INSERT

C- CANNULA

A   B   C

VIM- SILVERMAN NEEDLE
IN PLACE WITHIN CANNULA

Figure 5-2. Above is the renal biopsy site in relation to major anatomic markings. *A* is the obturator, *B* the Vim-Silverman insert, and *C* the thin-walled needle. The circular insert shows the grooved prongs which grip the plug of tissue, cut off by rotating the needle over the insert.

witnessed demonstrations of both the Vim-Silverman and the aspiration technic and had tried both on animal tissues and in a mock procedure on cadavers.

The needles that have been used in the larger series include the Iversen needle [12], the Turkel needle [31], the Franklin modification [15] (the tips of the Vim-Silverman needle are filled with metal), the Schreiner modification of the Vim-Silverman [42] (17-gauge, thin-walled needle with pin lock without depth attachment: overall shaft length is $8\frac{1}{4}$ inches with a shaft length of 7 inches; overall blade length is $9\frac{1}{4}$ inches with a blade length of $8\frac{1}{8}$ inches; the ends are filled; and the protrusion length is $1\frac{3}{16}$ inches), the Ross modification [37] (milled sliding head acts as depth stop), and the Lindholm [22] needle (conical tip modification of Iversen). The problem of sharpening and sterilization has recently been approached by the development of a disposable needle.* The sliding outer jacket cuts over a notched obturator rod, and the needle has two parts instead of three. The stop on the handle slide acts as an automatic

---

* Pediatric ($3\frac{1}{2}$ inch) and adult (6 inch) size disposable biopsy needles may be obtained from Travenol Laboratories, Inc., Morton Grove, Ill.

depth gauge. We have used this needle successfully, and its use has been reported on 22 pediatric patients [21]. A T-tube head to provide for aspiration has been reported by Radner [36].

Technic for Percutaneous Renal Biopsy.

When the decision for biopsy has been made, and after a discussion of the procedure and its risks has been completed, the voluntary signed permission of the patient is obtained. X-ray films of the patient's kidneys are reviewed to be sure that there are two renal shadows and that satisfactory localization is possible. The potential biopsy site is then localized in the lower pole of one kidney, as indicated in Figure 5-2. The expected area of disease is the first determinant of laterality. For example, a malformed or ectopic kidney on one side might direct one's choice to the opposite side when looking for diffuse parenchymal disease. A poorly functioning kidney on one side with a normal kidney on the other would generally direct one toward the poorly functioning kidney. In many renal diseases, however, such as the nephrotic syndrome, attention is rarely directed to one side in preference to the other. With the patient in the prone position it is generally more comfortable for a right-handed operator to biopsy the left kidney. Some physicians regularly choose the right kidney in order to avoid proximity to great vessels; however, since we have not yet hit a large vessel in over 1200 biopsies, it does not appear to be a significant risk. With splenomegaly, however, the right side is highly preferable. Simple blood studies, usually including the hematocrit, the bleeding, clotting, or plasma recalcification time, and prothrombin time, the platelet count, and, in patients who have severe azotemia, prothrombin consumption or an equivalent test, are performed. Two units of typed and crossmatched blood are held readily available.

The essential equipment for biopsy is contained in a presterilized renal biopsy tray (Fig. 5-3). The essential items are: one minor surgical drape, three sterile towels, one 10 ml. syringe, three needles (No. 19, 26, and 23 long), a No. 11 blade scalpel, a tongue depressor blade, the Vim-Silverman needle with Schreiner modifications, and in addition a stack of sterile 4 by 4 sponges, bottles of vari-

ous fixatives, skin sterilizing solution, broad adhesive or Elastoplast tape, atropine, procaine, and spirits of ammonia. The standard 19-gauge needle is used for withdrawing procaine from the vial. The small intradermal needle is used for making the initial skin wheal; the No. 23 long is used as a probe to locate the kidney and to inject procaine at the capsule and in the track of the biopsy needle.

We prefer to biopsy the patient in his own bed in order to avoid the psychologic trauma of an operating or procedure room, and in order to minimize the handling of the patient in the postbiopsy period. The patient is placed in a prone position over sandbags or a firm pillow, with a soft pillow on top. Care is taken to see that the body is bent forward at the level of the diaphragm, that the shoulders are down, and that the patient's head is turned away from the operator. Figure 5-4 shows the ideal patient position. It is imperative that the horizontal level of the shoulder girdle be absolutely parallel to the bed and that the spine be as straight as possible. The operator approaches the patient, discusses breathing maneuvers, and then reviews the x-ray films against a view box or window. The previous markings of the midspinal line, the outline

Figure 5-3. Kit for renal biopsy at Georgetown University Hospital. Special items are the long, thin-walled Vim-Silverman needle, No. 23 long procaine needle, scalpel, and minor surgical drape.

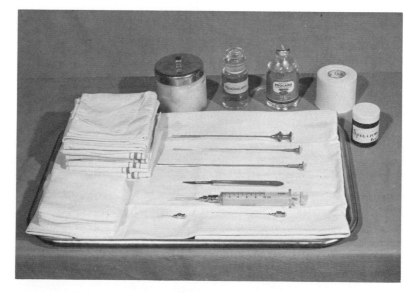

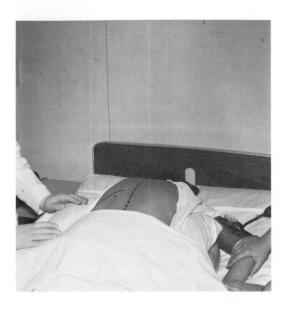

Figure 5-4.   Patient in position to be biopsied.

of the last rib, and the prospective biopsy site are all checked and are transferred by measurement from the x-ray films to the patient's back (Figs. 5-2, 5-4) with a small ruler and a skin-marking pencil. In the biopsy position the rib cage is cephalad, and the kidneys are thrown to a posterior position. The chosen biopsy site usually falls in the normal anatomic triangle formed by the lateral border of the sacrospinalis, the inferior border of the last rib, and the upper border of the quadratus lumborum. Only the thin fibers of the latissimus dorsi and serratus posterior muscles need be penetrated by the biopsy needle.

A blood pressure cuff is applied to the arm, and the pulse and blood pressure are recorded. Usually systemic sedation is not necessary, but for highly excitable persons, an oral tranquilizer, hours before as premedication, or 0.1 gm. of phenobarbital subcutaneously, a few minutes before beginning the biopsy preparations, may be employed. Local anesthesia is administered first as a skin wheal of procaine at the point where the measurement from the

midspinal line transects the descending measurement from the lower rib. A small linear incision is made about 1 cm. long, parallel to the midspinal line to allow free respiratory motion of the needles. The 23-gauge, 3-inch needle is then inserted and alignment is viewed by moving to the foot end of the bed and observing the needle hub. It must be in the exact saggital section, parallel to the spine, and directed neither medially nor laterally. The needle is inserted until the renal capsule is felt as a firm resistance. The patient is then asked to hold his breath while a small amount of procaine is injected at the renal capsule. With interruption of the procedure to allow one or two breaths, the procaine is then injected along the needle track as the needle is withdrawn. To standardize the respiratory motion, the patient is usually directed to "take a breath half way in to a deep breath." The same respiratory movement is reproduced upon insertion of the biopsy needle. We use the Schreiner modification of the Vim-Silverman needle.* We use this longer needle because the sensitivity of a lever is proportional to its length, and the short needles, when inserted, allow very little touch sensitivity in the hub, particularly in obese people. With the patient holding his breath, the needle with the obturator in place is inserted into the renal capsule; the operator is aware of the popping sensation when the capsule is perforated. Sensitivity of touch is critical for proper insertion of the biopsy needle. In most cases, one will observe a marked to-and-fro respiratory swing, as well as a vascular pulsation. *Under no circumstances and at no time during the biopsy procedure is the motion of a freely swinging needle to be restricted by the operator.*

The patient is asked to hold his breath in a mid-respiratory position and, as is shown in Figure 5-5, the obturator is removed and the

* Obtainable from the MacGregor Division of Travenol Laboratories, Morton Grove, Ill.

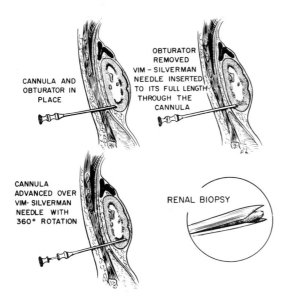

CANNULA AND
OBTURATOR IN
PLACE

OBTURATOR
REMOVED
VIM - SILVERMAN
NEEDLE INSERTED
TO ITS FULL LENGTH
THROUGH THE
CANNULA

CANNULA
ADVANCED OVER
VIM- SILVERMAN
NEEDLE WITH
360° ROTATION

RENAL BIOPSY

Figure 5-5. Sagittal sections illustrating the major steps in the technic of renal biopsy.

Vim-Silverman needle is inserted to its full length through the cannula. The patient is allowed to take a breath or two and is then warned that there may be a slight, painful sensation with the next maneuver. The patient is again asked to hold his breath in mid-inspiration, the cannula is advanced over the Vim-Silverman needle with 360° rotation, and the entire apparatus is swiftly removed from the patient.

The renal biopsy should be a gray-to-red plug of tissue in which there is a brighter red vascular line indicating the cortical-medullary junction where the arcuate blood vessels are transected. This is usually discernible to the naked eye or with a small hand lens. One may also identify the capsule with perirenal fat. The biopsy plug is placed immediately in a suitable fixative. For routine purposes we use a buffered formalin adjusted to pH 7.4. Other fixatives are used for electron microscopy, and fresh pieces of the biopsy are frozen for immunofluorescent staining. Absolute alcohol may be used for uric acid and other crystal preparations. If the plug is pre-

dominantly fat, it will float, but if the needle has been in the proper position and sufficient parenchyma has been obtained, the plug will immediately sink to the bottom of the fixative. From 20 to 30 mm. is a good length for this type of specimen, and with our thin-walled needle the average number of glomeruli is 16 per section, with a median of 13. We have obtained specimens with 50 to 70 glomeruli. Some operators use a dissecting microscope to split the biopsy lengthways. We find this very difficult to do at the bedside and usually place the biopsy on a sterile tongue depressor contained in the kit, and with a sharp No. 11 blade scalpel cut small sections of cortex and of medulla for electronmicroscopy and fluorescent microscopy while preserving the major specimen for light microscopy. If the patient is suspected of having an infectious process, the pronged insert and needle tip are used to stir a suitable liquid bacteriological or viral culture medium (or both). Immediately after the biopsy, pressure is exerted with 4 by 4 sponges for 20 minutes, and the patient is kept in the same prone position during this time. Pressure bandages are then applied to the site, and the patient is shifted to his back, permitted to use only one pillow to support his head, and maintained as quietly as possible for 4 hours, and in bed for 24 hours. He is instructed not to cough, smoke, or sneeze, or do anything that would cause him to hold his breath, tighten his abdominal muscles, or raise his venous pressure for the next 4 hours. The first urine specimen after the biopsy is examined for red blood cells, and the patient is kept at bed rest beyond the 24-hour period if hematuria is present, remaining there as long as it continues. The patient's pulse and blood pressure are taken every 15 minutes during the first hour after the biopsy, every 30 minutes during the second hour, and every 60 minutes throughout the subsequent 3 to 4 hours. About 6 per cent of the patients have hematuria continuing up to 24 hours. Patients are instructed not to do any heavy lifting for 10 days after the biopsy procedure, and then to resume normal activity. The 1 cm. incision is closed readily, and we never have had to employ sutures.

Value of Renal Biopsy

Renal biopsy would have to be considered one of the most important new diagnostic technics in the modern era of nephrology. Some of the advantages of renal biopsy are:

1. For accurate histologic diagnosis in a wide variety of pathologic states, e.g., nephrotic syndrome, collagen disease
2. For the separation of the proportional contribution of multiple renal diseases, e.g., Kimmelstiel-Wilson disease, hypertension, and pyelonephritis (often coexistent)
3. To follow serially progression of chronic renal disease
4. To follow the duration of and the degree of healing in reversible conditions
5. For the correct choice of therapy in, e.g., hypertension due to pyelonephritis, nephrotic syndrome, collagen disease, and renal lesions associated with subacute bacterial endocarditis.
6. To detect early phases of diseases not otherwise diagnosable, e.g., sarcoid granuloma, nephrocalcinosis
7. To achieve an estimate of prognosis
8. For the clinical investigation of renal histology and serial changes in both nonfatal and early disease processes, to achieve correlation between structure and function, and to employ new histochemical technics
9. For research in electron microscopy, enzyme localization, tissue metabolism, cell energetics, experimental cytology, immunofluorescence

Some of the contraindications to renal biopsy are:

1. Unilateral kidney
2. Abnormality in bleeding or coagulation tests rendering or creating an inordinate risk
3. Rapidly advancing uremia
4. Severe malignant hypertension except under carefully controlled conditions
5. Known malignancy or perinephritis
6. Marked congenital abnormalities of position or renal vasculature
7. Uncooperative patient, e.g., under the age of six, neurologic disorders, psychosis, severe debility, deforming skeletal defects, uncooperativeness, etc.
8. When death is imminent and no information beneficial to the patient is likely to be obtained
9. *Relative contraindications,* i.e., marked obesity, small kidneys, atypical position (high, low, rotated), pregnancy

SAMPLING ERROR

Still unknown to a large extent is the effect of sampling error on the interpretation of renal biopsies. Some reviews that give overall percentages are not too informative. Obviously there are some types of pathologic changes so characteristic that diagnosis may be made on a single glomerulus. For example, we have made the diagnosis of the renal complication of subacute bacterial endocarditis on a single glomerulus. In other conditions the sampling error may be very large when only a small number of glomeruli are obtained. The sampling error is presumably minimized if 10 or more glomeruli are contained in a section. In the case of diffuse disease, comparison of the biopsy specimen with a wedge section obtained later at autopsy has been reported to have generally good conformity, in the small series of Parrish and Howe [30], Vernier et al. [47], Muehrcke et al. [28], and Sala [38]. Kellow et al. [19] studied biopsies and wedge sections in 103 patients and found an 84 per cent correlation in diffuse renal disease, and a 51 per cent correlation in local renal disease.

EFFECTIVENESS OF THE BIOPSY PROCEDURE

Wide variations in the effectiveness of biopsy attempts have been published. The success of early series which provided satisfactory biopsies in 50 per cent of the cases has been markedly improved with the development of the technic. In our first 150 consecutive biopsies [42], we obtained renal tissue in 94 per cent which was satisfactory for diagnoses in 91 per cent. In our original series of 183 nephrotic patients, 180 biopsy attempts were made in 95 patients. Six attempts yielded inadequate tissue samples. There was, thus, an effectiveness in the procedure of 94 per cent. In this particular series, all biopsies were done after the renal evaluation was otherwise complete, and in 68 instances, the biopsy interpretation supported the clinical diagnosis. There was disagreement between the clinical and the histologic diagnosis in 21 instances. Five of these involved the distinction between amyloid and glomerulonephritis; five, the differentiation of diabetic glomerulosclerosis from glomerulonephritis; and one, the differentiation of amyloidosis from diabetic glomerulosclerosis. In the remaining patients the discrepancies were merely between various stages of glomerulonephritis. In Welt's questionnaire, the collected data were as follows: of 6017 biopsies done on patients older than the age of 14, 89.8 per cent yielded renal tissue; in the 1292 biopsies done on those younger than the age of 14, the yield was 93.5 per cent.

MORTALITY FROM RENAL BIOPSY

It is the general experience of nephrologists and experienced clinicians that the mortality rate from renal biopsy at each stage of its development has been considerably less than other accepted biopsy procedures — for example, that of liver biopsy. In Welt's questionnaire there was a mortality rate of 0.07 per cent. White [48], in a review of the literature, found a reference to 17 deaths among over 10,000 renal biopsies, with an estimated mortality of 0.17 per cent. We have had no deaths in our own series of over 1200 biopsies; the contraindications listed previously have been taken into account.

COMPLICATIONS

One of the most frequent complications is gross hematuria which, according to Dodge et al. [6], occurred in 5.2 per cent, flank or loin pain in 2.2 per cent, perirenal hematoma in 0.4 per cent, bleeding requiring transfusion in 0.8 per cent, and bleeding requiring nephrectomy in 0.1 per cent of the patients. In Welt's compilation there were 16 hematomas, five nephrectomies, one repair of a laceration of the liver, and two splenectomies. Also reported were perforations of the gallbladder, ureter, colon, a pneumothorax, and the production of five arteriovenous fistulas. Complications reported in the literature are renal infection, ureteral colic from blood clots, and paralytic ileus. Other tissues that have been obtained include bowel, spleen, liver, pancreas, adrenal gland, and, of course, muscle and fascia. Some misadventures which are complications (on formal grounds) turn out to have values in other forms. In one instance we solved a diagnostic dilemma on a patient who had been evaluated for fever of undetermined origin for a period of three years, before she developed the nephrotic syndrome. Inadvertent sampling of the spleen revealed Sternberg-Reed cells and led to the diagnosis of abdominal Hodgkin's disease. In another patient we penetrated an intrarenal abscess filled with purulent material. We cultured *Proteus* from the abscess and successfully drained it through the biopsy needle (Fig. 5-6).

Summary and Conclusions

In summary, renal biopsy is a serious procedure that should be performed only by those with experience, with the exception of those who are learning this procedure for a serious purpose, and then only under the direct super-

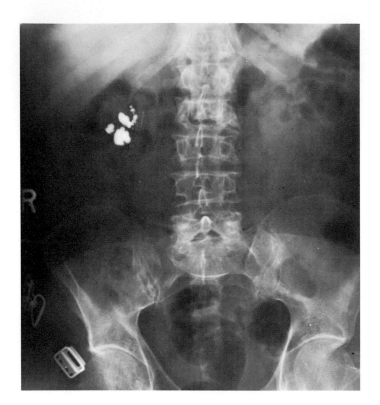

Figure 5-6. Lipoidal in abscess within renal parenchyma.

vision of their mentors. The morbidity rate is substantially lower in experienced hands; in our laboratory we confine biopsy experience to second-year fellows in nephrology who are learning the procedure to use as a lifetime tool.

In all patients the blood should be typed and cross-matched for the small risk of bleeding. If one carefully selects the patients, keeping the contraindications in mind, the mortality rate from the procedure can be very low. Although the total accurate statistics on mortality may not be known, the three published compilations of 0.07 per cent ($\overline{N}$ 8081), 0.12 per cent ($\overline{N}$ 4000), and 0.17 per cent ($\overline{N}$ 10,000) suggest that the mortality rate is substantially less than the 0.3 per cent seen in association with liver biopsy procedure [43], and is probably within medically acceptable limits when done for good indication [13, 29]. Failure to obtain kidney tissue may not be solely the fault of the operator. In our experience a repeated failure has been most often caused by excessive anterior mobility of the kidney. In the patients who have had repeated biopsies in our series, an initial failure is often followed by additional failure, but an initial success is almost invariably followed by successful biopsy attempts thereafter. Some of the rare conditions that we have encountered utilizing percutaneous biopsy include nephrocalcinosis, platelet thrombosis in renal venules, sarcoid granuloma and calcification, Fabry's disease, sickle-cell nephropathy, familial nephritis, cystinosis, ethylene glycol poisoning, myeloma kidney in patients without overt clinical myeloma, gouty nephropathy, aspergillosis, focal cortical necrosis, scleroderma, Wegener's granulomatosis, kaliopenic nephropathy, hemosiderosis, leukemic infiltration, mycosis fungoides, extramedullary erythropoiesis, lipomatosis of the kidney, Goodpasture's syndrome, and toxic nephropathies due to a wide range of nephrotoxins [40, 41].

In recent years we have become aware that patients who have nonspecific findings on light microscopy may have more specific findings on electron microscopy (e.g., the intermembranous and subendothelial deposits of complexes in lupus nephritis), and that definitive information may be obtained from immunofluorescent staining (e.g., the linear deposits of globulin in Goodpasture's syndrome). We continue to predict that in the future most renal biopsies will be examined by all three modalities when a serious diagnostic problem arises and that additional technical aids such as special histochemical staining for enzymes may further enhance the diagnostic yield in this interesting new procedure.

Acknowledgment

From the Department of Medicine and the Renal and Electrolyte Division, Georgetown University School of Medicine, Washington, D.C. Supported in part by the John A. Hartford Foundation, Inc., the Georgetown University Kidney Research Fund, and T01 HE 05256–09. We are pleased to acknowledge the assistance of our colleague, Dr. John F. Maher, and our Editorial Assistant, Miss Joan P. Ryan.

References

1. Alwall, N. Aspiration biopsy of the kidney. *Acta Med. Scand.* 143:430, 1952.
2. Berlyne, G. M. Ultrasonics and renal biopsy: An aid to determination of kidney position. *Lancet* 2:750, 1961.
3. Brun, C., and Raaschou, F. Kidney biopsies. *Amer. J. Med.* 24:676, 1958.
4. Castleman, B., and Smithwick, R. H. The relation of vascular disease to the hypertensive state based on a study of renal biopsies from 100 hypertensive patients. *J.A.M.A.* 12:1256, 1943.
5. DiGaddo, M., Torsoli, A., and Righini, E. Tecnica della biopsia renale mediante agopunctura transentanio. *Urologe* 21:376, 1954.
6. Dodge, W. F., Daeschner, C. W., Jr., Brenna, J. C., Rosenberg, H. S., Travis, L. B., and Hopps, H. C. Percutaneous renal biopsy in children: I. General considerations. *Pediatrics* 30:287, 1962.
7. Edelmann, C. M., Jr., and Greifer, I. A modified technique for percutaneous needle biopsy of the kidney. *J. Pediat.* 70:81, 1967.
8. Fiaschi, E., Ercoli, G., and Torsoli, A. La biopsia rénale médiante agopunctura transcutanea; rilievi anatomo-clinici. *Minerva Med.* 2:1, 1953.
9. Ginsberg, I., Durant, J. R., and Mendoz, L. Percutaneous renal biopsy under direct radiologic direction. *J.A.M.A.* 181:211, 1962.
10. Haddad, J. K., and Mani, R. L. Percutaneous renal biopsy: An improved method using television monitoring and high-dose infusion pyelography. *Arch. Intern. Med.* (Chicago) 119:157, 1967.
11. Heptinstall, R. H. Renal biopsies in hypertension. *Brit. Heart J.* 16:133, 1954.
12. Iverson, P., and Brun, C. Aspiration biopsy of the kidney. *Amer. J. Med.* 11:324, 1951.
13. Jungmann, E. Über chronische streptokokkeninfektionen. *Deutsch. Med. Wschr.* 50:71, 1924.
14. Kark, R. M. Needle biopsy of the kidney. (Letters to the Editor.) *Lancet* 1:51, 1956.
15. Kark, R. M. Renal biopsy. *J.A.M.A.* 205:220, 1968.
16. Kark, R. M., and Buenger, R. E. Television-monitored fluoroscopy in percutaneous renal biopsy. *Lancet* 1:904, 1966.
17. Kark, R. M., and Muehrcke, R. C. Biopsy of the kidney in the prone position. *Lancet* 1:1047, 1954.
18. Kark, R. M., Muehrcke, R. C., Pollak, V. E., Pirani, C. L., and Kiefer, J. H. An analysis of five hundred percutaneous renal biopsies. *A.M.A. Arch. Intern. Med.* 101:439, 1958.

19. Kellow, W. F., Cotsonas, N. J., Jr., Chomet, B., and Zimmerman, H. J. Evaluation of the adequacy of needle-biopsy specimens of the kidney: An autopsy study. *A.M.A. Arch. Intern. Med.* 194:353, 1959.

20. Kipnis, G. P., Jackson, G. G., Dallenbach, F. D., and Schoenberger, J. A. Renal biopsy in pyelonephritis: Correlative study of kidney morphology, bacteriology, and function in patients with chronic urinary tract infection. *A.M.A. Arch. Intern. Med.* 95: 445, 1955.

21. Lavastida, M. T., Musil, G., and Hewlitt, W. H. A disposable needle for percutaneous renal biopsy. *Clin. Pediat.* (Phila.) 7: 170, 1968.

22. Lindholm, T., Hagstam, K. E., and Kjellstrand, C. M. Some instrumental and methodological modifications of the technique for percutaneous renal biopsy. *Acta Med. Scand.* 181:245, 1967.

23. Lusted, L. B., Mortimore, G. E., and Hopper, J., Jr. Needle renal biopsy under image amplifier control. *Amer. J. Roentgen.* 75:953, 1956.

24. Merrill, A. J. The nephrotic syndrome. *Amer. Heart J.* 53:305, 1957.

25. Merrill, A. J., and Mitchell, G. L. Continuous ACTH therapy of nephrotic syndrome in children. *J. Clin. Invest.* 32:589, 1953.

26. Merrill, A. J., Wilson, J., and Timberlake, L. F. Nephrotic syndrome in children. *A.M.A. Arch. Intern. Med.* 94:925, 1954.

27. Mertz, J. H. O., Lang, E., and Klingerman, J. J. Percutaneous renal biopsy utilizing cinefluoroscopic monitoring. *J. Urol.* 95:618, 1966.

28. Muehrcke, R. C., Kark, R. M., and Pirani, C. L. Biopsy of the kidney in the diagnosis and management of renal disease. *New Eng. J. Med.* 253:537, 1955.

29. Needle biopsy of the kidney. (Leading Article.) *Lancet* 2:1231, 1955.

30. Parrish, A. E., and Howe, J. S. Needle biopsy as an aid in diagnosis of renal disease. *J. Lab. Clin. Med.* 42:152, 1953.

31. Parrish, A. E., and Howe, J. S. Serial renal biopsies and function in acute glomerulonephritis. *Clin. Res. Proc.* 4:139, 1956.

32. Parrish, A. E., Watt, M. F., and Howe, J. S. Membranous glomerulonephritis. *A.M.A. Arch. Intern. Med.* 100:620, 1957.

33. Payet, M., Pene, P., Camain, R., Gouaze, A., and Calvez, F. La biopsie du rein à l'aiguille. *Presse Med.* 61:989, 1953.

34. Perez Ara, A. La biopsia punctural del rinon no megalico considerationes generales y aportacion de un nuevo metodo. *Bol. Liga Contra el Cáncer, Habana.* 25:121, 1950.

35. Posen, G. A., Kaye, M., and Rosenthal, L. Radioisotope localisation for renal biopsy. (Letters to Editor.) *Lancet* 1:1043, 1964.

36. Radner, S. Another type of biopsy needle. *Scand. J. Clin. Lab. Invest.* 14:656, 1962.

37. Ross, J. H. Techniques of renal biopsy. (Letters to Editor.) *Lancet* 2:214, 1967.

38. Sala, A. M. Value of renal biopsy determined by autopsy control. Third International Congress of Clinical Pathology, Brussels, July, 1957.

39. Saltz, M., Sommers, S. C., and Smithwick, R. C. Clinical pathologic correlations of renal biopsies from essential hypertensive patients. *Circulation* 16:207, 1957.

40. Schreiner, G. E. Toxic Nephropathy. In Becker, E. L. (Ed.), *Structural Basis of Renal Disease.* New York: Hoeber Med. Div., Harper & Row, 1968. Pp. 703–756.

41. Schreiner, G. E. Toxic Nephropathy. In Beeson, P. B., and McDermott, W. (Eds.), *Cecil-Loeb Textbook of Medicine.* Philadelphia: Saunders, 1968. Pp. 818–824.

42. Schreiner, G. E., and Berman, L. B. Experience with 150 consecutive renal biopsies. *Southern Med. J.* 50:733, 1957.

43. Sherlock, S. *Diseases of the Liver and Biliary System.* New York: Oxford, 1955.

44. Simon, A. I. Normal renal size: An absolute criterion. *Amer. J. Roentgen.* 92:270, 1964.

45. Telfer, N., Ackroyd, A. E., and Stock, S. L. Radioisotope localisation by renal biopsy. *Lancet* 1:132, 1964.

46. Vernier, R. L., Farquhar, M. C., Brunson, J. G., and Good, R. A. Renal biopsy in the study of chronic renal disease in children by light and electron microscopy. *Univ. Minnesota M. Bull.* 28:58, 1956.

47. Vernier, R. L., Farquhar, N. G., Brunson, J. G., and Good, R. A.   Chronic renal disease in children: Correlation of clinical findings with morphologic characteristics seen by light and electron microscopy. *A.M.A. J. Dis. Child.* 96:306, 1958.

48. White, R. H. R.   Observations on percutaneous renal biopsy in children. *Arch. Dis. Child.* 38:260, 1963.

1. The kidney hypertrophies, increasing GFR by approximately 60 per cent [41].
2. Glomerulotubular balance is reset at a very different level — the ratios $\frac{C_{PAH}}{GFR}$ and $\frac{Tm_{PAH}}{GFR}$ are reduced, as well as the per cent reabsorption of water and a variety of solutes (urea, sodium phosphate, urate) [35, 39, 228, 254].
3. The glucose titration curve becomes markedly splayed [246].
4. There is limited ability to conserve sodium and to form a hypertonic urine.

These changes occurred to the same extent in those kidneys whose mass was reduced by hemi-infarction (or partial nephrectomy) as in those damaged by pyeloncphritis and glomerulonephritis.

The diseased kidney in the uremic environment is functionally different in many ways. The behavior of the ratios $\frac{C_{PAH}}{GFR}$, $\frac{Tm_{PAH}}{GFR}$, $\frac{Tm_{G}}{GFR}$ in the uremic environment is of particular importance. These ratios are one index of glomerulotubular balance. It has been shown by Kolberg [158, 159] that marked reduction in nephron mass, where the remaining kidney fragment is normal and can prevent uremia, is associated with an increase in the ratio $\frac{Tm_{PAH}}{GFR}$, both in dogs and man.

Since subtotal nephrectomy is known to increase GFR, the increased ratio indicated greater tubular than glomerular hypertrophy. However, in a uremic environment, the ratios are reduced. This cannot be due to a reduction in GFR per nephron, since nephron filtration rate actually rises further when uremia supervenes [41]. Nor is it likely that a rise in GFR per se might reduce the ratios. In other cir-

cumstances — for example, pro...
drugs — marked increases in GF...
if any effect on glomerulotub...
[176]. Clearly, uremia must so...
a suppression of tubular activity...
be principally an expression of i...
diuresis per nephron, because...
tubular activity involves a v...
transport functions which are ...
influenced by osmotic diuresis.

ROLE OF INCREASED EFFECTIVE EX...
VOLUME IN RESETTING GLOMERU...
BALANCE IN UREMIA

It is likely that the resetting...
tubular balance caused by a...
tubular activity results from ad...
physiologic factors involved i...
sodium excretion. In the prese...
nephron mass, the dietary i...
represents a relatively small...
logic control mechanism, th...
that each nephron rejects app...
cent of its filtered sodium. If...
is kept constant and the nur...
reduced to 10 per cent of n...
imbalance between intake...
ensue, expanding extracellu...
physiologic control mechan...
reset at a different level, an...
now reject 10 per cent of th...
[209]. A new steady state su...
intake and output are onc...
effective extracellular volu...
overexpanded, oscillating...
provides a more-or-less c...
to suppress sodium reabsor...
of the filtered load. In a...
ducing the number of neph...
increasing the salt load t...
of nephrons by an infusio...

The infusion of saline...
the fraction of glomerula...
in the proximal tubule [6...
also exert an inhibitory...
nephron, although this...

change in th...
(ionized cal...
dling of ano...
To assess...
the distorted...
environment...
devised an...
renal diseas...
nucleoside n...
been the exp...
induce rena...
were under...
[36–39, 42–4...
used to per...
from the dis...
normal one...
ney served to...
of the extrac...
mize hypert...
preparation...
function of...
eased kidne...
vironment...
contralateral...
This facilita...
tion of the...
havior of th...
205, 227, 228...

FUNCTION O...
NORMAL ENV...

In the pr...
volume and...
diseased kic...
contralateral...
conserve soc...
concentrate...
served. The...
renal plasm...
for PAH...
phosphate (...
various sub...
were all rec...
in a propor...
viding these...

6

Consequences of Renal Failure and Their Management

Donald W. Seldin, Norman W. Carter, and Floyd C. Rector, Jr.

The clinical course of chronic renal disease is intimately linked with the nature of the underlying pathogenic process in two ways. In general, derangements may arise, quite apart from the kidney, which are attributable to the systemic effects of the basic disease: The course of chronic pyelonephritis may be punctuated by evidences of infection; lupus nephritis may be associated with symptoms referable to a systemic disorder of connective tissue. More specifically, the pathologic process may cause renal disturbances of a characteristic type, such as early loss of concentrating power and marked polyuria in the case of nephrocalcinosis, or massive proteinuria in the case of chronic glomerulonephritis and diabetic renal disease. Nevertheless, the multitude of pathologic processes which are responsible for chronic progressive renal disease show a common pattern of deranged renal excretory and regulatory function which ultimately terminates in the clinical picture of uremia. In this sense, it has been proposed that the term *chronic Bright's disease* be used to refer to all forms of chronic progressive renal pathology [33, 42]. The following discussion concerns itself chiefly with the manifestations of chronic Bright's disease, defined in this manner.

Nephron Mass and Nephron Function

Every facet of renal function is markedly deranged in the end stage of chronic renal disease. Renal plasma flow and glomerular filtration rate (GFR) are both diminished, more or less proportionately to the reduction in renal mass. The functional capacity of the tubules, estimated from the maximal ability

211

to sec
to rea
duced
tubula
is ma
Tm i
of fil
cium,
crease
abilit
dilute
acid,
gluco
splay,
funct
units.

Th
abnoi
contr
in fu
in th
inevi
disea
of Ol
that
rons
bizar
and
but
norm
tubul
tubul
singl
area

Th
an as
the r
form
spect
electi
vanc
of ar
conc

In
evolv

pendent on an intact renal architecture — that is, concentrating and diluting ability — are notably deranged.

The interpretation of these studies has recently been challenged by Biber and his associates [31]. These investigators found that in single nephrons of kidneys acutely damaged by either potassium dichromate or mercuric chloride the ratio of TF/P_{inulin}* to TF/P_{PAH} was the same as in single nephrons of normal kidneys; normalization of a tubular function by factoring by GFR, therefore, does not exclude the existence of tubular damage. Biber et al. have criticized the use of clearance ratios on the basis that the urine volume term cancels out, leaving two U/P or TF/P terms, both of which are tubular rather than glomerular functions.

In answer to this objection, the following points have been raised [35]: In the first place, many of the indications of functional integrity of the unilaterally diseased kidney (i.e., acidification, concentration, and dilution of the urine, low urine sodium concentration, glucose-free urine) are not dependent on factoring by GFR. Secondly, the normal ratio of TF/P_{PAH} to TF/P_{inulin} in the damaged nephrons studied by Biber et al. [31] may have been due to the use of isotopic PAH. The damaged nephron might be able to extract isotopic PAH completely, but not chemical amounts of PAH. Bricker et al., using chemical PAH (1.0 to 1.5 mg. per 100 ml.), were unable to confirm Biber's results. Finally, a U/P or TF/P ratio is a function of two processes — the manner in which the substance is added to tubular urine and the tubular reabsorption of water. If the U/P ratios of two substances are compared, the effects of water reabsorption will be identical on both and can be ignored. The comparative ratios, therefore, will reflect only the relative magnitude of the

* The term TF/P refers to the concentration ratio in tubular fluid to plasma of a substance, which is designated by a subscript. Hence, TF/P_{inulin} refers to the concentration ratio of inulin in tubular fluid to plasma.

processes by which the
added to, or removed fr
comparison of the clea
glomerular substance, s
substance secreted by the
does, in fact, give an es
balance between glomer
tions.

If the clearance ratio
truly normal in damag
an artifact arising fro
PAH, then this would i
aged nephrons are cap
appropriate level of glo
and that the presenc
ratios cannot be used
normal nephrons are
urine in the unilate
However, this in no
major point of Bri
namely, that the chr
in a normal environ
sentially normal fash
the many distortion
served in similarly
setting of uremia.
nephrons are contri
they cannot account
function. Rather, it
the uremic environ
function in both
nephrons.

FUNCTION OF DISEAS
UREMIC ENVIRONME

That it is enviro
the diseased kidne
function is best ill
which the unilater
studied in the pre
lateral kidney and
ney is removed. In
kidney, the disea
essentially normal
After removing t
striking changes

unsettled at the present time. The suppression of proximal reabsorption during saline diuresis is relatively nonspecific. Micropuncture studies have demonstrated that isotonic, isohydric expansion of extracellular fluid volume suppresses proximal reabsorption, not only of sodium chloride and water but also of potassium, calcium, bicarbonate, and phosphate [109, 161]. Clearance studies show an increased excretion of water, sodium, calcium [32, 187, 278], magnesium [187], bicarbonate [164], phosphate [269], and uric acid [268]. In addition, saline infusions depress both Tm_{PAH} and Tm_G and cause marked splaying of glucose titration curves [231].

Activation of the physiologic control mechanism to an extent sufficient to maintain sodium balance in the face of a greatly reduced nephron mass, therefore, may suppress all proximal tubular functions in a nonspecific fashion and thus account for many peculiar features of renal function seen in uremia. The disturbed transport of PAH and glucose may well be attributable to this hypothesis.

Reduced Tm_{PAH}. When renal mass is reduced by subtotal nephrectomy [158, 159], both GFR and Tm_{PAH} are reduced, but the ratio Tm_{PAH} to GFR is increased. In uremic patients, however, Tm_{PAH} is disproportionately reduced, so that the Tm_{PAH}/GFR ratio is very low; in some instances Tm_{PAH} may approach zero [34, 191]. The low Tm_{PAH} has been interpreted as evidence of tubular damage. There are two alternative explanations, however; Preuss et al. [213] have found that uremic plasma inhibits PAH uptake by isolated dog tubules and have suggested that some circulating inhibitor is responsible for the disproportionately low Tm_{PAH}. More recently, Bricker and his associates [40] have found that saline infusions depress Tm_{PAH}, and more importantly, that plasma from saline-loaded dogs contains a substance which inhibits PAH uptake by kidney slices. They have found a similar inhibitor of PAH uptake in plasma of uremic patients. This may also

be the same factor identified by Preuss et al. in uremic plasma. The profound depression of Tm_{PAH}, therefore, may merely be an expression of the capacity of expanded extracellular volume to inhibit proximal tubular transport.

Glycosuria, Decreased Tm_G, *and Splaying of Glucose Titration Curves.* Patients with chronic nephritis may exhibit nondiabetic glucosuria [185, 227]. Two types of renal glucosuria have been described in patients without underlying chronic renal disease. In one type the maximum capacity to reabsorb glucose (Tm_G) is normal, but the plasma level at which glucose reabsorption becomes incomplete (renal threshold) is greatly reduced. In the second and more common type both the Tm_G and the threshold for glucose are reduced. In patients with chronic renal insufficiency the Tm_G is reduced but not to the extent that the GFR is lowered; as a matter of fact, the ratio of Tm_G to GFR tends to be modestly elevated [185, 227]. Thus, the glucosuria in chronic nephritis cannot be attributed to relative reduction in the glucose reabsorptive capacity. Glucose titration curves, however, are markedly abnormal and reveal that the plasma concentration or threshold at which glucose reabsorption becomes incomplete is markedly reduced, despite the normal or elevated reabsorptive capacity per unit GFR.

Normally, the Tm_G is approximately 230 mg. per 100 ml. GFR, and the splay point (ratio of filtered load to Tm at point where reabsorption becomes incomplete and excretion begins) is 0.8; this represents a renal threshold for glucose of approximately 190 mg. per 100 ml. In chronic renal insufficiency the Tm_G is increased to approximately 350 mg. per 100 ml. GFR and the splay point is reduced to 0.2 to 0.6, depending on the severity of the renal disease; those patients with glomerular filtration rates below 15 ml. per minute have splay points between 0.2 and 0.4, while those with rates above 15 ml. per minute have splay points between 0.4 and 0.6. The renal threshold in chronic renal insufficiency, therefore, ranges from 60 to 80 mg. per 100 ml.

One possibility for these findings is marked heterogeneity of the nephron population, with some nephrons (? damaged) having very low Tm_G/GFR ratios and other nephrons (? hypertrophied) having very high Tm_G/GFR ratios. During a glucose titration study, glucose will be excreted by the nephrons with low Tm_G/GFR at low plasma concentrations, before the nephrons with higher Tm_G/GFR are saturated, giving a markedly splayed curve. The overall Tm_G/GFR can be low, normal, or high depending on the relative proportions of nephrons with low and high Tm_G/GFR. Mudge [194], on the other hand, has pointed out that competitive inhibition of glucose transport may cause splaying of the glucose titration curve without altering the Tm. Studies by Shankel and his associates [246] show that the unilaterally diseased kidney, in the presence of a normal contralateral kidney, has a normal glucose titration curve. Only after removal of the opposite kidney and development of uremia does the diseased kidney exhibit the abnormal splay of the glucose titration curve. This suggests that the splaying is not the consequence of nephron heterogeneity but rather the result of the presence of some factor of the uremic environment, possibly some competitive inhibitor. Of particular interest are the recent studies of Robson et al. [231] demonstrating that large saline infusions in normal animals alter the glucose titration curves in a fashion that is at least partially similar to that seen in uremia. This finding raises the possibility that suppression of fractional reabsorption of filtrate in the proximal tubule necessary to maintain sodium homeostasis in the presence of reduced renal mass is responsible for the abnormal kinetics of glucose reabsorption in uremia.

ROLE OF ALTERED PLASMA COMPOSITION IN CHANGING PHYSIOLOGIC CONTROL SYSTEMS

In the case of phosphate, the main determinant of its behavior seems to be the greatly exaggerated stimulation of a physiologic control system, parathyroid activity. During the course of progressive renal disease serum phosphorus does not rise until the glomerular filtration rate has fallen to about 25 ml. per minute. When finally the filtration rate falls below 25 ml. per minute, phosphorus clearance falls and serum phosphorus rises until a new steady state is reached in which intake and excretion are equal [120]. Since the dietary intake of phosphorus is roughly constant, the normal plasma concentration despite a falling glomerular filtration rate must be due to diminishing tubular reabsorption of phosphate.

Several lines of evidence suggest that low per cent tubular reabsorption of phosphate (TRP) in uremia is not the consequence of specific damage to the transport system. First, in dogs with unilateral kidney disease, the per cent TRP in the diseased kidney is normal when the contralateral normal kidney is present; however, the per cent TRP is sharply reduced (40 to 50 per cent) when the opposite kidney is removed and uremia supervenes [254]. Second, the per cent TRP in uremic patients can be increased into the normal range by suppressing parathyroid activity with a prolonged infusion of calcium [94] or administration of vitamin D [255]. This suggests that secondary hyperparathyroidism (secondary to vitamin D resistance and the concomitant hypocalcemia), rather than tubular damage, is the primary factor responsible for the diminished per cent TRP in uremia.

ROLE OF SOLUTE DIURESIS IN INFLUENCING VOLUME AND CONCENTRATION OF URINE

In addition to the elevated GFR per nephron and suppressed proximal reabsorption in the uremic kidney, the glomerular filtrate contains high concentrations of poorly reabsorbable solutes (urea, sulfate, phosphate, etc.). These three factors combine to flood the distal tubule with large amounts of filtrate containing high concentrations of poorly reabsorbable solutes. Excessive solute excretion in

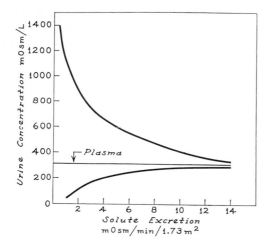

Figure 6-1. Concentration and dilution of the urine during solute diuresis in normal subjects. The data are drawn from the studies of Rapoport, Brodsky, and their associates [49, 216] on normal human subjects and plotted in the manner of Bull [51]. It has subsequently been demonstrated that extreme osmotic diuresis during hydropenia results in the formation of hypotonic urine in the dog (which can be greatly exaggerated by salt restriction [122]) and isotonic urine in man [215].

normal subjects results in an increase in urine flow and a fall or rise in urinary osmotic pressure toward that of plasma, depending on whether the subject is hydropenic or under maximal water diuresis (Fig. 6-1).

Since patients with advanced renal disease always display some degree of impairment in concentrating and diluting ability, Platt [210] developed in detail the hypothesis that these disturbances were the consequence of excessive solute excretion through remaining, presumably normal, nephrons. Apart from the analogy with osmotic diuresis in normal subjects, several lines of evidence in support of this hypothesis were advanced. Hayman and his associates [137] and Platt [210] demonstrated in normal dogs and rats, respectively, that subtotal nephrectomy impaired concentrating ability even when plasma composition did not change greatly. Since the remaining nephrons were normal, the impaired concentrating

power was attributed not to any intrinsic defect in the tubular system, but rather to the increased solute excretion per remaining nephron. The increased solute excretion, in turn, results primarily from increased filtration rate per nephron and suppression of sodium reabsorption. These factors could therefore account for isosthenuria even when plasma composition is not greatly altered. With greater renal destruction there is, in addition, a change in plasma composition, principally a rise in urea, which further augments solute excretion per nephron. The observation that reduction in blood pressure, and therefore presumably a fall in filtration rate and solute excretion, increases urine osmolality [137] supports the thesis that the impaired concentrating power of the kidney fragment is the consequence of solute diuresis.

To answer the question whether the diseased kidney behaves in the same way as the normal kidney fragment, the overall concentrating and diluting powers of the kidney can be examined in two ways. The maximal concentrating or diluting gradient the normal kidney can establish can be tested during conditions of normal solute excretion, and is usually expressed as maximal or minimal urinary osmolality (or, more properly, as the ratio of urine to plasma osmolality, U_{OSM}/P_{OSM}).

In advanced renal disease, total solute excretion is normal if the patient is eating reasonably well, but since the number of functioning nephrons is drastically reduced, each nephron is exposed to an increased solute load. Even if the remaining units are completely normal, the solute diuresis per nephron would prevent the concentrating or diluting mechanism from developing the maximal gradients of which it is capable. To compare, therefore, the maximal and minimal osmolalities of the normal and diseased kidney, it is necessary to determine these functions when solute excretion per nephron is comparable. By assuming that the glomerular filtration rate is an approximate estimate of nephron mass, the solute load of the diseased kidney per nephron can be made comparable to that of the normal kidney: normal GFR/observed GFR $\times$ observed rate of solute excretion = predicted rate of solute excretion with normal renal mass. The expression, therefore, permits a comparison of maximal and minimal urinary osmolalities when solute excretion per nephron is comparable.

Similarly, the maximal concentrating ($T^C_{H_2O}$) and diluting (C_{H_2O}) capacities of the normal and diseased kidneys can only be compared if correction is made for nephron mass:

$$\frac{C_{H_2O}}{\text{Observed GFR}} \times 100 = \text{Free water clearance per 100 ml. glomerular filtrate}$$

$$\frac{T^C_{H_2O}}{\text{Observed GFR}} \times 100 = \text{Free water reabsorption per 100 ml. glomerular filtrate}$$

It should be noted that this correction for nephron mass by factoring with GFR assumes that the relation between GFR and tubular function per nephron is the same in the normal and diseased kidney, an assumption which is highly questionable. Nevertheless, a rough estimate of nephron integrity in the diseased state can be obtained in this manner.

The impaired ability to form a dilute urine in renal disease appears to be attributable to the increased solute load per nephron. When free water clearance is corrected for glomerular filtration rate (C_{H_2O}/GFR) and solute excretion, a normal value is obtained. Similarly, minimal urinary osmolality is normal when corrected for solute excretion per nephron [154].

Impaired concentrating ability is less easily attributed solely to osmotic diuresis. To examine maximal urine osmolality, solute excretion can be corrected as described above to give the equivalent solute excretion for a normal glomerular filtration rate, and then compared with the maximal osmotic U/P ratio attained by normal subjects at the same rate of solute excretion [83, 154]. The values obtained indicate a significantly lower maximal urinary osmolality in patients with renal disease.

If solute diuresis alone were responsible for impaired concentrating ability, it should be possible, by reducing the filtered load of solute, to increase maximal urinary osmolality. Franklin et al. [104] could find no increase in maximal osmotic U/P ratios, despite reductions in osmolar clearance by about 58 per cent, produced either by lowering GFR with hypotensive agents or by lowering serum urea with dialysis. Similarly, Levitt and his associates [173] could demonstrate only very slight rises in maximal urinary osmotic pressure when the GFR was acutely lowered. These data do not involve factoring for GFR and solute excretion, and therefore circumvent some of the pitfalls involved in these corrections. The findings could mean that factors other than solute load are responsible for the concentrating defect. On the other hand, if solute excretion per nephron were extreme, the kidney would be functioning on a portion of the curve relating solute excretion to osmotic pressure (see Fig. 6-1) which is quite flat and near isotonicity. If this were so, even marked reductions in solute excretion might have little effect on urinary osmolality.

The maximum urinary concentrating capacity ($T^C_{H_2O}$) has also been studied extensively in renal failure. For comparative purposes $T^C_{H_2O}$ must be corrected for reduced renal mass by factoring by GFR. In the study by Baldwin and his associates [11] $T^C_{H_2O}$ was found to be normal in most patients with chronic nephritis and decreased in a few; however, Dorhout Mees [84] uniformly noted marked decreases.

Although these results indicate that factors in addition to osmotic diuresis are contributing to the impaired concentrating powers of the diseased kidney, it should be noted that in the presence of glomerular hyperperfusion of the remaining nephrons in renal failure, the glomerular filtration rate represents an overestimation of nephron mass [41]. Therefore, correction of $T^C_{H_2O}$ for GFR would give falsely low values, which could account in part for the finding of seemingly impaired concentrating capacity of the remaining nephrons. In addition, disproportionate destruction of long nephrons, alteration of renal circulation, and retardation of diffusion by exudate and scarring could diminish medullary hypertonicity, and thereby reduce concentrating ability, independent of injury to discrete segments of the nephron. Although tubular damage as a contributing factor to the disturbance in diluting and concentrating capacity cannot be excluded, the combined effects of osmotic diuresis and distorted renal architecture are sufficient to explain the defect without invoking the additional factor of more specific tubular injury.

The hypothesis may be ventured, by way of summary, that the kidney in renal failure displays a pattern of water and electrolyte excretion determined principally by the influence of a uremic environment on a reduced number of nephrons in a setting of distorted renal architecture. If uremia is prevented by the presence of a contralateral normal kidney, glomerulotubular balance is, on the whole, well maintained. If the contralateral normal kidney is removed and uremia allowed to supervene, glomerulotubular balance is disrupted and fractional reabsorption in the proximal tubule appears to be sharply reduced. Admittedly, nephron damage may be present. The salient feature of the uremic kidney, however, is its remarkably preserved regulatory function in the face of extreme reduction in nephron mass. This suggests that *overall nephron balance or regulation* is well preserved because the resetting of glomerular-

tubular balance ensures adequate delivery of filtrate out of the proximal tubule, thereby furnishing sufficient materials to the more distal nephron where reabsorption can be adjusted to maintain external balance. If nephrons are damaged, this must mean that they have nevertheless largely retained their capacity to respond to physiologic stimuli in such a manner as to preserve homeostatic functions.

Failure of Renal Function: Electrolyte Derangements

AZOTEMIA AND GLOMERULAR FILTRATION RATE

The concentration of urea in blood is the most commonly used clinical index of glomerular filtration rate. Goldring and Chasis [121] pointed out that the relationship between the blood urea nitrogen (BUN) and glomerular filtration rate is hyperbolic, as indicated in Figure 6-2. The three curved lines describe the relation of the BUN to GFR at three different levels of protein intake. The urinary excretion rate of urea nitrogen was

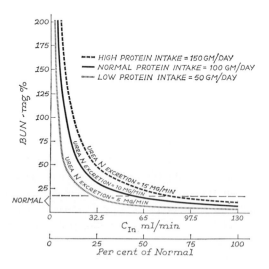

Figure 6-2. Relation of BUN to glomerular filtration rate at different levels of protein intake.

assumed to be 85 per cent of the protein nitrogen intake.

In a steady state, urea excretion must equal urea production. Assuming that urea production is constant, it follows that as nephrons are destroyed and GFR falls, the excretion of urea will fall transiently, resulting in a rise in BUN to a level at which excretion and production once again become equal and a new steady state is established. The rate of rise of the steady-state concentration of urea is very slow at first, since a 50 per cent reduction in GFR will only approximately double the BUN. Consequently, more than 60 per cent of the kidney must be destroyed before the BUN rises definitely outside the normal range. At this point, small absolute changes in GFR produce marked changes in BUN, and the latter becomes a sensitive index of GFR.

Although the BUN is used as an index of GFR, two other factors influence it: urine flow and urea loads. In patients with polyuria, moderate water restriction may raise the BUN without altering GFR. More commonly, water loads are sometimes given to patients, not necessarily because they are dehydrated, but because of the mistaken impression that the fall in BUN such a procedure may induce indicates an improvement in renal function.

The influence of changes in urine flow on urea excretion is determined, in part, by the site in the nephron where fluid is being reabsorbed. The proximal tubule is highly permeable to urea, and is the principal site of its passive reabsorption. The distal nephron is relatively impermeable to urea, even in the presence of antidiuretic hormone. If everything else is constant, salt depletion will tend to produce more azotemia at the same low urine flow than will water reduction, because salt depletion accelerates proximal reabsorption while water restriction accelerates reabsorption principally in the distal nephron [123].

These considerations also bear on the behavior of the BUN as renal failure advances.

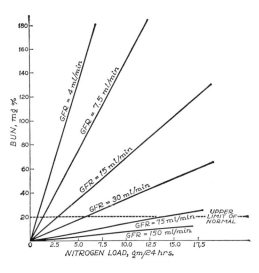

Figure 6-3. Relation of nitrogen load to the BUN at various levels of renal function.

Under such circumstances, fractional reabsorption in the proximal nephron is reduced; therefore, there is less back-diffusion of urea, and the BUN becomes a better index of glomerular filtration rate.

Variations in urea load also influence the BUN, as Figure 6-2 indicates. In Figure 6-3, the effect of nitrogen loads on the BUN at different levels of GFR is plotted. It is apparent the greater the reduction in GFR, the greater is the sensitivity of the BUN to changes in urea load. The rate of urea production is determined by the nitrogen intake on the one hand and tissue breakdown on the other.

Nitrogen loads can be influenced by internal bleeding, accelerated tissue catabolism, or dietary changes. Gastrointestinal bleeding may elevate the BUN, not alone because the reduced blood volume lowers GFR but also because of the digestion of red blood cells and plasma proteins. The BUN may rise because of increased tissue breakdown associated with the stress of severe infection in an otherwise well-nourished patient [235]. Administration of adrenal steroids may increase the nitrogen load and, consequently, elevate the BUN, by virtue of their antianabolic action. Tetracycline antibiotics also exert an antianabolic action and may cause severe azotemia, particularly in patients who accumulate high concentrations of the drug because of renal insufficiency [249]. Acute hyponatremia may also tend to augment azotemia by eliciting, through unknown mechanisms, a catabolic response [169, 177]. Variations in dietary intake are equally important. Patients with advanced renal disease may improve clinically with the correction of such disturbances as salt depletion and heart failure, yet at times the BUN may rise instead of fall, because an enhanced appetite and increased ingestion of protein masks any small rise in GFR. On the other hand, clinical deterioration may not be reflected in a rise in BUN because impaired appetite may lower protein intake. With the use of a high biologic quality protein diet the BUN may become completely disassociated from the level of GFR. The nitrogen constituents of these diets, consisting of a very high fraction of essential amino acids, are so effectively incorporated into tissue that urea load becomes very small; consequently the BUN may fall into the normal range despite no improvement or even further reduction in the GFR.

Creatinine excretion is relatively uninfluenced by diet [82] and consequently the serum creatinine concentration should be a better index of GFR than the BUN. However, recent studies have shown that creatinine, as well as urea, excretion is influenced by the rate of urine flow. More importantly, in renal insufficiency creatinine is produced at a lower-than-normal rate (perhaps because of malnutrition and wasting) and is secreted to a variable extent by the renal tubule [29]. These factors would tend to blunt the rise in serum creatinine concentration as GFR progressively falls during the course of renal disease. Despite these difficulties, the serum creatinine and endogenous creatinine clearance, although not a quantitatively accurate measure of GFR, are useful in following the level of renal function in any given patient [182].

URINE FLOW AND URINE CONCENTRATION

Impairment of concentrating ability occurs comparatively early in chronic renal disease, even before significant azotemia supervenes [137]. Evidence has been presented in a preceding section which suggests that the principal factor in the concentrating defect is the increased solute load per nephron. Pyelonephritis seems to impair concentrating ability earlier and to a greater extent than other disorders [47, 48, 214]. This may be the consequence of early and more severe destruction of the few nephrons that penetrate all the way to the tip of the papilla and are responsible for concentrating the papillary interstitial fluid, which furnishes the osmotic gradient for abstraction of the final increment of solute-free water from all the nephrons [195]. In addition, scarring and inflammation of the medulla may impair the countercurrent function of the capillary loops, and may cause shunting of blood through the medulla, which in turn would result in dissipation of medullary and papillary hypertonicity. Since pyelonephritis has a high predilection for the medulla, it is not unreasonable to anticipate earlier and more severe impairment of concentrating ability in this disorder without necessarily invoking discrete tubular damage as the mechanism.

In contrast to the early impairment of concentrating power, ability to form a dilute urine is relatively well preserved until renal disease is advanced. In fact, the capacity to form free water may be elevated for each nephron. Nevertheless, the absolute free-water clearance is usually low, because there are so few nephrons. Consequently, the ability to excrete a water load may be markedly impaired, rendering these patients extremely vulnerable to acute dilutional hyponatremia if given excess water. The administration of large quantities of water to patients with advanced renal failure in an attempt to reduce azotemia may precipitate water intoxication. As a result, severe central nervous system symptoms can supervene, simulating uremia.

Despite the impaired ability to concentrate urine, polyuria is not a common feature of renal failure. The frequent occurrence of nocturia is the consequence, not of polyuria, but of a reversal of the diurnal variation [77, 210]. In a few instances, however, a type of acquired nephrogenic diabetes insipidus has been encountered with amyloidosis, pyelonephritis, polycystic kidney disease, medullary cystic disease, hydronephrosis, and nephrocalcinosis [23, 56, 85, 155, 156, 233]. The mechanism is not understood, but it appears to be associated with those diseases that might either reduce the permeability of the collecting duct to water (amyloidosis, nephrocalcinosis) or produce disproportionate destruction of the renal medulla [267]. This latter process, by reducing the number of long nephrons and distorting the architecture of the medulla, would reduce medullary tonicity and the osmotic gradient responsible for water reabsorption from the collecting ducts, while at the same time causing redistribution of filtrate to more superficial cortical nephrons. These alterations will augment the excretion of dilute urine in two ways. First, the abstraction of water from the descending limb of Henle's loop will be markedly reduced; the resulting augmentation of fractional delivery of filtrate to more distal diluting segments will enhance the formation of solute-free water and will accelerate the rate of tubular flow through the normal osmotic equilibrating sites (distal convoluted tubule, cortical collecting ducts). Recent studies in dogs [60] and monkeys [19] have shown that osmotic equilibration in the distal convoluted tubule normally may be incomplete; therefore, acceleration of tubular flow through this segment may sweep large volumes of dilute fluid into the medullary collecting ducts. Second, due to absence of medullary hypertonicity and possibly abnormal

surface-volume relationships in dilated collecting ducts, the abstraction of solute-free water by the collecting ducts will be reduced. The combination of these factors, which tend to occur more commonly in hydronephrosis and other diseases selectively damaging the renal medulla, may give rise to a syndrome of nephrogenic diabetes insipidus, despite serious reduction in overall glomerular filtration rate.

SODIUM

Patients with severe renal disease exhibit a remarkable ability to regulate sodium balance in the face of modest variations in intake [209, 210]. As the functioning mass of the kidney is reduced by chronic diseases and the dietary intake of salt remains in the normal range, a greater fraction of filtered sodium must escape reabsorption if sodium balance is to be maintained. In contrast to normal subjects, who excrete only 0.5 to 1.0 per cent of their filtered sodium on a normal intake, patients with glomerular filtration rates of approximately 4 ml. per minute will excrete 8 per cent of their filtered sodium while on a diet of 3.5 gm. of NaCl. and 16 per cent of filtered sodium when given 7.0 gm. of NaCl. If these patients are given an isotonic saline infusion, the fractional sodium excretion may increase up to 40 per cent of the filtered load [253].

Variations in sodium intake have little, if any, effect on GFR in normal subjects, but produce marked changes in GFR in patients with chronic renal disease [197]. Although these changes in GFR may participate in the regulation of sodium balance, they are not the primary factor. Slatapolsky et al. [253] found that in uremic patients a rise in GFR induced by injections of parathormone increased sodium excretion slightly, but not to the extent occurring with similar increments in GFR produced by saline infusions. Thus, expansion of extracellular fluid volume accelerates sodium excretion primarily by inhibiting tubular reabsorption of sodium.

These changes in tubular reabsorption are

clearly not mediated by variations in aldosterone levels. In Slatapolsky's studies infusion of saline suppressed tubular reabsorption despite administration of the potent mineralocorticoid, 9-alpha-fluorohydrocortisone. Of particular note in this respect is the fact that uremic patients on a normal diet (approximately 100 mEq. of sodium) have high aldosterone excretory and secretory rates, yet are excreting 10 to 15 per cent of their filtered sodium.

The factors responsible for maintaining sodium balance not only are activated to maintain a high fractional excretion on a normal salt diet but also respond appropriately to changes in salt intake. Despite the persistence of this normal control mechanism, uremic patients have difficulty in adjusting to extreme variations in intake, either excessive salt loads or rigid restriction.

Patients in advanced renal failure are vulnerable to salt retention and venous congestion. The reasons for this are not always clear. In careful balance studies, Slatapolsky and his associates [253] have shown that a patient with a GFR of the order of 5 ml. per minute can excrete up to 35 per cent of the filtered sodium, and should therefore be able to handle 330 mEq. per day. Clearly, this is not the case. Scribner and his associates [241] have emphasized the vulnerability of patients with renal failure to develop edema on free access to salt, and this is our experience as well. It is likely that activity and the erect posture limit the capacity of the uremic kidney to suppress sodium reabsorption. In addition, acute acidosis, by causing venoconstriction [136] and impairing the ventricular response curve [287], may render the uremic patient susceptible to salt retention and pulmonary congestion. Patients with advanced renal failure appear to lack the normal capacity to maintain sodium balance — they often become salt-depleted on a restricted intake and overexpanded on a normal intake. For this reason, most patients

in advanced renal failure should be maintained on a moderate sodium intake (2 to 4 gm. NaCl per day).

On the other hand, almost all patients with advanced renal disease waste salt under appropriate circumstances. Three forms of salt wastage have been described. First, there is a very mild salt-wasting syndrome which virtually all patients with advanced renal failure display when subjected to rigid sodium restriction [63]. Second, there is a rare, massive salt-wasting syndrome which tends to occur in those patients with renal diseases causing disproportionate medullary destruction [103, 274]. Both of these salt-wasting states tend to be unrelenting until circulatory collapse develops. A third form of salt wastage represents a more transient disorder in which salt wastage appears to stop after extracellular volume is sharply reduced [13, 55].

The cause of the mild salt-wasting syndrome appears to be the inability of patients with chronic renal disease to reduce the urinary sodium concentration below a relatively high fixed value [63]. Tubular damage does not seem to be responsible for the defect, since reducing the osmotic load by drug-induced hypotension reduced urinary sodium concentration. The cause of the high minimal urinary sodium concentration (ranging approximately from 10 to 15 mEq. per liter) is most likely solute diuresis through remaining nephrons. If oral sodium chloride intake is reduced below about 20 millimoles (mM) per day, it is clear that salt wastage will usually appear [63]. The provision of 2 to 3 gm. (35 to 50 mM) of NaCl in the diet is sufficient to maintain sodium balance in most patients.

In rare instances, renal salt wastage may be extreme, simulating Addison's disease, but differing from the latter in that adrenal cortical function is intact and desoxycorticosterone acetate does not correct the defect [103, 209, 274]. Such patients seem to be suffering from diseases which disproportionately destroy the medulla — for example, polycystic kidney disease, hydronephrosis, medullary cystic disease, analgesic-abuse nephritis, and pyelonephiritis [103, 265, 274]. It is possible that these disorders, by destroying nephrons with long loops and a high capacity for sodium reabsorption, produce a flooding of the remaining nephrons with short loops, as a result of which their reabsorptive capacity is quickly exceeded and salt wastage ensues.

Finally, Bartter's syndrome [13], consisting of juxtaglomerular hyperplasia, very high plasma renin levels with normal blood pressure, high aldosterone, and hypokalemic alkalosis, may be a peculiar form of renal salt wastage [158] in which the propensity to excrete sodium, when extracellular volume is normal, is so great that restoration to a normal volume is difficult. In consequence, the patients appear to be in a steady state in which extracellular volume is chronically contracted, thereby activating the renin-angiotensin-aldosterone system. In this steady state, sodium is not wasted. By giving massive amounts of saline so as to ensure a correction of volume deficits, it has been possible to correct the disorder [286].

The presence of salt wastage does not ensure against salt retention under different circumstances. Certain patients who develop mild salt depletion on salt restriction may also develop edema and congestion when given salt loads. An appropriate salt intake must be sought between these limits.

POTASSIUM

The ability to excrete potassium is usually well maintained despite severe renal disease. Ordinarily, severe elevations in serum potassium (greater than 7.0 mEq. per liter) are uncommon until the terminal stages of renal failure with marked oliguria [91, 151]. Since most of these patients are on a normal diet, the potassium intake is also approximately nor-

mal; consequently, potassium excretion, despite profound reduction in the filtration rate, must also have been normal. This suggests that the excretion of potassium is relatively independent of the amount filtered, and is a result instead of tubular activity. Indeed, a number of studies have demonstrated that in advanced renal disease potassium clearance may exceed inulin clearance by two to six times [168, 194, 209].

These findings in renal disease are in accord with the general conceptual framework regarding potassium secretion as elaborated by Berliner and his associates. They have demonstrated that in normal animals excreted potassium is relatively independent of filtered potassium [21]. Filtered potassium is thought to be completely reabsorbed in the proximal portion of the nephron, and urinary excretion is entirely derived from tubular secretion of potassium in exchange for reabsorbed sodium in the distal exchange sites [22, 70]. The nephron mass is normally sufficiently great so that, unlike in the patient with advanced renal failure, potassium clearance is usually well below inulin clearance, but under appropriate circumstances the clearance of potassium in normal dogs may exceed that of inulin [20].

The normal excretion of potassium in renal failure, then, must represent an adaptive change in the residual nephrons involving the progressive utilization of the latent capacity to secrete potassium in exchange for sodium. Two critical points follow from this theory. First, since the potassium secretory system is functioning at near-capacity levels, there is very little reserve with which to respond to additional potassium loads. Therefore, the reduced renal mass, although usually adequate to handle the normal dietary intake of potassium, may be unable to excrete any additional increments. Second, since the secretory system is functioning near capacity and is critically dependent on sodium reabsorption, any reduction in the amounts of sodium reaching the exchange site, such as may occur as a result of salt restriction, could produce potassium retention. Both factors are responsible for episodes of hyperkalemia in patients with renal disease.

Increased potassium loads may result from several factors. The transfusion of old blood (where potassium has leaked out of the red cells and accumulated in plasma) can result in acute hyperkalemia. Potassium salts are often added to the diet to prevent an anticipated potassium deficiency in patients receiving diuretic agents. In advanced renal disease, diuresis is not likely to occur, but the potassium salts may precipitate potassium intoxication. Finally, a severe catabolic response to stress may result in the liberation of large amounts of potassium from cells [263], with consequent potassium intoxication.

The second factor responsible for episodes of hyperkalemia involves the reduced delivery of sodium to the distal tubular exchange site. Restriction of dietary salt intake, in the treatment of hypertension or edema, may result in the development of mild hyperkalemia. Far more important, however, is the salt depletion produced by vomiting and diarrhea, as a result of which filtration rate falls sharply and severe hyperkalemia may supervene.

Finally, metabolic acidosis will increase the concentration of serum potassium for any given level of total body potassium [52, 240, 252]. Presumably, extracellular hydrogen ions penetrate tissue cells in exchange for potassium which is extruded into the extracellular fluid. Since acidosis will increase serum potassium in normal subjects as well as in uremic patients, it is evident that renal failure is not a necessary condition for the hyperkalemia; apparently, during acidosis, the proportion of total body potassium which is in the extracellular fluid is increased irrespective of the state of renal function. However, in renal failure this effect may well be exaggerated because of the inability of the kidneys to excrete any portion of the additional potassium. The magni-

tude of the rise in serum potassium during acidosis is impressive: an increase of from 0.4 to 1.2 mEq. per liter may occur with each 0.1 unit fall in blood pH [52, 240]. These findings serve to emphasize the importance of correcting acidosis if hyperkalemia is present, and also explain why some patients, whose serum potassium was initially normal or only slightly elevated, develop hypokalemia as acidosis recedes.

Hypokalemia during the course of advanced renal disease may develop because of losses associated with vomiting and diarrhea. Although these extrarenal losses may be adequate to explain most instances of potassium deficiency, data are not available from patients with advanced renal disease which delineates their capacity to conserve potassium.

On rare occasions potassium deficiency develops during the course of renal disease as a result of renal potassium wastage. It seems likely that the accelerated losses of potassium are the consequence, not of a specific tubular lesion that interferes with potassium reabsorption, but rather result from enhanced potassium secretion. This is often due to secondary aldosteronism. In the syndrome of salt-losing nephritis [263], the depletion of extracellular volume may elicit enhanced aldosterone output, which, in the presence of increased delivery of sodium to the exchange site, can augment potassium secretion and lead to severe deficiency. Patients with malignant hypertension or unilateral renal disease may develop a form of secondary aldosteronism [166] which is the consequence of chronic stimulation of the juxtaglomerular apparatus, thereby leading to activation of the renin-angiotensin system and through it oversecretion of aldosterone [275]. As a consequence, hypokalemia and alkalosis may develop.

Primary aldosteronism may be complicated by the development of renal disease as a result of potassium deficiency, which can produce nephropathy [221, 281], hypertension, or pyelonephritis. In rare instances the distinction between primary aldosteronism with secondary renal disease on the one hand and renal artery disease and malignant hypertension with secondary aldosteronism on the other may be exceedingly difficult to make. In several of the early cases of "potassium-losing nephritis" the patients may well have been suffering from primary aldosteronism [65]. Usually, alkalosis rather than acidosis, the lack of azotemia, and a fairly benign-appearing urinary sediment serve to exclude primary renal disease as the cause of the potassium deficit. However, if secondary renal disease becomes a prominent feature of primary aldosteronism or secondary aldosteronism a prominent feature of renal disease, the differences tend to disappear [86, 281].

Finally, it should be mentioned that although azotemic renal failure occurring as the consequence of the ordinary causes of chronic Bright's disease does not appear to result in a specific lesion that promotes potassium loss, renal potassium wastage is a regular feature of hyperchloremic renal tubular acidosis [3]. Here, too, the excessive loss of potassium does not seem to be the result of a specific lesion in the potassium transport system of the nephron. Rather, potassium secretion appears to be augmented because, owing to a disturbance in hydrogen secretion in the distal nephron, increased amounts of tubular sodium are reabsorbed in exchange for potassium. These patients usually have hyperchloremic acidosis (not hypochloremic alkalosis), little azotemia, and a defective ability to secrete an acid urine, and consequently they can readily be distinguished from patients with azotemic renal failure.

UREMIC ACIDOSIS

The acidosis associated with azotemic renal failure is of two varieties. The most common form is characterized by a fall in the concentration of plasma bicarbonate with a commensurate rise in undetermined anions, principally sulfate and phosphate, but also various organic acid anions [244]. Azotemia is marked and hyperkalemia not infrequent. The plasma chloride is usually normal. However, hypochloremia may supervene either because of water retention (in which case the plasma concentrations of sodium and chloride will be depressed proportionately) or because of vomiting (which will usually produce a proportionately greater reduction in plasma chloride than in plasma sodium concentration). In some patients with azotemic renal failure, acidosis is associated with hyperchloremia and little or no increase in undetermined anions. These patients, too, exhibit azotemia and a tendency to hyperkalemia [167].

These forms of acidosis must be the consequence of a defect in the renal excretion of acid. The *net effect* of renal activities serving to eliminate acid from the body is given by the algebraic sum of the urinary excretion of NH_4^+ + titratable acid − HCO_3^-. In a steady state, where food intake and cellular metabolism and composition are constant and plasma bicarbonate and extracellular volume stable, the rate of acid excretion must equal the rate at which acids are invading the extracellular fluid, the excretion of which by the kidneys preserves acid-base balance. Any fall in NH_4^+ + titratable acid − HCO_3^- will result in acidosis. Should reduced acid excretion continue, lethal acidosis might eventually supervene. Actually, patients with renal disease usually stabilize at different levels of acidosis. This seems to be the consequence of two factors: (1) some rise in net acid excretion as serum bicarbonate falls; and (2) continuous neutralization of some of the retained acid in tissues, presumably in bone [125, 170, 171], without the titration of extracellular buffers. Therefore, to explain the mechanisms responsible for renal acidosis, any theory must account not merely for its development but also for the factors responsible for the steady state.

To characterize the pattern of acid excretion in renal failure a variety of studies have been made on urine pH, ammonia, bicarbonate, and titratable acid excretion. When their plasma bicarbonate is normal or near normal, patients with azotemic renal acidosis do not acidify their urine well. When the plasma bicarbonate is depressed, it is apparent that they have the ability to lower urine pH maximally [206]. Despite the low urine pH in chronic acidosis, the excretion of ammonia is strikingly diminished [238, 290]. Since ammonia transport is determined by the trapping of NH_3 as NH_4^+ within the tubular lumen [204], these findings point to a diminution in NH_3 production. No data are available regarding the activity of the ammonia-producing enzyme systems in renal disease. However, the studies of Wrong and Davies [290] and Morrin and his associates [193] indicate that when ammonia excretion is corrected for glomerular filtration rate, the excretion of ammonia per nephron is normal. This suggests that the impaired ability to excrete ammonia in renal disease is the result, not of specific damage to the ammonia-producing enzyme systems, but rather of diminished nephron mass.

Since ammonia excretion is low at all levels of plasma bicarbonate and rises only slightly as urine pH falls, the elimination of acid is critically dependent on the ability to form titratable acid. Briggs and his associates [46] demonstrated increased titratable acid excretion in patients with uremic acidosis as contrasted with normal subjects. The failure of others [290] to demonstrate this increase, they attribute to poor food intake, since if urine pH is comparably reduced the amount of titratable acid excretion will be determined by the excretion of phosphate. However, the fall in urine pH and rise in titratable acid excretion, as plasma bicarbonate concentration declines, is very slow, and only becomes appreciable when systemic acidosis of some degree has supervened [238]. These findings suggest that uremic acidosis develops because the excretion of ammonia and titratable acid

is sharply reduced; the steady state is finally achieved when the augmented excretion of titratable acid and the additional contribution of titration of bone salts balance acid production.

In a minority of patients bicarbonate wastage is apparently responsible for the acidosis [238]. This bicarbonate loss is not the consequence of a diminished total hydrogen secretory capacity, since acute bicarbonate-loading experiments by Roberts and her associates [229] have demonstrated that the bicarbonate Tm is not reduced in uremic acidosis. Presumably, therefore, a slight trickle of bicarbonate into the urine, before the bicarbonate Tm is reached, may cumulate over a 24-hour period to an amount sufficient to produce acidosis in some patients.

From these observations on urinary acid excretion a tentative reconstruction of the events leading to uremic acidosis may be ventured. As nephron mass is reduced during the advance of renal disease, the capacity to excrete ammonia is profoundly depressed, probably because of a great diminution in tubular mass. Consequently, the elimination of acid becomes critically dependent on titratable acid excretion. However, urine pH falls and titratable acid excretion rises very slowly as the plasma bicarbonate declines, reaching a maximal value only when acidosis of some magnitude has supervened. Two factors may be responsible for the slow rise in titratable acid excretion.

First, the fall in glomerular filtration rate, by reducing the excretion of hydrogen acceptors, may be responsible, at least in part, for the laggard response of titratable acid excretion during the development of uremic acidosis. As GFR falls, the delivery of buffer anions (principally phosphate) as well as unreabsorbed anions of other types (such as sulfate) to the exchange sites of the nephron diminishes. Titratable acid excretion is a function of both buffer excretion and urine pH. Since the excretion of phosphate is reduced as

GFR falls, less titratable acid can be formed than if the filtered phosphorus were normal. Moreover, the pH of the urine tends to be high because of the reduced excretion of sodium salts of unreabsorbed anions; hence, less titratable acid is produced for any given level of phosphate excretion than if the urine were highly acid. There is abundant evidence that acid excretion is much greater if sodium salts of unreabsorbed anions are given than with equivalent loads of sodium chloride [12, 218, 243]. Micropuncture studies in rats have demonstrated that the administration of sodium sulfate produces a sharp rise in the distal transtubular potential difference of approximately — 15 millivolts (mv) [59]. It is likely, therefore, that if the mechanism for hydrogen secretion is a $Na^+ — H^+$ exchange pump, the increased transtubular potential difference augments urinary acidification by restraining the back-diffusion of H^+. The falling GFR, therefore, by diminishing the delivery of unreabsorbed anions and buffer anions to the exchange site, could contribute to the development of acidosis by reducing the excretion of titratable acid. As the plasma concentrations of these anions mount, their urinary excretion returns to normal and a new steady state is achieved; once again, sufficient sodium salts of unreabsorbed anions reach the exchange site to promote a sharp fall in urinary pH and a rise in phosphate excretion. Although ammonia excretion increases only minimally, the significant augmentation in titratable acid excretion is sufficient to facilitate a new steady state.

This explanation of the slow increase in titratable acid as plasma bicarbonate falls does not account for the failure of the acute administration of sodium bicarbonate to correct acidosis more than transiently. After sodium bicarbonate administration is stopped, acidosis rapidly reappears [238].

A second factor must therefore be operative in delaying this fall in urine pH and rise in titratable acid which is responsible in large part for the establishment of a steady state at low plasma concentrations of bicarbonate. It is likely that the surviving nephrons in renal disease are enormously overperfused. If the plasma bicarbonate concentration is raised toward normal, suppression of proximal tubular reabsorption (in the manner previously discussed) would result in the delivery of large amounts of alkaline fluid to the distal nephron. Exactly the same distal flooding would occur if a population of nephrons were destroyed by disease; this would result from a suppression of proximal fractional reabsorption in the remaining units. If the distal bicarbonate delivery were very great, the hydrogen secretory capacity of the distal nephron would be overwhelmed and bicarbonate wastage would ensue. More commonly, the increased bicarbonate delivery soaks up the secreted hydrogen, so that the urine pH is relatively high and titratable acid excretion is low. In both instances metabolic acidosis results. The plasma HCO_3^- will stabilize (at any given rate of metabolic acid production in excess of that titrated by body buffers [125, 170, 171]) when the concentration falls sufficiently to allow more complete reabsorption. This permits the distal nephron to lower urine pH and thereby facilitate the formation of maximal amounts of titratable acid.

It is apparent that suppression of proximal reabsorption during advancing renal disease will flood the distal nephron with alkaline fluid. In consequence, the intrinsic ability of this segment to perform acidifying functions will be masked. The capacity for net hydrogen secretion (titratable acid + NH_4^+ — HCO_3^-) and for the generation of pH gradients cannot emerge when distal hydrogen secretion, though greatly increased, is expended on bicarbonate reabsorption. Infusion of sodium sulfate into patients with chronic renal acidosis [242] lowered urine pH normally when plasma bicarbonate was low, but actually raised urine pH when plasma bicarbonate was normal. This suggests that the intrinsic acidifying capacity of the distal neph-ron is well preserved. Similarly, overall bi-carbonate reabsorption is normal in dogs with experimental renal disease. It is the uremic environment that results in a suppression of proximal reabsorption. The pattern of uremic acidosis can thus be explained [242] without invoking the hypothesis of discrete tubular damage which reduces hydrogen secretory capacity.

Acidosis may develop in the course of azotemic renal failure that is associated with hyperchloremia but with little or no rise in undetermined acids [167]. This disorder is often accompanied by hyperkalemia. As in uremic acidosis without hyperchloremia, these patients can elaborate a urine with a pH of maximum acidity. There is no evidence of a disturbance in bicarbonate reabsorption, as judged by titration studies in our laboratory. In Figure 6-4 the relation of plasma bicarbo-nate to bicarbonate reabsorption is plotted as plasma bicarbonate is raised from 10 to 35 mEq. per liter by an infusion of sodium bi-carbonate. It should be noted that the bicarbon-ate Tm is not depressed, nor is there any excessive bicarbonate spillage before the bi-carbonate Tm is reached, as indicated by the

superimposition of points on the theoretical line of 100 per cent bicarbonate reabsorption. These findings are similar to those observed in normal subjects and in patients with uremic acidosis without hyperchloremia.

What is the cause of the hyperchloremia? In Lathem's study, the underlying disease process was chronic pyelonephritis; azotemia was usually milder than in the ordinary type of uremic acidosis, the BUN and NPN rang-ing from 40 to 119 mg. per 100 ml. As the disease advanced, hyperchloremia tended to recede, and acidosis was associated with a rise in undetermined anions.

This pattern suggests that the cause of the hyperchloremia is unusually excessive filtra-tion in residual nephrons. It is reasonable to suppose that under such circumstances the reduction in the number of functioning neph-ron units may sharply reduce the total capac-ity of the kidney to secrete ammonia. Unde-termined acids, HR, which invade the blood, decompose the plasma bicarbonate in a nor-mal fashion, but since the glomerular filtra-tion rate is not drastically reduced, the acid anions are not retained in the blood, but are filtered into the tubular urine as NaR.

Under normal circumstances, Na^+ would be reabsorbed in exchange for H^+ and re-turned to the blood as $NaHCO_3$, while the anion would be excreted into the urine prin-cipally as NH_4R. In these patients, however, since the total ammonia-producing capacity of the kidneys is sharply reduced, some of the NaR filtered at the glomerulus is excreted into the urine. This loss of plasma $NaHCO_3$ as NaR, without commensurate loss of plasma Cl^-, will result in a reduction in extracellular volume, acidosis, and some hyperchloremia. The reduction in extracellular volume, in turn, will stimulate the retention of dietary NaCl. Since in normal extracellular fluid the ratio of sodium to chloride is about 1.4:1, the reexpansion of extracellular fluid by sodium chloride retention will increase the hyper-chloremia. Exactly the same mechanism, but

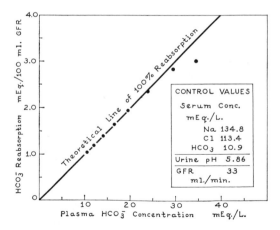

Figure 6-4. Relationship between HCO_3^- reab-sorption and plasma HCO_3^- concentration in ure-mic acidosis with hyperchloremia.

for different reasons, is responsible for the syndrome of hyperchloremic renal tubular acidosis. As renal disease advances and filtration rate falls, undetermined anions are retained in plasma and ordinary uremic acidosis without hyperchloremia supervenes.

Chronic pyelonephritis was responsible for the syndrome in all of Lathem's cases. However, we have commonly observed this disorder in chronic Bright's disease of all types.

Uremic acidosis, unless extraordinarily severe, does not usually give rise to dyspnea at rest or frank evidences of hyperventilation. Dyspnea on exertion, however, may be a prominent complaint, and is occasionally the presenting symptom of azotemic renal failure. Mild hyperkalemia may also appear as severe acidosis develops. It is possible that some of the lethargy and somnolence of severe renal failure may, in part, result from acidosis. For these reasons, measures to restore the acid-base pattern of plasma to normal are well worth while. However, the dramatic clinical features of ketonemic acidosis or acute ammonium chloride acidosis [223], such as marked mental confusion, hyperglycemia, or leukocytosis, are not commonly seen.

CALCIUM AND PHOSPHORUS

Derangements of calcium metabolism are common accompaniments of chronic renal disease and are summarized as follows:

A. Plasma
  1. Calcium
     a. Total and ionized [Ca] usually reduced
     b. Rarely, total [Ca] is elevated
     c. Tetany rare — occurs with alkalosis
  2. Phosphorus — elevated
  3. Alkaline phosphatase — sometimes elevated
B. Bone — azotemic renal osteodystrophy
  1. Osteomalacia or rickets
  2. Osteitis fibrosa or secondary hyperparathyroidism
  3. Osteosclerosis
C. Metastatic calcification
D. Pseudogout

These derangements are considered in detail in Chapter 8. The following remarks concern the plasma concentrations of phosphorus and calcium.

The serum phosphorus does not rise until the GFR has fallen to about 25 ml. per minute [120]. Since the dietary intake of phosphorus is roughly constant, the normal plasma concentration despite a falling GFR must be due to diminished tubular reabsorption of phosphate. Both inferential and direct evidence strongly indicate that the factor responsible for the progressive diminution in renal phosphate reabsorption is enhanced parathyroid secretion. If the serum calcium is raised, either by prolonged calcium infusions [94] or by chronic treatment with oral calcium, aluminum hydroxide gel, and vitamin D [255], the tubular reabsorption of phosphate rises into the normal range. This suggests that prolonged elevations of serum calcium suppress parathyroid secretion, an inference which has been confirmed by immunoassay studies, indicating that the concentration of the hormone rises as renal failure advances [30, 220].

It is likely that the secretion of parathormone is stimulated by a fall in the concentration of ionized calcium. From the destruction of the very first nephron, there must have been some phosphate retention, causing a slight fall in ionized calcium and eliciting parathyroid secretion. The latter, in turn, would accelerate urinary phosphate excretion, so that the plasma phosphate would fall and the ionized calcium rise. But the compensation cannot be complete, because as plasma phosphate approaches a normal value, the stimulus to parathormone secretion is removed. Plasma phosphate therefore stabilizes at a slightly increased concentration, depressing ionized calcium, thereby stimulating parathormone secretion. In consequence, with progressive nephron destruction there is a sustained, oscillating increase in parathyroid secretion [45, 220]. When the glomerular filtration rate falls below 25 ml. per minute, hyperphosphatemia supervenes. Presumably at this point, parathyroid secretion is at a maximum, and further nephron destruction elicits increasing hyperphosphatemia.

It is likely that factors in addition to phosphate influence the depression of ionized calcium. Kleeman and his associates have pointed out that in moderate renal insufficiency the plasma concentration of phosphate tends to be low in many patients. This suggests that other factors, perhaps other complexing anions, may contribute significantly to a reduction in ionized calcium.

Mild hypocalcemia is common in renal failure and severe hypocalcemia tends to appear in the terminal stages. Hypocalcemia usually coexists with hyperphosphatemia, although instances in which the serum calcium is normal despite an elevated phosphorus concentration are by no means rare. For instance, a serum phosphorus as high as 10.2 mg. per 100 ml. has been reported when the serum calcium was 10.3 mg. per 100 ml. [74].

Despite the frequency of hypocalcemia in azotemic renal failure, tetany is rare. The reasons for this are not apparent. Since only the ionized portion of the total calcium concentration is related to neuromuscular activity, it has been suggested that this component may be normal, irrespective of the level of total calcium. Two reasons have been advanced in support of this thesis: (1) as a consequence of hypoproteinemia, the protein-bound fraction might be diminished, leaving ionized calcium unchanged; and (2) acidosis might exert a protective action by diminishing the binding of calcium by plasma proteins. Several studies have attempted to explore this problem by determination of the concentration of the various calcium fractions in uremic plasma [95, 279].

The total calcium of plasma is divided into three main components: ionized, protein-bound, and complexed. Complexed calcium refers to that fraction which is ultrafiltrable but not ionized. This calcium is complexed to small diffusible molecules, such as citrate, phosphate, and sulfate. Fanconi and Rose [95] obtained the following values in normal subjects for the various calcium fractions, expressed per 100 mg. of plasma water: ionized, 5.88 to 6.51 mg. per 100 ml.; protein-bound, 3.35 to 3.93 mg. per 100 ml.; and complexed, 0.5 mg. per 100 ml. In two uremic patients with low total calciums [95], protein-bound calcium was reduced and complexed calcium increased, but the most striking finding was the profound reduction in ionized calcium to 3.0 to 3.5 mg. per 100 ml. Walser [279] also found severe depressions of ionized calcium in some uremic plasmas. Despite the low ionized calcium, the patients of Fanconi and Rose did not develop tetany. This is particularly noteworthy, since patients with hypoparathyroidism in the study regularly developed tetany when ionized calcium fell below 4.3 mg. per 100 ml. Fanconi and Rose suggest that the resistance to tetany in uremic patients with diminished ionized calcium may be due to the counteracting effect of high levels of serum magnesium. Walser [279] found that the concentration of free magnesium was increased in uremia in about one-third of the patients studied despite a simultaneous rise in magnesium complexes. However, the increase was only minor.

Although in an occasional patient neuromuscular hyperactivity may be due to tetany, particularly if large amounts of alkali are rapidly administered, it should be emphasized that disturbances in neuromuscular function are usually the manifestation of terminal uremia. Occasionally, mental disturbances, muscular twitching, and cramps may be due to water intoxication. Finally, severe hypertension may be responsible for a similar picture. In patients with azotemic renal failure, therefore, mental disturbances and neuromuscular hyperirritability should arouse suspicion of uremic encephalopathy, hypertensive encephalopathy, and acute dilutional hyponatremia, despite the presence of hypocalcemia, especially if there is no Trousseau sign.

MAGNESIUM

In normal persons, the mean concentration of magnesium in plasma is variously reported as ranging from 1.7 to 2.3 mEq. per liter [90]. Patients with chronic renal disease but no azotemia have normal or low serum concentrations [258]. These low values are presumably the consequence of starvation and gastrointestinal losses, although the suggestion has been made that in some instances urinary losses of magnesium may be excessive [90, 258], particularly in those patients with chronic renal disease who have polyuria. In only a few cases, however, has there been clinical evidence, such as neuromuscular hyperirritability, tremors, and convulsions, to suggest that the magnesium deficiency might be symptomatic [140, 258].

When the glomerular filtration rate falls below 30 ml. per minute, hypermagnesemia may supervene unless counteracting influences are present, such as starvation or accelerated urinary excretion due to diuretics [230]. The significance of these high values of total serum magnesium is difficult to assess, since only the ionized fraction is responsible for the physiologic action. Normally, about 25 to 35 per cent of the plasma magnesium is bound to protein; the remainder is present in the ionized form, except for a small fraction which is complexed to anions, such as citrate, phosphate, and sulfate [90, 170, 249]. Apparently, protein binding is mediated principally by albumin, approximately 0.012 to 0.013 mEq. of magnesium being bound to 1.0 gm. of albumin [66, 211].

As in the case of calcium, the proportion of total magnesium which is ionized should be influenced by changes in pH, the concentration of plasma proteins, and the concentrations of various complexing anions. For any given level of plasma magnesium, therefore, acidosis and hypoproteinemia should increase, while high concentrations of complexing anions should decrease, the concentration of ionized magnesium. Little quantitative information is available on the influence of pH and anions on magnesium binding. Moreover, in uremia opposing effects can be anticipated from the presence of both increased complexing anions and acidosis. Consequently, to ascertain the significance of the high total magnesium concentration in uremia, it is necessary to determine ionized magnesium directly. The data on this issue are meager, but Walser [279] found that despite an increase in magnesium complexes, the concentration of total magnesium was elevated in one-half and ionic magnesium was elevated in one-third of the patients studied. These findings, therefore, raise the question as to whether hypermagnesemia in renal failure may not give rise to clinical disorders, particularly to the somnolence and coma characteristic of advanced uremia.

Symptoms of magnesium intoxication include principally retardation of neuromuscular transmission, central nervous system depression, peripheral vasodilatation, and disturbances in cardiac conduction. The effects on the nervous system are related to the concentration of magnesium in serum [142]. Excess of magnesium ions blocks neuromuscular transmission mainly by decreasing the amount of acetylcholine liberated at the neuromuscular junction [73]. Simple twitches, such as the patellar reflex, disappear first, while respirations, which depend on tetany, disappear later as the concentration of magnesium continues to rise. When plasma levels of magnesium are raised to approximately 15 mEq. per liter, unconsciousness and central respiratory paralysis develop. These effects of hypermagnesemia on the nervous system can be corrected by the administration of large amounts of calcium. Magnesium is also a powerful peripheral vasodilator and may produce peripheral flushing and hypotension. Finally, direct effects on the heart, save for bradycardia, do not appear until the serum concentration exceeds 10 to 15 mEq. per liter, at which point the PR interval is lengthened, the QRS complex widens, and the heart may stop in diastole [256].

In uremic patients who are not given magnesium salts orally or parenterally, high values for total magnesium are encountered, especially in those instances where oliguria or coma exists [90, 258]. The values in a group of patients with uremia and somnolence ranged from 2.0 to 3.7 mEq. per liter [258]. Winkler and his associates [289] report some values as high as 4.9 mEq. per liter. Since failure of tendon reflexes does not appear until serum magnesium exceeds 10 mEq. per liter, while coma does not appear until plasma concentrations approach 15 mEq. per liter [257], it is unlikely that magnesium can be responsible for these features of the uremic state. Although it can be argued that the low values of ionized calcium can potentiate the depressant effects of high concentrations of magnesium, it should be remembered that ionized magnesium is not as high as would ordinarily be predicted from the total serum concentration, owing to the formation of magnesium complexes [279]. If the patellar reflex is intact, then coma as a result of magnesium intoxication is highly unlikely [257].

However, the administration of magnesium salts, either orally in the form of laxatives or antacids or parenterally to control convulsions, can raise the concentration of magnesium to very high levels at which serious central nervous system depression may develop [140, 289]. This risk seems unjustified, and therefore such procedures should be avoided if severe renal insufficiency is present.

Uremia

It has been pointed out repeatedly [33, 51] that the term uremia has been used to identify the symptom complex resulting from the failure of renal function. The term means "urine in the blood," and implies that the symptoms arise from retention of intoxicating agents. It is now clear that renal failure is associated with loss, as well as retention, of electrolytes, water, and other substances. Moreover, certain regulatory functions of the kidney concerned, to take two obvious examples, with the control of arterial blood pressure and erythropoiesis, are grossly abnormal yet the disturbances are not plainly due to either urinary loss or retention. It is clear, therefore, that the term uremia requires redefinition.

Bull [51] has proposed that uremia be defined as those states that occur "when the kidneys are unable to maintain a normal internal environment." This definition is extremely broad. The term could be applied to the asymptomatic patient with mild azotemia as well as to the person suffering from terminal renal failure, with pericarditis and coma. For purposes of the present discussion, a more restrictive definition is more useful.

The advance of chronic Bright's disease may be characterized in terms of four stages. First, there is the phase of *diminished renal reserve*. About 50 per cent of the nephrons may be destroyed without giving rise to any readily detectable abnormalities. It is true that the BUN rises, but this rise is within the normal range, and consequently identifiable azotemia is not present. The excretory and regulatory functions of the kidneys are well preserved.

Renal insufficiency is the second stage and is usually identified by the development of mild azotemia, when the patient is on a normal diet, and by impairment in urine concentrating ability. Nocturia is usually present. Mild anemia may appear. The precarious state of renal function is indicated by the ease with which stresses, such as mild salt depletion, infection, or surgery, may precipitate evidence of markedly deranged renal excretory and regulatory function.

The third stage is *renal failure*. Severe azotemia, acidosis, hyponatremia, hyperphosphatemia, and hypocalcemia tend to develop. Mild hyperkalemia may appear. The concentrating powers of the kidney are severely compromised, and impaired diluting ability may supervene. Anemia is severe.

The term *uremia* is reserved for the terminal stage. Two groups of clinical symptoms are present. First, symptoms referable to deranged renal excretory and regulatory function, characteristic of renal failure, are prominent. Second, a unique constellation of gastrointestinal, neuromuscular, and cardiovascular disturbances develops which is independent of, though often similar to concomitant disturbances caused by electrolyte abnormalities, hypertension, and hematologic disorders such as anemia and purpura. According to this definition, the second group of characteristic clinical features is necessary for the diagnosis of uremia, although other disturbances are usually present as well. It is significant that almost without exception the signs and symptoms of uremia can be relieved by dialysis.

CAUSES OF END-STAGE RENAL DISEASE

In the United States in 1964, the number of deaths due to primary kidney disease of all ages was as follows [226]:

Primary Kidney Disease	Number of Deaths
Nephritis and nephrosis	12,414
Infections of kidney	9,889
Polycystic diseases of kidney	3,981
Total	27,345

Crude death rate = 14.3/100,000 persons.

These figures were gathered from death certificates and are very crude. They nevertheless suggest that about one-third of patients dying

from uremia are suffering from some form of kidney infection which may be potentially either treatable or preventable.

A much more homogeneous study was reported by Hood and his associates [143] based on a scrutiny of all case records of deaths from uremia in Göteborg, Sweden, a city of about 400,000 people. Of 262 deaths from chronic uremia, in ages below 60, the diseases responsible were: nonobstructive pyelonephritis, 42 per cent; chronic glomerulonephritis, 21 per cent; diabetic renal disease, 18 per cent; obstructive pyelonephritis, 7 per cent; polycystic kidney disease, 5 per cent; malignant hypertension, 3 per cent; and various conditions, 4 per cent.

It is noteworthy that, of the 110 cases of nonobstructive pyelonephritis (42 per cent of total), 68 had papillary necrosis. Conceivably, analgesic abuse may have played a role here. If this group is subtracted, then the incidence of pyelonephritis as a cause of uremic death in this series is 16 per cent. This is still a fairly high fraction of the cause of death from uremia. In other pathologic studies, pyelonephritis is the most frequent cause of death from uremia, being several times more common than glomerulonephritis [47, 111, 196].

Freedman [107, 108] has recently challenged this view, and has argued that autopsy studies overestimate the incidence of chronic nonobstructive pyelonephritis as a cause of uremia. On the basis of pathologic criteria alone, it is difficult or impossible to distinguish chronic nonobstructive pyelonephritis from nephrosclerosis, chronic glomerulonephritis, analgesic-abuse nephritis, etc., and critical review of the older literature suggests that these diseases had not been excluded [107, 108]. Moreover, pyelonephritis is frequently a secondary feature of glomerulonephritis or nephritis of analgesic abuse, and is assumed to be the cause of this end-stage kidney disease, whereas it may have been only a late complication.

Studies of the life history of nonobstructive pyelonephritis disclose an uncommon advance to terminal renal disease, at least in women with infection [107, 110]. This impression is supported by the sex differences in frequency of urinary tract infection during life and at autopsy. While women are affected six times more often than men during life, "pyelonephritis" at autopsy is about equal in both sexes [107, 110].

Finally, Gault and Dossetor [115] have reviewed the cause of terminal renal failure in 315 recipients of kidney transplants, and found a ratio of glomerulonephritis to pyelonephritis of 2.7:1. The figures may be difficult to interpret because patients with pyelonephritis may have been rejected as unsuitable for transplantation. Nevertheless, at centers with large renal clinics, where preselection does not seem to be a problem, the incidence of nonobstructive pyelonephritis as the primary disease responsible for uremia appears to be infrequent.

The studies of Little and his co-workers [178] and Jackson and his associates [146] suggest that pyelonephritis can cause permanent renal damage, but do not establish the frequency with which the damage progresses to the point of terminal renal failure. On the basis of the considerations cited above, it appears that uncomplicated, nonobstructive pyelonephritis is not a common cause for uremia.

ETIOLOGY OF UREMIA

Urea was early implicated as the cause of uremia [58]. The recent demonstration [128] that bilaterally nephrectomized dogs dialyzed by intermittent peritoneal lavage against high concentrations of urea developed weakness, anorexia, vomiting, hemorrhagic diarrhea, and coma after several days, despite a normal electrolyte composition of plasma, lends weight to this hypothesis. However, the concentrations of urea in extracellular fluid varied from 540 to 1690 mg. per 100 ml., levels considerably higher than that encountered in clin-

ical uremia. Perhaps the most cogent evidence against the toxic action of urea has been furnished by Merrill and his associates [190], who dialyzed chronic uremic patients by means of an artificial kidney against baths containing urea in sufficient amounts to prevent a fall in the concentration of urea in blood. Nevertheless, signs of uremia abated.

Phenols, present in high concentrations in blood and spinal fluid, have been held responsible for uremic symptoms [16]. Although phenol intoxication resembles some of the features of uremia [186], the evidence in favor of this hypothesis is tenuous. For the most part, the methods used to quantitate phenols have been nonspecific, and there has been no clear-cut correlation between blood or spinal fluid concentrations and the clinical state of the patient [133].

In 1915 Foster [99, 100] reported the isolation of an organic base, apparently guanidine [133], from the blood of uremic patients which, when injected into the peritoneal cavity of guinea pigs, caused rapid respirations, convulsions, and ultimately death. Although using somewhat nonspecific methods, Harrison and his co-workers [133, 134] and subsequently others [6] demonstrated increased concentrations of a guanidine-like material in blood and spinal fluid of experimentally uremic dogs and clinically uremic patients. Guanidine injected into laboratory animals produces muscle twitching, hyperexcitability, paresis, and convulsions, as well as hemorrhagic bowel lesions. Experimentally, therefore, guanidine can produce some of the features of the uremic syndrome. The actual role of guanidine as a uremic toxin, however, has not been established, in part because of the problems involved in its chemical analysis [186] and in part because the amounts required to produce lesions in animals are far in excess of those found in uremia. Moreover, the blood levels of guanidine and phenol actually found in uremic patients, in recent studies [202], although tending to increase as azotemia advances, are not correlated with central nervous system depression or gastrointestinal disturbances. However, other guanidinian compounds may be more potent. Recently, guanidinosuccinic acid has been isolated from the urine of uremic patients and could conceivably contribute to the picture of uremic toxicity.

Perhaps the most exciting and promising new development has been the demonstration by Welt and his associates [62, 283, 284] of a defect in red cell transport of uremic patients, characterized by high sodium concentrations in the red blood cells, low rates of active sodium transport, adequate levels of ATP, but diminished activity of ouabain-sensitive ATPase. This transport defect is not an intrinsic disturbance of the red cell membrane, since a similar disturbance can be induced in normal red cells by incubating them with plasma from patients with uremia and a high red cell sodium. The factor is not present in uremia generally, but only in those patients whose red cell sodium is high. It is not clear that this defect is specific for uremia, since a similar disorder has been demonstrated in desperately ill patients with a variety of different defects. The plasma factor has not as yet been identified.

IMPAIRED CARBOHYDRATE TOLERANCE IN UREMIA

The majority of patients with uremia, perhaps 75 per cent, have impaired glucose tolerance; in a small proportion of these patients, fasting hyperglycemia is also present [132, 207, 285]. Although severe hyperglycemia rarely occurs, the occasional extreme elevation in blood sugar encountered in patients undergoing peritoneal dialysis may represent an expression of the basic carbohydrate intolerance under circumstances of a carbohydrate load contained in dialysis fluid. Despite the impaired carbohydrate metabolism, basal levels of immunoreactive insulin are elevated [8]. Finally, elevated fasting levels of plasma triglycerides have been observed [8].

The presence of elevated levels of plasma insulin, together with hyperglycemia and impaired carbohydrate tolerance, suggests that the disturbance is the consequence, not of defective insulin secretion, but rather of insulin antagonism [132, 207, 285]. This inference is supported by the insensitivity to insulin of the uremic patient [132, 207, 285].

The factor responsible for insulin antagonism has not been identified. Potassium deficiency and metabolic acidosis are not responsible for the disorder, since it can occur in their absence. Bagdade and his associates [8] have recently proposed a hypothesis to explain lipemia and impaired carbohydrate tolerance. They suggest that, as a result of insulin antagonism, hyperglycemia and impaired glucose tolerance develop despite elevated basal insulin levels. Hypertriglyceridemia results from two mechanisms: (1) inhibition of lipoprotein lipase as a result of insulin antagonism, causing delayed triglyceride removal; and (2) increased hepatic triglyceride synthesis under the influence of elevated plasma insulin levels. It is noteworthy that impaired carbohydrate tolerance and lipemia can both be corrected by aggressive dialysis [4, 132].

IMPAIRED IMMUNOLOGIC RESPONSE IN UREMIA

Various observations indicate that certain immunologic mechanisms are suppressed in uremia. The survival of homotransplanted kidney [145] and skin homografts [69] is prolonged in uremic patients as compared to normal individuals. Delayed hypersensitivity reactions seem to be impaired in some uremic patients. Susceptibility to bacterial infections appears to be increased.

The cause of these defects is uncertain. Production of circulating antibodies is well maintained. Serum complement levels are normal. It has been suggested, on the basis of animal studies, that the uremic defect is a disturbance in antibody production to a primary stimulation, since antibody response to antigens encountered before uremia supervened is unimpaired [126].

Anorexia, nausea, and vomiting are common in uremia and occasionally constitute the first symptoms of renal disease. Typically, anorexia first develops in a characteristic pattern: the patient is hungry up to the point of actually seeing or smelling the food, when he becomes nauseated [97]. Vomiting then develops, often occurring particularly in the morning when the patient arises. Hiccoughs may also be prominent.

In some patients vomiting becomes pernicious and results in severe deficits of sodium and potassium. The reduction in extracellular volume, in turn, causes further worsening of renal function. If the patient drinks fluids while he is vomiting, severe dilutional hyponatremia may ensue, and symptoms of water intoxication may be superimposed on those arising from salt depletion and increasing renal failure. Characteristically, metabolic acidosis becomes increasingly severe, doubtless because of the further deterioration of renal function secondary to the volume deficit. Occasionally, however, severe vomiting in uremia may eventuate in metabolic alkalosis [135].

Though patients in uremia may have little or no free hydrochloric acid in gastric juice, this is not necessarily a result of a failure in hydrochloric acid production. Rather it develops because of the increased formation in gastric juice of ammonia which then neutralizes gastric acidity. Accelerated ammonia production, in turn, has been attributed to the high levels of blood urea which elevate the concentration of urea in gastric juices where it is hydrolyzed, under the influence of urease, to ammonia [175]. The hydrolysis of urea to ammonia is probably responsible for the ammoniacal taste and odor in uremia.

Although constipation is more common, diarrhea, often bloody, tends to appear in the later stages of renal failure. It causes severe depletion in extracellular volume as well as potassium deficiency. Anemia is often greatly aggravated. It should be borne in mind that bleeding originates anywhere in the gastrointestinal tract, not only in the colon. The stomach and duodenum are frequent additional sites. The bleeding usually occurs from ulcers of the mucosa, although at times only ill-defined mucosal hemorrhages are observed.

Mucosal ulcerations also occur in the mouth. The ulcers may be small and punctate on the gums, but they can attain large size, particularly on the lips and at the corners of the mouth. Although salivation may be increased as ulcers develop, most patients complain of dryness of the mouth.

Severe abdominal pain, sometimes with generalized tenderness, develops especially in those patients with severe vomiting and diarrhea. The pain could come from ulcerative lesions, but it is also possible that it is a result of pancreatic involvement, since inspissation of secretions and flattened acinous epithelium are frequently found at autopsy [9], and serum amylase levels are sometimes high.

The cause of the gastrointestinal disorders is not clear. Anorexia, nausea, and vomiting have been attributed to central nervous system disturbances. Ulcerative lesions may be responsible for diarrhea and perhaps, to some extent, for vomiting as well. Guanidine, which can produce such lesions in laboratory animals, is thought by some investigators to be responsible for the ulcers. They have also been thought to result from the high ammonia content brought about by action of bacterial flora on urea. In normal subjects at least one-fourth of the urea pool is continuously acted upon by intestinal flora [280]; in uremia, far greater amounts of ammonia should be produced because of the greatly increased size of the urea pool. Increased ammonia is present in both gastric contents [175] and stool [288] of uremic patients.

NEUROMUSCULAR MANIFESTATIONS OF UREMIA

Mental disturbances are common, and frequently display a characteristic pattern. Early there is drowsiness that progresses to profound lethargy. The patient becomes disinterested in all aspects of his environment. Inability to concentrate and a lack of facility in abstract thinking are readily brought out by the failure of the patient to sum numbers accurately or to count backward. Psychiatric disturbances may be prominent [10]. Delusions are more common, in our experience, than auditory and visual hallucinations, and may be a manifestation of severe mental confusion [180]. Patients may become manic, depressed, or euphoric, and occasionally paranoid tendencies develop.

Lethargy and apathy are frequently intermingled with profound restlessness. Sleep is almost always fitful, disturbed, and often accompanied by agitating dreams. As uremia deepens, consciousness is lost, and coma supervenes.

Muscular twitching is a common manifestation of neuromuscular hyperirritability [97]. Fibrillar twitchings appear early, but later large muscle groups are involved. Sometimes, what appears to be a positive Chvostek sign is observed, but the Trousseau sign, almost without exception, is absent (unless intense alkali therapy has produced alkalosis). Deep tendon reflexes are active or hyperactive, but pathologic reflexes do not appear [97, 203]. Sporadically, muscular twitching may increase to involve the major muscle groups of all extremities and mimic a convulsive seizure. However, these episodes are not as severe or as prolonged as typical hypertensive convulsions; they are not followed by the occurrence of pathologic reflexes or a postconvulsive state. In uremia without hypertension, grand mal convulsions are very rare, in contrast to their comparative frequency when uremia is accompanied by hypertension [88]. This distinction between uremic encephalopathy and hypertensive encephalopathy, originally drawn by Oppenheimer and Fishberg [203], is important, since uremic encephalopathy, but not hypertensive encephalopathy, can be corrected by dialysis. It should be stressed that, in the nonhypertensive uremic patient who convulses, every effort should be made to delineate the cause of convulsion before it is ascribed to uremia per se.

Another interesting finding with regard to the central nervous system and uremia is an apparent breakdown of the blood-brain barrier [106]. This abnormality has been shown to be corrected by dialysis with decrease in uremic signs [106].

Uremia is frequently accompanied by a polyneuropathy [7]. It tends to be a symmetrical sensorimotor disturbance. The neuropathy may at first be manifested only by shooting or burning pains, but in later stages it can be a crippling paralysis. The distal medullated nerve fibers are first affected; in a subclinical state, the entity can be recognized by increased nerve conduction times [212]. It appears that the progression of the neuropathy may be arrested by adequate dialysis [148]. Neurogenic bladder has occasionally been reported [189]. A flapping tremor, in the absence of significant hepatic or pulmonary disease, has also been noted [64, 259].

The mental clouding and neuromuscular hyperirritability of uremia must be distinguished from other disturbances that are frequent accompaniments of the uremic state. Hypertensive encephalopathy, water intoxication, and rarely tetany can closely simulate uremic encephalopathy. Since all these disturbances require different forms of treatment, the specific identification of the cause of the syndrome is of great importance. For a more detailed discussion of these problems see Chapter 9.

CARDIOPULMONARY MANIFESTATIONS OF UREMIA

Pericarditis is the most characteristic manifestation of uremia, occurring in about half the patients who die [277]. Pain, which is of the same type as that found in other kinds of acute pericarditis, is present less frequently than in benign idiopathic pericarditis, occurring in about one-third of the cases [277]; this may in part reflect the inability of a patient in an obtunded state to appreciate and report various sensory disturbances. Usually, typical electrocardiographic evidences of pericarditis develop [152]. There is little evidence of myocardial involvement in uremia, except for that which may occur immediately adjacent to an inflamed pericardium [165].

Although hemopericardium was reported in the past in uremia, it was usually a postmortem finding. In 1957 the first two cases were reported in which an antemortem diagnosis was made and successful treatment was instituted [129]. There followed a series of reports describing this condition [15, 130, 188, 271] and suggesting that hemopericardium with tamponade was a more frequent life-threatening complication than previously thought. Although patients have been successfully treated with simple pericardiocentesis, recurrence of effusions or inability to remove fluid by a needle may necessitate a partial or complete pericardiectomy. Moreover, dialysis, which is specific therapy for pericarditis, is slow in correcting hemopericardium. The use of regional heparinization for dialysis has been recommended in cases of pericarditis to avoid provoking bleeding because of anticoagulation [15]. However, late clotting difficulties have been associated with this procedure [131].

Although it is doubtful that the heart fails as a pump as a result of uremia per se, congestion of the circulation is extremely common and may arise from several factors. First, classic myocardial failure may supervene as a sequela of hypertensive cardiovascular disease. Second, the retention of excessive amounts of salt from an ordinary diet containing liberal amounts of salt can produce, not only edema but also severe venous congestion [89], with high venous pressure, cardiac dilatation, and pulmonary congestion; the cir-

culation time tends to be normal or rapid, in contrast to the prolongation encountered in myocardial failure. Third, a similar state of venous congestion can develop as a result of severe anemia. Not infrequently, all three types of disturbances are present simultaneously.

It is particularly important to analyze the nature of the factors responsible for the congestive state, since not only is the therapy different in each instance, but measures designed to correct one type of disorder may actually aggravate another. For example, if myocardial failure is mistaken for anemia with congestion, the administration of blood may precipitate frank pulmonary edema.

The cause of the striking pulmonary findings noted at autopsy and on x-ray films of some patients with uremia has been the subject of considerable debate. The terms uremic lung and uremic pneumonitis have been applied to an x-ray picture characterized by a bilateral butterfly infiltration of the lungs, radiating out from the hilus, with a peripheral clear zone of emphysema. Histologic study discloses the presence of edema which is rich in protein, extensive fibrin deposition in the alveoli, and some macrophages [14, 144]. In the more recent studies no evidence of arteritis has been found [144].

Although some observers have interpreted this x-ray and pathologic picture to be specific for uremia, the findings are quite similar to those of typical pulmonary edema secondary to left ventricular failure, except perhaps that the periphery of the lung fields tends to be clear. Dock [79] has suggested that the peripheral clear zones seen on x-ray may be the result of hyperventilation secondary to metabolic acidosis, which would expand the periphery of the lungs more than the central areas, thereby preventing the collection of fluid in the peripheral alveoli.

It has been repeatedly pointed out that this pulmonary picture does not occur in every patient with uremia, that its occurrence cannot be correlated with the degree of azotemia, that evidence of left-sided heart failure or non-myocardial venous congestion is present in patients who do manifest the characteristic x-ray findings [5, 75, 81, 189, 224], and that clearing of the x-ray findings is paralleled by a reduction in body weight owing to fluid loss [5]. Doniach [81] and Rendich et al. [224] have emphasized that the x-ray picture may be found in some patients with heart disease without azotemia. It seems very doubtful that the uremic lung can develop in the absence of left ventricular failure or fluid overload, although admittedly various aspects of the uremic state may impart certain characteristic features [116, 138].

Fibrinous pleuritis, unassociated with evidence of underlying pulmonary disease, appears to be a specific manifestation of uremia [198]. Pleuritic pain is usually present, but mild.

FUNCTIONAL RENAL FAILURE OR REVERSIBLE UREMIA

The advance of chronic Bright's disease from the early stage of diminished renal reserve to the final termination in uremia describes the consequences of the pathologic process within the kidneys. However, the patient with chronic renal disease is extremely vulnerable, because of diminished renal reserve, to a further deterioration in renal function due to extrarenal factors. These extrarenal disturbances probably influence the kidney by causing a reduction in renal blood flow sufficient to reduce renal function drastically, but they probably do not produce anatomic injury. The extrarenal disturbances, therefore, are potentially reversible. Consequently, the renal decompensation has been termed reversible uremia [92] or functional renal failure.

Salt depletion, dehydration, and blood loss are particularly frequent factors responsible for renal decompensation, owing to the frequency of vomiting, diarrhea, and gastrointestinal bleeding in renal failure. We have

noted that renal function in patients with renal disease who have sustained a significant volume loss does not quickly return to the previous state when that volume is adequately replaced. Occasionally, renal function in a patient with severe renal disease will return only after a period of from 5 to 10 days following replacement of the volume loss. The reasons for this rather marked delay are not altogether clear. It is probably not due to the development of tubular necrosis, since patients who cannot adequately concentrate their urine probably cannot develop acute tubular necrosis [270, 282]. It is, therefore, not unusual for patients with renal disease who have sustained volume deficits due to vomiting or diarrhea to require a period of acute peritoneal or hemodialysis to tide them over until their renal function returns.

Congestive heart failure and infection, especially of the kidneys, can suddenly diminish renal function [199]. Potassium deficiency might be expected to aggravate renal failure owing to its capacity to produce renal lesions [221, 222]. In addition, potassium deficiency may have an adverse effect on the overall circulatory system as the result of its action on the heart. Sharp falls in renal blood flow and glomerular filtration rate can result from urinary tract obstruction, often resulting from: (1) ureteral calculi [92]; (2) prostatism [199]; (3) atonic bladder secondary to neurologic disturbances of uremia; (4) semistupor or coma in a bedridden patient. A meticulous search should be made for all these causes of reversible uremia since their correction may permit the remaining kidney tissue to maintain a reasonable degree of homeostasis.

Treatment of Renal Insufficiency and Renal Failure

Patients in early stages of chronic Bright's disease, in which renal reserve is diminished but excretory and regulatory functions are well maintained, require no therapy directed specifically at the kidney. As renal insufficiency and then renal failure supervene, nocturia, azotemia, disturbances in electrolyte and water metabolism, hypertension, and anemia make their appearance.

The clinical course of azotemic renal failure is commonly punctuated by episodes of insidious or abrupt deterioration in renal function characterized by increased azotemia, metabolic acidosis, and commonly oliguria. Mental, neuromuscular, and gastrointestinal features of uremia may appear. Severe hyperkalemia can develop. It is particularly important to ascertain whether the episode of renal decompensation has been precipitated by a complicating disturbance or is simply the expression of progressive unrelenting intrinsic renal disease. This issue can be resolved only by a careful search for the factors known to precipitate reversible uremia and by appropriate therapeutic trials designed to correct postulated disturbances.

Salt depletion, with contraction of the extracellular volume, is a common precipitating factor. Vomiting and diarrhea, to which the uremic patient is extraordinarily vulnerable, may be responsible. On the other hand, the insidious development of renal failure may be precipitated by renal salt wastage brought about by a rigid salt-free diet (usually prescribed to treat hypertension) in a nonedematous patient. Dehydration, blood loss, congestive heart failure, infection, especially of the kidneys, and potassium deficiency are other well-recognized causes of reversible uremia. The important role of urinary tract obstruction is perhaps less well appreciated [92]. Renal function may improve dramatically when chronic partial bladder obstruction secondary to prostatism or uretheral stricture is relieved [199]. In addition, the obtunded, bedridden patient in chronic renal failure may be unable to empty his bladder, a disturbance that can be corrected at times with such an agent as bethanechol or furtrethonium [92].

Finally, the possibility of ureteral obstruction from calculi should be explored by radiographic examination of the abdomen. Intravenous pyelography is the safest and most helpful procedure, and is usually satisfactory if the serum creatinine is below 10 mg. per 100 ml., although large amounts of contrast material and abdominal compression may be necessary to obtain satisfactory roentgenograms. If intravenous pyelography is unsatisfactory, owing to severe renal failure, cystoscopy and retrograde pyelography may have to be undertaken. Obviously these are hazardous procedures because of danger of inducing urinary tract infection or bacteremia; they should be reserved for those patients in whom the presence of obstruction is a strong likelihood.

LOW-PROTEIN DIET

The protein content of the diet influences not merely the magnitude of azotemia but also the development of hyperkalemia and metabolic acidosis. In addition, many of the symptoms of uremia seem to be related to the accumulation of waste products of protein breakdown. For these reasons, low-protein diets have been employed in the treatment of renal failure when azotemia and symptoms of uremia begin to appear. This is usually when the filtration falls below about 20 ml. per minute. Restriction of protein intake had the dual aim, therefore, of a reduction to a minimum of the breakdown products of protein metabolism at the same time that sufficient protein was furnished to preserve nitrogen balance and thereby avoid protein malnutrition.

To avoid a negative nitrogen balance, diets containing about 0.5 gm. of protein per kilogram of body weight per day, or about 40 gm. of protein per day, were usually prescribed [139]. This represented a compromise between the requirements for protein restriction to relieve uremic symptoms and the magnitude of protein intake necessary for nitrogen balance. Such programs were not strikingly beneficial, although they did tend to reduce azotemia and mitigate acidosis.

A major improvement in dietary therapy was introduced by Giordano [117], who demonstrated that if essential amino acids were the only source of protein, nitrogen balance could be maintained on an amount equivalent to about 12 gm. of protein per day. The supply of adequate calories in the form of fat and carbohydrate, together with a small amount of essential amino acids, would preserve nitrogen balance because the utilization of urea would furnish sufficient nitrogen for the synthesis of nonessential amino acids. Although Giordano thought that urea could be utilized directly to form amino acids, the laboratory studies of Richards et al. [225] and others suggest that urea is first broken down to ammonia and the latter is then incorporated into amino acids. It is likely that bacterial flora are required to hydrolyze urea to ammonia, although this is not certain.

Giovannetti and Maggiore [118] subsequently substituted small amounts of a high-quality protein for essential amino acids and found that nitrogen balance could be maintained when as little as 20 gm. per day of protein, derived from eggs, and a calorically adequate diet was furnished. Berlyne, Shaw, and their co-workers [24, 25, 28, 247] adapted the diet for Anglo-Saxon tastes. The protein is derived from eggs and milk. In very severe renal failure (GFR of 3 ml. per minute or less), the protein intake is set at 18 gm.; with a GFR of 5 ml. per minute, at 25 to 30 gm.; and with a GFR of 10 ml. per minute, at 40 gm. [24].

The key points in the dietary program are these. First, not merely the amount but also, and perhaps more important, the quality of the protein is critical. For this reason, vegetable proteins and meat are avoided. Indeed, it appears that somewhat larger amounts of protein may be tolerated if the protein is of high biologic value. Moreover, losses of protein into the urine or into peritoneal fluid in patients undergoing dialysis require that protein be added to the diet to balance these losses. Second, adequate calories must be furnished from carbohydrate or fat to prevent the breakdown of protein to satisfy caloric requirements. Although 100 gm. of carbohydrate per day will prevent ketosis and exert some protein-sparing effect [113], at least 2000 calories, principally as carbohydrate, are required to achieve nitrogen balance when protein intake is adequate. Herndon and his co-workers [139] have suggested a caloric intake of 30 calories per kilogram of body weight per day with a carbohydrate to fat ratio of 3:1. Anabolic steroids have been advocated by some to facilitate the promotion of positive nitrogen balance. In a very careful study Thaysen [273] could demonstrate only a very transient effect; therefore, there is no reason to give these agents on a long-term basis. Third, the diet is monotonous and unpalatable, and therefore requires great patience on the part of the physician to encourage its acceptance [25, 260]. Indeed, it is often wise to start the diet when symptoms are severe, so that the clinical improvement will outweigh the dietary unpalatability. On the other hand, some patients may be too sick to start this diet and require an initial period of dialysis before the treatment is initiated. Finally, B complex vitamins should be provided, since the diet is deficient in them.

Clinical improvement is often very heartening. The blood urea nitrogen falls, gastrointestinal symptoms recede, there is an improvement in appetite and sense of well-being; frequently, patients can return to a productive life or at least to a more active existence. If renal failure is very severe, the diet can be supplemented by occasional peritoneal dialysis [172].

Complications of the dietary program include acidosis and severe hyperkalemia. The cause of the acidosis is not clear. It may be a consequence of the low neutral phosphate and sulfate content of the diet. A reduction in the delivery of these nonreabsorbable and buffer anions to the distal nephron would limit the secretion of hydrogen and potassium, in exchange for sodium, and thereby predispose to acidosis and hyperkalemia [102]. Acidosis can be controlled by administration of alkali. Hyperkalemia will be mitigated by the correction of acidosis; in addition, cation-exchange resins may be required.

In patients whose glomerular filtration rate is less than 2 ml. per minute, the dietary program is unlikely to be successful, but it should certainly be tried, either alone or with occasional dialysis [172].

ACIDOSIS

Some degree of metabolic acidosis will develop in every patient, particularly if the protein intake is high. Usually, the acidosis is fairly mild, with the plasma bicarbonate stabilized above 15 mEq. per liter, and asymptomatic. If the plasma bicarbonate falls below 15 to 18 mEq. per liter and does not respond to a low-protein diet, the administration of alkali appears to be beneficial for several reasons. First, acidosis, at least in normal subjects, is associated with anorexia and nausea and may contribute to these disturbances in patients with renal disease. Second, hyperkalemia is exaggerated by acidosis [52, 240]. Third, chronic metabolic acidosis appears to result in a titration of bone salts and thereby probably contributes to the development of renal osteodystrophy [179]. Fourth, although classic Kussmaul respirations are unusual in chronic uremic acidosis, it is not uncommon to find mild dyspnea on exertion developing because of it. Fifth, metabolic acidosis induces two derangements in the circulation which render the patient vulnerable to pulmonary edema: (1) venoconstriction, which reduces the capacity of the circulation [136]; and (2) depression of myocardial contractility [287]. The combination of these two disturbances makes patients with severe metabolic acidosis susceptible to pulmonary edema when given salt loads. Sixth, acidosis may be responsible for some of the somnolence and lethargy of uremic patients. Finally, a low plasma bicarbonate in a steady state makes the patient vulnerable to a profound decompensated acidosis of life-threatening proportions, if additional alkali loss (diarrhea) or acid load is imposed.

The clinical use of oral sodium bicarbonate is frequently associated with much abdominal bloating and belching. A more satisfactory alkalizing salt is sodium citrate, usually given in the form of Shohl's solution [250]: 140 gm. of citric acid, and 98 gm. of hydrated crystalline salt of sodium citrate are dissolved in water to a final volume of 1 liter. The original purpose of the citric acid was to enhance calcium absorption in the intestine by providing an acid buffer. It also makes the solution more palatable. In the body sodium citrate is converted to sodium bicarbonate while the citric acid is dissipated as CO_2 and water. Shohl's solution, made up in this manner, contains sodium in a concentration of 1 mEq. per milliliter of solution. Usually a total of 40 to 90 ml. is given daily in three divided doses. The solution should be diluted before being given. Generally, it is acceptable when diluted with plain water. However, to many it becomes more palatable when taken in a carbonated beverage or in fruit juice.

The serum bicarbonate should be checked occasionally to make certain that metabolic alkalosis has not been induced. Edema, if it forms, is not usually the consequence of the administration of bicarbonate loads; rather, it is almost invariably due to the concomitant intake of chloride. Should edema form, sodium chloride should be rigidly restricted from the diet and Shohl's solution continued unchanged. We have not observed edema in patients with chronic renal failure given Shohl's solution when they had no access to chloride. For this reason, alkali can be given even in the presence of congestive failure.

Clarkson and his associates [61] have employed calcium carbonate ($CaCO_3$) to correct metabolic acidosis. The alkalinizing effect results from the conversion of $CaCO_3$ to $CaCl_2$ in acid gastric juice, and then the reconversion of most of the $CaCl_2$ back to $CaCO_3$ in the alkaline intestine:

$$CaCO_3 + 2HCl \rightarrow CaCl_2 + H_2O + CO_2$$

$$CaCl_2 + 2NaHCO_3 \rightarrow$$
$$CaCO_3 + 2NaCl + H_2O + CO_2$$

In addition to correcting alkalosis, $CaCO_3$ will raise serum calcium and neutralize excess hydrochloric acid produced by some patients in renal failure. The authors indicate that the prolonged administration of $CaCO_3$ poses the hazards of soft tissue and renal calcification [61]. Except for special problems, $CaCO_3$ should probably not be used for long-term correction of metabolic acidosis.

POTASSIUM

It has been pointed out in a previous section that in patients with azotemic renal failure deficits or excesses of potassium may develop. Potassium deficiency is usually the consequence of extrarenal losses resulting from vomiting and diarrhea. In addition, in occasional patients with salt-losing nephritis or secondary aldosteronism associated with unilateral renal disease or malignant hypertension the potassium level may become low because of renal losses. Judicious therapy with potassium chloride, bearing in mind the danger of excessive administration, is indicated.

Mild hyperkalemia (serum concentrations slightly in excess of 5.5 mEq. per liter) is common in renal insufficiency but seldom gives rise to clinical evidences of potassium intoxication. For the most part, restriction of dietary protein and treatment of metabolic acidosis by the administration of alkali are sufficient to correct this disturbance. Not infrequently, the institution of a rigid salt-free diet, for the treatment of either edema or hypertension, may be associated with an insidious rise in the concentration of serum potassium, probably because of the delivery of inadequate amounts of sodium to the exchange site in the distal portions of the nephron. If restriction of protein intake is not sufficient to correct the disturbance and alkali cannot be given because there is no associated acidosis, we have administered about 3 to 5 gm. of sodium sulfate daily in divided doses. This augments renal potassium secretion without magnifying edema formation and may be all that is required.

Severe hyperkalemia (serum potassium greater than 7.0 mEq. per liter) with electrocardiographic and other evidences of potassium intoxication, may develop spontaneously in the terminal phases of renal failure, usually when there is marked oliguria. The administration of potassium salts, massive tissue breakdown associated with a catabolic response to stress, and severe metabolic acidosis may all precipitate severe potassium intoxication. Comparatively simple measures should be immediately instituted:

1. Exogenous potassium intake should be stopped.

2. Infusion of 1 liter of a solution containing 100 gm. of glucose and 2.0 gm. of calcium gluconate should be given. The glucose load results in the transfer of potassium from the extracellular to the intracellular phase as glycogen is deposited, while calcium antagonizes the cardiotoxic effects of potassium. It is doubtful whether insulin should be routinely administered to nondiabetic patients, since hyperglycemia elicits endogenous insulin output. If undue hyperglycemia develops following glucose loads, perhaps because of impaired carbohydrate tolerance, about 20 units of regular insulin can be given intravenously.

3. If metabolic acidosis is severe, an infusion of 5 per cent sodium bicarbonate, the amount varying from 100 to 1000 ml. or more depending on the magnitude of the acidosis and the

gravity of the hyperkalemia, may dramatically ameliorate potassium intoxication [239]. If acidosis is not severe, the cardiotoxic effects of hyperkalemia can often be corrected by injecting 1 liter of ⅙ M lactate containing 100 gm. of glucose and 2 gm. of calcium lactate. Calcium salts cannot be given in sodium bicarbonate solutions owing to precipitation.

4. To reduce body stores of potassium, a cation-exchange resin should be given. Kayexalate (Winthrop Laboratories), a sodium-cycle polystyrene resin, is most conveniently given as a suspension of 100 gm. of resin to 300 ml. of water or ginger ale, the average daily amount being 20 to 60 gm. in divided doses. Assuming that 1 gm. of resin binds approximately 1 mEq. of potassium and that 20 mEq. of potassium daily are released from cells if glucose is given to repress protein catabolism, Flinn et al. [98] recommend the larger dose to lower serum potassium and the smaller dose for maintenance. Sorbitol, given simultaneously by mouth, in doses of 20 ml. of a 70 per cent solution three or four times daily, is poorly absorbed and serves to propel the resin through the gastrointestinal tract. Mineral oil and cascara can also be used for laxative action. Should nausea and vomiting prevent oral therapy, 50 gm. of resin can be suspended in 200 ml. of 5 per cent glucose in water and instilled into the rectum as a retention enema. After four to six hours, a cleansing enema is given, followed by a fresh instillation of resin. In this manner, several hundred grams of resin can be given daily. To prevent hypokalemia during resin therapy, daily determinations of serum potassium should be obtained.

This program has proved extraordinarily effective in controlling hyperkalemia [98, 237, 264], although an occasional patient will still require dialysis, either because the extreme degree of potassium intoxication requires a very rapid form of therapy or because the catabolic release of potassium exceeds the rate of uptake by the resin [237].

Berlyne and his associates [26] have pointed out that patients given Kayexalate absorb about 2.0 to 3.1 mEq. of sodium for each gram of resin taken. If the daily dose is 15 to 60 gm., between 30 to 180 mEq. of sodium salts will be absorbed. This has led to edema, heart failure, and hypertension. For this reason, a resin in the calcium cycle appears to be more suitable [27].

CLINICAL SIGNIFICANCE OF HYPOKALEMIA
AND HYPERKALEMIA

Potassium depletion, particularly when the serum potassium concentration falls below 2.5 mEq. per liter, may produce a variety of disturbances in neuromuscular function, such as drowsiness, fatigue, weakness, decreased reflexes, and flaccid paralysis (including muscles of respiration). The electrocardiogram during potassium depletion may display a depressed S-T segment, depressed or inverted T wave, prolongation of the Q-T interval, and a prominent U wave [18].

In contrast, retention of potassium only rarely produces neuromuscular symptoms. However, when these symptoms do appear, usually as the serum potassium concentration rises above 8 mEq. per liter, they include muscular irritability, hyperactive reflexes, and on rare occasions, flaccid paralysis not unlike that seen with extreme hypokalemia. Changes in the electrocardiogram during hyperkalemia include peaked T waves, followed by prolongation of the QRS interval. There may be prolongation of the P-R interval with eventual disappearance of the P waves. Finally, complete heart block with eventual ventricular fibrillation or ventricular arrest may occur [17].

The frequency and severity of these changes in neuromuscular excitability during both potassium deficit and excess are only roughly correlated with the serum concentration of potassium. Neuromuscular excitability is a function, not of the serum concentration alone, but of the ratio of intracellular to extracellu-

Table 6-1. Neuromuscular Excitability as a Function of the Ratio of Intracellular and Extracellular Potassium (K) Concentrations

Resting Conditions	Normal	K Deficiency		K Intoxication	
		Acute	Chronic	Acute	Chronic
$[K]_i$ $\overline{}$ $[K]_e$	160 $---$ 4.5 35	140 $---$ 2.0 70	90 $---$ 2.0 45	160 $---$ 12.5 13	170 $---$ 8 21
K equil. pot., E_K $= -61.5 \log \dfrac{[K]_i}{[K]_e}$	-95 mv	-113 mv	-102 mv	-68 mv	-82 mv
Membrane pot., F_m $= -61.5 \log \dfrac{[K]_i + 0.01\,[Na]_i}{[K]_e + 0.01\,[Na]_e}$	-88 mv	-100 mv	-88 mv	-65 mv	-77 mv
Excitability $= E_m - E_t$	$88 - 65$ 23 mv	$100 - 65$ 35 mv	$88 - 65$ 23 mv	$65 - 65$ 0	$77 - 65$ 12
Electrochemical excitation	Normal	Hyperpolarization block: paralysis	Normal	Depolarization block: paralysis	Partial depolarization: hyperexcitability

The values given for $[K]_i$ and $[K]_e$ under various circumstances are illustrative only and do not represent actual data. The potassium equilibrium potential, E_K, is estimated from the Nernst equation, and closely approximates the membrane potential, E_m. The latter is more accurately estimated from the Goldman equation, which takes into account the effects of other ions on the potential.

lar potassium. Since intracellular potassium concentration normally averages about 160 mEq. per liter while extracellular concentration averages about 4.5 mEq. per liter, it is apparent that the ratio $\dfrac{[K]_i}{[K]_e}$ will be influenced predominantly by the denominator (where $[K]_i$ = intracellular potassium concentration and $[K]_e$ = extracellular potassium concentration). In Table 6-1 a model is constructed to depict the possible effects of variations in the ratio on neuromuscular activity.

The excitability of neuromuscular tissue is defined as the difference between the membrane potential (E_m) and the threshold potential (E_t). E_m is determined principally by the ratio of intracellular to extracellular potassium. The relationship between the concentration gradient of potassium and the potential it can generate, assuming the membrane is impermeable to all other ions, is given by the Nernst equation:

$$E_K = -61.5 \log \frac{[K]_i}{[K]_e}$$

However, since the resting membrane has a small but measurable permeability to sodium, the equilibrium potential for potassium, (E_K), as given by the Nernst equation, does not completely define the resting membrane potential [2]. A more complete description is afforded by the Goldman equation:

$$E_m = -61.5 \log \frac{[K]_i + 0.01\,[Na]_i}{[K]_e + 0.01\,[Na]_e},$$

where 0.01 is the relative permeability of Na to K [141]. During excitation the discharge of acetylcholine at synaptic junctions and motor end-plates depolarizes the membrane and lowers E_m. When E_m is reduced to about -65 mv (the threshold potential), the tissue is activated. Therefore, any factor that increases E_m or decreases E_t will render the tissues less excitable, while factors that lower E_m or raise E_t will enhance excitability.

Alterations in potassium affect membrane excitability only through changes in the resting membrane potential and do not alter the threshold potential [245]. In general, hypokalemia increases the membrane potential, producing a hyperpolarization block, while hyperkalemia decreases the membrane potential, giving hyperexcitability. These effects, however, can be greatly modified by the state of total body potassium stores, which in turn appear to be dependent to a large extent on the speed with which hypokalemia or hyperkalemia develop.

During acute potassium depletion, as might occur after severe vomiting or fulminant diarrhea, the serum potassium concentration falls much more rapidly than the intracellular concentration, so that the ratio $\dfrac{[K]_i}{[K]_e}$ rises (Table 6-1); consequently, the membrane potential also increases, causing a hyperpolarization block with symptoms of weakness and, if severe, paralysis. In contrast, a similar degree of hypokalemia, if developed slowly, might be associated with a commensurate fall in the intracellular concentration of potassium; consequently, there may be little or no change in either the ratio $\dfrac{[K]_i}{[K]_e}$ or the E_m, and therefore little or no clinical derangements will appear.

A similar consideration also applied to potassium intoxication (Table 6-1). A rapid rise in serum potassium, as might be seen in crush injuries, may be associated with only minor changes in intracellular concentration. The ratio $\dfrac{[K]_i}{[K]_e}$ will, therefore, fall sharply, as will the E_m. If E_m falls below the value for E_t, a complete depolarization block with paralysis and ventricular conduction defects will result. On the other hand, a gradual retention of potassium will cause some increase in intracellular potassium so that for any serum concentration of potassium the ratio $\dfrac{[K]_i}{[K]_e}$ will be higher than during acute potassium intoxication, and consequently the severity of symptoms will be far less pronounced.

The critical role of the ratio of intracellular to extracellular potassium concentration serves to explain the numerous discrepancies between serum concentrations of potassium on the one hand and clinical disturbances on the other. We have observed a patient with acute tubular necrosis, increased tissue breakdown, and a serum potassium concentration rapidly rising to 10 mEq. per liter develop flaccid paralysis and complete heart block with a sine wave on the electrocardiogram. The development of flaccid paralysis with hyperkalemia, as well as with hypokalemia, has been observed by others [184, 272], and requires, in ambiguous cases, that the concentration of serum potassium be measured before therapy is instituted. On the other hand, a patient with severe chronic renal failure whose serum potassium rose slowly to 9.5 mEq. per liter over a period of several weeks had no symptoms or electrocardiographic changes referable to hyperkalemia.

In addition to the various factors that influence neuromuscular excitability through their effects on the resting membrane potential, other factors may be altered in renal failure which change the threshold potential, thus obviating or augmenting the effects mediated through the resting potential. Although a number of drugs are known to affect the threshold potential, the principal physiologic factor is the concentration of ionized calcium [245]. Hypocalcemia raises the threshold potential, decreasing the difference between E_m and E_t, and thus increases excitability. Hypocalcemia, therefore, would aggravate the effects of hyperkalemia. Hypercalcemia, on the other hand, lowers E_t, and renders the membrane less excitable. Rapidly raising serum calcium with intravenous injections of calcium salts, by its action on E_t, is an effective means of counteracting the potentially lethal effects of hyperkalemia. Factors other than calcium — for example, possibly magnesium — may also influence E_t, but these are not well understood.

The net effect of all these interacting factors, through their action on both the resting membrane potential and the threshold potential, makes it very difficult to obtain any straightforward correlation between the serum concentration of potassium and the neuromuscular symptoms or electrocardiographic changes. If, however, the serum potassium is interpreted with respect to anticipated changes in the concentration of intracellular potassium and extracellular ionized calcium, a much more satisfactory correlation will be forthcoming.

SALT DEPLETION, HYPONATREMIA, EDEMA

Salt depletion is an important cause of reversible uremia. Severe reduction in extracellular volume can develop dramatically in association with vomiting and diarrhea, or, very rarely, because of massive renal salt wastage. On the other hand, a slow insidious deficit may develop in patients placed on rigid salt-free diets (usually for the treatment of hypertension) who are unable to conserve sodium efficiently. Studies in the authors' laboratory [63] disclose that virtually all patients with advanced renal failure waste salt when placed on rigid low-sodium diets. The magnitude of this obligatory salt loss is small,

ranging from about 10 to 20 mEq. per day when a steady state of sodium excretion is attained. Should the dietary intake be below this level, clinically significant salt depletion would eventuate. Glomerular filtration rate fell and hyponatremia uniformly developed when a diet very low in salt was administered for 10 to 20 days. Only several grams of sodium chloride daily are required to prevent this deficit.

There is, however, a small group of patients with chronic renal disease in whom massive salt wasting occurs. Their obligatory renal salt loss may amount to as much as 40 gm. of sodium chloride per day [274]. The underlying renal diseases are usually those which disproportionately destroy the medulla — chronic hydronephrosis, medullary cystic disease, polycystic disease, analgesic-abuse nephritis, and chronic pyelonephritis [103, 265]. Usually, the restriction of salt in these patients is accompanied by dramatic deterioration of the circulation owing to loss of extracellular volume. We have, however, seen two children with medullary cystic disease in whom the magnitude of the obligatory salt loss was not at first appreciated. The usual features of diminished effective extracellular volume, such as lowered blood pressure, orthostatic hypotension, tachycardia, and hyponatremia, were not present. Nevertheless, there was a dramatic increase in glomerular filtration rate and well-being when salt supplements of 10 gm. daily were added to the diet.

Extrarenal salt loss or renal salt wastage may result in marked depletion of extracellular volume. Increased azotemia, acidosis, and hyperkalemia may supervene. If the patient drinks fluids as he becomes depleted, hyponatremia also develops. Hyponatremia can best be treated by restriction of fluid intake together with isotonic replacement of extracellular volume. If acidosis is appreciable, isotonic sodium bicarbonate, rather than sodium chloride, should be used. Hypertonic sodium chloride (5 per cent) solutions are seldom required, save, perhaps, in the very rare instances of severe symptomatic hyponatremia. In some instances, during far-advanced renal failure, the diseased kidney will not respond to volume replacement by promptly excreting the excess water. A congestive state may then result, particularly if severe metabolic acidosis is present. Peritoneal dialysis is a very efficient and safe way to correct the volume deficit, hyponatremia, and acidosis simultaneously.

Hyponatremia develops in some patients, not in association with salt loss, but rather because excessive water loads are given, usually in the mistaken impression that the reduction in azotemia that results indicates improvement in renal function [51, 291]. It has previously been pointed out that a reduction in azotemia under such circumstances may be due solely to increased urine volume, without any change in glomerular filtration rate. The water intoxication that may result is preferably treated by water restriction alone, although hypertonic saline or dialysis may be required if extreme hyponatremia is producing major central nervous system derangements.

Hyponatremia is very common in edematous patients with renal failure. Occasionally, the water excess is due to acute water loads, parenterally or orally, and may produce evidence of water intoxication. If the symptoms are not extreme, restriction of water is the best form of treatment, providing the patient can elaborate adequate amounts of urine. Hypertonic salt solutions may precipitate pulmonary edema and should therefore be avoided if possible. In most patients with edema, hyponatremia produces no symptoms. The treatment is not cessation of salt restriction, but rather a sharp reduction in water intake. Hyponatremia tends to be asymptomatic in virtually all instances in which it develops slowly, is of long duration, and is unassociated with salt loss.

Edema may develop for a variety of reasons in azotemic renal failure. In some instances it is virtually asymptomatic, producing no detectable cardiovascular disturbances. Hypoalbuminemic edema, arising because of a nephrotic syndrome or severe malnutrition, is of this sort. In occasional patients, successful hypotensive therapy with drugs may result in edema formation, presumably because the fall in blood pressure reduces renal blood flow and glomerular filtration rate. If significant evidences of deteriorating renal function also supervene, hypotensive therapy must then be discontinued.

Far more serious is the development of edema with venous congestion. Myocardial failure, on the basis of hypertensive cardiovascular disease, is a common cause. As in most forms of chronic myocardial failure, digitalis, salt restriction, and bed rest constitute the basis of treatment. However, certain features of the uremic state complicate the management of this disorder. Hyperkalemia may diminish the sensitivity of the myocardium to digitalis and necessitate larger doses. Should the serum potassium then fall as a result, in part, of a successful response, digitalis intoxication may ensue. The administration of calcium salts to correct hypocalcemia, particularly if given intravenously, may also cause digitalis intoxication.

The selection of a proper dose of a digitalis preparation requires special care. Most active glycosides in human subjects are excreted principally by the kidney as the unchanged glycoside (digoxin, lanatoside C, ouabain) or in the form of metabolites (digitoxin). In the case of digoxin, impaired renal function results in a prolongation of the half-life and elevated plasma concentrations. Therefore, digoxin doses should be reduced by one-third to one-half when the BUN reaches levels of 70 to 80 mg. per 100 ml. [80]. About 40 per cent of the usual digoxin dose is recommended in anuria [149]. The reduction in the dose of digitoxin is less, because renal excretion is more involved with the elimination of metabolites of digitoxin rather than with the active glycoside. A reduction of the usual dose of digitoxin by about one-third is recommended in advanced renal failure. There seems little doubt that hyperkalemia protects many patients from overt toxicity. The occasional precipitation of digitalis intoxication by dialysis appears to be related to the correction of potassium intoxication. Digoxin is not removed from the body, either by peritoneal dialysis or by hemodialysis, not because of protein binding, but rather because of low plasma levels and relatively inaccessible tissue stores [1].

In addition to salt restriction, bed rest, and digitalis, the potent diuretics, furosemide and ethacrynic acid, are of distinct benefit. Ethacrynic acid should not be used intravenously in advanced renal failure because it can produce deafness [208]. Both ethacrynic acid and furosemide can be used orally, in large doses; their capacity to induce salt loss depends not only on inhibiting sodium reabsorption in the kidney but also on their inhibitory action on sodium reabsorption in the gut, an action which may result in abdominal cramps and diarrhea.

In many instances, edema and heart failure persist despite the most aggressive medical measures. Dialysis can be extremely effective in removing edema and improving cardiac function. Once edema has been removed, cardiovascular function may improve to a degree sufficient to permit reasonable activity.

Not infrequently, patients develop edema and venous congestion for reasons other than myocardial failure. Severe anemia can lead to salt retention and a high-output state very similar in many respects to myocardial failure. In still other patients salt retention develops simply because of the inability of the diseased kidney to excrete salt loads. Here, too, severe venous congestion may develop. Finally, Bricker et al. [42] have suggested that severe acidosis alone may be responsible for a high-output state. This may well be an expression of the venoconstriction [136] and diminished ventricular function [287] that acidosis induces. Although special hemodynamic features serve to distinguish these disorders from chronic myocardial failure [89], only the history and the rapid circulation time are of much clinical utility. In some patients the coexistence of severe anemia, hypertension, and plentiful salt intake poses a serious problem. Not infrequently such patients are already digitalized. If the circulation time is normal or rapid, it is safest first to remove the edema fluid with peritoneal dialysis and then transfuse the patient so as partially to correct the anemia. In this manner, the danger of precipitating pulmonary edema by blood transfusion is mitigated. Peritoneal dialysis will benefit all three forms of venous congestion and permit the institution of additional measures when cardiopulmonary function may be much improved.

CALCIUM AND RENAL OSTEODYSTROPHY

Although hypocalcemia and reduced concentrations of ionized calcium are usually present in the late stages of chronic Bright's disease, it has been emphasized that tetany is exceedingly rare. Renal osteodystrophy, although a frequent finding at autopsy, is not commonly symptomatic in adults, even when detectable on x-ray examination. The occasional patient with symptomatic bone disease — bone pain, pathologic fractures, displaced epiphyses — may be benefited by measures designed to correct the deranged calcium metabolism, particularly if osteomalacia predominates as the bony lesion.

To overcome vitamin D resistance, calciferol (vitamin D_2) can be given in doses ranging from 1 to 10 mg. daily (40,000 to 400,000 international units). Since the action of vitamin D persists for about two weeks, the amount given is not changed rapidly. After the hypocalcemia and osteomalacia have been corrected, the dose can be reduced to about 0.25 mg. daily. The dietary intake of calcium is ordinarily supplemented with calcium salts, such as calcium lactate, in amounts of 15 to 30 gm. daily. The correction of metabolic acidosis with Shohl's solution will reduce calcium losses and bring about calcium balance, but it does not produce a positive balance [179]. Until prolonged studies have been performed to delineate the role of acidosis, it is probably well to keep the plasma bicarbonate near normal.

The hazards of this program should be clearly recognized. Metastatic calcification in eyes, blood vessels, joints, and bursa tends to appear whenever the product of the plasma concentrations of calcium and phosphorus exceeds 70. Coronary occlusion, intermittent claudication, and peripheral ischemia may occur as expressions of calcification of the coronary arteries and the aorta or its large branches. Precipitation of calcium pyrophosphate crystals in the joint may produce pseudogout. To prevent metastatic calcification, the plasma phosphate should be reduced by administration of aluminum hydroxide, 30 to 50 ml. with each meal, and removal of milk from the diet before vitamin D is started. If the serum calcium level is normal or near normal because of severe secondary hyperparathyroidism, it is particularly important to lower the phosphate before treatment is initiated.

Massive doses of vitamin D and calcium can induce serious hypercalcemia. As a consequence anorexia, lassitude, and thirst may develop, renal function may deteriorate further, and metastatic calcification may supervene [74, 261]. It is mandatory, therefore, to follow patients on such a program with frequent determinations of serum calcium, especially since the presence of advanced underlying renal disease, by preventing hypercalciuria, renders unreliable the urinary calcium as an index of the serum calcium. Aluminum hydroxide gel given for prolonged periods can produce phosphorus deficiency, thereby aggravating renal osteomalacia [74]. It should therefore be given

only as long as hyperphosphatemia persists.

If the osseous disease is principally symptomatic secondary hyperparathyroidism, vitamin D is contraindicated because of the grave danger of metastatic calcification. The plasma calcium tends to be near normal, and the hyperphosphatemia does not respond well to phosphate restriction or dialysis. Subtotal parathyroidectomy may be necessary to control severe bone disease or hypercalcemia [96, 262]. After parathyroid surgery, vitamin D and calcium are required to promote skeletal healing and correct hypocalcemia. Intractable pruritus, which does not respond to dialysis, recedes following subtotal parathyroidectomy, but the mechanism responsible for the improvement is unclear [157]. (See Chapter 8 for a more detailed discussion of these problems.)

ANEMIA AND BLEEDING

Eventually, all patients with azotemic renal failure acquire anemia regardless of the cause of the renal disease. If major blood loss does not supervene, the anemia is normocytic and normochromic in character [54, 181]. It is generally agreed that in the terminal stages of renal failure, anemia is of great severity and carries an ominous prognosis [50, 54]. In the earlier stages, the magnitude of anemia may correlate in a very general way with the degree of azotemia [50, 54, 232], but exceptions are numerous [76]. The red cell volume, as the disease slowly advances, tends to stabilize for long periods at a constant low level, to which it will return after an episode of bleeding [276].

The primary cause of the anemia appears to be deficient erythropoiesis. Despite the presence of normal red cell precursors in the bone marrow of most patients with chronic Bright's disease [54], a number of investigators have contended, on the basis of the demonstration of diminished utilization of radioactive iron [75, 150, 181], that red cell production is profoundly reduced. This failure of erythropoiesis is usually attributed to the inadequate production of erythropoietin by the diseased kidney. The demonstration by Goldstein and Jacobson and their associates [124, 147] that intact and ureteral-ligated animals produce a humoral agent, in response to cobalt, bleeding, and hypoxia, that stimulates erythropoiesis, whereas nephrectomized animals lose this ability, forms the basis of this hypothesis. The failure of Gallagher and his associates [112] to demonstrate, by bioassay, significant levels of erythropoietin in anemic patients with renal disease lends strong support to this hypothesis.

A second factor contributing to the anemia is a shortened life span of the red cell [76, 150, 181]. The cause of the hemolysis appears to be an extracorpuscular hemolytic factor and not any abnormality in the uremic red cells, since red cells from patients with renal disease have a normal life span when transfused into healthy recipients, while normal red cells have a shortened life span when transfused into uremic recipients [76, 150, 181]. The negative Coombs test argues against an autoimmune mechanism as the basis for the hemolytic process [150, 181, 276]. Hemolysis is absent or mild in most patients until the terminal stages, when it may become severe [76, 150, 181]. The more significant factor in the anemia is the deficient red cell production which is invariable. A virtual arrest of erythropoiesis may occur terminally [276]. In addition to the deficient red cell production and hemolytic process, the hemoglobin concentration may be further reduced by blood loss and hemodilution associated with heart failure [276]. In instances where active infection may be present (e.g., pyelonephritis), anemia of infection may play a role. Finally, those patients with necrotizing vascular disease may develop a hemolytic anemia in association with a red cell fragmentation syndrome.

In patients with renal failure undergoing adequate chronic hemodialysis, anemia may eventually lessen and the blood transfusion requirement may dramatically fall [57, 93]. Although erythropoiesis appears to increase significantly, red cell survival still tends to be decreased. The eventual rise in hematocrit incident to adequate dialysis can apparently be blunted by the overzealous use of transfusions, which should therefore be minimized.

The only uniformly effective means of correcting the anemia is blood transfusion. However, normal red cells in a uremic recipient tend to have a shortened life span, so that the rise in hemoglobin concentration may be quite transient. Moreover, repeated transfusions involve the hazards not only of homologous serum hepatitis and hemolytic and febrile reactions but also of precipitating pulmonary edema in the patient whose cardiovascular function is marginal. There is little reason, therefore, to transfuse patients unless symptoms referable to anemia supervene. When the hemoglobin concentration falls below 8 or 9 gm. per 100 ml., fatigue and dyspnea on exertion may develop. Transfusions may then be tried. If the rise in hemoglobin is sustained for a reasonable period of time and this is associated with the relief of symptoms, transfusions may be repeated at intervals. Since the object is to relieve symptoms and not to restore the hemoglobin to a normal value, levels of 8 to 9 gm. per 100 ml. may be quite satisfactory. In the terminal stages of Bright's disease, the hemoglobin may fall below 7 gm. per 100 ml. In such patients edema and venous congestion may develop as a result of anemia. This state must be distinguished carefully from myocardial failure and salt retention due to salt loads. If such a distinction cannot be made, it is wise to treat the patient for myocardial failure, and then, if no improvement ensues, to try small blood transfusions. Gardner [114] has advocated the use of cobalt, which stimulates erythropoietin production, and Gallagher and his associates [112] have noted an occasional patient who seems to respond. However, the results in most patients are disappointing; moreover, gastrointestinal disturbances are frequent. For these reasons, cobalt therapy seems to be of little value in the majority of patients.

Bleeding may be a prominent feature in uremia. Apart from the gastrointestinal bleeding associated with ulcerative lesions, a definite bleeding tendency sometimes develops. Cutaneous ecchymoses and oozing from mucous membranes may be prominent. Several defects appear to contribute to the bleeding tendency. Thrombocytopenia has been noted in some patients [174, 217], but it is usually comparatively mild. Increased capillary fragility has also been noted [160], and may possibly be attributable to the low serum serotonin values almost consistently found [174]. However, the most likely cause of the bleeding tendency is a qualitative defect in the platelets [53, 174, 217], as evidenced by abnormal prothrombin consumption and thromboplastin generation. Indeed, a specific defect in the activity of platelet factor 3 has been observed [53]. The cause of these disturbances is unknown; they are not produced by urea.

Gastrointestinal bleeding is an almost constant finding in uremia. Fortunately, it is generally of small magnitude and does not require major replacement of red cells. The bleeding is probably caused chiefly by ammonia burns of the intestinal mucosa brought about by the high intestinal pNH_3 resulting from the enteric breakdown of urea. In addition, however, the platelet defects of uremia probably play a role in blood loss from all bleeding sites [53].

Major bleeding in uremia generally is gastrointestinal and is the result of a specific lesion, not necessarily related directly to uremia, such as peptic ulceration [236]. An exception would be the stress ulcer that is occasionally seen in patients with terminal renal failure. (See Chapter 7 for an extensive discussion of these problems.)

HYPERTENSION

Although not invariable, hypertension is a leading feature of chronic renal failure from any cause. Since hypertension may generate severe symptoms, cause cerebral disease, precipitate cardiac failure, and accelerate the advance of renal failure, it should be treated aggressively.

Treatment of hypertension in chronic renal failure is complicated by three special problems: (1) The overexpansion of extracellular volume, so common in advanced renal failure, renders the patients resistant to the hypotensive action of drugs; (2) renal failure predisposes to retention of the drug, so that cumulative toxicity is common; and (3) successful hypotensive therapy may generate distressing side effects (orthostatic hypotension), serious complications (cerebral accident, coronary ischemia), or further deterioration in renal function. These considerations do not outweigh the potential benefits, but simply constitute therapeutic hurdles.

Measures to reduce extracellular volume are usually necessary. Salt restriction is helpful. In mild renal failure, thiazide diuretics should be used; severe renal failure requires the use of a more potent agent, such as furosemide. In addition, a hypotensive agent should be given. Alpha-methyl dopa and guanethidine are the most useful; either can be given with the diuretic. The slow renal excretion of these drugs makes cumulative toxicity common. To circumvent this, the drug dose should be increased very slowly. Alpha-methyl dopa should be started in a dose of 250 mg. three times daily and can be increased very slowly to a total dose of 2 gm. daily. If high doses are required, somnolence and lethargy tend to appear. Guanethidine has the advantage of not producing somnolence or lethargy. Therapy should be started with a small dose, 12.5 to 25.0 mg. per day, and very slowly increased until the blood pressure has been reduced. Orthostatic hypotension is a major problem.

It is imperative to distinguish salt depletion from hypotensive drug action as the cause of this disorder. Generally, this can be accomplished by adding a small amount of salt to the diet if the patient is not overexpanded.

Fulminant hypertension may develop, either as an exacerbation of preexisting milder hypertension or in a previously normotensive individual. Hypertensive encephalopathy, with convulsions, blindness, visual disturbances, heart failure, or accelerated renal failure, may rapidly appear. Sodium amytal, in a dose of 0.5 to 1.0 gm. intravenously, is effective in controlling convulsions. Hydralazine, in doses of 25 to 400 mg. intramuscularly per day, is particularly useful. In some instances hypertension is not appropriately corrected by hydralazine. Reserpine can then be given. Usually, the blood pressure can be abruptly lowered by the intramuscular administration of 0.5 to 1.0 mg. in a single injection; occasionally, as much as 2.5 mg. is needed. If large doses of reserpine are required, lethargy and even frank stupor may result. Since these symptoms may be difficult to distinguish from those produced by the underlying hypertensive vascular disease, hydralazine, which does not produce mental depression, is probably the hypotensive agent of choice to start with. If refractory edema is present, dialysis can be very helpful in removing excess fluid and thereby rendering the patient sensitive to the hypotensive agents. In the rare patient who does not respond, trimethaphan (Arfonad) should be given as a slow infusion at a concentration of 500 mg. per liter; the blood pressure must be carefully monitored to prevent undue hypotension.

ANTIBIOTICS AND INFECTION

Infections of the urinary tract are common in chronic renal failure from whatever cause, in part, no doubt, because of the frequency of catheterization, cystoscopy, retrograde pyelography, and the impaired bladder emptying so frequent in these patients. Systemic infections also appear to be common, although the incidence is hard to document [192]. The frequent use of indwelling venous catheters, arteriovenous shunts, and peritoneal dialysis contributes to the high prevalence of infection. In addition, a variety of factors associated with chronic renal failure — for example, steroids and immunosuppressive agents, debility and malnutrition, and the suppression of immunologic defenses characteristic of the uremic state — seem to increase the susceptibility to infection by interfering with immunologic defenses.

Administration of antibiotics to patients with renal failure is associated with two types of complications: (1) those which arise as a consequence of direct pharmacologic toxicity; and (2) hypersensitivity reactions. Both of these processes may manifest themselves in the form of systemic reactions or nephrotoxicity. In the case of direct toxicity with tetracycline, for example, high blood levels, such as may occur when the drug is given in large doses parenterally for the treatment of the pyelonephritis of pregnancy, may produce not only striking azotemia (owing to the antianabolic action of the drug) but also pancreatitis and fulminant hepatic necrosis, which may be lethal. Sulfonamides can cause a systemic angiitis as a manifestation of hypersensitivity. In general, pharmacologic toxicity is a dose-dependent phenomenon, while hypersensitivity may be accompanied by other characteristic signs, such as eosinophilia and skin rashes. Nephrotoxicity owing to hypersensitivity is comparatively uncommon, but in its severe form, as in hypersensitivity angiitis associated with sulfonamides, it may be irreversible. The usual cause of nephrotoxicity is pharmacologic toxicity owing to excessive blood levels. The antibiotics causing nephrotoxicity are usually those whose main route of excretion is through the kidney. Nephrotoxic reactions in patients with advanced renal disease may not be readily

Table 6-2. Antibiotic Usage in Patients with Renal Insufficiency

Group	Antibiotic	Serum Half-Life (hours)		Recommended Dosage for Adults (70 kg.)			Serious Adverse Effects[a]
		Normal Subject	Anuric Patient	Normal Renal Function	Serum Creatinine 2–10 mg./100 ml.	Serum Creatinine 10 mg./100 ml.	
I. Major reduction in dosage	Amphotericin B	Prolonged	?	Up to 1 mg./kg./day (IV)	Up to 0.5 mg./kg. every 2–3 days[b]	Up to 0.5 mg./kg. every 3–7 days[b]	Nephrotoxicity
	Colistimethate	2–3	48–72	1.00–1.25 mg./kg. every 6 hr. (IM)	1.00–1.25 mg./kg. every 24 hr.[b,c]	1.00–1.25 mg./kg. every 48–72 hr.[c]	Nephrotoxicity; paresthesia
	Demethylchlortetracycline	12	?	0.3 gm. every 6 hr. (po)	0.3 gm. every 24–48 hr.[b,c]	0.3 gm. every 72–96 hr.[b,c]	Hepatotoxicity
	Gentamicin	2	48–72	80 mg. every 8 hr. (IM)	80 mg. every 12–24 hr.	80 mg. every 48 hr.	Nephrotoxicity; ototoxicity (vestibular)
	Kanamycin	3	72–96	7 mg./kg. every 12 hr. (IM)	7 mg./kg. every 36–72 hr.[b,c]	7 mg./kg. every 96 hr.[b,c]	Nephrotoxicity; ototoxicity (cochlear)
	Oxytetracycline	10	?	0.5 gm. every 6 hr. (po); 8 mg./kg. every 6 hr. (IV)	0.5 gm. every 24–48 hr.[b]	0.5 gm. every 72–96 hr.[b]	Hepatotoxicity
	Polymyxin B	6	48–72	0.8 mg./kg. every 8 hr. (IM)	0.8 mg./kg. every 24–72 hr.[b,c]	0.8 mg./kg. every 72–95 hr.[b,c]	Nephrotoxicity; paresthesia
	Streptomycin	2–3	52–100	0.5 gm. every 6 hr. (IM)	0.5 gm. every 36–48 hr.[b,c]	0.5 gm. every 72 hr.[b,c]	Ototoxicity (vestibular)
	Tetracycline	8.5	57–108	0.5 gm. every 6 hr. (po); 8 mg./kg. every 6 hr. (IV)	0.5 gm. every 24–48 hr.[b]	0.5 gm. every 72–96 hr.	Hepatotoxicity
	Vancomycin	6	?	7 mg./kg. every 6 hr. (IV)	7 mg./kg. every 24–48 hr.[b,c]	7 mg./kg. every 72–96 hr.[b,c]	Ototoxicity (cochlear)

II. Moderate reduction in dosage	Carbenicillin	0.5–1.0	12.5	1.0 gm./hr. (IV)	1.0 gm. every 2–4 hr.[b]	2.0 gm. every 8 hr.	Urticaria Asymptomatic ↑SGOT
	Cephaloridine	1.5	20–23	12.5 mg./kg. every 6 hr. (IM)	12.5 mg./kg. every 12 hr.[b]	12.5 mg./kg. every 24 hr.	Hypersensitivity; nephrotoxicity
	Cephalothin	0.5	3–18	15–35 mg./kg. every 4 hr. (IV)	20 mg./kg. every 6–8 hr.[b]	20 mg./kg. every 24 hr.	Hypersensitivity
	Penicillin G	0.5	7–10	Up to 2,000,000 units every 2 hr. (IV)	Up to 2,000,000 units every 4–12 hr.[b]	Up to 2,000,000 units every 12 hr.	Hypersensitivity; seizures
III. None or minor reduction in dosage	Ampicillin	0.5–1.0[d]	?	15–30 mg./kg. every 4–6 hr. (po or IV)	At 30 mg./kg. reduce to every 6 hr.[e]	At 30 mg./kg. reduce to every 8 hr.[b]	Hypersensitivity; seizures
	Chloramphenicol Active	2–3	3–4	3.5–10.0 mg./kg. every 6 hr. (po or IV)	Not required	Not required	Hematotoxicity
	Conjugate	4–5	70–150				
	Cloxacillin	0.5–1.0[d]	?	7–20 mg./kg. every 4–6 hr. (po or IV)	Not required	Not required	Hypersensitivity
	Erythromycin	1.4	5–6	7 mg./kg. every 6 hr. (po or IV)	Not required	Not required	Phlebitis
	Isoniazid	1–4	?	3–5 mg./kg./day (po); usually 300 mg.	Probably should not exceed 300 mg./day[b]	Probably should not exceed 300 mg./day[b]	Peripheral neuropathy

Table 6-2. (Continued)

Group	Antibiotic	Serum Half-Life (hours)		Recommended Dosage for Adults (70 kg.)			Serious Adverse Effects[a]
		Normal Subject	Anuric Patient	Normal Renal Function	Serum Creatinine 2-10 mg./100 ml.	Serum Creatinine 10 mg./100 ml.	
	Lincomycin	4.5	10-13	7 mg./kg. every 6 hr. (po, IM, or IV)	Not required	7 mg./kg. every 8-12 hr.	Gastrointestinal
	Methicillin	0.5	4	20-40 mg./kg. every 4-6 hr. (IV)	Not required	Probably should not exceed 12 gm./day[b]	Hypersensitivity; nephrotoxicity
	Nafcillin	0.5-1.0[d]	?	7-20 mg./kg. every 4-6 hr. (po or IV)	Not required	Not required	Hypersensitivity
	Novobiocin	2	?	7 mg./kg. every 6 hr. (po or IV)	Not required	Not required	Skin rash; jaundice
	Oxacillin	0.5	2	7-20 mg./kg. every 4-6 hr. (po or IV)	Not required	Not required	Hypersensitivity
IV. Agents that should not be used	Bacitracin	1.5	?	25,000 u every 6 hr. (IM)	Use alternative agent	Use alternative agent	Nephrotoxicity
	Chlortetracycline	5.6	6.8-11.0	0.5 gm. every 6 hr. (po)	Use alternative agent[e]	Use alternative agent[e]	—

[a] Adverse effects may be either frequent or infrequent.
[b] Recommendations represent estimates which seem reasonable; actual confirmatory studies have not been done.
[c] An initial "loading dose" of twice the dosage listed is recommended in serious infections.
[d] Estimated from published disappearance curves.
[e] Metabolic effects may occur despite rapid inactivation.
SOURCE: Data from many sources, but predominantly from Kunin, C. M. [162].

identifiable since proteinuria, cylindruria, hematuria, and azotemia attributable to the drug may not be readily distinguished from that attributable to the underlying renal disease. Finally, it should be remembered that nephrotoxicity may generate a vicious cycle in which the renal damage caused by the drug may produce disproportionately higher blood levels, therefore causing further renal damage.

The use of antibiotics in renal failure is fraught with hazards, since impaired renal clearance may cause the excessive accumulation of those drugs whose principal route of elimination is through the kidney, and thereby promote pharmacologic toxicity. The data presented in Table 6-2 are drawn from many sources, but especially from Kunin [162, 163] and Sanford [234], and provide a guide to the selection and dose of appropriate agents.

The magnitude of renal failure as well as the extent to which the drug is eliminated by the kidney determine the modification of antibiotic dosage. Patients whose plasma creatinine is above 10 mg. per 100 ml. (creatinine clearance of less than 10 ml. per minute) can be considered virtually anuric [162]. More modest degrees of renal failure (serum creatinine of 2 to 10 mg. per 100 ml.) also require some reduction of drug dosage. If serum creatinine is normal or only slightly elevated (< 2 mg. per 100 ml.), ordinary therapeutic doses can be given. No matter what the degree of renal failure, the initial dose is given in the full amount recommended for patients without renal failure; it is only the frequency of subsequent maintenance doses that is modified. Table 6-2 lists the amount and frequency of the maintenance dose recommended for different antibiotics in the presence of various states of renal function.

In any drug whose dose is lowered to prevent toxic accumulation in plasma, the normal plasma concentrations will permit effective treatment of parenchymal infections. However, the urinary excretion of the drug on the reduced dosage will be low; eradication of bacteriuria may therefore be difficult.

Kunin [162] suggests that the antibiotic or antibiotic combination be chosen with respect to therapeutic efficacy against the infection, without regard to potential toxicity. However, if equally good agents are available, it is best to avoid, where possible, the agents in group I, which are eliminated principally by the kidney and require major modifications in drug dosage. To the agents listed in group IV, which should be avoided in renal failure, nitrofurantoin (Furadantin) and methenamine mandelate (Mandelamine) should be added. Group II lists the drugs where only a moderate modification in dosage may be required. Group III includes those drugs where a modification of the frequency of the maintenance dose is either slight or not required. Some disagreement exists in the case of chloramphenicol. Bone-marrow toxicity in patients with renal failure given 2 gm. daily has been reported by some [266] but not by others [183]. Serum iron and reticulocyte counts should be followed to detect early bone-marrow depression.

Peritoneal dialysis or hemodialysis influence the antibiotic program to the extent that the drug is dialyzable, since this will require an increase in the dose; in addition, dialysis may afford a means of treating serious toxicity if the antibiotic can be appreciably removed. Kanamycin is significantly removed; maintenance dose during peritoneal dialysis is therefore increased to 250 mg. daily [127]. Streptomycin is also dialyzable, and hemodialysis has been used to treat acute toxicity [87]. Colistimethate is partially dialyzable; the maintenance dose is increased to 2 mg. per kilogram of body weight daily [127]. Tetracycline, chloramphenicol, and methicillin are not removed significantly during peritoneal dialysis, and therefore necessitate no adjustment in drug dosage [127].

Tetracycline, as well as several nephrotoxic antibiotics, is absorbed in significant amounts when added to peritoneal dialysis solutions [248]. Cumulative toxicity may result. Appropriate adjustment of the amount of drug incorporated in peritoneal solutions is required if their use is mandatory for the treatment of peritonitis [248].

In patients with bacteriuria, recurrence after treatment with broad-spectrum antibiotics occurs in the majority of patients [105]. In one study, 88 per cent of the patients were bacteria-free when treatment was discontinued, but recurrence occurred in 86 per cent of the group in a 13-month follow-up period [105]. If continuous therapy was instituted after initial suppression with broad-spectrum antibiotics, recurrences could be prevented in the majority of patients. Only if the initial treatment was successful, however, was continuous therapy effective. Methenamine mandelate was the most effective agent; nitrofurantoin and sulfamethizole were less successful. Although exacerbations were prevented, no data are available concerning the influence of this treatment on renal function.

STEROIDS, ANTIMETABOLITES, AND HEPARIN

Steroids alone or with antimetabolites have been effectively used in the treatment of the nephrotic syndrome of glomerulonephritis. Proteinuria can be eliminated or sharply reduced in a significant number of patients. A number of investigators have contended that these forms of treatment not only control proteinuria but also influence favorably the course of the underlying renal disease. Indeed, antimetabolites such as azathioprine, cyclophosphamide, and methotrexate are increasingly used to treat advancing glomerulonephritis without the nephrotic syndrome. Unfortunately, there are no controlled studies which clearly delineate the efficacy of these agents. Since steroids and antimetabolites have serious toxic potentialities of their own, it is critical to know if they are beneficial and to what extent their beneficial effects outweigh their toxicity. Until such information is forthcoming, the use of these agents in the treatment of progressive glomerulonephritis must be regarded as experimental.

More recently, heparin has been advocated for the treatment of a wide variety of acute renal disorders caused by diffuse vascular or glomerular lesions. The underlying diseases include oliguric glomerulonephritis, thrombotic thrombocytopenic purpura, and the hemolytic-uremic syndrome. In many instances, a microangiopathic hemolytic anemia is present. It has been suggested that the basic lesion is an immunologic injury of endothelial cells, secondary to which fibrin deposits, ultimately forming thrombi. Heparin is given for 2 to 6 weeks in doses sufficient to keep the coagulation time between 25 and 40 minutes. Although large controlled studies are not available, the results look promising [153].

References

1. Ackerman, G. L., Doherty, J. E., and Flanigan, W. J. Peritoneal dialysis and hemodialysis of tritiated digoxin. *Ann. Intern. Med.* 67:718, 1967.

2. Adrian, R. H. The effect of internal and external potassium concentration on the membrane potential of frog muscle. *J. Physiol.* (London) 133:631, 1956.

3. Albright, F., Burnett, C. H., Parsons, W., Reifenstein, E. C., and Roos, A. Osteomalacia and late rickets. *Medicine* (Balt.) 25: 399, 1946.

4. Alfrey, A. C., Sussman, K. E., and Holmes, J. H. Changes in glucose and insulin metabolism induced by dialysis in patients with chronic uremia. *Metabolism* 16:733, 1967.

5. Alwall, N., Lunderquist, A., and Olsson, O. Studies on electrolyte-fluid retention: I. Uremic lung — fluid lung? On patho-

genesis and therapy. *Acta Med. Scand.* 146: 157, 1953.

6. Andes, J. E., Linegar, C. R., and Myers, B. A. Guanidine-like substances in the blood: II. Blood guanidine in nitrogen retention and hypertension. *J. Lab. Clin. Med.* 22:1209, 1937.

7. Asbury, A. K., Victor, M., and Adams, R. D. Uremic polyneuropathy. *Arch. Neurol.* (Chicago) 8:413, 1963.

8. Bagade, J. D., Porte, D., Jr., Curtis, F. K., and Bierman, E. L. Uremic lipemia: An unrecognized abnormality in triglyceride synthesis and removal. *Trans. Ass. Amer. Physicians* 81:190, 1968.

9. Baggenstoss, A. J. The pancreas in uremia: A histopathologic study. *Amer. J. Path.* 24:1003, 1948.

10. Baker, A. B., and Knutson, J. Psychiatric aspects of uremia. *Amer. J. Psychiat.* 102: 683, 1946.

11. Baldwin, D. S., Berman, H. J., Heinemann, H. O., and Smith, H. W. The elaboration of osmotically concentrated urine in renal disease. *J. Clin. Invest.* 34:800, 1955.

12. Bank, N., and Schwartz, W. B. The influence of anion penetrating ability on urinary acidification and the excretion of titratable acid. *J. Clin. Invest.* 39:1516, 1960.

13. Bartter, F. C., Pronove, P., Gill, J. R., and MacCardle, R. C. Hyperplasia of the juxtaglomerular complex with hyperaldosteronism and hypokalemic alkalosis. *Amer. J. Med.* 33:811, 1962.

14. Bass, H. E., Greenberg, D., Singer, E., and Miller, M. A. Pulmonary changes in uremia. *J.A.M.A.* 148:724, 1952.

15. Beaudry, C., Nakamoto, S., and Kolff, W. J. Uremic pericarditis and cardiac tamponade in chronic renal failure. *Ann. Intern. Med.* 64:990, 1966.

16. Becher, E. Pathogenese, Symptomatologie und Therapie der Urämie. *Ergebn. Ges. Med.* 18:51, 1933.

17. Bellet, S. The electrocardiogram in electrolyte imbalance. *A.M.A. Arch. Intern. Med.* 96:618, 1955.

18. Bellet, S., Steiger, W. A., Nadler, C. S., and Gazes, P. C. Electrocardiographic patterns in hypopotassemia: Observations on 79 patients. *Amer. J. Med. Sci.* 219:542, 1950.

19. Bennett, C. R., Brenner, B. M., and Berliner, R. W. Micropuncture study of nephron function in the rhesus monkey. *J. Clin. Invest.* 47:203, 1968.

20. Berliner, R. W., and Kennedy, T. J., Jr. Renal tubular secretion of potassium in the normal dog. *Proc. Soc. Exp. Biol. Med.* 67: 542, 1948.

21. Berliner, R. W., Kennedy, T. J., Jr., and Hilton, J. G. Renal mechanisms for excretion of potassium. *Amer. J. Physiol.* 162:348, 1950.

22. Berliner, R. W., Kennedy, T. J., Jr., and Orloff, J. Relationship between acidification of the urine and potassium metabolism. *Amer. J. Med.* 11:274, 1951.

23. Berlyne, G. M. Distal tubular function in chronic hydronephrosis. *Quart. J. Med.* n. s. 30:339, 1961.

24. Berlyne, G. M. Medical management of chronic renal failure. *Practitioner* 201:452, 1968.

25. Berlyne, G. M., Gaan, D., and Ginks, W. R. Dietary treatment of chronic renal failure. *Amer. J. Clin. Nutr.* 21:547, 1968.

26. Berlyne, G. M., Janabi, K., and Shaw, A. B. Dangers of resonium A in the treatment of hyperkalemia in renal failure. *Lancet* 1: 167, 1966.

27. Berlyne, G. M., Janabi, K., Shaw, A. B., and Hocken, G. G. Treatment of hyperkalemia with a calcium-resin. *Lancet* 1:169, 1966.

28. Berlyne, G. M., Shaw, A. B., and Nilwarangkur, S. Dietary treatment of chronic renal failure. *Nephron* 2:129, 1965.

29. Berlyne, G. M., Varley, H., Nilwarangkur, S., and Hoerni, M. Endogenous creatinine clearance and the glomerular filtration rate. *Lancet* 2:874, 1964.

30. Berson, S. A., and Yalow, R. S. Parathyroid hormone in plasma in adenomatous hyperparathyroidism, uremia, and carcinoma. *Science* 154:907, 1966.

31. Biber, T. U. L., Mylle, M., Baines, A. D., Gottschalk, C. W., Oliver, J. R., and MacDowell, M. C. A study of micropuncture

and microdissection of acute renal damage in rats. *Amer. J. Med.* 44:664, 1968.

32. Blythe, W. B., Gitelman, J. J., and Welt, L. G. Effect of expansion of the extracellular space on the rate of urinary excretion of calcium. *Amer. J. Physiol.* 214:52, 1968.

33. Bradley, S. E. *The Pathologic Physiology of Uremia in Chronic Bright's Disease.* Springfield, Ill.: Thomas, 1948.

34. Bradley, S. E., Bradley, G. P., Tyson, C. J., Curry, J. J., and Blake, W. D. Renal function in renal diseases. *Amer. J. Med.* 9:766, 1950.

35. Bricker, N. S. On the meaning of the intact nephron hypothesis. *Amer. J. Med.* 46:1, 1969.

36. Bricker, N. S., Dewey, R. R., Lubowitz, H., Stokes, J., and Kirkensgaard, T. Observations on the concentrating and diluting mechanisms of the diseased kidney. *J. Clin. Invest.* 38:516, 1959.

37. Bricker, N. S., Kime, S. W., Jr., and Morrin, P. A. F. The Functional Integrity of the Pyelonephritic Kidney. In Quinn, E. L., and Kass, E. H. (Eds.), *Biology of Pyelonephritis.* (Henry Ford Hospital International Symposium.) Boston: Little, Brown, 1960. P. 331.

38. Bricker, N. S., Kime, S. W., Jr., Morrin, P. A. F., and Orlowski, T. The influence of glomerular filtration rate, solute excretion and hydration on the concentrating mechanism of the experimentally diseased kidney in the dog. *J. Clin. Invest.* 39:864, 1960.

39. Bricker, N. S., Klahr, S., Lubowitz, H., and Rieselbach, R. E. Renal function in chronic renal disease. *Medicine* (Balt.) 44:263, 1965.

40. Bricker, N. S., Klahr, S., Purkerson, M., and Schultze, R. G. On an in vitro assay system for a humoral substance in plasma and serum during extracellular fluid volume expansion and uremia. *Nature* (London) 219:1058, 1968.

41. Bricker, N. S., Klahr, S., and Rieselbach, R. E. The functional adaptation of the diseased kidney: I. Glomerular filtration rate. *J. Clin. Invest.* 43:1915, 1964.

42. Bricker, N. S., Morrin, P. A. F., and Kime, S. W., Jr. The pathologic physiology of chronic Bright's disease. *Amer. J. Med.* 28:77, 1960.

43. Bricker, N. S., Orlowski, T., Kime, S. W., Jr., and Morrin, P. A. F. Observations on the functional homogeneity of the nephron population in the chronically diseased kidney of the dog. *J. Clin. Invest.* 39:1771, 1960.

44. Bricker, N. S., Stokes, J. M., Lubowitz, H., Dewey, R. R., Bernard, H. R., and Hartroft, P. M. Experimentally induced permanent unilateral renal disease in dogs. *J. Lab. Clin. Med.* 52:571, 1958.

45. Bricker, N. S., Slatapolsky, E., Reiss, E., and Avioli, L. V. Calcium, phosphorus, and bone in renal disease and transplantation. *Arch. Intern. Med.* (Chicago) 123:543, 1969.

46. Briggs, A. P., Waugh, W. H., Harms, W. S., and Findley, T. Pathogenesis of uremic acidosis as indicated by urinary acidification on a controlled diet. *Metabolism* 10:749, 1961.

47. Brod, J. Chronic pyelonephritis. *Lancet* 1:973, 1956.

48. Brod, J., Prat, V., and Dejdar, R. Early Functional Diagnosis of Chronic Pyelonephritis with Some Remarks on the Pathogenesis of the Pyelonephritic Contracted Kidney. In Quinn, E. L., and Kass, E. H. (Eds.), *Biology of Pyelonephritis.* (Henry Ford Hospital International Symposium.) Boston: Little, Brown, 1960. P. 311.

49. Brodsky, W. A., and Rapoport, S. The mechanism of polyuria of diabetes insipidus in man: The effect of osmotic loading. *J. Clin. Invest.* 30:282, 1951.

50. Brown, G. E., and Roth, G. M. Prognostic value of anemia in chronic glomerular nephritis. *J.A.M.A.* 81:1948, 1923.

51. Bull, G. M. The uraemias. *Lancet* 1:731, 777, 1955.

52. Burnell, J. M., Villamil, M. F., Uyeno, B. T., and Scribner, B. H. Effect in humans of extracellular pH change on the relationship between serum potassium concentration and intracellular potassium. *J. Clin. Invest.* 35:935, 1956.

53. Cahalane, S. F., Johnson, S. A., Monto,

R. W., and Caldwell, M. J. Acquired thrombocytopathy; observations on the co-agulation defect in uremia. *Amer. J. Clin. Path.* 30:507, 1958.

54. Callen, I. R., and Limarzi, L. R. Blood and bone marrow studies in renal disease. *Amer. J. Clin. Path.* 20:3, 1950.

55. Cannon, P. J., Leeming, J. M., Sommers, S. C., Winters, R. W., and Laragh, J. H. Juxtaglomerular cell hyperplasia and secondary hyperaldosteronism (Bartter's syndrome): A reevaluation of the pathophysiology. *Medicine* (Balt.) 47:107, 1968.

56. Carone, F. A., and Epstein, F. H. Nephrogenic diabetes insipidus caused by amyloid disease. *Amer. J. Med.* 29:539, 1960.

57. Carter, R. A., Hawkins, J. B., and Robinson, B. H. B. Iron metabolism in the anemia of chronic renal failure: Effects of dialysis and of parenteral iron. *Brit. Med. J.* 3:206, 1969.

58. Christison, R. Observations on the variety of dropsy which depends on diseased kidneys. *Edinburgh Med. J.* 32:262, 1829.

59. Clapp, J. R., Rector, F. C., Jr., and Seldin, D. W. Effect of unreabsorbed anions on proximal and distal transtubular potentials in rats. *Amer. J. Physiol.* 202:781, 1962.

60. Clapp, J. R., and Robinson, R. R. Osmolality of distal tubular fluid in the dog. *J. Clin. Invest.* 45:1847, 1966.

61. Clarkson, E. M., McDonald, S. J., and de Wardener, H. E. The effect of a high intake of calcium carbonate in normal subjects and patients with chronic renal failure. *Clin. Sci.* 30:425, 1966.

62. Cole, C. H., Balfe, J. W., and Welt, L. G. Induction of an ouabain-sensitive ATPase defect by uremic plasma. *Trans. Ass. Amer. Physicians* 81:213, 1968.

63. Coleman, A. J., Arias, M., Carter, N. W., Rector, F. C., Jr., and Seldin, D. W. The mechanism of salt wastage in chronic renal disease. *J. Clin. Invest.* 45:1116, 1966.

64. Conn, H. O. Asterixis in non-hepatic disorders. *Amer. J. Med.* 29:647, 1960.

65. Conn, J. W., and Louis, L. H. Primary aldosteronism, a new clinical entity. *Ann. Intern. Med.* 44:1, 1956.

66. Copeland, B. E., and Sunderman, F. W. Studies in serum electrolytes: XVIII. The magnesium binding property of the serum proteins. *J. Biol. Chem.* 197:331, 1952.

67. Cortney, M. A., Mylle, M., Lassiter, W. E., and Gottschalk, C. W. Renal tubular transport of water, solute, and PAH in rats loaded with isotonic saline. *Amer. J. Physiol.* 209:1199, 1965.

68. Damadian, R. V., Shwayni, E., and Bricker, N. S. On the existence of non-urine forming nephrons in the diseased kidney of the dog. *J. Lab. Clin. Med.* 65:26, 1965.

69. Dammin, G. J., Couch, N. P., and Murray, J. E. Prolonged survival of skin homografts in uremic patients. *Ann. N.Y. Acad. Sci.* 64:967, 1957.

70. Davidson, D. G., Levinsky, N. G., and Berliner, R. W. Maintenance of potassium excretion despite reduction of glomerular filtration during sodium diuresis. *J. Clin. Invest.* 37:548, 1958.

71. Davis, J. O., Ayers, C. R., and Carpenter, C. C. J. Renal origin of an aldosterone-stimulating hormone in dogs with thoracic caval constriction and in sodium-depleted dogs. *J. Clin. Invest.* 40:1466, 1961.

72. Davis, J. O., Carpenter, C. C. J., Ayers, C. R., Holman, J. E., and Bahn, R. C. Evidence for secretion of an aldosterone-stimulating hormone by the kidney. *J. Clin. Invest.* 40:684, 1961.

73. del Castillo, J., and Engbaek, L. The nature of the neuromuscular block produced by magnesium. *J. Physiol.* (London) 124:370, 1954.

74. Dent, C. E., Harper, C. M., and Philpot, G. R. The treatment of renal-glomerular osteodystrophy. *Quart. J. Med.* 30:1, 1959.

75. DePass, W. S., Stein, J., Poppel, M. H., and Jacobson, H. G. Pulmonary congestion and edema in uremia. *J.A.M.A.* 162:5, 1956.

76. Desforges, J. F., and Dawson, J. P. The anemia of renal failure. *A.M.A. Arch. Intern. Med.* 101:326, 1958.

77. de Wardener, H. E. Polyuria, *J. Chronic Dis.* 11:199, 1960.

78. Dirks, J. H., Cirksena, W. J., and Berliner, R. W. The effect of saline infusion on sodium reabsorption by the proximal tubule of the dog. *J. Clin. Invest.* 44:1160, 1965.

79. Dock, W. The evil sequelae of complete bed rest. *J.A.M.A.* 125:1083, 1944.

80. Doherty, J. E., Perkins, W. H., and Wilson, M. C. Studies with tritiated digoxin in renal failure. *Amer. J. Med.* 37:536, 1964.

81. Doniach, I. Uremic edema of the lungs. *Amer. J. Roentgen.* 58:620, 1947.

82. Doolan, P. D., Alpen, E. L., and Theil, G. B. A. A clinical appraisal of the plasma concentration and endogenous clearance of creatinine. *Amer. J. Med.* 32:65, 1962.

83. Dorhout Mees, E. J. Role of osmotic diuresis in impairment of concentrating ability in renal disease. *Brit. Med. J.* 1:1156, 1959.

84. Dorhout Mees, E. J. Relation between maximal urine concentration, maximal water reabsorption capacity, and mannitol clearance in patients with renal disease. *Brit. Med. J.* 1:1159, 1959.

85. Dorhout Mees, E. J. Reversible water losing state, caused by incomplete ureteric obstruction. *Acta Med. Scand.* 168:193, 1960.

86. Eales, L., and Linder, G. C. Potassium-losing pyelonephritis and malignant hypertension: A case report with balance studies. *Metabolism* 8:445, 1959.

87. Edwards, K. D. G., and Whyte, H. M. Streptomycin poisoning in renal failure. An indication for treatment with the artificial kidney. *Brit. Med. J.* 1:752, 1959.

88. Effersøe, P. Signs and symptoms in chronic renal failure: II. Vomiting, twitching, hemorrhagic diathesis, convulsions, itching and diarrhea. *Acta Med. Scand.* 160: 417, 1958.

89. Eichna, L. W. Circulatory congestion and heart failure. *Circulation* 22:864, 1960.

90. Elkinton, J. R. The role of magnesium in the body fluids. *Clin. Chem.* 3:319, 1957.

91. Elkinton, J. R., Tarail, R., and Peters, J. P. Transfers of potassium in renal insufficiency. *J. Clin. Invest.* 28:378, 1949.

92. Epstein, F. H. Reversible uremic states. *J.A.M.A.* 161:494, 1956.

93. Eschbach, J., Funk, D., Adamson, J., Kuhn, I., Scribner, B. H., and Finch, C. A. Erythropoiesis in patients with renal failure undergoing chronic dialysis. *New Eng. J. Med.* 276:653, 1967.

94. Falls, W. F., Jr., Carter, N. W., Rector, F. C., Jr., and Seldin, D. W. The mechanism of impaired phosphate reabsorption in chronic renal disease. *Clin. Res.* 9:74, 1966.

95. Fanconi, G., and Rose, G. A. The ionized complexed, and protein-bound fractions of calcium in plasma. *Quart. J. Med.* 27:463, 1958.

96. Felts, J. H., Whitley, J. E., Anderson, D. D., Carpenter, H. M., and Bradshaw, H. H. Medical and surgical treatment of azotemic osteodystrophy. *Ann. Intern. Med.* 62:1272, 1965.

97. Fishberg, A. M. *Hypertension and Nephritis* (5th ed.). Philadelphia: Lea & Febiger, 1954.

98. Flinn, R. B., Merrill, J. P., and Welzant, W. R. Treatment of the oliguric patient with a new sodium-exchange resin and sorbitol: A preliminary report. *New Eng. J. Med.* 264:111, 1961.

99. Foster, N. B. The isolation of a toxic substance from the blood of uremic patients. *Trans. Ass. Amer. Physicians* 30:305, 1915.

100. Foster, N. B. Uremia. *J.A.M.A.* 76:281, 1921.

101. Franklin, S. S., Gordon, A., Kleeman, C. R., and Maxwell, M. H. Use of a balanced low-protein diet in chronic renal failure. *J.A.M.A.* 202:141, 1967.

102. Franklin, S. S., Kleeman, C. R., Vilamill, M., Maxwell, M. H., and Gerstein, A. J. Effect of the Giordano-Giovannetti low-protein diet on the renal response of normal subjects to acute potassium and acid loads. *Clin. Res.* 14:377, 1966.

103. Franklin, S. S., and Merrill, J. P. The kidney in health; the nephron in disease. *Amer. J. Med.* 28:1, 1960.

104. Franklin, S. S., Niall, J. F., and Merrill, J. P. The influence of solute load on the isosthenuria of renal disease. *J. Clin. Invest.* 38:1005, 1959.

105. Freeman, R. B., Bronner, L., Brancato, F., Cohen, S. I., Garfield, C. E., Griep, R. J., Hinman, E. J., Richardson, J. A., Thurm, R. H., Urner, C., and Smith, W. M. Prevention of recurrent bacteriuria with con-

tinuous chemotherapy. *Ann. Intern. Med.* 69:655, 1968.

106. Freeman, R. B., Sheff, M. F., Maher, J. F., and Schreiner, G. E. The blood-cerebrospinal fluid barrier in uremia. *Ann. Intern. Med.* 56:233, 1962.

107. Freedman, L. R. Prolonged Observations on a Group of Patients with Acute Urinary Tract Infections. In Quinn, E. L., and Kass, E. H. (Eds.), *Biology of Pyelonephritis.* (Henry Ford Hospital International Symposium.) Boston: Little, Brown, 1960. P. 345.

108. Freedman, L. R. Chronic pyelonephritis at autopsy. *Ann. Intern. Med.* 66:697, 1967.

109. Frick, A., Kunau, R., Rector, F. C., Jr., and Seldin, D. W. Unpublished observations.

110. Fry, J., Dillane, J. B., Joiner, C. L., and Williams, J. D. Acute urinary infections: Their course and outcome in general practice with special reference to chronic pyelonephritis. *Lancet* 1:1318, 1962.

111. Gall, E. A. Pyelonephritis. *Bull. N.Y. Acad. Med.* 37:367, 1961.

112. Gallagher, N. I., McCarthy, J. M., Hart, K. T., and Lange, R. D. Evaluation of plasma erythropoietic-stimulating factors in anemic uremic patients. *Blood* 14:662, 1959.

113. Gamble, J. L. Physiological information gained from studies on life raft ration. *Harvey Lect.* 42:247, 1946–1947.

114. Gardner, F. H. The use of cobaltous chloride in the anemia associated with chronic renal disease. *J. Lab. Clin. Med.* 41:56, 1953.

115. Gault, M. H., and Dossetor, J. B. Chronic pyelonephritis: Relative incidence in transplant recipients. *New Eng. J. Med.* 275:813, 1966.

116. Gibson, D. G. Hemodynamic factors in the development of acute pulmonary edema in renal failure. *Lancet* 2:1217, 1966.

117. Giordano, C. Use of exogenous and endogenous urea for protein synthesis in normal and uremic subjects. *J. Lab. Clin. Med.* 62:231, 1963.

118. Giovannetti, S., and Maggiore, Q. A low-nitrogen diet with proteins of high biological value for severe chronic uremia. *Lancet* 1:1000, 1964.

119. Goldman, D. E. Potential, impedance and rectification in membranes. *J. Gen. Physiol.* 27:37, 1943.

120. Goldman, R., and Bassett, S. H. Phosphorus excretion in renal failure. *J. Clin. Invest.* 33:1623, 1954.

121. Goldring, W., and Chasis, H. *Hypertension and Hypertensive Disease.* New York: Commonwealth Fund, 1944.

122. Goldsmith, C., Beasley, H. K., Whalley, P. J., Rector, F. C., Jr., and Seldin, D. W. The effect of salt deprivation on the urinary concentrating mechanism in the dog. *J. Clin. Invest.* 40:2043, 1961.

123. Goldstein, M. H., Lenz, P. R., and Levitt, M. F. Effect of urine flow rate on urea reabsorption in man: Urea as a "tubular marker." *J. Appl. Physiol.* 26:594, 1969.

124. Goldwasser, E., Fried, W., and Jacobson, L. O. Studies in erythropoiesis: VIII. The effect of nephrectomy on the response to hypoxic anoxia. *J. Lab. Clin. Med.* 52:375, 1958.

125. Goodman, A. D., Lemann, J., Jr., Lennon, E. J., and Relman, A. S. Production, excretion, and net balance of fixed acid in patients with renal acidosis. *J. Clin. Invest.* 44:495, 1965.

126. Gowland, G., and Smiddy, F. G. The effect of acute experimental uremia on the immunological responses of the rabbit to bovine serum albumin. *Brit. J. Urol.* 34:274, 1962.

127. Greenberg, P. A., and Sanford, J. P. Removal and absorption of antibiotics in patients with renal failure undergoing peritoneal dialysis. *Ann. Intern. Med.* 66:465, 1967.

128. Grollman, E. F., and Grollman, A. Toxicity of urea and its role in the pathogenesis of uremia. *J. Clin. Invest.* 38:749, 1959.

129. Guild, W. R., Bray, G., and Merrill, J. P. Hemopericardium with cardiac tamponade in chronic uremia. *New Eng. J. Med.* 257:230, 1957.

130. Hager, E. B. Clinical observations on five patients with uremic pericardial tamponade. *New Eng. J. Med.* 273:304, 1965.

131. Hampers, C. L., Blaufox, M. D., and Merrill, J. P. Anticoagulation rebound after

hemodialysis. *New Eng. J. Med.* 275:776, 1966.

132. Hampers, C. L., Soeldner, J. S., Doak, P. B., and Merrill, J. P. Effect of chronic renal failure and hemodialysis on carbohydrate metabolism. *J. Clin. Invest.* 45:1719, 1966.

133. Harrison, T. R., and Mason, M. F. The pathogenesis of the uremic syndrome. *Medicine* (Balt.) 16:1, 1937.

134. Harrison, T. R., Mason, M. F., and Resnik, H. Observations on the mechanism of muscular twitchings in uremia. *J. Clin. Invest.* 15:463, 1936.

135. Harrison, T. R., and Perlzweig, W. A. Alkalosis, not due to administration of alkali, associated with uremia. *J.A.M.A.* 84:671, 1925.

136. Harvey, R. M., Enson, Y., Lewis, M. L., Greenough, W. B., Ally, K. M., and Panno, R. A. Hemodynamic effects of dehydration and metabolic acidosis in Asiatic cholera. *Trans. Ass. Amer. Physicians* 79:177, 1966.

137. Hayman, J. M., Jr., Shumway, N. P., Dumke, P., and Miller, M. Experimental hyposthenuria. *J. Clin. Invest.* 18:195, 1939.

138. Henkin, R. I., Maxwell, M. H., and Murray, J. F. Uremic pneumonitis: A clinical, physiological study. *Ann. Intern. Med.* 57:1001, 1962.

139. Herndon, R. F., Freeman, S., and Cleveland, A. S. Protein requirements in chronic renal insufficiency patients. *J. Lab. Clin. Med.* 52:235, 1958.

140. Hirschfelder, A. D. Clinical manifestations of high and low plasma magnesium; dangers of epsom salt purgation in nephritis. *J.A.M.A.* 102:1138, 1934.

141. Hodgkin, A. L. Ionic movements and electrical activity in giant nerve fibers. *Proc. Roy. Soc.* (London) Series B. 148:1, 1957.

142. Hoff, H. E., Smith, P. D., and Winkler, A. W. Effects of magnesium on nervous system in relation to its concentration in serum. *Amer. J. Physiol.* 130:292, 1940.

143. Hood, B., Falkheden, T., and Carlsson, M. Trends and pattern of mortality in chronic uremia. *Acta Med. Scand.* 181:561, 1967.

144. Hopps, H. C., and Wissler, R. W. Uremic pneumonitis. *Amer. J. Path.* 31:261, 1955.

145. Hume, D. M., Merrill, J. P., Miller, B. F., and Thorn, G. W. Experiences with renal homotransplantation in the human: Report of nine cases. *J. Clin. Invest.* 34:327, 1955.

146. Jackson, G. G., Dallenbach, F. D., and Kipnis, G. P. Pyelonephritis. *Med. Clin. N. Amer.* 39:297, 1955.

147. Jacobson, L. O., Goldwasser, E., Fried, W., and Pizak, L. Role of the kidney in erythropoiesis. *Nature* (London) 179:633, 1957.

148. Jebsen, R. H., Tenchoff, H., and Horst, J. C. Natural history of uremic polyneuropathy and effects of dialysis. *New Eng. J. Med.* 277:327, 1967.

149. Jelliffe, R. W., and Blankenhorn, D. A. Improved method of digitalis therapy in patients with reduced renal function. *Circulation* 36(Suppl. 2):150, 1967.

150. Joske, R. A., McAlister, J. M., and Prankerd, T. A. J. Isotope investigations of red cell production and destruction in chronic renal disease. *Clin. Sci.* 15:511, 1956.

151. Keith, N. M., and Burchell, H. B. Clinical intoxication with potassium: Its occurrence in severe renal insufficiency. *Amer. J. Med. Sci.* 217:1, 1949.

152. Keith, N. M., Pruitt, R. D., and Baggenstoss, A. H. Electrocardiographic changes in pericarditis associated with uremia. *Amer. Heart J.* 31:527, 1946.

153. Kincaid-Smith, P., Saker, B. M., and Fairley, K. F. Anticoagulants in "irreversible" acute renal failure. *Lancet* 2:1360, 1968.

154. Kleeman, C. R., Adams, D. A., and Maxwell, M. H. An evaluation of maximal water diuresis in chronic renal disease: I. Normal solute intake. *J. Lab. Clin. Med.* 58:169, 1961.

155. Kleeman, C. R., and Epstein, F. H. An illustrative case of chronic pyelonephritis with persistently hypotonic urine. *Amer. J. Med.* 23:488, 1957.

156. Kleeman, C. R., Hewitt, W. L., and Guze, L. B. Pyelonephritis. *Medicine* (Balt.) 39:3, 1960.

157. Kleeman, C. R., Massry, S. G., Popovtger, M. M., Makoff, D. L., Maxwell, M. H., and Coburn, J. The disappearance of intractable pruritus after parathyroidectomy in uremic patients with secondary hyperparathy-

roidism. *Trans. Ass. Amer. Physicians* 81: 203, 1968.

158. Kolberg, A. Altered influence of acetate on excretion of para-aminohippurate in hypertrophic renal tubular epithelium. *Acta Med. Scand.* 153:315, 1956.

159. Kolberg, A. Relations of renal tubular and glomerular function as influenced by 75 per cent reduction of nephron number. *Scand. J. Clin. Lab. Invest.* 11(Suppl. 41): 1, 1959.

160. Kuhlback, B. The bleeding tendency in chronic renal failure. *Acta Med. Scand.* 157: 173, 1957.

161. Kunau, R. T., Jr., Frick, A., Rector, F. C., Jr., and Seldin, D. W. Micropuncture study of the proximal tubular factors responsible for the maintenance of alkalosis during potassium deficiency in the rat. *Clin. Sci.* 34:223, 1968.

162. Kunin, C. M. A guide to use of antibiotics in patients with renal disease: A table of recommended doses and factors governing serum levels. *Ann. Intern. Med.* 67:151, 1967.

163. Kunin, C. M. Nephrotoxicity of antibiotics. *J.A.M.A.* 202:204, 1967.

164. Kurtzman, N. A. Regulation of renal bicarbonate reabsorption by extracellular volume. *J. Clin. Invest.* 49:586, 1970.

165. Langendorf, R., and Pirani, C. L. The heart in uremia. *Amer. Heart J.* 33:282, 1947.

166. Laragh, J. H., Ulick, S., Januszewicz, V., Deming, Q. B., Kelley, W. G., and Lieberman, S. Aldosterone secretion and primary and malignant hypertension. *J. Clin. Invest.* 39:1091, 1960.

167. Lathem, W. Hyperchloremic acidosis in chronic pyelonephritis. *New Eng. J. Med.* 258:1031, 1958.

168. Leaf, A., and Camara, A. A. Renal tubular secretion of potassium in man. *J. Clin. Invest.* 28:1526, 1949.

169. Leaf, A., and Couter, W. T. Evidence that renal sodium excretion by normal human subjects is regulated by adrenal cortical activity. *J. Clin. Invest.* 28:1067, 1949.

170. Lemann, J., Lennon, E. J., Goodman, A. D., Litzow, J. R., and Relman, A. S. The net balance of acid in subjects given large loads of acid or alkali. *J. Clin. Invest.* 44:507, 1965.

171. Lemann, J., Jr., Litzow, J. R., and Lennon, E. J. The effects of chronic acid loads in normal man: Further evidence for the participation of bone mineral in the defense against chronic metabolic acidosis. *J. Clin. Invest.* 45:1608, 1966.

172. Levin, S., and Winhelstein, J. A. Diet and infrequent peritoneal dialysis in chronic anuric uremia. *New Eng. J. Med.* 277:619, 1967.

173. Levitt, M. F., Levy, M. S., and Polemeros, D. The effect of a fall in filtration rate on solute and water excretion in hydropenic man. *J. Clin. Invest.* 38:463, 1969.

174. Lewis, J. H., Zucker, M. B., and Ferguson, J. H. Bleeding tendency in uremia. *Blood* 11:1073, 1956.

175. Lieber, S. C., and LeFèvre, A. Ammonia as a source of gastric hypoacidity in patients with uremia. *J. Clin. Invest.* 38:1271, 1959.

176. Lindheimer, M. D., Lalone, R. C., and Levinsky, N. G. Evidence that an acute rise in glomerular filtration has little effect on sodium excretion in the dog unless extracellular volume is expanded. *J. Clin. Invest.* 46:256, 1967.

177. Linhart, J. W., and Welt, L. G. The effect of hyponatremia and cellular dilution on tissue catabolism in the rat. *Trans. Ass. Amer. Physicians* 76:184, 1963.

178. Little, P. J., McPherson, D. R., and de Wardener, H. E. The appearance of the intravenous pyelogram during and after acute pyelonephritis. *Lancet* 1:1186, 1965.

179. Litzow, J. R., Lemann, J., Jr., and Lennon, E. J. The effect of treatment of acidosis on calcium balance in patients with chronic azotemic renal disease. *J. Clin. Invest.* 46: 280, 1967.

180. Loche, S., Merrill, J. P., and Tyler, H. R. Neurologic complications of acute uremia. *Arch. Intern. Med.* (Chicago) 108:519, 1961.

181. Loge, J. P., Lange, R. D., and Moore, C. V. Characterization of the anemia associated with chronic renal insufficiency. *Amer. J. Med.* 24:4, 1958.

182. Lubowitz, H., Slatapolsky, E., Shankel, S., Rieselbach, R. E., and Bricker, N. S. Glomerular filtration rate: Determination in patients with chronic renal disease. *J.A.M.A.* 199:252, 1967.

183. McCurdy, P. R. Plasma concentrations of chloramphenicol and bone marrow suppression. *Blood* 21:363, 1963.

184. McNaughton, R. A., and Burchell, H. B. Paralysis with potassium intoxication in renal insufficiency. *J.A.M.A.* 145:481, 1951.

185. McPhaul, J. J., Jr., and Simonaitis, J. J. Observations on the mechanisms of glucosuria during glucose loads in normal and nondiabetic subjects. *J. Clin. Invest.* 47:702, 1968.

186. Mason, M. F., Resnik, H., Jr., Minot, A. S., Rainey, J., Pilcher, C., and Harrison, T. R. Mechanism of experimental uremia. *Arch. Intern. Med.* 60:312, 1937.

187. Massry, S. G., Coburn, J. W., Chapman, L. W., and Kleeman, C. R. The effect of NaCl infusion on urinary Ca and Mg during reduction in their filtered loads. *Amer. J. Physiol.* 213:1218, 1967.

188. Merihas, G., Samartzis, M., and Marhetos, S. Massive cardiac tamponade in uremic pericarditis with complete recovery. *New Eng. J. Med.* 266:1089, 1962.

189. Merrill, J. P. *The Treatment of Renal Failure.* New York: Grune & Stratton, 1965.

190. Merrill, J. P., Legrain, M., and Hoigne, R. Observations on the role of urea in uremia. *Amer. J. Med.* 14:519, 1953.

191. Michie, A. J., Michie, C. R., and Ragni, M. C. Kidney function in unilateral pyelonephritis: II. Physiologic interpretations. *Amer. J. Med.* 22:190, 1957.

192. Montgomerie, J. Z., Kalmanson, G. M., and Guze, L. B. Renal failure and infection. *Medicine* (Balt.) 47:1, 1968.

193. Morrin, P. A. F., Bricker, N. S., and Kime, S. W., Jr. An evaluation of the acidifying capacity of the chronically diseased kidney in the experimental animal. *J. Clin. Invest.* 39:1013, 1960.

194. Mudge, G. H. Disorders of renal tubular function. *Amer. J. Med.* 20:448, 1956.

195. Mudge, G. H. General Discussion. In Quinn, E. L., and Kass, E. H. (Eds.), *Biology of Pyelonephritis.* (Henry Ford Hospital International Symposium.) Boston: Little, Brown, 1960. P. 361.

196. Nesson, H. R., and Robbins, S. L. Glomerulonephritis in older age groups. *Arch. Intern. Med.* (Chicago) 105:23, 1960.

197. Nickel, J. F., Lowrance, P. B., Leifer, E., and Bradley, S. E. Renal function, electrolyte excretion and body fluids in patients with chronic renal insufficiency before and after sodium deprivation. *J. Clin. Invest.* 32:68, 1953.

198. Nidus, B. D., Matalon, R., Cantacyzino, D., and Eisinger, R. P. Uremic pleuritis — a clinico-pathological entity. *New Eng. J. Med.* 281:255, 1969.

199. Olbrich, O., Woodford-Williams, E., Irvine, R. E., and Webster, D. Renal function in prostatism. *Lancet* 1:1322, 1957.

200. Oliver, J. When is the kidney not a kidney? *J. Urol.* 63:373, 1950.

201. Oliver, J., Bloom, F., and MacDowell, M. Structural and functional transformations in the tubular epithelium of the dog's kidney in chronic Bright's disease and their relation to mechanisms of renal compensation and failure. *J. Exp. Med.* 73:141, 1941.

202. Olsen, N. S., and Bassett, J. W. Blood levels of urea nitrogen, phenol, guanidine and creatinine in uremia. *Amer. J. Med.* 10:52, 1951.

203. Oppenheimer, B. S., and Fishberg, A. M. Hypertensive encephalopathy. *Arch. Intern. Med.* 41:264, 1928.

204. Orloff, J., and Berliner, R. W. The mechanism of the excretion of ammonia in the dog. *J. Clin. Invest.* 35:223, 1956.

205. Orlowski, T., and Bricker, N. S. The relationship between renal function and the direct glomerular count in normal dogs. *Acta Med. Pol.* 5:247, 1964.

206. Palmer, W. W., and Henderson, L. J. A study of the several factors of acid excretion in nephritis. *Arch. Intern. Med.* 16:109, 1915.

207. Perkoff, G. T., Thomas, G. L., Newton, J. D., Sellman, J. C., and Tyler, F. H. Mechanism of impaired glucose tolerance in uremia and experimental hyperazotemia. *Diabetes* 7:375, 1958.

208. Pillay, V. K. G., Schwartz, F. D., Aimi, K., and Kark, R. M. Transient and permanent deafness following treatment with ethacrynic acid in renal failure. *Lancet* 1: 77, 1969.

209. Platt, R. Sodium and potassium excretion in chronic renal failure. *Clin. Sci.* 9:367, 1950.

210. Platt, R. Structural and functional adaptation in renal failure. *Brit. Med. J.* 1:1313, 1372, 1952.

211. Prasad, A. S., Flink, E. B., and Zinneman, H. H. The base binding property of the serum proteins with respect to magnesium. *J. Lab. Clin. Med.* 54:357, 1959.

212. Preswick, G., and Jeremy, D. Subclinical polyneuropathy in renal insufficiency. *Lancet* 2:731, 1964.

213. Preuss, H. G., Massry, S. G., Maher, J. F., Gilliece, M., and Schreiner, G. E. Effects of uremic sera on renal tubular p-aminohippurate transport. *Nephron* 3:265, 1966.

214. Raaschou, F. *Studies of Chronic Pyelonephritis.* Copenhagen: Ejnar Munksgaard, 1948.

215. Raisz, L. G., Au, W. Y., and Scheer, R. L. Studies on the renal concentrating mechanism: IV. Osmotic diuresis. *J. Clin. Invest.* 38:1725, 1959.

216. Rapoport, S., Brodsky, W. A., West, C. D., and Mackler, B. Urinary flow and excretion of solutes during osmotic diuresis in hydropenic man. *Amer. J. Physiol.* 156:433, 1949.

217. Rath, C. E., Mailliard, J. A., and Schreiner, G. E. Bleeding tendency in uremia. *New Eng. J. Med.* 257:808, 1957.

218. Rector, F. C., Jr., and Seldin, D. W. Influence of unreabsorbed anions on renal threshold and Tm for bicarbonate. *Amer. J. Physiol.* 202:313, 1962.

219. Rector, F. C., Jr., Sellman, J. C., Martinez-Maldonado, M., and Seldin, D. W. The mechanism of suppression of proximal tubular reabsorption by saline infusions. *J. Clin. Invest.* 46:47, 1967.

220. Reiss, E., Canterbury, J. M., and Egdahl, R. H. Experience with a radioimmunoassay of parathyroid hormone in human sera. *Trans. Ass. Amer. Physicians* 21:104, 1968.

221. Relman, A. S., and Schwartz, W. B. The nephropathy of potassium depletion: A clinical and pathological entity. *New Eng. J. Med.* 255:195, 1956.

222. Relman, A. S., and Schwartz, W. B. The kidney in potassium depletion. *Amer. J. Med.* 24:764, 1958.

223. Relman, A. S., Shelburne, P. F., and Talman, A. Profound acidosis resulting from excessive ammonium chloride in previously healthy subjects: A study of two cases. *New Eng. J. Med.* 264:848, 1961.

224. Rendich, R. A., Levy, A. H., and Cove, A. M. Pulmonary manifestations of azotemia. *Amer. J. Roentgen.* 46:802, 1941.

225. Richards, P., Metcalfe-Gibson, A., Ward, E. E., Wrong, O., and Houghton, B. J. Utilization of ammonia nitrogen for protein synthesis in man, and the effect of protein restriction and uremia. *Lancet* 2:845, 1967.

226. Report of *The Committee on Chronic Dialysis* ("Gottschalk" Report). Sept. 1967.

227. Rieselbach, R. E., Shankel, S. W., Slatapolsky, E., Lubowitz, H., and Bricker, N. S. Glucose titration studies in patients with chronic progressive renal disease. *J. Clin. Invest.* 46:157, 1967.

228. Rieselbach, R. E., Todd, L., Rosenthal, M., and Bricker, N. S. The functional adaptation of the diseased kidney: II. Maximum rate of transport of PAH and the influence of acetate. *J. Lab. Clin. Med.* 64:724, 1964.

229. Roberts, K. E., Randall, H. T., Vanamee, P., and Poppell, J. W. Renal mechanisms involved in bicarbonate reabsorption. *Metabolism* 5:404, 1956.

230. Robinson, R. R., Murdaugh, H. V., Jr., and Peschel, E. Renal factors responsible for the hypermagnesemia of renal disease. *J. Lab. Clin. Med.* 53:572, 1959.

231. Robson, A. M., Srivastava, P. L., and Bricker, N. S. The influence of saline loading on renal glucose reabsorption. *J. Clin. Invest.* 47:329, 1968.

232. Roscoe, M. H. Anaemia and nitrogen retention in patients with chronic renal failure. *Lancet* 1:444, 1952.

233. Roussak, J. J., and Oleesky, S. Water losing nephritis — a syndrome simulating diabetes insipidus. *Quart. J. Med.* 23:147, 1954.

234. Sanford, J. P. Personal communication, 1969.

235. Sanford, J. P., and Belli, J. A. The occurrence of azotemia in pneumococcal pneumonia. *Amer. Rev. Resp. Dis.* 83:704, 1961.

236. Scalettar, R., Rubini, M. E., and Meroney, W. H. Report of two cases of massive hemorrhage resulting from causes other than uremic enterocolitis. *New Eng. J. Med.* 257:211, 1957.

237. Scherr, L., Ogden, D. A., Mead, A. W., Spritz, N., and Rubin, A. L. Management of hyperkalemia with a cation exchange resin. *New Eng. J. Med.* 264:115, 1961.

238. Schwartz, W. B., Hall, P. W., Hays, R. M., and Relman, A. S. On the mechanism of acidosis in chronic renal disease. *J. Clin. Invest.* 38:39, 1959.

239. Schwarz, K. C., Cohen, B. D., Labash, G. D., and Rubin, A. L. Severe acidosis and hyperpotassemia treated with sodium bicarbonate infusion. *Circulation* 19:215, 1959.

240. Scribner, B. H., and Burnell, J. M. Interpretation of the serum potassium concentration. *Metabolism* 5:468, 1956.

241. Scribner, B. H., Fergus, E. B., Boen, S. T., and Thomas, E. D. Some therapeutic approaches to chronic renal insufficiency. *Ann. Rev. Med.* 16:285, 1965.

242. Seldin, D. W., Coleman, A. J., Carter, N. W., and Rector, F. C., Jr. The effect of Na_2SO_4 on urinary acidification in chronic renal disease. *J. Lab. Clin. Med.* 69:893, 1967.

243. Seldin, D. W., Welt, L. G., and Cort, J. H. The role of sodium salts and adrenal steroids in the production of hypokalemic alkalosis. *Yale J. Biol. Med.* 29:229, 1956.

244. Seligson, D., Bluemle, L. W., Jr., Webster, G. D., Jr., and Senesky, D. Organic acids in body fluids of the uremic patient. *J. Clin. Invest.* 38:1042, 1959.

245. Shanes, A. M. Electrochemical aspects of physiological and pharmacological action in excitable cells: II. The action potential and excitation. *Pharmacol. Rev.* 10:165, 1958.

246. Shankel, S. W., Robson, A. M., and Bricker, N. S. On the mechanism of the splay in the glucose titration curve in advanced experimental renal disease in the rat. *J. Clin. Invest.* 46:164, 1967.

247. Shaw, A. B., Bazzard, F. F., Booth, E. M., Nilwarangkur, S., and Berlyne, G. M. The treatment of chronic renal failure by a modified Giovannetti diet. *Quart. J. Med.* 34:237, 1965.

248. Shear, L., Shinaberger, J. J., and Barry, K. G. Peritoneal transport of antibiotics in man. *New Eng. J. Med.* 272:666, 1965.

249. Shils, M. E. Renal disease and the metabolic effects of tetracycline. *Ann. Intern. Med.* 58:389, 1963.

250. Shohl, A. T. The effect of the acid-base content of the diet upon the production and cure of rickets with special reference to citrates. *J. Nutr.* 14:69, 1937.

251. Silverman, S. H., and Gardner, L. J. Ultrafiltration studies on serum magnesium. *New Eng. J. Med.* 250:938, 1954.

252. Simmons, D. H., and Avedon, M. Acid-base alterations and plasma potassium concentration. *Amer. J. Physiol.* 197:319, 1959.

253. Slatapolsky, E., Elkan, I. O., Weerts, C., and Bricker, N. S. Studies on the characteristics of the control system governing sodium excretion in uremic man. *J. Clin. Invest.* 47:521, 1968.

254. Slatapolsky, E., Gradowska, L., Kashemsant, C., Keltner, R., Manley, C., and Bricker, N. S. The control of phosphate excretion in uremia. *J. Clin. Invest.* 45:672, 1966.

255. Slatapolsky, E., Robson, A. M., Elkan, I., and Bricker, N. S. Control of phosphate excretion in uremic man. *J. Clin. Invest.* 47:1865, 1968.

256. Smith, P. K., Winkler, A. W., and Hoff, H. E. Electrocardiographic changes and concentration of magnesium in serum following intravenous injection of magnesium salts. *Amer. J. Physiol.* 126:720, 1939.

257. Smith, P. K., Winkler, A. W., and Hoff, H. E. The pharmacological actions of par-

enterally administered magnesium salts: A review. *Anesthesiology* 3:323, 1942.

258. Smith, W. O., and Hammarsten, J. F. Serum magnesium in renal disease. *A.M.A. Arch. Intern. Med.* 102:5, 1958.

259. Smythe, C. M., and Baroody, N. B. Hepatic-type "flapping tremor" occurring in patients without hepatic disease. *J.A.M.A.* 165:31, 1957.

260. Sorensen, M. K., and Kopple, J. D. Assessment of adherence to protein restricted diets during conservative management of uremia. *Amer. J. Clin. Nutr.* 21:631, 1968.

261. Stanbury, S. W. Azotaemic renal osteodystrophy. *Brit. Med. Bull.* 13:57, 1957.

262. Stanbury, S. W., Lumb, G. A., and Nicholson, W. F. Elective subtotal parathyroidectomy for renal hyperparathyroidism. *Lancet* 1:793, 1960.

263. Stanbury, S. W., and Mahler, R. F. Salt-wasting renal disease. *Quart. J. Med.* 28:425, 1959.

264. Steinmetz, P. R., and Kiley, J. E. Hyperkalemia in renal failure. *J.A.M.A.* 175:689, 1961.

265. Strauss, M. B. Clinical and pathological aspects of cystic disease of the renal medulla: An analysis of eighteen cases. *Ann. Intern. Med.* 57:373, 1962.

266. Suhrland, L. G., and Weisberger, A. S. Chloramphenicol toxicity in liver and renal disease. *Arch. Intern. Med.* (Chicago) 112:747, 1963.

267. Suki, W., Eknoyan, G., Rector, F. C., Jr., and Seldin, D. W. Patterns of nephron perfusion in acute and chronic hydronephrosis. *J. Clin. Invest.* 45:122, 1966.

268. Suki, W. N., Hull, A. R., Rector, F. C., Jr., and Seldin, D. W. Mechanism of the effect of thiazide diuretics on calcium and uric acid. *Clin. Res.* 15:78, 1967.

269. Suki, W. N., Martinez-Maldonado, M., Rouse, D., and Terry, A. Effect of expansion of extracellular fluid volume on renal phosphate handling. *J. Clin. Invest.* 48:1888, 1969.

270. Swan, R. C., and Merrill, J. P. The clinical course of acute renal failure. *Medicine* (Balt.) 32:215, 1953.

271. Symons, H. S., and Wrong, O. M. Uremic pericarditis with cardiac tamponade: A report of four cases. *Brit. Med. J.* 1:605, 1964.

272. Teschan, P. E., Post, R. S., Smith, L. H., Jr., Abernathy, R. S., Davis, J. H., Gray, D. M., Howard, J. M., Johnson, K. E., Klapp, E., Mundy, R. L., O'Meara, M. P., and Rush, F. B. Post-traumatic renal insufficiency in military casualties: I. Clinical characteristics. *Amer. J. Med.* 18:172, 1955.

273. Thaysen, J. H. Anabolic Steroids in the Treatment of Renal Failure. In Gross, F. (Ed.), *Protein Metabolism.* Berlin: Springer-Verlag, 1962.

274. Thorn, G. W., Koepf, G. F., and Clinton, M., Jr. Renal failure simulating adrenocortical insufficiency. *New Eng. J. Med.* 231:76, 1944.

275. Tobian, L. Interrelationship of electrolytes, juxtaglomerular cells and hypertension. *Physiol. Rev.* 40:280, 1960.

276. Verel, D., Turnbull, A., Tudhope, G. R., and Ross, J. H. Anaemia in Bright's disease. *Quart. J. Med.* 28:491, 1959.

277. Wacker, W., and Merrill, J. P. Uremic pericarditis in acute and chronic renal failure. *J.A.M.A.* 156:764, 1954.

278. Walser, M. Calcium clearance as a function of sodium clearance in the dog. *Amer. J. Physiol.* 200:1099, 1961.

279. Walser, M. The separate effects of hyperparathyroidism, hypercalcemia of malignancy, renal failure and acidosis on the state of calcium, phosphate, and other ions in plasma. *J. Clin. Invest.* 41:1454, 1962.

280. Walser, M., and Bodenlos, L. J. Urea metabolism in man. *J. Clin. Invest.* 38:1617, 1959.

281. Welt, L. G., Hollander, W., Jr., and Blythe, W. B. The consequences of potassium depletion. *J. Chronic Dis.* 11:213, 1960.

282. Welt, L. G., and Peters, J. P. Acute renal failure; lower nephron nephrosis. *Yale J. Biol. Med.* 24:221, 1951.

283. Welt, L. G., Sachs, J. R., and McManus, T. J. An ion transport defect in erythrocytes from uremic patients. *Trans. Ass. Amer. Physicians* 77:169, 1964.

284. Welt, L. G., Smith, E. K. M., Dunn, M. J., Czerwinski, N., Proctor, H., Cole, C., Balfe, J. W., and Gitelman, H. J. Membrane transport defect: The sick cell. *Trans. Ass. Amer. Physicians* 80:217, 1967.

285. Westervelt, F. B., Jr., and Schreiner, G. E. The carbohydrate intolerance of uremic patients. *Ann. Intern. Med.* 57:266, 1962.

286. White, M. G. Bartter's syndrome (BS): A manifestation of primary renal tubular reabsorptive defects. *Clin. Res.* 18:67, 1970.

287. Wildenthal, K., Mierzwiak, D. S., Myers, R. M., and Mitchell, J. H. Effects of acute lactic acidosis on left ventricular perfor-mance. *Amer. J. Physiol.* 214:1352, 1968.

288. Williams, J. L., and Dich, G. F. The excretion of nonprotein nitrogen by the intestine. *J.A.M.A.* 100:484, 1933.

289. Winkler, A. W., Smith, P. K., and Hoff, H. E. Intravenous magnesium sulfate in the treatment of nephritic convulsions in adults. *J. Clin. Invest.* 21:207, 1942.

290. Wrong, O., and Davies, H. E. F. The excretion of acid in renal disease. *Quart. J. Med.* 28:259, 1959.

291. Wynn, V., and Rob, C. J. Water intoxication: Differential diagnosis of the hypotonic syndromes. *Lancet* 1:587, 1954.

7

Hematologic Aspects of Renal Failure

A. J. Erslev and S. S. Shapiro

Pallor and purpura are two of the most visible and dramatic manifestations of chronic renal failure. For years they have served both as valuable diagnostic clues for the clinician and as challenges for the pathophysiologist. Recent experimental and clinical observations have provided a great deal of information about the pathogeneses of pallor and of purpura, and they have shown the existence of close pathophysiologic relationships between kidney function, red cell kinetics, and blood coagulation. In this chapter an attempt is made to describe and document these relationships under the headings "Anemia and Renal Failure" and "Fibrin Deposition and Renal Failure."

Anemia and Renal Failure

Among the many signs and symptoms of chronic renal failure, anemia stands as a hallmark. It is almost invariably present, and it is directly related to the extent of renal impairment [135]. Figure 7-1 relates the hematocrit to the blood urea nitrogen (BUN) value in patients with chronic renal failure [82, 96, 136, 146, 160, 165, 263], and it shows a rough linear relationship at BUN levels of less than 100 mg. per 100 ml. A similar relationship has been found between hematocrit and creatinine or creatinine clearance [135]. However, at BUN levels above 100 mg. per 100 ml., the anemia does not become progressively more severe. This flattening of the hematocrit-BUN curve may be due in part to the fact that severely anemic patients tend to be treated with transfusions. Nevertheless, even untransfused patients reach a certain baseline hematocrit which appears to be maintained regardless of the degree of uremia.

The reduction in hematocrit is associated with a proportional reduction in hemoglobin concentration and red blood cell count, and on smear the red blood cells are usually normochromic and normocytic. Occasional cells may appear dense and deformed, exhibiting spicules, indentations, and intracellular blebs.

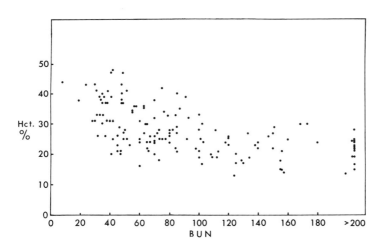

Figure 7-1. Relationship between BUN and hematocrit in 152 cases taken from references 82, 96, 136, 146, 160, 165, 263.

Such cells have been designated as "helmet cells," "triangular cells," or "Burr cells." Bell [17] has shown convincingly that these deformities are caused by the bursting of submembraneous vacuoles with loss of both volume and surface area of red cells. The deformities are more evident on dry blood smears than on wet preparations and may in part be caused by the mechanical trauma inherent in preparing a blood smear [56]. Reticulocytes are present, but in subnormal numbers when correlated to the degree of anemia, and the bone marrow likewise fails to disclose an appropriate increase in the number of nucleated red cells.

The total and differential leukocyte counts as well as the platelet count are usually normal in chronic renal failure and total hematopoiesis as judged from bone marrow smears, and sections do not appear substantially different from normal [42]. However, since renal failure can be caused by a great number of illnesses and be associated with many diverse complications, it is not surprising that the hematologic picture may vary considerably. The picture may be influenced by inflammatory changes as in pyelonephritis, by hypersplenism as in disseminated lupus erythematosus, by low serum iron as after uremic bleeding, or by protein derangements as in multiple myeloma or ne-

phrosis. Nevertheless, the anemia in patients with chronic renal failure appears to have a common denominator. In all cases the bone marrow fails to compensate adequately for an increased demand for red cells. The increased demand is believed to be caused by a shortened red cell life span and to a lesser extent by blood loss, while the inadequate bone marrow compensation is believed to be caused by a lack of erythropoietin. Recent observations on the effect of nephrectomy and dialysis suggest that hemolysis and blood loss are related to impaired renal excretory function, while the lack of erythropoietin is related to impaired renal endocrine function. Although each of these functions may be only moderately impaired, their combined action will invariably lead to the characteristic anemia of chronic renal failure.

EFFECTS OF IMPAIRED RENAL EXCRETORY
FUNCTION

Experimental and clinical studies of renal failure have suggested that uremia per se is responsible for a shortening in red cell life span, for an increased bleeding tendency, for bone marrow ineffectiveness, and for various other hematologic complications. A particular severe combination of hemolysis and bleeding tendency, the so-called hemolytic-uremic syndrome, may be caused by fibrin deposition rather than by azotemia, and is discussed separately.

Hydremia. The maintenance of a stable plasma volume depends at least in part on renal excretory function. In renal failure, the plasma volume may fluctuate rapidly, and the hematocrit becomes a better measure of dehydration or hypervolemia than of the total red cell mass. However, since oxygen transferred to the tissues depends both on hematocrit and on total blood volume [254], the low hematocrit in hydremia is offset by the corresponding increase in blood volume, and fluid-induced fluctuations in hematocrit are of little clinical consequence.

Decreased Red Blood Cell Life Span. Uremia appears to provide a particularly unfavorable environment for mature erythrocytes. The metabolic activities and life span of leukocytes are not known to be compromised, while erythrocytes often show morphologic changes, metabolic impairment, and shortened life span.

The presence of spicules and burr cells have already been referred to. These could be the consequence of toxic interference with the structural integrity of the red cell membrane. However, no known waste product retained has been shown to cause physical membrane alterations, and recent observations have suggested a mechanical cause. Normal red cells exposed to strong shearing stress will become deformed and fragmented [194], and the diffuse vascular changes frequently present in patients with hypertensive renal disease could expose circulatory red cells to undue mechanical stress. However, it does not seem reasonable to relate the presence of occasional burr cells in chronic renal failure to the shortening in red cell life span. Most investigators relate this shortening to changes in pH, ionic concentration, and solute composition in the environment of circulating red cells. Since mature erythrocytes have a limited capacity for detoxification and cytoplasmic renewal, their

survival is adversely influenced by such changes [101, 126, 184, 186]. Welt and co-workers [51, 269] have shown that uremic serum both in vivo and in vitro induces a reversible alteration in membrane ATPase and in the sodium pump. It has also been shown that glutathione stability is reduced [249] despite an apparently normal pentosephosphate shunt activity. These changes may not be very pronounced, but they indicate that a uremic environment can have an adverse effect on membrane stability and consequently on red cell survival.

It could be anticipated that the impairment in red cell metabolism and in red cell viability would be directly proportional to the severity of uremia. Indeed, Kurayanagi [145], Ragen et al. [208], Shaw [233], and Adamson et al. [3] have recently presented impressive data showing that the red cell life span depends directly on the BUN. However, many other studies of red cell life span in chronic renal disease do not suggest a linear relationship, and when 221 cases from the literature are tabulated (Fig. 7-2), the relationship becomes quite unconvincing [3, 48, 82, 136, 145, 146, 160, 208, 233, 240, 263]. The reason for the variable results is not clear, but it seems to be in accord with the literature on anemia of chronic renal disease, which since the days of Richard Bright has been characterized by confusing data. Although Figure 7-2 does not induce much confidence in the hypothesis that red cell life span depends on the degree of uremia, this hypothesis has received strong support from cross-transfusion studies. Red cells from uremic patients have been shown to survive normally in a healthy recipient, while normal red cells have a shortened life span in uremic recipients [63, 133]. In a few cases, it also appears that intensive dialysis tends to improve red cell viability [20]. In conclusion, it appears that most recent studies indicate that the red cell life span is inversely proportioned to the impairment in renal ex-

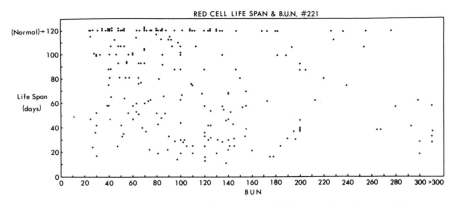

Figure 7-2. Relationship between BUN and calculated red cell life span from data on 221 cases provided by references 3, 48, 82, 136, 145, 146, 160, 208, 233, 240, 263.

cretory function, but that the accumulated data do not rule out the possibility that other still unknown factors may influence red cell viability in chronic renal disease.

Ineffective Red Cell Production. In many cases, erythrokinetic studies show decreased red cell utilization of radioactive iron despite normal turnover rates [160, 163]. Intensive long-term dialysis tends to improve the rate of utilization and also to raise the hematocrit and decrease transfusion requirements [82]. These results have in general been interpreted as suggesting that azotemia decreases the viability not only of mature red cells but also of red cell progenitors and causes ineffective red cell production [160]. However, Eschbach and co-workers [82] have suggested that the low iron utilization reflects increased parenchymal uptake of radioactive iron and that the improvement observed after intensive dialysis is not caused by less intramedullary destruction of red cells but by an actual increase in erythropoietic activity. The reason for such an erythropoietic stimulation is not clear, and it must be emphasized that both iron turnover and iron utilization may be perfectly normal despite severe azotemia.

Responsiveness to Erythropoietin. Administration of the erythropoietic hormone, erythropoietin, to uremic laboratory animals has

been shown to cause a subnormal response [28, 74]. It has also been noted in the few uremic human subjects who have received erythropoietin, that the erythropoietic effect appeared to be less than anticipated [150, 258]. Since this decreased responsiveness, at least in rabbits, is related to degree of uremia, it seems possible that the beneficial effect of chronic dialysis on red cell production [82] could in part be due to an increased effectiveness of remaining erythropoietin.

Lack of Iron, Folic Acid, and Transferrin. In patients with chronic renal failure, the disease process itself or the therapeutic management may lead to deficiencies which have an adverse effect on red cell production. In many cases of pyelonephritis, the inflammatory process may lead to a suppression of red cell production, ineffective iron utilization, and a low serum iron [25]. Low serum iron has also been encountered in patients who regularly lose small amounts of blood at each hemodialysis [3]. In addition, hemodialysis may lead to the loss of dialyzable folic acid and to megaloblastic anemia [114]. In a rare case, the urinary loss of transferrin in patients with the nephrotic syndrome has been reported to cause anemia [215]. Otherwise, nephrosis is not associated with development of an anemia similar to the anemia of chronic renal failure.

Bleeding Tendency. A hemorrhagic tendency is a common complication of severe azotemia, occurring in from one-third to one-half of all patients with renal failure [47, 65, 207, 226, 242]. Although often manifest only by minor purpuric lesions, abnormal bleeding may be of serious proportions, involving the gastrointestinal tract or the central nervous system, and has been held responsible for 6 per cent of deaths in acute renal failure [24, 164]. In addition, even a minor bleeding diathesis may interfere with proper management by preventing or complicating the use of diagnostic renal biopsy [33] and therapeutic hemodialysis [243].

Alterations in various components of the hemostatic mechanism have been reported in uremia. Changes in the plasma coagulation factors seem variable, and cannot account for the hemorrhagic tendency in the majority of cases [49, 65, 68, 137, 149, 157, 265, 271]. Approximately 20 per cent of patients with renal failure are thrombocytopenic, but platelet levels rarely fall below 50,000 per cubic millimeter and, in any case, do not correlate well with bleeding [42, 65, 83, 141, 198, 241, 242]. Since the platelet life span in nontransfused patients with uremia is normal [47, 241], it seems reasonable to assume that thrombocytopenia most often is due to a mild decrease in platelet production [137]. Whether this is to be ascribed to a direct toxic effect on the bone marrow, or to depressed production of a thrombopoiesis-stimulating factor [211, 229] is presently unknown. In some situations, particularly the hemolytic-uremic syndrome, thrombocytopenia may be related to intravascular coagulation and consequent peripheral overutilization of platelets. Because of its unusual pathogenetic mechanism, this syndrome is discussed more fully in a subsequent section.

Abnormal platelet *function* appears to be the major cause of the hemorrhagic tendency in uremia [41, 47, 49, 65, 124, 137, 141, 149, 157, 205, 207, 210, 226, 242, 265, 271]. In the normal individual, platelet aggregation is one of the earliest reactions to vascular damage [197]. At the site of vessel injury platelets rapidly adhere to exposed subintimal connective tissue. The adherent platelets release aggregating agents, primarily adenosine diphosphate (ADP), which mediate further growth of the platelet plug. Platelet plug formation is the primary mechanism of hemostasis in small-vessel injury, and it is this function of the circulating platelet which is measured clinically with the bleeding time. In somewhat larger vessels, complete hemostasis is also dependent upon the further action of the blood coagulation mechanism, and the eventual formation of fibrin. In these reactions, as well, the platelet serves an essential role through the release of a phospholipid complex — platelet factor 3 — required in several steps of the coagulation sequence [59]. This function of platelets is measured by the prothrombin consumption test, or by specific tests for platelet factor 3 [124, 207]. Platelet adhesiveness appears to depend upon integrity of the platelet membrane [166]. Although platelet factor 3 can be obtained in the test tube from nonviable platelets, physiologic release of this material may require, or at least be enhanced by, prior platelet aggregation [116] and thus may also depend in some way on membrane structure [166].

Both platelet aggregating ability and platelet factor 3 release are depressed in uremia [41, 47, 49, 65, 124, 137, 141, 149, 157, 205, 207, 210, 226, 242, 265, 271]. Using the Ivy technic, measured on the forearm, bleeding times are abnormal in nearly two-thirds of patients with renal failure, and are prolonged in nearly all patients with uremia who are bleeding [47, 226, 242]. The Duke bleeding time, measured on the ear lobe, has proved to be an insensitive test [47, 242] and probably should not be used. Adhesion of platelets to glass beads [225] and to cut surfaces [26] and platelet aggregation in response to ADP [27] also are subnormal in a majority of patients [47, 65, 205, 226, 242].

Release of platelet factor 3 is suboptimal in nearly 75 per cent of patients with renal failure, whether measured by the prothrombin consumption technic [226, 242, 265] or by more specific methods [47, 124, 207, 242]. It is necessary to standardize these tests carefully with respect to platelet numbers and to ensure optimal concentrations of plasma coagulation factors, if valid results are to be obtained. Diminished release of platelet factor 3 appears to be somewhat more common, but more poorly correlated with bleeding [207, 226, 242], than prolongation of the bleeding time, suggesting that the former represents a milder hemostatic defect than that induced by platelet adhesion-aggregation defects.

Poor clot retraction has been found in more than half of all patients with uremia [47, 207, 242]. The phenomenon of clot retraction is mediated by the ATP-dependent contraction of the platelet contractile protein, thrombasthenin [21], compacting the fibrin-platelet network of the clot. This platelet function, although differing in mechanism from those previously discussed, also requires a metabolically viable platelet. Despite its great biochemical interest, however, the physiologic importance of clot retraction remains unproved.

Several lines of evidence suggest that the abnormalities in platelet function seen in uremia are related to interaction of platelets with one or more abnormal components of uremic plasma. Thus, incubation of normal platelets with uremic plasma has been reported to cause defective ADP-induced platelet factor 3 release [124], and prolonged incubation of normal platelet extracts with uremic plasma is said to inactivate platelet factor 3 [41]. Furthermore, the bleeding tendency as well as the measured abnormalities in platelet function can be corrected by peritoneal or hemodialysis and by renal transplantation [47, 205, 207, 242].

Attempts to identify the abnormal plasma components have not yet proved successful. Although incubation of platelets in high concentrations of urea was reported to alter plate-

let activities [117], recent studies have failed to substantiate this finding [124, 226, 242]. Acute elevation of serum urea to 200 mg. per 100 ml. in normal subjects also failed to produce alterations in platelet function [47]. Finally, very little correlation has been found between defective platelet function and serum urea concentration [124, 242]. Creatinine and urate have also been investigated in vitro and found without effect on platelets [242].

Guanidino compounds have been shown to be inhibitors of ADP-induced platelet aggregation [132], and guanidinosuccinic acid has been found in increased concentrations in uremic urine [192]. Although some investigators report inhibition of ADP-induced platelet factor 3 release by this compound [124], others, using a slightly different technic, find it without effect [207].

In view of the ADP-dependent, membrane-mediated nature of platelet aggregation and platelet factor 3 release, the observation in patients with uremia of an erythrocyte-membrane defect associated with altered membrane-ATPase activity [51, 269] takes on added significance. Similar studies with platelets from normal subjects and patients with uremia would be of great interest.

Therapy of the uremic bleeding tendency is best accomplished by dialysis. Peritoneal dialysis and hemodialysis appear equally effective, although peritoneal dialysis may have fewer complications in this situation [242]. Clinical improvement usually is seen after a single dialysis [47, 242, 265], but platelet abnormalities may respond at variable rates, and multiple dialyses may be required before total correction occurs [207]. Both platelet numbers and function respond to this therapy, and the blood platelet concentration may continue to rise for several days after dialysis [25, 207, 242, 265]. In cases of severe bleeding it may be prudent to prepare the patient for dialysis with fresh platelet concentrates, especially when hemodialysis is planned. Occasionally, when a coagulation factor deficiency exists, stored or fresh-frozen plasma may also be indicated.

Screening of patients with renal failure for a hemorrhagic tendency is always requested prior to contemplated renal biopsy or hemodialysis. As has been indicated, the most common abnormalities among the more readily available hemostatic tests are a prolonged bleeding time, poor clot retraction, and deficient prothrombin consumption. Unfortunately, the frequency of abnormal results greatly exceeds the incidence of clinical bleeding, limiting somewhat the usefulness of screening procedures. Of any single test, the bleeding time appears to correlate best with the hemorrhagic tendency. Normal results are useful in ruling out a hemorrhagic diathesis, whereas uniformly abnormal results would probably contraindicate renal biopsy.

Perhaps with further refinements of testing and with a better understanding of the precise mechanism of the acquired platelet defects in uremia, adequate screening procedures will be developed. Until that time, however, clinical judgment, based upon close observation of the patient for hemorrhagic phenomena and for the presence of complicating factors such as hypertension, remains decisive in the management of bleeding complications in renal failure.

EFFECTS OF IMPAIRED RENAL
ENDOCRINE FUNCTION

In 1957 Jacobson and co-workers [127] reported that nephrectomized, uremic rats fail to respond to blood loss with a reticulocytosis, while ureter-ligated and equally uremic rats respond in an almost normal manner. This important observation established the kidney as a crucial link in the feedback chain controlling the rate of red cell production and the size of the red cell mass. It also suggested that the anemia of chronic renal failure could be caused by a decreased production or release of a renal erythropoietic hormone.

Physiologic Control of Red Cell Production. The red cell mass is an organ designed almost exclusively for the purpose of carrying oxygen from the lungs to the tissues. It is maintained at a functionally optimal size by the bone marrow which is tuned to the body's need for oxygen. Since the classic observations at the turn of the century by Bert, by Mischer, and by Carnot and Deflanders [87], it has been recognized that this tuning must be initiated by the tissue tension of oxygen and may be mediated by a hormone. More recent studies [87] have established that low tissue tension of oxygen results in the appearance of a humoral erythropoietic factor, named erythropoietin, and that this factor probably is responsible for the physiologic adjustment of red cell production to the demands for oxygen-carrying capacity [73, 128]

Erythropoietin was first demonstrated and quantitated by its capacity to induce a reticulocytosis in normal animals [72]. The present method of measurement is still a bioassay, but it is more sophisticated [54]. In order to abolish endogenous erythropoietin production the assay animals, i.e., mice or rats, are first rendered polycythemic by transfusion or exposure to hypoxia; starvation can also be used but is less reliable. The erythropoietic response to the assayed material is then measured most conveniently and accurately by determining the red cell utilization of radioactive iron. Using this technic, a linear relationship has been demonstrated between hemoglobin concentration and erythropoietin titers at hemoglobin levels below 10 gm. per 100 ml. [259]. At hemoglobin levels above 10 gm. per 100 ml. there is no detectable erythropoietic activity of serum, suggesting that erythropoietin may not be involved in the fine adjustments of red cell production. However, assays of appropriately concentrated urine have established a proportional relationship between 24-hour excretion of erythropoietin and hemoglobin concentrations ranging from polycythemic to anemic values [3]. At normal hemoglobin concentration "normal" men excrete about 2.8 units per day, while "normal" women excrete 0.9 units per day [5]. It has also been demonstrated that the administration of antierythropoietin to normal mice reduces the rate of red cell production [228]. These findings indicate that the level of erythropoietin in plasma determines the rate of red cell production not only in severe anemia but at all hemoglobin concentrations.

In the bone marrow, erythropoietin is believed to act primarily, if not exclusively, on a pool of self-sustaining, erythropoietin-sensitive stem cells [8, 75, 86]. In vitro and in vivo studies of the kinetics of red cell renewal suggest that erythropoietin is responsible for the production of a messenger RNA which initiates both a differentiation and a division of these stem cells [76, 140]. The differentiation transforms stem cells into hemoglobin-synthesizing pronormoblasts, and the division prevents the stem cell pool from becoming depleted. The further proliferation and maturation of erythroid cells do not appear to be controlled by erythropoietin. Intense erythropoietic stimulation appears to lead to an early release of large reticulocytes which may have a shorter-than-normal life span [245]. However, this inappropriate response may be a pharmacologic rather than a physiologic effect of erythropoietin since less intense exposure to erythropoietin leads to the formation of normal red cells with a normal life span [257].

In conclusion, the physiologic control of red cell production appears to involve a feedback loop between the bone marrow and the kidney, mediated in one direction by red-cell-bound oxygen and in the opposite by erythropoietin.

Erythropoietin: Biochemical Structure. Extensive purification of erythropoietin has so far not led to a biochemically well-defined compound [161]. However, recent studies have suggested strongly that it is a protein or carried by a protein with a molecular weight of 65,000 [199]. It contains sialic acid, is electrophoretically an interalpha globulin, and has been found to be quite stable when stored at $-20°$ or $4°C.$ [104]. It retains most of its biologic activity after heating to $100°C.$ for a few minutes. Erythropoietin isolated from urine may be less stable than erythropoietin isolated from plasma, but evidence for the existence of a stabilizing carrier protein in plasma is still not too convincing [183].

Erythropoietin: Production and Metabolism. As mentioned above, it is generally accepted that erythropoietin is produced in the kidneys [108]. Nephrectomized animals and human beings do not release erythropoietin in response to tissue hypoxia, and patients with chronic renal failure do not as a rule have measurable amounts of erythropoietin in plasma or urine despite even severe anemia [35, 96, 112, 188]. Kidney transplantation in anephric human beings has also been shown to be followed by resumption in the production of erythropoietin and by an accelerated rate of red cell production [1, 62].

The production or release of erythropoietin has been linked to the renal tissue tension of oxygen. Reduction in arterial blood supply to the kidneys may both experimentally [90, 115] and clinically [125, 162] lead to erythropoietin release and to erythrocytosis. However, the inconsistency with which this occurs, makes it seem possible that other changes in the renal parenchyma play a modifying or contributory role. Such changes have also been invoked to explain conflicting results from studies of in vitro perfusion of isolated kidneys [81, 88, 144, 212]. It has been suggested that the physiologic release of erythropoietin is too gradual to be measurable in a short time experiment and only when hypoxia is severe enough to cause tissue injury is it possible experimentally to demonstrate renal release of erythropoietin. Such injury may occur after injection of plastic microspheres into the renal artery [2], or after inducing parenchymal pressure by injecting plastic under the renal capsule [179]. This hypothetical mechanism may also be invoked to explain an increase in erythropoietin which often heralds rejection of a transplanted kidney [270] or the inappropriate production of erythropoietin in renal cysts, renal hydronephrosis, and renal neoplasms [266].

Erythropoietin is released in excessive amounts immediately after a hypoxic or anemic exposure, but the plasma level returns to only moderately elevated values 48 to 72 hours later. The reason for the initial overshoot is unknown, but it has been claimed that the subsequent reduction in plasma concentration is caused by an increased consumption by the activated erythroid tissue [246]. The decrease is probably not due to urinary loss since the renal clearance of erythropoietin is quite small. Weintraub and co-workers [268] were able to recover less than 5 per cent of injected sheep erythropoietin in the urine of a dog, and they calculated erythropoietin clearance to be from 0.1 to 0.6 ml. per minute, very similar to the clearance rate determined by Rosse and Waldmann on endogenous human erythropoietin [221]. These latter two authors also estimated the half-life of erythropoietin in humans to be 25 hours, with a range from 7 to 42 hours.

Erythropoietin: Cellular Site of Production. The site of erythropoietin production in the kidney is still unknown. Due to its generous perfusion rate, the renal cortex is maintained at a high oxygen pressure and would not be expected to be particularly sensitive to changes in oxygen-carrying capacity of blood. However, the medulla is less favored, and since it also has a considerable oxygen consumption, it theoretically would be an area suitable as an "oxygen-stat" [108]. Nevertheless, most attention has been directed at the cortex and here at the juxtaglomerular

cells (J.G. cells). Several authors have claimed a possible relationship between the production and release of renin and that of erythropoietin, [61, 120, 178]. The granularity of the J.G. cells has been reported by some to be increased after both blood loss and exposure to low oxygen tension, while others believe that the increase in granularity reflects a loss of blood volume, not a change in oxygen tension [103]. An attempt to use fluorescin-labeled antierythropoietin to pinpoint the cellular site of production merely revealed that the glomerular tuft, the site of possible erythropoietin filtration, shows fluorescence [16, 91]. Studies by Gordon and co-workers [108] indicate that the nuclear fraction or more specifically the light mitochondrial fraction of a kidney homogenate contains an enzyme capable of generating erythropoietin from an inactive circulating plasma factor. Although the site of production of this renal enzyme has not been determined, the activation procedure is so similar to that of the renin-angiotensin system that it is tempting to locate the site of production in the J.G. apparatus. However, these studies as well as similar studies by Kuratowska [143] are difficult to interpret or duplicate since they deal with the demonstration of small amounts of erythropoietin in a system which may contain a strong erythropoietin inhibitor. Erslev and Kazal have recently confirmed the work by Fisher and co-workers [89], and shown that renal homogenates contain a factor which in a nonenzymatic manner inactivates erythropoietin [79]. The possible physiologic significance of this factor is not clear. It has been suggested that it may contribute to the anemia of chronic renal disease by being released from the injured kidney [89]. However, its presence in liver and spleen extracts [79], the lack of inactivating property in most sera from uremic patients, and the similarities between the anemia in anephric and in nephritic patients make this suggestion somewhat untenable. It seems more likely that this inhibitor is responsible for the lack of success which has characterized almost all attempts to isolate erythropoietic material from kidney extracts.

Erythropoiesis in the Anephric Patient. The recent perfection of shunt dialysis has made it possible to evaluate erythropoietic function in the absence of renal erythropoietin. It was early realized that bilateral nephrectomy in rabbits or rats does not lead to erythroid aplasia [77, 213]. A low, constant rate of red cell production remains unresponsive to conditions which in the normal animal cause an increase or decrease in the rate of red cell production. A similar low constant level of erythropoiesis remains if endogenous erythropoietin production is suppressed by hypertransfusion [78]. The attainment of an autonomous baseline production of red cells has been shown most clearly in the anephric patient who has been kept in good condition, with minimal azotemia, for long periods [193]. In 2 anephric patients Erslev and co-workers found that induced changes in hemoglobin concentration from a low of 5 gm. per 100 ml. to a high of 18 gm. per 100 ml. did not change the rate of red cell production as assesed by absolute reticulocyte counts and iron turnover rates [80]. However, the conclusion that the bone marrow in the absence of renal erythropoietin reverts to a constant autonomous rate of red cell production has been challenged. In one anephric patient reported on by Nathan and co-workers [193], a severe acute blood loss appeared to cause an appropriate increase in red cell production, while transfusions to anephric patients by Naets and Wittek [189] appeared to decrease the percentage of normoblasts in the bone marrow. In patients with renal disease on chronic renal dialysis, Adamson and co-workers [3] found a suppression of erythropoiesis in response to transfusion, a response that they believed was not mediated by the nonfunctioning kidney. Further studies on anephric patients are obviously needed to determine whether or not there is an extrarenal regulatory system, possibly mediated by extrarenal erythropoietin.

Inappropriate Secretion of Erythropoietin. Erythrocytosis secondary to inappropriate secretion of erythropoietin has been reported with increasing frequency. Renal neoplasms, particularly hypernephromas [58, 266] but also a few cases of Wilms' tumor [187], and benign tumors [60] have been associated causally with erythrocytosis. The frequency of this complication in hypernephromas appears to be about 2 to 4 per cent, but in only a much smaller number has it been possible to demonstrate high levels of erythropoietin in blood or tumor extract [266]. In one case we found increased concentration of erythropoietin in extract from the tumor, but not in extract from the adjoining kidney tissue, suggesting initially that the release of erythropoietin comes from the tumor and not from compressed "hypoxic" normal kidney. However, as mentioned above, the presence of a strong erythropoietin inhibitor in normal kidney extract makes this conclusion untenable. The association of erythrocytosis with polycystic kidney disease [67, 95, 214, 222], with solitary renal cysts [264], and with hydronephrosis [53, 71, 131, 151, 167] also emphasizes the fact that we still do not know the source of the inappropriate secretion of erythropoietin. Erythrocytosis, presumably caused by inappropriate renal secretion of erythropoietin, has been reported in a few patients with arteriosclerotic renal artery stenosis [125, 162] and in some patients after renal transplantation [123, 195]. The rare association of uterine tumor with erythrocytosis [93, 175] may be caused by physical interference with the renal blood supply, but uterine production of erythropoietin has not been ruled out. Extrarenal, inappropriate secretion of an erythropoietin-like material has been reported in 2 anephric patients [80, 191] as well as in a number of patients with neoplasms, especially hepatomas [36] and cerebellar hemangioblastomas [118,

220]. It appears as if a number of tissues can elaborate erythropoietin-like material, but whether or not this is of physiologic significance is still an open question.

MANAGEMENT

Anemia in chronic renal failure is usually of only moderate severity, but because of associated hypertension, diffuse vascular disease, or fluid retention, it may become symptomatic at levels otherwise well tolerated. Several studies of patients in whom hemoglobin concentration has been restored to normal by means of intensive transfusion therapy have suggested that a normal oxygen-carrying capacity of blood does not benefit renal function in patients with chronic renal disease [34, 174]. On the contrary, in a few transfused patients there may even be an aggravation of renal impairment, possibly related to a reduction in effective renal plasma flow. Consequently, the optimal hemoglobin concentration for a patient with chronic renal disease appears to be that concentration which will cause the least subjective discomfort and can be maintained with the least therapeutic effort.

In renal failure hemoglobin concentrations of less than 7 to 8 gm. per 100 ml. are often symptomatic as gauged by the subjective benefits derived from transfusions. At present, the judicious use of a single unit of packed red cells appears to be the optimal treatment. Whole blood, whether "fresh" or "old," should as far as possible be avoided since the infused plasma is not sufficient to correct possible coagulation defects and may be harmful because of the calcium-binding anticoagulant and because of blood volume expansion. Even single units of packed red cells can be dangerous for a patient with borderline cardiac decompensation, and all transfusion therapy has to be carefully planned and competently executed.

It is obviously imperative, before transfusion therapy is contemplated, to rule out all treatable conditions that could contribute to the anemia. As mentioned before, dialysis in some patients leads to a loss of iron and folic acid, and in other patients iron deficiency may occur because of uremic bleeding or iron malabsorption [3]. On the other hand, iron overload may follow multiple transfusion and attempts to remove iron by chelation with desferrioxamine have been claimed to be a worthwhile procedure [255].

Since azotemia plays an important role in the pathogenesis of the anemia, treatment with peritoneal or hemodialysis would be anticipated to ameliorate the anemia. Eschbach and co-workers [82] have shown that intensive dialysis is of considerable benefit, not only by correcting premature red cell destruction but also by rendering the bone marrow more efficient. In addition, other authors have reported that correction of an elevated BUN will diminish platelet dysfunction and the excessive bleeding tendency [25, 207, 242, 265]. It seems almost certain that the increasing use of regular home-dialysis technics will render the anemia far more manageable and will diminish the need for therapeutic transfusions.

However, the elimination of anemia in chronic renal failure will, at least in theory, not be accomplished until erythropoietin is available for therapeutic use. Only a few patients with renal failure have received therapeutic trials with this hormone [150, 258], but the clinical data from these cases support the conclusions drawn from animal work that erythropoietin eventually will be the specific and preferred agent for the treatment of anemia in chronic renal failure. At the present, erythropoietin in adequate amounts is available only as impure preparations obtained from the plasma of anemic sheep [202] or from the urine of patients with aplastic anemia or hookworm anemia [110]. All preparations contain pyrogens and need much further purification before being suitable for clinical trials.

In lieu of exogenous erythropoietin, an attempt to induce endogenous erythropoietin production by means of cobalt and testosterone has been made. The exact mode of action of either drug is unknown, but recent data suggest that they promote erythropoiesis via the release of renal erythropoietin. Consequently their usefulness depends on the residual endocrine function of the failing kidney, and they cannot be expected to be of use in end-stage kidney disease or in the anephric patient.

Cobalt chloride has been shown to cause an erythrocytosis in laboratory animals as well as an increase in erythropoietin titer and an increase in the oxygen tension of a subcutaneous air pocket. These three pieces of data have been correlated with the known suppressive action of cobalt on several oxidative enzymes [201], and it is now believed that cobalt causes cellular hypoxia by blocking a pathway in the utilization of available oxygen, leading in turn to the release of renal erythropoietin and stimulation of red cell production [105]. This effect was first used 15 years ago to accelerate red cell production in renal disease [97], and although it was frequently successful in raising hemoglobin concentration, the beneficial effect to the patient may not have been greater than that caused by deliberately exposing the patient to low oxygen pressure. Of more immediate concern were the many side effects, particularly nausea and vomiting; at present the use of cobalt chloride has no place in the management of the anemia of chronic renal failure [57].

In regard to testosterone action, much recent evidence points to a direct effect on the erythropoietin-releasing mechanism in the kidney [94, 190]. Testosterone and some of its synthetic equivalents have been shown to have striking erythropoietic effects when used in pharmacologic doses and have been reported to be of benefit in children with aplastic anemia and in adults with myelofibrosis [98]. However, the effect in patients with chronic renal disease has been discouraging and has not justified the side effects such as masculinization, fluid retention, and jaundice.

In conclusion, the use of cobalt and testosterone have not been rewarding, and until erythropoietin is available, the anemia of renal failure is best managed by the careful use of small transfusions with packed cells and by the correction of azotemia.

Fibrin Deposition and Renal Failure

In recent years evidence has accumulated suggesting that the inappropriate generation of fibrin and its deposition on vascular surfaces and within vessel walls may represent a major mechanism of human disease [122, 169]. When the rate of fibrin deposition is rapid, acute localized or disseminated vascular plugging may occur, with attendant general hemodynamic changes and local tissue necrosis. When fibrin deposition is slow, it can produce a disease of some chronicity and progressive disability. Until recently, the diagnosis of excessive fibrin deposition rested solely upon *post facto* pathologic evidence. Newer immunologic methods and refined blood coagulation tests, together with the increased utilization of biopsy procedures, have produced a clearer picture of the various clinical syndromes and have offered some insight into the dynamics of the disease process.

In terms of their renal consequences, the two most pertinent examples of abnormal fibrin deposition are probably the hemolytic-uremic syndrome and thrombotic thrombocytopenic purpura. However, morphologic and experimental evidence strongly indicates that intravascular coagulation may play an important, although perhaps not causal, role in the development of a wide spectrum of glomerular disease [261]. In addition, localized fibrin deposition has been recognized as a hallmark of renal homograft rejection [32, 239], even though its etiologic significance in the rejection phenomenon remains unclear. Because of its increasing importance as a mechanism of disease and because its recognition may have therapeutic implications, the pathophysiology of disseminated intravascular coagulation and fibrin deposition will be discussed in some detail.

In 1955 Gasser and his colleagues [99] drew attention to a disease occurring in infants and young children characterized by severe hemolytic anemia, thrombocytopenia, and renal failure, to which they gave the name "hemolytic-uremic syndrome." Since that time several hundred cases have been reported [100, 111, 158, 204], together with suggestions that the incidence of this syndrome may be increasing [100, 204]. Males and females are equally affected, with 90 per cent of reported cases occurring in children below the age of 4 years. Typically, the disease begins a few days to two weeks after an episode of gastroenteritis or an upper-respiratory-tract infection, and first becomes manifest by the rather abrupt appearance of pallor, jaundice, weakness, purpura, and oliguria or anuria. The majority of patients also have neurologic manifestations, coma and convulsions being observed in almost half.

Physical findings include evidence of severe anemia and, usually, mild jaundice. Bleeding into the skin is very common, and gastrointestinal bleeding is not unusual. Hypertension is present in approximately 50 per cent of patients. Splenomegaly and hepatomegaly are uncommon, being observed in less than one-quarter of the cases.

Hematologic studies support the diagnosis of a severe hemolytic anemia, with low hemoglobin, reticulocytosis, absent serum haptoglobin, and, occasionally, hemoglobinuria. The platelet count is depressed in most patients, and is less than 50,000 per cubic millimeter in half the cases. Bone marrow aspiration shows erythroid hyperplasia and plentiful megakaryocytes. The white blood cell count is often moderately elevated. Examination of the peripheral blood reveals a characteristic picture (Fig. 7-3) of fragmented erythrocytes, so-called "Burr cells" [230], microspherocytes, and occasional nucleated red blood cells. Although small numbers of distorted cells, less than 1 or 2 per cent, may be seen in uremia from any cause [230], in the hemolytic-uremic syndrome commonly as many as a third of all erythrocytes are morphologically abnormal. These striking abnormalities of red blood cell morphology have been referred to as "microangiopathic" changes [29, 247] and are also seen in hemolytic states in some persons receiving cardiac prostheses [227] and in occasional patients with carcinomatosis [29]. Not only the patient's red cells, but also transfused normal donor cells are destroyed rapidly [204, 234]. Since tests for antierythrocyte antibodies are almost invariably negative, it is reasonable to conclude that the hemolytic process is due to an extracorpuscular, nonimmunologic mechanism. Similar data are not available with respect to platelet survival, but the presence of abundant megakaryocytes in the bone marrow clearly suggests excessive peripheral destruction as the cause of the characteristic thrombocytopenia.

Patients invariably show elevated blood concentrations of urea and creatinine, and the urine contains moderate to massive quantities of protein, red cells, white cells, and granular, hyaline and red cell casts. Some degree of oliguria is present in all patients, half of all affected persons having total anuria.

The course of the disease is variable. Recovery, when it occurs, generally takes place within two to five weeks. The presence of hypertension, either as an initial finding or as a complication during the disease, is a poor prognostic sign. Overall mortality has been close to 40 per cent. An additional 10 per cent of children recover from the acute episode but remain chronically hypertensive, or have persistent renal disease. Occasional patients in whom acute neurologic manifestations were marked are left with neurologic deficits [100]. Follow-up studies of the apparently fully re-

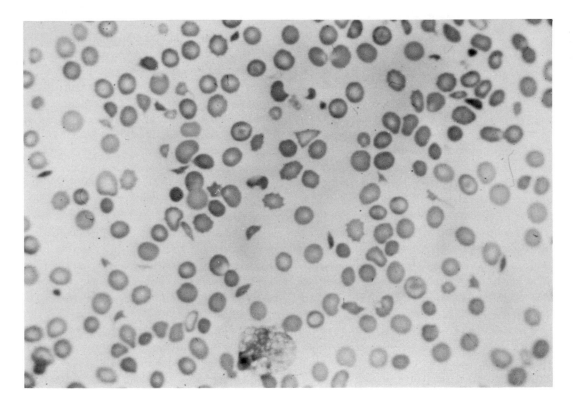

Figure 7-3. Blood smear from patient with the hemolytic-uremic syndrome. The red cells show the characteristic "microangiopathic" changes.

covered patients have not yet been long enough to be certain that there is not an increased frequency of arterial hypertension or renal disease as a late sequel of the acute illness.

The prodromal manifestations and the occurrence of outbreaks in epidemic form [100, 172] suggest an infectious component in the etiology of the hemolytic-uremic syndrome. Nevertheless, it has not been possible to identify an infectious agent in most cases. In the epidemic outbreak reported by Gianantonio et al. [100] a viral agent, apparently related to the virus of Argentinian hemorrhagic fever [12, 177], was isolated from the blood of 5 patients, and a rising antibody titer to this virus was demonstrated in 15 additional patients in whom paired serum specimens were available. Glasgow and Balduzzi [102] isolated

a Coxsackie virus Group A, Type 4 from the stool of one infant, who also showed a serum antibody rise to the same agent, and Piel and Phibbs [204] recovered an ECHO 29 virus from the stool of one of their patients. Several isolations of gram-negative bacteria have been reported from the urine [92, 155, 159, 180], blood [180], or stool [155, 235] of individual cases, but their number is small. Although no etiologic pattern has emerged from these studies, further efforts are clearly indicated. It would appear most useful, for example, to collect acute-phase and convalescent-phase serum specimens from all patients with this syndrome for possible viral or bacterial antibody screening.

Renal biopsy specimens taken during the acute phase of the disease [15, 111, 134, 158,

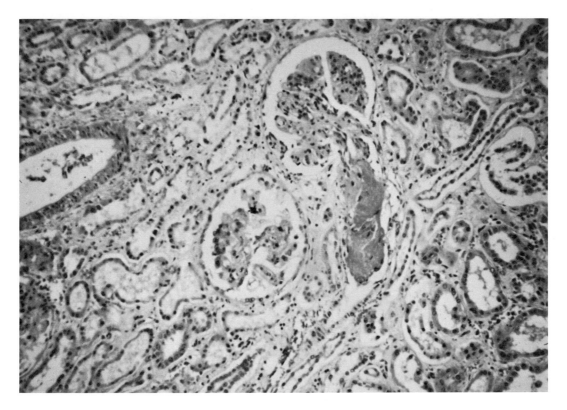

Figure 7-4. Renal biopsy from patient with acute hemolytic-uremic syndrome.

204] show focal occlusion of glomerular capillaries and afferent arterioles by homogeneous, eosinophilic, hyaline thrombi (Figs. 7-4, 7-5), which also take up the periodic acid–Schiff stain. Thrombi may be present in only a few glomeruli or may involve parts of all glomeruli in the specimen. There is usually some proliferative crescent formation and glomerular hyalinization. In severe cases necrosis of glomeruli is seen. Postmortem studies show the acute renal lesion to vary from the microscopic picture described above to gross bilateral renal cortical necrosis [100, 111, 155, 159, 173]. In addition, however, in fully 25 per cent of fatal cases extrarenal hyaline thrombi are present, as well as occasional intramural deposits of similar staining material, primarily in arterioles of the heart, lungs, pancreas, spleen, adrenal glands, or skeletal muscle [111, 158, 173, 204].

The widespread occurrence of amorphous, eosinophilic thrombi and intramural hyaline deposits in the terminal arterioles of many organs has long been considered the characteristic pathology of thrombotic thrombocytopenic purpura (TTP). This disease was first described by Moschcowitz [185] in 1925, since which time nearly 300 additional cases have been recorded [e.g., 9, 44, 46, 66, 69, 70, 129, 156, 181, 196]. Most cases have occurred between 10 and 40 years of age, with a distinct female sex preponderance [9]. Clinical manifestations typically include fever, hemolytic anemia, thrombocytopenic purpura, neurologic manifestations, and evidence of renal disease. The hemolytic anemia is of the "micro-

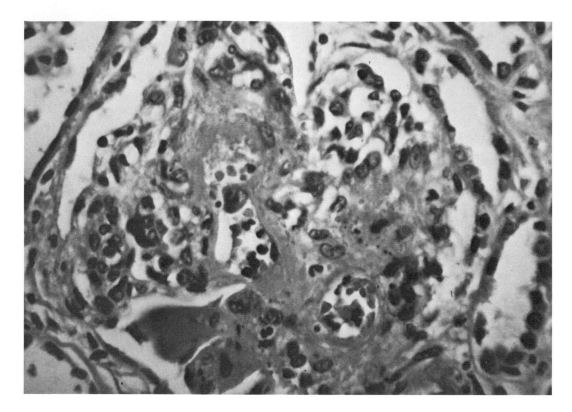

Figure 7-5. Renal biopsy from patient with acute hemolytic-uremic syndrome. Note characteristic focal changes in glomerular capillaries.

angiopathic" type, with a peripheral blood picture identical to Figure 7-3. In addition to purpura, retinal, gastrointestinal, and genitourinary hemorrhages are common. Central nervous system manifestations are prominent, although not infrequently transient [9], and include coma, convulsions, paresis, and aphasia. Renal abnormalities are the rule, but are usually mild; however, anuria may occur in an occasional case [70].

No typical prodromal phase precedes the onset of TTP, and no epidemics of this disease have occurred. There seems to be a disproportionate incidence of TTP in pregnancy [9, 44]. In a fraction of patients there is a history of febrile illness [66, 70] or of exposure to hair dyes [9] or drugs [156]. A number of cases have arisen in persons suffering from malignancies [46]. Despite the similarities in clinical characteristics and tissue findings, it seems safe to assume that multiple triggering factors will be found for this disease process.

The disease usually runs a rapidly progressive course, with death occurring in 75 per cent of affected individuals within 3 months of onset. Death is most commonly due to severe neurologic damage or to hemorrhage [9]. In some cases a more prolonged course, characterized by multiple remissions and exacerbations over a period of years is seen [40]. Less than 10 per cent of reported cases can be considered long-term cures [9]. It is not yet possible to ascertain whether recent therapeutic attempts (discussed below) have altered this grave prognosis.

The pathologic lesions in TTP have been

investigated by light and electron microscopy and by immunohistochemical technics [55, 85, 200, 260]. Thrombotic, subendothelial, and deeper intramural vascular lesions are seen, often accompanied by aneurysmal dilatation at arteriolar-capillary junctions [85, 200]. In involved areas the endothelial cells are usually considerably swollen [85]. The lesions stain brightly when reacted with fluorescein-tagged antifibrin or antifibrinogen antiserum, but not when reacted with antiplatelet antiserum [55, 85, 260]. One group of investigators also observed specific staining, of moderate intensity, with anti-IgG antiserum but no reaction with antiserum to the β_1C-globulin component of human complement [85]. In antigen-antibody mediated disease in which complement is fixed in vivo, both immunoglobulin and complement may be detected by immunologic means on endothelial surfaces and within vessel walls [84, 147, 256]. The significance of this finding for the understanding of TTP is unclear. Ultrastructurally, the hyaline thrombi and intramural hyaline deposits consist of bundles of fibrils having the same size and texture as fibrin, but lacking its characteristic cross-striations. Difficulty in visualizing striations in fibrin in tissue sections has been noted by others [244, 267] and may be related to the observation that when fibrin is formed slowly in vitro, using dilute thrombin solutions, no striations are seen [113].

A comparison of the pathologic findings in the hemolytic-uremic syndrome and TTP leads to the conclusion that the two diseases differ more in extent and distribution of vascular involvement than in the nature of the lesions themselves. Furthermore, it is difficult to differentiate these two syndromes on clinical or pathological grounds, since TTP has been reported in infants [181] and persons with widespread vascular lesions, but the clinical presentation of the hemolytic-uremic syndrome has occurred in adolescents [45] and adults [70]. Unfortunately, to date no immunohistochemical studies, and only a single

ultrastructural investigation [15], of the hemolytic-uremic syndrome have been published.

PATHOPHYSIOLOGY OF ABNORMAL FIBRIN DEPOSITION

The major experimental model for disseminated intravascular coagulation has been the generalized Shwartzman reaction [11, 236]. In rabbits pretreated with intravenous bacterial endotoxin [38, 252], or in which reticuloendothelial blockade has been produced by a variety of means [107, 237], a subsequent intravenous injection of endotoxin causes the rapid and widespread appearance of amorphous eosinophilic thrombi in arterioles, capillaries, and venules in many organs, but most prominently in the kidney. Renal lesions develop largely in the glomerular capillaries and afferent arterioles and are of sufficient magnitude to cause gross bilateral renal cortical necrosis in 60 to 80 per cent of exposed animals [38, 107]. A single dose of endotoxin may produce a small number of hyaline thrombi in many organs, but glomerular thrombi are found only in animals receiving two injections of endotoxin [37, 38, 171]. Histochemically [170] and by electron microscopy [203] the thrombotic lesions are composed of fibrinogen or fibrin, and seem to contain little antigenically identifiable platelet material. At the time of maximum fibrin deposition the animals develop thrombocytopenia and hypofibrinogenemia [171], as well as other evidence suggestive of an episode of diffuse intravascular coagulation [171, 216]. The fall in fibrinogen correlates roughly with the degree and extent of the vascular thrombi [171]. It is an unexplained fact that renal cortical necrosis is more easily produced in young animals [252]. The typical response to the provoking dose of endotoxin can be abolished by pretreatment of the animals with heparin [106] or a coumarin compound [232]. It is difficult to escape the conclusion that during the generalized Shwartzman reaction the coagulation mechanism is activated throughout the flowing blood, causing widespread fibrin formation and its deposition in multiple sites.

Intravenous injections of thrombin [152, 262], thromboplastic tissue extracts [262], or activated factor X [218] can produce a pathological picture identical to the Shwartzman reaction, including bilateral renal cortical necrosis, provided that animals are suitably prepared. "Preparation" may consist in inhibiting the fibrinolytic mechanism by the administration of epsilon-aminocaproic acid (EACA) [152, 262], or by producing reticuloendothelial blockade [262]. Without such preparation only scattered renal lesions are visible by light microscopy, although small amounts of fibrin-like material can regularly be identified with the electron microscope [262] within the glomerular basement membrane. Both fibrin aggregates [154] and activated coagulation components [238] are cleared by the reticuloendothelial system, and it seems reasonable to assume that prevention of phagocytosis might allow prolonged circulation, at increased concentration, of activated coagulation components and of fibrin, thereby increasing the number and severity of hyaline thrombi. Administration of EACA might allow the development of lesions that would otherwise be removed by the physiologic action of the fibrinolytic system. In addition to endotoxin and active coagulation factors, soluble antigen-antibody complexes can provoke a Shwartzman-like reaction in prepared animals [153, 168]. Two other circumstances that serve to sensitize animals to intravenous endotoxin are pregnancy [272] and cortisone administration [251]. The mechanism in these instances is not clear, but it is thought due in the former to depressed fibrinolytic activity and in the latter, to reticuloendothelial blockade. However, the functional state of the reticuloendothelial and fibrinolytic systems during pregnancy is a subject of some disagreement, and the effect of adrenal steroids on phagocytosis and on the Shwartzman reaction is complex, and may be dose-related.

The similarities between the hemolytic-ure-mic syndrome, TTP, and the Shwartzman reaction are striking, and include the morphology of the pathologic lesions, the thrombocytopenia, and the tendency for severe renal lesions to occur more frequently in young animals and humans. It was not appreciated, however, until the studies of Brain and co-workers [30, 31] indicated that hemolytic anemia is an important component of the generalized Shwartzman reaction. Infusion of endotoxin or thrombin into Thorotrast-treated animals regularly produces hemoglobinemia [31] of a degree closely correlated with the intensity and extent of small-vessel thrombi [30]. The hemoglobinemia as well as the vascular thrombi can be prevented by pretreatment with heparin [30]. The hemolysis is associated with the appearance in the circulation of fragmented, distorted red blood cells [30], morphologic abnormalities identical to the microangiopathic changes seen in the hemolytic-uremic syndrome and thrombotic thrombocytopenic purpura. Phase-contrast studies of circulating red cells show them adhering to fibrin strands and to microclots and undergoing distortion in the fluid stream, and subsequent lysis [224]. Furthermore, products of red cell lysis may produce a hypercoagulable state, especially when reticuloendothelial function is depressed [206], and may perpetuate the process.

Thus, the major biochemical and pathological findings of the hemolytic-uremic syndrome and thrombotic thrombocytopenic purpura can be produced by an episode of diffuse intravascular coagulation. It is important to recognize that in neither condition do we know the triggering stimulus for this calamitous process. With this major limitation in mind, we shall turn to a discussion of therapeutic approaches in these two diseases.

MANAGEMENT OF THE HEMOLYTIC-UREMIC SYNDROME AND THROMBOTIC THROMBOCYTOPENIC PURPURA

Rationale for therapy in the hemolytic-uremic syndrome and TTP is based on the analogy with the Shwartzman reaction. Thus it becomes essential to document the existence of a state of abnormal fibrin deposition during the course of these diseases. Morphologic evidence may be obtained by biopsy [15, 111, 134, 158, 204], but it is well to remember that immunohistochemical technics cannot differentiate between deposits of fibrinogen and of fibrin [55, 85, 170, 260]. Although direct precipitation of fibrinogen appears unlikely, in vitro and in vivo evidence suggests that such a phenomenon may occur, and this mechanism has been proposed to play a part in the development of the Shwartzman reaction [250, 253]. Whether or not such an initiating stimulus is operative, prevention of the reaction by sodium warfarin [232] indicates the involvement of the entire coagulation mechanism. The changes in the coagulation parameters during a period of intravascular coagulation resemble those occurring in vitro when blood clots [209, 217], and may be thought of as a tendency for the circulating plasma to resemble serum. They represent important criteria by which the clinical diagnosis of diffuse intravascular coagulation is made, and include depressed levels of platelets, fibrinogen, and to a variable extent factor V and factor VIII. In addition, evidence of secondary activation of the fibrinolytic system is usually present in the form of decreased plasminogen levels and circulating split-products produced by the action of plasmin on fibrin [176]. Few complete investigations of this type are available [156, 182], and no studies of platelet or fibrinogen turnover have been reported in either disease. Heparin, alone or with other agents, has been used with some success by a number of investigators to treat the hemolytic-uremic syndrome [14, 64, 139, 142, 204]. Platelet and fibrinogen levels begin to rise within 24 hours after starting therapy, but may not reach normal values for one week. Dosages of heparin adequate for treatment of disseminated intravascular coagulation should probably be in the range of 500 to 600 units per kilogram of body weight per day given intravenously [7, 10,

121]. In at least one case heparin therapy was discontinued in spite of an effective platelet response, due to excessive bleeding from venipuncture sites [204]. Since occasional cases of the hemolytic-uremic syndrome clear rapidly without treatment [182], care must be exercised in interpreting the efficacy of heparin therapy.

Although possible contraindications to the use of adrenal steroids exist [22, 251], these agents have been employed in the hemolytic-uremic syndrome. Success has been reported in some cases [109, 130, 158, 204], but the same and other authors have observed no beneficial effects [14, 100, 130, 158]. Since dosage schedules have not always been recorded, it is not possible to determine what part variations in dose may play in the clinical response.

Heparin has also been used in the treatment of TTP [4, 6, 13, 18, 19, 43, 219]. In several patients no improvement resulted [4, 6], while in others remissions were brought about [6, 13, 18, 43, 219]. In one case relapse occurred 20 months after successful heparin therapy [18] at which time the patient died despite the use of heparin [19]. In many of these reports heparin was used in conjunction with other drugs, especially adrenal steroids, so that conclusions regarding the effectiveness of anticoagulant treatment must be guarded. By analogy with its effect in preventing the Shwartzman phenomenon [52], streptokinase has been used in a single case of TTP [50]. Unfortunately, due to the very short term of treatment, it was impossible to judge the usefulness of this agent. It would appear very worthwhile to study the effect of fibrinolytic agents in this disease.

The common denominator in the largest number of successfully treated cases of TTP is the use of adrenal steroids in high dose [9, 39, 66, 119, 156, 181, 231, 248]. The rationale for such an approach is unknown. In some cases steroids were combined with splenectomy [66, 119, 231, 248], in others with heparin [219]. In one case [156] high-molecular-weight dextran was used in conjunction with steroids because of its known effectiveness in coating vascular surfaces [23] and platelets [223], and interfering with platelet aggregating ability [148]. In another case, low-molecular-weight dextran alone proved ineffective in altering the course of the disease [43]. Steroids appear to be useful in doses equivalent to 2 to 10 mg. of prednisone per kilogram of body weight per day. In the majority of cases the drug has been administered intravenously. Often steroids have been continued for several months.

Thus it appears that heparin therapy may be the treatment of choice in the hemolytic-uremic syndrome. Thrombotic thrombocytopenic purpura, on the other hand, may be treated best with very high dosage steroids, perhaps in conjunction with heparin, dextran, or splenectomy. In both diseases biochemical data are in short supply, and further trials, especially in TTP, will be necessary to determine finally the effectiveness of any of these agents.

General management in these diseases includes drug therapy of hypertension when indicated, and dialysis for severe uremia. Anticonvulsant therapy may be useful when convulsions are not due to severe uremia or hypertension. Unfortunately, until more is known about the cause of these diseases, treatment of the ensuing fibrin deposition remains a symptomatic approach only.

GRAFT REJECTION AND FIBRIN DEPOSITION

The acute rejection of a renal homograft is accompanied by the deposition of "fibrinoid" thrombi in glomeruli and their afferent arterioles [138, 239]. These lesions have been compared to those of thrombotic thrombocytopenic purpura [138] and identified as a Shwartzman reaction [239]. Local activation of the fibrinolytic system secondary to intravascular coagulation is demonstrated by the finding of fibrin split-products in the urine during the phase of rejection [32]. Although the etiologic importance of intravascular coagulation in the rejection phenomenon is quite unknown, there can be no doubt that, once initiated, abnormal fibrin deposition is an important factor in the development of the renal lesions. Efforts are presently underway to modify acute rejection by the use of agents interfering with platelet aggregation, such as phenylbutazone and sulfinpyrazone, and by the use of heparin and streptokinase [138]. These are promising approaches, and results will be awaited with great interest.

Acknowledgments

From the Cardeza Foundation for Hematologic Research, Department of Internal Medicine, Jefferson Medical College, Philadelphia, Pennsylvania. Supported in part by N.I.H. Grants H 4612 and H 09163.

References

1. Abbrecht, P. H., and Greene, J. A., Jr. Serum erythropoietin after renal homotransplantation. *Ann. Intern. Med.* 65:908, 1966.

2. Abbrecht, P. H., Malvin, R. L., and Vander, A. J. Renal production of erythropoietin and renin after experimental infarction. *Nature* (London) 211:1318, 1966.

3. Adamson, J. W., Eschbach, J., and Finch, C. A. The kidney and erythropoiesis. *Amer. J. Med.* 44:725, 1968.

4. Adelson, E., and Stefanini, M. Studies on

platelets: VI. Demonstration and characterization of a heterologous (Forssman) platelet agglutinin. *Blood* 7:700, 1952.

5. Alexanian, R. Urinary excretion of erythropoietin in normal men and women. *Blood* 28:344, 1966.

6. Allanby, K. D., Huntsman, R. G., and Sacker, L. S. Thrombotic microangiopathy: Recovery of a case after heparin and magnesium therapy. *Lancet* 1:237, 1966.

7. Allen, D. M. Heparin therapy of purpura fulminans. *Pediatrics* 38:211, 1966.

8. Alpen, E. L., and Cranmore, D. Observations on the Regulation of Erythropoiesis and on Cellular Dynamics by ^{59}Fe Autoradiography. In Stohlman, F., Jr. (Ed.), *The Kinetics of Cellular Proliferation.* New York: Grune & Stratton, 1959. P. 290.

9. Amorosi, E. L., and Ultmann, J. E. Thrombotic thrombocytopenic purpura: Report of 16 cases and review of the literature. *Medicine* (Balt.) 45:139, 1966.

10. Antley, R. M., and McMillan, C. W. Sequential coagulation studies in purpura fulminans. *New Eng. J. Med.* 276:1287, 1967.

11. Apitz, K. A study of the generalized Shwartzman phenomenon. *J. Immun.* 29:255, 1935.

12. Arribalzaga, R. A. Una nueva enfermedad epidemica a germen desconocido: Hipertermia nefrotoxica, leukopenica y enantematica. *Día Méd.* 27:1204, 1955.

13. Ata, M., and Jones, M. B. S. Heparin in thrombotic microangiopathy. *Lancet* 2:281, 1966.

14. Barnard, P. J., and Kibel, M. The haemolytic-uraemic syndrome of infancy and childhood: A report of eleven cases. *Cent. Afr. J. Med.* 11:31, 1965.

15. Bartman, J., Jacques, M., and Dustin, P., Jr. Anémie hémolytique, purpura thrombocytopénique et nephropathie aigue chez un nourisson: Étude au microscope électronique des lésions rénales. *Rev. Belg. Path.* 30:5, 1964.

16. Baum, J., Suki, W., and Frenkel, E. P. Localization of erythropoietin in the kidney by immunofluorescence. *Clin. Res.* 13:268, 1965.

17. Bell, R. E. The origin of "Burr" erythrocytes. *Brit. J. Haemat.* 9:552, 1963.

18. Bernstock, L., and Hirson, C. Thrombotic thrombocytopenic purpura: Remission on treatment with heparin. *Lancet* 1:28, 1960.

19. Bernstock, L., and Hirson, C. Heparin in thrombotic microangiopathy. *Lancet* 2:281, 1966.

20. Berry, E. R., Rambach, W. A., Alt, H. L., and Del Greco, F. Effect of peritoneal dialysis on erythrokinetics and ferrokinetics of azotemic anemia. *Trans. Amer. Soc. Artif. Intern. Organs* 10:415, 1965.

21. Bettex-Galland, M., and Lüscher, E. F. Thrombosthenin, the contractile protein from blood platelets and its relation to other contractile proteins. *Advances Protein Chem.* 20:1, 1965.

22. Blix, S., and Jacobsen, C. D. Intravascular coagulation, a possible accelerating effect of prednisone. *Acta Med. Scand.* 180:723, 1966.

23. Bloom, W. L., Harmer, D. S., Bryant, M. F., and Brewer, S. S. Coating of vascular surfaces and cells: A new concept in the prevention of intravascular thrombosis. *Proc. Soc. Exp. Biol. Med.* 115:384, 1964.

24. Bluemle, L. W., Jr., Webster, G. D., Jr., and Elkington, J. R. Acute tubular necrosis: Analysis of one hundred cases with respect to mortality, complications and treatment with and without dialysis. *A.M.A. Arch. Intern. Med.* 104:180, 1959.

25. Bock, H. F., Nieth, N., and Solth, K. Anemia in renal failure. *Deutsch. Med. Wschr.* 87:573, 1962.

26. Borchgrevink, C. F. A method for measuring platelet adhesiveness in vivo. *Acta Med. Scand.* 168:157, 1960.

27. Born, G. V. R. Aggregation of blood platelets by adenosine diphosphate and its reversal. *Nature* (London) 194:927, 1962.

28. Bozzini, C. E., Devoto, F. C. H., and Tomio, J. M. Decreased responsiveness of hematopoietic tissue to erythropoietin in acutely uremic rats. *J. Lab. Clin. Med.* 68:411, 1966.

29. Brain, M. C., Dacie, J. V., and O'Hourihane, D. O'B. Microangiopathic haemolytic anaemia: The possible role of vascular

lesions in pathogenesis. *Brit. J. Haemat.* 8: 358, 1962.

30. Brain, M. C., Esterly, J. R., and Beck, E. A. Intravascular haemolysis with experimentally produced vascular thrombi. *Brit. J. Haemat.* 13:868, 1967.

31. Brain, M. C., and O'Hourihane, D. O'B. Microangiopathic haemolytic anaemia: The occurrence of haemolysis in experimentally produced vascular disease. *Brit. J. Haemat.* 13:135, 1967.

32. Braun, W. E., and Merrill, J. P. Urine fibrinogen fragments in human renal allografts. *New Eng. J. Med.* 278:1366, 1968.

33. Brewer, D. B. *Renal Biopsy.* Baltimore: Williams & Wilkins, 1965. P. 3.

34. Brod, J., and Hornych, A. Effect of correction of anemia on the glomerular filtration rate in chronic renal failure. *Israel J. Med. Sci.* 3:53, 1967.

35. Brown, R. Plasma erythropoietin in chronic uremia. *Brit. Med. J.* 2:1036, 1965.

36. Brownstein, M. H., and Ballard, H. S. Hepatomas associated with erythrocytosis. *Amer. J. Med.* 40:204, 1966.

37. Brunson, J. G., Gamble, C. N., and Thomas, L. Morphologic changes in rabbits following the intravenous administration of meningococcal toxin: I. The effect produced in young and mature animals by a single injection. *Amer. J. Path.* 31:489, 1955.

38. Brunson, J. G., Thomas, L., Gamble, C. N. Morphologic changes in rabbits following the intravenous administration of meningococcal endotoxin: II. Two appropriately spaced injections; the role of fibrinoid in the generalized Shwartzman reaction. *Amer. J. Path.* 31:655, 1955.

39. Burke, H. A., and Hartmann, R. C. Thrombotic thrombocytopenic purpura: Two patients with remission associated with the use of large amounts of steroids. *A.M.A. Arch. Intern. Med.* 103:105, 1959.

40. Cahalane, S. F., and Horn, R. C., Jr. Thrombotic thrombocytopenic purpura of long duration. *Amer. J. Med.* 27:333, 1959.

41. Cahalane, S. F., Johnson, S. A., Monto, R. W., and Caldwell, M. J. Acquired thrombocytopathy — observations on the co-agulation defect in uremia. *Amer. J. Clin. Path.* 30:507, 1958.

42. Callen, I. R., and Limarzi, L. R. Blood and bone marrow studies in renal disease. *Amer. J. Clin. Path.* 20:3, 1950.

43. Carmichael, D. S., and Medley, D. R. K. Heparin in thrombotic microangiopathy. *Lancet* 1:1421, 1966.

44. Case Records of the Massachusetts General Hospital (Case 50–1966). *New Eng. J. Med.* 275:1125, 1966.

45. Case Records of the Massachusetts General Hospital (Case 37–1967). *New Eng. J. Med.* 277:536, 1967.

46. Case Records of the Massachusetts General Hospital (Case 24–1968). *New Eng. J. Med.* 278:1336, 1968.

47. Castaldi, P. A., Rozenberg, M. C., and Stewart, J. H. The bleeding disorder of uremia, a qualitative platelet defect. *Lancet* 2: 66, 1966.

48. Chaplin, H., Jr., and Mollison, P. L. Red cell lifespan in nephritis and in hepatic cirrhosis. *Clin. Sci.* 12:351, 1953.

49. Cheney, K., and Bonnin, J. A. Haemorrhage, platelet dysfunction, and other coagulation defects in uremia. *Brit. J. Haemat.* 8:215, 1962.

50. Clinicopathologic conference. Thrombotic thrombocytopenic purpura. *Amer. J. Med.* 27:115, 1959.

51. Cole, C. H., Balfe, J. W., and Welt, L. G. Induction of a ouabain-sensitive ATPase defect by uremic plasma. *Trans. Ass. Amer. Phys.* 81:213, 1968.

52. Condie, R. M., Hong, C. Y., and Good, R. A. Reversal of the lesions of the generalized Shwartzman phenomenon by treatment of rabbits with streptokinase. *J. Lab. Clin. Med.* 50:803, 1957.

53. Cooper, W. M., and Tuttle, W. B. Polycythemia associated with a benign kidney lesion: Report of a case of erythrocytosis with hydronephrosis, with remission of polycythemia following nephrectomy. *Ann. Intern. Med.* 47:1008, 1957.

54. Cotes, P. M. Quantitative estimation of erythropoietin. *Ann. N.Y. Acad. Sci.* 149: 12, 1968.

55. Craig, J. M., and Gitlin, D. The nature of

the hyaline thrombi in thrombotic thrombocytopenic purpura. *Amer. J. Path.* 33:251, 1957.

56. Dacie, J. V. *The Haemolytic Anaemias* (2d ed.). New York: Grune & Stratton, 1967.

57. Dameshek, W. (Ed.). Panels in therapy V. The use of cobalt and cobalt-iron preparations in the therapy of anemia. *Blood* 10:852, 1955.

58. Damon, A., Holub, D. A., and Melicow, M. M. Polycythemia and renal carcinoma. *Amer. J. Med.* 25:182, 1958.

59. Davey, M. G., and Lüscher, E. F. Biochemical aspects of platelet function and hemostasis. *Seminars Hemat.* 5:5, 1968.

60. DeMarsh, Q. B., and Warmington, W. J. Polycythemia associated with a renal tumor. *Northwest Med.* 54:976, 1955.

61. Demopoulos, H. B., Highman, B., Altland, P. D., Gerving, M. A., and Kaley, G. Effects of high altitude on granular juxtaglomerular cells and their possible role in erythropoietin production. *Amer. J. Path.* 46:497, 1965.

62. Denny, W. F., Flanigan, W. J., and Zukoski, C. F. Serial erythropoietin studies in patients undergoing renal homotransplantation. *J. Lab. Clin. Med.* 67:386, 1966.

63. Desforges, J. F., and Dawson, J. P. The anemia of renal failure. *A.M.A. Arch. Intern. Med.* 101:326, 1958.

64. Desmit, E. M., and Hart, H. Ch. Behandeling van het hemolytisch-uremisch syndroom. *Nederl. T. Geneesk.* 110:355, 1966.

65. Deutsch, E., and Fischer, M. Hämostase und urämie. *Thromb. Diath. Haemorrh.* 19 (Suppl. 25):155, 1968.

66. Distenfeld, A., and Oppenheim, E. The treatment of acute thrombotic thrombocytopenic purpura with corticosteroids and splenectomy. *Ann. Intern. Med.* 65:245, 1966.

67. Donati, R. M., Lange, R. D., and Gallagher, N. I. Nephrogenic erythrocytosis. *Arch. Intern. Med.* (Chicago) 112:198, 1963.

68. Donner, L., and Neuwirtova, R. The hemostatic defect of acute and chronic uremia. *Thromb. Diath. Haemorrh.* 5:319, 1961.

69. Duhamel, G., Vergoz, D., and André, R.

La maladie de Moschcowitz. Réflexions cliniques biologiques et histologiques à propos d'une observation. *Hémostase* 6:7, 1966.

70. Dunea, G., Muehrcke, R. C., Nakamoto, S., and Schwartz, F. D. Thrombotic thrombocytopenic purpura with acute renal failure. *Amer. J. Med.* 41:1000, 1966.

71. Ellis, H. Polycythaemia due to hydronephrosis. *Proc. Roy. Soc. Med.* 54:157, 1961.

72. Erslev, A. J. Humoral regulation of red cell production. *Blood* 8:349, 1953.

73. Erslev, A. J. Physiologic control of red cell production. *Blood* 10:954, 1955.

74. Erslev, A. J. Erythropoietic function in uremic rabbits. *A.M.A. Arch. Intern. Med.* 101:407, 1958.

75. Erslev, A. J. The effect of anemic anoxia on the cellular development of nucleated red cells. *Blood* 14:386, 1959.

76. Erslev, A. J. Erythropoietin in vitro: II. Effect on "stem cells." *Blood* 24:331, 1964.

77. Erslev, A. J. The role of erythropoietin in the control of red cell production. *Medicine* (Balt.) 48:661, 1964.

78. Erslev, A. J. Compensated anemia caused by over-work hyperplasia of the stem cell pool. *Int. Soc. Hemat.*, N.Y. 1968.

79. Erslev, A. J., and Kazal, L. A. Inactivation of erythropoietin by tissue homogenates. *Proc. Soc. Exp. Biol. Med.* In press.

80. Erslev, A. J., McKenna, P. J., Capelli, J. P., Hamburger, R. J., Cohn, H. E., and Clark, J. E. Rate of red cell production in two nephrectomized patients. *Arch. Intern. Med.* (Chicago) 122:230, 1968.

81. Erslev, A. J., Solit, R. W., Camishion, R. C., Amsel, S., Ioda, J., and Ballinger, W. F., II. Erythropoietin in vitro: III. Perfusion of a lung-kidney preparation. *Amer. J. Physiol.* 208:1153, 1965.

82. Eschbach, J. W., Funk, D., Adamson, J., Kuhn, I., Scribner, B. H., and Finch, C. A. Erythropoiesis in patients with renal failure undergoing chronic dialysis. *New Eng. J. Med.* 276:653, 1967.

83. Favre-Gilly, J., and Durand, J. De l'existence d'un purpura thrombocytopénique hémorrhagique au cours de la néphrite azotémique. *Sang* 21:755, 1950.

84. Feldman, J. D., Mardiney, M. R., and

Shuler, S. Immunology and morphology of acute poststreptococcal glomerulonephritis. *Lab. Invest.* 15:283, 1966.

85. Feldman, J. D., Mardiney, M. R., Unanue, E. R., and Cutting, H. The vascular pathology of thrombotic thrombocytopenic purpura: An immunohistochemical and ultrastructural study. *Lab. Invest.* 15:927, 1966.

86. Filmanowicz, E., and Gurney, C. W. Studies on erythropoiesis: XVI. Response to a single dose of erythropoietin in polycythemic mouse. *J. Lab. Clin. Med.* 57:65, 1961.

87. Fisher, J. W. Introduction to a conference on erythropoietin. *Ann. N.Y. Acad. Sci.* 149:9, 1968.

88. Fisher, J. W., and Birdwell, B. J. The production of an erythropoietic factor by the in situ perfused kidney. *Acta Haemat.* 26:224, 1961.

89. Fisher, J. W., Match, F. E., Roh, B. L., Allen, R. C., and Kelley, B. J. Erythropoietin inhibitor in kidney extracts and plasma from anemic uremic human subjects. *Blood* 31:440, 1968.

90. Fisher, J., and Samuels, A. J. Relationship between renal blood flow and erythropoietin production. *Proc. Soc. Exp. Biol. Med.* 125:482, 1967.

91. Fisher, J. W., Taylor, G., and Porteous, D. D. Localization of erythropoietin in glomeruli of sheep kidney by fluorescent antibody technique. *Nature* 205:611, 1965.

92. Fison, T. N. Acute glomerulonephritis in infancy. *Arch. Dis. Child.* 31:101, 1956.

93. Fleming, A. R., and Markley, J. C. Polycythemia associated with uterine myomas. *Amer. J. Obstet. Gynec.* 74:677, 1957.

94. Fried, W., and Gurney, C. W. The erythropoietic-stimulating effects of androgens. *Ann. N.Y. Acad. Sci.* 149:356, 1968.

95. Friend, D. G., Hoskins, R. G., and Kirkin, M. W. Relative erythrocythemia (polycythemia) and polycystic kidney disease, with uremia. *New Eng. J. Med.* 264:17, 1961.

96. Gallagher, N. I., McCarthy, J. M., and Lange, R. D. Observations on erythropoietic-stimulating factor (E.S.F.) in the plasma of uremic and non-uremic anemic patients. *Ann. Intern. Med.* 52:1201, 1960.

97. Gardner, F. H. The use of cobaltous chloride in the anemia associated with chronic renal disease. *J. Lab. Clin. Med.* 41:46, 1953.

98. Gardner, F. H., and Pringle, J. C. Androgens and erythropoiesis. *Arch. Intern. Med.* (Chicago) 107:846, 1961.

99. Gasser, C., Gautier, E., Steck, A., Siebenmann, R. E., and Oechslin, R. Hämolytisch-urämische syndrome: Bilaterale nierenrindennekrosen bei akuten erworbenen hämolytischen anämien. *Schweiz. Med. Wschr.* 85:906, 1955.

100. Gianantonio, C., Vitacco, M., Mendilaharzu, F., Rutty, A., and Mendilaharzu, J. The hemolytic-uremic syndrome. *J. Pediat.* 64:478, 1964.

101. Giovannetti, S., Balestri, P. L., and Cioni, L. Spontaneous in vitro autohaemolysis of blood from chronic uraemic patients. *Clin. Sci.* 29:407, 1965.

102. Glasgow, L. A., and Balduzzi, P. Isolation of Coxsackie virus group A, type 4, from a patient with hemolytic-uremic syndrome. *New Eng. J. Med.* 273:754, 1965.

103. Goldfarb, B., and Tobian, L. Relationship of erythropoietin to renal juxtaglomerular cells. *Proc. Soc. Exp. Biol. Med.* 112:65, 1963.

104. Goldwasser, E. Biochemical Control of Erythroid Cell Development. In Moscond, A. A., and Monroy, A. (Eds.), *Current Topics in Developmental Biology.* New York: Academic, 1966. P. 173.

105. Goldwasser, E., Jacobson, L. O., Fried, W., and Plzak, L. F. Mechanism of the erythropoietic effect of cobalt. *Blood* 13:55, 1958.

106. Good, R. A., and Thomas, L. Inhibition by heparin of local and generalized Shwartzman reactions. *J. Lab. Clin. Med.* 40:804, 1952.

107. Good, R. A., and Thomas, L. Studies on the generalized Shwartzman reaction: II. The production of bilateral cortical necrosis of the kidneys by a single injection of bacterial toxin in rabbits previously treated with Thorotrast or trypan blue. *J. Exp. Med.* 96:625, 1952.

108. Gordon, A. S., Cooper, G. W., and Zanzani, E. D. The kidney and erythropoiesis. *Seminars Haemat.* 4:337, 1967.

109. Griffiths, J., and Irving, K. G. A haemo-lytic-uraemic syndrome in infancy. *Arch. Dis. Child.* 36:500, 1961.

110. Gutnisky, A., Malgor, L., Nohr, M. L., and Van Dyke, D. Collection of erythropoietin from urine of patients with anemia secondary to hookworm. *Ann. N.Y. Acad. Sci.* 149:564, 1968.

111. Habib, R., Mathieu, H., and Royer, P. Le syndrome hémolytique et urémique de l'enfant. *Nephron* 4:139, 1967.

112. Hacrardsholm, F. P. Erythropoietin production in fetal hypoxia and in anemic, uremic patients. *Ann. N.Y. Acad. Sci.* 149:497, 1968.

113. Hall, C. E. Electron microscopy of fibrinogen and fibrin. *J. Biol. Chem.* 179:857, 1949.

114. Hampers, C. L., Streiff, R., Nathan, D. K., Snyder, D., and Merrill, J. P. Megaloblastic hematopoiesis in uremia and in patients on long-term hemodialysis. *New Eng. J. Med.* 276:551, 1967.

115. Hansen, P. Polycythemia produced by constriction of the renal artery of the rabbit. *Acta Path. Microbiol. Scand.* 60:465, 1964.

116. Hardisty, R. M., and Hutton, R. A. Platelet aggregation and the availability of platelet Factor 3. *Brit. J. Haemat.* 12:764, 1966.

117. Hellem, A. J., Odegaard, A. E., and Skolkegg, B. A. Platelet adhesiveness in chronic renal failure. Tenth Congress Internat. Soc. Hemat., Stockholm, 1964.

118. Hennessy, T. G., Stern, W. E., and Herrick, S. E. Cerebellar hemangioblastoma: Erythropoietic activity by radioiron assay. *J. Nucl. Med.* 8:601, 1967.

119. Hill, J. M., and Loeb, E. Massive hormonal therapy and splenectomy in acute thrombotic thrombocytopenic purpura. *J.A.M.A.* 173:778, 1960.

120. Hirashima, K., and Takaku, F. Experimental studies on erythropoietin: II. The relationship between juxtaglomerular cells and erythropoietin. *Blood* 20:1, 1962.

121. Hjort, P. F., Rapaport, S. I., and Jorgensen, L. Purpura fulminans: Report of a case successfully treated with heparin and hydrocortisone; review of 50 cases from literature. *Scand. J. Haemat.* 1:169, 1964.

122. Hjort, P. F., and Rapaport, S. I. Shwartzman reaction: Pathogenetic mechanisms and clinical manifestations. *Ann. Rev. Med.* 16:135, 1965.

123. Hoffman, G. S. Human erythropoiesis following kidney transplantation. *Ann. N.Y. Acad. Sci.* 149:504, 1968.

124. Horowitz, H. I., Cohen, B. D., Martinez, P., and Papayoanou, M. F. Defective ADP-induced platelet Factor 3 activation in uremia. *Blood* 30:331, 1967.

125. Hudgson, P., Pearce, J. M., and Yeates, W. K. Renal artery stenosis with hypertension and high hematocrit. *Brit. Med. J.* 1:18, 1967.

126. Hurt, G. A., and Chanutin, A. Organic phosphate compounds of erythrocytes from individuals with uremia. *J. Lab. Clin. Med.* 64:675, 1964.

127. Jacobson, L. O., Goldwasser, E., Fried, W., and Plzak, L. Role of the kidney in erythropoiesis. *Nature* (London) 179:633, 1957.

128. Jacobson, L. O., Goldwasser, E., Gurney, C. W., Fried, W., and Plzak, L. Studies on erythropoietin: The hormone regulating red cell production. *Ann. N.Y. Acad. Sci.* 77:551, 1959.

129. James, T. N., and Monto, R. W. Pathology of the cardiac conduction system in thrombotic thrombocytopenic purpura. *Ann. Intern. Med.* 65:37, 1966.

130. Javett, S. N., and Senior, B. Syndrome of hemolysis, thrombopenia, and nephropathy in infancy. *Pediatrics* 29:209, 1962.

131. Jaworski, Z. F., and Hirte, W. E. Polycythemia (erythrocytosis) and non-neoplastic renal disease. *Canad. Med. Ass. J.* 84:1421, 1961.

132. Jerushalmy, Z., Skoza, L., Zucker, M. B., and Grant, R. Inhibition by guanidino compounds of platelet aggregation induced by adenosine diphosphate. *Biochem. Pharmacol.* 15:1791, 1966.

133. Joske, R. A., McAlister, J. M., and Prankerd, T. A. J. Isotope investigations of red cell production and destruction in chronic renal disease. *Clin. Sci.* 15:511, 1956.

134. Kaplan, M., Grumbach, R., and Drapeau, P. Nephroanémie thrombopénique aigue:

Étude d'une forme curable avec biopsies rénales. *Sem. Hôp. Paris* 37:3572, 1961.

135. Kasanen, A., and Kalliomaki, J. L. Correlation of some kidney function tests with hemoglobin in chronic nephropathies. *Acta Med. Scand.* 158:213, 1957.

136. Kaye, M. The anemia associated with renal disease. *J. Lab. Clin. Med.* 52:83, 1958.

137. Kendall, A. G., Lowenstein, L., and Morgan, R. D. The hemorrhagic diathesis in renal disease (with special reference to acute uremia). *Canad. Med. Ass. J.* 85:405, 1961.

138. Kincaid-Smith, P. Histological diagnosis of rejection of renal homografts in man. *Lancet* 2:849, 1967.

139. Koller, F. The treatment of disseminated intravascular coagulation and fibrinolysis. *Thromb. Diath. Haemorrh.* Suppl. 26:359, 1967.

140. Krantz, S. B., and Goldwasser, E. On the mechanism of erythropoietin-induced differentiation: II. The effect on RNA synthesis. *Biochem. Biophys. Acta* 103:325, 1965.

141. Kuhlback, B. Bleeding tendency in chronic renal failure. *Acta Med. Scand.* 157:173, 1957.

142. Künzer, W., and Aalam, F. Treatment of the acute hemolytic-uremic syndrome with heparin. *Lancet* 1:1106, 1964.

143. Kuratowska, Z. The renal mechanism of the formation and inactivation of erythropoietin. *Ann. N.Y. Acad. Sci.* 149:128, 1968.

144. Kuratowska, Z. B., Lewartowski, B., and Michalski, E. Studies on the production of erythropoietin by isolated perfused organs. *Blood* 18:527, 1961.

145. Kuroyanagi, T. Anemia associated with chronic renal failure with special reference to kinetics of the erythron. *Acta Haemat. Jap.* 24:156, 1961.

146. Kurtides, E. S., Rambach, W. A., Alt, H. L., and Del Greco, F. Effects of hemodialysis on erythrokinetics in anemia of uremia. *J. Lab. Clin. Med.* 63:469, 1964.

147. Lachmann, P. J. Müller-Eberhard, H. J., Kunkel, H. G., and Paronetto, F. The localization of in vivo bound complement in tissue sections. *J. Exp. Med.* 115:63, 1962.

148. Langdell, R. D., Adelson, E., Furth, F. W., and Crosby, W. H. Dextran and prolonged bleeding time. *J.A.M.A.* 166:346, 1958.

149. Larrain, C., and Adelson, E. The hemostatic defect in uremia: I. Clinical investigation of three patients with acute post-traumatic renal insufficiency. *Blood* 11:1059, 1956.

150. Larsen, O. A., Josephsen, P., and Lassen, N. A. Nefrogen anaemi behandlet med erythropoietin. *Ugeskr. Laeg.* 125:435, 1963.

151. Lawrence, J. H., and Donald, W. G., Jr. Polycythemia and hydronephrosis or renal tumors. *Ann. Intern. Med.* 50:959, 1959.

152. Lee, L. Reticuloendothelial clearance of circulating fibrin in pathogenesis of the generalized Shwartzman reaction. *J. Exp. Med.* 115:1065, 1962.

153. Lee, L. Antigen-antibody reaction in pathogenesis of bilateral renal cortical necrosis. *J. Exp. Med.* 117:365, 1963.

154. Lee, L., and McCluskey, R. T. Immunohistochemical demonstration of the reticuloendothelial clearance of circulating fibrin aggregates. *J. Exp. Med.* 116:611, 1962.

155. Leikin, S. L. Hematologic aspects of renal disease. *Pediat. Clin. N. Amer.* 11:667, 1964.

156. Lerner, R. G., Rapaport, S. I., and Meltzer, J. Thrombotic thrombocytopenic purpura. *Ann. Intern. Med.* 66:1180, 1967.

157. Lewis, J. H., Zucker, M. B., and Ferguson, J. H. Bleeding tendency in uremia. *Blood* 11:1073, 1956.

158. Lieberman, E., Heuser, E., Donnell, G. N., Landing, B. H., and Hammond, G. D. Hemolytic-uremic syndrome: Clinical and pathological considerations. *New Eng. J. Med.* 275:227, 1966.

159. Lock, S. P., and Dormandy, K. M. Red-cell fragmentation syndrome: A condition of multiple etiology? *Lancet* 1:1020, 1961.

160. Loge, J. P., Lange, R. D., and Moore, C. V. Characterization of the anemia associated with chronic renal insufficiency. *Amer. J. Med.* 24:4, 1958.

161. Lowy, P. H., and Keighley, G. The fractionation of erythropoietin from anemic and normal human urine. *Ann. N.Y. Acad. Sci.* 149:59, 1968.

162. Luke, R. G., Kennedy, A. C., and Stirling,

W. B.   Renal artery stenosis, hypertension and polycythaemia. *Brit. Med. J.* 1:164, 1965.

163. Magid, E., and Hilden, M. Ferrokinetics in patients suffering from chronic renal disease and anemia. *Scand. J. Haemat.* 4:33, 1967.

164. Maher, J. F., and Schreiner, G. E.   Cause of death in acute renal failure. *Arch. Intern. Med.* (Chicago) 110:493, 1962.

165. Mann, D. L., Donati, R. M., and Gallagher, N. I.   Erythropoietin assay and ferrokinetic measurements in anemic uremic patients. *J. Amer. Med. Ass.* 194:1321, 1965.

166. Marcus, A. J., and Zucker, M. B.   *The Physiology of Blood Platelets.* New York: Grune & Stratton, 1965.

167. Martt, J. M., Sayman, A., and Neal, M. P.   Polycythemia and hydronephrosis. *Ann. Intern. Med.* 54:790, 1961.

168. McCluskey, R. T., Benacerraf, B., Potter, J. L., and Miller, F.   Pathologic effects of intravenously administered soluble antigen-antibody complexes: I. Passive serum sickness in mice. *J. Exp. Med.* 111:181, 1960.

169. McKay, D. G.   *Disseminated Intravascular Coagulation.* New York: Hoeber Med. Div., Harper & Row, 1965.

170. McKay, D. G., Gitlin, D., and Craig, J. M.   Immunochemical demonstration of fibrin in the generalized Shwartzman reaction. *A.M.A. Arch. Path.* 67:270, 1959.

171. McKay, D. G., and Shapiro, S. S.   Alterations in the blood coagulation system induced by bacterial endotoxin: I. In vivo (generalized Shwartzman reaction). *J. Exp. Med.* 107:353, 1958.

172. McLean, M. M., Jones, C. H., and Sutherland, D. A.   Haemolytic-uremic syndrome: A report of an outbreak. *Arch. Dis. Child.* 41:76, 1966.

173. McQuiggan, M. C., Oliver, W. J., Littler, E. R., and Cerny, J. C.   Hemolytic uremic syndrome. *J.A.M.A.* 191:787, 1965.

174. Melvin, K. E. W., Farrelly, R. O., and North, J. D. K.   Effect of blood transfusion on renal excretory function in chronic renal failure. *Lancet* 2:537, 1963.

175. Menzies, D. H.   Fibromyomata and poly-cythemia. *J. Obstet. Gynec. Brit. Comm.* 68:505, 1961.

176. Merskey, C., Johnson, A. J., Kleiner, G. J., and Wohl, H.   The defibrination syndrome: Clinical features and laboratory diagnosis. *Brit. J. Haemat.* 13:528, 1967.

177. Mettler, N., Buckley, S., and Casals, J.   Propagation of Junin virus, the etiological agent of Argentinian hemorrhagic fever, in Hela cell cultures. *Proc. Soc. Exp. Biol. Med.* 107:684, 1961.

178. Mitus, W. J., Toyama, K., and Braner, M. J.   Erythrocytosis, juxtaglomerular apparatus (JGA) and erythropoietin in the course of experimental unilateral hydronephrosis in rabbits. *Ann. N.Y. Acad. Sci.* 149:107, 1968.

179. Mitus, W. J., Galbraith, P., Gallerken, M., and Toyama, K.   Experimental renal erythrocytosis: I. Effects of pressure and vascular interference. *Blood* 24:343, 1964.

180. Monnens, L. A. H., and Retera, R. J. M.   Varianten van het hemolytisch-uremisch syndroom. *Maandschr. Kindergeneesk.* 33:205, 1965.

181. Monnens, L. A. H., and Retera, R. J. M.   Thrombotic thrombocytopenic purpura in a neonatal infant. *J. Pediat.* 71:118, 1967.

182. Monnens, L. A. H., and Schretlen, E.   Intravascular coagulation in an infant with the hemolytic-uremic syndrome. *Acta Paediat. Scand.* 56:436, 1967.

183. Moores, R. R., Gardner, E., Jr., Wright, C. S., and Lewis, J. P.   Potentiation of purified erythropoietin with serum proteins: II. Serial dose response relationships. *Proc. Soc. Exp. Biol. Med.* 123:618, 1966.

184. Morgan, J. M., and Morgan, R. E.   Study of the effect of uremic metabolites on erythrocyte glycolysis. *Metabolism* 13:629, 1964.

185. Moschcowitz, E.   An acute febrile pleiochromic anemia with hyaline thrombosis of terminal arterioles and capillaries: An undescribed disease. *Arch. Intern. Med.* 36:89, 1925.

186. Muirhead, E. E., and Jones, F.   Lowered glucose utilization, phosphate uptake, and reduced glutathione content of erythrocytes following bilateral nephrectomy. *J. Lab. Clin. Med.* 51:49, 1958.

187. Murphy, G. P., Mirand, E. A., Johnson,

G. S., Gibbons, R. P., Jones, R. L., and Scott, W. W. Erythropoietin release associated with Wilms' tumor. *The Johns Hopkins Med. J.* 120:26, 1967.

188. Naets, J. P., and Hense, A. F. Measurement of erythropoietin stimulating factor in anemic patients with and without renal lesions. *J. Lab. Clin. Med.* 60:365, 1962.

189. Naets, J. P., and Wittek, M. Erythropoiesis in anephric man. *Lancet* 1:941, 1968.

190. Naets, J. P., and Wittek, M. The mechanisms of action of androgens on erythropoiesis. *Ann. N.Y. Acad. Sci.* 149:366, 1968.

191. Naets, J. P., and Wittek, M. Presence of erythropoietin in the plasma of one anephric patient. *Blood* 31:249, 1968.

192. Natelson, S. I., Stein, I. M., and Bonas, J. E. Improvements in the methods of separation and identification of guanidino organic acids by column chromatography: Isolation and identification of guanidino succinic acid from human urine. *Microchem. J.* 8:371, 1964.

193. Nathan, D. G., Schupak, E., Stohlman, F. J., and Merrill, J. P. Erythropoiesis in anephric man. *J. Clin. Invest.* 43:2158, 1964.

194. Nevasil, C. G., Lynch, E. C., Alfrey, C. P., and Hellums, J. D. Erythrocyte damage and destruction induced by shearing stress. *J. Lab. Clin. Med.* 71:784, 1968.

195. Nies, B. A., Cohn, R., and Schrier, S. L. Erythremia after renal transplantation. *New Eng. J. Med.* 273:785, 1965.

196. Norkin, S. A., Freedman, H. H., and Evans, G. W. Thrombotic thrombocytopenic purpura in siblings. *Amer. J. Med.* 43:294, 1967.

197. O'Brien, J. R. Platelet stickiness. *Ann. Rev. Med.* 17:275, 1966.

198. O'Grady, J. A. Bleeding tendency in uremia. *J.A.M.A.* 169:1727, 1959.

199. Olesen, H., and Fogh, J. Apparent molecular weight of erythropoietin determined by gel filtration. *Scand. J. Haemat.* 5:211, 1968.

200. Orbison, J. L. Morphology of thrombotic thrombocytopenic purpura with demonstration of aneurysms. *Amer. J. Path.* 28:129, 1952.

201. Orten, J. M., and Bucciero, M. C. Effect of cysteine, histidine and methionine on production of polycythemia by cobalt. *J. Biol. Chem.* 176:961, 1948.

202. Painter, R. H., Bruce, W. R., and Goldwasser, E. The commercial production of erythropoietin from anemic sheep plasma. *Ann. N.Y. Acad. Sci.* 149:71, 1968.

203. Pappas, G., Ross, M. H., and Thomas, L. Studies on the generalized Shwartzman reaction: VIII. The appearance by electron microscopy of intravascular fibrinoid in the glomerular capillaries during the reaction. *J. Exp. Med.* 107:333, 1958.

204. Piel, C. F., and Phibbs, R. H. The hemolytic-uremic syndrome. *Pediat. Clin. N. Amer.* 13:295, 1966.

205. Pitney, W. R., and Potter, M. Retention of platelets by glass bead filters. *J. Clin. Path.* 20:710, 1967.

206. Rabiner, S. F., and Friedman, L. H. The role of intravascular haemolysis and the reticuloendothelial system in the production of a hypercoagulable state. *Brit. J. Haemat.* 14:105, 1968.

207. Rabiner, S. F., and Hrodek, O. Platelet Factor 3 in normal subjects and patients with renal failure. *J. Clin. Invest.* 47:901, 1968.

208. Ragen, P. A., Hagedorn, A. B., and Owen, C. A. Radioisotopic study of anemia in chronic renal disease. *Arch. Intern. Med.* (Chicago) 105:518, 1960.

209. Rapaport, S. I., Hjort, P. F., Patch, M. J., and Jeremic, M. Consumption of serum factors and prothrombin during intravascular clotting in rabbits. *Scand. J. Haemat.* 3:59, 1966.

210. Rath, C. E., Mailliard, J. A., and Schreiner, G. E. Bleeding tendency in uremia. *New Eng. J. Med.* 257:808, 1958.

211. Reiquam, C. W., and Prosper, J. C. Fresh plasma transfusions in the treatment of acute thrombocytopenic purpura. *J. Pediat.* 68:880, 1966.

212. Reissmann, K. R., and Nomura, T. Erythropoietin Formation in Isolated Kidneys and Liver. In Jacobson, H., and Doyle, M. (Eds.), *Erythropoiesis.* New York: Grune & Stratton, 1962. P. 71.

213. Reissmann, K. R., Nomura, T., Gunn, R. W., and Brosius, F. Erythropoietic re-

sponse to anemia or erythropoietin injection in uremic rats with and without functioning renal tissue. *Blood* 16:1411, 1960.

214. Reksten, K. R., Jr. Nephrogenic erythrocytosis. *Acta Med. Scand.* 176:757, 1964.

215. Rifkind, D., Kravetz, H. M., Knight, V., and Schade, A. L. Urinary excretion of iron-binding protein in the nephrotic syndrome. *New Eng. J. Med.* 265:115, 1961.

216. Rodríguez-Erdmann, F. Studies on pathogenesis of generalized Shwartzman reaction: I. Alterations in coagulation system during generalized Shwartzman reaction of pregnant rabbit. *Thromb. Diath. Haemorrh.* 12:452, 1964.

217. Rodríguez-Erdmann, F. Bleeding due to increased intravascular blood coagulation. *New Eng. J. Med.* 273:1370, 1965.

218. Rodríguez-Erdmann, F., and Naimi, S. Studies on the pathogenesis of the generalized Shwartzman reaction: IV. Production of a Shwartzman-like phenomenon with autoprothrombin-C. *Thromb. Diath. Haemorrh.* 17:156, 1967.

219. Rodríguez-Erdmann, F., Rubin, A. D., and Dameshek, W. Heparin in thrombotic microangiopathy. *Lancet* 1:1033, 1966.

220. Rosse, W. F., Berry, R. J., and Waldmann, T. A. Some molecular characteristics of erythropoietin from different sources determined by inactivation by ionizing radiation. *J. Clin. Invest.* 42:124, 1963.

221. Rosse, W. F., and Waldmann, T. A. The metabolism of erythropoietin in patients with anemia due to deficient erythropoiesis. *J. Clin. Invest.* 43:1348, 1964.

222. Rosse, W. F., Waldmann, T. A., and Cohen, P. Renal cysts, erythropoietin and polycythemia. *Amer. J. Med.* 34:76, 1963.

223. Rothman, S., Adelson, E., Schwebel, A., and Langdell, R. D. Adsorption of carbon-14 dextran to human blood platelets and red blood cells, in vitro. *Vox Sang.* 2:104, 1957.

224. Rubenberg, M. L., Bull, B. S., Regoeczi, E., Dacie, J. V., and Brain, M. C. Microangiopathic haemolytic anemia: Experimental production of the syndrome in vivo. *Blood* 30:850, 1967. (Abstract.)

225. Salzman, E. W. Measurement of platelet adhesiveness. *J. Lab. Clin. Med.* 62:724, 1963.

226. Salzman, E. W., and Neri, L. L. Adhesiveness of blood platelets in uremia. *Thromb. Diath. Haemorrh.* 15:84, 1966.

227. Sayed, H. M., Dacie, J. V., Handley, D. A., Lewis, S. M., and Cleland, W. P. Haemolytic anaemia of mechanical origin after open heart surgery. *Thorax* 16:356, 1961.

228. Schooley, J. C., and Garcia, J. F. Immunologic studies on the mechanism of action of erythropoietin. *Proc. Soc. Exp. Biol. Med.* 110:636, 1962.

229. Schulman, I., Pierce, M., Lukens, A., and Currimbhoy, Z. Studies in thrombopoiesis: I. A factor in normal human plasma required for platelet production; chronic thrombocytopenia due to its deficiency. *Blood* 16:943, 1960.

230. Schwartz, S. O., and Motto, S. A. The diagnostic significance of "Burr" red blood cells. *Amer. J. Med. Sci.* 218:563, 1949.

231. Shapiro, H. D., Doktor, D., and Churg, J. Thrombotic thrombocytopenic purpura: Report of a case with remission after splenectomy and steroid therapy. *Ann. Intern. Med.* 47:582, 1957.

232. Shapiro, S. S., and McKay, D. G. Prevention of generalized Shwartzman reaction with sodium warfarin. *J. Exp. Med.* 107:377, 1958.

233. Shaw, A. B. Haemolysis in chronic renal failure. *Brit. Med. J.* 2:213, 1967.

234. Shumway, C. N., Jr., and Miller, G. An unusual syndrome of hemolytic anemia, thrombocytopenic purpura and renal disease. *Blood* 12:1045, 1957.

235. Shumway, C. N., Jr., and Terpian, K. L. Hemolytic anemia, thrombocytopenia and renal disease in childhood: The hemolytic-uremic syndrome. *Pediat. Clin. N. Amer.* 11:577, 1964.

236. Shwartzman, G. *Phenomenon of Local Tissue Reactivity.* New York: Paul B. Hoeber, 1937.

237. Smith, R. T., Thomas, L., and Good, R. A. Generalized Shwartzman reaction: V. Intravenous injection of colloidal iron or carbon on response of rabbits to meningococcal

toxin. *Proc. Soc. Exp. Biol. Med.* 82:712, 1953.

238. Spaet, T. H., Horowitz, H. I., Zucker-Franklin, D., Cintron, J., and Biezenski, J. J.   Reticuloendothelial clearance of blood thromboplastin by rats. *Blood* 17:196, 1961.

239. Starzl, T. E., Lerner, R. A., Dixon, F. J., Groth, C. G., Brettschneider, L., and Terasaki, P. I.   Shwartzman reaction after human renal homotransplantation. *New Eng. J. Med.* 278:642, 1968.

240. Stewart, J. H.   Haemolytic anaemia in acute and chronic renal failure. *Quart. J. Med.* 36:85, 1967.

241. Stewart, J. H.   Platelet numbers and life span in acute and chronic renal failure. *Thromb. Diath. Haemorrh.* 17:532, 1967.

242. Stewart, J. H., and Castaldi, P. A.   Uremic bleeding: A reversible platelet defect corrected by dialysis. *Quart. J. Med.* 36:409, 1967.

243. Stewart, J. H., Tuckwell, L. A., Sinnett, P. F., Edwards, K. D. G., and Whyte, H. M.   Peritoneal and hemodialysis: A comparison of their morbidity, and of the mortality suffered by dialysed patients. *Quart. J. Med.* 35:407, 1966.

244. Still, W. J. S., and Boult, E. H.   Electron microscopic appearance of fibrin in thin sections. *Nature* (London) 179:868, 1957.

245. Stohlman, F., Jr.   Humoral regulation of erythropoiesis: VII. Shortened survival of erythrocytes produced by erythropoietin or severe anemia. *Proc. Soc. Exp. Biol. Med.* 107:884, 1961.

246. Stohlman, F., Jr., and Brecher, G.   Humoral regulation of erythropoiesis: V. Relationship of plasma erythropoietin level to bone marrow activity. *Proc. Soc. Exp. Biol. Med.* 100:40, 1959.

247. Symmers, W. St. C.   Thrombotic microangiopathic haemolytic anaemia (thrombotic microangiopathy). *Brit. Med. J.* 2:897, 1952.

248. Taub, R. N., Rodríguez-Erdmann, F., and Dameshek, W.   Intravascular coagulation, the Shwartzman reaction, and the pathogenesis of T.T.P. *Blood* 24:775, 1964.

249. Theil, G. B., Brodine, C. E., and Doolan, P. D.   Red cell glutathione content and sta-

bility in renal insufficiency. *J. Lab. Clin. Med.* 58:736, 1961.

250. Thomas, L., Brunson, J. G., and Smith, R. T.   Studies on the generalized Shwartzman reaction: VI. Production of the reaction by the synergistic action of endotoxin with three synthetic acid polymers. *J. Exp. Med.* 102:249, 1955.

251. Thomas, L., and Good, R. A.   The effect of cortisone on the Shwartzman reaction. *J. Exp. Med.* 95:409, 1952.

252. Thomas, L., and Good, R. A.   Studies on the generalized Shwartzman reaction: I. General observations concerning the phenomenon. *J. Exp. Med.* 96:605, 1952.

253. Thomas, L., Smith, R. T., and Von Korff, R.   Studies on the generalized Shwartzman reaction: VII. The role of fibrinogen in the deposition of fibrinoid after combined injections of endotoxin and synthetic acid polymer. *J. Exp. Med.* 102:263, 1955.

254. Thorling, E. B., and Erslev, A. J.   The relationship between tissue oxygen tension and hematocrit. *Blood* 31:332, 1968.

255. Tisher, C. C., Barnett, B. M. S., Finch, C. A., and Scribner, B. H.   Treatment of iron overload in patients with renal failure. *Clin. Sci.* 33:539, 1967.

256. Unanue, E., and Dixon, F. J.   Experimental glomerulonephritis: IV. Participation of complement in nephrotoxic nephritis. *J. Exp. Med.* 119:695, 1964.

257. Van Dyke, D. C., and Berlin, N. I.   Production of normal-lived erythrocytes with erythropoietin. *Proc. Soc. Exp. Biol. Med.* 104:573, 1960.

258. Van Dyke, D., Keighley, G., and Lawrence, J.   Decreased responsiveness to erythropoietin in a patient with anemia secondary to chronic uremia. *Blood* 22:838, 1963.

259. Van Dyke, D. C., Larysse, M., Lawrence, J. H., Garcia, J. F., and Pollycove, M.   Relation between severity of anemia and erythropoietin titer in human beings. *Blood* 18:187, 1961.

260. Vasquez, J. J., and Dixon, F. J.   Immunohistochemical analysis of lesions associated with "fibrinoid" change. *A.M.A. Arch. Path.* 66:504, 1958.

261. Vassalli, P., and McCluskey, R. I. The coagulation process and glomerular disease. *Amer. J. Med.* 39:179, 1965.

262. Vassalli, P., Simon, G., and Rouiller, C. Electron microscopic study of glomerular lesions resulting from intravascular fibrin formation. *Amer. J. Path.* 43:579, 1963.

263. Verel, D., Turnbull, A., Tudhope, G. R., and Ross, J. H. Anemia in Bright's disease. *Quart. J. Med.* 28:491, 1959.

264. Vertal, R. M., Morse, B. S., and Princi, J. E. Remission of erythropoiesis after drainage of a solitary renal cyst. *Arch. Intern. Med.* (Chicago) 120:54, 1967.

265. Von Kaulla, K. N., Von Kaulla, E., Wasantapruck, S., Marchioro, T. L., and Starzl, T. E. Blood coagulation in uremic patients before and after hemodialysis and transplantation of the kidney. *Arch. Surg.* (Chicago) 92:184, 1966.

266. Waldmann, T. A., Rosse, W. F., and Swarm, R. L. The erythropoiesis-stimulating factors produced by tumors. *Ann. N.Y. Acad. Sci.* 149:509, 1968.

267. Weiner, J., and Spiro, D. Electron microscopic studies in experimental thrombosis. *Exp. Molec. Path.* 1:554, 1962.

268. Weintraub, A. H., Gordon, A. S., Becker, E. L., Camiscoli, J. F., and Contrera, J. F. Plasma and renal clearance of exogenous erythropoietin in the dog. *Amer. J. Physiol.* 207:523, 1964.

269. Welt, L. G., Sachs, J. R., and McManus, T. J. An ion transport defect in erythrocytes from uremic patients. *Trans. Ass. Amer. Physicians* 77:169, 1964.

270. Westerman, M. P., Jenkins, J. L., Dekker, A., Krentner, A., and Fisher, B. Significance of erythrocytosis and increased erythropoietin secretion after renal transplantation. *Lancet* 2:755, 1967.

271. Willoughby, M. L. N., and Crouch, S. J. An investigation of the hemorrhagic tendency in renal failure. *Brit. J. Haemat.* 7:315, 1961.

272. Wong, T. C. A study on the generalized Shwartzman reaction in pregnant rats induced by bacterial endotoxin. *Amer. J. Obstet. Gynec.* 84:786, 1962.

8

Calcium and Phosphorus Metabolism in Renal Failure

S. W. Stanbury

The easily ascertainable biochemical facts concerning disordered calcium and phosphorus metabolism in chronic renal failure are few, well known, and — unless interpreted in conjunction with the available biologic facts — relatively uninformative. The biologic situation is immensely complicated (see Fig. 8-1) and imperfectly understood. The clinical features and natural history of renal osteodystrophy [35, 137, 140], its clinical roentgenology [35, 36, 140, 148], the biochemical changes in the plasma [140, 149], the external mineral balances [35, 63, 81, 82, 90, 145, 153], and the morbid anatomy of the bone [10, 12, 13, 21, 51, 52, 55, 56, 64, 101, 137, 140] and parathyroid glands [56], can be found described elsewhere.

An awareness of the pattern of the external calcium balance in chronic renal failure is crucial to an appreciation of the problems involved. The phosphorus balance is less immediately relevant, since it is largely dependent on the balances of calcium and nitrogen [148].

In chronic renal failure the fecal calcium is high [35, 63, 82, 90, 145, 148, 153], and, with natural diets containing between 200 and 1200 mg. per day, the fecal and dietary calcium have been found to be approximately equivalent [145, 150]; the absorption of orally administered radiocalcium is reduced [28, 64, 113]. This high fecal calcium is interpreted by some workers [30, 82, 94] as an adaptive reduction in calcium absorption determined by the low level of calcium in the urine, which rarely exceeds 100 mg. and is commonly 20 to 60 mg. per day [88, 140, 148]. Others [35, 50, 83, 91, 100, 137–151, 153], following the lead of Liu and Chu [90], consider the high fecal calcium to result from impaired intestinal absorption, probably due to lack of vitamin D action; this view is later elaborated in detail. But, disregarding the precise reason for the high fecal calcium, the critical point is that the *pattern of the calcium balance is always found to be essentially the same; irrespective of the state of the plasma chemistry and of the prevailing pathologic condition of the bone, the external balance is close to equilibrium or negative in minor degree* [89, 90, 145, 146, 148, 151, 153]. As a close approximation, this implies, firstly, that the plasma level of calcium is virtually independent of the urinary calcium and the dietary intake, and secondly, that the external calcium balance has little relevance to the principal anatomic events occurring in the bones. In other words, the patient with chronic renal failure can be regarded as effectively isolated from his nutritional environment in terms of calcium; his problems involve *internal* shifts and redistributions of minerals between bone, the extracellular fluids, and the soft tissues.

As in the normal person [106, 155], the plasma calcium in renal failure depends on biologic equilibria, between the bone and the extracellular fluid, controlled chiefly by the parathyroid hormone. Since the extracellular fluid is supersaturated with respect to the bone mineral [106], any increase of plasma phosphate will increase the rate of deposition in bone of both phosphate and calcium, thereby necessitating increased parathyroid activity to maintain the plasma calcium. But hypocalcemia not attributable to a reduced plasma albumin can occur in renal failure when the plasma phosphate is normal [81, 140, 148, 149]. This state of affairs is associated statistically with the presence of osteomalacic changes in the bone [149], which are probably directly responsible for the ineffectiveness of parathyroid action (see p. 308). It is thus evident that hypocalcemic stimulation to increased parathyroid activity can arise through two independent mechanisms (Fig. 8-1), the *physicochemical* effect of hyperphosphatemia and a *biologic* failure of response in the target organ.

The difficulties involved in explaining the actual pathogenesis of azotemic osteomalacia [138, 141, 146, 148, 150] are unlikely to be resolved until it is finally established whether or not vitamin D acts directly on bone to facilitate its mineralization. Osteomalacia, however, is probably the earliest and commonest [12, 52, 64] bone lesion to develop in renal failure, and this cardinal fact must be taken into account in any consideration of the pathogenesis of renal osteodystrophy. Such considerations have been notably lacking in the recent revival of interest in metabolic acidosis as a factor in the development of uremic bone disease [63, 87, 89, 123]. In a small group of uremic patients, correction of metabolic acidosis restored a minor negative calcium balance to equilibrium [89]; and it is argued that even a trivial calcium loss attributable to acidosis would, if prolonged, inevitably lead to attenuation of the skeleton [87, 123]. This argument is irrefutable, *but* calcium loss would not produce osteomalacia [110]; nor at the rate of loss observed, which is no greater than that seen in many normal individuals [98, 99, 145], would it be likely to cause osteitis fibrosa. The development of osteitis fibrosa in relation to calcium deficiency is a function of the rate and severity of calcium loss [77, 110]. The most to be expected from a slow, prolonged loss of calcium is the development of osteoporosis; but osteopenia (as distinct from osteitis fibrosa with net loss of bone) has not featured significantly in the systematic surveys made of bone from patients dying of uremia [13, 21, 51, 52, 55], whereas hyperostosis is a commonplace [55, 81, 141]. Prolonged metabolic acidosis in adult rats *with intact renal function* produced a minor loss of bone matrix as well as mineral, suggesting that acidosis may influence cellular mechanisms responsible for bone removal [15]. Such an action might hypothetically potentiate the action of parathyroid hormone, but, on present evidence, it is considered that metabolic acidosis plays at most a secondary or subsidiary role in the pathogenesis of azotemic bone disease. For this reason, it does not feature in the schema of Figure 8-1.

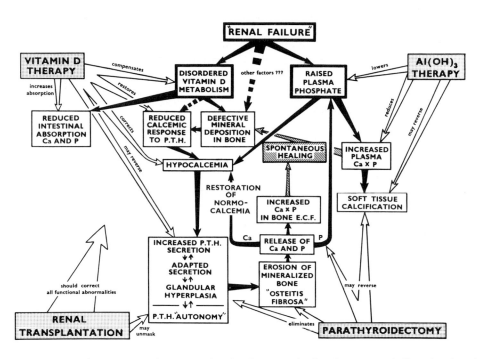

Figure 8-1. A simplified scheme of the disordered calcium and phosphorus metabolism in chronic renal failure and of the effects of specific therapy. Consequential pathogenetic events are linked by black arrows, which are broken when the step is considered to be unproved or of doubtful significance. The effects of therapy are indicated by white arrows and spontaneous healing by crosshatched arrows. No direct consequence of the failure of intestinal absorption of calcium is depicted, since this particular abnormality is regarded solely as a conveniently measurable index of lack of vitamin D action. Metabolic acidosis is also not featured, since there is no direct evidence that this plays any part in the production of azotemic bone disease, and its net effects on calcium and phosphorus metabolism are regarded as trivial. *E.C.F.*, extracellular fluid; *P.T.H.*, parathyroid hormone.

The Apparent Vitamin D Resistance of Renal Failure

There is now a general acceptance of the view that the uremic state is associated with an increased requirement for vitamin D or an acquired "resistance" to its biologic effects [9, 35, 50, 64, 83, 89–91, 100, 137–151, 153, 163]. It is firmly established that defective mineralization of the growth cartilage and of lamellar osteoid occurs commonly in uremic patients [10, 12, 13, 50–52, 55, 64, 137]. The resulting azotemic rickets or osteomalacia can be completely cured by treatment with vitamin D alone [35, 141, 144, 148, 150]; the ultimate

relapse of this bone disease, if therapy is completely withdrawn [141, 148, 150], suggests that there is a continued requirement for increased amounts of the vitamin. The curative effect of vitamin D is invariably associated with an increased intestinal net absorption of calcium and phosphorus [35, 140, 148, 150]. The clinical response to the larger doses of vitamin D usually required [91, 141, 146, 148, 150] resembles in all respects the response of nutritional rickets or osteomalacia to treatment with physiologic amounts of the vitamin. In addition to healing the defective mineralization, effective treatment with vitamin D will correct hypocalcemia, apparently reverse the accompanying secondary hyperparathyroidism [35, 140, 148], and restore power to the weakened proximal limb muscles of the uremic patient [143].

The occurrence of hypocalcemia in patients with azotemic rickets or osteomalacia has been regarded as collateral evidence for a state of effective vitamin D deficiency [149, 150]. In such patients, a low plasma calcium may be associated with normal levels of plasma phosphate and albumin [81, 141, 149]. Statistical examination of the plasma chemistry in a large collection of cases showed no significant inverse correlation between the levels of calcium and phosphate [149]. As in nutritional deficiency of vitamin D [122], hypocalcemia in uremic patients is uninfluenced by administration of parathyroid extract in amounts sufficient to produce a rise of plasma calcium in normal individuals [39, 149].

Although the impaired intestinal net absorption of calcium in uremia is also regarded as evidence for apparent resistance to vitamin D [137–151], it probably plays little or no part in the production of hypocalcemia. A similar intestinal abnormality is found in uremic patients with normal or even elevated levels of plasma calcium [151]. Moreover, in patients with severe azotemic osteomalacia, vitamin D treatment may sometimes promote the intestinal absorption and skeletal retention of 500 to 600 mg. of calcium per day for many weeks *without restoring the plasma calcium to normal* [148]. Such an observation is not readily compatible with the concept of a biochemical "permissive" effect of vitamin D in the calcemic action of parathyroid hormone [122], for it would imply that the therapy had overcome resistance to the vitamin in the alimentary tract but not in the bone. These phenomena, however, do fit with the old view of Albright and Reifenstein [4] that the hypocalcemia of vitamin D deficiency is attributable to the presence of excessive osteoid [80] or, alternatively, to a calcium-deficient bone matrix or bone cell [8]. This is of more than theoretical interest. Continued treatment of azotemic osteomalacia with effective amounts of vitamin D produces clinical and roentgenographic improvement, accompanied by a progressive fall in the level of alkaline phosphatase [148]. When normal levels of alkaline phosphatase are reached and the skeletal deficit of mineral is presumably replenished, a previously low plasma calcium may rise rapidly [91, 92]. If the plasma phosphate is elevated, a dangerously high plasma Ca $\times$ P product (see p. 311) can result; if therapy with vitamin D is continued, hypercalcemia may develop.

Vitamin D Metabolism

Oral treatment with calciferol increases the level of biologically assayable vitamin D activity in the plasma of uremic patients [91, 146, 150]; with a dose of 2.5 mg. (100,000 I.U.) per day, the plasma activity has reached a level of some five to ten times the average found in normal adults [91, 150]. In some patients with azotemic osteomalacia and advanced renal failure (creatinine clearance of 3 to 10 ml. per minute), it has been shown that this dose neither improved the bone disease nor promoted the intestinal absorption of calcium; larger doses given to the same patient were curative [91, 148, 150]. It is thus evident that in uremia the intestine may be unresponsive to a considerably increased level of biologically assayable vitamin in the plasma (see Fig. 8-2). While such observations serve to establish the concept of "resistance" to vitamin action in the gut, the magnitude of the curative dose might suggest that one is dealing with a pharmacologic effect of vitamin D rather than with the compensation of a disordered metabolism of vitamin D. Recent personal studies [91] of azotemic rickets in adolescent patients with less severe renal impairment (creatinine clearance of 20 to 30 ml. per minute) have demonstrated that a typical metabolic response can occur with daily doses of vitamin D_3 or vitamin D_2 as low as 100 to 225 μg. (4000 to 9000 I.U.). Increased intestinal absorption of calcium occurred in these patients with levels of assayed plasma vitamin D activity between 1.5 and 3.0 I.U. per milliliter. In my laboratory, the average vitamin D activity in the plasma of healthy British adults is 0.8 I.U. per milliliter, with a range of 0.3 to 1.6 I.U. per milliliter [91, 150]; almost identical values have been reported from London [158]. Thus, in these patients with less severe renal failure, responsiveness to vitamin D was associated with assayed levels of vitamin D activity in the plasma little more than three times the average, or twice the highest, levels in the indigenous healthy population. These moderately elevated levels of plasma vitamin D activity are apparently within the range encountered in healthy adults of the better vitaminized population of North America, where values of up to 4 I.U. per milliliter of plasma are accepted as normal [16, 17, 105]. This may bear on a previously unexplained difference between the natural history of renal osteodystrophy in Britain and in the United States. The dietary intake of vitamin D in Britain and parts of Europe is sometimes notoriously low [7, 42, 96], and although generally this appears to have little deleterious effect, nutritional osteomalacia is not rare in elderly persons secluded from sunlight [41, 65]. If, as the above data suggest, moderately severe renal impairment produces a moderate increase in the requirement for vitamin D, a state of effective vitamin deficiency may develop in a British patient when an American cousin with comparable renal involvement remains protected by his luxus consumption of the vitamin. In slowly progressive renal failure, as in patients with congenital renal hypoplasia and a normal blood pressure [136, 137], the bones of the British patient may thus be exposed to the effects of vitamin D deficiency for many years. This could explain the frequency with which florid azotemic rickets and

osteomalacia have been reported from Europe [10, 12, 14, 21, 35, 50, 56, 64, 67, 101, 137–150], as compared with their apparent relative rarity in the United States. The same mechanism could account for the severe rickets and osteomalacia encountered by Snapper [136] in patients with chronic renal failure in North China.

It is not possible to predict the requirement for vitamin D in the individual uremic patient [140, 150]. Because of the tedious procedure involved [91], it is unlikely that sufficient data will be accumulated to establish a firm relationship between the vitamin requirement and some parameter of renal failure. It is my impression, nonetheless, that the individual requirement for vitamin D increases with the severity of renal failure. If this is true, it is evident that all uremic patients will at some time develop effective vitamin D deficiency, irrespective of their national or individual habits of vitamin consumption. This is borne out by the frequent finding of osteomalacia in the histologic surveys made of uremic persons in many countries. But, if effective vitamin D deficiency develops relatively late in the course of renal failure, the patient may not survive long enough to develop clinically obvious rickets or osteomalacia.

An increased requirement that is initially measured in micrograms rather than in milligrams is much more acceptable evidence for a possible metabolic abnormality involving vitamin D. Avioli and Slatapolsky [9] have described an apparently abnormal vitamin D metabolism in patients with chronic renal failure which, they believe, would account for the phenomenon of vitamin D resistance. Using tritiated vitamin D_3, they found in renal failure a decreased intestinal absorption of the vitamin, an increase in its fractional turnover rate, and an increase in its degradation to biologically inactive polar metabolites. Such abnormalities could obviously increase the requirement for the vitamin and contribute to the low-normal levels of assayable activity found in the plasma of uremic patients [16, 91]. In addition, Mawer [102] has found that patients with gross proteinuria excrete unchanged vitamin D in the urine. Avioli's observations with isotopically labeled vitamin D were continued over a period of only some three or four days and produced a plasma half-life measured in hours. For this reason, it is perhaps premature to accept them as a complete description of the situation. If observations are extended in time, there is found in man [103] and in the rat [117] a second, slow phase in the decay of plasma radioactivity; in this decay phase, the half-life of unchanged vitamin D and of its polar metabolites is measured in weeks rather than in hours.

It is, however, more difficult to invoke these mechanisms to explain the requirement of some patients [91, 148, 150] for a daily intake as high as 2.5 to 7.5 mg. of vitamin D_2. As already indicated, these patients may exhibit no evidence of the biologic effects of vitamin D when their plasma contains considerably increased amounts of biologically assayable "vitamin D activity" (see Fig. 8-3). Although this plasmatic material is demonstrably biologically active in the vitamin D-deficient assay rat, its chemical nature is unknown. It could consist entirely of the unchanged vitamin alcohol, or admixture of this with one or more biologically active metabolites [34, 93, 112]. The recent studies of DeLuca and his collaborators [34, 93, 112] suggest that the biologically active form of vitamin D may be a more polar metabolite, formed in vivo, and now identified as 25-hydroxycholecalciferol [24]. If this transformation were defective in the uremic state, free (or esterified) vitamin D in the plasma might be biologically inert in the uremic patient; yet, in the biologic assay, it would be metabolized by the recipient rat and thereby measured as "plasma vitamin D activity." Compatible with the concept of an impaired transformation of the vitamin, is the fact that the vitamin D resistance of uremic patients can invariably be overcome if the amount of administered vitamin is increased sufficiently [140–150]. If an abnormal metabolic pathway led to "an increased formation of biologically inactive polar metabolites" [9], the mass effect of a greater dose of vitamin D might produce enough of the *active* metabolite (or metabolites) to establish vitamin D action in the patient. Preliminary observations in my laboratory would fit with this hypothesis; but elucidation of these problems will require more intensive study of vitamin D and its principal metabolites in uremic plasma and tissues.

It is also possible that the results obtained using tracer doses of radioisotopically labeled vitamin D_3 [9, 103] cannot be applied directly to patients receiving relatively massive dosages. Twenty years ago, in patients who had received prolonged high dosages of ergocalciferol as treatment for rheumatoid arthritis, Warkany and his co-workers [160, 161] showed that the biologically assayed level of "vitamin D activity" in the plasma remained high long after cessation of therapy. In patients with azotemic osteodystrophy similarly treated, Lumb, Mawer, and Stanbury [91] have found the biologically assayed "vitamin D activity" in the plasma to decay, after stopping treatment, with a half-life exceeding six months; levels as high as three to five times the average normal have been assayable four years later. This rate of disappearance is even slower than the slow phase of radioisotopic decay already mentioned; it suggests the operation of some other aspect of vitamin D metabolism and may be related to body storage of the vitamin. The conventional belief that vitamin D is not stored significantly in the body has been proved incorrect; both the vitamin and its polar metabolites have been found in most human tissues examined [91]. By virtue of its total mass, voluntary muscle may be quantitatively the most important site of storage in man [91], but significant amounts of the vitamin are stored also in adipose tissue. In patients receiving therapeutic amounts of vitamin D orally, the concentration of the bioassayed activity in the plasma increases as a power function of the daily dose administered [91]. It seems probable that as the plasma level is increased by such therapy a significant fraction of the absorbed vitamin is transferred from the plasma to the tissues. Transfer of stored vitamin from tissues back to blood might similarly explain the prolonged persistence of vitamin D activity in the plasma after cessation of therapy [91, 161]. Thus after the end of treatment with vitamin D, a considerable time may elapse before the patient escapes from the biologic effects of the vitamin. If such therapy is resumed, residual tissue stores of the vitamin may predispose the patient more readily to the development of intoxication through overdosage.

Because one is uncertain what fraction of the assayed activity in the plasma is functionally active in the patient (page 310), interpretation of these biologic vitamin assays must necessarily be tentative. Nonetheless, the very slow fall in plasma activity after stopping treatment would explain the long delay that may elapse before the rickets or osteomalacia relapses clinically [140, 141]. Resumption of treatment after relapse may then produce a very rapid rise in assayable plasma activity, even if a smaller daily dose is used [91]. *Until more precise measurements become possible, the data presented can serve as a reminder of the potential and real hazards attending therapy with vitamin D.*

VITAMIN D RESISTANCE AND METABOLIC ACIDOSIS

The metabolic responses to the required dose of vitamin D in azotemic osteomalacia and to physiologic amounts of the vitamin in nutritional osteomalacia are identical [35, 135, 148, 156]; intestinal net absorption of calcium is increased and the mineral balance becomes positive, with a proportionate retention of calcium and phosphorus in the skeleton. If the increased requirement and abnormal metabolism of vitamin D were directly attributable to uremic acidosis, correction of the acidosis should initiate a similar metabolic response and lead ultimately to healing of the osteodystrophy. It has been claimed that treatment with alkalis benefits azotemic osteodystrophy [4], but this claim was not documented, nor has it been substantiated subsequently [35, 148]. Control of the metabolic acidosis has been shown to produce a trivial improvement in the minimally negative calcium balance of uremic subjects [89]; but *the mineral balance was not rendered positive, and the fecal calcium remained approximately the same as the dietary calcium.* Moreover, vitamin D will produce its metabolic and curative effects in azotemic rickets and osteomalacia when the prevailing metabolic acidosis remains untreated [140, 148]. This was equally true of the cases previously discussed that required no more than 100 to 300 μg. of vitamin D per day [91]. It thus seems unlikely that metabolic acidosis is the cause of the vitamin D resistance in renal failure.

BIOLOGIC INHIBITORS OF CALCIFICATION, VITAMIN D, AND THE PLASMA Ca $\times$ P PRODUCT

Urine contains inhibitors capable of preventing both the precipitation of calcium phosphate from solution [47] and the nucleation of mineralization by biologic agents such as collagen or rat epiphyseal cartilage [47, 48, 164]. Uremic plasma also contains inhibitor (or inhibitors), demonstrated by the capacity of plasma ultrafiltrates to increase the product of calcium and phosphate ions (Ca $\times$ P product) required to produce in vitro calcification of ricketic rat cartilage [164]. Since azotemic rickets and osteomalacia may be associated with abnormally high values of the plasma Ca $\times$ P product (Fig. 8-2), it has been suggested that retention of such urinary inhibitors in the plasma might account for the defective mineralization in the skeleton [109, 164]. Of the identified urinary inhibitors, pyrophosphate is also a normal constituent of plasma [45], but its concentration has not been found consistently increased in renal failure [126]. The turnover of the minute amounts of pyrophosphate in plasma is extremely rapid [126], and pyrophosphate is also formed and destroyed locally in bone [126]. It would therefore be possible to have a disturbed pyrophosphate metabolism in bone, potentially capable of retarding mineralization, without this being reflected by a change of plasma pyrophosphate concentration. Pyrophosphate and other polyphosphates, added to the medium in relatively high concentration, will inhibit the calcification of living bone in culture [49].

Another group of urinary inhibitors has been identified as polypeptides of low molecular weight [73], and their concentration in uremic plasma may be greatly increased [157]. As yet, nothing is known of the origin, fate, and possible physiologic role of these potent substances, but they could prove to be of considerable importance in normal and morbid calcium metabolism.

There is no predictable relationship between the plasma Ca × P product and the *presence* of defectively mineralized bone [149]. For the group of cases shown in Figure 8-2, the mean value of this product was normal, but in some cases the values were very high and in others, so low as to fall in the range conventionally associated with defective mineralization. Because of this latter group of cases, it is difficult to refute the suggestion [111] that the actual *development* of defective mineralization might always occur in association with low values of plasma Ca × P product at an early, and probably unobserved, stage of the renal failure. In that event, the pathogenesis of azo-

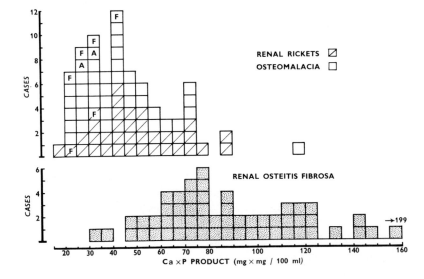

Figure 8-2. The plasma Ca × P product in patients with azotemic osteodystrophy. Patients with renal tubular acidosis are designated as A here while F designates those with the Fanconi syndrome; all these patients also had advanced renal failure. *Above,* 79 cases with defective mineralization and varying degrees of accompanying osteitis fibrosa. Mean plasma Ca, 7.63 mg. per 100 ml. (S.D. 1.47 mg./100 ml.); mean plasma P, 6.03 mg. per 100 ml. (S.D. 2.25 mg./100 ml.). *Below,* 55 cases with generalized osteitis fibrosa *and no defect of mineralization.* Mean plasma Ca, 10.05 mg. per 100 ml. (S.D. 1.25 mg./100 ml.); mean plasma P, 8.79 mg. per 100 ml. (S.D. 2.74 mg./100 ml.). (From Stanbury, S. W., and Lumb, G. A. [149].)

temic rickets and osteomalacia would conform with orthodox views of the significance of this product, and there would be no need to invoke the operation of biologic inhibitors of calcification. There is no evidence available, however, that the plasma Ca $\times$ P product is commonly subnormal in early renal failure, and the data of Figure 8-2 indicate that establishment of a normal or moderately increased Ca $\times$ P product does not alone suffice for the *healing* of defective mineralization. During treatment of azotemic osteodystrophy with vitamin D, the occurrence of mineral retention has been documented at all levels of the plasma Ca $\times$ P product from 25 to 75 [141, 148], and, in the individual patient, with no change in the product prevailing before treatment started [141]. This suggests that the curative effects of vitamin D in this situation are effected through some action other than the conventional one of regulating the plasma Ca $\times$ P product. There is some evidence that the vitamin may act directly on bone to facilitate its mineralization [26, 152]. Despite the circumstantial evidence provided by in vitro studies of ricketic "healing," it could yet prove that the plasma changes accompanying therapy with vitamin D are mere epiphenomena to a more fundamental action of the vitamin on the bone cell.

Since vitamin D can promote healing of azotemic rickets without producing significant change of plasma Ca $\times$ P product [141] and as no particular, "critical" value of this product appears to be required for healing [92, 141], it follows that inhibitors of mineralization cannot be active during effective therapy with the vitamin [141, 146, 148]. Either inhibitors are not involved in the production of defective mineralization, or their effects are overwhelmed by some action of vitamin D that does not involve the plasma Ca $\times$ P product, or effective therapy with vitamin D in some way causes their inactivation or destruction. There is obvious scope for measurement of the effect of vitamin D ther-

apy on the plasma level of peptide inhibitors, not only in uremia but also in other states associated with defective skeletal mineralization. The classic "alkaline phosphatase" apparently functions as a pyrophosphatase [126a], and its plasma level rises on the institution of vitamin D therapy [135]. Conceivably, the activation of osteoblast pyrophosphatase by vitamin D could facilitate mineralization by destroying pyrophosphate at the calcification front. Until more data are accumulated and more is known of the role of these inhibitors in controlling normal mineralization, comment on their significance in renal failure is purely speculative.

VITAMIN D RESISTANCE AND SECONDARY HYPERPARATHYROIDISM

Because hypocalcemia in chronic uremia is associated statistically with defective mineralization [149], it is sometimes implied that the effective vitamin D deficiency renders the bone "insensitive to parathyroid hormone" [83, 100]. As an unqualified statement this is incorrect. Unquestionably, the prevailing rate of parathyroid secretion is ineffective in maintaining a normal serum calcium; the reasons for this homeostatic failure have not been fully elucidated (see page 308). But in most, perhaps in all, cases of azotemic rickets and osteomalacia there is an associated osteitis fibrosa of variable severity [12, 55]. All available evidence indicates that this destructive lesion in the premorbid, mineralized bone is attributable to an increased secretion of parathyroid hormone [137–151]. The plasma level of parathyroid hormone, as measured by radioimmunoassay, is increased in azotemic patients with hypocalcemia, and it can be reduced by raising the plasma calcium artificially by calcium infusion [22]. There is also evidence that the effect of secondary hyperparathyroidism on the diseased kidney limits the increase in plasma phosphate caused by reduced glomerular filtration [43, 133, 134] and thereby contributes to the normal or near normal plasma phosphate levels not infrequently found in azotemic rickets and osteomalacia [81, 140, 149].

The functional state is analogous to that of simple vitamin D deficiency, where the effects of secondary hyperparathyroidism on the kidney produce hypophosphatemia [109] and in the bone, osteitis fibrosa [74]. In both azotemic [35, 36, 140, 148] and nutritional [74, 154] rickets or osteomalacia, there may be roentgenographic evidence of hyperparathyroidism in the form of typical subperiosteal erosions on the digital phalanges. Especially in the former disease, such changes may be found when there are no other roentgenographic abnormalities and, more especially, no specific signs of osteomalacia [140]. This is important for two reasons: (1) such findings may be misinterpreted to signify that the bone lesions are purely those of hyperparathyroidism, whereas bone biopsy could reveal a combination of osteomalacia and osteitis fibrosa [11, 55]; and (2) the radiographic evidence of hyperparathyroidism will disappear when the osteomalacia is treated with vitamin D [35, 140, 148], and it shows no tendency to recur rapidly when therapy is withdrawn. Although the point has yet to be proved by measurements of parathyroid hormone secretion rate, it appears that this treatment inhibits the secondary hyperparathyroidism and its erosive action on the bone [141, 148]. In this respect, also, the uremic state is analogous to that of simple vitamin D deficiency [74].

A feature of the natural history of untreated azotemic osteodystrophy, documented by both osteopathologic [56] and clinical roentgenologic [137] studies, is the fact that the ricketic lesions may heal spontaneously as the severity of the associated secondary hyperparathyroidism increases. Effectively the whole of the dietary calcium is recovered in the feces at all stages in the evolution of the disease [141, 151]. Consequently, secondary hyperparathyroidism does not produce spontaneous healing by the supposed action of parathyroid hor-

mone on the intestinal absorption of dietary calcium [31]. Moreover, in primary hyperparathyroidism, which is associated with a statistically increased absorption of calcium [145, 147], the development of secondary renal failure leads to failure of calcium absorption; the external mineral balance then becomes indistinguishable from that of primary renal disease [147]. The only alternative source of mineral salt for the process of healing is the calcified bone removed under the influence of increased parathyroid activity. In his pathologic material, Gilmour [56] considered the extent of spontaneous healing to be correlated roughly with the degree of osteitis fibrosa and parathyroid hyperplasia. Similar results were obtained by Garner and Ball [55].

As secondary hyperparathyroidism intensifies, progressive amounts of lamellar bone are replaced by woven bone [12], which tissue has been shown to mineralize when biochemical conditions are unfavorable for the mineralization of lamellar osteoid [54]. But lamellar osteoid is relatively resistant to erosive removal until it has been mineralized [79]; consequently, the process of spontaneous healing must involve the mineralization of existing osteoid. This implies that secondary hyperparathyroidism creates conditions that permit mineralization, in spite of the persistence of a state of apparent vitamin D deficiency [151]. Mineralization in osteomalacic states is not arrested but greatly slowed in rate, so that the life span of the osteoid seam is abnormally prolonged [53]. For purely physicochemical reasons [106, 155], any increase in the activity product of calcium and phosphate ions in the extracellular fluid at the calcification front would inevitably accelerate this process. The plasma Ca $\times$ P product in cases of azotemic osteodystrophy without defectively mineralized bones greatly exceeds, sometimes by a factor of several times, the values associated with rickets and osteomalacia (Fig. 8-2). The erosion of calcified bone caused by secondary hyperparathyroidism must release calcium and phosphate ions to the extracellular fluid of bone adjacent to the erosion sites. Especially in the presence of an increased plasma Ca × P product (Fig. 8-2), the local ion product within bone fluid could thus be boosted to very high levels, and, it is suggested, these would suffice to mineralize the osteoid seam (see Fig. 8-1).

SIGNIFICANCE OF THE SEVERITY AND THE
DURATION OF RENAL IMPAIRMENT

It is not known what degree of renal impairment is needed to produce the biochemical syndrome of apparent vitamin D resistance; nor is there evidence to indicate whether loss of renal tissue mass or of some specific renal function is responsible. The characteristic changes can develop when azotemia is minimal [88, 140] and their development is not prevented by the Giordano-Giovanetti type of low-protein diet [18]. Some evidence suggests that similar metabolic changes may occur in *acute* renal failure: the absorption of a standard oral test dose of calcium is reduced [162a], and temporary hypocalcemia may occur during the early phase of recovery, even when the plasma phosphate is normal or low [25, 139]. Metabolic balance studies have been made in the particular form of acute renal impairment caused by hypercalcemic crisis in patients with primary hyperparathyroidism [147]. In one such patient, with classic bone disease, no net absorption of calcium was observed after parathyroidectomy when the creatinine clearance was 22 ml. per minute; as renal function improved spontaneously, calcium absorption increased progressively to become equivalent to 43 per cent of the dietary intake when the creatinine clearance reached 40 ml. per minute. In a second case, the creatinine clearance after parathyroidectomy did not exceed 10 ml. per minute; despite the presence of severe bone disease, there was no net absorption of the dietary calcium, either spontaneously or in response to a daily

dose of 2.5 mg. (100,000 I.U.) of vitamin D_2 that increased the assayable plasma level of vitamin D activity to 5.6 I.U. per milliliter.

It thus appears to be the severity of the renal disease, rather than its duration, that causes the initial development of apparent vitamin D resistance. Subsequent events will depend on the tempo of evolution of the renal failure. Slow progression may permit the development of overt rickets or osteomalacia (see page 307). With progressive reduction of glomerular filtration, the plasma phosphate will rise; ultimately the phosphaturic action of secondary hyperparathyroidism becomes ineffective [61], and gross hyperphosphatemia ensues. This will contribute to the healing of defective mineralization as already discussed. If the intake of vitamin D were sufficient to meet the increased requirement (pages 308–311), significant osteomalacia might never develop and the bony changes would be those of hyperparathyroidism attributable to the action of hyperphosphatemia (Fig. 8-1; pages immediately following).

Secondary Hyperparathyroidism: The Vicious Circle of Hyperphosphatemia

The secretion of parathyroid hormone is regulated by the plasma level of ionic calcium [29, 132], and it has been established that the parathyroid glands do not respond directly to an increase in plasma phosphate [131]. If hypocalcemia in azotemic rickets depends on the presence of excess osteoid (pages 313–315), secondary hyperparathyroidism would fail to restore a normal plasma calcium until the defect of mineralization was repaired. Thus, in spite of an increased rate of hormonal secretion, the stimulus of hypocalcemia would persist ("hypocalcemic hyperparathyroidism"). It is not known how the human parathyroid gland responds to sustained hypocalcemia.

Judging from the response to chronic hypo-calcemia in the lactating cow [118, 120], there is likely to be an "adaptive" increase of hormonal secretion. A moderate degree of chief cell hyperplasia of the glands is well documented in cases of azotemic rickets [56]; (see Fig. 8-1). To the extent that increased parathyroid activity resulted in healing of the osteomalacia (pages 313–315), it should tend to correct the hypocalcemia; but there is no way of assessing the degree of spontaneous healing in the individual patient. The degree of osteitis fibrosa accompanying azotemic rickets and osteomalacia, whether assessed histologically [12, 21, 51, 52, 55, 64] or roentgenographically [35, 36, 148], varies enormously from case to case; this alone suggests that the parathyroid response may be correspondingly variable. Similarly, although defective mineralization is associated *statistically* with hypocalcemia, the plasma calcium in individual patients may range from very low to normal levels [149]; and it has been noted that patients with azotemic osteomalacia and very low levels of plasma calcium tend to show the least radiographic evidence of secondary hyperparathyroidism [148]. It is therefore likely that the prevailing rate of parathyroid secretion in these patients will depend not only on the degree of hypocalcemia [29, 132] but also on its duration, the degree of glandular hyperplasia, and the pathologic state of the bones.

In patients with chronic renal failure, an induced elevation of the plasma phosphate causes depression of the plasma calcium [35, 90, 100]. In so doing, it accelerates the deposition of mineral in bone [106, 155] and simultaneously perpetuates or intensifies the stimulus to increased parathyroid secretion. The spontaneous, progressive rise of plasma phosphate with deterioration of renal function must inevitably produce similar effects. In rickets and osteomalacia, which tend to develop at an earlier stage of renal failure, when the parathyroid response is still capable of maintaining a near-normal plasma phosphate

[134], this indirect stimulation to the parathyroid glands may not be operating. More recent observations by Reiss and his collaborators [122a] suggest that secondary hyperparathyroidism may develop very early in the course of renal disease and increase progressively with the progression of renal impairment. In animals with experimentally induced renal failure and severe uremia, these workers were apparently able to prevent the development of secondary hyperparathyroidism by measures of phosphate deprivation that prevented the usual elevation of the serum phosphate [134a]. In generalized renal osteitis fibrosa *without an associated defect of mineralization,* renal failure is further advanced and the plasma phosphate conspicuously higher than in azotemic rickets or osteomalacia [149]. In Figure 8-2, the supranormal values of the plasma Ca $\times$ P product in the 55 cases of generalized osteitis fibrosa were largely attributable to the height of the plasma phosphate [149]. But, paradoxically, in the presence of such hyperphosphatemia, the group as a whole was statistically normocalcemic: the mean plasma total calcium was 10 mg. per 100 ml. (S.D. 1.25 mg. per 100 ml.), and in one-fifth of the cases it was 11 mg. per 100 ml. or higher. This effective maintenance of a "normal" plasma calcium may simply reflect the magnitude of the parathyroid response; or it could be related to the absence of osteomalacia in this group of patients. In either event, hyperphosphatemia must contribute to this response by facilitating the healing of defective mineralization and by potentiating the stimulation of parathyroid secretion.

With the establishment of an apparently normal level of plasma calcium, one might expect a cessation of excessive parathyroid activity and an involution of glandular hyperplasia. In fact, the parathyroid glands in generalized osteitis fibrosa are usually greatly, or even enormously, enlarged [3, 37, 56, 71, 116, 149], and their continued secretory activity has been proved by parathyroidectomy

[6, 44, 149, 151, 163] and by their functional performance after successful renal homotransplantation [72, 95, 97, 163]. One possible reason for such sustained secondary hyperparathyroidism would be that the normocalcemia is only apparent or inconstantly maintained. The complexed fraction of calcium is increased in uremia [159] and a normal plasma total calcium need not imply a normal ionic fraction. Whereas Stanbury and Lumb [149] found no relationship between the plasma levels of phosphate and total calcium in their collection of cases, there was a significant inverse correlation between phosphate and directly measured ionic calcium in the patients of Kleeman et al. [83]. A plasma calcium that was normal in the fasting state might be depressed by the rise of plasma phosphate following a meal; and adequate assessment of the state of plasma ionic calcium might require serial measurements throughout the day. Indeed, any process that appreciably increased the plasma phosphate would tend to depress the ionic calcium [134]. In addition to eating, these would include episodes of dehydration or increasing acidosis and increased protein catabolism; phosphate released by erosion of mineralized bone may also contribute to the hyperphosphatemia [100, 149, 151]. At very high levels of $Ca \times P$ product, the plasma itself is physically supersaturated with calcium phosphate [71, 109], and calcium is lost from the extracellular fluid by its deposition in the soft tissues as well as in bone. In patients depositing masses of metastatic calcification, sizable spontaneous changes in plasma calcium have been recorded. Since the diseased kidney is itself one of the most common sites of metastatic calcification [70], physical supersaturation of the plasma may intensify the renal damage and, by further increasing the hyperphosphatemia, perpetuate the vicious circle. It is to be noted that this vicious circle is broken, at least temporarily, when the levels of both plasma calcium and phosphate are simultaneously depressed by parathyroidec-tomy [151]. The plasma becomes physically unsaturated (although it remains "supersaturated with respect to bone mineral" [106]), metastatic calcification may resorb [37, 44, 142, 163], and it has been possible to document a shift of calcium from the soft tissues to bone [142]. There is no evidence, however, that parathyroidectomy is followed by measurable improvement of renal function.

The sequence of events attributed to increasing hyperphosphatemia is likely to remain operating in patients treated by chronic intermittent hemodialysis. Such therapy is usually reserved for patients in the preterminal phase of renal failure; the glomerular filtration rate is already minimal, and it falls further in the course of treatment. The individual dialysis is usually effective in restoring a normal plasma phosphate, but hyperphosphatemia will develop during the interdialytic period in proportion to the dietary intake of phosphorus. While this tendency may be limited by the use of orally administered phosphate-binding agents, it is evident that such therapy is not always effective in practice. Reasons for this include the patients' intolerance of aluminum salts given in the gel form and their apparent failure to continue to take the prescribed amount, when binding agents are given in tablet form. It is not known what plasma levels of calcium and phosphate prevail during the greater part of the dialyzed patient's life. From the frequent description of metastatic calcification in the periarticular [27] and ocular issues [1] of dialyzed patients, it is evident that the plasma $Ca \times P$ product must be significantly elevated for a considerable time. Actual measurements made during the interdialytic periods indicate that the plasma calcium may fall to subnormal levels as hyperphosphatemia redevelops [18]. It thus seems likely that the parathyroid glands of patients treated by intermittent hemodialysis are perfused by hypocalcemic blood for a greater part of the time. Compatible with this concept of continued stimulation of the parathyroid glands is the frequency with which severe osseous hyperparathyroidism has been reported in such patients [82a, 115, 128].

Significance of the Mass of Hyperplastic Parathyroid Tissue: Parathyroid Autonomy

An alternative explanation for the sustained normocalcemia or minimal hypercalcemia [149] in hyperphosphatemic patients with generalized osteitis could be the development of secretory autonomy in the parathyroid glands. This was suggested by the finding of apparent adenomatous transformation in some cases [151], but it was not possible on histologic grounds alone to determine whether the often sizable, circumscribed nodules of oxyphil cells or acinar formation [56, 141, 151] represented the formation of adenomas. There is now no doubt that autonomy of hormonal secretion does sometimes occur, but its expression as overt hypercalcemia is prevented by the accompanying high plasma phosphate. Among the patients with advanced renal failure who underwent successful renal homotransplantation, the complete biochemical syndrome of "primary" hyperparathyroidism has developed in several when adequate function was established in the transplanted kidney [72, 95, 97, 163]. This postoperative development of hypercalcemia clearly indicates failure of the feedback control of parathyroid secretion [29, 132]; the accompanying hypophosphatemia and renal phosphaturia are uninfluenced when the plasma calcium is further elevated by infusion of calcium salts [95, 97]. In other respects, this functional autonomy differs from that exhibited by the classic parathyroid adenoma. In some renal transplant patients, loss of homeostatic control has been transient [95]; in others, hypercalcemia has been intermittent or apparently suppressed by adrenocortical steroids [72, 95]. Because of the hazard of hypercalcemia to the transplanted

kidney, parathyroidectomy has usually been performed in these patients within a short time of its detection. Normal control of hormonal secretion might have been restored in some of them, given the provision of further time. It can safely be assumed that renal failure of a severity sufficient to warrant homotransplantation will always be associated with significant secondary hyperparathyroidism; yet the development of postoperative hypercalcemia is the exception rather than the rule [95]. This must imply either that the feedback control of parathyroid secretion was still operating at the time of renal transplantation [104], or that its function was restored very rapidly by the procedure [95]. In extreme contrast with this is the experience of de Graeff [66] with two cases of post-transplantational hypercalcemia. In one, hypercalcemia decreased slowly and homeostatic control was regained after approximately six months. The second patient was still hypercalcemic after six months, and subtotal parathyroidectomy was performed; it is questionable whether this patient would have behaved like the first patient had parathyroidectomy been still further delayed. Because of the unpredictable duration of this parathyroid autonomy, there is much to recommend the suggestion of Massry et al. [100] that such patients might be protected from the deleterious effects of hypercalcemia and hypercalciuria during the interim period by the use of phosphate supplements [62]. It could thereby be possible to delay or circumvent the further trauma of parathyroidectomy in these precariously balanced patients.

It appears to be established that the secondary parathyroid hyperplasia of chronic renal failure can be complicated by adenoma formation, which causes functional suppression of the initially hyperplastic tissue [108]. This occurrence is probably rare, and it will usually be difficult to distinguish from primary hyperparathyroidism complicated by secondary chronic renal failure [59]. Indeed, it is difficult to assess the concept of "tertiary hyperparathyroidism" as applied in certain case reports [33] that provide neither histologic description of the nonadenomatous parathyroid tissue nor assessment of its secretory status using cytologic and electron microscopic technics such as those of Roth and his associates [108, 124, 125]. The formation of "secondary" adenomas appears not to be involved in the state of parathyroid autonomy following renal homotransplantation. Parathyroid glands resected from these patients have shown chief cell hyperplasia only [80a, 95, 97, 163], and although specifically sought, no adenomas have been found [personal communications from various authors]. The glands are invariably large; in generalized renal osteitis fibrosa the combined parathyroid weight may be some five to one hundred times the average normal [3, 37, 116, 149, 151], and the suggestion has been made that hormonal secretion increases pari passu with size [100]. The parathyroid transplantation studies of Gittes and Radde [58] in the rat indicate that a massive increase in the amount of *normal* parathyroid tissue in the individual animal can cause sustained hypercalcemia and hypophosphatemia. In these circumstances, moderate hypercalcemia fails to cause total suppression of the secretion of parathyroid hormone. In the "nutritional secondary hyperparathyroidism" of domestic animals, generalized osteitis fibrosa is associated with massive chief cell hyperplasia of the parathyroid glands [78, 84–86]. This condition, which results from the consumption of diets of high P:Ca ratio [85, 86], provides a close analogy with the effects of hyperphosphatemia in renal failure [141, 146]. In some affected animals, the tendency to hypocalcemia is apparently overcompensated by the parathyroid response and hypercalcemia develops [78, 86]; but adenoma formation has not been described in the hyperplastic glands. It is open to question whether this development of hypercalcemia is a function of the sheer mass of *hyperplastic* parathyroid tissue, as with the mass of *normal* tissue in the experiments of Gittes and Radde

[58], or whether it reflects a change of parathyroid cell function that has no structural counterpart. The same question remains unresolved in the parathyroid autonomy of renal failure. The fact that this autonomy may be reversible after homotransplantation indicates a process of involution; the long delay sometimes required before normal homeostasis is restored (see above) further suggests the occurrence of structural involution.

What is presently known or inferred about parathyroid function in chronic renal failure has been derived without benefit of actual measurements of hormonal secretion rate. This can now be remedied with the availability of radioimmunoassay as a method of measurement [22, 131]. However, so many factors are involved in determining the level of parathyroid activity in renal failure that no simple picture is likely to emerge. Random or isolated measurements of plasma hormone are unlikely to be helpful; it is also unlikely that data from a group of patients will show the expected [29, 131] relationship between plasma levels of calcium and hormone. This heretical comment can perhaps be justified by listed recapitulation:

1. Hypocalcemic azotemic osteomalacia may be associated with functionally ineffective hyperparathyroidism (page 315).
2. The plasma phosphate may determine the level of parathyroid activity required to maintain normocalcemia (page 316).
3. The mass of parathyroid tissue will vary unpredictably among patients (page 316).
4. Adaptive increase of hormonal secretion, functional autonomy, and actual adenoma formation will occur unpredictably in a proportion of cases.

Nonetheless, just as chronic renal failure provides unique opportunities for study of the reactions of the human bone [137], it has a similar potential in the function and oncology of the human parathyroid gland.

Metastatic Calcification in Chronic Renal Failure

The development of metastatic calcification in extraosseous tissues is primarily a function of the activity product aCa^{2+} $aHPO_4^{2-}$ in the extracellular fluids [71]. With the concentration of both total calcium and phosphorus expressed in mg. per 100 ml., physical saturation of the plasma and spontaneous precipitation of calcium phosphate is associated with values of the Ca $\times$ P product in the region of 70 to 80 [71, 109]. Since values as high as this are exceptional in patients with defective mineralization (Fig. 8-2), visible metastatic calcification is unusual in such cases, whereas its association with generalized osteitis fibrosa (see Fig. 8-2) has long been recognized [3, 37, 116].

In addition to the prerequisite physicochemical conditions in the extracellular fluids, a variety of local factors in the tissue may determine the actual sites of calcium phosphate deposition [70]. Among such factors, a "tendency to tissue alkalinity" [162] has been recognized for many years as possibly responsible for selective calcification in the renal tubules, gastric mucosa, and interalveolar septa of the lungs [70]. A local reduction of pCO_2, with consequent reduction in the solubility of calcium phosphate, is probably responsible for calcific deposits in the exposed tissues of the eye [19, 20]. In addition to the well-known limbal arc calcification in the cornea, a more common occurrence is the deposition of discrete crystals in the superficial layers of the interpalpebral bulbar conjunctiva [19, 20]. While most easily defined by the corneal microscope [19, 20], these crystals impart a roughened granular appearance to the conjunctiva that can be recognized by the naked eye or with the use of a simple ophthalmoscope. Crystal depositions can cause transient inflammatory reddening of the eye [20]. Once these ocular appearances are known,

they can provide a crude but useful clinical index of the state of the plasma biochemistry.

The factors responsible for the localization of metastatic calcification at other sites, such as in the media of small and medium arteries, are unknown. In certain instances of metastatic deposition at unusual sites, the phenomenon of "calciphylaxis" [129] has been invoked. The trauma of scratching due to uremic pruritus was considered to act as "challenging agent" in a case of calcinosis cutis [38]; in an extremely obese uremic patient, the traumatic effect of pressure may have been responsible for a patchily distributed calcifying panniculitis [5]. The repeated trivial trauma of simple physical activity might similarly contribute to the frequent periarticular localization of metastatic calcification. In animals suitably conditioned by procedures likely to increase the plasma Ca $\times$ P product, metastatic calcification can be induced by factors as different as epilation or the injection of miscellaneous chemicals [129]. It is at least possible that an equally wide range of chemical and physical factors could operate in the uremic patient.

Metastatic calcification will absorb, if the degree of saturation of extracellular fluid with calcium phosphate can be reduced sufficiently by therapy with aluminum hydroxide [5] or by parathyroidectomy [37, 44, 142, 163]. The extent of resorption from a particular site will presumably depend on the extent to which the deposited mineral remains in exchange equilibrium with the extracellular fluid. Thus the often large, soft, and *wet* subcutaneous masses may absorb rapidly and completely [37, 142]. On the other hand, although arterial calcification has been observed to diminish [5], this is not so usual [80a].

Parenthetically, if *circulating* inhibitors of calcification were involved in the prevention of adequate mineralization of bone in uremia [164] they should function similarly in respect to calcification in the soft tissue. When appropriate allowances are made for the filtrability of plasma calcium and phosphate and for the effect of pH, the Ca $\times$ P product at which soft tissue calcification is observed corresponds approximately to the solubility product of secondary calcium phosphate [71, 109]. An effectively functioning inhibitor would be expected to increase appreciably the ion product at which deposition occurs.

Therapeutic Implications

It is perhaps trite to suggest that treatment should not be instituted unless the physician knows what he is treating and what his therapy is likely to achieve. But perusal of contemporary nephrological literature gives the impression that, in the management of disordered calcium and phosphorus metabolism, it is sometimes the plasma biochemistry rather than the patient that is treated.

Although adequate correction of metabolic acidosis might hypothetically limit a slowly progressive loss of body calcium [89], the use of alkalis or even peritoneal dialysis in a patient with hypocalcemia can cause convulsions that may be complicated by lethal fractures [141]. If the plasma Ca $\times$ P product is high, alkalinization will facilitate metastatic calcification. I have observed no *clinically detectable* detriment from metabolic acidosis that has reduced the plasma total carbon dioxide to between 14 and 20 millimoles per liter. Many patients have been observed with untreated, stable acidosis of this magnitude for periods of five or, exceptionally, ten years.

It has been shown that some fraction of a massive daily oral dose of calcium salts is absorbed by the uremic patient, with a resulting trivial rise in the plasma calcium [30]. This is a Pyrrhic victory if it causes metastatic calcification [50]. In contradistinction to the proportionate retention of calcium and phosphorus that occurs when vitamin D is used effectively for the treatment of azotemic rickets and osteomalacia (page 311), retention of orally administered calcium is not accompanied by

retention of phosphorus [30, 141]. While such calcium therapy might restore the carbonate fraction of bone mineral [114], there is no evidence that it will mineralize osteoid, and no obvious reason why it should. If absorbed calcium is not lodged in bone, it must find its way to soft tissue as in the milk-alkali syndrome [121].

Thus, indiscriminate correction of uremic acidosis has its dangers; calcium therapy by itself is probably useless. The effective measures available for management of mineral disorders in renal failure are fourfold: (1) vitamin D therapy; (2) the administration of phosphate-binding agents; (3) subtotal parathyroidectomy; and (4) renal homotransplantation. Their individual use is a matter for clinical judgment, and since this involves appraisal of the prevailing state of the bone disease [144], considerable assistance is provided by a suitably processed bone biopsy [12].

RENAL HOMOTRANSPLANTATION

Theoretically, successful renal homotransplantation should correct all the abnormalities of mineral metabolism of renal failure. Postoperative healing of bone disease has occurred without resort to treatment with vitamin D [95]; but the restoration of normal vitamin D sensitivity and intestinal absorption of calcium has not yet been directly demonstrated. Reference has been made to the unmasking of autonomous hyperparathyroidism and the measures required to deal with this (pages 318–319). Two other points are worth noting: (1) if a patient has been receiving large doses of vitamin D prior to transplantation, restoration of normal renal function might render him liable to vitamin D intoxication; and (2) "successful" homotransplantation may not restore normal renal function but a lesser degree of the renal failure that prevailed before operation. Although rendered viable, such patients could remain liable to the development of defective mineralization like any other patient with comparably mild renal failure.

VITAMIN D THERAPY

The primary indication for the use of vitamin D is to correct defective mineralization in symptomatic azotemic rickets and osteomalacia. Vitamin D will also cure the myopathic muscular weakness that may sometimes be the only clinical indicator of the presence of metabolic bone disease [143]. It is important to appreciate that effective treatment with vitamin D promotes increased intestinal absorption not only of calcium but also of phosphorus, in an approximately mole for mole ratio [148]. The molar ratio of Ca to P in bone is about 2.2:1 [2] and absorbed phosphorus that is superfluous to this requirement for mineralization of bone must tend to increase the phosphate concentration in the extracellular fluid. For this reason, a rise in plasma phosphate suggests that the administered dose of vitamin D is adequate; but this rise in concentration of phosphate in plasma may also tend to depress the plasma calcium, and *failure of the latter to rise is not an indication for increased dosage.* Especially in patients with a glomerular filtration rate between 15 and 30 ml. per minute, the initial dose of vitamin D should probably not exceed 10,000 I.U. per day (see pages 308–309); if this proves ineffective, the dose should be increased slowly. With this moderate degree of renal failure, the plasma phosphate is likely to be normal or only trivially raised, and treatment with vitamin D carries no significant risk of causing further renal damage or metastatic calcification. *It is, however, essential to stop treatment or reduce it to a small maintenance dose once the bone lesions have healed* (see page 311).

ADMINISTRATION OF PHOSPHATE-BINDING AGENTS

When azotemic rickets or osteomalacia is associated with significant hyperphosphatemia and a normal or increased plasma Ca $\times$ P product (see Fig. 8-2), or in those patients with a gross degree of accompanying osteitis fibrosa, more caution is needed. Any further increase in plasma phosphate and Ca $\times$ P product during treatment with vitamin D is then potentially dangerous. Such changes can be minimized by limiting the net absorption of phosphorus with binding agents such as aluminum hydroxide gel, or by increasing the Ca : P ratio of the diet with a supplement of nonphosphatic calcium salts [35]. In either instance, one may encounter an unpredictable snag; if too little phosphorus is absorbed in company with calcium under the influence of vitamin D, bone mineralization will not proceed and hypercalcemia may develop. As shown in Figure 8-3, when an effective dose of vitamin D was administered, the phosphorus in the patient's very low protein diet was insufficient for the calcium absorbed, and hypercalcemia developed rapidly in spite of the presence of florid osteomalacia. Management of these patients with more advanced renal failure must proceed empirically. They are likely to need a larger dose of vitamin D (page 309); the requirement for aluminum hydroxide, supplementary calcium, or even a phosphate supplement (Fig. 8-3) can be decided only by careful monitoring of the changes in plasma chemistry induced by vitamin D.

In patients with generalized osteitis fibrosa and no defect of mineralization (Fig. 8-2) these difficulties are compounded. It is certainly possible to improve skeletal mineralization, relieve bone pain, and increase muscular strength in these patients with vitamin D [35], but the risks are such that this should be considered only a palliative measure for patients in whom no further procedures are contemplated. Metastatic calcification in arteries can develop rapidly to a degree that may prejudice their subsequent use for hemodialysis or renal transplantation. The risks can be reduced if the plasma Ca $\times$ P product is lowered by parathyroidectomy before starting treatment with vitamin D [151]. But since generalized osteitis fibrosa is a disorder of the preterminal phase of renal failure, it is only in the exceptional patient that such surgical treatment can be justified [141, 144, 151].

Figure 8-3. Vitamin D resistance and effects of therapy in florid osteomalacia complicating advanced renal failure. Urea clearance 3 ml. per minute. Urinary output shown in white, fecal output crosshatched. Note that (1) the normal plasma phosphorus was attributable to the low dietary intake of phosphorus; (2) an increased calcium intake produced a temporary retention of calcium and small rise in plasma calcium — the fecal phosphorus increased, and plasma and urinary phosphorus diminished; (3) each increment of vitamin D_2 therapy produced corresponding increases of biologically assayed plasma vitamin D activity — doses up to 18,000 I.U. per day had no effect on the external calcium balance although they increased the plasma activity to about 5 times the average normal; (4) the dose of 100,000 I.U. per day promoted calcium absorption in excess of available phosphorus — the plasma calcium rose rapidly to 13 mg. per 100 ml., the plasma phosphorus fell to 1.7 mg. per 100 ml., and *phosphorus disappeared from the urine;* and (5) provision of an oral phosphate supplement increased the Ca:P ratio of the intake from 3:1 to 1.2:1 — the plasma calcium and phosphorus levels returned to normal, and when corrected for nitrogen, the retention of calcium and phosphorus was appropriate for deposition in bone.

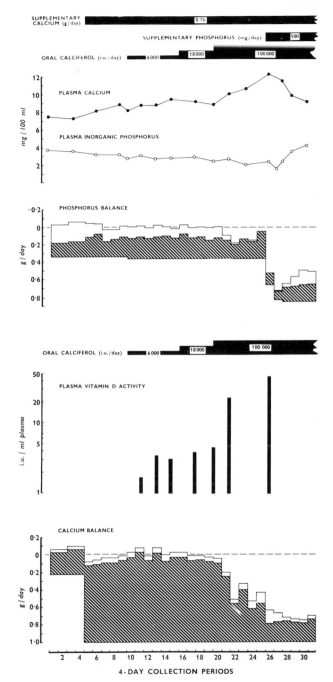

SUBTOTAL PARATHYROIDECTOMY

Apart from its occasional indication after renal transplantation (page 318), parathyroidectomy is likely to be required most frequently to control the deleterious effects of gross secondary hyperparathyroidism in patients treated by chronic hemodialysis [80a, 115, 128]. Because parathyroid autonomy is apparently rare, often reversible, and potentially manageable by medical means (see page 318), there is little to commend the suggestion [163] that parathyroidectomy should be performed routinely before undertaking renal transplantation. Moreover, if carried out after transplantation or in the chronically dialyzed patient awaiting this procedure, parathyroidectomy should probably always be subtotal. This involves accepting the trivial risk that the parathyroid remnant could remain permanently autonomous; but the alternative state of absolute hypoparathyroidism may not be easy to treat, and the use of vitamin D to control hypocalcemia could cause hypercalciuria potentially injurious to the transplanted kidney. If the chronically dialyzed patient can be offered no reasonable prospect of renal transplantation, a theoretical case can be made for *total* parathyroidectomy; with dialytic therapy in its present state, a partially resected gland would likely regenerate as life was prolonged. These comments are necessarily inductive since, apart from the report of Katz et al. [80a], there is no substantial experience on which to assess the role of parathyroid surgery in chronic dialytic therapy [128].

Because of a potentially impaired renal capacity to conserve sodium, the management of parathyroidectomy in renal failure calls for particular attention to the sodium balance during the immediate postoperative period. Postoperative hypocalcemia can be profound and prolonged [151, 163], sometimes necessitating massive infusion of calcium salts, but its effects can be mitigated if the metabolic acidosis is left untreated. Although parathyroidectomy in azotemic hyperparathyroidism presumably arrests the erosion of bone (Fig. 8-1), it does not alter the prevailing state of vitamin D resistance and dietary calcium is not utilized to reconstitute the skeleton [151]. If large subcutaneous deposits of metastatic calcification are present, the fall in plasma Ca × P product may permit their absorption, and a degree of osseous healing may be produced by a shift of minerals from soft tissues into bone [142]. Generally, however, osteoid formed after parathyroidectomy will not mineralize adequately — and hypocalcemia is unlikely to be con-

trolled — without the use of vitamin D [151]. An entirely analogous situation develops after parathyroidectomy in cases of *primary* hyperparathyroidism complicated by *secondary* renal failure [147]. In terms of the bone disease, parathyroidectomy effectively converts the lesions from generalized osteitis fibrosa to osteomalacia. Because such osteomalacia develops in association with more advanced renal failure than does spontaneously developing azotemic osteomalacia, it is correspondingly more difficult to treat safely with vitamin D (see above). These remarks apply primarily to parathyroidectomy in spontaneously developing azotemic hyperparathyroidism. In a patient treated by hemodialysis, there should be no problems with sodium balance; and, as discussed subsequently (page 325), the dialytic procedure may provide an extrinsic source of calcium sufficient to remineralize the skeleton without resource to vitamin D [80a].

The Special Case of the Chronically Dialyzed Patient

While hyperparathyroidism and the provision of additional *time* for its expression are probably chiefly responsible for the "devastating" bone disease of chronic dialysis [32, 115], there has been little systematic exploration of other possible contributory factors. Routine bone biopsy before admission to a dialytic program indicates that bone disease may already be established in many patients [18, 82a]. Insufficient attention has been given to the possibly critical concentration of ionic calcium used in dialysis fluids [123a]. Enquiry reveals that some dialysis units undertook dialysis for years without actually measuring calcium concentration in the made-up fluid — the literature of one commercial firm actually recommended a bath calcium of 10 mg. per 100 ml. A recent, statistically validated series of measurements [66] showed that the individual dialysis can produce either a net positive or a net negative body balance of calcium, depending on the calcium concentration of the dialysis fluid. A negative balance resulting from dialysis could only potentiate the negative bone balance produced by hyperparathyroidism; it is also possible that the action of parathyroid hormone on the bone is potentiated by the use of heparin as anticoagulant [60, 68]. Conversely, it is reasonable to expect that the production of a positive calcium balance by dialysis would limit the net destructive effect of hyperparathyroidism on the bone [123a, 147]. Ritz et al. [123a] documented the healing of renal osteitis fibrosa in the course of six months of hemodialysis treatment, in spite of persistent evidence of excessive secretion of parathyroid hormone. This was attributed to the establishment of a positive calcium balance by dialysis; and it is analogous to the healing of bone disease in patients with primary hyperparathyroidism treated by calcium salts [147]. In chronically dialyzed patients submitted to subtotal parathyroidectomy, healing of osteitis fibrosa has been observed postoperatively without recourse to vitamin D therapy [82a], which is required to remineralize the skeleton in the parathyroidectomized undialyzed patient [142, 148, 151]. The latter depends for remineralization on the *intrinsic* supply of minerals from his absorbing soft tissue calcification [142]; the former have an *extrinsic* source in their dialysis fluid [82a, 123a]. It must be emphasized, however, that, if hyperphosphatemia is inadequately controlled in the dialyzed patient, retained calcium would be shared between the bone and the soft tissues. If efficient hemodialysis eliminated the factor (or factors) responsible for vitamin D resistance, an intermittent increase of intestinal absorption might also contribute to a positive calcium balance. However, such measurements as have been made [23, 32] suggest that calcium absorption remains impaired during chronic dialysis; and metabolic studies in a few patients have shown that the fecal calcium level was high [32, 80a].

Since metabolic acidosis is well controlled in chronically dialyzed patients [115], the latter observations provide further evidence that acidosis itself is unlikely to be the cause of apparent vitamin D resistance (page 311). At the same time, since the tendency is to overcorrect the acidosis, this itself may contribute to development of metastatic calcification.

By now, clinically evident bone disease must have developed in some hundreds of chronically dialyzed patients, but no systematic study has been made of the actual bone lesions. An approach to this is made in a recent report by Kim et al. [82a], although the needle biopsy specimens obtained by them are unsuitable for an adequate assessment, especially of bone mass. From their data, from the roentgenographic descriptions provided by these and other authors [115], and from personal discussion with those encountering the problem, there is the suggestion that the bone disease is often a hypo-ostotic or osteopenic hyperparathyroidism. Such osteopenia could be a direct result of calcium deficiency (see above) but, even in default of the relevant information, there are therapeutic grounds for considering alternative mechanisms. Normally, in both primary [76] and spontaneously occurring azotemic secondary hyperparathyroidism [11], bone erosion is associated with reactive new bone formation; after parathyroidectomy, this is responsible for reconstitution of the bones. If chronic dialysis were to cause protein or amino acid deficiency [57, 130], or other specific nutritional abnormalities such as copper deficiency [69], the osteogenetic potential of the osteoblast could be impaired. Following parathyroidectomy, osteoid might thus fail to accumulate in the chronically dialyzed patient and he would be left with thin bones or osteoporosis. *In these circumstances, the enforced retention of calcium with vitamin D therapy could be directly harmful rather than beneficial.*

A potentially profitable approach to the problem of bone disease in the dialyzed patient would be the search for more effective methods for the sustained control of hyperphosphatemia. In the meantime, it can be anticipated that these patients will be submitted to various forms of experimental therapy. Its action in countering the osteolytic effects of parathyroid hormone [119] suggests calcitonin as an obvious candidate for trial; but its hypocalcemic action would tend to augment the effect of hyperphosphatemia. In nephrectomized rats, the administration of calcitonin appeared to increase the degree of secondary hyperparathyroidism [40]. The synthetic phosphonates and other polyphosphates [75, 126, 126a, 127] can prevent experimental metastatic calcification and also block the calcemic effect of parathyroid hormone; however, the latter action, like total parathyroidectomy, might produce hypo-

calcemia of a degree necessitating treatment with vitamin D.

At present the best prospect for control of disordered mineral metabolism and bone disease in the chronically dialyzed patient is renal homotransplantation. If this is available, the patient should not be poisoned by untried drugs, mutilated by unconsidered total parathyroidectomy, or have his arteries ruined by indiscriminate use of vitamin D. In a desperate clinical situation, it is always tempting to resort to any therapy that might conceivably be helpful. In this particular situation, what is first needed is an accurate documentation of the actual facts. Given this, it should be possible to devise appropriate animal experiments and then *controlled* trials of potentially useful therapy.

References

1. Abrams, J. D. Corneal and other ocular findings in patients on intermittent dialysis for renal failure. *Proc. Roy. Soc. Med.* 59: 533, 1966.
2. Agna, J. W., Knowles, H. C., and Alverson, G. The mineral content of normal human bone. *J. Clin. Invest.* 37:1357, 1958.
3. Albright, F., Drake, T. G., and Sulkowitch, H. W. Renal osteitis fibrosa cystica: Report of a case with discussion of metabolic aspects. *Bull. Johns Hopkins Hosp.* 60:377, 1937.
4. Albright, F., and Reifenstein, E. C. *The Parathyroid Glands and Metabolic Bone Disease.* London: Baillière, Tindall and Cox, 1948.
5. Anderson, D. C., Stewart, W. K., and Piercy, D. M. Calcifying panniculitis with fat and skin necrosis in a case of uraemia with autonomous hyperparathyroidism. *Lancet* 2:323, 1968.
6. Anderson, W. W., Mann, J. B., Kenyon, N., Farrell, J. J., and Hills, A. G. Subtotal parathyroidectomy in azotemic renal osteodystrophy. *New Eng. J. Med.* 268:575, 1963.
7. Arneill, G. C. Vitamin D as a public health problem. *Brit. Med. J.* 2:245, 1964.
8. Au, W. Y., and Raisz, L. G. Restoration of parathyroid responsiveness in vitamin D-deficient rats by parenteral calcium or dietary lactose. *J. Clin. Invest.* 46:1572, 1967.
9. Avioli, L. V., and Slatapolsky, E. The absorption and metabolism of vitamin D in chronic renal failure. *J. Clin. Invest.* 46: 1032, 1967.
10. Baker, S. L. The histopathology of porotic and malacic conditions of bone. *Brit. J. Radiol.* 27:604, 1954.
11. Ball, J. A simple method of defining osteoid in undecalcified sections. *J. Clin. Path.* 10:281, 1957.
12. Ball, J. Diseases of Bone. In Harrison, C. V. (Ed.), *Recent Advances in Pathology.* London: Churchill, 1960.
13. Ball, J., and Garner, A. Mineralization of woven bone in osteomalacia. *J. Path. Bact.* 91:563, 1966.
14. Barber, H. Renal dwarfism. A study of the course of the disease from seventeen cases. *Guy Hosp. Rep.* 76:307, 1926.

15. Barzel, U. S., and Jowsey, J. The effects of chronic acid and alkali administration on bone turnover in adult rats. *Clin. Sci.* 36:517, 1969.

16. Bell, N. H., and Bartter, F. C. Transient reversal of hyperabsorption of calcium and of abnormal sensitivity to vitamin D in a patient with sarcoidosis during episodes of nephritis. *Ann. Intern. Med.* 61:702, 1964.

17. Bell, N. H., Gill, J. R., and Bartter, F. C. On the abnormal calcium absorption in sarcoidosis. *Amer. J. Med.* 36:500, 1964.

18. Berlyne, G. M. Personal communication, 1968.

19. Berlyne, G. M. Microcrystalline conjunctival calcification in renal failure. *Lancet* 2: 366, 1968.

20. Berlyne, G. M., and Shaw, A. B. Red eyes in renal failure. *Lancet* 1:4, 1967.

21. Berner, A. Les osteodystrophies d'origine rénale: Étude systématique du squelette dans 138 cas de maladies rénales. *Helv. Med. Acta* 11:741, 1944.

22. Berson, S. A., and Yalow, R. S. Parathyroid hormone in plasma in adenomatous hyperparathyroidism, uremia and bronchogenic carcinoma. *Science* 154:907, 1966.

23. Blainey, J. D. In discussion of Stanbury [145].

24. Blunt, J. W., DeLuca, H., and Schnoes, H. K. 25-hydroxycalciferol, a biologically active metabolite of cholecalciferol. *Chem. Communic.* No. 14:801, 1968.

25. Botella, G., and Avendaño, H. Calcium plasma level in acute tubular necrosis. *Excerpta Med. Int. Cong. Series,* No. 67; 56, 1963.

26. Bordier, Ph., Matrajt, H., Hioco, D., Hepner, G. W., Thompson, G. R., and Booth, C. C. Subclinical vitamin D deficiency following gastric surgery. *Lancet* 1:437, 1968.

27. Caner, J. E. Z., and Decker, T. L. Recurrent acute (? gouty) arthritis in chronic renal failure treated by periodic hemodialysis. *Amer. J. Med.* 36:571, 1964.

28. Caniggia, A., and Gennari, P. Diagnostic différentiel des ostéomalacies par les études cinétiques a l'aide du calcium 45 et du calcium 47. In Hioco, D. J. (Ed.), *L'Ostéomalacie.* Paris: Masson, 1967.

29. Care, A. D., Sherwood, L. M., and Potts, J. T., Jr. Perfusion of the isolated parathyroid gland in the goat and sheep. *Nature* (London) 209:55, 1966.

30. Clarkson, E. M., McDonald, S. J., and de Wardener, H. E. The effect of a high intake of calcium carbonate in normal subjects and patients with chronic renal failure. *Clin. Sci.* 30:425, 1966.

31. Cramer, C. F. Quantitative Studies on the Absorption and Excretion of Calcium from Thiry-Vella Intestinal Loops in the Dog. In Wasserman, R. H. (Ed.), *The Transfer of Calcium and Strontium Across Biological Membranes.* New York: Academic, 1963.

32. Curtis, F. K., Davidson, R. C., and Pendras, J. P. Metabolic bone disease and chronic dialysis. *Abstracts Third International Congress of Nephrology.* 2:176, Washington, 1966.

33. Davies, D. R., Dent, C. E., and Watson, L. Tertiary hyperparathyroidism. *Brit. Med. J.* 2:395, 1968.

34. DeLuca, H. F. Mechanism of action and metabolic fate of vitamin D. *Vitamins Hormones* (N. Y.) 25:315, 1967.

35. Dent, C. E., Harper, C. M., and Philpot, G. R. Treatment of renal-glomerular osteodystrophy. *Quart. J. Med.* 30:1, 1961.

36. Dent, C. E., and Hodson, C. J. General softening of bones due to metabolic causes. Radiological changes associated with certain metabolic bone diseases. *Brit. J. Radiol. (N.S.)* 27:605, 1954.

37. Dreskin, E. A., and Fox, T. A. Adult renal osteitis fibrosa with metastatic calcification and hyperplasia of one parathyroid gland. *Arch. Intern. Med.* 86:533, 1950.

38. Eisenberg, E., and Bartholow, P. V. Reversible calcinosis cutis: Calciphylaxis in man. *New Eng. J. Med.* 268:1216, 1963.

39. Evanson, J. M. The response to infusion of parathyroid extract in hypocalcaemic states. *Clin. Sci.* 31:63, 1966.

40. Evanson, J. M., Garner, A., Holmes, A. M., Lumb, G. A., and Stanbury, S. W. Interrelations between thyrocalcitonin and parathyroid hormone in rats. *Clin. Sci.* 32:271, 1967.

41. Exton-Smith, A. N., Hodkinson, H. M.,

and Stanton, B. R. *Report on an Investigation into the Dietary of Elderly Women Living Alone.* King Edward's Hospital Fund, London, 1965.

42. Fahr, T. In Henke, F., and Lubarsch, O. *Handbuch der Speziellen Pathologischen Anatomie und Histologie.* Berlin: Springer, 1925.

43. Falls, W. F., Jr., Carter, N. W., Rector, F. C., Jr., and Seldin, D. W. The mechanism of impaired phosphate reabsorption in chronic renal disease. *Clin. Res.* 14:74, 1966.

44. Findley, T., Moore, J. D., and Brackney, E. L. Subtotal parathyroidectomy for renal hyperparathyroidism. (Letter to the editor.) *Lancet* 2:1150, 1961.

45. Fleisch, H., and Bisaz, S. Isolation from the plasma of pyrophosphate, an inhibitor of calcification. *Helv. Physiol. Pharmacol. Acta* 20:52, 1962.

46. Replaced by references 126 and 126a.

47. Fleisch, H., and Bisaz, S. Isolation from urine of pyrophosphate, a calcification inhibitor. *Amer. J. Physiol.* 203:671, 1962.

48. Fleisch, H., and Neuman, W. F. Mechanisms of calcification: Role of collagen, polyphosphates and phosphatase. *Amer. J. Physiol.* 200:1296, 1961.

49. Fleisch, H., Straumann, F., Schenk, R., Bisaz, S., and Allgower, M. Effect of condensed phosphates on calcification of chick embryo femurs in tissue culture. *Amer. J. Physiol.* 211:821, 1966.

50. Fletcher, R. F., Jones, J. H., and Morgan, D. B. Bone disease in chronic renal failure. *Quart. J. Med.* 32:321, 1963.

51. Follis, R. H., Jr. Renal rickets and osteitis fibrosa in children and adolescents. *Bull. Johns Hopkins Hosp.* 87:593, 1950.

52. Follis, R. H., Jr., and Jackson, D. A. Renal osteomalacia and osteitis fibrosa in adults. *Bull. Johns Hopkins Hosp.* 72:232, 1943.

53. Frost, H. M. The Dynamics of Human Osteoid Tissue. In Hioco, D. J. (Ed.), *L'Osteomalacia.* Paris: Masson, 1967.

54. Garner, A. Woven bone mineralisation in the rachitic rat. *J. Path. Bact.* 94:149, 1967.

55. Garner, A., and Ball, J. Quantitative observations on mineralised and unmineralised bone in chronic renal azotaemia and intestinal malabsorption syndrome. *J. Path. Bact.* 91:545, 1966.

56. Gilmour, J. R. *The Parathyroid Glands and Skeleton in Renal Disease.* London: Oxford Medical Publications, 1947.

57. Ginn, H. E., Frost, A., and Lacy, W. W. Nitrogen balance in hemodialysis patients. *Amer. J. Clin. Nutr.* 21:385, 1968.

58. Gittes, R. F., and Radde, I. C. Experimental hyperparathyroidism from multiple isologous parathyroid transplants: Homeostatic effect of simultaneous thyroid transplants. *Endocrinology* 78:1015, 1966.

59. Golden, A., Canary, J. J., and Kerwin, D. M. Concurrence of hyperplasia and neoplasia of the parathyroid glands. *Amer. J. Med.* 38:562, 1965.

60. Goldhaber, P. Heparin enhancement of factors stimulating bone resorption in tissue culture. *Science* 147:407, 1965.

61. Goldman, R., and Bassett, S. H. Phosphorus excretion in renal failure. *J. Clin. Invest.* 33:1623, 1954.

62. Goldsmith, R. S., and Ingbar, S. H. Inorganic phosphate treatment of hypercalcemia of diverse etiologies. *New Eng. J. Med.* 274:1, 1966.

63. Goodman, A. D., Lemann, J., Lennon, E. J., and Relman, A. S. Production, excretion and net balance of fixed acid in patients with renal acidosis. *J. Clin. Invest.* 44:495, 1965.

64. Gossmann, H. H., Baltzer, G., and Helms, H. Calciumstoffwechsel bei chronischer Niereninsuffizienz. *Klin. Wschr.* 46:497, 1968.

65. Gough, K. R., Lloyd, O. C., and Wills, M. R. Nutritional osteomalacia. *Lancet* 2: 1261, 1964.

66. de Graeff, J. Personal communication, 1968.

67. Graham, G., and Oakley, W. G. Treatment of renal rickets. *Arch. Dis. Child.* 13: 1, 1938.

68. Griffith, G. C., Nichols, G., Asher, J. D., and Flanagan, B. Heparin osteoporosis. *J.A.M.A.* 193:91, 1965.

69. Guggenheim, K. Copper and bones. *Israel J. Med. Sci.* 3:773, 1967.

70. Hass, G. M. Pathological Calcification. In

Bourne, G. H. (Ed.), *The Biochemistry and Physiology of Bone*. New York: Academic, 1956.

71. Herbert, F. K., Miller, H. G., and Richardson, G. O. Chronic renal disease, secondary parathyroid hyperplasia, decalcification of bone and metastatic calcification. *J. Path. Bact.* 53:561, 1941.

72. Herdman, R. C., Michael, A. F., Vernier, R. L., Kelly, W. D., and Good, R. A. Renal function and phosphorus excretion after human renal homotransplantation. *Lancet* 1:121, 1966.

73. Howard, J. E., Thomas, W. C., Barker, L. M., Smith, L. H., and Wadkins, C. L. The recognition and isolation from urine and serum of a peptide inhibitor to calcification. *Johns Hopkins Med. J.* 120:119, 1967.

74. Illig, von R., Uehlinger, E., and Prader, A. Sekundärer Hyperparathyreoidismus bei Vitamin-D-Mangel-Rachitis. *Helv. Paediat. Acta* 14:566, 1959.

75. Irving, J. T., Schibler, D., and Fleisch, H. Effect of condensed phosphates on vitamin D-induced aortic calcification in rats. *Proc. Soc. Exp. Biol. Med.* 122:852, 1966.

76. Jaffe, H. L. Hyperparathyroidism (Recklinghausen's disease of bone). *Arch. Path.* 16:63, 1933.

77. Jaffe, H. L., Bodansky, A., and Chandler, J. P. Ammonium chloride decalcification as modified by calcium intake: The relation between generalized osteoporosis and ostitis fibrosa. *J. Exp. Med.* 56:823, 1932.

78. Jeffree, G. M. Phosphatase activity in the limb bones of monkeys (*Lagothrix humboldti*) with hyperparathyroidism. *J. Clin. Path.* 15:99, 1962.

79. Johnson, L. C. Morphologic Analysis in Pathology: The Kinetics of Disease and General Biology of Bone. In Frost, H. M. (Ed.), *Bone Biodynamics*. Little, Brown, 1964.

80. Jowsey, J. Effect of parathyroid hormone in vitamin D or calcium-deficient puppies. To be published.

80a. Katz, A. I., Hampers, C. L., Wilson, R. E., Bernstein, D. S., Wachman, A., and Merrill, J. P. The place of subtotal parathyroidectomy in the management of patients with chronic renal failure. *Trans. Amer. Soc. Artif. Intern. Organs* 14:376, 1968.

81. Kaye, M., Pritchard, J. E., Halpenny, G. W., and Light, W. Bone disease in chronic renal failure with particular reference to osteosclerosis. *Medicine* (Balt.) 39:157, 1960.

82. Kaye, M., and Silverman, M. Calcium metabolism in chronic renal failure. *J. Lab. Clin. Med.* 66:535, 1965.

82a. Kim, D., Bell, N. H., Bundeson, W., Putong, P., Simon, N. M., Walker, C., and del Greco, F. Renal osteodystrophy in course of periodic dialysis for chronic uremia. *Trans. Amer. Soc. Artif. Intern. Organs* 14:367, 1968.

83. Kleeman, C. R., Better, O., Massry, S. G., and Maxwell, H. M. Divalent ion metabolism and osteodystrophy in chronic renal failure. *Yale J. Biol. Med.* 40:1, 1967.

84. Krook, L., and Barrett, R. B. Simian bone disease — a secondary hyperparathyroidism. *Cornell Vet.* 52:459, 1962.

85. Krook, L., Barrett, R. B., Usui, K., and Wolke, R. E. Nutritional secondary hyperparathyroidism in the cat. *Cornell Vet.* 53:224, 1963.

86. Krook, L., and Lowe, J. E. Nutritional secondary hyperparathyroidism in the horse. *Path. Vet.* (Basel) Suppl. 1, 1964.

87. Lemann, J., Litzow, J. R., and Lennon, E. J. The effects of chronic acid loads in normal man: Further evidence for the participation of bone mineral in the defense against chronic acidosis. *J. Clin. Invest.* 45:1608, 1966.

88. Lichtwitz, A., De Sèze, S., Parlier, R., Hioco, D., and Bordier, P. H. L'hypocalciurie glomérulaire. *Bull. Med. Hôp. Paris,* Nos. 3 & 4, 1960.

89. Litzow, J. R., Lemann, J., and Lennon, E. J. The effect of acidosis on calcium balance in patients with chronic renal disease. *J. Clin. Invest.* 46:280, 1967.

90. Liu, S. H., and Chu, H. I. Studies of calcium and phosphorus metabolism with special reference to pathogenesis and effect of dihydrotechysterol (A.T. 10) and iron. *Medicine* (Balt.) 22:193, 1943.

91. Lumb, G. A., Mawer, E. B., and Stanbury,

S. W.   The apparent vitamin D resistance
of chronic renal failure. A study of the
physiology of vitamin D in man. *Amer. J.
Med.* In press.

92. Lumb, G. A., and Stanbury, S. W.   The
treatment of azotemic rickets and osteomalacia; observations on the metabolism and
therapeutic hazards of vitamin D. (In preparation.)

93. Lund, J., and DeLuca, H. F.   Biologically
active metabolite of vitamin D_3 from bone,
liver and blood serum. *J. Lipid Res.* 7:739,
1966.

94. McDonald, S. J., Clarkson, E. M., and de
Wardener, H. E.   The effect of a large intake of calcium citrate in normal subjects
and patients with chronic renal failure.
Clin. Sci. 26:27, 1964.

95. McIntosh, D. A., Peterson, E. W., and Mc-
Phaul, J. J.   Autonomy of parathyroid func-
tion after renal homotransplantation. *Ann.
Intern. Med.* 65:900, 1966.

96. McNicholl, B.   Vitamin D as a public
health problem. *Brit. Med. J.* 2:245, 1964.

97. McPhaul, J. J., McIntosh, D. A., Hammond,
W. S., and Park, O. K.   Autonomous sec-
ondary (renal) parathyroid hyperplasia.
New Eng. J. Med. 271:1342, 1964.

98. Malm, O.   Calcium requirement and adaptation in adult man. *Scand. J. Clin. Lab. Invest.* Suppl. 36:1, 1958.

99. Malm, O.   Adaptations to Alteration in
Calcium Intake. In Wasserman, R. H.
(Ed.), *The Transfer of Calcium and Stron-
tium Across Biological Membranes.* New
York: Academic, 1963.

100. Massry, S. G., Coburn, J. W., and Kleeman,
C. R.   Bone mineral metabolism and osteodystrophy in uremia. *Amer. J. Clin. Nutr.*
21:457, 1968.

101. Matrajt, H., Bordier, Ph., and Hioco, D.
Mesures Histologiques Semi-quantitative
dans 17 Observations D'ostéomalacies Nu-
tritionelles et Rénales. Influence de la Vita-
mine D. In Hioco, D. J. (Ed.), *L'Ostéomalacie.* Paris: Masson, 1967.

102. Mawer, E. B.   Unpublished observations,
1968.

103. Mawer, E. B., and Stanbury, S. W.   Metab-

olism of vitamin D_3 in man. *Biochem. J.*
110:53 P, 1968.

104. Melick, R., and Martin, T. J.   Immunoassay of Parathyroid Hormone in Human
Plasma. In Talmage, R. V., Belanger, L. F.,
and Clark, I. (Eds.), *Parathyroid Hormone
and Thyrocalcitonin: Proceedings of the
Third Parathyroid Conference.* Amsterdam: Excerpta Med., 1968.

105. Morgan, H. G., Thomas, W. C., Jr., Had-
dock, L., and Howard, J. E.   Studies on the
mode of transport of vitamin D in human
serum. *Trans. Ass. Amer. Physicians* 71:93,
1958.

106. Neuman, W. F., and Neuman, M. W.
The Chemical Dynamics of Bone Mineral.
Chicago: University of Chicago Press, 1958.

107. Neuman, W. F., and Mulryan, B. J.   Synthetic hydroxyapatite crystals. III. The carbonate system. *Calcified Tissue Res.* 1:94,
1967.

108. Nichols, G., Jr., and Roth, S. I.   Chronic
renal disease and hypercalcemia. *New Eng.
J. Med.* 268:943, 1963.

109. Nordin, B. E. C.   Primary and secondary
hyperparathyroidism. *Advances Intern.
Med.* 9:81, 1958.

110. Nordin, B. E. C.   Osteoporosis and Cal-
cium Deficiency. In Rodahl, K., Nicholson,
J. S., and Brown, E. M. (Eds.), *Bone as a
Tissue.* New York: McGraw-Hill, 1960.

111. Nordin, B. E. C., and Smith, D. A.   Patho-
genesis and Treatment of Osteomalacia. In
Hioco, D. J. (Ed.), *L'Ostéomalacie.* Paris:
Masson, 1967.

112. Norman, A. W., Lund, J., and DeLuca,
H. F.   Biologically active forms of vitamin
D_3 in kidney and intestine. *Arch. Biochem.*
108:12, 1964.

113. Ogg, C. S.   The intestinal absorption of
^{47}Ca by patients in chronic renal failure.
Clin. Sci. 34:467, 1968.

114. Pellegrino, E. D., and Biltz, R. M.   The
composition of human bone in uremia.
Medicine (Balt.) 44:397, 1965.

115. Pendras, J. P., and Erickson, R. V.   Hemodialysis: A successful therapy for chronic
uremia. *Ann. Intern. Med.* 64:293, 1966.

116. Pollak, V. E., Schneider, A. F., Freund,
G., and Kark, R. M.   Chronic renal dis-

ease with secondary hyperparathyroidism. *A.M.A. Arch. Intern. Med.* 103:200, 1959.

117. Ponchon, G. Personal communication, 1968.

118. Potts, J. T., Jr., Buckle, R. M., Sherwood, L. M., Ramberg, C. F., Mayer, C. P., Kronfeld, D. S., Deftos, L. J., Care, A. D., and Aurbach, G. D. Control of Secretion of Parathyroid Hormone. In Talmage, R. V., Belanger, L. F., and Clark, I. (Eds.), *Parathyroid Hormone and Thyrocalcitonin: Proceedings of the Third Parathyroid Conference.* Amsterdam: Excerpta Med., 1968.

119. Raisz, L. G., and Niemann, I. Early effects of parathyroid hormone and calcitonin on bone in organ culture. *Nature* (London) 214:486, 1967.

120. Ramberg, C. F., Jr., Mayer, G. P., Kronfeld, D. S., Aurbach, G. A., Sherwood, L. M., and Potts, J. T., Jr. Plasma calcium and parathyroid hormone response to EDTA infusion in the cow. *Amer. J. Physiol.* 213:878, 1967.

121. Randall, R. E., Jr., Strauss, M. B., and McNeely, W. F. The milk-alkali syndrome: I. The diversity of the clinical manifestations. II. Pathogenesis. *Arch. Intern. Med.* (Chicago) 107:163, 1961.

122. Rasmussen, H., DeLuca, H., Arnaud, G., Hawker, C., and von Stedingk, M. The relationship between vitamin D and parathyroid hormone. *J. Clin. Invest.* 42:1940, 1963.

122a. Reiss, E., Canterbury, J. M., and Kanter, A. Circulating parathyroid hormone concentration in Chronic renal insufficiency. *Arch. Intern. Med.* (Chicago) 124:417, 1969.

123. Relman, A. S. Renal acidosis and renal excretion of acid in health and disease. *Advances Intern. Med.* 12:295, 1964.

123a. Ritz, E., Franz, H. E., and Jahns, E. The course of secondary hyperparathyroidism during chronic dialysis. *Trans. Amer. Soc. Artif. Intern. Organs* 14:385, 1968.

124. Roth, S. I., and Raisz, L. Effect of calcium concentration on the ultrastructure of rat parathyroid in organ culture. *Lab. Invest.* 13:331, 1964.

125. Roth, S. I., and Munger, B. L. The cytology of the adenomatous, atrophic and hyper-

plastic parathyroid glands of man: A light- and electron-microscopic study. *Virchow. Arch.* [*Path. Anat.*] 335:389, 1962.

126. Rusell, R. G. G., Bisaz, S., and Fleisch, H. Pyrophosphate and diphosphonates in calcium metabolism and their possible role in renal failure. *Arch. Intern. Med.* (Chicago) 124:571, 1969.

126a. Russell, R. G. G., and Fleisch, H. Pyrophosphate and Stone Formation. In Hodgkinson, A. and Nordin, B. E. C. (Eds.), *Renal Stone Research Symposium.* London: Churchill, 1969.

127. Schibler, D., and Fleisch, H. Inhibition of skin calcification (calciphylaxis) by polyphosphates. *Experientia* 22:367, 1966.

128. Scribner, B. H. Dialysis. In Black, D. A. K. (Ed.), *Renal Disease.* Oxford: Blackwell Scientific Publications, 1967.

129. Selye, H. *Calciphylaxis.* Chicago: University of Chicago Press, 1962.

130. Shinaberger, J. H., and Ginn, H. E. A Low Protein, High Essential Aminoacid Diet for Nitrogen Equilibrium in Chronic Dialysis. In Berlyne, G. M. (Ed.), *Nutrition in Renal Disease.* Edinburgh: Livingstone, 1968.

131. Sherwood, L. M., Mayer, G. P., Ramberg, C. F., Jr., Kronfield, D. S., Potts, J. T., Jr., and Aurbach, G. D. The relative importance of calcium and phosphate in the secretion of parathyroid hormone. *J. Clin. Invest.* 45:1072, 1966.

132. Sherwood, L. M., Potts, J. T., Jr., Care, A. D., Mayer, G. P., and Aurbach, G. D. Evaluation by radioimmunoassay of factors controlling the secretion of parathyroid hormone. *Nature* (London) 209:52, 1966.

132a. Slatapolsky, E., Cagler, S., Pennell, J. P., Taggert, D., Canterbury, J. M., Reiss, E., and Bricker, N. S. Pathogenesis of hyperparathyrodism in chronic renal disease. *J. Clin. Invest.* 49:89a, 1970.

133. Slatapolsky, E., Gradowska, L., Kashemsant, C., Keltner, R., Manley, C., and Bricker, N. S. The control of phosphate excretion in uremia. *J. Clin. Invest.* 45:672, 1966.

134. Slatapolsky, E., Robson, A. M., Elkan, I., and Bricker, N. S. Control of phosphate

excretion in uremic man. *J. Clin. Invest.* 47: 1865, 1968.

135. Smith, R., and Dick, M.   Total urinary hydroxyproline in osteomalacia and the effect upon it of treatment with vitamin D. *Clin. Sci.* 34:43, 1968.

136. Snapper, I.   *Medical Clinics on Bone Diseases.* New York: Interscience, 1943.

137. Stanbury, S. W.   Azotaemic renal osteodystrophy. *Brit. Med. Bull.* 13:57, 1957.

138. Stanbury, S. W.   Osteomalacia. *Schweiz. Med. Wschr.* 92:883, 1962.

139. Stanbury, S. W.   Metabolic Aspects of Renal Osteodystrophy. In Sissons, H. A. (Ed.), *Bone Metabolism in Relation to Clinical Medicine.* London: Pitman Medical Publishing Co. Ltd., 1962.

140. Stanbury, S. W.   Bony Complications of Renal Disease. In Black, D. A. K. (Ed.), *Renal Disease.* Oxford: Blackwell, 1962.

141. Stanbury, S. W.   Bony Complications of Renal Disease. In Black, D. A. K. (Ed.), *Renal Disease.* Oxford: Blackwell, 1967.

142. Stanbury, S. W.   Calcium and Phosphorus Metabolism in Chronic Renal Failure. In de Graeff, J., and Leijnse, B. (Eds.), *Water and Electrolyte Metabolism* (II). Western European Symposium on Clinical Chemistry, 3. Amsterdam: Elsevier, 1964.

143. Stanbury, S. W.   Muscle disorders of metabolic bone disease. *Manchester Med. Gaz.* 45:16, 1965.

144. Stanbury, S. W.   The treatment of renal osteodystrophy. *Ann. Intern. Med.* 65:1133, 1966.

145. Stanbury, S. W.   The Intestinal Absorption of Calcium in Normal Adults, Primary Hyperparathyroidism and Renal Failure. In Berlyne, G. M. (Ed.), *Nutrition in Renal Disease.* Edinburgh: Livingstone, 1968.

146. Stanbury, S. W.   Bone disease in uremia. *Amer. J. Med.* 44:714, 1968.

147. Stanbury, S. W.   Calcium metabolism in primary hyperparathyroidism; a problem in adaptation. In preparation.

148. Stanbury, S. W., and Lumb, G. A.   Metabolic studies of renal osteodystrophy: I. Calcium, phosphorus and nitrogen metabolism in rickets, osteomalacia and hyperparathyroidism complicating chronic uremia and

in the osteomalacia of the adult Fanconi syndrome. *Medicine* (Balt.) 41:1, 1962.

149. Stanbury, S. W., and Lumb, G. A.   Parathyroid function in chronic renal failure. *Quart. J. Med.* 35:1, 1966.

150. Stanbury, S. W., and Lumb, G. A.   The Osteomalacia of Renal Insufficiency. In Hioco, D. J. (Ed.), *L'Ostéomalacie.* Paris: Masson, 1967.

151. Stanbury, S. W., Lumb, G. A., and Nicholson, W. F.   Elective sub-total parathyroidectomy for renal hyperparathyroidism. *Lancet* 1:793, 1960.

152. Stauffer, M., and Rich, C.   Direct action of vitamin D and lactose on bone in osteomalacia. *J. Clin. Invest.* 46:1119, 1967.

153. Stickler, G. B., and Burke, E. C.   External calcium balances: A comparative study of renal disease and the celiac syndrome. *Amer. J. Dis. Child.* 106:154, 1962.

154. Taitz, L. S., and de Lacy, C. D.   Parathyroid function in vitamin D deficiency rickets. *Pediatrics* 30:875, 884, 1962.

155. Talmage, R. V., and Toft, R. J.   The Problem of the Control of Parathyroid Secretion. In Greep, R. O., and Talmage, R. V. (Eds.), *The Parathyroids.* Springfield, Ill.: Thomas, 1961.

156. Telfer, S. V.   Studies of calcium and phosphorus metabolism: V. Infantile rickets. The excretion and absorption of the mineral elements and the influence of fats in the diet on mineral absorption. *Quart. J. Med.* 20:7, 1926–1927.

157. Thomas, W. C.   Personal communication, 1968.

158. Thompson, G. R., Neale, G., Lewis, B., Watts, M., and Booth, C. C.   Plasma Vitamin D-like Activity and Vitamin D Absorption in Man. In Hioco, D. J. (Ed.), *L'Ostéomalacie.* Paris: Masson, 1967.

159. Walser, M.   The separate effects of hyperparathyroidism, hypercalcemia of malignancy, renal failure and acidosis on the state of calcium, phosphate and other ions in plasma. *J. Clin. Invest.* 41:1454, 1962.

160. Warkany, J.   Level of vitamin D in human blood serums. *Amer. J. Dis. Child.* 60:606, 1940.

161. Warkany, J., Guest, G. M., and Grabill,

F. J.   Vitamin D in human serum during and after periods of ingestion of large doses of vitamin D. *J. Lab. Clin. Med.* 27:557, 1942.

162. Wells, H. G.   *Chemical Pathology* (2d ed.). Philadelphia: Saunders, 1914.

162a. Williams, R. T.   Personal communication, 1968.

163. Wilson, R. E., Bernstein, D. S., Murray, J. E., and Moore, F. D.   Effects of para-thyroidectomy and kidney transplantation on renal osteodystrophy. *Amer. J. Surg.* 110: 384, 1965.

164. Yendt, E. R., Connor, T. B., and Howard, J. E.   *In vitro* calcification of rat cartilage in normal and pathological human sera with some observations on the pathogenesis of renal rickets. *Bull. Johns Hopkins Hosp.* 96:101, 1955.

9

Neurologic Complications of Uremia

H. Richard Tyler

Disorders of central nervous system and peripheral nerve function are not uncommon with advanced stages of renal failure. They occur in the acute and chronic disease states.

Abnormalities in cerebral function are the commonest finding in these patients. This often takes the form of chronic fatigue and irritability. The patient "doesn't feel well" and is not capable of prolonged intensive intellectual effort. If he is aware of the basic nature of this disease, significant psychologic factors, such as depression, may contribute to his poor intellectual performance. If the renal failure has been slow in its inception, surprisingly good mental function is possible. Rapid progression of renal failure is more likely to cause significant mental disturbances. Tests that require concentration and repetitive manipulation are especially sensitive in demonstrating these defects. Changes in recent and remote memory and fund of information occur much later.

Disorientation and confusion eventually appear, and it is not unusual to encounter delusions or hallucinatory behavior. Memory failure then becomes global.

Fixed attitudes, torpor, and other signs of toxic psychosis may occur. Periods of lucidity are often interspersed with pathologic behavior, and a patient may display striking insight into his illness, after statements or attitudes lead one to believe it lacking.

Among the most characteristic concomitants of this stage of the encephalopathy are myoclonus and fascicular twitching. Small fascicular twitching occurs at the same time gross generalized jerks are present. Facial twitching and fasciculations around lips and tongue are seen in the severer cases and often suggest a serious prognosis. When myoclonic movements are repetitive, they are difficult to separate from small seizures.

The lassitude, disorientation, and confusion pass into lethargy, and with progression stupor and subsequently coma supervene. Usually there is heightened muscle tone (rather than flaccidity). Decorticate postures (legs extended, arms flexed at wrists and elbows) are more common than decerebrate postures (legs extended, arms extended, hands inverted). Hyperventilation is characteristic of those patients with significant acidosis. In general the more rapid the development of the uremia, the more pronounced are the clinical changes. If the patient has a reversible renal lesion, improvement occurs in reverse order to loss. In patients in whom complete recovery occurs, there is amnesia for the period of disorientation and confusion.

Electroencephalographic disturbances usually parallel the clinical disorder. Most patients with a blood urea nitrogen (BUN) above 60 mg. per 100 ml. have some type of electroencephalographic abnormality [14]. In mild states, recordings are usually of a normal or a low-voltage type. This in turn is superseded by progressive slowing and disorganization, with intermittent paroxysms of much slower activity.

A small group of patients show a sensitivity to photic driving in the electroencephalogram. On rare occasions, either focal or generalized petit mal variants are noted. Focally abnormal electroencephalographic tracings usually mean focal disease.

It is difficult to correlate these clinical or electroencephalographic abnormalities with any single electrolyte abnormality. In any given patient, attention may be drawn to aberrations in BUN, sodium, potassium, calcium, chloride, phosphate, acid-base status, or osmolarity. There is no question that specific abnormalities may relate to disturbances in individual instances, but generalizations are difficult to make. Clinical states and electroencephalographic tracings often become "worse" if there is a rapid shift in electrolytes. Patients (and the EEG) may show marked improvement in the face of stable, abnormal blood chemistries.

It is evident that urea is not responsible for the clinical signs as shown by improvement following dialysis of patients with chronic uremia against a bath of high urea concentration [9].

Cerebral blood flow studies [6, 12] have demonstrated a defect in oxygen utilization which may occur in the face of normal, depressed, or elevated cerebral blood flow. Defects in permeability have also been noted [4]. This membrane defect, or defects in the sodium-potassium pump (or both), may result in a defect in oxygen utilization as has been measured in cerebral blood flow studies [17].

Studies attempting to correlate clinical states with cerebrospinal fluid changes rather than with serum electrolytes [5] have not clarified the situation, except to note that simple explanations such as osmolarity, acid-base changes, or electrolytic disturbances could not account for the clinical changes seen. At the present time, it appears likely that symptoms result from a diffuse dysfunction of the central nervous system at the neuronal level.

Other mental changes are seen but are much less specifically related to kidney failure. On occasion, a psychotic episode brings the patient to medical attention. This characteristically takes the form of an acute toxic psychosis. Almost every type of psychiatric illness has been mimicked. Korsakoff's psychosis and Wernicke's encephalopathy have been seen especially in the face of severe nutritional deficiencies. This is especially true with the restricted diets being used to treat uremic patients.

Asterixis has been characteristic of the metabolic encephalopathy seen in uremia [19]. Most descriptions of asterixis have included two or more entities: a striking, sudden lapse of position for which the term *asterixis* was coined, and a variously described tremulousness. The tremulousness often appears prior to the development of asterixis, and persists for a while following its disappearance. The usual position for testing for asterixis is dorsiflexion of the hand, but dorsiflexion of the foot or any sustained muscle contraction can evoke it. The abnormality appears to coincide with a lapse of electrical activity in the electromyogram, which occurs simultaneously in a set of contracting muscle groups. Asterixis is a nonspecific phenomenon seen in many conditions besides kidney disease. It appears to require a widespread disturbance of central nervous system function, usually metabolic in nature.

Convulsions are a late symptom of renal failure [12, 16]. In general, those patients with less severe renal failure who have seizures suffer from malignant hypertension. The many small lesions scattered throughout the cerebrum and brain stem seem to make these patients particularly vulnerable [15]. Some patients with a high BUN have their seizures following dialysis when rapid fall of the BUN is iatrogenically induced, or following diuresis when there may be a spontaneous fall in the BUN in a short time. Other factors that are particularly provocative are rapid changes in pH or shifts of electrolytes. It does not matter whether the shift is in the direction of improved serum electrolytes or not. The brain tolerates rapid adjustments of any kind poorly.

I have been unable to correlate seizures with any specific electrolyte abnormality. In any patient, one or more electrolytes could be abnormal, but there was no constancy from patient to patient. The potassium-calcium ratio is one of the better indications of seizure proneness.

Convulsions in acute anuria occur about the eighth to the eleventh day of renal failure, usually in association with severe encephalopathy. Frequently, seizures are a terminal event. In some patients they are secondary to cardiac arrhythmias. If clinical recovery is possible and the anuria has lasted four to six days, a seizure or a series of seizures frequently occurs just before or shortly after the onset of diuresis. They often correlate with striking shifts of BUN, water, or other electrolytes. These seizures are almost always generalized. Rare instances of focal seizures usually correlate with focal brain lesions, usually mild localized subarachnoid bleeding, or a focal area of encephalomalacia. A patient with a preexisting cerebral lesion or seizure tendency is most likely to have a seizure with the signs or lateralization originating from the focal characteristics of the original lesions at this time.

In chronic renal disease, seizures characteristically occur late in the course of the illness. It is extremely rare for the chronic uremic patient with normal electrolytes to have a seizure. Patients with a preexisting convulsive disorder frequently have convulsions in association with mild degrees of acidosis or water loading. The usual uremic convulsion occurs with moderate or severe acidosis or water intoxication, or a combination of both. This clearly is not the only factor, as many patients with similar disturbances in electrolytes do not convulse.

There is a significant group of patients with chronic renal disease who have their first and only seizure as a terminal or preterminal event. If they live long enough to be examined, the association of cardiac arrhythmia or myocardial infarction is impressive and probably is the cause of the seizures in these cases. Four out of five patients have a flurry of 3 to 7 seizures in a 12- to 36-hour period. Seizures rarely last more than two days, whether treated aggressively or not.

Not all patients have hypertension at the time of their seizures. Approximately one-third of the patients have a normal diastolic pressure. It should be noted that penicillin in high doses can cause seizures, especially in the patient with renal failure.

Abnormalities of Cranial Nerves

An acute loss of vision or "uremic amaurosis" occurs in a small number of patients. The fundi are normal, and the pattern of recovery is suggestive of cortical blindness.

Lesions in the retina occasionally cause scotoma, especially if the hemorrhage or exudate is near the macula. Hemianopic defects are only seen in the presence of focal lesions of the brain or following a focal seizure.

Other changes in other cranial nerves such as nystagmus, miosis, slight pupillary asymmetry, latent heterophoria and facial asymmetry are common, but are characterized by their fluctuation in intensity and evanescent character. A sixth nerve palsy is seen as an isolated phenomena in a small number of patients.

Deafness is not common in uncomplicated uremia though it is a frequent finding in the patients with hereditary interstitial nephritis. In two such cases, this was due to a degeneration of the cells in the ganglion of Corti [13]. In other cases deafness could be attributed to antibiotic medications such as streptomycin, neomycin, and colimycin.

Muscular Disorders

Muscular cramps occur frequently in patients with mildly decompensated renal disease. They usually occur nocturnally and tend to become recurrent and persistent. They can occur with normal sodium, chloride, bicarbonate, and potassium levels. Calcium levels are also usually normal, although as is true with most cases of renal failure, the phosphate levels are usually slightly elevated.

In general, cramping often disappears as a major symptom as progressive renal impairment leads to increasing inactivity. Rarely one sees a very severe tetanoid spasm of distal muscles, usually in a very ill patient. The mechanism of this is not clear.

Muscle irritability in the form of fasciculations are common, especially in the sick, decompensated patient. The fasciculations have electromyographic characteristics similar to the short tetanic bursts seen in nerve-root lesions.

The Chvostek and Trousseau signs indicative of clinical tetany and increased muscle tone are not uncommon. At times the hypertonicity may be so increased as to cause slight opisthotonos. Stiffness of the neck, or Kernig's sign, is frequently noted. The question of meningeal infection is often raised. This can be evaluated only by noting if the patient has a generalized tendency to extensor hypertonus and by examining the cerebrospinal fluid. The common denominator in most of these patients is moderate to severe acidosis or an elevated potassium-calcium ratio, or both.

On a few occasions one sees a flaccid paralysis associated with loss of stretch reflexes and of direct muscle excitability in uremic patients related to a very low serum potassium. I have not encountered a patient with paralysis and a high serum potassium as an isolated finding. Since other abnormalities are usually present, attributing the paralysis to hyperkalemia is usually an oversimplification.

It is not uncommon to see mild muscular weakness of proximal muscles and neck flexors in chronic uremia compatible with a mild polymyopathy. On rare occasions the muscular weakness may become a prominent part of the symptom complex. Muscle biopsies on such patients show minor changes — for example, sarcolemmal nuclei proliferation. On occasion, patchy and focal areas of muscle damage compatible with the diagnosis of polymyositis are seen.

Severe pain in proximal muscles often suggests the possibility of an underlying vasculitis. In a few patients acute muscular swelling develops with marked edema in the muscle compartments. Biopsy has shown severe segmental damage with evidence of regeneration. This disorder characteristically occurs with a history of seizures or excessive sedation, hypoxia, or hypotension. It has been suggested that this muscle infarction may relate to the hypoxia and hypotension.

Reactions to the phenothiazines, often in small doses, may include extrapyramidal syndromes such as torticollis and parkinsonian states. Neuromuscular paralysis of transient nature have also been noted with some antibiotics.

Marked variation in deep tendon reflexes is seen in almost all patients, ranging in a given individual from complete areflexia to marked hyperreflexia. Slight reflex asymmetries are not uncommon. Reflex loss may alert one to an early neuropathy.

Peripheral Neuritis

One of the earliest signs of peripheral neuritis is the restless-leg syndrome [2]. The patient notes a "difficult-to-describe" feeling which is usually relieved by moving the legs or by walking. The exact cause of this syndrome is not clear, but it is associated with a decreased motor nerve conduction rate.

A syndrome [1, 18] of painful, burning paresthesia of the feet often occurs independently, or following the restless-leg syndrome. It develops peripherally and quickly spreads to involve both dorsal and plantar surfaces of the feet. It is often associated with mild swelling and vasodilatation of the vessels of the skin. The patient finds any tactile or pain sensation very disagreeable, and ambulation is often severely curtailed. This syndrome is not associated with weakness or reflex suppression and is probably the result of the small nerve fibers being selectively damaged. In most cases a history will reveal severe and acute dietary deprivation. It is reversible by any treatment — for example, antiemetic agents, dialysis, intravenous fluids — that allows the patient to eat a normal diet. Symptoms can disappear in days, although one to two weeks are more usual. Vitamin supplements are helpful.

A severe distal neuropathy [1, 18], which involves all sensory modalities and motor function, and damages sympathetic fibers, often develops with a background of the burning-foot syndrome. The frequency of neuropathy has varied in most series from 13 to 86 per cent, depending on the nature of the clinic population and the definition of neuropathy. The neuropathy is fairly symmetrical, beginning first distally at the toes and spreading up the leg. The upper extremities are involved only in the face of severe lower-extremity involvement. The symmetry, severity, and distal emphasis separate it from most other types of neuropathy. On rare occasions a fulminant form leading to severe and total disability in two or three weeks is seen.

The pathologic findings [1, 8] consist of severe damage to the distal portions of the peripheral nerves. The type of damage to the neuron whereby the distal portion is primarily affected, and the Schwann cells supplying the terminal covering is selectively damaged, suggests that there is a defect in transport of some essential products from the nerve cell in the spinal cord to the distal segments.

Some clinics have claimed improvement with dialysis; others have not. Improvement does occur in the burning-foot sensory neuropathy and in motor nerve conduction times. Sensory nerve conduction times have also been shown to improve with dialysis. It is extremely rare to see recovery from a clinically significant neuritis with motor paralysis and sensory loss if dialysis is the only form of treatment. Renal transplantation, however, has been effective in handling this type of neuritis in most patients if the transplant functions well.

Nerve conduction studies usually show a depression in nerve conduction early in uremia even in the absence of any clinical or symptomatic evidence of neuritis. Rates that are 50 per cent normal are not unusual. Rates this slow are unusual for many other types of neuropathy and suggest a defect other than a "neuritis." The rapid fluctuation of motor nerve conduction rates suggests this is a physiologic rather than a structural defect.

Spinal Fluid and Pathology

The spinal fluid in uremia usually shows a slightly elevated pressure. The average pressure in my patients was 220 mm. of water. Protein levels in one series ranged from 32 to 108 mg. per 100 ml., with an average of 42 mg. per 100 ml. The cell count is usually normal.

The presence of xanthochromia may suggest an aneurysmal rupture, as in polycystic kidney disease, a necrotizing arteritis, as with polyarteritis nodosa, or most commonly, mild subarachnoid and meningeal bleeding associated with the bleeding diathesis of chronic renal disease.

Pathologically [4, 10] the most impressive finding in the central nervous system has been the paucity of gross lesions. The brain is usually a little pale, and the meninges slightly opacified. Small pial hemorrhages, scattered petechial white-matter lesions, and on rare occasions slightly larger ball hemorrhages, up to 6 or 7 mm. in diameter, have been noted.

The neurons are most frequently affected, showing such changes as chromatolysis, hyperchromaticity, vacuolation, varicose swelling in the dendrites, and loss of staining characteristics. If the course is subacute or chronic, changes may include pyknosis, fragmentation, cell shrinkage, and even areas of cellular depopulation.

There are no constant areas of predilection; changes in cortex, subcortical nuclei, brain-stem nuclei, cerebellum, and rarely, spinal cord have all been noted. Especially prominent in many reports have been the neuronal changes in the brain-stem nuclei (especially the tenth nerve nuclei and locus ceruleus).

There is often some glial proliferation and microglial nodules. Perivascular accumulation of small cells has often been conspicuous, although, occasionally, destruction of perivascular glia has also been noted. Small areas of demyelination have also been frequently reported. On rare occasions small areas of microinfarction have been noted. There may be mild meningeal reactions. Actual changes in the blood vessels, including changes in the endothelium, inner elastic membrane, and media, are often found. Changes such as desquamation and vacuolated cells in the choroid plexus have been emphasized by some.

Though in some patients there may be some degree of selectivity (i.e., emphasis in dentate nuclei and Purkinje cells), the changes in general have been widespread throughout the central nervous system. The changes for the most part are not specific for uremia, and other etiologic agents (i.e., toxins) could account for the pathologic changes noted above.

Complications of Treatment — Dialysis and Transplantation

Peritoneal dialysis and hemodialysis specifically have brought a number of problems that are relatively unique [4]. The major neurologic complications of peritoneal dialysis have been one or more convulsions and a toxic encephalopathy or psychosis. The incidence of seizures and toxic psychosis or encephalopathy is approximately 1 to 2 per cent. When a psychosis occurs it is often in a patient with a pre-existing unstable personality structure and could last up to two and one-half weeks.

Acute neurologic changes are seen more frequently following hemodialysis. It is not uncommon for patients to become somewhat sleepy as the procedure progresses. If it is prolonged, they often show signs of irritability. They may find it possible to engage in productive behavior such as reading, writing, or participating in games, but this is the exception rather than the rule.

The commonest complication is increased restlessness, often associated with headache, nausea, and rarely, vomiting. If dialysis is continued, the blood pressure tends to rise, and fasciculations, twitching, and asterixis are noted. On occasion, convulsions or coma may appear. There usually is a slow return to predialysis status over the next 24 to 36 hours. About 75 per cent of the time, electroencephalographic tracings deteriorate during the course of dialysis, returning to predialysis levels in one or two days. The more serious neurologic phenomena are more characteristic of long runs on the machine or rapid and extreme adjustments of either urea levels or acidosis. On occasion, such phenomena may be delayed 8 to 48 hours after the run for unexplained reasons. The more acutely ill and metabolically deranged the patient is, the less likely he is to tolerate acute dialysis well.

These phenomena were initially described as the "reverse urea syndrome" [11]. It was suggested that the urea in the brain was not freely removed during dialysis because of the blood-brain barrier. Lowering the blood urea nitrogen by increments to moderate levels, rather than trying to lower it to within the normal range, has been effective in moderating these complications. Patients now are also being dialyzed sooner than previously to prevent the necessity of lowering blood urea nitrogen radically. A similar situation occurs with rapid adjustments of acid-base regulation. A correction of serum pH of an acute nature usually accentuates the difference between pH of cerebrospinal fluid and blood. Under some circumstances, it may actually cause the cerebrospinal fluid to become more acid [3] (i.e., increasing central nervous system acidosis) and contribute to clinical deterioration. Most patients with such complications of dialysis will not demonstrate such changes in urea or acid-base metabolism, and other factors, as yet unrecognized, probably play a major role.

Two of the more prominent medical complications that arise in patients maintained with chronic dialysis are the burning-foot syndrome and the peripheral sensory motor neuropathy. These have previously been discussed. The importance of these complications should be emphasized, as many clinics have the potential for keeping patients alive for long periods. A useful and productive life is often severely interfered with by these neuritic complications. In contrast, patients with transplantation do much better in this regard. They rarely develop neuritis, and if one is present, it usually improves rapidly.

Neurologic complications may arise from the phenomena of rejection itself — that is, a patient with rejection of a transplanted kidney may show increasing hypertension and have an acute episode of hypertensive encephalopathy. If there is severe necrosis of the transplanted kidney, a toxic psychosis may develop. On the other hand, if the transplant functions extremely well, the sudden shifts of the electrolytes may precipitate a series of seizures. These usually will prove to be self-limiting over one or two days and rarely need aggressive treatment.

Since treatment is actively given to suppress the immunogenic reaction, one may also depress the hematopoietic system, and hemorrhage (intracerebral or extracerebral) may occur if the platelets are depressed. Rare examples of other disease states, such as central pontine myelinosis [4], have also been seen in the chronically ill uremic patient with a poor dietary intake.

The transplant cases may receive chronic high-dose steroid treatment, or drugs that depress their ability to respond with appropriate antibody responses or combat infection efficiently. There has been a high frequency of unusual infections in these patients. The clinician must be prepared to see unusual infections or a reexacerbation of quiescent infections.

Severe sodium depletion as a result of aggressive diuretic therapy, especially with the chlorothiazides [20], may lead to enough volume depletion to be associated with weakness and postural hypotension. On occasion, striking hyperkalemia may also be produced by these drugs.

Furadantin (nitrofurantoin) treatment [7] for renal infection has been associated with a diffuse symmetrical peripheral neuropathy in both uremic and nonuremic patients. Evidence of electromyographic abnormalities in patients treated with this drug have occurred

in almost two-thirds of the patients tested in one series.

References

1. Asbury, A. K., Victor, M., and Adams, R. D. Uremic polyneuropathy. *Arch. Neurol.* (Chicago) 8:413, 1963.
2. Callaghan, N. Restless legs syndrome in uremic neuropathy. *Neurology* (Minneap.) 16:359, 1966.
3. Cowie, J., Lambie, A. T., and Robson, J. S. The influence of extracorporeal dialysis on the acid-base composition of blood and cerebrospinal fluid. *Clin. Sci.* 23:397, 1962.
4. Fishman, R. A., and Raskin, N. H. Experimental uremic encephalopathy permeability and electrolyte metabolism of brain and other tissues. *Arch. Neurol.* (Chicago) 17:10, 1967.
5. Hampers, C. L., Doak, P. B., Callaghan, M. N., Tyler, H. R., and Merrill, J. P. The electroencephalogram and spinal fluid during hemodialysis. *Arch. Intern. Med.* (Chicago) 118:340, 1966.
6. Heyman, A., Patterson, J. L., Jr., and Jones, R. W., Jr. Cerebral circulation and metabolism in uremia. *Circulation* 3:558, 1951.
7. Lindholm, T. Electromyographic changes after nitrofurantoin (Furadantin) therapy in nonuremic patients. *Neurology* (Minneap.) 17:1017, 1967.
8. Marin, O. S. M., and Tyler, H. R. Hereditary interstitial nephritis associated with polyneuropathy. *Neurology* (Minneap.) 11:999, 1961.
9. Merrill, J. P., Legrain, M., and Hiogne, R. Observations on the role of urea in uremia. *Amer. J. Med.* 14:519, 1953.
10. Olsen, S. The brain in uremia. *Acta Psychiat. et Neurol. Scand.* 36(Suppl. 156):1, 1961.
11. Peterson, H., and Swanson, A. G. Acute encephalopathy occurring during hemodialysis. *Arch. Intern. Med.* (Chicago) 113:877, 1964.
12. Scheinberg, P. Effects of uremia on cerebral blood flow and metabolism. *Neurology* (Minneap.) 4:101, 1954.
13. Tyler, H. R. Unpublished observations.
14. Tyler, H. R. Convulsions and EEG changes in uremia. *Trans. Amer. Neurol. Ass.* 90:76, 1965.
15. Tyler, H. R. Neurological complications of dialysis, transplantation and other forms of treatment in chronic uremia. *Neurology* (Minneap.) 15:1081, 1965.
16. Tyler, H. R. Neurological Complications of Uremia. In Brest, A. N., and Moyer, J. H. (Eds.), *Renal Failure*. Philadelphia: Lippincott, 1967. Chap. 18, pp. 153–164.
17. Tyler, H. R. Neurological disorders in renal failure. *Amer. J. Med.* 44:734, 1968.
18. Tyler, H. R., and Gottlieb, A. . Peripheral neuropathy in uremia. *Proceedings of the Eighth International Congress of Neurology,* Vienna, 1965.
19. Tyler, H. R., and Leavitt, S. Studies in asterixis. *Arch. Neurol.* (Chicago) 10:360, 1964.
20. Walker, W. G., Looke, R. C., Iber, F. L., Lesch, M., and Caransos, G. J. Topics in clinical medicine. *Johns Hopkins Med. J.* 121:194, 1967.

IO

Dialysis

Lewis W. Bluemle, Jr.

Dialysis as it applies to clinical medicine may be defined as the removal of undesirable substances from the body fluids by diffusive transfer across a semipermeable membrane. Its importance in nephrology is that it affords a direct means for correcting the chemical and clinical abnormalities of severe uremia. Of historical significance, it represents man's first successful attempt to simulate the vital function of a complex living organ. In yet another sense, hemodialysis may be considered a fortuitous example of therapeutic empiricism where technology has outrun basic understanding of the condition being treated.

Development of Dialytic Technics

In 1861 Graham [106], the Scottish chemist, made the basic discovery that certain substances, such as gelatin and starch, passed through a membrane more slowly than others, such as inorganic salts. He called the former substances colloids, the latter crystalloids and the process for separating the two dialysis. One of the first mixtures dialyzed by Graham was urine, which "gave its crystalloidal constitu-

ents to the external water." From the dialysate he extracted urea "in so pure a condition as to appear in crystalline tufts . . ." [106]. This original concept of dialytic separation found important applications in chemistry and industry, but it required modification before it could be useful as a means for purifying uremic blood. *Selective* crystalloid removal and *substitution* were required, rather than complete crystalloid removal. This was accomplished easily by the addition of desired solutes in appropriate concentrations to the bath water.

EXTRACORPOREAL DIALYSIS (HEMODIALYSIS)

The first artificial kidney was conceived, built, and tested by Abel, Rowntree, and Turner, who published their results in 1913 [1, 2]. Their device, the prototype of all subsequent hemodialyzers, consisted of a series of handmade collodion tubes connected by glass manifolds and suspended in an isotonic bath flowing through a cylindrical jacket. Using hirudin extracted from leech heads as an anticoagulant, Abel and his colleagues succeeded in demonstrating that salicylate could be removed effectively from the circulating blood of rabbits. Their recognition of the significance of this observation was no less admirable than their inventive genius. That they foresaw the ultimate clinical value of hemodialysis is clearly attested to in the statement [1] "There are numerous toxic states in which the eliminating organs of the body, more especially the kidneys, are incapable of removing at an adequate rate the natural or unnatural substances whose accumulation is detrimental to life. In the hope of providing a substitute in such emergencies which might tide over a dangerous crisis as well as for the important information which it might be expected to provide . . . a method has been devised by which the blood of a living animal may be submitted to dialysis outside the body."

Over the next 30 years, sporadic attempts were made to augment Abel's observations and improve his device. In 1915 Haas [114a] utilized a similar apparatus for "Blutwaschung," and Van Hess [322] studied solubility characteristics of blood sugar by in vivo dialysis across collodion membranes. The principal defect of collodion, however, was that when cast too thin it would rupture, and when cast too thick, it became relatively impermeable. In 1920 Love [188] investigated animal intestine as an alternative membrane and concluded that cat, rabbit, chicken, or turkey gut provided better tensile strength. Three years later, Necheles [226] chose to explore parietal peritoneum, recognizing its comparative advantages of strength, thinness, and inertness as a transport surface. He dialyzed nephrectomized dogs with a device of his own design and noted symptomatic improvement. Later Necheles [227] modified his original model by supporting conical tubes of peritoneum on screens of wire gauze. This important innovation, which was to be exploited further in later years, provided for the first time a high surface-volume ratio.

Before hemodialysis could be developed as a safe and convenient clinical procedure, however, two additional advances had to be made.

First, a membrane had to be developed which was not only permeable and strong but also inexpensive and readily available in a convenient form. Fortunately, in the 1930's regenerated cellulose tubing (cellophane) became available. Since it was manufactured in large quantity as sausage casing, its cost was low. Secondly, a better anticoagulant than hirudin had to be discovered. Heparin, also a gratuitous contribution to dialysis from another field, solved this problem. The fact that neither heparin nor cellophane resulted from a search for improved dialysis methodology reflects an interesting characteristic of developments in this field — namely, a dependence on borrowed technology and enlightened improvisation. In 1938 Thalheimer [314] advanced the state of dialytic art by utilizing both heparin and cellophane in a device which he employed in conjunction with exchange transfusions to reduce azotemia.

It remained for Kolff and his associates [159, 160], however, to add the remaining ingredient for successful continuous hemodialysis as we know it today, a practical and reliable design in the form of a spiral of flattened cellophane tubing wound around a corrugated drum which revolved in a tub of dialyzing fluid. With the rotating drum dialyzer, which utilized the principle of Archimedes' screw to propel blood from inlet to outlet with minimal pressure drop, Kolff was the first to succeed in prolonging the life of patients with advanced uremia [157]. A fascinating account of this early work which laid the foundations for the use of the artificial kidney in clinical medicine was recorded two decades later [158]. Merrill et al. refined this device [217] and reported in 1950 on its first extensive clinical use in this country [216].

A major shortcoming of the rotating drum dialyzer, however, was that ultrafiltration for the removal of excess fluid could not be effected easily. Since the membrane tubing was constrained only on one side, hydrostatic pressure could not be utilized for this purpose.

Instead, an osmotic pressure gradient between blood and dializing fluid had to be generated by the addition of large amounts of glucose, an inconvenient and poorly controlled alternative. Several new models were developed in the late 1940's which surmounted this difficulty. The Alwall dialyzer employed two stationary, concentric, fluted cylinders as inside and outside supports for an interposed spiral of flattened cellophane tubing [3]. A similar apparatus was introduced by Murray [222]. In 1949 Skeggs and Leonards developed the first sheet-and-plate model [295, 296]. It consisted of a variable number of vertically stacked, rectangular rubber pads with longitudinal grooves on opposing surfaces, between each pair of which were held two sheets of membrane defining the blood flow path. This basic configuration was later modified by Kiil [155], who substituted longer, rigid boards for the elastomeric ones of Skeggs and Leonards and simplified the inlet and outlet adapters. Shortly thereafter, MacNeill and his associates [194] combined certain features of preceding models by utilizing flattened tubing in multiple, parallel arrangement with interposed plastic screen supports.

An extensive array of additional variants have been developed since 1950. Of these, the screen-coil unit of Watschinger and Kolff was one of the most innovative [163, 328]. Based on a prototype developed by Inouye and Engelberg [136], this design consisted of two parallel coils of cellophane tubing mounted between concentric layers of woven fiberglass screen wound about a central plastic core. Produced commercially as a sterile, disposable unit, it presented the great advantage of time-saving convenience in dialyzer preparation.

Along with the Kiil apparatus, the twin-coil unit has enjoyed wide acceptance for clinical use. Among the devices introduced more recently, perhaps several [298], utilizing multiple-point membrane supports developed by Bluemle [20–22], the Dialung, a compact sheet-and-plate unit developed by Esmond and

his co-workers [80, 81], and newer versions of the coil design [132, 153, 219] show the greatest promise.

Additional experimental models are currently undergoing clinical evaluation. Several of these present unique design features. The hollow-fiber dialyzer [186, 304, 305] utilizes thousands of extremely fine cellulosic tubes suspended as parallel blood paths between potted manifolds at either end of a transparent cylinder. This model is reminiscent of Abel's original design but on a micro scale. In addition to achieving an extremely high ratio of surface area to contained blood volume, the hollow-fiber dialyzer also obviates bulky membrane supports. It further poses the unique possibility of using far thinner membranes without compromising tensile strength, because of the inherent strength of fine tubes. Another promising design under development by Babb and Grimsrud [8] utilizes membrane supports made of metal foam, which combine optimal physical properties for atraumatic membrane constraint with turbulent dialyzing-fluid flow patterns.

INTRACORPOREAL DIALYSIS

Peritoneal Dialysis. The evolution of intracorporeal dialysis also covers about one century. In 1877 Wegner [330] made some preliminary explorations of the intact peritoneal membrane as a transfer surface. Based on Putnam's subsequent demonstration that the living peritoneum with its large surface area was an excellent dialyzing membrane [243], Ganter reported the first use of peritoneal dialysis as a clinical therapeutic procedure in 1923 [95]. Continuous peritoneal irrigation with fluid circulating through separate inlet and outlet catheters was explored further by Rosenak and Siwon [252] in 1926 and used in the treatment of acute renal failure by Frank and his co-workers [88, 89] in 1946. Because of frequent complications, however, particularly peritonitis, this technic was not widely adopted. Intermittent, short-term peritoneal irrigation was later shown by LeGrain and Merrill [174] to be an effective and safer procedure for removing solute and water from the oliguric patient. Refinements introduced by Doolan et al. [61] and Maxwell et al. [204] in 1959 were based largely on the use of a single, specially designed catheter and commercially prepared, sterile, and nonpyrogenic dialyzing fluid. Their technic, which has gained wide acceptance, calls for intermittent, rather than continuous, introduction, equilibration, and removal of fluid in batches of approximately 2 liters. The process is generally continued for 24 to 72 hours and repeated as necessary. Adequately detailed instructions for proper technic in peritoneal dialysis may be found in brochures enclosed in each carton of commercially prepared dialysis fluid.

The principal advantages of peritoneal dialysis over extracorporeal hemodialysis are simplicity and easy availability, without expensive or complex equipment. For these reasons, it has been widely used in smaller hospitals. Its principal disadvantage is poor transfer efficiency, necessitating longer or more frequent treatment. Abdominal discomfort, peritoneal inflammation, and excessive protein loss [307] may also be encountered, especially when peritoneal dialysis is continued over long periods. Peritonitis is not, however, an absolute contraindication to peritoneal dialysis, particularly since antimicrobial drugs can be introduced effectively via this route. In small children, peritoneal dialysis may be a safer and less cumbersome technic than extracorporeal dialysis. It has proved especially useful in the treatment of poisoning in children [278]. A comprehensive account of the history and kinetics of peritoneal dialysis has been presented by Boen [25].

Recent innovations in peritoneal dialysis have been directed toward two objectives: (1) enhanced solute transfer efficiency and (2) improved economy for long-term application. Henderson [128] demonstrated that faster removal of urea can be effected by augmenting diffusive transport with ultrafiltration induced by hypertonic glucose. Substitution of cotton seed oil or olive oil for aqueous dialyzing fluid has been shown experimentally to enhance removal of lipid-soluble drugs, such as glutethimide, but the hazard of transperitoneal lipid absorption makes this approach unsafe as yet for clinical use [292]. Albumin can serve a similar purpose for removing salicylate [83], as does THAM for barbiturate [156]. Secondary transfer systems have also been developed by which small volumes of recirculating peritoneal dialysis fluids can be repurified externally, either by an anion-exchange column [253] or by an artificial kidney [291]. Improved peritoneal access devices [311] and automated systems for fluid cycling [171] show promise for reducing both the complications and the cost of long-term peritoneal dialysis.

Intestinal Lavage. Although many body surfaces aside from the peritoneum have been explored as intracorporeal exchange membranes [57, 169, 258, 293], only the gut has provided a practical alternative to the peritoneum. The observation by Pendleton and West [234] that urea diffuses rapidly into intestinal fluid laid the groundwork for intestinal lavage as a treatment for uremia. Hamberger et al. [116, 117] utilized lavage of the small intestine through a Miller-Abbott tube. Gastric lavage, with or without an interposed cellophane bag, has also received attention [262, 276], although its usefulness is essentially limited to the correction of acidosis and hyperkalemia. Most attempts at continuous dialysis of the intact gut, however, were frequently complicated by edema as a result of active absorption of water and electrolytes [64, 187, 231]. Subsequently the technic was improved to avoid these difficulties by surgically isolating the segment of intestine to be perfused [85]. Clark [41, 42], who has reported an extensive experience with dialysis through isolated jejunal loops, confirmed previous observations of effective removal of urea but relatively slow removal of creatinine, urate, phosphate, and sulfate. He concluded that nightly jejunal dialysis was a valuable adjunct in the management of some patients with chronic renal failure. However, in end-stage uremia this therapeutic approach is insufficient to avoid peripheral neuropathy and increasing debility.

Functional Concept of Dialytic Transport

As in renal physiology, transport concepts, terminology, and methods for measuring efficiency have evolved for the artificial kidney. Clearance (C) for any given solute, a measurement of the minute volume of blood from which that solute is completely removed, may be determined as

$$C = Q_B \frac{C_{B_i} - C_{B_o}}{C_{B_i}}$$

where Q_B is blood flow in milliliters per minute, C_{B_i} is concentration of the solute in entering blood, and C_{B_o} is its concentration in exiting blood. Dialysance (D) is defined as

$$D = Q_B \frac{C_{B_i} - C_{B_o}}{C_{B_i} - C_{D_i}}$$

where C_{D_i} is concentration in entering dialysis fluid. This expression takes into account entering concentration gradient as a driving force.

Permeability (P), a measurement of solute transport per unit mean concentration gradient ($\Delta \overline{C}$) per unit membrane area (A), may be measured as

$$P = \left[\frac{QB}{A}\right]\left[\frac{C_{B_i} - C_{B_o}}{\Delta\overline{C}}\right]$$

For concurrent flow, $\Delta \overline{C}$ may be calculated as

$$\Delta\overline{C} = \frac{\ln\left[\dfrac{C_{B_i} - C_{D_i}}{C_{B_o} - C_{D_o}}\right]}{(C_{B_i} - C_{D_i}) - (C_{B_o} - C_{D_o})}$$

Permeability or its reciprocal, resistance to solute transport (R), may be defined in terms of each medium through which solute must pass during dialysis as

$$1/P = R_\Sigma = R_B + R_M + R_D$$

where R_Σ is total resistance, R_B is resistance to solute transport in the blood, R_M is resistance in the membrane, and R_D is resistance in the dialysis fluid. Methods for measuring each component of resistance have been elaborated [176, 178]. They have proved most useful in assessing major internal determinants of dialyzer behavior, particularly boundary layer conditions in fluid films adjacent to the membrane where solute movement by diffusion is relatively slow compared to convective movement in well-stirred areas.

A better understanding of the "physiology" of the artificial kidney and its close dependence on dialyzer "anatomy" has provided a rational basis for design improvement. Compiled data on the performance of various artificial kidneys indicates that under usual flow conditions, the major resistance to solute transport lies in the fluid films rather than in the membrane itself [49, 178]. Therefore, in addition to more permeable membranes [51, 179, 190–193, 202, 228, 336], design objectives have included thinner fluid flow paths, within the limits of tolerable pressure drop, and methods for inducing turbulence, short of erythrocyte damage. To achieve each objective, one must pay a predictable price. More permeable membranes demand more carefully constructed membrane supports. Thinner fluid flow paths result in higher pressure drops and may therefore force the use of multiple, short, parallel flow paths. These, in turn, impose the requirement of precise geometric uniformity in order to avoid maldistribution of blood or dialyzing fluid. Generally, any alteration of one design parameter necessitates change in others. The ultimate practical determinant of whether or not any sequence of changes should be pursued is a realistic appraisal of its probable net benefit compared to its total cost, including operating costs. This subject of dialyzer performance has been dealt with more quantitatively by Leonard and Bluemle [177] and Michaels [218], and comprehensively by others [21, 22, 94].

Indications for Dialysis

Severe uremia, whether irreversible or reversible, is the major indication for dialysis. Dialysis is also indicated in certain cases of acute poisoning. Since specific criteria for treatment differ materially according to the condition being treated, each will be discussed separately.

ACUTE RENAL FAILURE

In reviewing the evolution of the use of the artificial kidney in acute renal failure, one perceives a steady trend from conservatism to liberalism over the last 25 years. Shortly after Kolff's pioneering demonstration of its usefulness in severe uremia, the opinion was expressed that ". . . in spite of much effort and ingenuity, it is fair to say that the artificial kidney is still only an ideal and not an accomplished fact. It seems clear that until artificial kidneys become safer, they have no place in the treatment of acute renal failure" [70]. Dialytic procedures in their early days were indeed hazardous and complex. Results were variable, and convincing evidence that dialysis could reduce mortality rates was difficult to gather [24]. For these reasons, and because of an unfortunate polarization of attitudes among nephrologists, there was a tendency to pit dialysis against conservative management, which gave way only gradually to a more enlightened view of their close interdependence [209].

By 1957 it was generally agreed ". . . that some form of dialysis is indicated in patients who have not had a satisfactory diuresis by the seventh to tenth day of urinary suppression . . ." [166]. Merrill [210], however, advocated dialysis as a broadly elective procedure, employed not only in emergencies but according to specific indications in order to avoid, as well as to alleviate, the morbidity of severe uremia. Support for the early application of dialysis to prevent clinical deterioration was strengthened by an analysis of over 1000 cases of acute renal failure compiled by a study group organized in 1957 by Teschan [242]. Two years later, Teschan espoused the concept of "prophylactic daily dialysis" for severe, acute uremia [313]. He also devised a technic for avoiding frequent cutdowns through the use of indwelling arterial and venous catheters flushed hourly with heparin. His results in a modest series of patients so treated reflected decreased mortality, improved awareness and mobility, as well as decreased anorexia and malnutrition.

However, because of the practical difficulties and expense of daily dialysis, this regimen has not been followed rigidly in many centers. Nevertheless, the concept of early rather than late dialysis has gained wide support [69, 257, 269], especially following the advent of the arteriovenous shunt [274], which allows convenient access to the circulation for repeated dialysis until adequate renal function has returned. For additional information on dialysis in the management of acute renal failure, the reader is referred to Chapter 17.

As indicated previously, another application of dialysis is the removal of edema fluid, particularly when it accompanies renal failure [133]. To some degree, fluid removal is mandatory in the majority of dialyses conducted on oliguric patients, water being one of the substances retained in excessive amounts. Even in the absence of oliguria, the treatment of edema by ultrafiltration during dialysis has been utilized on occasion [161]. However, since the development of more potent diuretics, this relatively extreme therapeutic approach to edema without renal failure is seldom indicated.

POISONING

Another primary indication for dialysis is severe exogenous poisoning by certain substances of relatively low molecular weight. Notable examples are salicylates [62, 73, 82, 142, 195, 232, 264, 309, 316], certain barbiturates [16, 45, 130, 152, 168, 173, 185, 279], glutethimide [37, 58, 59, 92, 200], and methanol [75, 84, 201, 335]. Schreiner has presented four fundamental criteria for judging the applicability of dialysis in the treatment of acute poisoning [263]:

1. The poison molecule should diffuse through a dialysis membrane, such as cellophane, from plasma water and have a reasonable removal rate or "dialysance."
2. The poison must be sufficiently well distributed in accessible body fluid compartments. If substantial fractions of the absorbed poison are bound to protein, concentrated in inaccessible fluid compartments (e.g., cerebrospinal fluid), or attain a significant intracellular concentration, then effective dialysis will be sharply limited. This restriction can be diminished, however, if the "loculated" portion readily equilibrates with the plasma.
3. There should be a relationship between the blood concentration, the duration of the body's exposure to the circulating poison, and toxicity.
4. The amount of poison dialyzed must constitute a significant addition to the normal body mechanisms for dealing with the particular poison under consideration. This should include metabolism, conjugation, and elimination of the substance by the bowel and kidney.

Annually updated accounts of composite experience in the dialytic removal of poisons have been contributed by Maher and Schreiner as appendices in the *Transactions of the American Society for Artificial Internal Organs.* These reviews provide valuable guides in determining when and when not to dialyze in questionable cases.

CHRONIC RENAL FAILURE

During the last decade, the application of dialysis in chronic, irreversible uremia has assumed paramount importance because of the prevalence of progressive renal disease and mounting evidence that repeated dialysis can prolong life in otherwise fatal renal failure. The evolution of so-called chronic dialysis has been somewhat tortuous, partly because of sharply differing opinions and experience which have only recently achieved some degree of reconciliation. Prior to 1960, attempts to prolong life in patients with chronic renal failure by repeated dialysis were uniformly disappointing. Alwall et al. [5] succeeded in maintaining life in several irreversibly oliguric patients for as long as 116 days. Maher, Schreiner, and Waters [199] kept an oliguric patient alive for a record 181 days. The intervals between dialyses in these cases, however, were relatively long, and the severity of uremia tended to follow a jagged pattern in which the patients gradually deteriorated with malnutrition and frequent complications. The observation by Teschan et al. [313] that a smoother response could be achieved by daily dialysis in acute oliguria set the stage for the first concerted and successful attempt to restore useful life for an indefinite period in patients with obviously terminal, irreversible renal disease. This outstanding contribution made by Scribner and his colleagues [273] in 1960 was facilitated by the development of their ingeniously straightforward method for gaining access repeatedly to the circulation via a Teflon-Silastic shunt [127, 246]. No other technical innovation attests so clearly to the impact of creative bioengineering in this field.

Technic of Chronic Dialysis. A brief description of the technic of chronic dialysis is given below although more complete accounts can be found elsewhere [48, 125, 126]. Following implantation of the arteriovenous shunt, the patient is treated generally two to three times weekly for continuous periods of six to fourteen hours. Of the various types of dialyzers which can be used for this purpose, the Kiil dialyzer [47, 155, 241, 289] and the disposable twin-coil dialyzer [162, 233, 324] have been employed most widely. The dialyzing solution is generally identical to that used in the treatment of acute renal failure — that is, a slightly hypertonic solution containing all diffusible blood electrolytes in relatively normal concentrations in addition to glucose. Lactate or acetate [220] may be used instead of bicarbonate to maintain pH close to 7.4. A technical innovation developed specifically for chronic dialysis in order to prepare large volumes of dialyzing fluid for "single-pass" systems entails a constant proportioning pump which mixes small volumes of a stock concentrate with large volumes of tap water [46, 112, 236]. Centralized systems for this purpose are employed in many centers where a number of patients are treated simultaneously.

Survival Rates. Meaningful survival statistics have appeared only recently, owing to the relatively short duration of treatment in most cases and the variations in technic from time to time and from one center to another. It is anticipated that updated survival statistics will be made available through a registry for chronic dialysis patients [34] somewhat similar to the Kidney Transplantation Registry. The most comprehensive data to date have been provided by the Program Studies Section of the Kidney Disease Control Program, Public Health Service. Their data are based on an analysis of 478 patients in 34 centers supported through the Public Health Service or the Veterans Administration [104]. Of this total, 89 patients have died, yielding a crude survival rate of 81.5 per cent with a range of 100 per cent at 11 centers to 53.6 per cent at one center having 28 patients.

An analysis [104] of 302 patients receiving dialytic treatment of varying duration throughout a seven-year period ending in June, 1967, is presented graphically in Figure 10-1. Although the data on survival after five years is based on relatively few patients, it is not unreasonable to anticipate that approximately half of the patients now starting chronic dialysis at qualified American centers will remain alive at the end of seven years. A survey of 54 European dialysis centers involv-

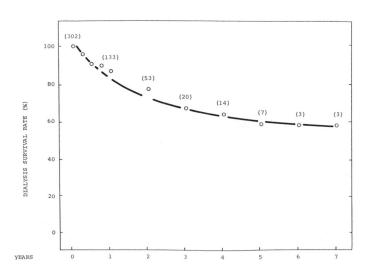

Figure 10-1. Cumulative seven-year survival rates for chronic dialysis patients. Numbers in parentheses indicate number of patients observed during each survival period.

ing 612 patients has been presented by Drukker et al. [65]; 75 of these patients received a kidney graft. Of the remaining 537 treated by dialysis alone, 70 per cent survived for the first six months, 61 per cent for one year, 56 per cent for two years, and 55 per cent for three years.

An analysis of survival according to age distribution [104] showed a gradually decreasing survival rate beyond the age of 35, suggesting that it is generally undesirable to initiate chronic dialysis in elderly patients. Exceptions, however, have been noted [137]. Few children have been treated by chronic hemodialysis, presumably because of their vulnerability to frequent medical and psychologic complications [287]. Kidney transplantation may be a preferable alternative in the majority of children with end-stage renal failure.

The success of long-term dialysis can be measured more critically in terms of restoration of *useful* life. Occupational rehabilitation and relief of symptoms have been the prime criteria. Pendras and Erickson [235] reported that of 19 patients treated at the Seattle Artificial Kidney Center, virtually none had gastrointestinal or other serious symptoms of uremia. The majority, however, continued to have moderate insomnia, pruritus, easy fatigability, and intermittent malaise. Hypertension was controlled in the vast majority of patients by sodium restriction and sodium and water removal during dialysis. Nutrition was well maintained despite moderate protein restrictions. Similarly favorable, and some unfavorable, results have been reported in a wide spectrum of experiences at other centers [32, 50, 52, 98, 99, 138, 165, 197, 206, 256, 267, 290, 338].

The degree of rehabilitation achievable during chronic dialysis has been assessed in several large series. Restoration to full activity was noted in 71 per cent of 79 patients under treatment for at least one year [104]. Of the remaining patients, 18 per cent were partially rehabilitated, while 11 per cent were restricted in activity or unable to work at all. An analysis of the employment status of another 172 patients under treatment at Veteran Administration Centers revealed that 26 per cent were fully employed and 60 per cent could work from 10 to 40 hours per week [104]. Compty, Baillod, Crockett, and Shaldon [50] reported 100 per cent rehabilitation in 23 of their 26 patients after 40 months of dialysis experience in a nurse-patient operated unit. All but one of Pendras' 19 patients were engaged in semisedentary occupations, working an average of 30 to 40 hours per week [235]. It is therefore reasonable to assume that the majority of patients undergoing long-term dialysis can be expected to resume relatively useful and productive lives.

Complications. The complications of chronic dialysis are at times difficult to distinguish from those of renal failure per se. Clearly, however, certain hazards have been recognized. These have been reviewed comprehensively by Maher and Schreiner [198], Hampers and Schupak [121], and Schreiner, Maher, Freeman, and O'Connell [266]. The most frequent complications have related to the arteriovenous cannulas. Notable are infection, clotting, thrombophlebitis, hemorrhages from cannula dislodgement or shunt separation, and erosion of subcutaneous tubing through the skin [39, 127, 223, 225, 235, 237, 244, 245, 267]. Occasionally, continuity of treatment has been threatened because of loss of cannula sites. Alternative technics for gaining access to the bloodstream have been proposed [40, 123, 182, 240, 249, 282, 283–285]. One of the most promising appears to be that of Brescia [27, 28, 208] utilizing a subcutaneous arteriovenous fistula with repeated percutaneous venipunctures.

Failure of automated machinery constitutes a rare but tragic complication with unique legal implications. On at least two occasions patients undergoing hemodialysis simultaneously at centers using central dialysis fluid systems have convulsed and died due to sudden hypernatremia related to malfunction of fluid-proportioning apparatus. More reliable pumps and control devices are under development [111, 113].

Hepatitis among patients and professional staff, probably transmitted through contaminated blood, has occurred with alarming frequency at some centers [43, 65, 93, 235, 268, 275]. Metabolic bone disease, including metastatic calcification, osteoporosis, pseudogouty arthritis, and secondary or tertiary hyperparathyroidism, has presented serious problems in some cases [36, 52a, 110, 124, 144, 145, 230, 277, 301, 302, 321, 337]. Variation in calcium content of tap water and its transport into blood by adsorption processes complicate these problems [52, 91, 323]. Peripheral neuropathy has been one of the most common causes of debility, particularly among patients whose dialytic treatment is inadequate [60, 151, 319, 320, 325]. Pulmonary embolism, hyperkalemia, septicemia [24, 43, 90, 154], malnutrition [65], pericarditis, and congestive heart failure with striking cardiomegaly [9, 15, 115, 327] have all been observed in patients undergoing repeated hemodialysis. Evidence for a causal relationship between these complications and dialysis is lacking, however. Anemia requiring multiple transfusions must be considered in part a consequence of dialysis when recovery of blood from the dialyzer is incomplete or when mechanical trauma to erythrocytes occurs [30, 135, 167, 288]. Heparinization, heparin rebound, and alteration of blood platelets can also predispose to blood loss [6, 35, 38, 74, 146, 172, 183, 247, 303, 326]. Hemosiderosis due to multiple transfusions [107] and absorption of iron from dialysis fluid [196] has been observed. Certain other complications noted frequently during the dialysis of patients with severe acute renal failure occur only rarely in chronic dialysis. For example, the disequilibrium syndrome [63, 67, 96, 118, 147, 149, 238, 239, 251, 270, 294], attributable in part to sudden changes in osmotic pressure gradients as high blood urea levels are rapidly reduced without concomitant reductions within fluid compartments of the central nervous system, seldom occurs in chronic dialysis where fluctuations of blood urea are less extreme.

Of special concern are the psychologic problems of these patients and their families [100, 109, 265, 339]. Sand, Livingston, and Wright [259] have described personality characteristics that influence the patient's reaction to various stresses imposed by cannula care, the threat of painful medical procedures or possible death, restrictions in activity and diet, financial reverses, job changes, and marital problems. In most cases, such stresses and losses can be handled by denial and projection with support through identification with others under treatment and open verbalization with interested persons at home or in the treatment unit. In the absence of such opportunities or if a strong determination for good self-care is missing, depression and continuous complications can be expected. Depressions, psychotic reactions, and schizophrenic-like episodes are particularly apt to occur in settings where skepticism about results is expressed overtly or covertly in the patient's presence or where professional interest seems focused more on research than on patient care [287].

Patient Selection and Indications for Chronic Dialysis. The primary indication for long-term dialysis is irreversible renal failure which has progressed to the stage where conservative measures can no longer maintain life. This stage is generally characterized by a creatinine clearance below 5 ml. per minute [44, 206, 235, 338]. Unfortunately, treatment capability is disproportionately low compared to the number of patients with end-stage renal failure. It has been estimated that about 35,000 Americans die each year with chronic renal failure, of whom about 7000 could benefit from chronic dialysis or kidney transplantation [104]. However, less than 1000 patients with advanced renal failure have access to long-term dialytic treatment in this country at the time of this writing [105]. Thus, the onerous task of patient selection must involve a consideration of factors other than the severity of uremia. There is as yet no universally acceptable set of criteria by which such decisions can be made, nor is one likely to evolve which is consistent with all values of civilized man [71, 72, 181, 211, 250, 308]. Human worth is not measurable except by arbitrary standards, with or without the aid of "selection committees" [122, 224]. Predictions of total response in any given case prior to clinical trial remains precarious.

Accordingly, a pragmatic approach to patient selection may be the least objectionable, if not the only recourse at the moment. Assuming it is desirable to invest limited dialysis resources in those patients who will tend to respond most favorably, age must be taken into account. The presence of other disease that might limit total benefit from dialysis also constitutes a contraindication [315], although severe hypertension, malnutrition, or other advanced complications of uremia, per se, may be excluded [97, 143, 235, 317]. In rare instances, severely uremic patients with diabetes [7], Goodpasture's syndrome [139], and lupus erythematosus [76] are said to have responded relatively well to chronic dialysis. Judgments regarding the patient's intelligence, discipline, motivation, family setting, ability to adapt to a new socioeconomic or employment status all tend to enter into the decision-making process, consciously or unconsciously [68, 71, 72, 100, 109, 121, 181, 211, 250, 265, 308, 339]. Without a reliable measurement of such qualities, the expedient of assessing prior ability or inability to follow a rigorous conservative program may serve as a practical guide of some predictable value.

Realistically, however, until dialysis capability can be expanded to meet the need [271], a major determinant of patient selection is whether or not a chronic dialysis program exists in the patient's environs and whether or not it can accept another patient. It has been ar-

gued that a "first come, first served" basis may be the only ethically acceptable one. Schupak et al. [268] concluded, on the basis of his experience with 26 "unselected" patients in a municipal-hospital program, that complete rehabilitation can be effected in some patients who superficially appeared to be poor candidates prior to therapy. Less favorable results with this approach have been reported with admirable candor by Retan and Lewis [248]. All 7 of their patients, chosen entirely at random in order of appearance, died within 2 to 22 months, generally after suffering many distressing complications. In this instance, however, inadequate facilities and lack of trained staff were contributory obstacles to optimal management.

Another determinant in patient selection is the likelihood of terminating dialysis through kidney transplantation [212]. When patient load is at the level of total capacity, additional commitments may be possible only for new patients awaiting transplantation. Of course, if the transplant fails, the question then arises as to whether the patient can be readmitted to an already saturated dialysis program. A close interrelationship between dialysis and transplantation has been emphasized by Scribner [271]. The alternative courses which any patient may follow between these two therapeutic modalities has been treated semiquantitatively by Rubini et al. [254] and by Greenberg [108] (Fig. 10-2).

Cost. The limiting factor to increased application of chronic dialysis is excessive cost, now estimated at $14,000 (range, $8,400 to $19,000) per patient per year [104]. Few patients can afford such treatment. Voluntary health insurance programs have offered partial support, but under restricted conditions. Even major medical insurance providing a maximum lifetime benefit of $25,000 ($100 deductible and co-insurance of 20 per cent) would provide only two years of dialysis (208 dialyses at $150 per dialysis), and then only at an additional cost to the patient of $6,200

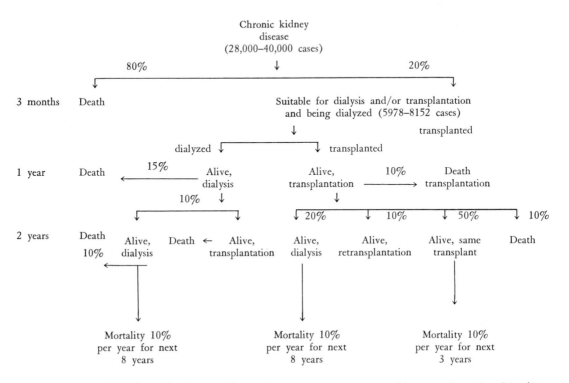

Figure 10-2. Probable flow of patients under varying treatment programs with expected survivorship. (From report of the Committee on Chronic Kidney Disease, Bureau of the Budget, 1967.)

[104]. Unfortunately, most insurance policies stipulate a limitation of benefits to a definite "spell of illness" which requires an interval between illnesses before payment can be resumed. Long-term intermittent dialysis does not fit this pattern.

Title 18 of the Social Security Act provides benefits only to patients 65 years of age or older, the age group least likely to be selected for treatment. To qualify under Title 19, a patient must be poor and remain poor for the duration of treatment according to the standards for medical indigency, which vary from state to state. Funds available through the Bureau of Vocational Rehabilitation to support restoration of patients to the labor force are applicable within budgetary restraints; however, benefits cease six months after employment has been obtained. At the present time, veterans are in a uniquely favorable position to qualify for federally supported dialysis treatment of unlimited duration in programs established within the Veterans Administration Hospital system.

In addition to the problem of financing patient care with existing facilities, there remains a question of funding the development of new programs to expand dialysis capability throughout the country. This question has been discussed in the context of general health planning [184], and analyzed in detail by national advisory groups [34, 104] and by authorities from various countries [4, 150, 271, 272, 315]. Concern has been expressed that a significantly larger allocation of medical resources and manpower for this purpose might have subtractive effects on other health programs and research activities [29, 34]. Recommendations for vastly expanded regional kidney disease programs have recently been submitted to appropriate federal agencies [34, 104]. They call for greater support of training and research activities as well as for expansion of chronic dialysis and transplantation programs in coordinated patterns across the country. One report projects a cost of $800,000,000 to $1,000,000,000 over a six-year period in order to bring treatment capability up to the level of demand [104]. In view of the vast number of social needs competing for federal support, however, some question remains as to when this particular one can be met.

Home Dialysis. The most significant step toward improved economy has been to remove chronic dialysis from its expensive hospital environment and conduct it in the patient's home. Initiated in 1964 [54, 120, 215, 281], home dialysis has grown from a cumbersome experimental procedure to a relatively safe and efficient one in which better chemical control of uremia can be accomplished in selected patients at about one-third the cost of that done at a medical center [10, 11, 13, 79, 119, 271]. Eschbach and his co-workers [77] attributes its success in 23 patients (2500 dialyses) to three factors: (1) thrice, instead of twice, weekly treatment, (2) thorough patient training, and (3) adequate but not oversolicitous patient support from his physician.

A basic requirement for home dialysis is a patient training unit. Following a short admission to the hospital for preliminary evaluation and implantation of an arteriovenous shunt in the leg, dialyses are conducted in the training unit, which need not be located in the hospital. After two to three weeks of supervised treatment, first for short periods during the day and then nocturnally for

periods of 8 to 10 hours, the patient gradually assumes more personal responsibilities for his own dialyses. When ambulatory, the patient and another member of his family learn how to clean, assemble, and sterilize the dialyzer, adjust monitor-alarms, order supplies, and become generally self-sufficient. The total training period usually lasts two months, during which the patient's own bedroom at home is modified to accommodate his equipment. Ideally, his family physician also becomes acquainted with the procedure and its possible complications, so the patient does not have to return to the training center or hospital except for major problems.

The success of home dialysis is directly dependent upon the ability of the patient and his family to cope with the inherent stresses and additional demands imposed on family life [286]. Poverty, inadequate living quarters, large family size, and emotional immaturity are but a few of the factors that may limit the application of home dialysis to perhaps half of the uremic population otherwise qualified for treatment. Nevertheless, its obvious cost-benefit advantages, not the least of which relates to reduced transfusion requirements with more frequent blood cleansing [78], makes home dialysis, integrated into the general practice of medicine, a practical and most promising possibility for expanded application at present [271].

Future Prospects

Improvements in the technology of dialysis and in alternative means for purifying the body fluids hold some promise for better efficiency and economy of operation. More compact dialyzers [23, 170, 180, 306] and secondary systems for purifying small volumes of recirculating dialyzing fluid [19, 56, 141, 164, 299, 300, 318, 329] may one day lead to the development of portable systems capable of operating continuously. While such systems are far from perfected at this time, they pose the theoretical advantages of more constant chemical control, greater patient mobility, and markedly reduced requirements in membrane area. More permeable membranes [51, 179, 189, 190–193, 202, 203, 207, 228, 229, 336] and technics for rendering them nonthrombogenic [87, 101–103, 134, 175, 214, 221, 332–334] are under investigation, as are new membrane supports which promote efficient solute transport [8, 22]. Lymph dialysis [260, 261, 331], hemosorption technics [56, 66, 340, 341], long-term peritoneal dialysis [12, 14, 26, 33, 86, 114, 131, 171, 205, 213, 255, 310–312], and isolated gut perfusion [41, 42] present certain advantages, but as yet, they have not been perfected as completely satisfactory alternatives to extracorporeal hemodialysis. Attempts to utilize external energy to accelerate solute transport have led to explorations of electro-hemodialysis [148, 239] and rapid blood filtration [18, 22, 31, 129].

Both technics have been shown to provide more rapid or more thorough solute transport in experimental studies. However, each presents unique problems that must be solved before either becomes clinically applicable.

In summary, extant technics and apparatus for cleansing the body fluids artificially, while of proved value, leave much to be desired in economy of operation and completeness of removal of toxic products of metabolism. With a more comprehensive knowledge of what these products are and the chemical pathways by which they cause the clinical abnormalities of uremia, a firmer foundation will be laid for new therapeutic approaches to renal failure. It is reasonable to assume, however, that there will always be a place for improved artificial methods for selective solute removal and that the living kidney will remain the model of excellence in this endeavor.

References

1. Abel, J. J., Rowntree, L. G., and Turner, B. B.   The removal of diffusible substances from the circulating blood by means of dialysis. *Trans. Ass. Amer. Physicians* 28:41, 1913.

2. Abel, J. J., Rowntree, L. G., and Turner, B. B.   On the removal of diffusible substances from the blood of living animals. *J. Pharmacol. Exp. Ther.* 5:275, 1914.

3. Alwall, N.   On the artificial kidney: I. Apparatus for dialysis of blood in vivo. *Acta Med. Scand.* 128:317, 1947.

4. Alwall, N.   Development of Dialysis Activities in Sweden, Need for Dialysis and Planning for the Future. In *Proceedings of the European Dialysis and Transplant Association.* Newcastle upon Tyne, England: Bolsten & Stols, 1966. Vol. 3, p. 149.

5. Alwall, N., Erlanson, P., Tornberg, A., Moëll, H., and Fajers, C. M.   Two cases of gross renal cortical necrosis in pregnancy with severe oliguria and anuria for 116 and 79 days respectively; clinical course, roentgenologic studies of the kidneys (size, outline and calcification), and post-mortem findings. *Acta Med. Scand.* 161:93, 1958.

6. Anderson, C. F., and DePalma, J. R.   Platelet counts and adhesiveness during hemodialysis. *Trans. Amer. Soc. Artif. Intern. Organs* 12:210, 1966.

7. Avram, M. D.   In *Proceedings of the Conference on Dialysis.* New York: National Dialysis Committee, 1966. P. 15.

8. Babb, A. L., and Grimsrud, L.   A new concept in hemodialyzer membrane support. *Trans. Amer. Soc. Artif. Intern. Organs* 10:31, 1964.

9. Bailey, G. L., Hampers, C. L., and Merrill, J. P.   Reversible cardiomyopathy in uremia. *Trans. Amer. Soc. Artif. Intern. Organs* 13:263, 1967.

10. Baillod, R. A., Comty, C., Ilahi, M., Konotey-Ahulu, F. I. D., Sevitt, L., and Shaldon, S.   Overnight Haemodialysis in the Home.

In *Proceedings of the European Dialysis and Transplant Association.* Newcastle upon Tyne, England: Bolsten & Stols, 1965. Vol. 2, p. 99.

11. Baillod, R. A., Comty, C., and Shaldon, S. Eighteen Months Experience with Chronic Peritoneal Dialysis. In *Proceedings of the European Dialysis and Transplant Association.* Newcastle upon Tyne, England: Bolsten & Stols, 1965. Vol. 2, p. 109.

12. Baillod, R. A., Comty, C. M., Crockett, R., and Shaldon, S. Experience with Regular Haemodialysis in the Home. In *Proceedings of the European Dialysis and Transplant Association.* Newcastle upon Tyne, England: Bolsten & Stols, 1966. Vol. 3, p. 125.

13. Barnett, B. M. S., Cole, J. J., Daly, S., Tyler, L., and Eschbach, J. W., Jr. A Report of Local and Remote Home Haemodialysis. In *Proceedings of the European Dialysis and Transplant Association.* Newcastle upon Tyne, England: Bolsten & Stols, 1966. Vol. 3, p. 132.

14. Barry, K. G., Schwartz, F. D., Harro, J. E., Schrier, R. W., and Canfield, C. Peritoneal Dialysis: Current Applications and Recent Developments. In *Proceedings of the Third International Congress of Nephrology,* Washington, D.C., 1967. Vol. 3, p. 288.

15. Beaudry, C., Nakamoto, S., and Kolff, W. J. Uremic pericarditis and cardiac tamponade in chronic renal failure. *Ann. Intern. Med.* 64:990, 1966.

16. Berman, L. B., Schreiner, G. E., Jeghers, H., and Pallotta, A. Hemodialysis: An effective therapy for acute barbiturate poisoning. *J.A.M.A.* 161:820, 1956.

17. Bier, M., Bruckner, G. C., and Roy, H. E. Blood electrodialysis. *Trans. Amer. Soc. Artif. Intern. Organs* 13:227, 1967.

18. Bixler, J. H., Nelson, L. M., and Bluemle, L. W., Jr. The development of a diafiltration system for blood purification. *Trans. Amer. Soc. Artif. Intern. Organs* 14:99, 1968.

19. Blaney, J. L., Lindan, O., and Sparks, R. E. Adsorption: A step toward a wearable artificial kidney. *Trans. Amer. Soc. Artif. Intern. Organs* 12:7, 1966.

20. Bluemle, L. W., Jr. The artificial kidney: Some approaches to improved design and function. *Med. Clin. N. Amer.* 50:1351, 1966.

21. Bluemle, L. W., Jr. Technical Aspects of Dialysis: New Apparatus. In *Proceedings of the Third International Congress of Nephrology,* Washington, D.C., 1967. Vol. 3, p. 256.

22. Bluemle, L. W., Jr., Dickson, J. G., Jr., Mitchell, J., and Podolnick, M. S. Permeability and hydrodynamic studies on the MacNeill-Collins dialyzer using conventional and modified membrane supports. *Trans. Amer. Soc. Artif. Intern. Organs* 6: 38, 1960.

23. Bluemle, L. W., Jr., Ushakoff, A., and Murphy, W. P., Jr. A compact blood dialyzer without membrane supports: Design and fabrication. *Trans. Amer. Soc. Artif. Intern. Organs* 11:157, 1965.

24. Bluemle, L. W., Jr., Webster, G. D., Jr., and Elkinton, J. R. Acute tubular necrosis; analysis of 100 cases with respect to mortality, complications and treatment with and without dialysis. *A.M.A. Arch. Intern. Med.* 104:180, 1959.

25. Boen, S. T. Kinetics of peritoneal dialysis: Comparison with artificial kidney. *Medicine* (Balt.) 40:243, 1961.

26. Boen, S. T., Mion, C. M., Curtis, F. K., and Shilipetar, G. Periodic peritoneal dialysis using the repeated puncture technique and an automatic cycling machine. *Trans. Amer. Soc. Artif. Intern. Organs* 10:409, 1964.

27. Brescia, M. J., and Cimino, J. E. Discussion on paper by Hayes, C. P., Gunnells, J. C., and Robinson, R. R. *Trans. Amer. Soc. Artif. Intern. Organs* 12:227, 1966.

28. Brescia, M. J., Cimino, J. E., Appel, K., and Hurwich, B. J. Chronic hemodialysis using venipuncture and a surgically created arteriovenous fistula. *New Eng. J. Med.* 275:1089, 1966.

29. Bricker, N. S. Presidential address to the American Society of Nephrology. Los Angeles, Calif., Oct. 18, 1967.

30. Brinsfield, D. B., Hopf, M. A., Geering, R. B., and Galletti, P. M. Hematologic changes in long-term perfusion. *J. Appl. Physiol.* 17:581, 1962.

31. Brown, C. E., and Kramer, N. C.   Factors in membrane design and selection as a step toward a wearable artificial kidney. *Trans. Amer. Soc. Artif. Intern. Organs* 14:36, 1968.

32. Brown, H. W., Maher, J. R., Lapierre, L., Bledsoe, F. H., and Schreiner, G. E.   Clinical problems related to prolonged artificial maintenance of life by hemodialysis in chronic renal failure. *Trans. Amer. Soc. Artif. Intern. Organs* 8:281, 1962.

33. Burns, R. E., Henderson, L. W., Hager, E. B., and Merrill, J. P.   Peritoneal dialysis. *New Eng. J. Med.* 267:1060, 1962.

34. Burton, B. T.   Report to the Surgeon General. Kidney Disease Program Analysis, 1967, Washington, D.C.

35. Cahalane, S. F., Johnson, S. A., Monto, R. W., and Caldwell, J. J.   Acquired thrombocytopathy: Observation on the coagulation defect in uremia. *Amer. J. Clin. Path.* 30:507, 1958.

36. Caner, J. E. Z., and Decker, J. L.   Recurrent acute (?gouty) arthritis in chronic renal failure treated with periodic hemodialysis. *Amer. J. Med.* 36:571, 1964.

37. Chandler, B. F., Meroney, W. H., Czarnecki, S. W., Herman, R. H., Cheitlin, M. D., Goldbaum, L. R., and Herndon, E. G.   Artificial hemodialysis in management of glutethimide intoxication. *J.A.M.A.* 170:914, 1959.

38. Cheney, K., and Bonnin, J. A.   Haemorrhage, platelet dysfunction and other coagulation defects in uremia. *Brit. J. Haemat.* 8:215, 1962.

39. Chisholm, G. D.   The Scribner arteriovenous fistula for hemodialysis. *Brit. Med. J.* 5:30, 1961.

40. Cimino, J. E., and Brescia, M. J.   Simple venipuncture for hemodialysis. *New Eng. J. Med.* 267:608, 1962.

41. Clark, J. E., Templeton, J. Y., III, Cohn, H. E., and Soricelli, R. R.   Isolated small bowel dialysis in 23 patients. *Trans. Amer. Soc. Artif. Intern. Organs* 11:18, 1965.

42. Clark, J. E.   Discussion. *Trans. Amer. Soc. Artif. Intern. Organs* 13:33, 1967.

43. Clark, J. E.   Personal communication, 1965.

44. Clark, J. E., and Soricelli, R. R.   Indications for dialysis. *Med. Clin. N. Amer.* 49: 1213, 1965.

45. Clemmesen, C.   New line of treatment in barbiturate poisoning. *Acta Med. Scand.* 148:83, 1954.

46. Cole, J. J., Fritzen, J. R., Vizzo, J. E., van Paasschen, W. H., and Grimsrud, L.   One year's experience with a central dialysate supply system in a hospital. *Trans. Amer. Soc. Artif. Intern. Organs* 11:22, 1965.

47. Cole, J. J., Pollard, T. L., and Murray, J. S. Studies on the modified polypropylene Kiil dialyzer. *Trans. Amer. Soc. Artif. Intern. Organs* 9:67, 1963.

48. Cole, J. J., Quinton, W. E., Williams, C., Murray, J. S., and Sherris, J. C.   The pumpless, low temperature hemodialysis system. *Trans. Amer. Soc. Artif. Intern. Organs* 8: 209, 1962.

49. Colton, C. K.   A review of the development and performance of hemodialyzers. Published by Artificial Kidney-Chronic Uremia Program, National Institute of Arthritis and Metabolic Diseases, National Institutes of Health, Bethesda, Md., 1967.

50. Comty, C. M., Baillod, R. A., Crockett, R., and Shaldon, S.   Forty Month's Experience with a Nurse-Patient Operated Chronic Dialysis Unit. In *Proceedings of the European Dialysis and Transplant Association.* Newcastle upon Tyne, England: Bolsten & Stols, 1966. Vol. 3, p. 68.

51. Connally, N. T., Jr.   Proceedings of the Conference on Hemodialysis. Nov. 9–10, 1964, Bethesda, Md., National Institutes of Health, 1965.

52. Curtis, F. K., Davidson, R. C., and Pendras, J. P.   Metabolic bone disease and chronic dialysis. (Abstract.) In Abstracts: II. Free Communications. Third International Congress of Nephrology, Washington, D.C., 1966. P. 176.

52a. Curtis, F. K., Davidson, R. C., and Pendras, J. P.   Metabolic Bone Disease in Chronic Dialysis. In *Proceedings of the Third International Congress of Nephrology,* Washington, D.C., 1967. Vol. 3, p. 176.

53. Curtis, J. R., Wing, A. J., and Coleman, J. C.   Bacillus cereus bacteremia: A compli-

cation of intermittent hemodialysis. *Lancet* 1:136, 1967.

54. Curtis, K., Cole, J. J., Fellows, B. L., Tyler, L. J., and Scribner, B. H. Hemodialysis in the home. *Trans. Amer. Soc. Artif. Intern. Organs* 11:7, 1965.

55. Dalla Rosa, C., Galanti, G., Ancona, G., Bruschi, E., and Confortini, P. Clinical Results of Treatment of Chronic Renal Insufficiency by Periodic Haemodialysis. In *Proceedings of the European Dialysis and Transplant Association.* Newcastle upon Tyne, England: Bolsten & Stols, 1966. Vol. 3, p. 107.

56. Dedrick, R. L., Vantoch, P., Gombos, E. A., and Moore, R. Kinetics of activated carbon kidney. *Trans. Amer. Soc. Artif. Intern. Organs* 13:236, 1967.

57. DeMorais, B., and DeCarvalo, S. Pleural dialysis. *Gaz. Med. Port.* 4:423, 1951.

58. DeMyttenaere, M. H., Maher, J. F., and Schreiner, G. E. Hemoperfusion through a charcoal column for glutethimide poisoning. *Trans. Amer. Soc. Artif. Intern. Organs* 13:190, 1967.

59. DeMyttenaere, M. H., Schoenfeld, L., and Maher, J. F. Treatment of glutethimide poisoning: A comparison of forced diuresis and dialysis. *J.A.M.A.* 203:885, 1968.

60. Dinapoli, R. P., Johnson, W. J., and Lambert, E. H. Experience with a combined hemodialysis-renal transplantation program: Neurologic aspects. *Mayo Clin. Proc.* 41:809, 1966.

61. Doolan, P. D., Murphy, W. P., Jr., Wiggins, R. A., Carter, N. W., Cooper, W. C., Watten, R. H., and Alpen, E. L. An evaluation of intermittent peritoneal lavage. *Amer. J. Med.* 26:831, 1959.

62. Doolan, P. D., Walsh, W. P., Kyle, L. H., and Wishinsky, H. Acetylsalicylic acid intoxication: A proposed method of treatment. *J.A.M.A.* 146:105, 1951.

63. Dosseter, J. B., Oh, J. H., Dayes, L., and Pappius, H. M. Brain urea and water changes with rapid hemodialysis of uremic dogs. *Trans. Amer. Soc. Artif. Intern. Organs* 10:323, 1964.

64. Dougherty, G. W., Odel, H. M., and Ferris, D. O. Continuous lavage of the colon as a means of treating renal insufficiency. *Proc. Mayo Clin.* 23:209, 1948.

65. Drukker, W., Alberts, Chr., Ode, A., Roozendall, K. J., and Wilmink, J. Report on Regular Dialysis Treatment in Europe: II. 1966. In *Proceedings of the European Dialysis and Transplant Association.* Newcastle upon Tyne, England: Bolsten & Stols, 1966. Vol. 3, p. 90.

66. Dunea, G., and Kolff, W. J. Clinical experience with Yatzidis charcoal artificial kidney. *Trans. Amer. Soc. Artif. Intern. Organs* 11:178, 1966.

67. Durr, F., Zysno, E., and Nieth, H. Influence of the extracorporeal hemodialysis on the electroencephalogram in acute and chronic renal failure. *Klin. Wschr.* 43:1140, 1965.

68. Dutz, H. Selection System for Patients. In *Proceedings of European Dialysis and Transplant Association.* Newcastle upon Tyne, England: Bolsten & Stols, 1966. Vol. 3, p. 146.

69. Easterling, R. E., and Forland, M. A five-year experience with prophylactic dialysis for acute renal failure. *Trans. Amer. Soc. Artif. Intern. Organs* 10:200, 1964.

70. Editorial. Treatment of uremia. *Lancet* 1:221, 1948.

71. Elkinton, J. R. Medicine and the quality of life. (Editorial.) *Ann. Intern. Med.* 64:711, 1966.

72. Elkinton, J. R. Moral problems in the use of borrowed organs, artificial and transplanted. (Editorial.) *Ann. Intern. Med.* 60:309, 1964.

73. Elliott, G. B., Crichton, J. U., and Miller, G. E. Peritoneal dialysis in salicylate poisoning. *Anesth. Analg.* (Cleveland) 42:338, 1963.

74. Erickson, R. V., Williman, M., and Pendras, J. P. A true hypercoagulability state in patients on chronic hemodialysis. *Trans. Amer. Soc. Artif. Intern. Organs* 12:205, 1966.

75. Erlanson, P., Fritz, H., Hagstam, K. E., Liljenberg, B., Tryding, H., and Voigt, G. Severe methanol intoxication. *Acta Med. Scand.* 177:393, 1965.

76. Eschbach, J. W., Jr. In *Proceedings of the*

Conference on Dialysis. New York: National Dialysis Committee, 1966.

77. Eschbach, J. W., Jr., Barnett, B. M. S., Daly, S., Cole, J. J., and Scribner, B. H. Hemodialysis in the home: A realistic and successful treatment for chronic uremia. *Ann. Intern. Med.* 67:1149, 1967.

78. Eschbach, J. W., Jr., Funck, D., Adamson, J., Kuhn, I., Scribner, B. H., and Finch, C. A. Erythropoiesis in patients with renal failure undergoing chronic dialysis. *New Eng. J. Med.* 276:653, 1967.

79. Eschbach, J. W., Jr., Wilson, W. E., Jr., Peoples, R. W., Wakefield, A. W., Babb, A. L., and Scribner, B. H. Unattended overnight home dialysis. *Trans. Amer. Soc. Artif. Intern. Organs* 12:346, 1966.

80. Esmond, W. G., Strauch, M., Clark, H., Lewitinn, A., and Moore, S. The Dialung artificial kidney: A compact, pumpless, low cost, hand portable, clinical hemodialysis system. Bulletin, University of Maryland School of Medicine, Jan., 1966.

81. Esmond, W. G., Strauch, M., Zapata, A., and Hernandez, F. Fourteen patient-years' experience with a simplified home-hospital chronic hemodialysis system. *Trans. Amer. Soc. Artif. Intern. Organs* 13:254, 1967.

82. Etteldorf, J. N., Dobbins, W. T., Summitt, R. L., Rainwater, W. T., and Fischer, R. L. Intermittent peritoneal dialysis using 5% albumin in the treatment of salicylate intoxication in children. *J. Pediat.* 58:226, 1961.

83. Etteldorf, J. N., Montolvo, J. M., Kaplan, S., and Sheffield, J. A. Intermittent peritoneal dialysis in the treatment of experimental salicylate intoxication. *J. Pediat.* 56:1, 1960.

84. Felts, J. H., Templeton, T. B., Wolff, W. A., Meredith, J. H., and Hines, J. Methanol poisoning treated by hemodialysis. *Southern Med. J.* 55:46, 1962.

85. Fine, J., Frank, H. A., and Seligman, A. M. The treatment of acute renal failure by peritoneal irrigation. *Ann. Surg.* 124:857, 1946.

86. Flanigan, W. J., Henderson, L. W., and Merrill, J. P. The clinical application and technique of peritoneal dialysis. *GP* 29:98, 1963.

87. Fourt, L., Schwartz, A. M., Quasius, A., and Bowman, R. L. Heparin-bearing surfaces and liquid surfaces in relation to blood coagulation. *Trans. Amer. Soc. Artif. Intern. Organs* 12:155, 1966.

88. Frank, H. A., Seligman, A. M., and Fine, J. Treatment of uremia after acute renal failure by peritoneal irrigation. *J.A.M.A.* 130:703, 1946.

89. Frank, H. A., Seligman, A. M., and Fine, J. Further experiences with peritoneal irrigation for acute renal failure. *Ann. Surg.* 128:561, 1948.

90. Freake, R., Nayman, J., and Gurr, F. W. A review of the incidence of septicaemia as a complication in 85 cases of acute and chronic renal failure. *Med. J. Aust.* 2:507, 1966.

91. Freeman, R. B., Maher, J. F., and Schreiner, G. E. The affinity of synthetic membranes for calcium. *Trans. Amer. Soc. Artif. Intern. Organs* 11:99, 1965.

92. Frey, W. G. Acute glutethimide poisoning managed by peritoneal dialysis. *J. Maine Med. Ass.* 59:3, 1968.

93. Friedman, E. A., and Thompson, G. E. Hepatitis complicating chronic hemodialysis. *Lancet* 2:675, 1966.

94. Galletti, P. M. Theoretical Considerations About Artificial Kidneys. In *Proceedings of the Third International Congress of Nephrology,* Washington, D.C. 1967. Vol. 3, p. 256.

95. Ganter, G. Ueber die Beseitigung giftiger Stoffe aus dem Blute durch Dialyse. *Munchen. Med. Wschr.* 70:1478, 1923.

96. Gilliland, K. G., and Hegstrom, R. M. The effect of hemodialysis on cerebrospinal fluid pressure in uremic dogs. *Trans. Amer. Soc. Artif. Intern. Organs* 9:44, 1963.

97. Ginn, H. E., Frost, A., and Lacy, W. W. Nitrogen balance in hemodialysis patients. *Amer. J. Clin. Nutr.* 21:385, 1968.

98. Gombos, E. A., Lee, T. H., Harton, M. R., and Cummings, J. W. One year's experience with an intermittent dialysis program. *Ann. Intern. Med.* 61:462, 1964.

99. Gonzalez, F. M., Pabico, R. C., Brown, H. W., Maher, J. F., and Schreiner, G. E. Further experience with the use of routine

intermittent hemodialysis in chronic renal failure. *Trans. Amer. Soc. Artif. Intern. Organs* 9:11, 1963.

100. Goodey, J., and Kelly, J. Social and economic effects of regular dialysis. *Lancet* 2:147, 1967.

101. Gott, V. L. Techniques of applying a graphite-benzalkonium-heparin coating to various plastics and metals. *Trans. Amer. Soc. Artif. Intern. Organs* 10:213, 1964.

102. Gott, V. L., and Whiffen, J. D. Effect of various surface active agents on heparin binding and clot formation on graphite surfaces. *Proc. Soc. Exp. Biol. Med.* 116:314, 1964.

103. Gott, V. L., Whiffen, J. D., and Dutton, R. C. Heparin bonding on colloidal graphite surfaces. *Science* 142:1297, 1963.

104. Gottschalk, C. W. Report of the Committee on Chronic Kidney Disease, Bureau of the Budget, 1967.

105. Gottschalk, C. W. Personal communication, 1968.

106. Graham, T. Chemical and Physical Researches. T. and A. Constable, Printers to Her Majesty at the Edinburgh University Press, 1876.

107. Gral, T., Sokal, A., and Rubini, M. E. Iron Overload in Patients on Chronic Hemo-Dialysis (CD): Role of Dialysate iron. (Abstract.) In *Proceedings of the Third International Congress of Nephrology*, Washington, D.C., 1967.

108. Greenberg, B. Statistical treatment of information provided to Committee on Chronic Renal Disease. Bureau of the Budget, Washington, D.C., 1967.

109. Greene, W. A. Psychological aspects of dialysis and transplantation. Unpublished report submitted to Committee on Chronic Renal Disease, Bureau of the Budget, Washington, D.C., 1967.

110. Griffith, G. C., Nichols, G., Asher, J. D., and Flannagan, B. Heparin osteoporosis. *J.A.M.A.* 193:91, 1965.

111. Grimsrud, L., Cole, J. J., Eschbach, J. W., Babb, A. L., and Scribner, B. H. Safety aspects of hemodialysis. *Trans. Amer. Soc. Artif. Intern. Organs* 13:1, 1967.

112. Grimsrud, L., Cole, J. J., Lehman, G. A.,

Babb, A. L., and Scribner, B. H. A central system for the continuous preparation and distribution of hemodialysis fluid. *Trans. Amer. Soc. Artif. Intern. Organs* 10:107, 1964.

113. Grimsrud, L., Lorentzen, O., and Coppelen, C. A truly portable, fully automatic, fluid preparation and control unit for hemodialysis. *Trans. Amer. Soc. Artif. Intern. Organs* 14:160, 1968.

114. Gutch, C. E. Peritoneal dialysis. *Trans. Amer. Soc. Artif. Intern. Organs* 10:406, 1964.

114a. Haas, G. Cited by Kolff, W. J. *The Artificial Kidney*. Kampen, Holland: J. H. Kok, N.V., 1946.

115. Hager, E. B. Clinical observations on five patients with chronic uremia. *New Eng. J. Med.* 273:304, 1965.

116. Hamberger, J., Halpern, B., and Mathe, G. Étude expérimentale de la perfusion intestinale chez le chien et de ses conséquences, en particulier sur l'equilibre hydrique de l'organisme. *Sem. Hop. Paris* 75:1, 1950.

117. Hamberger, J., Mathe, G., and Crosnier, J. La perfusion intestinale dans le traitement de l'insuffisance rénale aigue. *Bull. Mem. Soc. Med. Hop. Paris* 66:1716, 1950.

118. Hampers, C. L., Doak, P. B., Callighan, M. N., Tyler, H. R., and Merrill, J. P. The electroencephalogram and spinal fluid during hemodialysis. *Arch. Intern. Med.* (Chicago) 118:340, 1966.

119. Hampers, C. L., and Merrill, J. P. Hemodialysis in the home — 13 months' experience. *Ann. Intern. Med.* 64:276, 1966.

120. Hampers, C. L., Merrill, J. P., and Cameron, E. Hemodialysis in the home — a family affair. *Trans. Amer. Soc. Artif. Intern. Organs* 11:3, 1965.

121. Hampers, C. L., and Schupak, E. *Long-term Hemodialysis*. New York: Grune & Stratton, 1967.

122. Haviland, J. W. Experiences in establishing a community artificial kidney center. *Trans. Amer. Clin. Climatol. Ass.* 77:125, 1965.

123. Hayes, C. P., Jr., Gunnells, J. C., and Robinson, R. R. Percutaneous insertion of Teflon needles for hemodialysis. *Trans.*

Amer. Soc. Artif. Intern. Organs 12:215, 1966.

124. Hayes, C. P., Jr., Metz, E. N., Robinson, R. R., and Rundles, R. W. The use of allopurinol (HPP) to control hyperuricemia in patients on chronic intermittent hemodialysis. *Trans. Amer. Soc. Artif. Intern. Organs* 11:247, 1965.

125. Hegstrom, R. M., Murray, J. S., Pendras, J. P., Burnell, J. M., and Scribner, B. H. Hemodialysis in the treatment of chronic uremia. *Trans. Amer. Soc. Artif. Intern. Organs* 7:136, 1961.

126. Hegstrom, R. M., Murray, J. S., Pendras, J. P., Burnell, J. M., and Scribner, B. H. Two years' experience with periodic hemodialysis in treatment of chronic uremia. *Trans. Amer. Soc. Artif. Intern. Organs* 8: 266, 1962.

127. Hegstrom, R. M., Quinton, W. E., Dillard, D. H., Cole, J. J., and Scribner, B. H. One year's experience with the use of indwelling Teflon cannulas and bypass. *Trans. Amer. Soc. Artif. Intern. Organs* 7:47, 1961.

128. Henderson, L. W. Enhanced urea transfer using hypertonic peritoneal dialysis fluid. *J. Clin. Invest.* 45:950, 1966.

129. Henderson, L. W., Besarab, A., Michaels, A., and Bluemle, L. W., Jr. Blood purification by ultrafiltration and fluid replacement (diafiltration). *Trans. Amer. Soc. Artif. Intern. Organs* 13:216, 1967.

130. Henderson, L. W., and Merrill, J. P. Treatment of barbiturate intoxication: With a report of recent experience at Peter Bent Brigham Hospital. *Ann. Intern. Med.* 64: 876, 1966.

131. Henderson, L. W., Merrill, J. P., and Crane, C. Further experience with the inlying plastic conduit for peritoneal dialysis. *Trans. Amer. Soc. Artif. Intern. Organs* 9: 108, 1963.

132. Hoeltzenbein, J. A new, no-prime, no-blood loss, efficient and inexpensive hemodialysis system, potentially useful for home dialysis. *Trans. Amer. Soc. Artif. Intern. Organs* 14:89, 1968.

133. Holmes, J. H., and Nakamoto, S. Removal of fluid from the patient during

hemodialysis. *Trans. Amer. Soc. Artif. Intern. Organs* 5:58, 1959.

134. Indeglia, R. A., Dorman, F. D., Casteneda, A. R., Varco, R. L., and Bernstein, E. F. Use of GBH-coated Tygon tubing for experimental prolonged perfusions without systemic heparinization. *Trans. Amer. Soc. Artif. Intern. Organs* 12:166, 1966.

135. Indeglia, R. A., Shea, M. A., Forstrom, R., and Bernstein, E. F. Influence of mechanical factors on erythrocyte sublethal damage. *Trans. Amer. Soc. Artif. Intern. Organs* 14:264, 1968.

136. Inouye, W. Y., and Engelberg, J. Simplified artificial dialyzer and ultrafilter. *Surg. Forum* 4:438, 1953.

137. Johnson, W. J. In *Proceedings of the Conference on Dialysis.* New York: National Dialysis Committee, 1966. P. 5.

138. Johnson, W. J., Wagoner, R. D., Hunt, J. C., Mueller, G. J., and Hallenbeck, G. A. Long-term intermittent hemodialysis for chronic renal failure. *Mayo Clin. Proc.* 41: 73, 1966.

139. Jones, M. P. In *Proceedings of the Conference on Dialysis.* New York: National Dialysis Committee, 1966. P. 19.

140. Jorgensen, H. E., and Wieth, J. O. Dialysable poisons. Hemodialysis in the treatment of acute poisoning. *Lancet* 1:81, 1963.

141. Jutzler, G. A., Keller, H. E., Klein, J., Carius, J., Floss, K., Dyckmans, J., Fürsattel, L., and Leppla, W. Physico-chemical Investigations in Regeneration of the Dialysis Fluid. In *Proceedings of the European Dialysis and Transplant Association.* Newcastle upon Tyne, England: Bolsten & Stols, 1966. Vol. 3, p. 265.

142. Kallen, R. J., Zaltzman, S. Coe, F. L., and Metcoff, J. Hemodialysis in children: Technique, kinetic aspects related to varying body size, and application to salicylate intoxication, acute renal failure and some other disorders. *Medicine* (Balt.) 45:1, 1966.

143. Kaye, M., and Comty, C. Nutritional repletion during dialysis. *Amer. J. Clin. Nutr.* 21:583, 1968.

144. Kaye, M., Mangel, R., and Neubauer, E. Studies in Calcium Metabolism in Patients

on Chronic Haemodialysis. In *Proceedings of the European Dialysis and Transplant Association*. Newcastle upon Tyne, England: Bolsten & Stols, 1966. Vol. 3, p. 17.

145. Kaye, M., Silverman, M., Frueh, A. J., and Salmna, T. A study of vertebral bone powder from patients with chronic renal failure. (Abstract.) In Abstracts: II. Free Communications. Third International Congress of Nephrology, Washington, D.C., 1966. P. 219.

146. Kendall, A. G., Lowenstein, I., and Morgan, R. O. The hemorrhagic diathesis in renal disease. *Canad. Med. Ass. J.* 85:405, 1961.

147. Kennedy, A. C., Linton, A. L., and Eaton, J. C. Urea levels in cerebrospinal fluid after hemodialysis. *Lancet* 1:410, 1962.

148. Kennedy, A. C., Linton, A. L., Luke, R. G., and Renfrew, S. Electroencephalographic changes during haemodialysis. *Lancet* 1: 408, 1963.

149. Kennedy, A. C., Linton, A. L., Renfrew, S., Luke, R. G., and Dinwoodie, A. The pathogenesis and prevention of cerebral dysfunction during dialysis. *Lancet* 1:790, 1964.

150. Kerr, D. N. S. Planning for the Future in the United Kingdom. In *Proceedings of the European Dialysis and Transplant Association*. Newcastle upon Tyne, England: Bolsten & Stols, 1966. Vol. 3, p. 153.

151. Kerr, D. N. S., Barwick, D. D., Elliott, R. W., Horn, D. B., and Osselton, J. W. Persistence of uraemic features during intermittent haemodialysis: Evaluation of some screening procedures including EEG and nerve conduction time. (Abstract.) *Nephron* 3:69, 1966.

152. Kessel, M., Ibe, K., Neuhaus, G., Remmer, H., and Weller, H. Die extracorporale Dialyse von Luminal. *Klin. Wschr.* 40:580, 1962.

153. Khastagir, B., Erben, J., Shimizu, A., Rose, F., Nose, Y., Van Dura, D., and Kolff, W. J. The four-coil artificial kidney for home dialysis. *Trans. Amer. Soc. Artif. Intern. Organs* 13:14, 1967.

154. Kidd, E. E. Bacterial contamination of dialyzing fluid of artificial kidney. *Brit. Med. J.* 1:880, 1964.

155. Kiil, F. Development of a parallel-flow artificial kidney in plastics. *Acta Chir. Scand.* 253 (Suppl.):142, 1960.

156. Knochel, J. R., and Barry, K. G. THAM dialysis: An experimental method to study diffusion of certain weak acids in vivo: II. Secobarbital. *J. Lab. Clin. Med.* 65:361, 1965.

157. Kolff, W. J. The artificial kidney; past, present, and future. *Circulation* 15:285, 1957.

158. Kolff, W. J. First clinical experience with the artificial kidney. *Ann. Intern. Med.* 62: 608, 1965.

159. Kolff, W. J., and Berk, H. T. J. Artificial kidney, dialyzer with great area. *Acta Med. Scand.* 117:121, 1944.

160. Kolff, W. J., Berk, J. T. J., ter Welle, M., van der Ley, A. J. W., van Dijk, E. C., and van Noordwijk, J. Een Dialysator met groot Oppervlak. *Geneesk. Gids* 21:409, 1943.

161. Kolff, W. J., and Leonards, J. R. Reduction of otherwise intractable edema by dialysis or filtration. *Cleveland Clin. Quart.* 21: 61, 1954.

162. Kolff, W. J., and Watschinger, B. Further development of a coil kidney: A disposable artificial kidney. *J. Lab. Clin. Med.* 47:969, 1956.

163. Kolff, W. J., Watschinger, B., and Vertes, V. Results in patients treated with the coil kidney (disposable dialyzing unit). *J.A.M.A.* 161:1433, 1956.

164. Kolobow, T., and Dedrick, R. L. Dialysate capacity augmentation at ultra-low flow rates with activated carbon slurry. *Trans. Amer. Soc. Artif. Intern. Organs* 12: 1, 1966.

165. Kretchmar, L. H., Greene, W. M., Waterhouse, C. W., and Parry, W. L. Repeated hemodialysis in chronic uremia. *J.A.M.A.* 184:1030, 1963.

166. Kupfer, S. The place of dialysis procedures in clinical management. *Amer. J. Med.* 22:511, 1957.

167. Kusserow, B. K., Machanic, B., Collins, F. M., Jr., and Clapp, J. F., III. Changes observed in blood corpuscles after prolonged perfusions with two types of blood pumps.

Trans. Amer. Soc. Artif. Intern. Organs 11: 122, 1965.

168. Kyle, L. H., Jeghers, H., Walsh, W. P., Doolan, P. D., Wishinsky, H., and Pallotta, A. The application of hemodialysis to the treatment of barbiturate poisoning. *J. Clin. Invest.* 32:364, 1953.

169. Kylstra, J. A. Lavage of the lung. *Trans. Amer. Soc. Artif. Intern. Organs* 5:23, 1959.

170. Landé, A. J., Parker, B., Subramanian, V., Carlson, R. G., and Lillehei, C. W. Methods for increasing the efficiency of a new dialyzer-membrane oxygenator. *Trans. Amer. Soc. Artif. Intern. Organs* 14:227, 1968.

171. Lasker, N., McCauley, E. P., and Passarotti, C. T. Chronic peritoneal dialysis. *Trans. Amer. Soc. Artif. Intern. Organs* 12:94, 1966.

172. Lawson, L. J., Crawford, N., Edwards, P., Dawson, J., and Blainey, J. D. Platelet Destruction and Serotonin Release During Hemodialysis. In *Proceedings of the European Dialysis and Transplant Association*. Newcastle upon Tyne, England: Bolsten & Stols, 1965. Vol. 2, p. 63.

173. Lee, H. A., and Ames, A. C. Hemodialysis in severe barbiturate poisoning. *Brit. Med. J.* 1:1217, 1965.

174. LeGrain, M., and Merrill, J. P. Short-term, continuous, transperitoneal dialysis. *New Eng. J. Med.* 248:125, 1953.

175. Leininger, R. I., Epstein, M. M., Falb, R. D., and Grode, G. A. Preparation of non-thrombogenic plastic surfaces. *Trans. Amer. Soc. Artif. Intern. Organs* 12:151, 1966.

176. Leonard, E. F., and Bluemle, L. W., Jr. Factors influencing permeability in extracorporeal hemodialysis. *Trans. Amer. Soc. Artif. Intern. Organs* 4:4, 1958.

177. Leonard, E. F., and Bluemle, L. W., Jr. Engineering in medicine: Design of an artificial kidney. *Trans. N.Y. Acad. Sci.* (Ser. II.) 21:585, 1959.

178. Leonard, E. F., and Bluemle, L. W., Jr. The permeability concept as applied to dialysis. *Trans. Amer. Soc. Artif. Intern. Organs* 6:33, 1960.

179. Leonard, E. F., and Bluemle, L. W. Eval-uation of dialysis membranes. *Trans. Amer. Soc. Artif. Intern. Organs* 8:182, 1962.

180. Leonard, E. F., Moffsky, R. M., Casterline, J. E., and Cascone, R. F. A new tidal-flow dialyzer: In vivo, in vitro and mathematical assessment. *Trans. Amer. Soc. Artif. Intern. Organs* 13:208, 1967.

181. Letters and comments: Moral problems of artificial and transplanted organs. *Ann. Intern. Med.* 61:355, 1964.

182. Lewis, H. Y., and Retan, J. W. A new technique of bypass cannulation for intermittent hemodialysis. *Trans. Amer. Soc. Artif. Intern. Organs* 9:62, 1963.

183. Lewis, J. H., Zucker, M. B., and Ferguson, J. H. Bleeding tendency in uremia. *Blood* 11:1073, 1956.

184. Linnenberg, C. C., Jr. Economics in program planning for health. *Public Health Rep.* 81:1085, 1966.

185. Linton, A. L., Luke, R. G., Speirs, I., and Kennedy, A. C. Forced diuresis and haemodialysis in severe barbiturate intoxication. *Lancet* 1:1008, 1964.

186. Lipps, B. J., Steward, R. D., Perkins, H. A., Holmes, G. W., McLain, E. A., Rolfs, M. R., and Oja, P. D. The hollow fiber artificial kidney. *Trans. Amer. Soc. Artif. Intern. Organs* 13:200, 1967.

187. Lorenzini, L. Water-electrolyte distribution during peritoneal dialysis: Perfusion of colon in anuria. *Chir. Pat. Sper.* 4:1020, 1956.

188. Love, G. R. Vividiffusion with intestinal membranes. *Med. Rec.* 98:649, 1920.

189. Luthinger, M., Cooper, C. W., and Leininger, R. I. Preparation of novel hemodialysis membranes. *Trans. Amer. Soc. Artif. Intern. Organs* 14:5, 1968.

190. Lyman, D. J. Investigation of synthetic membrane for hemodialysis. *Trans. Amer. Soc. Artif. Intern. Organs* 9:92, 1963.

191. Lyman, D. J. New synthetic membranes for the dialysis of blood. *Trans. Amer. Soc. Artif. Intern. Organs* 10:17, 1964.

192. Lyman, D. J., Bock, H. L., and Muir, W. M. New synthetic membranes for the dialysis of blood: III. The concept of liquid partition of biological molecules by means of mem-

branes. *Trans. Amer. Soc. Artif. Intern. Organs* 11:91, 1965.

193. Lyman, D. J., Muir, W. M., and Lee, I. J. The effect of chemical structure and surface properties of polymers on the coagulation of blood: I. Surface free energy effects. *Trans. Amer. Soc. Artif. Intern. Organs* 11: 301, 1965.

194. MacNeill, A. E., Doyle, J. E., Anthone, R., and Anthone, S. Technic with parallel flow, straight tube blood dialyzer. *New York J. Med.* 59:1437, 1959.

195. Maher, J. F. Hemodialysis and peritoneal dialysis: A review of their use in renal insufficiency and acute poisoning. *Ohio Med. J.* 60:235, 1964.

196. Maher, J. F., Freeman, R. B., Schmidt, G., and Schreiner, G. E. Adherence of metals to cellophane membranes and removal by whole blood: A mechanism of solute transport during hemodialysis. *Trans. Amer. Soc. Artif. Intern. Organs* 11:104, 1965.

197. Maher, J. F., Freeman, R. B., and Schreiner, G. E. Hemodialysis for chronic renal failure: II. Biochemical and clinical aspects. *Ann. Intern. Med.* 62:535, 1965.

198. Maher, J. F., and Schreiner, G. E. Medical Progress: Hazards and complications of dialysis. *New Eng. J. Med.* 273:370, 1965.

199. Maher, J. H., Schreiner, G. E., and Waters, T. J. Successful intermittent hemodialysis —longest reported maintenance of life in true oliguria (181 days). *Trans. Amer. Soc. Artif. Intern. Organs* 6:124, 1960.

200. Maher, J. F., Schreiner, G. E., and Westervelt, F. B. Acute glutethimide intoxication: I. Clinical experience (22 patients) compared to acute barbiturate intoxication (62 patients). *Amer. J. Med.* 33:70, 1962.

201. Marc-Aurele, J., and Schreiner, G. E. The dialysance of ethanol and methanol: A proposed method for the treatment of massive intoxication by ethyl or methyl alcohol. *J. Clin. Invest.* 39:892, 1960.

202. Markle, R. A., Falb, R. D., and Leininger, R. I. Development of improved membranes for artificial kidney dialysis. *Trans. Amer. Soc. Artif. Intern. Organs* 12:22, 1964.

203. Mason, N. S., Lindan, O., and Sparks, R. E. Reinforced cellulose acetate dialysis membranes. *Trans. Amer. Soc. Artif. Intern. Organs* 14:31, 1968.

204. Maxwell, M. H., Rockney, R. E., Kleeman, C. R., and Twiss, M. R. Peritoneal dialysis. I. Technique and applications. *J.A.M.A.* 170:917, 1959.

205. McDonald, H. P., Jr. Automatic Peritoneal Dialysis. In *Proceedings of the European Dialysis and Transplant Association.* Newcastle upon Tyne, England: Bolsten & Stols, 1965. Vol. 2, p. 118.

206. McDonald, H. P., Jr., Friedman, E. A., Waterhouse, K., and Thomson, G. E. One Thousand Dialyses in a 15-Bed Hemodialysis Unit. In *Proceedings of the European Dialysis and Transplant Association.* Newcastle upon Tyne, England: Bolsten & Stols, 1966. Vol. 3, p. 111.

207. Meltzer, T. H., Gutfreund, K., Kulshrestha, V. K., and Stake, A. M. Optimized cellulose membranes for the artificial kidney dialysis applications. *Trans. Amer. Soc. Artif. Intern. Organs* 14:12, 1968.

208. Menno, A. D., Zizzi, J., Hodson, J., and McMahon, J. An evaluation of the radial arteriovenous fistula as a substitute for the Quinton shunt in chronic hemodialysis. *Trans. Amer. Soc. Artif. Intern. Organs* 13: 62, 1967.

209. Merrill, J. P. The artificial kidney. *New Eng. J. Med.* 246:17, 1952.

210. Merrill, J. P. The Treatment of Renal Failure. In *Therapeutic Principles in the Management of Acute and Chronic Uremia.* New York: Grune & Stratton, 1955.

211. Merrill, J. P. Clinical experience is tempered by genuine human concern. *J.A.M.A.* 189:626, 1964.

212. Merrill, J. P. The Treatment of Chronic Renal Failure. In *Therapeutic Principles in the Management of Acute and Chronic Uremia.* (2d ed.) New York: Grune & Stratton, 1965.

213. Merrill, J. P., Sabbaga, E., Henderson, L. W., Welzant, E., and Crane, C. The use of an inlying plastic conduit for chronic

peritoneal irrigation. *Trans. Amer. Soc. Artif. Intern. Organs* 8:252, 1962.

214. Merrill, E. W., Salzman, E. W., Lipps, B. J., Jr., Gilliland, E. R., Austen, W. G., and Joison, J. Antithrombogenic cellulose membranes for blood dialysis. *Trans. Amer. Soc. Artif. Intern. Organs* 12:139, 1966.

215. Merrill, J. P., Schupak, E., Cameron, E., and Hampers, C. L. Hemodialysis in the home. *J.A.M.A.* 190:468, 1964.

216. Merrill, J. P., Smith, S., III, Callahan, E. J., III, and Thorn, G. W. Use of an artificial kidney: Clinical experience. *J. Clin. Invest.* 29:425, 1950.

217. Merrill, J. P., Thorn, G. W., Walter, C. W., Callahan, E. J., III, and Smith, L. H., Jr. Use of artificial kidney: Technic. *J. Clin. Invest.* 29:412, 1950.

218. Michaels, A. S. Operating parameters and performance criteria for hemodialyzers and other membrane separation devices. *Trans. Amer. Soc. Artif. Intern. Organs* 12: 387, 1966.

219. Miller, F. W., Clark, J. E., Jones, C. P., Smeltzer, K. L., and Bluemle, L. W., Jr. A new Cuprophan®, no-prime disposable cartridge dialyzer. *Trans. Amer. Soc. Artif. Intern. Organs* 14:126, 1968.

220. Mion, C. M., Hegstrom, R. M., Boen, S. T., and Scribner, B. H. Substitution of sodium acetate for sodium bicarbonate in the bath fluid for hemodialysis. *Trans. Amer. Soc. Artif. Intern. Organs* 10:110, 1964.

221. Murphy, P., Holly, F., van Someren, L., Bankole, M., Singh, S., and Bernhard, W. F. Antithrombogenic properties of electrified polymers. *Trans. Amer. Soc. Artif. Intern. Organs* 13:131, 1967.

222. Murray, G. Development of an artificial kidney: Experimental and clinical experience. *Arch. Surg.* 55:505, 1947.

223. Murray, J. S., Pendras, J. P., Lindholm, D. D., and Erickson, R. V. Twenty-five months' experience in the treatment of chronic uremia at an outpatient community hemodialysis center. *Trans. Amer. Soc. Artif. Intern. Organs* 10:191, 1964.

224. Murray, J. S., Tu, W. H., Albers, J. B., Burnell, J. M., and Scribner, B. H. A community hemodialysis center for the treat-

ment of chronic uremia. *Trans. Amer. Soc. Artif. Intern. Organs* 8:315, 1962.

225. Nakamoto, S., Brandon, J. M., Franklin, M., Rosenbaum, J., and Kolff, W. J. Experience with A-V shunt cannulas for repeated dialysis. *Trans. Amer. Soc. Artif. Intern. Organs* 7:57, 1961.

226. Necheles, H. Über dialysieren des stromenden Blutes am Lebenden. *Klin. Wschr.* 2:1257, 1923.

227. Necheles, H. A. A method of vivi-dialysis. *Chin. J. Physiol.* 1:69, 1927.

228. Nishihara, T., Rubin, A. L., and Stanzel, K. H. Biologically derived collagen membranes. *Trans. Amer. Soc. Artif. Intern. Organs* 13:243, 1967.

229. Odian, M., and Leonard, E. F. Synthesis and evaluation of graded poly vinyl alcohol membranes. *Trans. Amer. Soc. Artif. Intern. Organs* 14:19, 1968.

230. Ogden, D. A., and Holmes, J. H. Changes in total and ultrafilterable plasma calcium and magnesium during hemodialysis. *Trans. Amer. Soc. Artif. Intern. Organs* 12: 200, 1966.

231. Oppenheimer, G. D. Irrigation of the intestine in the treatment of certain types of uremia. *J. Mount Sinai Hosp. N.Y.* 14:908, 1948.

232. Parsons, F. M. The Use of the Artificial Kidney in Salicylate Poisoning. In Dixon, A. St. J., Martin, B. K., Smith, M. J. H., and Wood, P. H. N. (Eds.), *Salicylates, an International Symposium, Empire Rheumatism Council*. Boston: Little, Brown, 1963. P. 281.

233. Patel, R., Vertes, V., Bloomfield, D., and Levy, M. Improvements in use of the twin coil kidney for chronic dialysis in a large center. *Trans. Amer. Soc. Artif. Intern. Organs* 13:5, 1967.

234. Pendleton, W. R., and West, F. E. The passage of urea between blood and the lumen of the small intestine. *Amer. J. Physiol.* 101:391, 1932.

235. Pendras, J. P., and Erickson, R. V. Hemodialysis: A successful therapy for chronic uremia. *Ann. Intern. Med.* 64:293, 1966.

236. Pendras, J. P., Smith, F. R., and Field, D. C. One year's experience with an Archimedes

screw central dialysate production system. *Trans. Amer. Soc. Artif. Intern. Organs* 13: 10, 1967.

237. Pendras, J. P., and Smith, M. P.   The Silastic-Teflon arteriovenous cannula. *Trans. Amer. Soc. Artif. Intern. Organs* 12:222, 1966.

238. Deleted in proof.

239. Peterson, H., and Swanson, A. G.   Acute encephalopathy occurring during renal hemodialysis — the reverse urea effect. *Arch. Intern. Med.* (Chicago) 113:877, 1964.

240. Piazza, A., Chaname, W., and Cauti, D.   Double lumen percutaneous cannula for dialysis with the artificial kidney. *Trans. Amer. Soc. Artif. Intern. Organs* 10:136, 1964.

241. Pollard, T. L., Barnett, B. M. S., Eschbach, J. W., and Scribner, B. H.   A technique for storage and multiple reuse of the Kiil dialyzer and blood tubing. *Trans. Amer. Soc. Artif. Intern. Organs* 13:24, 1967.

242. Proceedings of Study Group on Acute Renal Failure held at U.S. Army Surgical Research Unit, Brooke Army Medical Center, Fort Sam Houston, Texas, Oct. 14–16, 1957 (unpublished).

243. Putnam, T. J.   The living peritoneum as a dialyzing membrane. *Amer. J. Physiol.* 63: 548, 1923.

244. Quinton, W. E., Dillard, D. H., Cole, J. J., and Scribner, B. H.   Possible improvements in the technique of long-term cannulation of blood vessels. *Trans. Amer. Soc. Artif. Intern. Organs* 7:60, 1961.

245. Quinton, W. E., Dillard, D. H., Cole, J. J., and Scribner, B. H.   Eight months' experience with Silastic-Teflon bypass cannulas. *Trans. Amer. Soc. Artif. Intern. Organs* 8: 236, 1962.

246. Quinton, W. E., Dillard, D. H., and Scribner, B. H.   Cannulation of blood vessels for prolonged hemodialysis. *Trans. Amer. Soc. Artif. Intern. Organs* 6:104, 1960.

247. Rath, E., Malliard, J. A., and Schreiner, G. E.   Bleeding tendency in uremia. *New Eng. J. Med.* 275: 808, 1957.

248. Retan, J. W., and Lewis, H. Y.   Repeated dialysis of indigent patients for chronic renal failure. *Ann. Intern. Med.* 64:284, 1966.

249. Reus, W. F., and Heetderks, D.   Use of double lumen catheter in extracorporeal dialysis. *J. Mich. Med. Society* 61:971, 1962.

250. Robin, E. D.   Rapid scientific advances bring new ethical questions. *J.A.M.A.* 189: 624, 1964.

251. Rosen, S. M., O'Connor, K., and Shaldon, S.   Haemodialysis disequilibrium. *Brit. Med. J.* 2:672, 1964.

252. Rosenak, S. S., and Siwon, P.   Experimentelle Untersuchungen neber die peritoneale Ausscheidung hornpflichtiger Substarzen aus dem Blute. *Mitt. Grenzgeb. Med. Chir.* 39:391, 1926.

253. Rosenbaum, J. L., and Mandanas, R.   Treatment of phenobarbital intoxication in dogs with an anion-recirculation peritoneal dialysis technique. *Trans. Amer. Soc. Artif. Intern. Organs* 13:183, 1967.

254. Rubini, M. E., Goldman, K. L., Agre, K. L., Koppel, M. H., Koppel, J. D., Gral, T., Shinaberger, J. H., and Sokol, A.   Dialysis and transplantation: Some interactions and comparisons. *Trans. Amer. Soc. Artif. Intern. Organs* 14:355, 1968.

255. Rubini, M., Sokol, A., Gaynor, S., Coburn, J., McCray, J., and Gordon, S.   Some preliminary experience with chronic peritoneal dialysis. *Clin. Res.* 12:72, 1964.

256. Rubini, M. E., Wolfram, J. G., and Sokol, A.   An analysis of a Veterans Administration dialysis unit. *Trans. Amer. Soc. Artif. Intern. Organs* 12:376, 1966.

257. Salisbury, P. F.   Timely versus delayed use of the artificial kidney. *A.M.A. Arch. Intern. Med.* 101:690, 1958.

258. Salisbury, P. F., Briggs, J. N., Hamel, N. C., Cross, C. E., and Rieben, P. A.   Pulmonary lavage: The use of lung, in situ, as an "artificial kidney." *Trans. Amer. Soc. Artif. Intern. Organs* 5:32, 1959.

259. Sand, P., Livingston, G., and Wright, R. G.   Psychological assessment of candidates for a hemodialysis program. *Ann. Intern. Med.* 64:602, 1966.

260. Sarles, H. E., Artz, C. P., Smith, G. H.,

Hargest, T. S., and Remmers, A. R., Jr. Observations concerning the use of lymph for extracorporeal dialysis. *Trans. Amer. Soc. Artif. Intern. Organs* 11:165, 1965.

261. Sarles, H. E., Smith, G. H., Jr., Fish, J. C., Artz, C. P., Hargest, T. S., and Remmers, A. R., Jr. Further observations concerning the use of lymph for extracorporeal dialysis. *Trans. Amer. Soc. Artif. Intern. Organs* 12:33, 1966.

262. Schloerb, P., and Carr, M. H. Dialysis of gastric secretion in vivo with a semipermeable dialyzing balloon. *Surg. Gynec. Obstet.* 3:531, 1960.

263. Schreiner, G. E. The role of hemodialysis (artificial kidney) in acute poisoning. *A.M.A. Arch. Intern. Med.* 102:896, 1958.

264. Schreiner, G. E., Berman, L. B., Griffin, J., and Feys, J. Specific therapy for salicylism. *New Eng. J. Med.* 253:213, 1955.

265. Schreiner, G. E., and Maher, J. F. Hemodialysis for chronic renal failure: III. Medical, moral and ethical, and socioeconomic problems. *Ann. Intern. Med.* 62:551, 1965.

266. Schreiner, G. E., Maher, J. F., Freeman, R. B., and O'Connell, J. M. B. Problems of Hemodialysis. In *Proceedings of the Third International Congress of Nephrology,* Washington, D.C., 1967. Vol. 3, p. 316.

267. Schupak, E., and Merrill, J. P. Experience with long-term intermittent hemodialysis. *Ann. Intern. Med.* 62:509, 1965.

268. Schupak, E., Sullivan, J. F., and Lee, D. Y. Chronic hemodialysis in "unselected" patients. *Ann. Intern. Med.* 67:708, 1967.

269. Scribner, B. H. Role of the artificial kidney in the management of acute renal failure. *Northwest Med.* 58:555, 1959.

270. Scribner, B. H. Discussion. *Trans. Amer. Soc. Artif. Intern. Organs* 8:195, 1962.

271. Scribner, B. H. Hemodialysis in the Treatment of Chronic Uremia. In *Proceedings of the Third International Congress of Nephrology,* Washington, D.C. 1967. Vol. 3, p. 305.

272. Scribner, B. H. Planning for the Future in the U.S. In *Proceedings of the European Dialysis and Transplant Association.* Newcastle upon Tyne, England: Bolsten & Stols, 1966. Vol. 3, p. 156.

273. Scribner, B. H., Buri, R., Caner, J. E. Z., Hegstrom, R., and Burnell, J. M. The treatment of chronic uremia by means of intermittent hemodialysis: A preliminary report. *Trans. Amer. Soc. Artif. Intern. Organs* 6:114, 1960.

274. Scribner, B. H., Caner, J. E. Z., Buri, R., and Quinton, W. The technique of continuous hemodialysis. *Trans. Amer. Soc. Artif. Intern. Organs* 6:88, 1960.

275. Scribner, B. H., Fergus, E. B., Boen, S. T., and Thomas, E. D. Some therapeutic approaches to chronic renal insufficiency. *Ann. Rev. Med.* 16:285, 1965.

276. Scribner, B. H., Koreski, W. R., Marr, T. A., and Burnell, J. M. Gastrodialysis in treatment of acute renal insufficiency. *Clin. Res.* 6:295, 1958.

277. Seegmiller, J. E., Grayzel, A. I., Howell, R. R., and Plato, C. The renal excretion of uric acid in gout. *J. Clin. Invest.* 41:1094, 1962.

278. Segar, W. E. Peritoneal dialysis in the treatment of boric acid poisoning. *New Eng. J. Med.* 282:798, 1960.

279. Setter, J. G., Maher, J. F., and Schreiner, G. E. Barbiturate intoxication: Evaluation of therapy including dialysis in a large series selectively referred because of severity. *Arch. Intern. Med.* (Chicago) 117:224, 1966.

280. Setter, J. G., Singh, R., Brackett, N. C., Jr., and Randall, R. E., Jr. Studies on the dialysis of methanol. *Trans. Amer. Soc. Artif. Intern. Organs* 13:178, 1967.

281. Shaldon, S. In *Proceedings of the Working Conference on Chronic Dialysis.* Seattle, Wash.: University of Washington, 1964. P. 66.

282. Shaldon, S., Chiandussi, L., and Higgs, D. Hemodialysis by percutaneous catheterization of femoral artery and vein with regional heparinization. *Lancet* 2:857, 1961.

283. Shaldon, S., Rae, A. I., Rosen, S. M., Silva, H., and Oakley, S. R. N. Refrigerated femoral venous-venous hemodialysis with coil preservation for rehabilitation of terminal uremic patients. *Brit. Med. J.* 1:1716, 1963.

284. Shaldon, S., Silva, H., Pomeroy, J., Rae, A. I., and Rosen, S. M. Percutaneous femoral venous catheterization and reusable dia-

lyzer in the treatment of acute renal failure. *Trans. Amer. Soc. Artif. Intern. Organs* 10: 133, 1964.

285. Shaldon, S., Silva, H., and Rosen, S. M. Technique of refrigerated coil preservation hemodialysis with femoral venous catheterization. *Brit. Med. J.* 2:411, 1964.

286. Shambaugh, P. W., Hampers, C. L., Baily, G. L., Snyder, D., and Merrill, J. P. Hemodialysis in the home — emotional impact on the spouse. *Trans. Amer. Soc. Artif. Intern. Organs* 13:41, 1967.

287. Shea, E. J., Bogdan, D. F., Freeman, R. B., and Schreiner, G. E. Hemodialysis for chronic renal failure: IV. Psychological considerations. *Ann. Intern. Med.* 62:558, 1965.

288. Shea, M. A., Indeglia, R. A., Dorman, F. D., Haleen, J. F., Blackshear, P. L., Varco, R. L., and Bernstein, E. B. The biologic response to pumping blood. *Trans. Amer. Soc. Artif. Intern. Organs* 13:116, 1967.

289. Shibagaki, M., and Kolff, W. J. In vitro and clinical studies of fluid removal with the Kiil dialyzer and subatmospheric pressure dialysate circuit. *Cleveland Clin. Quart.* 32: 157, 1963.

290. Shimizu, A. G., Kaye, M., and Innes, B. J. Chronic hemodialysis for terminal renal failure. *Canad. Med. Ass. J.* 94:311, 1966.

291. Shinaberger, J. H., Shear, L., and Barry, K. G. Increasing efficiency of peritoneal dialysis: Experience with peritoneal extracorporeal recirculation dialysis. *Trans. Amer. Soc. Artif. Intern. Organs* 11:76, 1965.

292. Shinaberger, J. H., Shear, L., Clayton, L. E., Barry, K. G., Knowlton, M., and Goldbaum, L. R. Dialysis for intoxication with lipid soluble drugs: Enhancement of glutethimide extraction with lipid dialysate. *Trans. Amer. Soc. Artif. Intern. Organs* 11: 173, 1965.

293. Shumway, N. E. Pleural dialysis in the uremic dog. *J. Urol.* 81:567, 1959.

294. Sitprija, V., and Holmes, J. H. Preliminary observations on the change in intracranial pressure and intraocular pressure during hemodialysis. *Trans. Amer. Soc. Artif. Intern. Organs* 8:300, 1962.

295. Skeggs, L. T., Jr., and Leonards, J. R. Studies on artificial kidney: 1. Preliminary results with new type of continuous dialyzer. *Science* 108:212, 1948.

296. Skeggs, L. T., Jr., Leonards, J. R., and Heisler, C. R. Artificial kidney: 2. Construction and operation of improved continuous dialyzer. *Proc. Soc. Exp. Biol. Med.* 72:539, 1949.

297. Smith, A. L., Berkowitz, H. D., and Bluemle, L. W., Jr. Electrodialysis of blood: Evaluation of a high capacity unit. *Trans. Amer. Soc. Artif. Intern. Organs* 10:273, 1964.

298. Someren, T., Geering, R. B., Kern, G., Martinez, F. J., and Galletti, P. M. A simple, no prime, pumpless artificial kidney: A preliminary report. *Trans. Amer. Soc. Artif. Intern. Organs* 9:73, 1963.

299. Sparks, E., and Lindan, O. Design problems in the artificial kidney. Design Engineering Conference, American Society of Mechanical Engineers, Chicago, Ill., May, 1966.

300. Sparks, R. E., Blaney, J. L., and Lindan, O. Adsorption of Nitrogenous Waste Metabolites from Artificial Kidney Dialyzing Fluid. In Chemical Engineering Progress Symposium Series, New York, 1966. American Institute of Chemical Engineers. No. 66, vol. 62, p. 1.

301. Stanbury, S. W. Bone disease in uremia. *Amer. J. Med.* 44:714, 1968.

302. Stanbury, S. W., and Lumb, G. A. Metabolic studies of renal osteodystrophy: I. Calcium, phosphorus and nitrogen metabolism in rickets, osteomalacia and hyperparathyroidism complicating chronic uremia and in osteomalacia of the adult Fanconi syndrome. *Medicine* (Balt.) 41:1, 1962.

303. Stewart, J. H., and Castaldi, P. A. Uremic bleeding: A reversible platelet defect corrected by dialysis. *Quart. J. Med.* 36:409, 1967.

304. Stewart, R. D., Baretta, E. D., Cerny, J. C., and Mahon, H. I. An artificial kidney made from capillary fibers. *Invest. Urol.* 3: 614, 1966.

305. Stewart, R. D., Cerny, J. C., and Mahon, H. I. The capillary "kidney": Preliminary

report. *Univ. Mich. Med. Cent. J.* 30:116, 1964.

306. Stewart, R. D., Lipps, B. J., Baretta, E. D., Piering, W. R., Roth, D. A., and Sargent, J. A. Short-term hemodialysis with the capillary kidney. *Trans. Amer. Soc. Artif. Intern. Organs* 14:121, 1968.

307. Strauch, M., Walzer, P., v.Henning, G. E., Roettger, G., and Christ, H. Factors influencing protein loss during peritoneal dialysis. *Trans. Amer. Soc. Artif. Intern. Organs* 13:172, 1967.

308. Stumpf, S. E. Some moral dimensions of medicine. *Ann. Intern. Med.* 64:460, 1966.

309. Sussman, S. Severe salicylism and acute pancreatitis. *Calif. Med.* 99:29, 1963.

310. Tenckhoff, H., and Boen, S. T. Long-term Peritoneal Dialysis in the Home: The First One and One-half Years. In *Proceedings of the European Dialysis and Transplant Association.* Newcastle upon Tyne, England: Bolsten & Stols, 1965. Vol. 2, p. 104.

311. Tenckhoff, H., and Schecter, H. A bacteriologically safe peritoneal access device. *Trans. Amer. Soc. Artif. Intern. Organs* 14:181, 1968.

312. Tenckhoff, H., Shilipetar, G., and Boen, S. T. One year's experience with home peritoneal dialysis. *Trans. Amer. Soc. Artif. Intern. Organs* 11:11, 1965.

313. Teschan, P. E., Baxter, C. R., O'Brien, T. F., Freyhof, J. N., and Hall, W. H. Prophylactic hemodialysis in the treatment of acute renal failure. *Ann. Intern. Med.* 53:992, 1960.

314. Thalheimer, W. Experimental exchange transfusions for reducing azotemia: Use of an artificial kidney for the purpose. *Proc. Soc. Exp. Biol. Med.* 37:641, 1938.

315. Thaysen, J. H. The Need for Treatment of Terminal Renal Failure. In *Proceedings of the European Dialysis and Transplant Association.* Newcastle upon Tyne, England: Bolsten & Stols, 1966. Vol. 3, p. 138.

316. Thomsen, A. C., and Dalgard, O. Z. Hemodialysis in acute acetylsalicylic acid poisoning. *Amer. J. Med.* 25:484, 1958.

317. Toussaint, Ch., Cremer, M., Heuse, A., Vereerstraeten, P., Van Geertruyden, J.,

Cuykens, J. J., and Vernoiry, A. L'hypertension artérielle maligne incontrôlable, indication à la néphrectomie bilatérale dans le mal de Bright au stade ultime. In *Proceedceedings of the European Dialysis and Transplant Association.* Newcastle upon Tyne, England: Bolsten & Stols, 1966. Vol. 3, p. 65.

318. Twiss, E. E., and Poulssen, M. M. P. Dialysis System Incorporating the Use of Activated Charcoal. In *Proceedings of the European Dialysis and Transplant Association.* Newcastle upon Tyne, England: Bolsten & Stols, 1966. Vol. 3, p. 262.

319. Tyler, H. R. Neurological complications of dialysis, transplantation and other forms of treatment in chronic uremia. *Neurology* (Minneap.) 15:1081, 1965.

320. Tyler, H. R. Neurological disorders in renal failure. *Amer. J. Med.* 44:734, 1968.

321. Vanelon, J., Perrin, D., Zingraff, J. L., and Funck-Brentano, J. L. Calcifications keratoconjunctivales an cours des traitements par hemodialyse periodique. In *Proceedings of the European Dialysis and Transplant Association.* Newcastle upon Tyne, England: Bolsten & Stols, 1966. Vol. 3, p. 24.

322. Van Hess, C. L., and McGuigan, H. The condition of the sugar in the blood. *J. Pharmacol. Exp. Ther.* 6:45, 1914–15.

323. Verberckmoes, R. Dosage de la fraction ultrafilterable du calcium par une méthode utilisant le rein artificiel de type twin coil. In *Proceedings of the European Dialysis and Transplant Association.* Newcastle upon Tyne, England: Bolsten & Stols, 1966. Vol. 3, p. 28.

324. Versaci, A. A., Nakamoto, S., and Kolff, W. J. Comparison of the twin coil, single coil, and small twin coil artificial kidneys in vivo. *Trans. Amer. Soc. Artif. Intern. Organs* 10:186, 1964.

325. Versaci, A. A., Olsen, K. J., McMain, P. B., Nakamoto, S., and Kolff, W. J. Uremic polyneuropathy and motor nerve conduction velocities. *Trans. Amer. Soc. Artif. Intern. Organs* 10:328, 1964.

326. Von Kaulla, K. N., Von Kaulla, E., Wasantapruck, S., Marchioro, T. L., and Stazl,

T. E. Blood coagulation in uremic patients before and after hemodialysis and transplantation of the kidney. *Arch. Surg.* (Chicago) 92:184, 1966.

327. Wacker, W., and Merrill, J. P. Uremic pericarditis in acute and chronic renal failure. *J.A.M.A.* 156:764, 1954.

328. Watschinger, B., and Kolff, W. J. Further development of the artificial kidney of Inouye and Engelberg. *Trans. Amer. Soc. Artif. Intern. Organs* 1:37, 1955.

329. Weber, W. J., Jr., and Morris, J. C. Kinetics of adsorption on carbon from solution. Proc. Amer. Soc. Civil Engin., *J. Sanit. Engin. Div.* 89:31, 1963.

330. Wegner, G. Chirgische Bernerkungen über die Peritonealhöhle, mit besonderer Berücksichtigung der Ovariotomie. *Arch. Klin. Chir.* 20:51, 1877.

331. Weinstein, A. B., Wen, S. F., Shelp, W. D., and Pellett, J. R. Dextran gel filtration of uremic thoracic duct lymph. *Trans. Amer. Soc. Artif. Intern. Organs* 12:26, 1966.

332. Whiffen, J. D., Dutton, R. C., and Young, W. P. Heparin application to graphite-coated intravascular prostheses. *Surgery* 56: 8, 1964.

333. Whiffen, J. D., and Gott, V. L. Effect of various surface active agents on heparin binding and clot formation on graphite surfaces. *Proc. Soc. Exp. Biol. Med.* 116:134, 1964.

334. Whiffen, J. D., Young, W. P., and Gott, V. L. Stability of the thrombus-resistant graphite-benzalkonium-heparin surface in an anti-heparin environment. *J. Thorac. Cardiovasc. Surg.* 48:317, 1964.

335. Wieth, J. O., and Jorgensen, H. E. Treatment of methanol and ethanol by poisoning by hemodialysis. *Danish Med. Bull.* 8:103, 1961.

336. Wilcox, C., Freeman, R. B., Maher, J. F., and Schreiner, G. E. Comparison of physical properties and permeabilities of six cellulose membranes. *Trans. Amer. Soc. Artif. Intern. Organs* 12:44, 1966.

337. Wilson, R. E., Bernstein, D. S., Murray, J. E., and Moore, F. D. Effects of parathyroidectomy and kidney transplantation on renal osteodystrophy. *Amer. J. Surg.* 110: 384, 1965.

338. Wing, A. J., Curtis, J. R., de Wardener, H. E., and Evans, D. B. Two Years' Experience in Intermittent Hemodialysis. In *Proceedings of the European Dialysis and Transplant Association.* Newcastle upon Tyne, England: Bolsten & Stols, 1966. Vol. 3, p. 102.

339. Wright, R. G., Sand, P., and Livingston, G. Psychological stress during hemodialysis for chronic renal failure. *Ann. Intern. Med.* 64: 611, 1966.

340. Yatzidis, H. Recherches sur l'épuration extra-renale à l'aide du charbon actif. *Nephron* 1:310, 1964.

341. Yatzidis, H. Further experience with the charcoal artificial kidney. (Abstract.) In Abstracts: II. Free Communications. Third International Congress of Nephrology, Washington, D.C., 1966. P. 299.

II

Pathogenesis of Glomerulonephritis

Alfred J. Fish, Alfred F. Michael, and Robert A. Good

W ithin recent years increasing attention has been focused on immunologic mechanisms in the pathogenesis of glomerulonephritis. This interest has been stimulated by two important observations associated with clinical forms of glomerulonephritis. Firstly, it has been recognized for over 50 years [29, 69, 82, 173] that in many cases of glomerulonephritis there is a marked depression of serum complement levels, complement being an important effector mechanism of the immune response. Secondly, in 1956 Mellors et al. [98] demonstrated by immunofluorescent microscopy that immunoglobulins are deposited on the glomeruli in systemic lupus erythematosus and chronic membranous glomerulonephritis.

Current understanding of the pathogenesis and immunopathology of the various forms of glomerulonephritis observed clinically has been derived from numerous experimental studies of glomerulonephritis in animals. In this chapter a review of the experimental approach to glomerulonephritis is made, and the important relationships of these experimental studies to the pathogenesis of diffuse glomerular disease in man are considered.

Soluble Antigen-Antibody Complexes in Experimental Glomerulonephritis

When a given amount of antibody is reacted with a small amount of antigen, an insoluble macromolecular-complex precipitate is formed. However, when the same amount of antibody is reacted with an excess of antigen, the resulting precipitate is considerably less, and the supernate contains soluble macromolecular complexes of antigen and antibody. Extensive studies have revealed that soluble antigen-antibody complexes are biologically active: when injected intradermally into the skin, increased vascular permeability and inflammation result [65]; when applied to isolated strips of ileum or uterine smooth muscle, contraction occurs [150]; and when injected intravenously into guinea pigs, anaphylaxis regularly develops with marked depression of serum complement [42].

It has been shown by Ishizaka et al. [64, 66] that soluble antigen-antibody complexes of low molecular weight, those formed in very great antigen excess, bind the least amount of complement in vitro and, in general, have low biologic activity. In contrast, antigen-antibody complexes formed in slight antigen excess and closer to equivalence contain less antigen with proportionately more antibody and have an overall larger molecular weight; these complexes possess more potent biologic activity and bind more complement.

The relationship of antigen-antibody complexes to the various forms of glomerulonephritis is shown below:

1. Exogenous antigen release:
   a. Acute serum sickness nephritis
   b. Chronic serum sickness nephritis
2. Endogenous antigen release:
   a. Kidney-in-adjuvant nephritis (Heymann)
   b. Spontaneous SLE nephropathy in NZB mice
   c. Viral infection and nephritis
3. Soluble immune complex injury in man:
   a. Acute poststreptococcal glomerulonephritis
   b. Systemic lupus erythematosus

ACUTE SERUM SICKNESS NEPHRITIS

For more than 50 years it has been recognized that proliferative glomerulonephritis occurs during the course of serum sickness resulting from the administration of large doses of heterologous serum proteins in laboratory animals and man [89]. Numerous experiments were performed by Rich and Gregory [128, 129], who administered large doses of horse serum to rabbits and observed the development of diffuse proliferative glomerulonephritis and vascular lesions similar to those of polyarteritis nodosa. Subsequent studies by Hawn and Janeway [53] showed that similar

experimental lesions could be produced with the use of purified serum proteins such as bovine serum albumin (BSA) and bovine IgG.

The morphologic changes of serum sickness characteristically occur between seven and nine days after the administration of a foreign protein when circulating antigen is disappearing and before the appearance of antibody to this antigen [40]. At this time in the course of experimental serum sickness there is a depression in serum complement [132] and deposition of gamma globulin in the glomerulus [96]. Dixon et al. [21] subsequently showed that following the intravenous administration of a large dose of BSA in rabbits, small amounts of antibody are released into the circulation and complex with available antigen to form soluble antigen-antibody complexes. Between the sixth and the tenth day after the administration of antigen there is continuing release of antibody which complexes with the circulating antigen, and the resulting soluble antigen-antibody complexes are removed from the circulation as the complexes increase in size. At the time when all soluble complexes disappear from the circulating blood, the pathologic alterations of serum sickness become manifest, and IgG, β_1C globulin, and antigen may be demonstrated in a granular distribution along the glomerular capillaries (Fig. 11-1). Light microscopy shows endothelial cell proliferation with polymorphonuclear leukocyte infiltration. Studies by Fish et al. [37] revealed that during the healing phase of this experimental form of glomerulonephritis large nodular deposits of IgG and β_1C globulin can be demonstrated in a discrete fashion on the epithelial side of the glomerular basement membrane. Examination of these lesions by electron microscopy reveals characteristic "hump"-like deposits of electron-dense material along the epithelial side of the glomerular basement membrane (Fig. 11-2). These lesions are indistinguishable from the immunopathologic changes observed

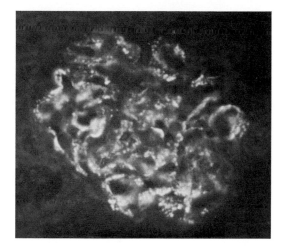

Figure 11-1. Immunofluorescent photomicrograph of a rabbit glomerulus during acute serum sickness nephritis showing a granular and finely nodular deposition of IgG.

in acute poststreptococcal glomerulonephritis in man [36, 37].

CHRONIC SERUM SICKNESS NEPHRITIS

Elaborating on initial experimental observations by McLean et al. [92], a model of chronic serum sickness nephritis in the rabbit was comprehensively studied and delineated by Dixon et al. [19]; purified bovine serum albumin (BSA) was given intravenously to rabbits almost every day in an effort to maintain a state of slight antigen excess in the circulation over a period of six weeks to two months. Rabbits which were poor antibody producers did not develop glomerular lesions, whereas those which produced large quantities of antibody either died from anaphylaxis or experienced acute serum sickness-like reactions from which they recovered. However, in a third group of rabbits, those which were moderate antibody producers, and in which it was possible to achieve a state of slight antigen excess over a long period, chronic membranoproliferative glomerulonephritis developed. BSA, IgG, and β_1C globulin were present as large discrete deposits within the glomerular

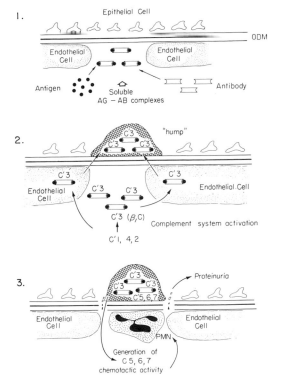

Figure 11-2. Diagrammatic representation of the development of glomerular injury by soluble antigen-antibody complexes. Step 1: Antibody is released into the circulation in an environment of antigen excess, and soluble complexes are formed. Step 2: Soluble complexes activate the complement system, pass through the glomerular capillary endothelium, and localize as discrete subepithelial humps. Step 3: Generation of chemotactic factor results in polymorphonuclear leukocyte (PMN) migration and further damage.

basement membrane and in a subepithelial locus. By electron microscopy prominent dense deposits in the subepithelium were present. These deposits were shown by Andres et al. [6], who used immunoferritin technics to contain IgG, β_1C globulin, and BSA. This disease may progress to uremia even if antigen administration is stopped. It has been shown by Valdes et al. [160] that if, in the late stages of chronic serum sickness nephritis, larger daily doses of antigen, 50 times the amount used to induce the disease, are then administered intravenously, the immune deposits appear to undergo dissolution, with resultant regression of the glomerular disease. Presumably in this situation of large antigen excess at the level of the glomerulus, deposited complexes are "solubilized."

In these models of acute and chronic serum sickness nephritis the kidney is damaged as an innocent bystander by biologically active antigen-antibody complexes which localize in the glomerulus. Several observations suggest certain important predisposing mechanisms for the glomerular or vascular localization of antigen-antibody complexes in serum sickness. Cochrane and Hawkins [14] demonstrated that antigen-antibody complexes of low molecular weight — that is, those complexes formed in presence of large antigen excess — did not localize to blood vessels of guinea pig lung which had been previously damaged by pretreatment with histamine resulting in increased vascular permeability. However, soluble antigen-antibody complexes of larger molecular weight, those formed in presence of slight antigen excess, with sedimentation coefficients greater than 19S were capable of localizing in pulmonary vessel walls. Studies by Pincus et al. [123] have shown, however, that the circulating soluble antigen-antibody complexes in chronic serum sickness nephritis are comprised chiefly of "nonprecipitating antibody," have less tendency for clearance by the reticuloendothelial system, and, by virtue of their slower clearance, have a greater propensity to localize in the kidney. Evidence that physiologic mechanisms of glomerular filtration and renal plasma flow may be important in the localization of complexes was provided by Germuth et al. [41], who showed that narrowing of the renal artery or unilateral ureteral occlusion in experimental serum sickness nephritis diminished localization of complexes, and the resultant glomerular injury was minimal.

When soluble antigen-antibody complexes

are phagocytosed by glomerular capillary endothelial cells, there is cellular proliferation and capillary-loop narrowing. It appears that tissue damaging, biologically active, soluble antigen-antibody complexes move from the endothelial cell into a subendothelial location and then cross the glomerular basement membrane where they are sequestered as discrete masses in the subepithelial zone (see Fig. 11-2). It is of considerable interest that these macromolecular complexes should be handled in this way and inevitably cause severe glomerular damage, whereas it has been shown by other workers [31, 83, 100] that macromolecules such as ferritin and colloidal particles are transported by glomerular mesangial cells, a network of cells which supports the glomerular capillaries. It has been shown by Michael, Fish, and Good [103] that when large doses of aggregated human IgG (a macromolecular complex with identical biologic properties to soluble antigen-antibody complexes) is injected intravenously in mice, there is glomerular localization, chiefly within the mesangial apparatus, and subsequent clearance from the glomerulus via the mesangium with no evidence of glomerular injury. Germuth et al. [43] have recently shown that in acute and chronic serum sickness nephritis when cortisone is administered to rabbits, the localization of soluble antigen-antibody complexes is shifted from the glomerular capillary endothelium to the mesangium. In this situation in which there appears to be no reduction in antigen-antibody complex formation per se, there is an alternate site of complex localization in the glomerulus with a marked reduction in the extent of glomerular injury. By immunofluorescent microscopy the antigen-antibody complexes seem to be localized within the mesangium and in that locus are less able to induce glomerular injury. It appears that corticosteroid therapy prevents glomerulonephritis by blocking the transport of antigen-antibody complexes across the capillary wall.

KIDNEY-IN-ADJUVANT NEPHRITIS

In the experimental studies of acute and chronic complex nephritis described above, the antigen is usually an exogenous or foreign protein such as bovine serum albumin. Several other forms of experimental glomerulonephritis have been recognized in which the antigen participating in complex formation is endogenous or autologous. Since the host's own antigens are participating in an immune reaction leading to tissue destruction, these phenomena could correctly be termed "auto immune." Hunter, Hackel, and Heymann [63] were able to induce progressive chronic glomerulonephritis in rats by repeated intraperitoneal injections of rat kidney incorporated in complete Freund's adjuvant. Proteinuria, edema, and the classic features of the nephrotic syndrome regularly developed in rats treated in this manner. By immunofluorescent microscopy it was observed that the glomeruli in these animals have granular, lumpy deposits of both IgG and $\beta_1 C$ globulin which are present within the glomerular basement membrane [59, 112]. Electron microscopic examination of the glomeruli in these rats revealed small, discrete electron-dense deposits in a subepithelial distribution [20]. These findings provide strong evidence that the glomerular injury was mediated by the action of soluble antigen-antibody complexes.

Elegant investigation of this model (described above) by Edgington and his co-workers [26, 28] revealed that the antigen taking part in soluble complex formation resided in the brush border of epithelial cells lining the proximal convoluted tubule. In these experiments, rabbit antisera against antigens in the brush border of proximal convoluted tubular epithelial cells were rendered specific by absorption of the antisera with normal rat serum and other fractions of the rat kidney. To detect the renal tubular epithelial antigen within the immune deposits in the glomerulus using these fluorescein-labeled antisera, it was found necessary to partially elute the deposited IgG using 2.5 M potassium thiocyanate, thereby exposing free antigenic sites within the glomerular immune deposits with which the antitubular epithelial antigen serum could react. Having identified the antigen in this fashion, it has been possible to induce this disease primarily using as little as 3 μg. N of purified antigen from the brush border of the proximal tubular epithelial cells, administered intraperitoneally in complete Freund's adjuvant [27]. It has been shown that minute quantities of this antigen are present at extremely low concentrations within the circulation of normal animals. Following immunization with the antigen, autoantibodies are formed and combine with normally circulating autologous antigen to form soluble antigen-antibody complexes which are subsequently deposited within the glomerulus [46].

In an analogous situation, Weigle and High [171] produced autoantibodies to thyroglobulin by immunizing rabbits with heterologous thyroglobulin or other preparations of homologous thyroglobulin chemically altered by the addition of haptenic groups. Glomerulonephritis, with localization of antigen-antibody complexes, was induced in these animals by administering a large dose of radioactive iodine (^{131}I) which damages the thyroid gland, releasing large amounts of thyroglobulin into the circulation. The latter complexes with circulating antithyroglobulin antibody, forming soluble antigen-antibody complexes that localize in the glomerulus and produce glomerulonephritis.

SPONTANEOUS SLE NEPHROPATHY IN NZB MICE

The spontaneous development of a systemic lupus erythematosus-like (SLE-like) syndrome in an inbred strain of New Zealand black mice was recognized and described by Bielschowsky, Helyer, and Howie [10]. These animals were noted to have autoimmune hemolytic anemia and a progressive form of glomerulonephritis. Helyer and Howie [54] described the development of glomerulonephritis in the F_1 hybrids of NZB and NZW mice. In these animals a lupus-like syndrome was characterized by the development of positive antinuclear antibody titers and the occurrence of LE cells. The disease occurs spontaneously at the age of five to six months, and the development of kidney lesions shows rapid progression with death in 98 per cent of female mice before the age of one year [62]. The development of this autoimmune process is accelerated by neonatal thymectomy.

Ajax mice also develop antinuclear antibodies, Coombs-positive hemolytic anemia, and a progressive SLE-like renal disease; this syndrome is also accelerated by neonatal thymectomy [148]. Immunofluorescent microscopy examination of the glomerular lesions reveals the deposition of host IgG and β_1C globulin as granular deposits along the glomerular basement membrane and within the glomerular mesangium [1, 95].

Lambert and Dixon [78] completely eluted the IgG from glomerular deposits of NZB/NZW mice and demonstrated that the eluate contained antinuclear antibody activity. In addition, immunofluorescent studies were performed on NZB/NZW kidney biopsies which had been treated with 2.0 M sodium chloride solution to partially remove some of the deposited IgG, and then stained with fluorescein-labeled antiserum to DNA; positive staining was obtained in this situation indicating that immune deposits in the glomeruli in these animals contained deoxyribonucleic acid (DNA). In additional experiments, young NZB/NZW mice which had significant antibody titers to DNA but no evidence of kidney disease were given daily intravenous injections of DNA. In this situation, soluble antigen-antibody complexes between the administered DNA and the circulating antibody to DNA occurred with the subsequent development of glomerular injury identical to that which occurs spontaneously later in life in these ani-

mals. Mellors and Huang [97] have presented evidence that a virus infection in New Zealand black mice is responsible for this phenomenon. The development of anti-DNA antibodies may represent antibody against viral DNA or autoantibody against denatured host DNA occurring as a result of tissue injury.

VIRAL INFECTION AND NEPHRITIS

Oldstone and Dixon [113, 114] have studied mice with long-standing viral infections due to lymphocytic choriomeningitis (LCM) virus and demonstrated glomerulonephritis with IgG, β_1C globulin, and LCM viral antigen deposited within the glomerular lesions. Although these laboratory animals were believed to be tolerant to the LCM virus, they formed small amounts of antibody to the virus which were detected only in the kidney and were presumably deposited there as a result of trapping of virus-antibody complexes within the glomeruli. Although less well documented, a similar mechanism is probably active in the production of glomerular lesions associated with Aleutian disease in mink [55, 72, 124] and in glomerulonephritis of mice experimentally infected with ECHO 9 virus [13]; perhaps numerous other viruses can produce this type of renal injury.

Glomerular Injury by Soluble Antigen-Antibody Complexes in Man

ACUTE POSTSTREPTOCOCCAL GLOMERULONEPHRITIS

In 1907 Schick [131] noted and compared the delay in appearance of symptoms of serum sickness with the latent period following streptococcal infections and the onset of acute glomerulonephritis. It has been recognized for many years that in acute glomerulonephritis there is marked depression of serum complement titers [69, 82, 173], and more recently Michael et al. [101] observed that in this disease IgG and β_1C globulin are deposited within glomeruli as discrete fine nodular deposits adjacent to the glomerular basement membrane (Figs. 11-3, 11-4). By electron microscopy, accumulations of electron-dense material (i.e., "humps") are found in acute poststreptococcal nephritis in a subepithelial distribution. Kimmelstiel [71], Movat [109], Andres [4], Michael [101], Osawa [115], and Herdson [58] and their co-workers have demonstrated that these ultrastructural changes in acute nephritis are indistinguishable from the findings in laboratory animals in which acute serum sickness nephritis was induced with heterologous serum proteins [36]. Although these observations present compelling evidence in support of the hypothesis that the glomerular lesions associated with acute poststreptococcal glomerulonephritis in man is mediated by soluble antigen-antibody complexes, thus far it has not been possible to isolate circulating antigen-antibody

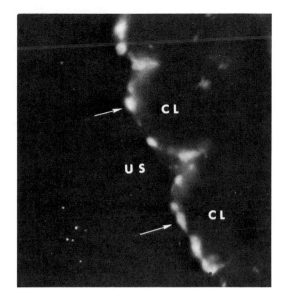

Figure 11-4. High magnification, oil immersion, immunofluorescent photomicrograph revealing discrete subepithelial immune deposits (*arrows*) of β_1C in two peripheral glomerular capillary loops in acute poststreptococcal glomerulonephritis. The glomerular capillary lumen (CL) and the urinary space (US) are identified.

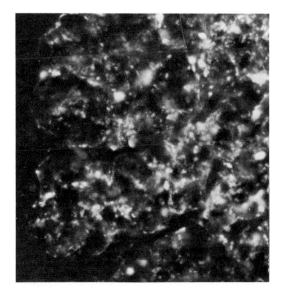

Figure 11-3. A portion of the glomerulus in acute poststreptococcal glomerulonephritis showing discrete nodular deposits of IgG along the glomerular capillary loops.

complexes from the serum of these patients. Inability to find antigen-antibody complexes in sera from patients with acute nephritis may result from examining serum specimens too late in the course of the disease, at a time when complexes have already disappeared from the circulation and have been deposited within the glomeruli. Interestingly enough, Palmer and his associates [118] have demonstrated the development of unilateral acute glomerulonephritis when the contralateral kidney was "protected" by renal-artery stenosis. This observation nicely parallels the experimental studies of Germuth and his associates [41] when localization of soluble complex was similarly blocked. In addition, there have been reports by Michael et al. [101] and by Seegal and her co-workers [133] of the presence of streptococcal antigens within the glomerulus in acute poststreptococcal glomerulonephritis. Streptococcal antigens have not consistently been observed within the glomeruli, and on those occasions when streptococcal products have been detected, their distribution has not paralleled the nature and distribution of IgG and β_1C globulin localization.

Feldman et al. [33], in studies of patients with poststreptococcal glomerulonephritis, failed to demonstrate nodular deposits of IgG and β_1C globulin; in those studies focal linear deposits of immunoproteins along the glomerular basement membrane were detected. Fish et al. [35], who investigated an epidemic of acute glomerulonephritis during the summer and fall of 1966 on the Red Lake Indian Reservation, demonstrated that a percentage of the patients, those with the severest clinical findings of glomerulonephritis, showed the classic immunopathologic changes, with nodular immunoprotein deposits on their glomeruli. The remaining patients with milder forms of the disease were found only to have focal interrupted linear deposition of β_1C globulin along the glomerular basement membrane and within the mesangium, and no immune deposits were observed. In this study, for the first time, it was possible to investigate the entire clinical spectrum of acute glomerulonephritis to include the mild asymptomatic forms as well as the severe classic cases of the disease.

Following the demonstration by Rammelkamp et al. [126, 144] that acute glomerulonephritis was associated with type 12 beta-hemolytic streptococcal pharyngitis, numerous efforts were made experimentally to induce glomerulonephritis in laboratory animals with streptococcal infection. In studies by Reed and Matheson [127], Hinkle et al. [61], Kelly and Winn [70], and Tan et al. [146], beta-hemolytic streptococci were administered subcutaneously and intraperitoneally in Millipore chambers. Significant glomerular alteration was not found, although in many cases the animals developed varying degrees of tubular degeneration. Lindberg et al. [87] reported a high frequency of proteinuria in rats receiving the intraperitoneal chambers containing type 12 beta-hemolytic streptococci; although no evidence of glomerulonephritis was found by light microscopy, focal mesangial and glomerular basement membrane deposition of IgG and complement, along with M protein antigen, were observed. More recently Holm and his co-workers [61] reported that a single intravenous injection of a cell-free streptococcal autolysate in rabbits consistently appeared to induce proliferative glomerulonephritis. In another recent study by Becker and Murphy [7], group A beta-hemolytic streptococci were repeatedly injected intravenously into rabbits, resulting in the development of proliferative glomerulonephritis. Immunofluorescent microscopy was not performed in the majority of these studies, and consequently there is no possibility of comparing the immunopathologic processes with those mentioned in this review.

Treser et al. [151] reported recently that the serum from patients with acute poststreptococcal glomerulonephritis and some serum from "normal" subjects contained antibody in the IgG fraction of the serum which fixes focally to the glomerular basement membrane and the mesangium of glomeruli from patients with acute poststreptococcal glomerulonephritis when studied by immunofluorescent microscopy. These antibodies did not stain normal glomeruli or glomeruli in biopsies from other forms of subacute or chronic glomerulonephritis. The authors suggest that in acute poststreptococcal glomerulonephritis antigenic determinants within the basement membrane and mesangium of the glomerulus are exposed during the acute injury. It was also shown that the antibody activity in the serum cross-reacted with antigenic determinants in the plasma membrane of beta-hemolytic streptococci. The significance of these observations must await further investigation.

In acute poststreptococcal glomerulonephritis whole-complement titers are low; analysis of complement components by Gewurz et al. [44] reveals that C′3 (β_1C) and the terminal complement components are depressed, although C′1, C′4, and C′2 are normal. The significance of these observations is discussed on page 387 along with a comparison of the changes in serum complement components in systemic lupus erythematosus.

SYSTEMIC LUPUS ERYTHEMATOSUS

In 1957, Mellors et al. [99] demonstrated that immunoglobulins are deposited within the glomeruli in systemic lupus erythematosus (SLE). With the previous demonstration of depression in the serum complement titer in the majority of patients with SLE and the observation by Lachmann et al. [77] that C′3 (β_1C globulin) is also deposited on the glomerulus in this disease, cogent evidence was at hand that immunologic mechanisms play an important role in the pathogenesis of SLE nephropathy (Fig. 11-5). It has been recognized for some time that the serum of patients with SLE contains antibodies directed against nuclear components, specifically against nucleoprotein and DNA. Freedman and Markowitz [38], with the use of citrate buffer at low pH, eluted immunoglobulins from isolated glomeruli obtained from SLE kidneys at autopsy and demonstrated that the eluted immunoglobulin possessed antinuclear antibody activity similar to that found in serum from patients with SLE. By electron microscopy, the glomerular capillary loops in SLE contain prominent electron-dense deposits within subendothelial and subepithelial loci as well as within the glomerular basement membrane; these alterations of ultrastructure are indistinguishable from those found in experimental chronic antigen-antibody complex nephritis [49]. Patients with SLE in the acute stage,

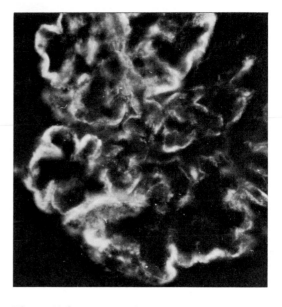

Figure 11-5. Segment of a glomerulus in SLE showing granular deposits of IgG within the glomerular basement membrane. In some areas the deposits have become confluent with focal thickening of the glomerular basement membrane, giving rise to the "wire-loop" lesion seen by light microscopy.

before treatment or during exacerbation, have elevated antibody titers to DNA. Tan et al. [147] demonstrated that in some patients during the acute phase of the disease anti-DNA antibodies are not present, and in this situation small amounts of DNA are detectable within the circulation; it is assumed that the detected DNA within the circulation is present in the form of a soluble antigen-antibody complex, as DNA–anti-DNA. Further evidence that lupus nephritis is due to soluble antigen-antibody complexes was recently shown by Koffler and Kunkel [74, 76], who demonstrated that the deposited IgG could be removed from the glomerulus by treating the frozen-tissue sections with deoxyribonuclease; this suggests that the immunoglobulin bound in SLE glomeruli is associated with DNA antigen and is thereby released with this form of enzymatic treatment. Partial elution of the deposited IgG with 2.0 M sodium chloride revealed DNA antigen within the glomerular deposits in two patients when the sections were stained with fluorescein-labeled antibody to DNA. These observations provide some clues to the pathogenesis of SLE nephritis and bear strong resemblance to the findings described above of SLE-like nephropathy in NZB/NZW mice [78]. Current knowledge points strongly toward a chronic antigen-antibody complex pathogenesis of the renal lesions in SLE. At present it is not known whether the anti-DNA activity in these patients is directed against viral DNA or host DNA released from tissues undergoing inflammatory or other tissue-damaging processes.

As in acute poststreptococcal glomerulonephritis, whole-serum complement titers in SLE are low, but complement-component analysis by Gewurz et al. [44] has revealed that C′1, C′4, C′2, and C′3 are all depressed. This pattern of complement alteration relates most closely to that observed in experimental antigen-antibody complex nephritis, and is correlated with the observation of Hanauer and Christian [51] that in SLE C′1q (an 11S component of C′1) is low. Tojo and Friou [149] have shown that among SLE patients nephritis develops only in those showing high complement-fixing activity of antibodies to nuclear antigens.

It is of considerable interest that in acute poststreptococcal glomerulonephritis and in hypocomplementemic chronic glomerulonephritis (see page 389) that a different complement profile is observed [44], featured by relative sparing of C′1, C′4, and C′2 with depression of the six terminal components including C′3 (β_1C). This may reflect a different pathogenetic mechanism of immune injury in these forms of glomerulonephritis. Other examples of C′3 activation without the earlier components may be found in the reaction of guinea pig gamma-1 immunoglobulin [116], and the lysis of sheep red blood cells by bacterial endotoxin [45].

Glomerulonephritis Mediated by Antibodies to Glomerular Basement Membrane

The types of glomerulonephritis mediated by antibodies to glomerular basement membrane are:

1. Heteronephrotoxic serum nephritis
2. Autoimmune antiglomerular basement membrane nephritis
3. Autoimmune glomerulonephritis in man; Goodpasture's syndrome

NEPHROTOXIC NEPHRITIS

The administration of heteronephrotoxic antikidney serum to the laboratory animal causes severe glomerulonephritis and the nephrotic syndrome, and may lead to uremia and death. This model of experimental glomerulonephritis was studied by Masugi in 1933 in rabbits and rats, and has been produced in many other animals including rats, dogs, rabbits, monkeys, and mice; the findings in these species are covered in review articles by Unanue and Dixon [154] and Michael et al. [102] (Fig. 11-6).

During the past decade a major contribution to our understanding of the pathogenesis of this form of experimental nephritis has been made by Dixon and associates. Nephrotoxic serum nephritis occurs in two distinct phases: the first involves the immediate fixation of the heteronephrotoxic antibody to the glomerular basement membrane (GBM) which results in immediate proteinuria; and the second, which starts four or five days later, when the animal develops antibody to the heterologous immunoglobulin deposited along the glomerular basement membrane. This se-

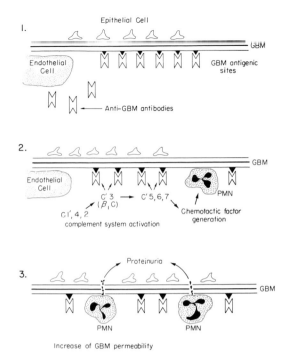

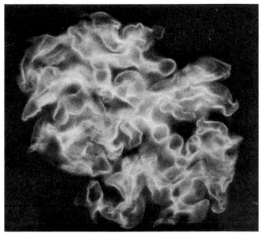

Figure 11-7. Fluorescent photomicrograph showing diffuse linear deposition of rabbit IgG along the glomerular basement membranes of a rat glomerulus following intravenous administration of rabbit anti-rat glomerular basement membrane serum.

Figure 11-6. Diagrammatic representation of the development of glomerular injury by anti-glomerular basement membrane (*anti-GBM*) antibodies. Step 1: Fixation of anti-GBM antibodies to antigenic sites on the GBM. Step 2: Activation of the complement system follows with β_1C deposition and generation of chemotactic factor. Step 3: Release of enzymes from polymorphonuclear leukocytes (PMN) contributes to GBM damage and increased permeability.

quence was clearly elucidated by Hammer and Dixon [50] in rats decomplemented by the administration of aggregated immunoglobulin. These animals did not develop immediate proteinuria and had mild glomerulonephritis. The pathogenesis of the second stage of nephrotoxic nephritis was shown by using rats made tolerant to rabbit IgG at birth and then given rabbit antirat nephrotoxic serum at a later date; immediate proteinuria occurred, but the second stage of the disease was blocked with absence of prolonged proteinuria.

In nephrotoxic nephritis the administered heterologous immunoglobulin, host IgG, and β_1C globulin of complement are deposited in a diffuse fine linear fashion along the glomerular basement membrane when examined by fluorescent microscopy (Fig. 11-7). These observations are the hallmark of immunologic glomerular injury due to antiglomerular basement membrane antibodies. This pattern is in complete contrast to that described above where glomerular injury is mediated by soluble antigen-antibody complexes and the immunopathologic alteration consists of granular and nodular deposits of immunoproteins. In nephrotoxic nephritis, the earliest electron microscopic changes observed consist of separation of the glomerular capillary endothelial cells from the glomerular basement membrane. Using nephrotoxic IgG labeled with ferritin, which appears as an electron-dense particle (due to the iron moieties on the ferritin molecule), Andres et al. [5] and Vogt et al. [168] were able to demonstrate that the first localization of nephrotoxic antibodies in this form of experimental nephritis occurred on the subendothelial side of the glomerular basement membrane. There is eventual complete separation of glomerular endothelial cells as polymorphonuclear leukocytes marginate along the denuded glomerular basement membrane adjacent to the sites of antibody fixation as the prominent feature of the ultrastructural alteration in nephrotoxic nephritis [32].

Nephrotoxic serum nephritis is a progressive ongoing destructive process leading to death and uremia. The mechanism by which ongoing glomerular destruction takes place over several weeks is not clearly understood. It has been shown by Unanue and his associates [157] that none of the IgG deposited late in the course of the disease was autoantibody to glomerular basement membrane; these findings are in contrast to the observations of Pfeiffer and his co-workers [120] and Lange and his associates [81], who demonstrated transmission of nephritis to a normal rat parabiosed with a nephritic rat given rabbit nephrotoxic serum. Vassalli and McCluskey [161–163] showed that deposition of fibrin within the glomeruli was a prominent feature during the ongoing later phases of this disease in rabbits, and they were able to alter significantly the degree of glomerular

damage and mortality by prolonged anticoagulation with warfarin.

Considerable attention has been focused by many workers [67, 134, 152] on the production of nephrotoxic antisera derived from animals immunized with membrane fractions from nonkidney sources. Antisera made especially against lung and placenta, and to a lesser extent against heart, spleen, and muscle, possess cross-reacting kidney-fixing, nephritogenic properties.

AUTOIMMUNE ANTIGLOMERULAR BASEMENT MEMBRANE NEPHRITIS

In 1962 Steblay described the induction of experimental severe progressive glomerulonephritis in sheep by the administration of multiple injections of homologous or heterologous (but not autologous) glomerular basement membrane in complete Freund's adjuvant [138]. Glomerular basement membrane from man, monkey, dog, rabbit, and rat when administered in this fashion regularly induced glomerulonephritis in recipient sheep. These animals have an ultralinear deposition of host IgG and β_1C globulin along the glomerular basement membrane [139, 140] (Fig. 11-8). From these observations, it was suggested that an autoimmune process may be active, with

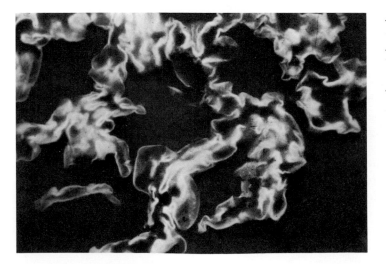

Figure 11-8. Deposition of IgG in a diffuse linear fashion along the glomerular basement membrane of a glomerulus from a sheep immunized with heterologous glomerular basement membrane. (Photomicrograph generously provided by Dr. Raymond Steblay.)

antibody formation against the glomerular basement membrane of the host. This concept was strengthened by Steblay's [141] observation that by performing cross-circulation experiments between a normal sheep and a nephritic sheep previously injected with glomerular basement membrane in adjuvant, there was immediate development of glomerulonephritis in the normal partner, with transfer of antibody to the glomerular basement membranes. In spite of these observations, it was not possible at any time to detect circulating antibody to glomerular basement membrane in the nephritic sheep. Lerner and Dixon [84] were successful in detecting circulating antiglomerular basement membrane antibodies by performing bilateral nephrectomies in nephritic sheep, thereby removing the "sink" or target organ for autoantibodies produced against glomerular basement membrane. These authors transferred this form of autoimmune experimental nephritis into normal sheep by using plasma from the nephrectomized nephritic sheep. Similar forms of autoimmune glomerulonephritis were induced in rabbits by Unanue and Dixon [155] and Unanue et al. [156], using heterologous and homologous renal antigens, and in monkeys by Paronetto and Koffler [119], using homologous glomerular basement membrane. Interestingly enough, Steblay and Rudofsky [142] have reported the development of autoimmune glomerulonephritis in sheep induced by immunization with human lung in complete Freund's adjuvant. This appears to be the first autoimmune disease induced by antigens that are not organ specific [143].

Lerner and Dixon [85] have recently observed that significant amounts of glomerular basement membrane-like material is excreted in the urine of normal rabbits. When this material was concentrated and reinjected into rabbits in complete Freund's adjuvant, autoimmune glomerulonephritis resulted. In all the above situations where autoimmune glomerulonephritis was induced by one means or another, a common observation was made in each instance — namely, that the IgG and β_1C globulin of the host animal are deposited in a linear fashion diffusely along the glomerular basement membrane.

Markowitz et al. [90, 91] have demonstrated cross-reactivity between antigens in the plasma membrane of beta-hemolytic streptococci and human glomerular basement membrane. Following passive immunization with sheep antiserum to these cross-reacting antigens of the glomerular basement membrane, glomerulonephritis ensued; immunofluorescent microscopy of these lesions revealed linear deposition of host immunoproteins along the glomerular basement membrane. Since studies of the pathogenesis of acute poststreptococcal glomerulonephritis in man suggests injury mediated by soluble antigen-antibody complexes, as discussed above, the significance of these findings by Markowitz and his co-workers will require further study and elucidation.

THE ROLE OF ANTIGLOMERULAR BASEMENT MEMBRANE ANTIBODY IN THE PATHOGENESIS OF HUMAN GLOMERULONEPHRITIS

The immunopathologic finding of diffuse ultralinear deposition of IgG and β_1C globulin along the glomerular basement membrane in human kidney biopsy material is rarely found. Goodpasture's syndrome is characterized clinically by recurrent pulmonary hemorrhages associated with the development of progressive and usually fatal glomerulonephritis. Duncan et al. first reported [23] that there is diffuse linear deposition of IgG and β_1C globulin along the glomerular basement membrane (Fig. 11-9). It is recognized from experimental studies that cross-reactivity exists between lung and kidney glomerular basement membrane antigens, and that glomerulonephritis may be induced experimentally using lung basement membrane. It is postulated that in Goodpasture's syndrome the primary process within the lung results in an alteration in lung basement membrane, with subsequent

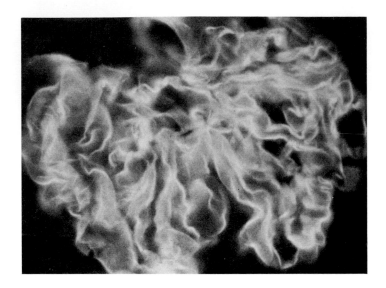

Figure 11-9. Fluorescent photomicrograph showing diffuse linear deposition of IgG along the glomerular basement membrane in Goodpasture's syndrome.

formation of autoantibodies against altered lung basement membrane which cross-react with glomerular basement membrane and damage the kidney. Immunofluorescent studies of lung tissue in some cases of this disease have not revealed the presence of IgG or β_1C deposition along the alveolar capillary basement membrane [23]. However, in a recent report, Beirne et al. [8] demonstrated localization of IgG and β_1C globulin along the alveolar basement membrane and capillaries of a patient with classic immunopathologic features of Goodpasture's syndrome in the kidney. Koffler and Kunkel [75] described similar findings in the lung and showed that the antibody eluted from lung tissue had specificity for lung and glomerular basement membranes.

In a recent study, Lerner et al. [86] treated the isolated glomeruli from autopsy kidney specimens in Goodpasture's syndrome at low pH with citrate buffer. In vitro studies of the immunoglobulin eluted in this manner were performed by overlaying the eluates on normal human kidney. When examined by immunofluorescent microscopy, there was extensive localization of eluted Goodpasture antibody to the glomerular basement membrane, Bowman's capsule, and tubular basement membrane. The eluted antibody was also administered intravenously to squirrel monkeys and resulted in the onset of immediate proteinuria leading to severe nephrotic syndrome, proliferative glomerulonephritis, and uremia. These in vivo studies with eluted Goodpasture antibody demonstrated localization to the glomerular basement membrane in the diseased kidneys of squirrel monkeys. These studies and the results of other experimental forms of autoimmune nephritis provide evidence that glomerulonephritis associated with Goodpasture's syndrome is mediated on an autoimmune basis with antibody activity directed against host glomerular basement membrane. Preliminary observations suggest that in a few patients with severe progressive subacute glomerulonephritis the eluted antibody from these glomerular lesions possesses similar antiglomerular basement membrane activity. Also, in a few isolated cases, circulating antiglomerular basement membrane antibody has been demonstrated in the plasma of patients with subacute glomerulonephritis only in the period following bilateral nephrectomy, prior to renal homotransplantation. The frequency and significance of these findings in patients with various forms of progressive glomerulonephritis must await further investigation. At present, however, these preliminary observations are of great importance, particularly with reference to the development of immunologic injury to the glomerular basement membranes of normal transplanted kidneys.

Humoral and Cellular Mediators of Immune Injury

It has been shown by Hammer and Dixon [50] that in decomplemented rats the initial phase of glomerular basement membrane injury, with the sudden onset of proteinuria in nephrotoxic nephritis, does not occur. It was also shown by Lange [79], who administered avian (duck) heteronephrotoxic antibody against rabbit kidney, that the first phase of glomerular injury did not occur and the onset of proteinuria was delayed approximately four days until the beginning of the second phase of the disease. Inability to produce immediate renal disease is thought to be related, in part, to the inability of avian antisera to fix mammalian complement [68].

When antibody is fixed to red blood cell membrane or glomerular basement membrane surfaces, there is a sequential activation of the complement system. Activation of C′3 (β_1C) and the next three complement components (C′5, C′6, and C′7) provide a stimulus for the localization of polymorphonuclear leukocytes to the glomerulus [110]. By observing the migration of polymorphonuclear leukocytes through the micropore filter of a modified Boyden chamber, Ward et al. [169] established the chemotactic properties of C′5 and C′6. These observations were subsequently extended to include C′7 as well in the complement-component complex responsible for polymorphonuclear leukocyte chemotaxis [16]. Recent studies by Snyderman et al. [135] have shown that chemotactic factor is probably derived from C′5 and has a molecular weight of 15,000. The complement-dependent migration of polymorphonuclear leukocytes (PMN), with localization of leukocytes in close proximity to the glomerular basement membrane in nephrotoxic nephritis, appears to be important in the development of proteinuria in these animals (see Fig. 11-6). Cochrane et al. [15] showed that in animals depleted of polymorphonuclear leukocytes (by treatment with anti-PMN antisera or with nitrogen mustard) there was complete absence of polymorphonuclear leukocyte infiltration within the glomeruli, and no proteinuria was found in these animals. Hawkins and Cochrane [52] have recently shown that the increased permeability of the glomerular basement membrane in nephrotoxic nephritis is due, in part, to the direct action of acid proteases (cathepsins) which directly damage the glomerular basement membrane with liberation of glomerular basement membrane material into the urine. The role of complement and polymorphonuclear leukocytes as mediators or effectors of the immune response in nephrotoxic nephritis may be applied in the same fashion to explain the pathogenesis of the immune injury associated with soluble antigen-antibody complexes (see Fig. 11-2). Soluble complexes bind complement and consequently have a strong chemotactic potential.

It should be mentioned that vasoactive amines such as histamine and serotonin cause marked alteration in vascular permeability and contribute significantly to the development of various forms of immune injury [73]. There has been increasing attention focused on the role of kinins in producing increased vascular permeability. Following incubation of normal serum with antigen-antibody precipitates, the serum develops vascular permeability-enhancing activity [107, 108, 153]. Activation of the kinin system in this manner is dependent upon complement and factor XII (Hageman factor). The role of kinins in immune injury of the glomerulus seems likely and remains to be further elucidated.

Immunologic Injury in Other Forms of Glomerulonephritis

In the foregoing sections current concepts of the pathogenesis of the glomerular injury occurring in poststreptococcal glomerulonephritis, systemic lupus erythematosus, and Goodpasture's syndrome have been presented. There are, in addition, numerous other types of glomerulonephritis associated with distinct clinical entities in which the injury to the glomerulus appears to be mediated by immunologic mechanisms (Table 11-1); precise delineation of these processes has not been achieved. General review of the immunopathologic findings in human kidney biopsy material has been presented by Michael [102], Drummond [22], Vernier [165], Lange [80], and McCluskey [93] and their co-workers. In a recent study Herdman et al. [56] examined the nature of the light (L) chains found in glomerular deposits of IgG in a variety of diseases. They observed that the ratio of kappa-to-lambda L chains in circulating plasma IgG does not coincide with the qualitative frequency and appearance of L-chain determinants of deposited IgG in the glomerular lesions. This suggests that there is not merely a nonspecific utilization of circulating IgG in these reactions, but that a select and specific population of immunoglobulin molecules is being deposited in the glomeruli.

Idiopathic Nephrosis

Idiopathic nephrosis, seen frequently in children and less commonly in adults, is characterized by the nephrotic syndrome with normal renal function, normal serum complement, and normal or minimal glomerular changes by light microscopy [22]. Eighty-five

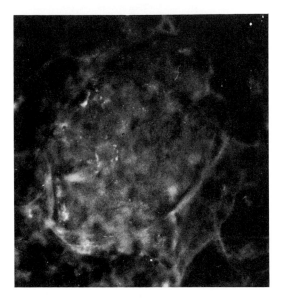

Figure 11-10. Glomerulus from a patient with childhood idiopathic nephrosis showing no significant deposition of IgG.

per cent of these patients respond completely to steroid therapy. There is minimal or no deposition of IgG or $\beta_1 C$ globulin in the glomerulus (Fig. 11-10), and levels of $\beta_1 C$ globulin in the serum are generally normal [173]. It seems unlikely that immunologic mechanisms play a role in the pathogenesis of this disorder.

Chronic Membranoproliferative Glomerulonephritis with Hypocomplementemia

Among the many cases of chronic glomerulonephritis seen clinically, West [172] and Gotoff [48] and their associates first observed that certain patients seem to represent a distinct clinical and pathological entity with persistently low serum complement or $\beta_1 C$ globulin and characteristic light microscopic findings of lobular membranoproliferative glomerulonephritis. West et al. [172] described splitting of the glomerular basement membrane with zones of nonargyrophilia.

Table 11-1. Immunofluorescence in Nephrotic Syndrome

Immunofluorescence	Glomerular Pathology			Serum Complement	Proteinuria	Renal Function	Response to Steroid Therapy
	Light Microscopy	Fluorescent Microscopy					
		Predominant Distribution	Character of Immunopathology				
Negative							
Idiopathic nephrosis	Normal (or minimal changes)		Negative	Normal	Selective[a]	Normal	Good
Positive							
Poststreptococcal glomerulonephritis	Abnormal	GBM[b] & extra-GBM	Nodular	Low	Nonselective	Normal or low	?
Systemic lupus erythematosus	Abnormal	GBM & extra-GBM	Granular & focal linear	Low	Nonselective	Normal or low	Moderate
Membranous glomerulonephritis	Abnormal	Intra-GBM	Granular & nodular	Normal	Nonselective	Normal or low	None
Membranoproliferative glomerulonephritis	Abnormal	Intralobular & peripheral lobular GBM	Granular & focal linear	Low or normal	Nonselective	Normal or low	None
Anaphylactoid nephritis	Abnormal	Focal GBM & mesangial	Arborized mesangial	Normal	Nonselective	Normal or low	None
Goodpasture's syndrome	Abnormal	GBM	Diffuse linear	Normal	Nonselective	Normal or low	None

[a] Selective proteinuria refers to urinary excretion of serum proteins of low molecular weight like albumin, and nonselective proteinuria includes the urinary excretion of higher molecular serum proteins in addition to albumin (Blainey et al. [12]).
[b] Glomerular basement membrane.

The features of hypocomplementemic glomerulonephritis have been described as well by Ogg [111], Herdman [57], Michael [104] and their co-workers.

In the study by Michael et al. [104], 23 patients with this disease were investigated. The average age of onset was 9.6 years (range, 4 to 14½ years), and slightly more females than males were affected. Onset of the disease was characterized clinically by gross hematuria in nine patients, asymptomatic proteinuria in seven, and insidious edema in nine. Seventeen patients had the nephrotic syndrome sometime in the course of the disease. Total serum hemolytic complement activity remained low for many years in most patients with occasional fluctuation toward normal. In many of the patients who survived into adult life, there was gradual return of the serum complement levels to normal values.

Numerous abnormalities of the complement system in this disease have been reported. West et al. [174] demonstrated low $C'3$ (β_1C globulin) levels with increased amounts of α_2D globulin, a breakdown product of $C'3$. Gewurz et al. [44] have described a complement-component profile in these patients similar to that observed in acute poststreptococcal glomerulonephritis and distinctly different from that observed in SLE. Whereas in the latter, depression of total complement and all the complement components has been demonstrated, in acute glomerulonephritis and chronic membranoproliferative glomerulonephritis total complement and $C'3$ (β_1C) are low, but $C'1$, $C'4$, and $C'2$ are normal or very minimally depressed. Page et al. [117] have demonstrated that these patients have an impaired polymorphonuclear leukocyte response when examined by the skin-window technic of Rebuck, as well as an inhibitor of leukocyte chemotaxis as studied in the Boyden chamber. Recently Pickering et al. [122] observed the presence of an inhibitor of total hemolytic complement activity in some of these patients, which may be accounted for by an increase in one of the complement inhibitors normally present in serum, or by other factors such as circulating complexes of antigen and antibody which utilize complement. The serum complement inhibitor is also present in patients with acute poststreptococcal glomerulonephritis as well, and it remains to be ascertained whether this factor is related to or caused by the renal disease. Recent studies by Pickering [121], and Alper and Rosen [2, 3] measuring the disappearance rate of radiolabeled β_1C from the circulation in chronic membranoproliferative glomerulonephritis indicate increased metabolism. The latter workers have also suggested that there may be decreased synthesis of β_1C in this disorder.

Herdman et al. [57] report that the clinical course of hypocomplementemic nephritis is slowly progressive and variable. In an observation of 145 patient years, one patient died, four received renal homotransplants because of renal failure (one of these patients had persistent hypocomplementemia after renal homotransplantation, and in spite of immunosuppressive therapy chronic nephritis developed in the transplanted organ). Significant loss in renal function usually develops after five years; however, the oldest patient had a normal glomerular filtration rate 13 years after the onset of the disease. By light microscopy, lobular glomerulonephritis, with marked hyperplasia and proliferation of glomerular mesangial cells, was a prominent feature. Silver methenamine stains demonstrated splitting of the glomerular basement membrane with deposition of nonargyrophilic material. Examination of frozen-tissue sections by immunofluorescence revealed a specific immunopathologic lesion. Early in the course of the disease IgG and β_1C are deposited along the glomerular basement membrane in an intralobular fashion (Fig. 11-11). Serial biopsies demonstrate staining of only the peripheral lobular aspects of the glomerular basement membrane for β_1C alone (Fig. 11-12). By electron microscopy extensive hyperplasia of the

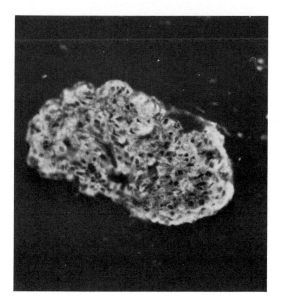

Figure 11-11. Glomerulus from a patient early in the course of chronic membranoproliferative glomerulonephritis with hypocomplementemia, showing intralobular deposition of β_1C.

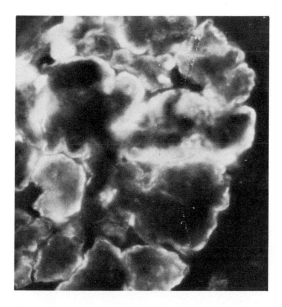

Figure 11-12. Portion of a glomerulus showing peripheral lobular deposition of β_1C focally along the glomerular basement membrane late in the course of membranoproliferative glomerulonephritis with hypocomplementemia.

mesangium, with increased mesangial matrix, is observed. There appears to be extension of mesangial cell cytoplasmic processes which project around the capillary in a subendothelial position and which contain material similar to mesangial matrix. These abnormalities in the glomerular ultrastructure account for the splitting of the basement membrane observed by light microscopy. Electron-dense deposits are occasionally seen in a subendothelial position around the glomerular capillaries. At present, the pathogenesis of this form of glomerulonephritis is not completely understood, although an antigen-antibody complex mechanism appears most probable. The distinctive features described above suggest that a single process will eventually be described to account for these findings.

Systemic Infection Associated with Glomerulonephritis

Before the advent of antibiotic therapy, the association of diffuse proliferative subacute glomerulonephritis was described by Bell [9] and others [39] in patients with subacute bacterial endocarditis. More recently Williams and Kunkel [175] have described patients with subacute bacterial endocarditis who have depression in serum complement titers. Vernier and Urizar [166], Cordeiro and his co-workers [18] and Michael and his associates [104] have performed immunofluorescent microscopy on kidney biopsy material from two patients with subacute bacterial endocarditis and have found granular nodular deposits of immunoglobulin and complement on the glomeruli. Recently Black et al. [11] and Stickler and his co-workers [145] have described the development of nephrotic syndrome and proliferative glomerulonephritis in infants having chronic bacteremia due to infected ventriculoatrial shunts that were inserted to correct obstructive hydrocephalus. In several of these patients kidney biopsies studied by immunofluorescent microscopy showed significant deposition of immunoglobulins and complement. At least one of these patients is known to have had depression of serum complement.

Soothill and Hendrickse [136] have reported a depression in $\beta_1 C$ globulin in Nigerian children with nephrotic syndrome due to chronic infection with plasmodium malaria. Protein complexes containing $\beta_1 C$ globulin were eluted in the first peak on G-200 sephadex column chromatography of serum from these patients. These findings suggest chronic circulating antigen-antibody complexes. Recent studies by Ward and Kibukamusoke [170] have demonstrated nodular thickening of the glomerular basement membrane with deposition of IgG and $\beta_1 C$ globulin in the same distribution, and these investigators were able to detect malarial antigen on the glomerular basement membrane in two out of 12 of these patients.

The nephrotic syndrome has been described during the course of secondary syphilis by Falls et al. [30] and by Spargo [137]. In each of these cases electron microscopic study of the glomeruli revealed discrete nodular deposits of electron-dense material on the epithelial side of the glomerular basement membrane (Fig. 11-13). The evidence presented in the above situations suggests that

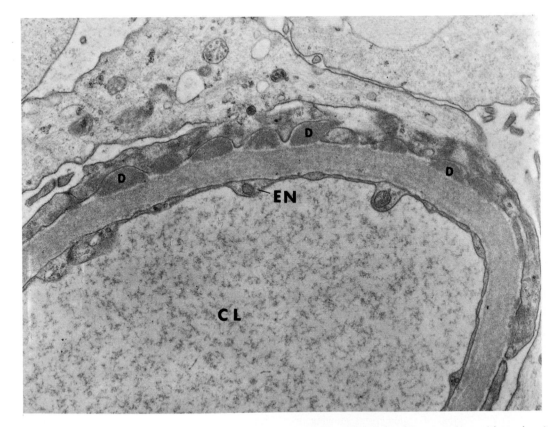

Figure 11-13. Electron photomicrograph showing a segment of a glomerulus from a patient with nephrotic syndrome due to secondary syphilis. Numerous electron-dense deposits (D) are present on the epithelial side of the glomerular basement membrane. Narrowing of the glomerular capillary lumen (CL) and endothelial cell (EN) proliferation are absent. (Photomicrograph generously provided by Dr. Benjamin Spargo.)

the mechanisms of glomerular injury in many of these instances is mediated by soluble antigen-antibody complexes, with antigens being released from the various infecting agents.

Anaphylactoid Nephritis

It has been recognized that focal proliferative glomerulonephritis develops in up to 50 per cent of patients with Henoch-Schönlein purpura [167]. Immunofluorescent studies by Urizar et al. [159] have revealed wedge-like deposits of IgG and β_1C globulin in the glomerular mesangium (Fig. 11-14). A prominent feature of this disease is the deposition of fibrin in a similar distribution in the glomerular mesangium. Ultrastructural analysis of these glomerular lesions reveals predominantly mesangial deposition with fibrin localization. In a recent study by Urizar and Herdman [158], three patients with anaphylactoid purpura who lacked clinical evidence of renal disease, with the absence of hematuria or albuminuria, were found to have significant

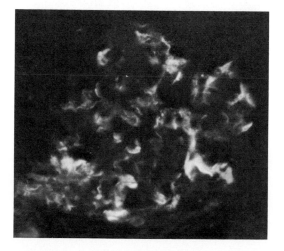

Figure 11-14. Immunofluorescent photomicrograph in anaphylactoid nephritis showing an arborized mesangial distribution of deposited IgG within the glomerulus.

deposition of fibrin within the glomerular mesangium. These observations suggest that a primary initiating process in the pathogenesis of this disease involves glomerular deposition of fibrin. Of interest, Morris [106] and Vassalli [164] and their associates have reported fibrin deposition in the glomerular lesions associated with toxemia of pregnancy.

Membranous Glomerulonephritis and Renal Vein Thrombosis

In membranous glomerulonephritis immune deposits of IgG and β_1C globulin are observed in a densely packed, finely beaded distribution within the glomerular basement membrane (Fig. 11-15). With progression of the disease, the glomerular basement membrane becomes thickened and serrated along its epithelial border (Fig. 11-16). Membranous glomerulonephritis and renal vein thrombosis occur together in a high frequency. In some cases it appears that the nephritis is present first, and the thrombosis develops secondarily. In other cases, nephrotic syndrome and nephritis occur after the thrombosis (which often is associated with trauma).

Duncan and Fish [24], who studied, by immunofluorescent microscopy, four patients with unilateral renal vein thrombosis, observed the same immunopathologic findings in both kidneys — fine microgranular fluorescence in the glomerular basement membrane (Fig. 11-17). Similar observations have been made by Cohn et al. [17]. In spite of the morphologic similarity of this lesion with Heymann's nephritis, Edgington and Fish [25] were unable to detect proximal tubular epithelial antigens in the glomerular deposits. It remains a puzzling issue to explain how a mechanical injury such as renal vein thrombosis can lead to glomerular damage most likely mediated by antigen-antibody complexes.

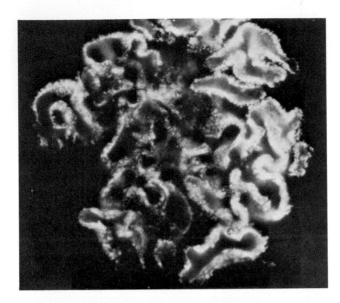

Figure 11-15. Immunofluorescent photomicrograph early in the course of membranous glomerulonephritis showing fine granular deposits of IgG within the glomerular basement membrane.

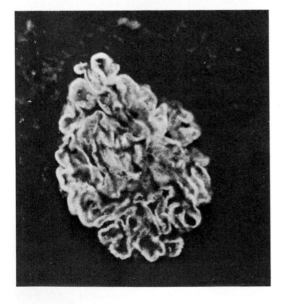

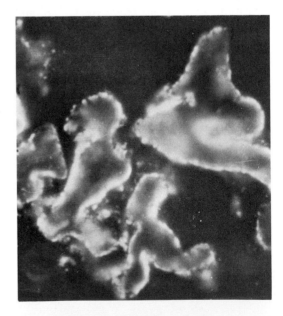

Figure 11-16. Immunofluorescent photomicrograph late in membranous glomerulonephritis showing confluence of intramembranous IgG deposits and overall thickening of the glomerular basement membrane.

Figure 11-17. High magnification, oil immersion, immunofluorescent photomicrograph showing numerous delicate granular intramembranous deposits of IgG in the glomerulus of a patient with unilateral renal vein thrombosis and nephrotic syndrome of two weeks' duration; biopsies from both kidneys revealed the same immunopathologic alteration, and were normal by light microscopic examination.

Renal Homograft Transplantation Reaction

Although hyperacute rejection of renal homografts may occur due to humoral antibodies, homograft rejection in general is mediated by cellular immunity with perivascular round cell infiltration. Considerable variation exists among the reported findings of the immunopathologic alterations in transplanted kidneys. Rosenau [130], Fish [34], and Lindquist [88] and their co-workers have observed minimal deposition of β_1C and IgG focally along the glomerular basement membrane and within the mesangium. In contrast, Porter et al. [125] and McKenzie and Whittingham [94] describe deposition of IgM, IgG, and β_1C in the majority of patients examined. Over 80 per cent of the patients reported by Porter et al. [125] have membranous or proliferative glomerulonephritis as the original kidney disease leading to transplantation; it seems likely that the glomerular immunoprotein deposits in the transplanted kidney represent transmission of the original kidney disease, partially altered by concurrent immunosuppressive therapy. Glassock et al. [47] report similar, but more severe, alterations in renal isografts in identical twin transplants with development of the original kidney disease in the transplanted organ.

In this review we have outlined an extensive body of knowledge currently accumulated which has shed considerable insight into the pathogenesis of several forms of glomerulonephritis. As an outgrowth of these studies new methods of therapy including immunosuppression (Michael et al. [105]) have been devised in an effort to alter the course in many of these situations, which otherwise would develop into progressive and life-threatening forms of advanced renal disease. It is anticipated that with further critical examination of many of the unexplored aspects of glomerulonephritis over the coming decade, new concepts in the pathogenesis of proliferative glomerulonephritis will emerge.

Acknowledgments

Aided by grants from The Minnesota Heart Association, American Heart Association, U.S. Public Health Service (HE 06314, HE 05662, AI 08677, AM 12375), and The National Foundation.

Dr. Fish is an Established Investigator of the American Heart Association.

References

1. Aarons, I. Renal immunofluorescence in NZB/NZW mice. *Nature* (London) 203: 1080, 1964.
2. Alper, C. A., Levin, A. S., and Rosen, F. S. β_1C globulin: Metabolism in glomerulonephritis. *Science* 153:180, 1966.
3. Alper, C. A., and Rosen, F. S. Studies of the in vivo behavior of human C'3 in normal subjects and patients. *J. Clin. Invest.* 46: 2021, 1967.
4. Andres, G. A., Accinni, L., Hsu, K. C., Zabriskie, J. B., and Seegal, B. C. Electron microscopic studies of human glomerulonephritis with ferritin-conjugated antibody: Localization of antigen-antibody complexes in glomerular structures of patients with acute glomerulonephritis. *J. Exp. Med.* 123: 399, 1966.
5. Andres, G. A., Morgan, C., Hsu, K. C., Rifkind, R. A., and Seegal, B. C. Electron microscopic studies of experimental nephritis with ferritin-conjugated antibody: The basement membranes and cisternae of the visceral epithelial cells in nephritic rat glomeruli. *J. Exp. Med.* 115:929, 1962.
6. Andres, G. A., Seegal, B. C., Hsu, K. C.,

Rothenberg, M. S., and Chapeau, M. L. Electron microscopic studies of experimental nephritis with ferritin-conjugated antibody. Localization of antigen-antibody complexes in rabbit glomeruli following repeated injections of bovine serum albumin. *J. Exp. Med.* 117:691, 1963.

7. Becker, C. G., and Murphy, G. E.   The experimental induction of glomerulonephritis like that in man by infection with group A streptococci. *J. Exp. Med.* 127:1, 1968.

8. Beirne, G. J., Octaviano, G. N., Kopp, W. L., and Burns, R. O.   Immunohistology of the lung in Goodpasture's syndrome. *Ann. Intern. Med.* 69:1207, 1968.

9. Bell, E. T.   Glomerulonephritis. In *Renal Diseases*. Philadelphia: Lea & Febiger, 1946. P. 153.

10. Bielschowsky, M., Helyer, B. J., and Howie, J. B.   Spontaneous hemolytic anemia in mice of the NZB/Bl strain. *Proc. Univ. Otago Med. Sch.* 37:9, 1959.

11. Black, J. A., Challacombe, D. N., and Ockenden, B. G.   Nephrotic syndrome associated with bacteremia after shunt operations for hydrocephalus. *Lancet* 2:921, 1965.

12. Blainey, J. D., Brewer, D. B., Harwicke, J., and Soothill, J. F.   The nephrotic syndrome: Diagnosis by renal biopsy and biochemical and immunological analyses related to the response to steroid therapy. *Quart. J. Med.* 29:235, 1960.

13. Burch, G. E., Chu, K. C., and Sohal, R. S.   Glomerulonephritis induced in mice by ECHO 9 virus. *New Eng. J. Med.* 279:1420, 1968.

14. Cochrane, C. G., and Hawkins, D.   Studies on circulating immune complexes: III. Factors governing the ability of circulating complexes to localize in blood vessels. *J. Exp. Med.* 127:137, 1968.

15. Cochrane, C. G., Unanue, E. R., and Dixon, F. J.   A role of polymorphonuclear leukocytes and complement in nephrotoxic nephritis. *J. Exp. Med.* 122:99, 1965.

16. Cochrane, C. G., and Ward, P. A.   The Role of Complement in Lesions Induced by Immunologic Reactions. In Grabar, P., and Miescher, P. A. (Eds.), *Immunopathology.*

Fourth International Symposium. New York: Grune & Stratton, 1965. P. 433.

17. Cohn, L. H., Lee, J., Hopper, J., and Najarian, J. S.   The treatment of bilateral renal vein thrombosis and nephrotic syndrome. *Surgery* 64:387, 1968.

18. Cordeiro, A., Costa, H., and Laginha, F.   Immunologic phase of subacute bacterial endocarditis. *Amer. J. Cardiol.* 16:477, 1965.

19. Dixon, F. J., Feldman, J. D., and Vazquez, J. J.   Experimental glomerulonephritis: The pathogenesis of a laboratory model resembling the spectrum of human glomerulonephritis. *J. Exp. Med.* 113:899, 1961.

20. Dixon, F. J., Unanue, E. R., and Watson, J. I.   Immunopathology of the Kidney. In Grabar, P., and Miescher, P. A. (Eds.), *Immunopathology. Fourth International Symposium.* New York: Grune & Stratton, 1965. P. 363.

21. Dixon, F. J., Vazquez, J. J., Weigle, W. O., and Cochrane, C. G.   Pathogenesis of serum sickness. *A.M.A. Arch. Path.* 65:18, 1958.

22. Drummond, K. N., Michael, A. F., Good, R. A., and Vernier, R. L.   The nephrotic syndrome of childhood: Immunologic, clinical and pathologic correlations. *J. Clin. Invest.* 45:620, 1966.

23. Duncan, D. A., Drummond, K. N., Michael, A. F., and Vernier, R. L.   Pulmonary hemorrhage and glomerulonephritis: Report of six cases and study of the renal lesion by fluorescent antibody technique and electron microscopy. *Ann. Intern. Med.* 62:920, 1965.

24. Duncan, D. A., and Fish, A. J.   Unpublished observations, 1969.

25. Edgington, T. S., and Fish, A. J.   Unpublished results, 1967.

26. Edgington, T. S., Glassock, R. J., and Dixon, F. J.   Autologous immune-complex pathogenesis of experimental allergic glomerulonephritis. *Science* 155:1432, 1967.

27. Edgington, T. S., Glassock, R. J., and Dixon, F. J.   Autologous immune complex nephritis induced with renal tubular antigen: I. Identification and isolation of the pathogenetic antigen. *J. Exp. Med.* 127:555, 1968.

28. Edgington, T. S., Glassock, R. J., Watson,

J. I., and Dixon, F. J. Characterization and isolation of specific renal tubular epithelial antigens. *J. Immun.* 99:1199, 1967.

29. Ellis, H. A., and Walton, K. W. Variations in serum complement in the nephrotic syndrome and other forms of renal disease. *Immunology* 1:234, 1958.

30. Falls, W. F., Ford, K. L., Ashworth, C. T., and Carter, N. W. The nephrotic syndrome in secondary syphilis: Report of a case with renal biopsy findings. *Ann. Intern. Med.* 63:1047, 1965.

31. Farquhar, M. G., and Palade, G. E. Functional evidence for the existence of a third cell type in the renal glomerulus: Phagocytosis of filtration residues by a distinctive "third" cell. *J. Cell. Biol.* 13:55, 1962.

32. Feldman, J. D. Pathogenesis of Ultrastructural Glomerular Changes Induced by Immunologic Means. In Grabar, P., and Miescher, P. A. (Eds.), *Immunopathology. Third International Symposium.* Basel: Schwabe and Company, 1963. P. 263.

33. Feldman, J. D., Mardiney, M. R., and Shuler, S. E. Immunology and morphology of acute post-streptococcal glomerulonephritis. *Lab. Invest.* 15:283, 1966.

34. Fish, A. J., Herdman, R. C., Kelly, W. D., and Good, R. A. Glomerular changes in well-functioning human renal homografts. *Transplantation* 5:1338, 1967.

35. Fish, A. J., Herdman, R. C., Michael, A. F., Pickering, R. J., and Good, R. A. Epidemic acute glomerulonephritis associated with type 49 streptococcal pyoderma: II. Correlative study of light, immunofluorescent and electron microscopic findings. *Amer. J. Med.* 48:28, 1970.

36. Fish, A. J., Michael, A. F., Good, R. A., and Vernier, R. L. Correlation of Experimental Serum Sickness Nephritis in Rabbits with Acute Poststreptococcal Glomerulonephritis in Man. In Metcoff, J. (Ed.), *Acute Glomerulonephritis. Proceedings, Seventh Annual Conference on the Kidney.* Boston: Little, Brown, 1967. P. 227.

37. Fish, A. J., Michael, A. F., Vernier, R. L., and Good, R. A. Acute serum sickness nephritis in the rabbit: An immune deposit disease. *Amer. J. Path.* 49:997, 1966.

38. Freedman, P., and Markowitz, A. S. Isolation of antibody-like gammaglobulin from lupus glomeruli. *Brit. Med. J.* 1:1175, 1962.

39. From, A. H. L., Wang, Y., Eliot, R. S., Stone, N. H., and Edwards, J. E. Aortic valvular bacterial endocarditis in tetralogy of Fallot following Blalock anastomosis. *Dis. Chest* 49:321, 1966.

40. Germuth, F. G. A comparative histologic and immunologic study in rabbits of induced hypersensitivity of the serum sickness type. *J. Exp. Med.* 97:257, 1953.

41. Germuth, F. G., Kelemen, W. A., and Pollack, A. D. Immune complex disease: II. The role of circulatory dynamics and glomerular filtration in the development of experimental glomerulonephritis. *Johns Hopkins Med. J.* 120:252, 1967.

42. Germuth, F. G., and McKinnon, G. E. Studies on the biological properties of antigen-antibody complexes: I. Anaphylactic shock induced by soluble antigen-antibody complexes in unsensitized normal guinea pigs. *Bull. Johns Hopkins Hosp.* 101:13, 1957.

43. Germuth, F. C., Valdes, A. J., Senterfit, L. B., and Pollack, A. D. A unique influence of cortisone on the transit of specific macromolecules across vascular walls in immune complex disease. *Johns Hopkins Med. J.* 122:137, 1968.

44. Gewurz, H., Pickering, R. J., Mergenhagen, S. E., and Good, R. A. The complement profile in systemic lupus erythematosus, acute glomerulonephritis and hypocomplementemic chronic glomerulonephritis. *Int. Arch. Allerg.* 34:557, 1968.

45. Gewurz, H., Shin, H. S., and Mergenhagen, S. E. Interactions of the complement system with endotoxic lipopolysaccharide: Consumption of each of the six terminal complement components. *J. Exp. Med.* 128:1049, 1968.

46. Glassock, R. J., Edgington, T. S., Watson, J. I., and Dixon, F. J. Autologous immune complex nephritis induced with renal tubular antigen: II. The pathogenetic mechanism. *J. Exp. Med.* 127:573, 1968.

47. Glassock, R. J., Feldman, D., Reynolds, E. S., Dammin, G. J., and Merrill, J. P.

Human renal isografts: A clinical and pathologic analysis. *Medicine* (Balt.) 47: 411, 1968.

48. Gotoff, S. P., Fellers, F. X., Vawter, G. F., Janeway, C. A., and Rosen, F. S. The β_1C globulin in childhood nephrotic syndrome. Laboratory diagnosis of progressive glomerulonephritis. *New Eng. J. Med.* 273:524, 1965.

49. Grishman, E., Porush, J. C., Rosen, S. M., and Churg, J. Lupus nephritis with organized deposits in the kidneys. *Lab. Invest.* 16:717, 1967.

50. Hammer, D. K., and Dixon, F. J. Experimental glomerulonephritis: II. Immunologic events in the pathogenesis of nephrotoxic serum nephritis in the rat. *J. Exp. Med.* 117:1019, 1963.

51. Hanauer, L. B., and Christian, C. L. Clinical studies of hemolytic complement and the 11S component. *Amer. J. Med.* 42:882, 1967.

52. Hawkins, D., and Cochrane, C. G. Glomerular basement membrane damage in immunological glomerulonephritis. *Immunology* 14:665, 1968.

53. Hawn, C. V. Z., and Janeway, C. A. Histological and serological sequences in experimental hypersensitivity. *J. Exp. Med.* 85:571, 1947.

54. Helyer, B. J., and Howie, J. B. Renal disease associated with positive lupus erythematosus tests in a cross-breed strain of mice. *Nature* (London) 197:197, 1963.

55. Henson, J. B., Gorham, J. R., and Tanaka, Y. Renal glomerular ultrastructure in mink affected by Aleutian disease. *Lab. Invest.* 17:123, 1967.

56. Herdman, R. C., Hong, R., Michael, A. F., and Good, R. A. Light chain distribution in immune deposits on glomeruli of kidneys in human renal disease. *J. Clin. Invest.* 46: 141, 1967.

57. Herdman, R. C., Pickering, R. J., Michael, A. F., Vernier, R. L., Fish, A. J., Gerwurz, H., and Good, R. A. Chronic glomerulonephritis associated with low serum complement activity (chronic hypocomplementemic glomerulonephritis). *Medicine* (Balt.) 49:207, 1970.

58. Herdson, P. B., Jennings, R. B., and Earle, D. P. Glomerular fine structure in poststreptococcal acute glomerulonephritis. *Arch. Path.* (Chicago) 81:117, 1966.

59. Heymann, W., Kmetec, E. P., Wilson, S. G. F., Hunter, J. L. P., Hackel, D. B., and Cuppage, F. Experimental Autoimmune Renal Disease in Rats. In Grabar, P., and Miescher, P. A. (Eds.), *Immunopathology. Third International Symposium.* Basel: Schwabe and Company, 1963. P. 240.

60. Hinkle, N. H., Partin, J., and West, C. D. Nephropathy in mice after exposure to Group A Type 12 streptococci. *J. Lab. Clin. Med.* 56:265, 1960.

61. Holm, S. E., Jönsson, J., and Zettergren, L. Experimental streptococcal nephritis in rabbits. *Acta Path. Microbiol. Scand.* 69:417, 1967.

62. Holmes, M. C., and Burnet, F. M. The natural history of autoimmune disease in NZB mice: A comparison with the pattern of human autoimmune manifestations. *Ann. Intern. Med.* 59:265, 1963.

63. Hunter, J. L. P., Hackel, D. B., and Heymann, W. Nephrotic syndrome in rats produced by sensitization to rat kidney proteins: Immunologic studies. *J. Immun.* 85: 319, 1960.

64. Ishizaka, K. Gamma Globulin and Molecular Mechanisms in Hypersensitivity Reactions. In Kallos, P., and Waksman, B. (Eds.), *Progress in Allergy.* Basel: S. Karger, 1963. Vol. 7, p. 32.

65. Ishizaka, K., Ishizaka, T., and Campbell, D. H. The biological activity of soluble antigen-antibody complexes: II. Physical properties of soluble complexes having skin-irritating activity. *J. Exp. Med.* 109:127, 1959.

66. Ishizaka, K., Ishizaka, T., and Campbell, D. H. Biological activity of soluble antigen-antibody complexes: III. Various antigen-antibody systems and the probable role of complement. *J. Immun.* 83:105, 1959.

67. Katz, D. H., Unanue, E. R., and Dixon, F. J. Nephritogenic properties of cross-reacting kidney-fixing antibodies to heart, spleen and muscle. *J. Immun.* 98:260, 1967.

68. Kay, C. F. The mechanism by which experimental nephritis is produced in rabbits injected with nephrotoxic duck serum. *J. Exp. Med.* 72:559, 1940.

69. Kellett, C. E., and Thomson, J. G. Complement activity of blood serum in nephritis. *J. Path. Bact.* 48:519, 1939.

70. Kelly, D. K., and Winn, J. F. Renal lesions produced by Group A Type 12 streptococci. *Science* 127:1337, 1958.

71. Kimmelstiel, P., Kim, O. J., and Beres, J. Studies on renal biopsy specimens, with the aid of the electron microscope: II. Glomerulonephritis and glomerulonephrosis. *Amer. J. Clin. Path.* 38:280, 1962.

72. Kindig, D., Spargo, B., and Kirsten, W. H. Glomerular response in Aleutian disease of mink. *Lab. Invest.* 16:436, 1967.

73. Kniker, W. T., and Cochrane, C. G. The localization of circulating immune complexes in experimental serum sickness: The role of vasoactive amines and hydrodynamic forces. *J. Exp. Med.* 127:119, 1968.

74. Koffler, D., and Kunkel, H. G. Mechanisms of renal injury in systemic lupus erythematosus. *Amer. J. Med.* 45:165, 1968.

75. Koffler, D., Sandson, J., Carr, R., and Kunkel, H. G. Immunologic studies concerning the pulmonary lesion in Goodpasture's syndrome. *Amer. J. Path.* 54:293, 1969.

76. Koffler, D., Schur, P. H., and Kunkel, H. G. Immunological studies concerning the nephritis of systemic lupus erythematosus. *J. Exp. Med.* 126:607, 1967.

77. Lachmann, P. J., Müller-Eberhard, H. J., Kunkel, H. G., and Paronetto, F. The localization of in vivo bound complement in tissue sections. *J. Exp. Med.* 115:63, 1962.

78. Lambert, P. H., and Dixon, F. J. Pathogenesis of the glomerulonephritis of NZB/W mice. *J. Exp. Med.* 127:507, 1968.

79. Lange, K. In Metcoff, J. (Ed.), *Proceedings of the Ninth Annual Conference on the Nephrotic Syndrome.* New York: National Kidney Foundation, 1958. P. 13.

80. Lange, K., Treser, G., Sagel, I., Ty, A., and Wasserman, E. Routine immunohistology in renal diseases. *Ann. Intern. Med.* 64:25, 1966.

81. Lange, K., Wachstein, M., and McPherson, S. E. Immunologic mechanism of transmission of experimental glomerulonephritis in parabiotic rats. *Proc. Soc. Exp. Biol. Med.* 106:13, 1961.

82. Lange, K., Wasserman, E., and Slobody, L. B. The significance of serum complement levels with the diagnosis and prognosis of acute and subacute glomerulonephritis and lupus erythematosus disseminatus. *Ann. Intern. Med.* 53:636, 1960.

83. Latta, H., and Maunsbach, A. B. Relations of the central lobular region of the glomerulus to the juxtaglomerular apparatus. *J. Ultrastruct. Res.* 6:562, 1962.

84. Lerner, R. A., and Dixon, F. J. Transfer of ovine experimental allergic glomerulonephritis (EAG) with serum. *J. Exp. Med.* 124:431, 1966.

85. Lerner, R. A., and Dixon, F. J. The induction of acute glomerulonephritis in rabbits with soluble antigens isolated from normal homologous and autologous urine. *J. Immun.* 100:1277, 1968.

86. Lerner, R. A., Glassock, R. J., and Dixon, F. J. The role of antiglomerular basement membrane antibody in the pathogenesis of human glomerulonephritis. *J. Exp. Med.* 126:989, 1967.

87. Lindberg, L. H., Vosti, K. L., and Raffel, S. Experimental streptococcal glomerulonephritis in rats. *J. Immun.* 98:1231, 1967.

88. Lindquist, R. R., Guttmann, R. D., Merrill, J. P., and Dammin, G. J. Human renal allografts: Interpretation of morphologic and immunohistochemical observations. *Amer. J. Path.* 53:851, 1968.

89. Longscope, W. T. The production of experimental nephritis by repeated protein intoxication. *J. Exp. Med.* 18:678, 1913.

90. Markowitz, A. S., Clasen, R., Nidus, B. D., and Ainus, H. Streptococcal related glomerulonephritis: II. Glomerulonephritis in rhesus monkeys immunologically induced both actively and passively with a soluble fraction from human glomeruli. *J. Immun.* 98:161, 1967.

91. Markowitz, A. S., and Lange, C. F. Streptococcal related glomerulonephritis: I. Isolation, immunochemistry and comparative chemistry of soluble fractions from Type 12

nephritogenic streptococci and human glomeruli. *J. Immun.* 92:565, 1964.

92. McClean, C. R., Fitzgerald, J. D. L., Young-
husband, O. Z., and Hamilton, J. D. Diffuse glomerulonephritis induced in rabbits
by small intravenous injections of horse
serum. *A.M.A. Arch. Path.* 51:1, 1951.

93. McCluskey, R. T., Vassalli, P., Gallo, G.,
and Baldwin, D. S. An immunofluorescent
study of pathogenic mechanisms in glomerular diseases. *New Eng. J. Med.* 274:695,
1966.

94. McKenzie, I. F. C., and Whittingham, S.
Deposits of immunoglobulin and fibrin in
human allografted kidneys. *Lancet* 2:1313,
1968.

95. Mellors, R. C. Autoimmune disease in
NZB/Bl mice: I. Pathology and pathogenesis of the model system of spontaneous
glomerulonephritis. *J. Exp. Med.* 122:25,
1965.

96. Mellors, R. C., Arias-Stella, J., Siegel, M.,
and Pressman, D. Analytical pathology:
II. Histopathologic demonstration of glo-
merular-localizing antibodies in experimental glomerulonephritis. *Amer. J. Path.*
31:687, 1955.

97. Mellors, R. C., and Huang, C. Y. Immunopathology of NZB/Bl mice: VI.
Virus separable from spleen and pathogenic
for Swiss mice. *J. Exp. Med.* 126:53, 1967.

98. Mellors, R. C., and Ortega, L. G. Analytical pathology: III. New observations on
the pathogenesis of glomerulonephritis,
lipoid nephrosis, periarteritis nodosa and
secondary amyloidosis in man. *Amer. J.
Path.* 32:455, 1956.

99. Mellors, R. C., Ortega, L. G., and Holman,
H. R. Role of gamma globulins in pathogenesis of renal lesions in systemic lupus
erythematosus and chronic membranous
glomerulonephritis, with an observation on
the lupus erythematosus cell reaction. *J.
Exp. Med.* 106:191, 1957.

100. Menefee, M. G., Mueller, C. B., Bell, A. L.,
and Myers, J. K. Transport of globin by
the renal glomerulus. *J. Exp. Med.* 120:
1129, 1964.

101. Michael, A. F., Drummond, K. N., Good,
R. A., and Vernier, R. L. Acute poststrep-

tococcal glomerulonephritis: Immune deposit disease. *J. Clin. Invest.* 45:237, 1966.

102. Michael, A. F., Drummond, K. N., Vernier,
R. L., and Good, R. A. Immunologic basis
of renal disease. *Pediat. Clin. N. Amer.* 11:
685, 1964.

103. Michael, A. F., Fish, A. J., and Good, R. A.
Glomerular localization and transport of
aggregated proteins in mice. *Lab. Invest.*
17:14, 1967.

104. Michael, A. F., Herdman, R. C., Fish,
A. J., Pickering, R. J., and Vernier, R. L.
Chronic membranoproliferative glomer-
ulonephritis with hypocomplementemia.
Transplant. Proc. 1:925, 1969.

105. Michael, A. F., Vernier, R. L., Drummond,
K. N., Levitt, J. I., Herdman, R. C., Fish,
A. J., and Good, R. A. Immunosuppres-
sive therapy of chronic renal disease. *New
Eng. J. Med.* 276:817, 1967.

106. Morris, R. H., Vassalli, P., Beller, F. K.,
and McCluskey, R. T. Immunofluorescent
studies of renal biopsies in the diagnosis of
toxemia of pregnancy. *Obstet. Gynec.* 24:32,
1964.

107. Movat, H. Z., and DiLorenzo, N. L. Activation of the plasma kinin system by antigen-antibody aggregates: I. Generation of
permeability factor in guinea pig serum.
Lab. Invest. 19:187, 1968.

108. Movat, H. Z., DiLorenzo, N. L., and Tre-
loar, M. P. Activation of the plasma kinin
system by antigen-antibody aggregates: II.
Isolation of permeability-enhancing and
kinin-releasing fractions from activated
guinea pig serum. *Lab. Invest.* 19:201, 1968.

109. Movat, H. Z., Steiner, J. W., and Huhn, D.
The fine structure of the glomerulus in
acute glomerulonephritis. *Lab. Invest.* 11:
117, 1962.

110. Müller-Eberhard, H. J., Nilsson, U. R.,
Dalmasso, A. P., Polley, M. J., and Calcott,
M. A. A molecular concept of immune
cytolysis. *Arch. Path.* (Chicago) 82:205,
1966.

111. Ogg, C. S., Cameron, J. S., and White,
R. H. R. The C′3 component of complement (β_1C globulin) in patients with heavy
proteinuria. *Lancet* 2:78, 1968.

112. Okuda, R., Kaplan, M. H., Cuppage, F. E.,

and Heymann, W. Deposition of autologous gamma globulin in kidneys of rats with nephrotic renal disease of various etiologies. *J. Lab. Clin. Med.* 66:204, 1965.

113. Oldstone, M. B. A., and Dixon, F. J. Lymphocytic choriomeningitis: Production of antibody by "tolerant" infected mice. *Science* 158:1193, 1967.

114. Oldstone, M. B. A., and Dixon, F. J. Pathogenesis of chronic disease associated with persistent lymphocytic choriomeningitis viral infection: I. Relationship with antibody production to disease in neonatally infected mice. *J. Exp. Med.* 129:483, 1969.

115. Osawa, G., Beres, J., and Kimmelstiel, P. Glomerulonephritis: Observations by light and electron microscopy. *Amer. J. Clin. Path.* 46:295, 1966.

116. Osler, A. G., Oliveira, B., Shin, H. S., and Sandberg, A. L. The fixation of guinea pig complement by γ_1 and γ_2 immunoglobulins. *J. Immun.* 102:269, 1969.

117. Page, A. R., Gewurz, H., Pickering, R. J., and Good, R. A. The Role of Complement in the Acute Inflammatory Response. In Miescher, P. A., and Grabar, P. (Eds.). *Immunopathology. Fifth International Symposium.* New York: Grune & Stratton, 1967. P. 221.

118. Palmer, J. M., Eversole, S. L., and Stamey, T. A. Unilateral glomerulonephritis: Virtual absence of nephritis in a kidney with partial occlusion of the main renal artery. *Amer. J. Med.* 40:816, 1966.

119. Paronetto, F., and Koffler, D. Autoimmune proliferative glomerulonephritis in monkeys. *Amer. J. Path.* 50:887, 1967.

120. Pfeiffer, E. F., et al. Studien zur "Übertragung" der Masuginephritis der Ratte: II. Die Übertragung durch Parabiose genetisch gleichartiger Partner. *Z. Ges. Exp. Med.* 132:436, 1960.

121. Pickering, R. J. In preparation.

122. Pickering, R. J., Gewurz, H., and Good, R. A. Complement inactivation by serum from patients with acute and hypocomplementemic chronic glomerulonephritis. *J. Lab. Clin. Med.* 72:298, 1968.

123. Pincus, T., Haberkern, R., and Christian, C. L. Experimental chronic glomerulitis. *J. Exp. Med.* 127:819, 1968.

124. Porter, D. D., and Larson, A. E. Aleutian disease of mink: Infectious virus-antibody complexes in the serum. *Proc. Soc. Exp. Biol. Med.* 126:680, 1967.

125. Porter, K. A., Andres, G. A., Calder, M. W., Dossetor, J. B., Hsu, K. C., Rendall, J. M., Seegal, B. C., and Starzl, T. E. Human renal transplants: II. Immunofluorescent and immunoferritin studies. *Lab. Invest.* 18:159, 1968.

126. Rammelkamp, C. H., Jr., and Weaver, R. S. Acute glomerulonephritis: The significance of the variations in the incidence of the disease. *J. Clin. Invest.* 32:345, 1953.

127. Reed, R. W., and Matheson, B. H. Experimental nephritis due to type-specific streptococci: I. The effect of a single exposure to type 12 streptococci. *J. Infect. Dis.* 95:191, 1954.

128. Rich, A. R., and Gregory, J. E. The experimental demonstration that periarteritis nodosa is a manifestation of hypersensitivity. *Bull. Johns Hopkins Hosp.* 72:65, 1943.

129. Rich, A. R., and Gregory, J. E. Experimental evidence that lesions with basic characteristics of rheumatic carditis can result from anaphylactic hypersensitivity. *Bull. Johns Hopkins Hosp.* 73:239, 1943.

130. Rosenau, W., Lee, J. C., and Najarian, J. S. A light, fluorescence, and electron microscopic study of functioning human renal transplants. *Surg. Gynec. Obstet.* 128:62, 1969.

131. Schick, B. Nachkrankheiten des Scharlach. *Jahrb. Kinderheilk.* 65:132, 1907.

132. Schwab, L., Moll, F. C., Hall, T., Brean, H., Kirk, M., Van Zandt, C., Hawn, M. D., and Janeway, C. A. Experimental hypersensitivity in the rabbit: Effect of inhibition of antibody formation by x-radiation or nitrogen mustards on the histologic and serologic consequences, and on the behavior of serum complement, following single large injections of foreign proteins. *J. Exp. Med.* 91:505, 1950.

133. Seegal, B. C., Andres, G. A., Hsu, K. C., and Zabriskie, J. B. Studies on the pathogenesis of acute and progressive glomerulo-

nephritis in man by immunofluorescein and immunoferritin techniques. *Fed. Proc.* 24: 100, 1965.

134. Seegal, B. C., Hasson, M. W., Gaynor, E. C., and Rothenberg, M. S. Glomerulonephritis produced in dogs by specific antisera: I. The course of the disease resulting from the injection of rabbit antidog-placenta serum or rabbit antidog-kidney serum. *J. Exp. Med.* 102:789, 1955.

135. Snyderman, R., Shin, H. S., Phillips, J. K., Gewurz, H., and Mergenhagen, S. E. A neutrophil chemotactic factor derived from C′5 upon interaction of guinea pig serum with endotoxin. *J. Immun.* 103:413, 1969.

136. Soothill, J. F., and Hendrickse, R. G. Some immunological studies of the nephrotic syndrome of Nigerian children. *Lancet* 2:629, 1967.

137. Spargo, B. Personal communication, 1968.

138. Steblay, R. W. Glomerulonephritis induced in sheep by injections of heterologous glomerular basement and Freund's complete adjuvant. *J. Exp. Med.* 116:253, 1962.

139. Steblay, R. W. Glomerulonephritis induced in monkeys by injections of heterologous glomerular basement membrane and Freund's adjuvant. *Nature* (London) 197: 1173, 1963.

140. Steblay, R. W. Glomerulonephritis Induced in Sheep and Monkeys by Injections of Heterologous Glomerular Basement Membrane and Freund's Adjuvant. In Grabar, P., and Miescher, P. A. (Eds.), *Immunopathology. Third International Symposium.* Basel: Schwabe and Company, 1963. P. 252.

141. Steblay, R. W. Transfer of nephritis from sheep with autoimmune nephritis to recipient sheep by artery-to-artery cross circulation. *Fed. Proc.* 23:449, 1964. (Abstract.)

142. Steblay, R. W., and Rudofsky, U. Autoimmune glomerulonephritis induced in sheep by injections of human lung and Freund's adjuvant. *Science* 160:204, 1968.

143. Steblay, R. W., and Rudofsky, U. In vitro and in vivo properties of autoantibodies eluted from kidneys of sheep with autoimmune glomerulonephritis. *Nature* (London) 218:1269, 1968.

144. Stetson, C. A., Rammelkamp, C. H., Krause, R. M., Kohen, R. J., and Perry, W. D. Epidemic acute nephritis: Studies on etiology, natural history and prevention. *Medicine* (Balt.) 34:431, 1955.

145. Stickler, G. B., Shin, M. H., Burke, E. C., Holley, K. E., Miller, R. H., and Segar, W. E. Diffuse glomerulonephritis associated with infected ventriculo-atrial shunt. *New Eng. J. Med.* 279:1077, 1968.

146. Tan, E. M., Hackel, D. B., and Kaplan, M. H. Renal tubular lesions in mice produced by Group A streptococci grown in intraperitoneal diffusion chambers. *J. Infect. Dis.* 108:107, 1961.

147. Tan, E. M., Schur, P. H., Carr, R. I., and Kunkel, H. G. Deoxyribonucleic acid (DNA) and antibodies to DNA in the serum of patients with systemic lupus erythematosus. *J. Clin. Invest.* 45:1732, 1966.

148. Teague, P. O., Yunis, E. J., Rodey, G. E., Fish, A. J., Stutman, O., and Good, R. A. Autoimmune phenomena and renal disease in inbred mice: Role of thymectomy aging and involution of immunologic capacity. *Lab. Invest.* 22:121, 1970.

149. Tojo, T., and Friou, G. J. Lupus nephritis: Varying complement-fixing properties of immunoglobulin G antibodies to antigens of cell nuclei. *Science* 161:904, 1968.

150. Trapani, I. L., Garvey, J. S., and Campbell, D. H. Stimulating action of soluble antigen-antibody complexes in normal guinea pig smooth muscle. *Science* 127:700, 1958.

151. Treser, G., Semar, M., McVicar, M., Franklin, M., Ty, A., Sagel, I., and Lange, K. Antigenic streptococcal components in acute nephritis. *Science* 163:676, 1969.

152. Tsuzuku, O., Yagi, Y., and Pressman, D. Highly specific lung localizing antibodies. *J. Immun.* 99:1, 1967.

153. Tucker, E. S., and Wuepper, K. D. Contact factor (CF) activation of rabbit kininogenase. *Fed. Proc.* 28:363, 1969.

154. Unanue, E. R., and Dixon, F. J. Experimental Glomerulonephritis: Immunopathological Events and Pathogenic Mechanisms. In Dixon, F. J., and Humphrey, J. H. (Eds.), *Advances in Immunology.* New York: Academic, 1967. Vol. 6, p. 1.

155. Unanue, F. R., and Dixon, F. J. Experimental allergic glomerulonephritis induced in the rabbit with heterologous renal antigens. *J. Exp. Med.* 125:149, 1967.

156. Unanue, E. R., Dixon, F. J., and Feldman, J. D. Experimental allergic glomerulonephritis induced in rabbits with homologous renal antigens. *J. Exp. Med.* 125:163, 1967.

157. Unanue, E. R., Lee, S., Dixon, F. J., and Feldman, J. D. Experimental glomerulonephritis: VII. The absence of an autoimmune antikidney response in nephrotoxic serum nephritis. *J. Exp. Med.* 122:565, 1965.

158. Urizar, R. E., and Herdman, R. C. Anaphylactoid purpura: III. Early morphologic glomerular changes. *Amer. J. Clin. Path.* 53:258, 1970.

159. Urizar, R. E., Michael, A. F., Sisson, S., and Vernier, R. L. Anaphylactoid purpura: II. Immunofluorescent and electron microscopic studies of the glomerular lesions. *Lab. Invest.* 19:437, 1968.

160. Valdes, A. J., Senterfit, L. B., Pollack, A. D., and Germuth, F. G. The effect of antigen excess on chronic immune complex glomerulonephritis. *Johns Hopkins Med. J.* 124:9, 1969.

161. Vassalli, P., and McCluskey, R. T. The pathogenic role of fibrin deposition in immunologically induced glomerulonephritis. *Ann. N.Y. Acad. Sci.* 116:1052, 1964.

162. Vassalli, P., and McCluskey, R. T. The pathogenic role of the coagulation process in rabbit Masugi nephritis. *Amer. J. Path.* 45:653, 1964.

163. Vassalli, P., and McCluskey, R. T. The coagulation process and glomerular disease. *Amer. J. Med.* 39:179, 1965.

164. Vassalli, P., Morris, R. H., and McCluskey, R. T. The pathogenic role of fibrin deposition in the glomerular lesions of toxemia of pregnancy. *J. Exp. Med.* 118:467, 1963.

165. Vernier, R. L., Tinglof, B., Urizar, R., Litman, N., and Smith, F., Jr. Immunofluorescence Studies in Renal Disease. In *The Proceedings of the Third International Congress of Nephrology.* (Washington, 1966.) Basel/New York: Karger, 1967. Vol. 3, p. 83.

166. Vernier, R. L., and Urizar, R. E. Personal communication, 1969.

167. Vernier, R. L., Worthen, H. G., Peterson, R. D. A., Colle, E., and Good, R. A. Anaphylactoid purpura: I. Pathology of the skin and kidney and frequency of streptococcal infection. *Pediatrics* 27:181, 1961.

168. Vogt, A., Bockhorn, H., Kozima, K., and Sasaki, K. Electron microscopic localization of the nephrotoxic antibody in the glomeruli of the rat after intravenous application of purified nephritogenic antibody-ferritin conjugates. *J. Exp. Med.* 127:867, 1968.

169. Ward, P. A., Cochrane, C. G., Müller-Eberhard, H. J. The role of serum complement in chemotaxis of leukocytes in vitro. *J. Exp. Med.* 122:327, 1965.

170. Ward, P. A., and Kibukamusoke, J. W. Evidence for soluble immune complexes in the pathogenesis of glomerulonephritis of quartan malaria. *Lancet* 1:283, 1969.

171. Weigle, W. O., and High, G. L. The behaviour of autologous thyroglobulin in the circulation of rabbits immunized with either heterologous or altered homologous thyroglobulin. *J. Immun.* 98:1105, 1967.

172. West, C. D., McAdams, A. J., McConville, J. M., Davis, N. C., and Holland, N. H. Hypocomplementemic and normocomplementemic persistent (chronic) glomerulonephritis; clinical and pathologic characteristics. *J. Pediat.* 67:1089, 1965.

173. West, C. D., Northway, J. D., and Davis, N. C. Serum levels of beta$_1$C globulin, a complement component, in the nephritides, lipoid nephrosis and other conditions. *J. Clin. Invest.* 43:1507, 1964.

174. West, C. D., Winter, S., Forristal, J., McConville, J. M., and Davis, N. C. Evidence for in vivo breakdown of β_1C globulin in hypocomplementemic glomerulonephritis. *J. Clin. Invest.* 46:539, 1967.

175. Williams, R. C., and Kunkel, H. G. Rheumatoid factor, complement, and conglutinin aberrations in patients with subacute bacterial endocarditis. *J. Clin. Invest.* 41:666, 1962.

12

Pathology of Acute Glomerulonephritis

R. H. Heptinstall

The clinical syndrome of acute glomerulonephritis is attended by a surprisingly consistent histologic picture — that is, an acute inflammatory reaction in the glomeruli. The adjective acute is appropriate for both the clinical and the histologic picture. This is unique when the whole spectrum of glomerulonephritis is considered, for in general, one is confronted by a bewildering array of terms.

In this brief chapter the pathologic picture of acute *diffuse* glomerulonephritis is described, the type that follows group A streptococcal infection being taken as the model. This is the type that has received the greatest attention from clinician, pathologist, epidemiologist, and immunologist alike. No discussion of focal glomerulonephritis is given here since this is adequately discussed in Chapter 14. In addition, an account is given of the pathology of the various courses that acute glomerulonephritis might take.

Pathology of Acute Poststreptococcal Glomerulonephritis

The advent of the renal biopsy has contributed greatly to our knowledge of the pathology of glomerulonephritis, but it should be remembered that the pathology of acute glomerulonephritis was well characterized, at least from the point of view of light microscopy, as a result of autopsy studies. The biopsy, however, has permitted the study of the disease process at different stages in its evolution, and because of the freshness of the tissue, has permitted studies such as electron microscopy and immunofluorescence to be carried out.

MACROSCOPIC APPEARANCE

The kidneys are enlarged up to twice normal size. They may be pale or dark, with a cut surface that bulges because of interstitial edema; the subcapsular surface is smooth. The glomeruli can usually be made out as gray dots, although in some cases the eye of faith may be required to perceive this.

LIGHT MICROSCOPIC APPEARANCE

Glomeruli. With the light microscope, the main abnormalities are in the glomeruli, all of which are affected, usually to an equal degree. The capillary tufts are somewhat enlarged, appear more solid than usual, and contain large numbers of nuclei. The capillary lumina lack their usual patency. Most of the increased cells are either endothelial or mesangial, the latter causing the lobules to be somewhat club-shaped, with varying numbers of polymorphonuclear leukocytes in both the mesangium and the capillary lumina (Fig. 12-1). Epithelial cells of the tuft may be more conspicuous than usual, mainly because they are swollen; they are not greatly increased in numbers. The capillary basement membranes of the tuft are not appreciably thickened, and there is usually no proliferation of the cells lining Bowman's capsule with crescent formation, although crescents may be seen, particularly in the severe cases. With a Heidenhain stain, Jennings and Earle [25] have described small red dots along the outer side of the capillary basement membranes, and using Gomori's trichrome method, Strunk et al. [47] have described red dots against green basement membranes. These dots — which may also be seen in favorable circumstances in toluidine blue-stained, 0.5 micron, plastic-embedded sections — correspond to the electron-dense deposits seen by electron microscopy on the epithelial side of the lamina densa, the so-called humps.

There has long been a controversy about

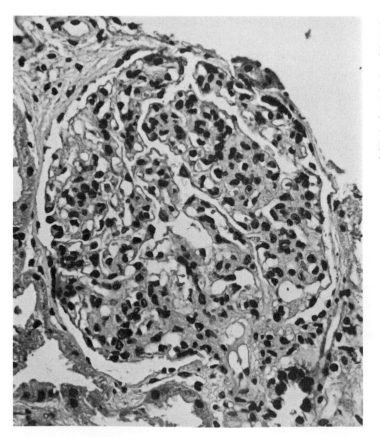

Figure 12-1. Renal biopsy from a 24-year-old woman with acute poststreptococcal glomerulonephritis. The glomerulus shows a broadening of the lobules, increase in cellularity, with moderate numbers of polymorphs, and reduction of the capillary lumina. Complete clinical recovery took place in a period of weeks. Hematoxylin and eosin. ×400.

the type of cell involved in the cellular increase in the glomeruli. Langhans [32] originally considered endothelial cells to be the main component, but the predominantly mesangial distribution of the cells raises the possibility of mesangial or even nonindigenous mononuclear cells taking part in the increase [20, 27]. Polymorphonuclear leukocytes vary considerably in their numbers, and in general there may be very large numbers of them in a form referred to as the exudative (Fig. 12-2) and regarded by Jennings and Earle [25] as being likely to lead to "subacute" glomerulonephritis.

Changes other than an increase in cells take place in the mesangium. MacCallum [35] described exudation into the mesangium — or intercapillary space, as he referred to it — and how this exudate could become organized in those cases of the disease entering a chronic stage. McGregor [38] has described fine blue fibers situated between proliferating endothelial cells and polymorphonuclear leukocytes in Heidenhain-stained sections. These fibers increased in number and size, ending up as a hyaline mass in cases that failed to resolve. McGregor [38] considered the location of these fibers to be intracapillary — as did Bell [4, 5] — but neither of these authors believed in a mesangium, and it is probable that the fibers were in fact situated in what is now regarded as mesangium. Jones [27] has also described fibers in the mesangium, referring to them as fibromucin fibers. The importance of these various changes lies in their relation to the processes of resolution or progression to chronicity. In cases that progress into the stage of latent chronic glomerulonephritis, there is solidification in the mesangial area manifest as eosinophilic areas in the center of the lobules, a change referred to as centrolobular hyalinization. The question of the

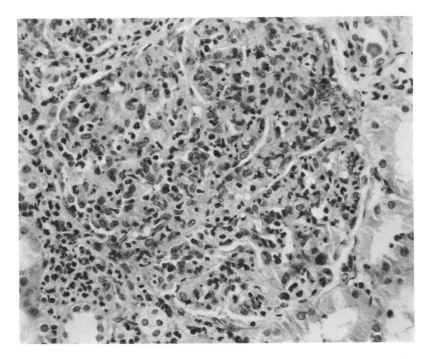

Figure 12-2. Acute glomerulonephritis with considerable polymorph "exudative" change. Hematoxylin and eosin. ×390.

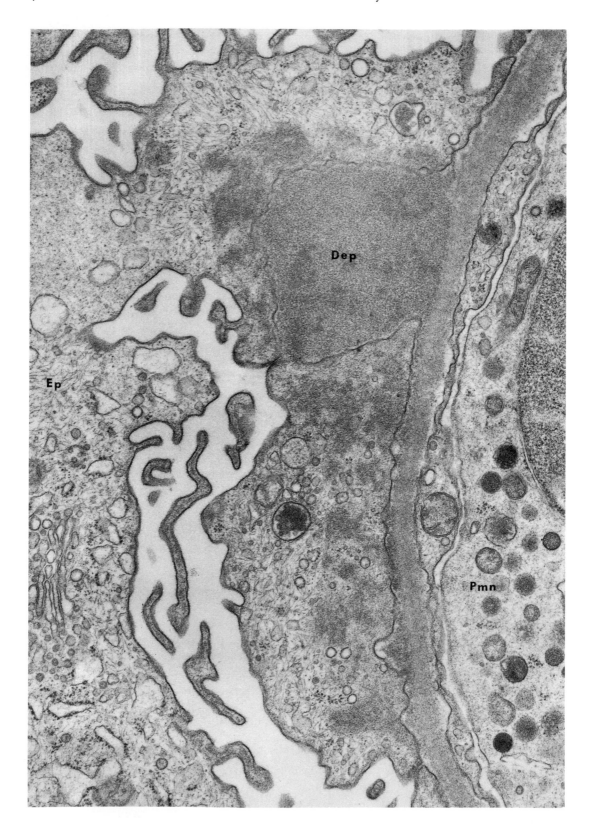

reversibility of areas characterized by centrolobular eosinophilic changes has not been completely resolved; reference is made to this later.

Tubules. Tubular changes are not usually very striking, but the epithelial cells sometimes appear swollen, and hyaline droplets may be observed. The lumina of the tubules may contain red blood cells which are often found in the presence of eosinophilic cast-like material. In cases with the pronounced polymorphonuclear leukocyte reaction in the glomeruli there are likely to be similar leukocytes in the lumen of proximal convoluted segments [7].

Some authors have been impressed with a change described as "advanced focal degeneration" [24]. This consisted of dilatation of distal convoluted tubules with degeneration of epithelium and sometimes disruption of the wall; the interstitium in adjacent areas showed a cellular reaction. Flattening of epithelium and dilatation of the lumen were also described as occurring in the proximal convoluted segment. The suggestion was made that the tubular changes were the result of a process similar to that producing the glomerular lesions rather than a consequence of ischemia. I have not been impressed with tubular changes except in rare cases where the clinical course has been more prolonged and glomerular damage has been severe; in such an event the proximal convoluted segment may exhibit focal loss, or dilatation with a change to a lower type of epithelium.

Epithelial vacuolation of both a fine and a coarse type has been described in the epithelium of the proximal convoluted tubules [53]. Tubular vacuolation is seen so frequently in diverse conditions in a busy renal-biopsy service that it is doubtful if any special significance can be attached to this observation.

Interstitium. The interstitium may show no dramatic changes, but in some instances there may be edema and scattered cellular foci; the cells may be polymorphonuclear leukocytes, mononuclears, or lymphocytes. As noted above, cellular infiltrates have been described in relation to tubular changes [24], and extensive lymphocytic infiltration has been noted in certain repeat biopsies by Kushner et al. [30]. When acute glomerulonephritis is found as part of a streptococcal septicemia — a seemingly rare event nowadays — there are large numbers of polymorphonuclear cells in the interstitium.

Vessels. Arteries and arterioles usually show little abnormality. Fordham et al. [17] have described polyarteritic changes in poststreptococcal glomerulonephritis, but this is a very rare event.

ELECTRON MICROSCOPIC FINDINGS

The most significant feature on electron microscopy is that of electron-dense deposits, the so-called humps, that are situated on the epithelial side of the lamina densa of the capillary wall (Fig. 12-3). These take the form of discrete mounds, and differ in their numbers from case to case. They are more frequent in relation to capillaries adjacent to the mesangium. They have been seen as early as eight days after onset of the disease [29], but are purely evanescent structures and invariably disappear by six weeks after onset [23]. Such deposits are also seen in the experimental serum sickness type of glomerulonephritis [9,

Figure 12-3. Glomerular capillary wall from a patient with acute glomerulonephritis. The visceral epithelial cell (Ep) is toward the left, and the capillary lumen containing a polymorphonuclear leukocyte (Pmn) is toward the right. The visceral epithelium exhibits loss of foot-process organization and along the basement membrane shows aggregates of material within the cell sap. At one point the epithelium is separated from the basement membrane by a large deposit (Dep). In the cytoplasm surrounding the deposit there are aggregates of the dense material in the cytoplasmic ground substance. The epithelial cell also exhibits microvilli along the cell surface. Specimen fixed in 2% OsO₄ buffered with s-collidine: section double stained with uranyl acetate and lead hydroxide. ×18,000. (Supplied by Dr. Glenn C. Faith.)

16], and in exacerbations of chronic glomeru-lonephritis [10]. The humps, as seen by elec-tron microscopy, are considered to correspond to the finely nodular nonlinear pattern of im-munofluorescence when the glomeruli are treated with fluorescent antiserum to im-munoglobulins, and beta-1-C (β_1C) globulin.

The endothelial pores may be decreased, and the endothelial cytoplasm eroded, with poly-morphonuclear leukocytes adherent to the denuded basement membrane [10]. The basement membrane is in general unaltered, but in localized areas it may show a patchy in-crease in density, simple thickening, or thick-ening with areas of rarefaction. Localized areas of fusion of foot processes may be found, and cytoplasmic droplets may be seen in epi-thelial cells of the glomerular tuft.

The cells in the expanded mesangial areas consist of mesangial cells and adjacent endo-thelial cells; processes of the former cells can often be seen extending out peripherally be-tween the basement membrane and the endo-thelium [14]. Some of the cells in the mesangial area are unidentified mononuclear cells [47], while polymorphonuclear cells are also found.

Fibrin is rarely seen in the glomeruli in acute poststreptococcal glomerulonephritis with the use of the light or the electron micro-scope; this fact initially is surprising in view of the frequency with which it can be dem-onstrated by immunofluorescent technics [37]. However, the fluorescent antifibrinogen serum used also stains precursors of fibrin which may not be visible to the electron micro-scope. Dodge et al. [10] have demonstrated fibrin in glomeruli in acute exacerbations of chronic glomerulonephritis, contrasting this with its rarity in initial attacks of acute post-streptococcal glomerulonephritis.

In cases proceeding to chronicity, as evi-denced clinically by persistent proteinuria, there is an increase of basement membrane-like material [10], presumably corresponding to the centrolobular hyaline change observed by light microscopy (see above) [4, 5, 35].

IMMUNOFLUORESCENCE

When the appropriate immunofluorescent technics are applied, it is found that with anti-body against the immunoglobulins and β_1C globulin there is a fine nodular fluorescence along the basement membranes [15, 31, 37, 39]. This corresponds to the "humps" seen on elec-tron microscopy. When similar technics are used with an antiserum prepared against fibrinogen, the distribution is much more widespread and is found within, and between, proliferating endothelial and mesangial cells, or in some instances along the basement mem-brane [37]. With fluorescent antialbumin, no fluorescence is seen in the glomeruli [31, 37]. When fluorescent antibody to streptococci or their products is used, there is no fluorescence [15, 31, 37] although Seegal et al. [43] have reported positive fluorescence to type 12 beta-hemolytic streptococci in 6 of the 10 cases studied.

Course of Poststreptococcal Glomerulonephritis

RESOLUTION

In the great majority of cases of acute post-streptococcal glomerulonephritis, especially in childhood, the lesion resolves completely, so that a biopsy performed at a later date reveals normal glomeruli. Polymorphonuclear leuko-cytes are the first cells to disappear during healing, but the cells in the mesangium per-sist longer (Fig. 12-4) and may be present in increased numbers — eventually to return to normal levels — in a renal biopsy after the clinical manifestations and urinary sediment have returned to normal. The electron-dense deposits on the outside of the lamina densa

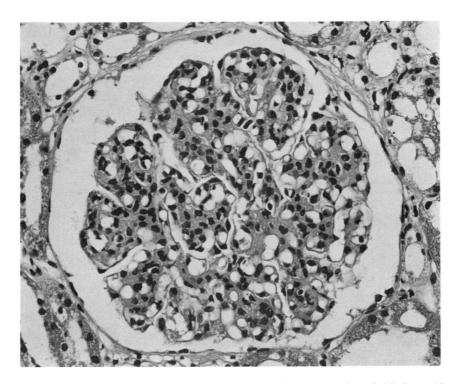

Figure 12-4. Glomerulus from a 23-year-old woman with resolving glomerulonephritis but with persistent hypercellularity in mesangium. The capillaries are widely patent. Hematoxylin and eosin. ×350.

("humps") also disappear early and are not seen after six weeks [23].

PROGRESSION TO LATENT CHRONIC STAGE

A certain proportion of patients with acute poststreptococcal glomerulonephritis exhibit persistent proteinuria, and sometimes abnormalities in the urinary sediment. Their disease is then considered to have passed into the latent chronic stage. The histologic picture in the kidneys shows a considerable decrease in the glomerular cellularity seen at the height of the infection, but abnormalities are seen in the mesangium. There is an accentuation of the lobular pattern of the glomerulus, with an increase in the amount of eosinophilic material in the centers of the lobules, attended in some cases by an increased number of mesangial cells (Fig. 12-5). The evolution of the centro-lobular lesion has been traced by McGregor [38] and by Bell [4, 5] from the fibers seen in the acute stage. With the electron microscope the mesangial increase is caused by an accumulation of material with the staining characteristics of basement membrane [10, 25]. Adhesions between glomerular tuft and Bowman's capsule, and epithelial crescents, either fresh or organized, may also be found in the latent chronic stage, but these changes are by no means constant.

One of the dilemmas facing the investigator is to determine how long one should wait for a clearing of proteinuria and a return of the urinary sediment to normal before declaring that a patient's disease has entered the latent chronic stage. Clearly, healing will take longer in some patients than in others — periods of 26 months [25], 24 months [7], and

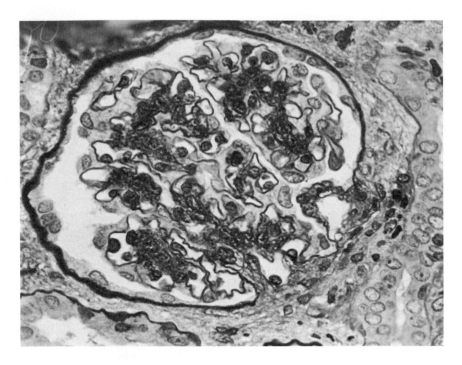

Figure 12-5. Glomerulus from patient in early stage of latent chronic glomerulonephritis. There is lobular stalk (mesangial) thickening and hypercellularity in this region. Periodic acid–Schiff (PAS) method with hematoxylin counterstain. ×500. (From Earle, D. P., and Jennings, R. B. In Wolstenholme, G. E. W., and Cameron, M. P. (Eds.), *Ciba Foundation Symposium on Renal Biopsy.* Boston: Little, Brown, 1962.)

15 months [24], have been recorded — so that if an arbitrary time period for recovery is set, and this is exceeded by a number of patients who will ultimately recover completely, erroneous statistics will result in published works that give a falsely high figure for the development of chronic glomerulonephritis. This dilemma could be resolved if the pathologist could say with absolute certainty that a given glomerular lesion was committed to a progressive course. In many cases this is possible, but the lesser degrees of centrolobular or mesangial thickening can certainly disappear [10, 36]. Using the epithelial crescent as a marker for chronicity is also erroneous because of the rapidity with which they can develop, and the fact that they can disappear [22, 36]. Persistence of immunofluorescence, when sections are treated with fluorescent antibody to im-

munoglobulins and β_1C globulin, may provide a clue to the continuation of activity in glomerulonephritis, and a recent study by Treser et al. [48] looks promising in this regard.

The relation of early hyalinization of the centrolobular or mesangial area and the condition of chronic lobular glomerulonephritis is of considerable interest. This particular form of chronic glomerulonephritis is found from time to time in a renal biopsy from patients presenting with a nephrotic syndrome. The glomeruli are almost universally involved and show an exaggeration of the lobular pattern, with the centrolobular or mesangial area replaced by eosinophilic, PAS-positive material, in fact an accentuation of the process seen in latent chronic glomerulonephritis (Fig. 12-6). Increased numbers of cells, par-

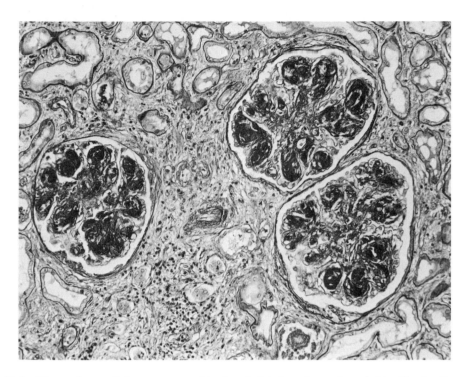

Figure 12-6. Three glomeruli from a man with chronic lobular glomerulonephritis. The hyaline material in the intercapillary or mesangial regions is strongly PAS positive. There is no crescent formation. Periodic acid–Schiff method. ×150.

ticularly in the mesangium, are almost invariably present. The increase in mesangium when seen with the electron microscope is made up of basement membrane-like material, with some collagen fibers demonstrable in certain cases [1]. There is evidence to show that some, at least, of these cases are a sequel to poststreptococcal glomerulonephritis [22, 23].

Earle and Jennings [11] have described a condition that they call chronic proliferative glomerulonephritis, in which the glomeruli show prominent lobulation of the tufts with increased mesangial cellularity. A high percentage of the 35 patients described with this condition showed antibodies to type 12 beta-hemolytic streptococci. If this condition can be regarded as an early stage of chronic lobular glomerulonephritis — which seems likely — further proof of a streptococcal background is provided.

Further studies are required to determine with certainty what proportion of cases of acute poststreptococcal glomerulonephritis progress to a chronic stage. Similarly, it is uncertain how many patients with end-stage chronic glomerulonephritis began their renal problems with an attack of poststreptococcal glomerulonephritis. These aspects are reviewed elsewhere [22].

EVOLUTION INTO RAPIDLY PROGRESSIVE
AZOTEMIC COURSE

Rapidly progressive glomerulonephritis is a term used to describe a fulminant, usually fatal, renal disease in which there is a quickly mounting blood urea nitrogen level, variable degrees of proteinuria and hypertension, and red blood cells in the urine. In some cases these findings are accompanied by considerable loss of protein with the production of a nephrotic syndrome, and many patients present with oliguria. The patients are usually in the third and fourth decades, with males predominating; death ensues over a period of weeks or months.

This condition has been referred to in the past as subacute glomerulonephritis [50], an unfortunate term because it has also been used to describe patients with a nephrotic syndrome extending over long periods. Löhlein's [34] name of stormy course is more appropriate, but a modification of Ellis's [13] term, rapidly progressive Type I glomerulonephritis, seems to be the most satisfactory of all. Acute oliguric glomerulonephritis [21] and acute anuric glomerulonephritis [6] have been used for the forms with oliguria or anuria.

Undoubtedly many of these cases have their origin in a poststreptococcal glomerulonephritis, but a considerable proportion give no evidence whatsoever of a previous streptococcal infection. Thus, less than 25 per cent of cases in my own experience have shown evidence of a previous streptococcal infection, and the work of Bacani et al. [2] shows how common the nonstreptococcal form is. On the other hand, Harrison et al. [21] found positive cultures for beta-hemolytic streptococci or raised antistreptolysin-O (ASO) titers in 9 out of 21 cases of the oliguric type, and Forland et al. [18] demonstrated evidence of streptococcal involvement in 4 out of 5 cases of the oliguric form. It is of interest that a better prognosis has attended those with a probable streptococcal etiology [21, 42]. A similar clinical course and comparable pathologic picture may be seen occasionally in the Schönlein-Henoch syndrome, and in most cases of lung hemorrhage and glomerulonephritis, the so-called Goodpasture's syndrome.

The pathologic findings in this condition, irrespective of the etiologic background, are remarkably uniform.

Macroscopic Appearance. The kidneys are enlarged and swollen with smooth subcapsular surfaces. They may be pale, or be dusky and rather congested, and petechial hemorrhages are frequently seen on the subcapsular surface. The cortex is widened, and the glomeruli can be seen as gray dots on the cut surface.

Microscopic Appearance. The *glomeruli* are virtually all involved. The glomerular tufts show increased numbers of cells, although not to the same extent as in acute glomerulonephritis. The tufts are frequently disorganized, but in some a pronounced lobular pattern, with increased numbers of cells in the mesangium, is present; this latter change occurs more frequently in those patients with a history of a streptococcal infection than in those without. Localized areas of necrosis, and scarred areas with adhesion to Bowman's capsule may be found in the tuft. Red cells, fibrin, and proteinaceous material are found in the capsular space, which is also filled by proliferating cells derived from those lining Bowman's capsule (Fig. 12-7). It is this proliferation of epithelial cells with the formation of epithelial crescents that is the most conspicuous feature of rapidly progressive glomerulonephritis, and in certain cases the increase in cells may be so great as to completely fill the capsular space. Mitotic figures are commonly seen in these areas of active cell production. It was because of this proliferation of cells outside the capillaries of the glomerular tuft that Volhard and Fahr [51] referred to this type of glomerulonephritis as the extracapillary form. The reason for crescent formation is not clear, but it is by no means a feature confined to this form of glomerulonephritis; crescents may be seen in the microscopic form of polyarteritis, in the malignant phase of essential hypertension, and even in glomeruli around the periphery of infarcts. Whether they arise as a response to the presence of fibrin in the capsular space (the traditionally held theory), because of ischemia, or because of some generalized stimulus for developmentally similar cells to proliferate — proximal tubular cell proliferation has been claimed to occur [19] — cannot be answered at present.

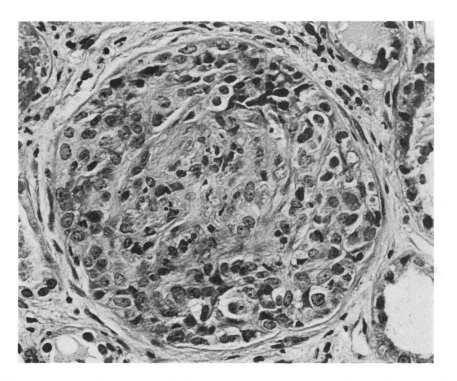

Figure 12-7. Extreme proliferation of cells lining Bowman's capsule in a 23-year-old man with oliguric form following a streptococcal infection. Hematoxylin and eosin. ×400.

The *tubules* may show hyaline-droplet change or atrophy and loss. Casts, red blood cells, and polymorphonuclear leukocytes may be found in the lumina. The *interstitial tissue* is often edematous, with lymphocytes and plasma cells occurring in variable numbers.

Arteries and arterioles may show no dramatic changes, but in some cases a fine collagenous thickening of the intima may be present. The latter change is likely to be found in the cases attended by significant increases in blood pressure.

ACUTE EXACERBATION IN CHRONIC
GLOMERULONEPHRITIS

In certain patients with chronic glomerulonephritis, acute exacerbations may occur. These are manifest by hematuria, increased proteinuria, transient impairment of renal function, and sometimes by increase in edema. They are brought on by infections and occur very shortly after the infection, in contrast to the delay that occurs in an initial attack of acute poststreptococcal glomerulonephritis. The infection may be brought about by a beta-hemolytic streptococcus, and this is the responsible organism in the majority of cases. However, nonspecific infections can also produce the exacerbation [12, 41, 49]. The exacerbation only occasionally causes significant permanent deterioration of renal function although this has been recorded [44, 54].

The diagnosis of an exacerbation may be difficult for the clinician if the patient is seen for the first time during such an event; similar difficulties may be encountered by the pathologist. The features of acute glomerulonephritis are present on biopsy, and "humps" on electron microscopy have been demonstrated [10]. In addition, however, there are glomeruli that may be completely solidified, partially scarred, or showing fibrosing crescents, together with tubular loss out of proportion to what would be expected in an initial attack of acute glomerulonephritis [10, 26, 49]. Clearly, considerable caution should be exercised before one makes a diagnosis of chronic renal damage. This is particularly true in those cases where biopsy is delayed, because it is now apparent that events can occur with great speed in the kidney.

Other Forms of Acute Diffuse Glomerulonephritis

The picture of diffuse proliferative glomerulonephritis has been described as an apparent sequel to other organisms, but without the common association that characterizes the so-called nephritogenic strains of group A streptococci. Because of the sporadic nature of these other cases, the pathologic picture is not so well worked out and accounts of the ultrastructural and immunologic aspects are lacking.

An acute diffuse proliferative glomerulonephritis has been described in subacute bacterial endocarditis caused by *Streptococcus viridans* [3, 8], accompanying ventriculoatrial shunts infected by staphylococci [46], virus infections [40, 55], and quartan malaria [28] in which soluble antigen-antibody complexes have been invoked [45, 52].

References

1. Anagnostopoulos, T., and de Montera, H. La glomérulite lobulaire. *Rev. Franc. Etud. Clin. Biol.* 9:934, 1964.
2. Bacani, R. A., Velasquez, F., Kanter, A., Pirani, C. L., and Pollak, V. E. Rapidly progressive (nonstreptococcal) glomerulonephritis. *Ann. Intern. Med.* 69:463, 1968.
3. Bell, E. T. Glomerular lesions associated with endocarditis. *Amer. J. Path.* 8:639, 1932.
4. Bell, E. T. *Renal Diseases* (2d ed.). Philadelphia: Lea & Febiger, 1950.
5. Bell, E. T., and Hartzell, T. B. The etiology and development of glomerulonephritis. *Arch. Intern. Med.* 29:768, 1922.
6. Berlyne, G. M., and Baker, S. B. de C. Acute anuric glomerulonephritis. *Quart. J. Med.* 33:105, 1964.
7. Callis, L., Castelló, F., and Garcia, L. Histopathological aspects of acute diffuse glomerulonephritis in children. *Helv. Paediat. Acta* 22:3, 1967.
8. Christian, H. A. The kidneys in subacute streptococcus viridans endocarditis. *J. Mount Sinai Hosp. N.Y.* 8:427, 1941–1942.
9. Dixon, F. J., Feldman, J. D., and Vazquez, J. J. Experimental glomerulonephritis: The pathogenesis of a laboratory model resembling the spectrum of human glomerulonephritis. *J. Exp. Med.* 113:899, 1961.
10. Dodge, W. F., Spargo, B. H., Bass, J. A., and Travis, L. B. The relationship between the clinical and pathologic features of poststreptococcal glomerulonephritis: A study of the early natural history. *Medicine* (Balt.) 47:227, 1968.
11. Earle, D. P., and Jennings, R. B. Post-streptococcal Glomerulonephritis. In Wolstenholme, G. E. W., and Cameron, M. P. (Eds.), *Ciba Foundation Symposium on Renal Biopsy*. Boston: Little, Brown, 1962. P. 156.
12. Earle, D. P., Seegal, D., Lyttle, J. D., Loeb, E. N., and Jost, E. L. The relation of the serum antistreptolysin titer to the exacerbation in chronic glomerulonephritis. *J. Clin. Invest.* 21:491, 1942.
13. Ellis, A. Natural history of Bright's disease: Clinical, histological and experimental observations. *Lancet* 1:1, 1942.
14. Faith, G. C., and Trump, B. F. The glomerular capillary wall in human kidney disease: Acute glomerulonephritis, systemic lupus erythematosus, and preeclampsia-eclampsia. *Lab. Invest.* 15:1682, 1966.
15. Feldman, J. D., Mardiney, M. R., and Shuler, S. E. Immunology and morphology of acute post-streptococcal glomerulonephritis. *Lab. Invest.* 15:283, 1966.
16. Fish, A. J., Michael, A. F., Vernier, R. L.,

and Good, R. A. Acute serum sickness nephritis in the rabbit. An immune deposit disease. *Amer. J. Path.* 49:997, 1966.

17. Fordham, C. C., Epstein, F. H., Huffines, W. D., and Harrington, J. T. Polyarteritis and acute post-streptococcal glomerulonephritis. *Ann. Intern. Med.* 61:89, 1964.

18. Forland, M., Jones, R. E., Easterling, R. E., and Forrester, R. H. Clinical and renal biopsy observations in oliguric glomerulonephritis. *J. Chronic Dis.* 19:163, 1966.

19. García-Cáceres, U. Histologic aspects of subacute glomerulonephritis, with special reference to proliferative alterations in the epithelium of renal tubules. *Amer. J. Path.* 35:755, 1959.

20. Grishman, E., and Churg, J. Acute glomerulonephritis: A histopathologic study by means of thin sections. *Amer. J. Path.* 33:993, 1957.

21. Harrison, C. V., Loughridge, L. W., and Milne, M. D. Acute oliguric renal failure in acute glomerulonephritis and polyarteritis nodosa. *Quart. J. Med.* 33:39, 1964.

22. Heptinstall, R. H. *Pathology of the Kidney.* Boston: Little, Brown, 1966.

23. Herdson, P. B., Jennings, R. B., and Earle, D. P. Glomerular fine structure in post-streptococcal acute glomerulonephritis. *Arch. Path.* (Chicago) 81:117, 1966.

24. Hutt, M. S. R., Pinniger, J. L., and de Wardener, H. E. The relationship between the clinical and the histological features of acute glomerular nephritis: Based on a study of renal biopsy material. *Quart. J. Med.* 27:265, 1958.

25. Jennings, R. B., and Earle, D. P. Post-streptococcal glomerulonephritis: Histopathologic and clinical studies of the acute, subsiding acute and early chronic latent phases. *J. Clin. Invest.* 40:1525, 1961.

26. Jennings, R. B., and Earle, D. P. Acute Glomerulonephritis. In Becker, E. L. (Ed.), *Structural Basis of Renal Disease.* New York: Hoeber Med. Div., Harper & Row, 1968. P. 271.

27. Jones, D. B. The nature of scar tissue in glomerulonephritis. *Amer. J. Path.* 42:185, 1963.

28. Kibukamusoke, J. W., and Hutt, M. S. R. Histological features of the nephrotic syndrome associated with quartan malaria. *J. Clin. Path.* 20:117, 1967.

29. Kimmelstiel, P., Kim, O. J., and Beres, J. Studies on renal biopsy specimens with the aid of the electron microscope: II. Glomerulonephritis and glomerulonephrosis. *Amer. J. Clin. Path.* 38:280, 1962.

30. Kushner, D. S., Armstrong, S. H., Dubin, A., Szanto, P. B., Markowitz, A., Maduros, B. P., Levine, J. M., River, G. L., Gynn, T. N., and Pendras, J. P. Acute glomerulonephritis in the adult: Longitudinal, clinical, functional and morphologic studies of rates of healing and progression to chronicity. *Medicine* (Balt.) 40:203, 1961.

31. Lange, K., Treser, G., Sagel, I., Ty, A., and Wasserman, E. Routine immunohistology in renal diseases. *Ann. Intern. Med.* 64:25, 1966.

32. Langhans, T. Ueber die Veränderung der Glomeruli bei der Nephritis nebst einigen Bemerkungen über die Entstehung der Fibrincylinder. *Virchow. Arch. Path. Anat.* 76:85, 1879.

33. Lawrence, J. R., Pollak, V. E., Pirani, C. L., and Kark, R. M. Histologic and clinical evidence of post-streptococcal glomerulonephritis in patients with the nephrotic syndrome. *Medicine* (Balt.) 42:1, 1963.

34. Löhlein, M. Über Nephritis nach dem heutigen Stande der pathologisch-anatomischen Forschung. *Ergebn. Inn. Med. Kinderheilk.* 5:411, 1910.

35. MacCallum, W. G. Glomerular changes in nephritis. *Bull. Johns Hopkins Hosp.* 55:416, 1934.

36. McCluskey, R. T., and Baldwin, D. S. Natural history of acute glomerulonephritis. *Amer. J. Med.* 35:213, 1963.

37. McCluskey, R. T., Vassalli, P., Gallo, G., and Baldwin, D. S. An immunofluorescent study of pathogenic mechanisms in glomerular diseases. *New Eng. J. Med.* 274:695, 1966.

38. McGregor, L. The cytological changes occurring in the glomerulus of clinical glomerulonephritis. *Amer. J. Path.* 5:559, 1929.

39. Michael, A. F., Drummond, K. N., Good, R. A., and Vernier, R. L. Acute poststrep-

tococcal glomerulonephritis: Immune deposit disease. *J. Clin. Invest.* 45:237, 1966.

40. Minkowitz, S., Wenk, R., Friedman, E., Yuceoglu, A., and Berkovich, S. Acute glomerulonephritis associated with varicella infection. *Amer. J. Med.* 44:489, 1968.

41. Murphy, F. D., and Schulz, E. G. Natural history of glomerular nephritis: A report of patients treated from 10 to 25 years after the acute stage. *A.M.A. Arch. Intern. Med.* 98: 783, 1956.

42. Nakamoto, S., Dunea, G., Kolff, W. J., and McCormack, L. J. Treatment of oliguric glomerulonephritis with dialysis and steroids. *Ann. Intern. Med.* 63:359, 1965.

43. Seegal, B. C., Andres, G. A., Hsu, K. C., and Zabriskie, J. B. Studies on the pathogenesis of acute and progressive glomerulonephritis in man by immunofluorescein and immunoferritin techniques. *Fed. Proc.* 24:100, 1965.

44. Seegal, D., Lyttle, J. D., Loeb, E. N., Jost, E. L., and Davis, G. On the exacerbation in chronic glomerulonephritis. *J. Clin. Invest.* 19:569, 1940.

45. Soothill, J. F., and Hendrickse, R. G. Some immunological studies of the nephrotic syndrome of Nigerian children. *Lancet* 2:629, 1967.

46. Stickler, G. B., Shin, M. H., Burke, E. C., Holley, K. E., Miller, R. H., and Segar, W. E. Diffuse glomerulonephritis associated with infected ventriculoatrial shunt. *New Eng. J. Med.* 279:1077, 1968.

47. Strunk, S. W., Hammond, W. S., and Benditt, E. P. The resolution of acute glomerulonephritis. An electron microscopic study of four sequential biopsies. *Lab. Invest.* 13:401, 1964.

48. Treser, G., Ehrenreich, T., Ores, R., Sagel, I., Wasserman, E., and Lange, K. Natural history of "apparently healed" acute poststreptococcal glomerulonephritis in children. *Pediatrics* 43:1005, 1969.

49. Vernier, R. L., Worthen, H. G., Wannamaker, L. W., and Good, R. A. Renal biopsy studies of the acute exacerbation in glomerulonephritis. *A.M.A. J. Dis. Child.* 98: 653, 1959.

50. Volhard, F. Die doppelseitigen hämatogenen Nierenerkrankungen (Bright'sche Krankheit). In Mohr, L., and Staehelin, R. (Eds.), *Handbuch der Inneren Medizin*. Berlin: Springer, 1918. Vol. 3, part 2, p. 1149.

51. Volhard, F., and Fahr, T. *Die Brightsche Nierenkrankheit*. Berlin: Springer, 1914.

52. Ward, P. A., and Kibukamusoke, J. W. Evidence for soluble immune complexes in the pathogenesis of the glomerulonephritis of quartan malaria. *Lancet* 1:283, 1969.

53. Watt, M. F., Howe, J. S., and Parrish, A. E. Renal tubular changes in acute glomerulonephritis. *A.M.A. Arch. Intern. Med.* 103:690, 1959.

54. Wilson, C. The Natural History of Nephritis. In Black, D. A. K. (Ed.), *Renal Disease*. Philadelphia: F. A. Davis, 1962. P. 188.

55. Yuceoglu, A. M., Berkovich, S., and Minkowitz, S. Acute glomerulonephritis associated with ECHO virus type 9 infection. *J. Pediat.* 69:603, 1966.

13

Clinical Aspects of Acute Poststreptococcal Glomerulonephritis

William B. Schwartz and Jerome P. Kassirer

Acute glomerulonephritis often comes to the attention of a physician because of striking clinical manifestations such as smoky urine, periorbital and peripheral edema, hypertension, and circulatory congestion. In its most florid form, seizures, pulmonary congestion, or anuria may be the dominant features. On the other hand, the disease may be so insidious in its onset and so subtle in its manifestations that the patient suffers no symptoms, and only the most careful investigation discloses its presence.

Only a minority of patients present the entire clinical syndrome considered characteristic of acute glomerulonephritis, but it nevertheless seems desirable to summarize briefly the features of the so-called classic case. Typically the illness begins with pharyngitis or tonsillitis accompanied by fever and malaise. Whether or not specific antibiotic therapy is given, respiratory symptoms and fever disappear after a few days, and the patient feels entirely well. One or two weeks after the onset of the illness, weakness and anorexia return, and the patient suddenly notices that his urine is scanty in amount and smoky in appearance. Upon awakening the next morning, he notes swelling around the eyes and complains of shortness of breath and headache.

When the patient is first seen by a physician, the blood pressure is found to be slightly elevated, the neck veins distended, and a few moist rales are heard at both lung bases. Despite the clinical evidence of circulatory congestion, the circulation time is normal. The urine has a high specific gravity, and the supernatant has a brownish discoloration. Microscopic examination of the sediment reveals numerous red cells, many white blood cells, and casts. Most of the casts are coarsely or finely granular in appearance, but some are composed entirely of intact or degenerating red blood cells. The throat culture reveals a few beta-hemolytic streptococci. A mild normochromic, normocytic anemia is present, and the protein concentration of the plasma is slightly diminished. Evaluation of renal function discloses a significant elevation of both serum creatinine and blood urea nitrogen concentrations.

After a few days, during which manifestations of the disease remain intense, the signs and symptoms gradually abate. A diuresis begins, hematocrit and plasma protein concentration rise, circulatory congestion disappears, and blood urea nitrogen concentration falls. Gross hematuria ceases, but proteinuria and microscopic hematuria persist. Hyaline, granular, and red blood cell casts are still easily found, but within several weeks the patient feels entirely well and is eager to return to his normal activities.

Six or seven months later the majority of such patients no longer have proteinuria, but often the urine still contains red blood cells and casts. The antistreptolysin-O (ASO) titer, if elevated during the acute episode, will in most cases have returned to normal. At the end of a year microscopic hematuria and cylinduria have usually disappeared.

As mentioned earlier, in some instances the illness has a more insidious character. A week or two after a respiratory infection the patient notes slight ankle edema, and examination of the urine reveals protein, red blood cells, and casts. After a brief period edema disappears, and the patient feels entirely well. Other patients have no symptoms or signs, the diagnosis being first suspected when urinary abnormalities are detected fortuitously during the course of a routine urinalysis. The subsequent demonstration of a high ASO titer gives evidence that the preceding infection was of streptococcal origin. The outcome of the illness that begins in this occult fashion is usually the same as that seen in association with more overt manifestations.

The underlying structural, hemodynamic, and metabolic alterations that are discussed in this chapter provide insight into many of the clinical features of acute glomerulonephritis and furnish a rational basis for treatment. It will be apparent, however, that because there is no way of altering the development, progression, or healing of the renal lesion, the role of the physician in this disease is largely limited to the prevention or treatment of the various complications.

Epidemiology

It has long been known that acute glomerulonephritis, like rheumatic fever, often follows beta-hemolytic streptococcal infections, but many features of its epidemiology have been poorly understood until recent years. In contrast to acute rheumatic fever, in which the attack rate after streptococcal infections is fairly constant at about 3 per cent [217], the attack rate of acute glomerulonephritis varies widely. In some follow-up studies of infections with group A streptococci there has been a negligible incidence of glomerulonephritis [216], whereas others have found that nephritis subsequently developed in as many as one-fifth of patients with streptococcal infections [260]. As might be anticipated from these findings, glomerulonephritis sometimes occurs sporadically and at other times assumes epidemic proportions [9, 91, 98, 137, 144, 180, 207, 208, 211, 218, 221], often striking several members of the same family [73, 76, 98, 100, 141, 253].

These puzzling aspects of the epidemiology of acute glomerulonephritis have been largely clarified by the demonstration that certain types of beta-hemolytic streptococci have specific nephritogenic properties. Types 12 and 4 have been the offending organisms in the majority of cases [23, 215, 216, 266], but other types, including types 1 and 49, have occasionally been implicated [9, 100, 223]. Although organisms cannot always be isolated during the acute illness, type-specific antibodies, chiefly to types 12 and 4, have frequently been identified in the serum during the convalescent phase [28, 49, 209, 215]. Conversely, acute glomerulonephritis is rarely seen as a sequel to infections with other types of beta-hemolytic streptococci [216].

In summary, it is now clear that the epidemiology of acute nephritis parallels the epidemiology of infection with certain specific types of streptococci; widespread outbreaks of the disease have, in every recorded instance, resulted from dissemination of a specific nephritogenic organism throughout the community.

It should be pointed out, however, that even after infection with organisms such as type 12 or type 4, the incidence of acute glomerulonephritis varies considerably [216, 235, 266]. This variation suggests that strain differences may occur within the individual types and that these strains in turn may differ in their nephritogenic capacities. For example, some strains of type 12 streptococci are apparently not nephritogenic [136] — that is, they have never been observed to precipitate an attack of acute nephritis.

Although beta-hemolytic streptococcal infections are responsible for nearly all cases of acute glomerulonephritis, the disease may also occur in association with subacute bacterial endocarditis and possibly with certain viral infections (see page 440).

AGE AND SEX

Acute glomerulonephritis is chiefly a disease of children and young adults. For reasons that are not clear, there is a definite predominance of males over females, the ratio sometimes approaching 2 : 1 [74, 172, 232]. The disease is commonest between the ages of 3 and 7 [114, 172], and is rare in children under the age of 2 years [89]. The predominance during the preschool and early school years probably can be attributed to the fact that at this time children are likely to have their first exposure to hemolytic streptococci. With each advancing decade, there are fewer cases than in the pre-

vious decade [191, 214, 232], but first attacks of glomerulonephritis even in older persons are not rare. For example, in several series patients over the age of 50 comprise 5 to 10 per cent of the total group [191, 214, 232]. Furthermore, evidence from a recent postmortem study demonstrates that the disease occurs in the older age group significantly more often than has generally been recognized by the clinician [198]. The data from this latter study indicate that even when patients have many of the signs of acute glomerulonephritis, including hypertension, edema, azotemia, and urinary abnormalities, the correct diagnosis may be missed in as many as three-quarters of the cases [198]. The frequency with which dyspnea and orthopnea dominate the clinical syndrome in the elderly probably accounts for many errors in diagnosis, the physician tending to be diverted from the primary renal problem by the dramatic pulmonary manifestations [232–234].

SITE OF PRECEDING INFECTION

It has generally been thought that the respiratory tract is the site of preceding infection in the great majority of cases of acute poststreptococcal glomerulonephritis. In most series pharyngitis, otitis media, or tonsillitis [34, 39, 110, 169, 173, 192, 242] was the common predisposing illness. Skin infections with the streptococcus have also been known to induce the disease but have usually been cited as the etiologic factor in only 5 to 10 per cent of cases. Several recent observations have indicated, however, that in certain epidemics skin infections are the dominant cause of the illness. In brief, it appears that earlier studies demonstrating a low incidence of skin infections were carried out in northern climes where respiratory infections are common and impetigo relatively infrequent. Recent observations in southern and tropical areas indicate that streptococcal skin infections in these regions act as the etiologic factor in from 30 to 80 per cent of cases of acute glomerulonephritis [26, 59, 179, 208, 210]. On the basis of these findings, it is now possible to account for the striking seasonal differences in the peak incidence of the disease in various geographical regions. In the North the peak incidence is in the winter and spring, corresponding to the period when respiratory infections are most common, whereas in the South the majority of cases occur in the summer, the time at which skin infections are most prevalent [59].

The foregoing considerations also seemingly account for another heretofore puzzling observation — namely, that though respiratory infections with the streptococcus occur much less often in the South than in the North, the overall incidence of acute glomerulonephritis is virtually the same at all latitudes [243]. It appears that the higher incidence of impetigo in warm climates is approximately balanced by the higher incidence of respiratory infections in colder regions, the net effect being a similar frequency of the disease in all parts of the United States.

The clinical picture and course of acute glomerulonephritis after impetigo is evidently no different from that observed after respiratory infections [26, 59, 208]. Perhaps the only distinguishing feature is that the ASO titer is elevated considerably less often after skin infections, a rise in titer occurring in only one-fourth of cases of impetigo as compared to three-fourths in those with respiratory infections [10, 59].

Clinical Immunology

Antibodies to the extracellular antigens of the hemolytic streptococcus confer little or no immunity on the patient infected with these organisms, but antibody levels are often useful diagnostically because a high titer indicates that a streptococcal infection has occurred. One or more of these antibodies, including antistreptolysin-O (ASO), antistreptokinase (ASK), antihyaluronidase (AH), and antidesoxyribonuclease (ADNase), usually increase in the serum. Of these, ASO is the most convenient to use as a model of the antibody response because it is easily titrated and is more likely to be elevated after a streptococcal infection than are the other antibodies to extracellular antigens.

The ASO titer ordinarily begins to rise one to three weeks after a hemolytic streptococcal infection and reaches a maximum (as high as several thousand units) in three to five weeks. Subsequently, there is a gradual decline, but the rate of fall is quite variable [168]. In about 50 per cent of patients the titer returns to normal within six months and in 75 per cent within one year [173]. In a few cases abnormal titers persist for as long as two years [173]. An elevated ASO titer provides unequivocal evidence of a previous streptococcal infection, but a normal titer does not exclude it; only 70 to 80 per cent of patients with proved streptococcal infections show significant increases in antistreptolysin-O levels [174, 263]. However, by the use of bacteriologic studies during the acute attack and ASO determinations both during and after the acute illness, evidence of a streptococcal infection can be obtained in almost all cases [23, 173].

The frequency of acute glomerulonephritis after streptococcal infections is the same whether or not the ASO titer rises. Furthermore, in patients who show an antibody response there is no correlation between the height of the titer and the incidence of renal disease [249]. In the cases in which glomerulonephritis develops, the ASO response does not appear to have any prognostic significance; there is no relation between the height of the titer and either the severity of the disease or the subsequent propensity of the process to heal [173].

Before the era of antibiotics, the finding of a persistently normal ASO titer argued against a previous streptococcal infection and thus against the diagnosis of acute glomerulonephritis. However, this correlation no longer holds true. In patients treated with penicillin early in the course of their infection, the frequency of an ASO response is reduced from the usual 70 to 80 per cent to between 10 and 15 per cent [140, 263]; as a result, in many patients with acute glomerulonephritis an elevated ASO titer never develops. A normal ASO titer can be taken as evidence against an antecedent streptococcal infection only if the patient has not been treated with antibiotics.

Antibodies form in response not only to the extracellular antigens of beta-hemolytic streptococci but also to the M protein, the cellular antigen that confers on the streptococcus its type specificity. Antibodies to the M protein develop slowly, some patients first showing an elevated titer as late as two months after the infection [56]. Such antibodies probably play the major role in the prolonged type-specific immunity that follows streptococcal infections [56, 174, 235]. It should be noted that type-specific antibodies may be found even in patients who do not have a rise in ASO titer [153]. Demonstrable type-specific antibody often disappears from the bloodstream within a few months [28, 245], but it may persist for many years after the initiating infection has occurred [156, 215, 245]. It seems, moreover, that type-specific immunity outlasts the presence of measurable antibody in the bloodstream; such persistent immunity has been attributed to the fixation of type-specific antibody to tissues.

The foregoing statements, which apply to patients with streptococcal infection in general, are also applicable to those in whom acute glomerulonephritis develops [28, 49, 215]. In patients who have had acute glomerulonephritis and in whom the type of the offending organism is unknown, it is often possible to detect antibodies to type 12, type 4, or other nephritogenic streptococci long after the acute illness [28, 49, 215]. Some patients are found to have type-specific antibodies to more than one nephritogenic organism (for

example, types 12 and 4 [49, 215] or type 12 and type 49 [28]). Although it is possible that these patients had infections with both types of streptococci, it seems more likely that antigenic properties shared by the several organisms produced these serologic findings. This view is supported by the observation that only one of the two elevated titers tends to persist over a prolonged period, presumably indicating the type of the infecting organism [28].

Antibiotic therapy not only aborts the antibody response to the extracellular antigens of the streptococcus but also interferes with the development of type-specific antibodies [50, 56]. Inhibition of the immune response is related to both the dose of antibiotic and the route of administration. For example, in patients given 250,000 units of penicillin twice daily parenterally for 10 days bacteriostatic antibodies do not develop; but if the same amount is given orally, or if a smaller amount is given either orally or parenterally, an antibody response occurs in a significant number of patients [50]. Thus, only prolonged and intensive antibiotic therapy will consistently inhibit antibody production. These considerations have clinical significance because the failure to develop type-specific antibodies increases the risk of subsequent infection by a homologous serologic type [33]. The implications of aborting the immune response will be discussed further under the heading *Prophylaxis*.

SERUM COMPLEMENT ACTIVITY

It is now well recognized that serum complement activity is almost always low in acute glomerulonephritis. Apparently these low titers do not result from losses of complement components in the urine but reflect the utilization of complement in the antigen-antibody reaction that follows the inciting streptococcal infection [86]. Complement levels usually return to normal within a month after the acute illness [87, 157].

Patients with the lowest initial complement levels have been reported to have a more prolonged and stormy course than those with only moderate reductions [157]. The persistence of a low serum complement level (presumably giving evidence of continued activity of the basic immunologic process) has also been said to augur a poor prognosis [157], but this correlation has not been observed by other investigators [87]. The possible usefulness of serum complement levels in predicting the outcome of the acute attack remains to be further evaluated.

Recent studies have demonstrated that the serum level of the third component of complement, $\beta_1 C$ globulin, more or less parallels the level of total complement activity during and after an attack of acute glomerulonephritis [104]. The low serum level of this protein characteristically seen during the acute illness is apparently the result of several factors including binding of the protein to the glomerular capillary walls [84, 104, 146, 187, 268], decreased synthesis [6], and an increased breakdown as the result of reaction with immune complexes [267]. Because of the convenience and simplicity of measurement of beta $_{1C}$ globulin, the concentration of this substance has come into widespread use as an index of the more difficult-to-measure serum complement activity.

Characteristics of the Latent Period

Between the onset of a streptococcal infection and the development of symptoms or signs of acute glomerulonephritis, there is a latent period that usually ranges between one and two weeks and that averages 10 days [201, 215, 273]. Latent periods shorter than a week are not uncommon, however, and occur in as many as one-fifth of the cases [201, 215, 273]. Only in an occasional patient does acute glomerulonephritis develop as long as three to four weeks after the inciting infection. Latent periods of more than one month have not been noted, and it is doubtful whether an infection that precedes the onset of renal abnormalities by such a period has a relation to subsequent renal disease.

If the urine is examined during the acute phase of the initial streptococcal infection, microscopic hematuria and proteinuria will be found in about a third of the patients [249]. These findings are analogous to those observed in a variety of febrile illnesses and may well be of a similar nonspecific origin. However, there is some evidence that if microscopic hematuria is present during an acute streptococcal infection, acute glomerulonephritis is more likely to develop than if hematuria is absent [249]. After the acute infection has subsided, microscopic hematuria and proteinuria usually disappear, only to recur at the onset of the acute attack one or two weeks later.

It is of interest that acute exacerbations of chronic glomerulonephritis ordinarily occur after a much shorter latent period than a first attack, usually within one to four days after the onset of a streptococcal infection. However, exacerbations occasionally occur after an interval of one to two weeks [244], and for this reason, the length of the latent period cannot in itself be taken as an absolute criterion for differentiating between an exacerbation and an initial attack.

Clinical Features

This section will consider in detail the usual systemic and renal manifestations of acute glomerulonephritis. However, before such a discussion is begun, some stress should be laid on the diverse ways in which the disease may manifest itself and on the diagnostic difficulties that may therefore arise. The diagnosis is most readily overlooked when the usual systemic manifestations such as edema or gross hematuria are not present or when symptoms are so minor that the individual does not seek medical advice [61, 269]. This problem is well illustrated by the finding of a high prevalence of glomerulonephritis in asymptomatic siblings of patients with the overt form of the disease [61]. Such "silent" cases of poststreptococcal nephritis probably contribute significantly to the reservoir of persons who, without an antecedent history of renal disease, are discovered to have chronic glomerulonephritis. It is therefore desirable to carry out a urinalysis on all persons who are known to have suffered a recent streptococcal infection (and all contacts of the index case) even though clinical signs are not present.

The diagnosis of acute glomerulonephritis may also be overlooked in the occasional case in which urinary abnormalities are slight or absent. Despite the presence of florid clinical manifestations such as hypertension, edema, and circulatory congestion, the urine may contain little or no protein, and the sediment may reveal only a few red blood cells or may be entirely unremarkable [3, 22, 26, 46, 62, 101, 119]. The evidence supporting the diagnosis in patients with such minimal urinary changes has been impressive. Infection with beta-hemolytic streptococci has been documented by culture or measurements of ASO titer (or both), renal biopsy has shown changes typical of the disease [3, 22, 26, 46, 101, 119], and the subsequent clinical course has been that of classic acute glomerulonephritis. In no case was another disease present that might have been expected to cause a glomerulitis. These observations clearly indicate that the physician must be alert to the possibility that a benign-appearing urine may occasionally conceal an instance of otherwise overt poststreptococcal glomerulonephritis.

SYSTEMIC SYMPTOMS

Many patients have no systemic symptoms, but some complain of lethargy, malaise, weakness, and anorexia. These symptoms usually disappear during the initial period of bed rest. In an occasional patient the outstanding symptom is marked weakness, which may persist for several months after the acute attack. High fever and chills do not occur commonly during the acute phase and when present usually indicate that the initial streptococcal infection is still present. It is not clear whether fever ever occurs simply as a response to the inflammatory reaction in the renal parenchyma.

HEMATURIA

Gross hematuria, one of the most common initial symptoms, occurs in more than one-third of the patients. The urine is often described as reddish-brown, smoky, rusty, tea-colored, or cloudy. In most cases, gross hematuria disappears after a few days, but it may continue for one or two weeks. Microscopic hematuria can, of course, be found for a much longer period and often persists even after significant proteinuria is no longer present. In some cases, hematuria has been observed for as long as several years after all other abnormalities have vanished [239]. The residual hematuria is probably of little significance; nearly all patients in whom urinary sediment abnormalities are the only remaining evidence of disease ultimately go on to complete healing [239].

EDEMA

Edema is found in the great majority of patients. It most often involves the face and is particularly prominent in the periorbital area. Puffiness of the face and eyelids, when combined with pallor, constitutes the so-called nephritic facies. Edema of the legs and sacrum is also common. In patients with massive retention of fluid, swelling of the genitalia, pleural effusions, and ascites may occur. However, now that sodium intake is restricted routinely in edematous patients, such massive fluid accumulation is rare.

The distribution of edema fluid is largely influenced by two factors: gravity and local tissue tension. The characteristic involvement of the face seems to be entirely the consequence of the patient's ability to assume the recumbent position without becoming orthopneic and of the ready distensibility of the soft tissues around the eyes. This view is borne out by the clinical observation that facial edema is most prominent on awakening and tends to disappear after the patient has been upright for a few hours. Patients with cardiac failure would presumably develop a similar distribution of edema were they not orthopneic and hence unable to lie flat.

Significant fluid retention may also be present in the absence of overt edema. Many patients who, on careful physical examination, have no evidence of fluid accumulation will later undergo an abrupt diuresis and a weight loss of 2 to 5 kg. In retrospect, it may sometimes become evident that slight but definite swelling of the face had been present. The relation of edema to disturbances of renal and cardiovascular function is discussed in later sections.

HYPERTENSION

Hypertension occurs in the majority of cases. With the exception of edema, it is the most common presenting clinical feature of the disease. The blood pressure in most cases is only moderately elevated, with typical systolic values ranging from 140 to 160 mm. Hg and diastolic from 90 to 110 mm. Hg. A few patients show a more pronounced increase, with diastolic pressures of 115 to 120 mm. Hg, but extreme hypertension with a blood pressure higher than 200/120 mm. Hg is uncommon. Blood pressure elevations in children are usually less striking than in adults, but when the values are interpreted in relation to the normal range for the patient's age, it will be found that hypertension occurs with about the same frequency and severity as in the older age group.

Hypertension, like edema, is often absent in mild cases. However, it may sometimes be overlooked because it is present only transiently, or because "normal" pressures recorded during the illness are not compared with readings taken after recovery. Although hypertension is usually present at the onset of the acute illness, it develops in an occasional patient only after the other signs of the disease are clearly evident. Hypertension ordinarily subsides concomitantly with the diuresis or with progressive improvement in the patient's renal status but rarely may persist for a considerably longer period. A sustained elevation of blood pressure in association with continued proteinuria suggests that the disease is entering a latent or chronic phase.

The cause of the elevated blood pressure is unknown. Hypertension has been variously attributed to expansion of intravascular or extracellular volume and to vasospasm resulting from either neurogenic or humoral influences.

CARDIOVASCULAR SYSTEM

Signs and Symptoms. The signs and symptoms of circulatory congestion are common. In the experience of most observers they occur in one-fifth of the patients [183, 192, 194, 230] but have been noted in as many as 70 per cent [270]. This wide divergence in the reported frequency of "heart failure" has probably resulted in large part from the use of different diagnostic criteria.

In some patients, symptoms can be elicited only by careful questioning, and the circulatory disturbance is manifested on physical examination solely by the presence of a few pulmonary rales. In others, dyspnea and cough are prominent complaints, there are many rales, and the neck veins are markedly distended. Basal or apical heart murmurs are frequently heard, and occasionally a gallop rhythm is present. Circulatory congestion usually occurs in company with overt peripheral edema, but now and then it may be seen in patients who are not edematous.

A few patients present the clinical picture of acute pulmonary edema; in these, severe dyspnea, orthopnea, and cyanosis may be the outstanding features of the illness. As a result, the underlying renal disorder may readily be overlooked; indeed, its presence is sometimes suspected only after a careful history has been obtained and the characteristic changes of acute glomerulonephritis have been observed in the urinary sediment. As mentioned earlier, the frequency of dyspnea and pulmonary edema is much higher in the older than in the younger age group [232, 233, 234], and it is therefore in the elderly that the predominance of congestive pulmonary symptoms is likely to create difficulties in diagnosis. The high incidence of pulmonary congestion can best be explained by the greater frequency of underlying cardiovascular disease in the elderly and the consequent predisposition for fluid to accumulate in the lungs during a period of excessive salt and water retention.

Roentgenographic Findings. X-ray films of the chest taken during the acute phase of the disease often reveal abnormal findings [143, 193, 204]. Frequently the heart is enlarged, and there is evidence of pulmonary congestion or even frank pulmonary edema. These radiographic changes are more common in patients who have peripheral edema than in those who do not [204]. As diuresis occurs, the cardiac silhouette returns to normal, usually within several days. In a few cases, the heart remains enlarged for as long as several months after the acute attack [143].

Sometimes pulmonary congestion is found in association with a heart that is of normal size as estimated from the cardiothoracic ratio [143]. In many such cases serial chest x-rays will nevertheless reveal a definite diminution in the transverse diameter of the heart, and in retrospect it will become apparent that cardiac enlargement was present initially [143]. On the other hand, the heart size may be unequivocally normal despite the presence of congested lungs.

Electrocardiographic Changes. Minor electrocardiographic abnormalities are present in the majority of patients and are most frequently found in those with hypertension or cardiac enlargement. Usually, the changes are limited to the T waves, which are generally flattened or inverted. Sometimes the QRS or Q-T interval is prolonged. Lengthening of the P-R interval, distortion of the P waves, and arrhythmias are also seen occasionally [12, 155, 183, 271].

Although the clinical syndrome of circulatory congestion in acute glomerulonephritis in many respects is similar to that seen in left-sided heart failure, a number of features are distinctive. These include edema of the face and eyelids, a normal or slow heart rate [52, 55], and the relatively infrequent occurrence of orthopnea [204, 270]. Furthermore, even in the presence of severe circulatory congestion, the circulation time usually remains normal [55, 70, 72, 154, 212]. The explanation for these peculiarities becomes apparent when they are considered in conjunction with physiologic data indicating that primary renal retention of salt and water, rather than myocardial failure, is responsible for the circulatory disturbances.

Pathophysiology of Circulatory Congestion and Edema. ROLE OF CAPILLARY PERMEABILITY, HYPERTENSION, AND MYOCARDITIS. Many theories have been proposed to explain the congestive phenomena that occur during the course of acute glomerulonephritis. Early investigators of the problem, taking note of the unusual distribution of the edema and its high protein content (as measured by the rather crude methods then available), ascribed edema to a generalized increase in capillary permeability. This theory no longer seems tenable, since later studies, using more exact methods, have shown that the protein content of the edema fluid is comparable to that found in a variety of transudates [261].

The congestive phenomena have also been ascribed to myocardial failure resulting from either hypertension [154, 194, 230] or myocarditis [102]. It seems unlikely, however, that the brief period of hypertension to which pa-

tients with acute glomerulonephritis are subjected could be an important factor in the
development of myocardial insufficiency; individuals with normal hearts can tolerate
severe hypertension for much longer periods
without cardiac decompensation. Furthermore, the degree of hypertension in acute glomerulonephritis correlates poorly with the
severity of the circulatory disturbance [52,
270], and in some cases circulatory congestion
is seen in the absence of hypertension [163,
193].

The view that myocarditis may be responsible for the circulatory congestion in acute
glomerulonephritis has been based on pathologic and electrocardiographic studies. Some
observers have reported a serous type of myocarditis, with interstitial edema, in approximately 10 per cent of patients coming to
postmortem examination [102]. These
changes, in conjunction with a high frequency
of electrocardiographic abnormalities, have
been taken as evidence of significant myocardial disease. However, the microscopic
changes in the myocardium are minor; there
is little evidence of muscle necrosis, of infiltration by inflammatory cells, or of other important histologic abnormalities. The myocardium, in fact, is unremarkable in appearance
in many patients who die as a result of circulatory congestion [102, 212, 270]. Furthermore, in such cases electrocardiographic
abnormalities may be absent and even when
present, as mentioned earlier, are usually minor and nonspecific. Thus, there is little evidence to support the contention that circulatory congestion is the consequence of
myocardial failure.

ROLE OF PRIMARY SALT AND WATER RETENTION.
There is convincing clinical evidence that all
the signs and symptoms of circulatory congestion, including dyspnea, peripheral edema,
pulmonary congestion, cardiac enlargement,
and increased venous pressure, are the result
of a primary defect in the renal excretion of
sodium and water and the consequent expansion of plasma volume. It is now well recog-

nized that an identical syndrome can be
produced in normal persons by the administration of sodium and water at a rate that
exceeds renal excretory capacity [4, 70]. The
syndrome also occurs in patients with acute
renal failure who are given excessive amounts
of fluids [93].

The weight of the physiologic evidence summarized below also indicates that the pattern
of altered circulatory function in acute glomerulonephritis is virtually identical with that
induced by primary fluid overload but is
strikingly different from that observed with
intrinsic myocardial failure. The characteristic changes in blood volume, circulatory dynamics, renal hemodynamics, and the response
to digitalis have served to clarify this complex
problem.

The presence of mild anemia and hypoalbuminemia and their prompt disappearance
after diuresis originally aroused suspicion that
plasma volume might be expanded in acute
glomerulonephritis [41, 227]. Studies with
Evans blue dye supported this concept [41,
227], but it was argued that the values yielded
by the dye method might be falsely high because of penetration of this substance into the
extravascular space. However, recent observations, using more reliable techniques, have
confirmed the presence of hypervolemia. Measurement of the volume of distribution of
radiochromium-tagged red blood cells has
shown not only that total blood volume is
significantly increased but also that the expansion is solely the result of an increase in
plasma volume [72]. During diuresis there is
a contraction of plasma volume unaccompa-
nied by a change in red cell mass [72]. (The
validity of these interpretations depends, of
course, on the assumption that venous hematocrit is a fair reflection of total body hematocrit.)

The contrast between circulatory congestion
in acute glomerulonephritis and that in myocardial failure is particularly striking when
these disorders are assessed in hemodynamic
terms. Typically, in congestive heart failure
caused by hypertension or coronary artery dis-

ease, the cardiac output is reduced and circulation time is prolonged. As a consequence of inadequate delivery of blood to the tissues, the arteriovenous oxygen difference is increased [34, 224, 248]. The same measurements made in patients with acute glomerulonephritis yield a distinctively different profile: cardiac output is normal or occasionally increased, and both circulation time and oxygen extraction are normal [52, 55, 70, 80, 90]. Similar changes are seen when the extracellular fluid volume of normal subjects is expanded by administration of steroids and salt [4]. The hemodynamic changes in acute glomerulonephritis are thus in no way suggestive of intrinsic myocardial disease.

The characteristic clinical response to digitalis in patients with myocardial failure is not usually seen in those with acute glomerulonephritis. The signs and symptoms of circulatory congestion continue unabated until the usual diuresis occurs, and hydremia is relieved. The clinical impression that digitalis has little therapeutic value in glomerulonephritis gains objective support from physiologic measurements carried out during the rapid intravenous infusion of the drug. The usual rise in cardiac output, fall in venous pressure, and narrowing of the arteriovenous oxygen difference seen in congestive heart failure are not produced by the drug in circulatory congestion secondary to acute glomerulonephritis [70, 90].

In summary, it appears justified to conclude that the circulatory congestion in acute glomerulonephritis is primarily the result of sodium and water retention. The possibility that underlying heart disease contributes to the clinical picture in an occasional case cannot, of course, be excluded.

ENCEPHALOPATHY

The syndrome of hypertensive encephalopathy has been reported to occur in about 5 to 10 per cent of patients with acute glomerulonephritis [35, 39, 74, 110, 214, 225]; it is found almost exclusively in those with severe hypertension. In recent years there has been a decrease in the frequency of this complication, probably because severe hypertension, when it occurs, usually is promptly controlled by means of the newer antihypertensive drugs.

The most frequent symptoms of hypertensive encephalopathy are severe headache and vomiting, and in some patients these may actually be the initial clinical manifestations of glomerulonephritis. An occasional patient will have more advanced neurologic abnormalities, including confusion, somnolence, coma, or repeated convulsions. Transient aphasia, mild paresis, hemiplegia, and decrease in visual acuity have all been described but are uncommon.

When the blood pressure falls, either spontaneously or under the influence of antihypertensive drugs, the neurologic symptoms disappear. As a rule, there are no residual abnormalities. The pathogenesis of the encephalopathy is not clear, but the suggestion has been made that cerebral vasospasm with anoxia is responsible. Salt and water retention, by predisposing to cerebral edema, may be a contributory factor. The therapy of neurologic complications is discussed under *Treatment*.

RETINOPATHY

The optic fundi are usually normal, and when retinopathy does occur, it is usually minimal [35, 88, 214, 259]. It seems likely that the low frequency of severe retinal changes can be explained by the short duration of the blood pressure elevation. Retinal arteriolar constriction and flame-shaped hemorrhages are found occasionally [88, 259], but papilledema is rare even in patients with hypertensive encephalopathy.

GENITOURINARY TRACT

Genitourinary complaints are not frequent. A few patients suffer from flank pain, which may radiate to the groin or testicle and which may also be accompanied by tenderness over the costovertebral angle. Others complain of dull back pain. The pathogenesis of the back and flank pain is not clear, but these symptoms have sometimes been attributed to stretching of the kidney capsule secondary to swelling of the renal parenchyma. Urgency and dysuria are rare in uncomplicated acute glomerulonephritis; when these symptoms occur, the presence of a superimposed urinary tract infection should be suspected.

In a few patients in whom urine cultures are originally negative, significant bacilluria will subsequently develop. Unfortunately, the urinary sediment is not a reliable guide to the presence or absence of urinary tract infection, because white blood cells and white-cell casts may be present solely as the result of the glomerulitis; conversely, these elements may be absent even in the presence of active infection. Several urine cultures should be obtained during and after the acute illness so that an asymptomatic infection will not be overlooked.

OTHER INVOLVEMENT

Not infrequently the patient complains of *gastrointestinal symptoms,* most often nausea but occasionally constipation or diarrhea. Abdominal pain is less usual. The *skin* frequently appears pale, even in the absence of marked anemia, probably as the result of distention of subcutaneous tissues with edema fluid. *Purpura* is said to occur in a small percentage of patients, but if this abnormality is present, the diagnosis of acute poststreptococcal glomerulonephritis should be viewed with suspicion. Most patients with purpura and nephritis do not have evidence of a preceding streptococcal infection, and frequently they will have signs of some other disease, such as necrotizing angiitis or anaphylactoid purpura (see section on *Differential Diagnosis*).

Joint involvement with pain and swelling is uncommon in uncomplicated poststreptococcal nephritis and is also suggestive of a widespread systemic disease. *Splenomegaly* is seen infrequently and, when present, is probably related to the original infection.

Acute rheumatic fever rarely occurs in association with acute glomerulonephritis, and it seems likely that the coexistence of the two diseases is fortuitous.

Renal Function and Electrolyte Disturbances

Some disturbance in renal function occurs in the majority of patients with acute glomerulonephritis. Even when the blood urea nitrogen and serum creatinine concentrations are not unequivocally elevated, precise measurements of glomerular filtration rate often reveal some degree of functional impairment [32]. Renal failure severe enough to produce overt clinical manifestations is seen infrequently.

A distinctive pattern of renal functional abnormalities has been demonstrated by many observers. In general, glomerular filtration rate as measured by inulin, creatinine, or urea clearance is moderately or markedly depressed [32, 66, 80]. Reductions in renal blood flow and renal plasma flow are uncommon (except when severe renal failure develops), and in some cases renal blood flow is actually higher than normal* [32, 42, 48]. Because renal plasma flow is ordinarily well maintained even when filtration rate is moderately reduced, the filtration fraction is characteristically low [32, 48, 66, 116]. This pattern of altered renal hemodynamics is strikingly different from that seen in both essential hypertension and congestive heart failure; in these disorders, renal plasma flow is usually reduced out of proportion to filtration rate, and the filtration fraction is thus increased [71, 112, 185]. The characteristic renal hemodynamic pattern of acute glomerulonephritis is usually maintained even in the face of significant hy-

---

* The low PAH clearances reported by some observers [66] are probably the result of a reduced extraction of PAH by the tubules [32] rather than a true reduction in renal plasma flow.

pertension or circulatory congestion [66, 80].

Tubular as well as glomerular function is commonly impaired. The extraction of para-aminohippuric acid (PAH) as well as the maximum tubular capacity for secretion of PAH and the reabsorption of glucose are both usually decreased [48, 65, 66]. In general, however, tubular function is less severely impaired than glomerular function [66]. Such a dissociation is often manifested clinically by an elevation of serum creatinine concentration in the face of little or no reduction in the excretion of phenolsulfonphthalein [32, 239].

Despite a normal or increased renal plasma flow, the renal arteriovenous oxygen difference and the total oxygen consumption of the kidneys are frequently reduced [42]. The reduction in oxygen consumption is probably due to the lowered glomerular filtration rate and the concomitant decrease in filtered sodium load. Because nearly all oxygen consumed by the kidney is utilized in the active transport of sodium from the tubular lumen, a reduction in the quantity of sodium presented for reabsorption is characteristically accompanied by a proportionate fall in the renal consumption of oxygen [139, 158]. The earlier hypothesis that oxygen intake is diminished in acute glomerulonephritis because of an impairment of tubular function no longer seems tenable.

The cause of the salt and water retention in acute glomerulonephritis remains uncertain. For many years it was thought that a reduction in glomerular filtration rate, and therefore in filtered sodium load, was responsible for the excessive reabsorption of sodium by the renal tubules. However, a number of clinical observations are at variance with this view. In some patients with glomerulonephritis, edema develops in the absence of a detectable reduction in inulin clearance. Moreover, in others in whom inulin clearance is abnormally low a diuresis occurs without a perceptible rise in filtration rate [66]. Physiologic studies also argue against the concept that a reduction in filtered sodium load is the prime determinant of edema formation. Chronic reductions in filtration rate induced by aortic clamping produce only a slight retention of sodium [54, 162], far too small to account for the sodium accumulation frequently observed in patients with acute glomerulonephritis. For these reasons, it seems almost certain that other factors must be at play; it is appealing to speculate, for example, that the inflammatory changes within the kidney influence sodium reabsorption by altering one or more of the physical determinants of sodium reabsorption, such as interstitial pressure, vasomotor tone, or oncotic pressure [67, 181, 182]. It is also possible that hormonal factors, such as changes in the rate of aldosterone secretion, are important, but further study of this problem will be necessary before the genesis of the salt and water retention can be determined.

During recovery from acute glomerulonephritis, there is a progressive rise in both glomerular filtration rate and filtration fraction and a restoration of normal tubular function. In most patients who are destined to heal, this improvement occurs within the first several weeks after the onset of symptoms [32, 66, 116], but in an occasional case a mild disturbance in renal function may persist for a longer time.

Impairment of renal function also occurs frequently during acute exacerbations of chronic glomerulonephritis. The hemodynamic changes are similar to those seen with a first attack of acute nephritis, both filtration rate and filtration fraction being reduced [66]. As the patient recovers from the acute exacerbation, renal function usually returns to the basal level determined by the severity of the preexisting renal disease [244].

Electrolyte Disturbances. In acute glomerulonephritis electrolyte disturbances are unusual since, as stated earlier, there is usually only modest impairment of renal function. Typically, plasma carbon dioxide content is normal and serum potassium concentration is normal or only slightly elevated. However, an occasional patient ingesting a diet high in potassium content may show moderate or severe hyperkalemia. This problem is discussed in the section on *Treatment* under "Diet."

In the presence of severe renal failure accompanied by oliguria or anuria, one may see the typical electrolyte disturbances that ensue in any form of acute renal sufficiency — namely, hyperkalemia, acidosis, hyperphosphatemia, and hypocalcemia. If, during the period of oliguria, fluid intake is not appropriately restricted, dilutional hyponatremia may also develop. Improvement in renal function and the onset of diuresis is followed by a prompt disappearance of all electrolyte abnormalities.

Laboratory Data

URINARY FINDINGS

Grossly, the urine is often reddish-brown or smoky in appearance. The supernatant in most cases has a characteristic rusty discoloration. This discoloration probably results from degeneration of red cells with a consequent liberation of hemoglobin, which is rapidly converted to acid hematin [115]. Even when the unspun urine is grossly clear, the spun urine may exhibit a small button of red blood cells at the bottom of the centrifuge tube. Often the urine volume is reduced, and the specific gravity, even after correction for the presence of protein, is high (usually greater than 1.015 or 1.020). If renal damage is severe, the specific gravity is usually lower (generally near 1.010). As would be expected, the specific gravity falls as urine volume increases during the period of diuresis.

Routine qualitative tests for protein commonly yield values of 1+ to 3+, but the 24-hour protein excretion varies considerably from patient to patient. In most cases it is less than 3 gm. per day, but it occasionally reaches a level of 5 to 15 gm. per day (see section on *Nephrotic Syndrome*).

Hematuria is the most obvious and striking abnormality on microscopic examination of the urinary sediment. The red blood cells are often crenated, and many ghost forms may be seen. A few white blood cells are almost always present, and in a rare case up to 40 or 50 white cells per high-power field may be found, even in the absence of active urinary tract infection.

A large number of casts are ordinarily present, often as many as 10 to 20 per low power field. Most of these are hyaline or granular in texture, but if the urine is examined meticulously, one will nearly always find a few red-cell casts (Fig. 13-1). This last finding is of particular importance when the diagnosis of acute glomerulonephritis is not obvious, because the red-cell cast provides strong evidence of the presence of a glomerulitis. Occasionally, casts containing renal tubular cells or mixtures of red blood cells and tubular cells may also be seen. In some cases white blood cell casts are encountered as well. Although this type of cast is ordinarily closely identified with pyelonephritis, one should remember that it may appear in other inflammatory diseases of the kidney, such as acute glomerulonephritis, lupus erythematosus, and anaphylactoid purpura. Fatty elements, including oval fat droplets, may also be seen from time to time but are usually present in only small numbers. No unfavorable prognostic significance is attached to the presence of such fatty elements.

EVOLUTION OF URINARY ABNORMALITIES

The duration of proteinuria is extremely variable. In some patients protein excretion returns to normal levels within a matter of days, whereas in others, in whom healing eventually takes place, it persists for weeks or months. Continued slight proteinuria will sometimes be overlooked if one relies only on qualitative examination of a random specimen. Failure to detect significant proteinuria

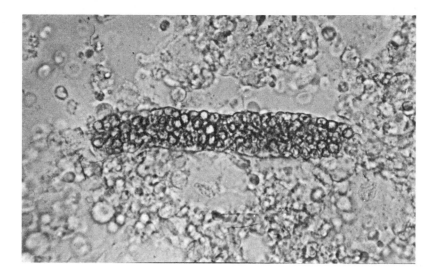

Figure 13-1. Typical red-cell cast from the urinary sediment of a patient with acute poststreptococcal glomerulonephritis. Multiple red blood cells are seen in the background. High power.

is particularly likely when protein excretion is in the range of 150 to 250 mg. per day (upper limit of normal in adults is 100 mg. per day), or when proteinuria is postural in nature. It is therefore desirable to measure the 24-hour excretion of urine in any suspected case in which proteinuria is not detected on examination of a random specimen. Quantitative values for protein excretion are also useful guides to the evolution of the disease, often giving evidence of improvement well before the healing process is reflected by qualitative examination of the urine.

Microscopic hematuria usually outlasts proteinuria by several weeks or months and may sometimes be present for as long as several years after the latter has disappeared. The urine of patients with persistent microscopic hematuria usually contains a few casts, including red blood cell casts, and these too may persist for prolonged periods [239].

A sudden transient increase in the degree of hematuria and proteinuria may occur in the convalescent patient in association with a new streptococcal infection, even when the infecting organism is not nephritogenic in character [178]. Similar exacerbations have also been reported after infections with viruses [39] and with bacteria other than streptococci [178].

IMPORTANT TECHNICAL CONSIDERATIONS IN EXAMINATION OF URINARY SEDIMENT

Certain simple precautions help to ensure that abnormalities of the urinary sediment will not be overlooked. The urine should be examined within 20 or 30 minutes after it is voided, because casts and, to a lesser degree, red blood cells are apt to deteriorate on prolonged standing. One should also try to obtain a specimen that has an acid pH; strongly alkaline urines are unlikely to reveal the number of formed elements that would otherwise be found, in part because cast formation in the distal portion of the tubule is inhibited by an alkaline pH, and also because casts, once formed, tend to disintegrate if the pH is high. It therefore cannot be assumed that the urinary sediment has yielded a maximum amount of information until several fresh, acid, and well-concentrated specimens have been meticulously examined.

As mentioned earlier, in cases in which one strongly suspects but cannot prove the diagnosis of acute glomerulonephritis, a particular effort should be made to determine if red-cell or hemoglobin casts are present. The likelihood of finding such casts will be enhanced if the sediment derived from several volumes of urine is examined. A concentrated sediment of this type can be obtained if the supernatant of a centrifuged specimen is decanted, replaced with unspun urine, and recentrifuged.

BACTERIOLOGY

Beta-hemolytic streptococci can be cultured from the nose and throat or from the skin in the majority of patients with untreated acute glomerulonephritis [23, 110, 173, 273]. In many patients, however, the infection will have disappeared spontaneously by the time glomerulonephritis appears, and in others the organisms are present in such small numbers or are buried so deeply in lymphoid tissue that they are difficult or impossible to isolate. If the initial culture is negative, it should be repeated at least once, because the probability of recovering the organism is thus considerably enhanced. Often when bacteriologic studies of the patient are negative, cultures of the nose and throat from members of the family or other close contacts will be positive. The implications of this finding are considered in the section on *Prophylaxis*.

HEMOGLOBIN AND HEMATOCRIT

Severe anemia is unusual, but slight reductions in hemoglobin and hematocrit concentrations occur in about half the cases. The anemia is primarily the result of sodium and water retention and the consequent expansion in plasma volume (see page 428). Commonly, the hemoglobin is reduced to a level of 11 to 12 gm. per 100 ml., and the hematocrit to approximately 35 per cent. As diuresis occurs (and plasma volume contracts), both hemoglobin concentration and hematocrit return

to normal levels. In nonedematous patients and in those who do not undergo a demonstrable diuresis, there is usually no anemia and the hematocrit remains constant throughout the illness [227].

It thus appears that the anemia is usually of a completely different origin from that seen in chronic renal failure, in which bone-marrow depression and hemolysis are the dominant etiologic factors [167, 238]. In only a few cases of acute glomerulonephritis has evidence been obtained that either of these latter factors is involved [44, 75, 134, 256].

SEDIMENTATION RATE

There is nearly always an increase in erythrocyte sedimentation rate in the early phase of the disease. Values between 30 and 60 mm. per hour (Westergren method) are common, and in a few cases the initial rate may exceed 100 mm. per hour [214, 239]. The level of the sedimentation rate during the acute illness has no prognostic significance; healing is as frequent whether it is mildly, moderately, or markedly elevated [214].

As the acute attack subsides, the sedimentation rate ordinarily returns slowly to normal. In most patients this change more or less parallels the healing of the renal lesion. In some, however, the sedimentation rate returns to normal before full recovery has taken place [231], and in others it remains elevated even after all clinical evidence of renal disease has disappeared [191]. Thus it appears that changes in the sedimentation rate have little prognostic value.

SERUM ALBUMIN CONCENTRATION

The serum albumin concentration is often slightly low [41, 114, 204]. This reduction appears to be largely the result of fluid retention and expansion of blood volume. As diuresis occurs and blood volume contracts, the albumin concentration ordinarily returns to normal [41]. The quantity of protein lost in the urine is usually relatively small and does not contribute significantly to the depression of serum albumin level. An occasional patient, however, may have massive proteinuria (5 to 15 gm. per day), and in such cases severe hypoalbuminemia may occur. Under such circumstances it may be difficult to decide whether the patient is suffering from acute glomerulonephritis or from the idiopathic nephrotic syndrome. This problem in diagnosis is discussed in a subsequent section.

CHOLESTEROL AND TOTAL LIPIDS

Approximately 40 per cent of patients with acute glomerulonephritis have a significant elevation of serum cholesterol concentration and of total serum lipids [114]. Hypercholesterolemia and hyperlipemia are found as often in those whose serum albumin concentration is normal as in those with low values [114]. Elevations in plasma concentration are seen as early as two to four days after the onset of the illness and usually disappear within three or four weeks.

Renal Histology

Serial renal biopsies have made it possible to demonstrate the earliest histologic changes that occur in acute glomerulonephritis and to clarify the relation between structural abnormalities and the subsequent clinical course. Furthermore, the application of technics such as electron and immunofluorescent microscopy has provided detailed information about ultrastructure that was unattainable by the use of traditional methods.

Early in the course of acute glomerulonephritis the glomeruli are hypercellular, and the capillary lumina, compressed by the cellular proliferation, are devoid of blood (Fig. 13-2) [60, 79, 84, 105, 113, 127, 142, 145, 190, 199, 251]. These changes are chiefly the result of hypertrophy and hyperplasia of capillary endothelial cells and mesangial cells, but an infiltration of leukocytes and macrophages

also contributes significantly [60, 84, 105, 113, 127, 142, 145, 190, 199, 251]; in an occasional case the leukocytic reaction is the dominant histologic feature [113, 127]. The abundant cellular proliferation and associated edema widens the waist of the axial stalk [113, 142, 190, 251], giving individual lobules a club-shaped appearance and accentuating the lobular pattern of each glomerulus (Figs. 13-2 and 13-3) [113, 199]. There is little alteration in the glomerular epithelial cells except for some cytoplasmic swelling. The foot processes may be plump and fused in some areas but, by contrast with the marked alterations seen in the idiopathic nephrotic syndrome, the changes are slight and patchy [82, 113, 142, 145, 190, 251]. Irregular swelling of the basement membrane is a nearly constant finding and has been shown to result from the accumulation of electron-dense material on the surface of the membrane or within the laminae. Two types of deposits have been identified: the focal and the diffuse. The first type of lesion, the focal accumulation, which is regularly found in patients with acute poststreptococcal glomerulonephritis [79, 84, 113, 142] is also sometimes encountered in "focal glomerulonephritis" [246]. These deposits are located on the epithelial side of the basement membrane, and protrude into the cytoplasm of the epithelial cells (Fig. 13-4) frequently opposing fused foot processes [79, 84, 113, 142]. Such focal accumulations are most often found in peripheral capillary loops and are seen almost exclusively during the first six weeks after the onset of the disease [113]. The second type of lesion results from the diffuse accumulation of electron-dense material beneath the endothelial or epithelial cells of the basement membrane or within the laminae [84, 142, 190, 199, 251]; it is this abnormality that is chiefly responsible for the distortion of the structure of the membrane [142, 190, 199, 251]. Similar diffuse deposits are found in a variety of diseases other than acute glomerulonephritis. Immunofluorescent studies of renal biopsy material

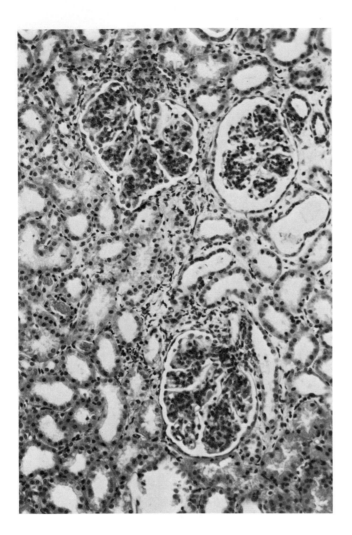

Figure 13-2. Renal biopsy demonstrating three glomeruli with abnormal lobulation, diffuse hypercellularity, narrowed tuft capillaries, and swelling of the glomerulus with decrease in Bowman's capsular space. Hematoxylin and eosin. ×120. (Courtesy of Dr. Sheldon C. Sommers.)

have demonstrated that both the focal and the diffuse electron-dense deposits contain β_1C globulin and gamma G globulin [84, 187]. The "lumpy-bumpy" pattern seen under immunofluorescence is indistinguishable from that observed in other forms of immune deposit disease.

Studies during the acute phase of the disease have shown a rough correlation between the severity of the glomerular lesion and the degree of impairment of glomerular function, as measured by inulin clearance [145, 202]. Patients with pronounced glomerular proliferation tend to have marked reductions in clearance, whereas those with minor changes usually have little or no change in function. There are, however, many exceptions to this general rule [122, 145].

The renal tubules are also affected in acute glomerulonephritis. Tubular dilatation and cloudy swelling, vacuolization, degeneration, and atrophy are frequently seen [122, 145, 262]. One also frequently finds red-cell casts within the tubular lumina [64, 127]. In the interstitial space there may be edema, fibrosis, and infiltration with inflammatory cells, but these changes are not usually prominent. No correlation has been noted between

Figure 13-3. Renal biopsy demonstrating axial hypercellularity (*arrows*) with crowded mesangial-cell nuclei that arborize from the hilus of the glomerulus. Hematoxylin and eosin. ×600. (Courtesy of Dr. Sheldon C. Sommers.)

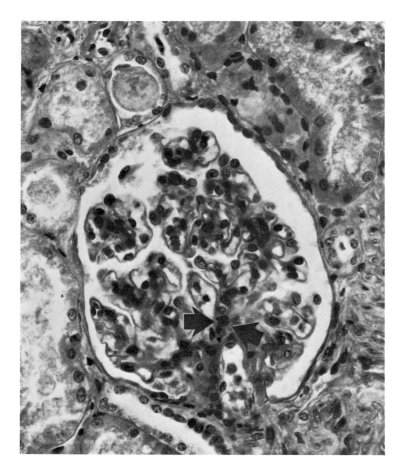

the severity of histologic abnormalities and changes in tubular function [262].

Serial biopsies done during recovery from the acute phase of the disease have demonstrated, as one might expect, that normal glomerular architecture is progressively restored. As the activity of the process subsides, glomerular swelling is reduced, capillaries reopen, and Bowman's space enlarges [60, 84, 113, 199, 251]. The time sequence of improvement in the histologic findings varies from patient to patient and probably depends on the initial severity of the glomerular lesion as well as on the inherent effectiveness of the patient's reparative processes.

When the severe proliferative response subsides, scattered residual abnormalities may be seen, including focal hypercellularity, scarring of the axial stalk, glomerular scars, and adhesions. These features can be found even in patients in whom all clinical and laboratory evidence of the disease has disappeared [60, 84, 152, 251]. Such slight residual evidences of the disease do not appear to have any clinical significance.

The histologic appearance of the kidney during the acute phase of the illness is often of value in foretelling the outcome of the disease. Severe abnormalities such as massive glomerular proliferation and extensive thrombosis and fibrinoid necrosis have an ominous prognostic significance; in most cases these lesions lead to oliguria, progressive renal failure, and death from uremia within a short time [36,

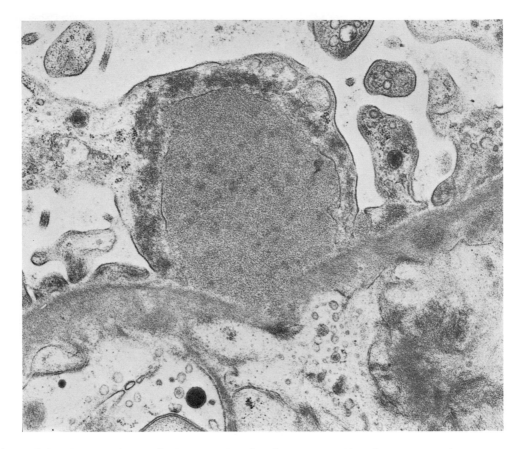

Figure 13-4. Electron micrograph demonstrating the glomerular capillary basement membrane extending across the midportion of the photograph. Bulging upward from the outer surface of the basement membrane is a prominent electron-dense deposit. Portions of epithelial cytoplasm are stretched over the periphery of the large deposit. ×22,500. (Courtesy of Dr. Jacob Churg.)

236]. Even less severe histologic abnormalities may augur ill for the patient; proliferative changes of a magnitude sufficient to elevate serum creatinine concentration to more than 10 mg. per 100 ml. usually herald, even in the absence of oliguria, the inexorable progression of the renal disease [161]. Death typically occurs within several months of the onset of the illness.

The biopsy also has considerable prognostic value in patients with slight or no impairment of function, serving as a useful guide to the likelihood of ultimate healing. Those who demonstrate hypercellularity of the glomeruli as the sole abnormality are likely to undergo complete recovery, whereas those who demonstrate abnormalities such as glomerular crescents and adhesions and interstitial fibrosis are more likely to develop chronic renal disease [64, 127]. There are, however, numerous exceptions to these generalizations. Even when glomerular hypercellularity is the only significant lesion, healing does not invariably occur. Conversely, the presence of mild and patchy glomerular hyalinization or even of a few crescents or scars [127, 234] does not preclude the possibility of complete clinical recovery.

Glomerulonephritis After Infections Not of Hemolytic Streptococcal Origin

SUBACUTE BACTERIAL ENDOCARDITIS

Two types of glomerular disease are encountered in patients with subacute bacterial endocarditis: One is a diffuse process indistinguishable from that seen in classic poststreptococcal glomerulonephritis; the other is a distinctive disorder in which the lesions, at least initially, involve only a portion of the glomerulus. The term *focal embolic glomerulonephritis* has usually been applied to the latter abnormality. The lesions just described have been found not only when *Streptococcus viridans* is the etiologic agent but also when the endocarditis is caused by gonococci, pneumococci, or the influenza bacillus [13, 15, 247]. The majority of patients with renal involvement have proteinuria, hematuria, and cylindruia [45, 103, 131, 184, 240, 254], but even when the urinalysis is normal, structural abnormalities of the kidney may be found at postmortem examination [45].

Studies early in this century suggested that the diffuse glomerular lesion rarely occurred in patients with positive blood cultures but instead was restricted almost exclusively to those in the "abacterial phase" [14, 164]. Subsequent observations (in the pre-penicillin era) did not confirm these findings. The frequency of diffuse glomerulonephritis is apparently similar in patients with or without demonstrable bacteremia; postmortem examination has revealed the lesion in approximately one-third to one-half of each group [17, 45, 135, 247, 257].

In focal embolic glomerulonephritis there are histologic alterations in only a single lobule, or in several lobules, of the affected glomeruli, and many glomeruli are spared entirely [17]. Two distinct types of lesions are found, the hyaline and the fibrous. The hyaline lesions consist chiefly of intracapillary thromboses with or without necrosis of capillary walls. Fibrous lesions, on the other hand, are characterized by thickening of the basement membrane and, in the most severe form, by obliteration of capillaries and the formation of dense fibrotic areas. Either the hyaline or the fibrous type may produce injury serious enough ultimately to obliterate the entire glomerulus [17, 30].

The origin of the focal lesions of focal embolic glomerulonephritis is obscure. Early workers ascribed them to bacterial emboli originating from the heart valves, but more recently it has been suggested that they are the result of an immunologic disorder similar to that proposed for the renal lesion of acute glomerulonephritis. The latter pathogenic mechanism has been proposed chiefly because focal embolic glomerulonephritis has been shown to occur in patients without positive blood cultures and also in those whose infection is limited to the right side of the heart [15, 16]. Furthermore, bacteria are rarely found in the glomerular lesions.

It has frequently been stated that renal insufficiency in subacute bacterial endocarditis is almost always the result of diffuse glomerulonephritis. However, uremia secondary to extensive focal embolic glomerulonephritis is not uncommon [17, 30, 257]; for this reason, it is difficult if not impossible to predict on clinical grounds the nature of the renal involvement in the azotemic patient. Furthermore, focal embolic glomerulonephritis and diffuse glomerulonephritis may coexist, each contributing to the impairment of renal function.

In the preantibiotic era uremia contributed to the fatal outcome in about 5 to 10 per cent of cases. Antibiotic therapy has markedly reduced the overall mortality rate from renal insufficiency [25, 38, 94, 184, 205, 212a, 226, 247, 255, 258], but renal failure continues to be a common cause of death among patients in whom the infection does not respond to treatment [129, 200]. In rare cases death from uremia has been reported even after bacteriologic cure [103, 129]. In patients dying despite therapy, diffuse and focal embolic lesions are seen with about the same frequency as in untreated patients studied in the prepenicillin era [129, 200].

Slight impairment of renal function is still encountered commonly, but if not present before the beginning of therapy, it is unlikely to appear later [129]. After appropriate antibiotic therapy, function usually returns to normal. Proteinuria and sediment abnormalities, which are frequently seen even in patients without renal dysfunction, ordinarily diminish or disappear during the course of treatment [200, 205]; clinical evidence of renal disease is thus rarely manifest for more than a few months [43]. On the other hand, residual histologic changes often persist indefinitely [228, 247].

It should be emphasized that renal failure is no longer a frequent clinical problem in subacute bacterial endocarditis. In fact, in the patient treated early and successfully for his underlying infection, renal insufficiency is a rare complication.

OTHER INFECTIONS

Clinical and histologic features typical of acute poststreptococcal glomerulonephritis have been noted to occur occasionally in patients with a variety of infections, both bacterial and viral. It has frequently been proposed, therefore, that the renal lesion generally held to be of poststreptococcal origin may, in fact, have multiple antecedents. Among the bacteria said to have nephritogenic properties, the pneumococcus has figured most prominently [24, 99, 197, 213, 241]. Among the viruses, those of influenza, coxsackie, ECHO, mumps, and measles have most often been singled out as the offending agents [128, 222]. The finding that exfoliated cells in the urine of patients with measles and cytomegalic inclusion disease often contain inclusion bodies [128, 222] has been adduced as specific evidence that

viral diseases may produce significant renal involvement.

It is apparent, on the other hand, that before one can conclude that acute nephritis is a direct consequent of any of the above infections, it is necessary to rule out the presence of a concomitant infection with a beta-hemolytic streptococcus. If negative throat (or skin) cultures and a persistently normal ASO titer are taken as minimum criteria for excluding a streptococcal infection, most of the reported instances of nonstreptococcal nephritis cannot be viewed as established cases. There are, however, a few well-studied cases of acute glomerulonephritis associated with mumps, varicella, and ECHO virus infections in which the data suggest that a streptococcal infection was not present [121, 188, 274, 275]. Even in these cases, however, the relation between the viral illness and the glomerulonephritis cannot be considered firmly established. Studies of antibodies to streptococci other than ASO, such as AH, ASK, and ADNase, were not performed, and it is conceivable that such observations would have provided evidence for a complicating streptococcal infection. Detailed immunologic observations in suspected cases of viral nephritis, combined with histologic examination by immunofluorescent and electron microscopy, should help determine if viral diseases can produce the syndrome of acute glomerulonephritis.

Clinical Course and Prognosis

MORTALITY IN THE ACUTE PHASE

Until recent years, the mortality rate in the acute phase of glomerulonephritis was approximately 5 to 10 per cent [5, 39, 47, 74, 96, 171, 172, 214]. Death was most often the result of either the original inciting infection, pulmonary edema, or hypertensive encephalopathy. In the last decade or two, this pattern has changed. The widespread use of antibiotics, sodium restriction, and antihypertensive drugs has appreciably reduced the number of fatalities. The occasional death that still occurs as the result of circulatory congestion or hypertensive encephalopathy is usually the consequence of a delay in obtaining adequate medical attention.

Now that most of the major complications of the disease are controllable, a lethal outcome is usually caused by severe glomerular damage. Irreversible renal failure occurs in 1 to 2 per cent of patients and manifests itself clinically by a prolonged period of severe oliguria or anuria. Although anuria of more than three or four days' duration usually presages a fatal outcome, such a result does not always follow. An occasional patient undergoes a diuresis and demonstrates considerable improvement of renal function even after periods of anuria ranging up to four or five weeks [8, 109, 132, 161, 175, 186]. Complete recovery — that is, restoration of normal renal function and disappearance of proteinuria — is rarely seen in adults but occasionally occurs in children [107, 109, 251]. On the basis of these prognostic considerations, it seems justified to dialyze the oliguric or anuric patient over a prolonged period before it is concluded that the renal damage is irreversible.

It has been proposed that the anuric form of poststreptococcal glomerulonephritis occurs with particular frequency in patients over the age of fifty [160], but it is not entirely clear that such a conclusion is warranted. In many cases the documentation of a preexisting streptococcal infection is lacking [20, 29, 109, 160], and in others a history of purpura or hemoptysis [20, 29] raises the possibility that a disease of small blood vessels was the underlying disorder. More detailed studies of patients over the age of fifty with "anuric acute glomerulonephritis" will be needed to determine how often this syndrome occurs as an aftermath of streptococcal infections.

In a few cases the acute phase of glomerulonephritis merges into a state of *subacute glomerulonephritis*. In such patients the florid changes initially present in the urinary sediment persist, and in some cases a frank nephrotic syndrome develops [21, 175]. Progression into the subacute form of the disease is an ominous prognostic sign because it is characterized by relentless deterioration of renal function [21, 74, 109, 161, 175], with death usually occurring in a period of six months to two years.

LONG-TERM PROGNOSIS

As is evident from the preceding paragraphs, the great majority of patients do not suffer from severe renal failure and recover from the acute phase of the illness in an uneventful fashion. However, even among those with mild or moderate renal insufficiency the magnitude of the functional changes has important implications for the likelihood of ultimate healing — that is, the less the reduction in filtration rate, the greater the probability of full recovery [161].

As discussed earlier, the histology of the kidney during the acute phase can also provide a useful prognostic guide. If a large proportion of the glomeruli demonstrate changes such as epithelial crescents and adhesions, the outlook for full recovery is not favorable [64, 127]. By contrast, proliferation of endothelial or mesangial cells, even when moderately severe, generally does not have unfavorable prognostic significance. It should be emphasized, however, that though these correlations have value for predicting the outcome in large groups of patients, they have only limited applicability to the individual case; full recovery sometimes takes place despite histologic changes of considerable magnitude, and persistent renal disease may develop even in the patient with what appears to be mild renal injury [64, 127, 234].

Except for the histologic and functional features already considered, the other manifestations of the disease have no prognostic significance. Such indices as the degree of hematuria, proteinuria, or hypertension, or the rapidity of the sedimentation rate do not foretell the likelihood of healing.

Observations in the preantibiotic era suggested that persistence of the streptococcal infection during an attack of acute glomerulonephritis was accompanied by an increased tendency to chronic renal disease [170, 172], but this view has been disputed [47, 63]. Such considerations are now largely academic, because prompt treatment with antibiotics has made persistent infection a rarity.

FREQUENCY OF COMPLETE RECOVERY

Complete recovery can be said to occur only when renal function has returned to normal, 24-hour protein excretion is less than 100 mg. per day, and abnormalities of the urinary sediment have disappeared.

The outlook for healing in *children* is excellent, disappearance of all urinary abnormalities generally having been reported in some 85 to 95 per cent of cases [2, 5, 39, 47, 53, 68, 95, 96, 106, 117, 126, 172, 177, 178, 206]. More recently, in fact, several authors have presented data suggesting that all children with acute glomerulonephritis recover completely [26, 165, 203]; the exact frequency of healing in childhood must therefore be viewed as a question yet to be resolved. In *adults,* on the other hand, it appears that only 50 to 75 per cent become free of all evidences of renal disease [19, 47, 64, 161, 214, 225, 323]. The explanation for this lower frequency of healing is not clear, but it may well reflect differences in immunologic or other host factors. Alternatively, it is possible that the inclusion of a large number of patients undergoing an acute exacerbation of an unrecognized latent glomerulonephritis has contributed significantly to the apparently less favorable outlook in adults than in children [111].

In a matter of four to six months after the acute attack the urines of approximately half the adults [225] and the great majority of children [2, 95, 117, 178, 231] are free of protein. Within 12 months most patients destined

to heal already have done so; if there is a continued abnormal excretion of protein beyond this time, there are reasonable grounds for concern that the patient has entered the latent phase. However, complete recovery sometimes takes place even when proteinuria has persisted for longer than a year [127, 175, 225, 239].

The demonstration that proteinuria, though persistent, has become postural in nature is of considerable prognostic significance, because it suggests that healing will ultimately occur. Even if postural proteinuria persists, it apparently has little clinical significance [57, 58, 239].

As mentioned earlier, microscopic hematuria and red-cell casts may be found for as long as several years after proteinuria has disappeared; these sediment abnormalities do not appear to have unfavorable prognostic implications and should not be interpreted as evidence that chronic renal disease will develop.

There is little evidence that *hypertension* occurs as a sequel to healed acute glomerulonephritis; long-term studies of patients who have recovered from acute glomerulonephritis indicate that persistent elevation of blood pressure is an uncommon finding [111, 214]. In addition, the incidence of hypertension in patients with healed nephritis and in control subjects has been found to be similar [232]. The only evidence favoring the existence of "postnephritic hypertension" is derived from observations on several patients in whom an elevated blood pressure persisted for as long as one to two years after proteinuria had disappeared [11].

Patients who do not heal and enter the so-called latent stage of glomerulonephritis often remain entirely well for many years. The only demonstrable abnormalities are persistent proteinuria, microscopic hematuria, and cylindruria. Eventually, progressive renal insufficiency slowly develops in many of these patients [19], but a few retain normal renal function for several decades or longer and ultimately succumb to an unrelated illness

NEPHROTIC SYNDROME

The nephrotic syndrome is an infrequent feature of acute glomerulonephritis, but it may occur at two points during the course of the disease. In an occasional case it appears concomitantly with the onset of the acute attack [175, 239, 272]; the development of the nephrotic syndrome at this stage of the illness has not been thought to alter the usual benign clinical course of acute glomerulonephritis [272], but a recent report suggests that it may, in fact, be associated with an increased incidence of progressive renal failure [175]. As mentioned earlier, the nephrotic syndrome may also appear several weeks after the onset of the acute attack, heralding the development of subacute glomerulonephritis.

In an occasional patient, the nephrotic syndrome develops long after the acute attack, in the course of the latent phase of the disease [1, 159]. The subsequent evolution may be into progressive renal failure, but a return to the latent phase can also take place.

Recurrences

Many years ago it was observed that patients who have fully recovered from an attack of acute glomerulonephritis rarely suffer a second attack even if they contract a subsequent infection with beta-hemolytic streptococci [166].* Before the recognition that only certain types of streptococci are nephritogenic there was no satisfactory explanation for this phenomenon. It now appears that the infrequency of recurrences is accounted for by type-specific immunity to the original organism together with the small statistical likelihood that the patient will become infected with a

second nephritogenic organism. Persons with healed glomerulonephritis probably have further immunologic protection against a potentially nephrotoxic reinfection because nephritogenic streptococci often share certain antigenic properties [28].

When penicillin is administered early in the course of a streptococcal infection, the type-specific antibody response is inhibited [50], and therefore the usual immunity to reinfection cannot be relied upon [33]. This fact may have important implications for the patient who has recovered from acute glomerulonephritis if, as just discussed, the rarity of second attacks is chiefly the consequence of prolonged type-specific immunity. The continued susceptibility to infection with the original nephritogenic organism (which is likely to be endemic in the community) in penicillin-treated patients would be expected to result in an increased frequency of such recurrences. Whether or not second attacks are occurring more often now than in the pre-antibiotic era is not possible to say, but future observations on the natural history of the disease should serve to answer this question.

Patients with chronic glomerulonephritis may have acute exacerbations that are closely similar to first attacks. Although an early study of this problem [244] indicated that such flare-ups occur in approximately one-fifth of patients with chronic disease, more recent experience suggests that the incidence is considerably lower. When exacerbations occur, they are characterized by a marked increase in hematuria and, in most cases, a reduction in renal function [244]. This element of renal dysfunction usually disappears as the acute illness subsides [244].

Differential Diagnosis

A variety of renal diseases share with acute glomerulonephritis one or more of its typical manifestations, and under some circumstances

---

* That second attacks occur at all has been questioned by some observers, but several reports appear to substantiate the existence of such recurrences [23, 31, 214].

these similarities may lead to difficult problems in diagnosis. In the present section the disorders most likely to create confusion are considered briefly, and the salient features that often serve to elucidate the diagnosis are summarized.

ACUTE EXACERBATIONS OF CHRONIC GLOMERULONEPHRITIS

Patients with an acute exacerbation of chronic glomerulonephritis may exhibit clinical features and changes in the urinary sediment identical with those of acute glomerulonephritis. For prognostic purposes it is obviously important to distinguish between these two entities, because healing cannot be anticipated if the episode represents an exacerbation of an underlying chronic process. As the first step in diagnosis, it should be determined whether the patient has suffered earlier from an illness suggestive of acute glomerulonephritis or if proteinuria has been found on previous examinations. Every effort should be made to obtain information concerning urinalyses performed in connection with examinations for military service, employment, life insurance, or previous hospitalizations. From these data alone it will often be possible either virtually to exclude the diagnosis of antecedent renal disease or to confirm its presence with a reasonable degree of confidence.

Another feature of the history that may be of help is the duration of the latent period. If only one or two days have elapsed from the onset of the streptococcal infection, there is a strong likelihood that the attack represents an acute recurrence in a patient with chronic disease [244].

When the history is inconclusive, several physical and laboratory findings may be of diagnostic value. Extensive changes in the optic fundi, such as hemorrhages and exudates, as well as clinical, electrocardiographic, or radiographic evidence of left ventricular hypertrophy, point to the existence of long-standing hypertension and thus to the presence of chronic renal disease. The demonstration of broad "renal-failure casts" in the urinary sediment also points to the diagnosis of chronic glomerulonephritis. Plain films of the abdomen may provide additional useful information because a reduction in renal mass is almost certainly indicative of chronic rather than of acute renal disease.

ACUTE TUBULAR NECROSIS

The patient with acute tubular necrosis may at times present a clinical picture difficult to distinguish from that seen in the oliguric patient with acute glomerulonephritis. In most cases, however, the history will provide valuable diagnostic information. In acute tubular necrosis there will usually be an obvious predisposing cause such as prolonged hypotension, trauma, a transfusion reaction, or exposure to nephrotoxic agents. Examination of the urine may also be helpful. Typically, in tubular necrosis there is a profusion of narrow hyaline and granular casts, and often many renal tubular cells are present. Hematuria is not usually a prominent feature unless the patient has been catheterized. By contrast, patients with acute glomerulonephritis are more likely to have marked microscopic hematuria and fewer casts. In both instances, hemoglobin casts may be present, although such casts are seen more frequently and in greater numbers in patients with acute glomerulonephritis. Red-cell casts rarely occur in acute tubular necrosis.

Additional diagnostic information may be obtained by measurement of urinary specific gravity and sodium concentration. In acute glomerulonephritis, the specific gravity is usually high during the oliguric phase (1.015 to 1.020 or more), and the sodium concentration is low [250]. In acute tubular necrosis, the specific gravity is ordinarily close to that of an ultrafiltrate of plasma (1.010), and the urine sodium concentration is high (greater than 40 mEq. per liter) [37]. None of the above laboratory measurements serve as absolute means of differentiation, but the combination of a careful history and appropriate studies of the urine will usually make it possible to arrive at the correct diagnosis.

FOCAL GLOMERULONEPHRITIS

Patients with focal glomerulonephritis commonly give a history of gross hematuria that has developed closely on the heels of a respiratory infection [27, 85, 108, 229, 246]. Urinalysis reveals a smoky urine containing red blood cells and red blood cell casts, changes characteristic of an acute glomerulitis. Although the clinical picture may be similar to that seen in acute glomerulonephritis, several distinctive features usually make it possible to arrive at the correct diagnosis. Typically, the interval between the preceding respiratory infection and the onset of hematuria in focal nephritis is only one or two days, whereas in acute poststreptococcal nephritis the latent period is generally one or two weeks. In addition, the respiratory infection in focal nephritis is usually not of streptococcal origin. These distinguishing features taken together with the absence of hypertension or edema usually serve to suggest the correct diagnosis.

Long-term observations will usually provide further help in clarifying the problem. Patients who have had poststreptococcal nephritis and have either recovered or entered the latent phase rarely have recurrent bouts of gross hematuria, whereas those with focal nephritis commonly have such recurrences. A renal biopsy will, of course, provide the most definitive information, the typical patchy lesions of focal glomerulonephritis standing in sharp contrast to the diffuse lesion of poststreptococcal nephritis. In an occasional case, however, the clinical syndrome of focal glomerulonephritis may occur in association with a diffuse renal lesion [85], and the exact classification and prognosis of such cases remains to be determined.

HEREDITARY NEPHRITIS

Although patients with hereditary nephritis usually do not have the clinical manifestations of acute poststreptococcal glomerulonephritis (edema, hypertension, circulatory congestion), they may have gross hematuria and changes in the urinary sediment identical to those seen in acute nephritis. There are some features, however, that are distinctive. *Recurrent* gross hematuria is common in hereditary nephritis but is rare in poststreptococcal nephritis. In addition, patients with hereditary nephritis frequently have a positive family history of nerve deafness and of death from renal failure. Furthermore, because of the dominant, nonsex-linked nature of the inheritance pattern, a large number of close relatives may be found to have hematuria, proteinuria, and evidence of impaired hearing. Thus, in any suspected case careful study of parents, siblings, and even aunts, uncles, and cousins is likely to be helpful in clarifying the diagnosis.

OTHER GLOMERULITIDES

Patients with diseases such as anaphylactoid purpura, polyarteritis nodosa, Wegener's granulomatosis, Goodpasture's syndrome, and rapidly progressive glomerulonephritis often have gross hematuria, proteinuria, cylindruria, and renal failure. Usually, however, there is no preceding history of a respiratory infection, the throat culture is negative, and the ASO titer is normal. In addition, the clinical manifestations are often notably different from those seen in poststreptococcal nephritis, the illness frequently being characterized by such features as gastrointestinal bleeding, purpura, arthralgia, fever, and pulmonary hemorrhage. Furthermore, the course of these disorders is often stormy with progressive renal failure developing within a few weeks or months.

The recent development of immunofluorescent methods applied to kidney biopsies offers considerable promise of clarifying the nosology of this group of renal diseases, and these technics have already been shown to have diagnostic value. A linear pattern of fluorescence of the glomerular capillary wall (presumably caused by antiglomerular basement membrane antibodies) has been identified as characteristic in patients with Goodpasture's syndrome and in some patients with rapidly progressive glomerulonephritis [59a]. By contrast, a lumpy, nodular pattern of fluorescence (presumably caused by deposition of immune complexes) is found in lupus nephritis and poststreptococcal glomerulonephritis [59a].

IDIOPATHIC NEPHROTIC SYNDROME

Patients with idiopathic nephrotic syndrome ("lipoid nephrosis," Ellis Type 2 glomerulonephritis) ordinarily do not have a previous history of a respiratory infection, their throat cultures are negative for beta-hemolytic streptococci, and their ASO titers are not elevated. Hypertension is uncommon, and both gross hematuria and clinical evidence of circulatory congestion are rarely if ever seen. Microscopic hematuria is usually slight (rarely exceeding 10 to 15 RBC/HPF), and red-cell casts, though sometimes present, are scanty in number. Even if the history and laboratory findings are inconclusive, continued observation will in most cases clarify the nature of the underlying disease. In patients with the idiopathic nephrotic syndrome, hypoalbuminemia, hypercholesterolemia, massive proteinuria, and edema ordinarily persist for many months. In the occasional patient in whom a nephrotic picture occurs as a feature of acute glomerulonephritis, the nephrotic syndrome is usually of short duration, typically lasting for only a few days or weeks. The nephrotic syndrome as it occurs in the course of acute glomerulonephritis is discussed in more detail under *Clinical Course*.

SUBACUTE BACTERIAL ENDOCARDITIS

Acute glomerulonephritis occurring as a complication of subacute bacterial endocarditis has been discussed in detail in an earlier section. The urinary findings are identical to those of poststreptococcal nephritis, but hypertension, edema, and gross hematuria are uncommon. Furthermore, there is ordinarily no history of a preceding respiratory infection, and the ASO titer is normal [138]. Because none of the above features offer an absolute means of distinguishing between the two disorders, the differentiation ultimately depends upon establishing the diagnosis of subacute bacterial endocarditis. Cardiac murmurs, persistent fever, splenomegaly, and splinter hemorrhages point to the latter disorder, and the demonstration of bacteremia confirms the clinical impression.

MALIGNANT HYPERTENSION

Malignant hypertension may present many features suggestive of acute glomerulonephritis. The elevated blood pressure is frequently accompanied by proteinuria, hematuria, and a mild or moderate degree of renal functional impairment, and in a few cases, the presence of red blood cell casts further serves to confuse the diagnosis. By careful evaluation of the entire clinical picture, it is usually possible to differentiate between the two disorders. An important feature is that the blood pressure uncommonly rises above 115 or 120 mm. Hg in the patient with acute glomerulonephritis, whereas it is characteristically elevated above this level in malignant hypertension. Furthermore, extreme elevations of blood pressure, even when they occur in acute glomerulonephritis, are usually of too brief duration to produce the retinal hemorrhages, exudates, and papilledema characteristic of malignant hypertension. A reduction in kidney size also indicates that the hypertension is of relatively long standing and is almost certainly not the result of acute nephritis.

Although slight or moderate renal failure may be present in both disorders, it usually disappears rather promptly in acute glomerulonephritis, whereas in malignant hypertension it tends to progress even after the blood pressure has been reduced by therapy. In the rare case in which the clinical picture and the natural history of the illness do not clarify the diagnosis, a renal biopsy will usually do so.

URINARY ABNORMALITIES INDUCED BY EXERCISE

Proteinuria, hematuria, and cylindruria are frequently encountered after strenuous exercise, often rendering the urine indistinguishable from that seen in acute glomerulonephritis [97]. These changes occur not only after contact sports such as football and boxing [92], in which there is direct trauma to the kidneys, but also after other vigorous activities such as swimming and rowing [7]. The abnormalities usually disappear within one or two days and have no clinical significance. The explanation for the urinary findings is readily arrived at by means of a carefully taken history and by reexaminations of the urine after the patient has avoided exercise for several days.

FEBRILE PROTEINURIA

Mild proteinuria and cylindruria occur commonly at the height of a variety of acute febrile illnesses. Indeed, proteinuria can readily be produced in normal persons by elevating the body temperature by physical means [265]. These abnormal urinary findings disappear promptly when fever subsides and ordinarily present no problem in diagnosis.

Prophylaxis

It is now well recognized that the incidence of acute glomerulonephritis can be sharply reduced if the dissemination of the nephritogenic streptococcus is halted; if penicillin prophylaxis is employed during an epidemic, it is promptly effective in aborting the spread of the disease [223]. This epidemiologic fact obviously has important implications for the physician dealing with a case of poststreptococcal acute nephritis; not only should the patient himself be treated (see page 449), but all those with whom he has been in intimate contact should be studied by bacteriologic means to identify those who are harboring hemolytic streptococci. Such persons should receive penicillin in amounts sufficient to eradicate the organism. A single injection of 600,000 units of benzathine penicillin appears to be adequate for this purpose.

DOES TREATMENT OF THE STREPTOCOCCAL INFECTION PREVENT ACUTE GLOMERULONEPHRITIS?

Acute glomerulonephritis often follows in the wake of a streptococcal infection even when the organism has been eradicated promptly by appropriate antibiotic therapy [18, 249, 264]. Whether prompt treatment of infection reduces the statistical likelihood of renal sequelae in patients infected with nephritogenic streptococci has, however, not been answered definitively. From the only controlled observations on this problem, it was concluded that such therapy does have a protective effect [249]. However, when the difference between the penicillin-treated and the control group was evaluated by means of the chi-square test, the results proved not to be statistically significant [133]. Further study will be necessary before any firm conclusion can be drawn concerning the efficacy of antibiotic therapy in reducing the frequency of subsequent renal disease.

Treatment

No therapeutic measure has been shown to influence either the speed with which recovery takes place or the probability of ultimate healing. Many forms of treatment, such as prolonged bed rest, a low-protein diet, and adrenocorticosteroid therapy, have been reported to influence favorably the course of the disease, but, as is discussed below, there is no convincing evidence to support the view that any of these is efficacious.

On the other hand, complications of the illness can be influenced or controlled by appropriate measures based on an understanding of the pathophysiologic mechanisms involved. Potentially fatal disorders, including hypertensive encephalopathy, pulmonary edema, and hyperkalemia, are amenable to therapy. Severe renal failure accompanied by oliguria or anuria cannot be dealt with by an attack on the underlying problem, but if life is prolonged by dialysis, an optimal opportunity can be provided for repair or healing of the renal lesion.

EDEMA AND CIRCULATORY CONGESTION

The single most important measure in control of edema and prevention of circulatory congestion is restriction of salt intake because (except in the severely oliguric or anuric patient) sodium retention is a prerequisite for fluid accumulation. Usually, no therapy other than salt restriction is necessary, but if edema is marked or there are signs and symptoms of pulmonary congestion, vigorous treatment with diuretics may be necessary. If significant azotemia is present, a diuretic such as furosemide should be employed; in contrast to most other agents this drug exhibits natriuretic properties even when the creatinine clearance is as low as 5 to 10 ml. per minute [195, 196]. The large doses of furosemide often required to achieve a satisfactory diuresis in the face of impaired renal function do not appear to carry a significant hazard of serious side effects [196, 223a]. If pulmonary congestion is severe, more urgent measures must be employed. The head of the bed should be elevated, or, if feasible, the patient should be placed in a cardiac chair. The resulting shift of fluid to the lower extremities may in itself produce a striking improvement in respiratory signs and symptoms. Additional benefit may be derived from the use of rotating tourniquets, positive-pressure ventilation, morphine, and oxygen. Venesection, with removal of 500 ml. of blood in adults and a proportionately smaller volume in children, may also be followed by marked improvement. If underlying heart disease is present, control of hypertension will prevent a deleterious effect of the elevated blood pressure on myocardial function.

There is no convincing evidence that

digitalis ordinarily has a favorable effect on the circulatory abnormalities (see page 429). However, if the patient is desperately ill, a trial with this drug is warranted because even the remote possibility of a beneficial effect outweighs the potential hazards of treatment. If there is evidence of underlying heart disease or of true cardiac failure (for example, if the circulation time is prolonged), it is more likely that digitalis will have therapeutic value. Preparations with a rapid onset of action such as digoxin, lanatoside C, or ouabain should be used.

HYPERTENSION AND HYPERTENSIVE ENCEPHALOPATHY

There is no evidence that mild hypertension has a deleterious effect on the clinical course, and therapy is therefore not necessary. However, a marked elevation of blood pressure, with diastolic values of 115 mm. Hg or more, is an indication for a prompt program of antihypertensive therapy. Such treatment becomes a matter of urgency if cerebral symptoms appear.

In past years magnesium sulfate was the drug most widely used for the treatment of hypertensive encephalopathy. However, hypertension is often not controlled by this agent even when the drug is used to the point of toxicity as reflected by absence of the knee jerks. In addition, the use of magnesium sulfate can be hazardous, because if the plasma magnesium level is raised excessively both stupor and respiratory paralysis may result [118, 219]. Patients with renal insufficiency are especially prone to such complications because of their inability to excrete magnesium at a normal rate [219].

The development of more effective and less toxic antihypertensive drugs such as reserpine and hydralazine have made magnesium sulfate therapy obsolete in the treatment of hypertensive encephalopathy. Reserpine, administered intramuscularly or intravenously, will nearly always induce a marked reduction in blood pressure within one or two hours.

Adolescents and adults should be given an initial injection of 1.0 to 2.5 mg. [120]. The initial dose in children is 0.05 to 0.10 mg. per kilogram of body weight [120]. Further quantities of the drug should be given at intervals of several hours as required. Often the amount necessary for control of the blood pressure diminishes rapidly after the original hypotensive effect is achieved. Mild side effects such as somnolence, nasal congestion, and weakness can be anticipated, but since treatment is usually necessary for only a few days, these symptoms rarely become a significant problem. More serious symptoms of reserpine toxicity, including depression, bizarre dreams, and the parkinsonian syndrome, are not likely to occur unless large doses of the compound are given for a long time.

Hydralazine is also effective in the treatment of severe hypertension. An initial parenteral dose of 20 mg. should ordinarily be employed in adults, and a dose of 0.25 to 0.50 mg. per kilogram of body weight should be given to children [78, 176]. Additional quantities of the drug may be used either orally or parenterally as necessary. Tachycardia, nausea, vomiting, dizziness, and orthostatic hypotension are common side effects of parenteral hydralazine therapy. When hydralazine and reserpine are used together, smaller doses of each drug are required, and the side effects of both can often be avoided [77].

Although control of hypertension is the keystone in the management of encephalopathy, other measures may be useful. In particular, administration of sedatives and of anticonvulsants such as diphenylhydantoin may be of great assistance in the prevention of recurrent seizures.

ANTIBIOTICS

Any patient with acute glomerulonephritis who is found to have beta-hemolytic streptococci in his throat or on his skin should receive a full therapeutic course of penicillin (or its equivalent) to eradicate the organism and also to protect against suppurative complications such as otitis media and peritonsillar abscess. Antibiotic therapy is probably warranted even if cultures are negative, because beta-hemolytic streptococci will not be detected in a small but significant number of patients who still harbor the organism. As discussed earlier, there is no evidence that administration of antibiotics or sulfonamides during the acute illness has any influence on the course or ultimate prognosis of the disease [91, 220].

Several facts suggest that penicillin prophylaxis (200,000 units twice daily by mouth) should be maintained during the period of convalescence. In patients treated intensively with penicillin early in the course of their infection, immunologic protection cannot be counted on to prevent a recurrent infection with the original nephritogenic organism (see page 423); continued antibiotic therapy thus serves to reduce the likelihood of an exacerbation of the nephritis. Protection is also afforded against streptococci that are ordinarily not nephritogenic but that on occasion may cause a flare-up of the disease [178].

DIET

If the patient is endematous or is tending to gain weight, the sodium intake should be limited to 200 to 300 mg. per day. Ordinarily, there are no special hazards attached to the ingestion of such a diet, but severe hyperkalemia has occasionally been noted to accompany a salt-restricted regimen. In most of these cases, it has been found that the diet contained liberal quantities of a low-sodium, high-potassium milk prepared by means of an ion-exchange process in which potassium is substituted for sodium [239]; one liter of the commercially available product contains approximately 60 mEq. of potassium. If low-sodium milk is to be incorporated into the diet, the remainder of the diet should be relatively low in potassium content.

Diets low in protein were once widely recommended for the treatment of patients with acute glomerulonephritis on the theory that reducing the nitrogen load diminished the work demanded of the kidneys and thus favored the healing process. Advocates of such a dietary program have pointed out that the life of a rat with experimental nephritis is prolonged by a diet low in protein and that the renal lesions in such animals are more likely to heal if the diet is protein-poor [83]. However, long-term observations in large groups of patients have given no hint that a restricted protein intake has a favorable influence on the healing process [69, 232]. Furthermore, well-controlled studies in which alternate patients were given diets low in protein indicate that the frequency with which complete recovery occurs is not significantly affected by the level of protein ingestion [124, 189]. On the basis of these data it seems fair to conclude that there is no advantage to be gained by providing other than a normal quantity of dietary protein. In the patient with severe oliguria or anuria there are, of course, problems in dietary management beyond those considered here. These are discussed on page 451.

BED REST

The time-honored treatment of acute glomerulonephritis consists of rest in bed, and there is general agreement that marked restriction of activity is desirable during the acute phase of the disease, i.e., when edema, gross hematuria, hypertension, and azotemia are present. Whether such a regimen should be continued after the acute signs and symptoms have subsided, however, has been a subject of controversy. The traditional view holds that bed rest is of critical importance in minimizing the likelihood that chronic renal disease will develop. On this basis, it has often been recommended that if proteinuria and sediment abnormalities persist, the patient should be kept in bed for as long as 6 to 12 months. There is, however, no evidence to support this view; even when patients are allowed to become active as soon as the acute stage of the disease has subsided, there are ordinarily

no signs of a deleterious effect on the healing process [2, 130, 178].

As a general rule, it seems that one should recommend bed rest only for as long as there is evidence of continued improvement of renal function or of a striking and progressive reduction in the excretion of protein and formed elements. Usually, this rapid improvement occurs within a few weeks. Persistent slight proteinuria and hematuria should not be considered a bar to the resumption of normal activity. If, however, a marked increase in protein and red-cell excretion follows closely upon increased activity, the patient should probably return to bed for an additional period of several weeks, after which ambulation can again be attempted.

Early ambulation has both psychologic and economic advantages. Often a family can be spared the serious financial and social problems that may be created by the prolonged absence of the father from his employment or of the mother from her household responsibilities. Early ambulation will also avert the emotional problems that frequently appear in children who are kept away from friends and school for a long interval.

ADRENOCORTICOSTEROIDS

There is no convincing evidence that administration of adrenocorticosteroids favorably influences the prognosis of acute glomerulonephritis. The scattered reports suggesting that these agents improve renal function and diminish urinary abnormalities [51, 81, 125] are difficult to evaluate because spontaneous recovery occurs so frequently. Furthermore, some studies have suggested that these agents, may, in fact, have a deleterious effect [40, 252]. On the basis of available data there appears to be no justification for the use of adrenocorticosteroids, particularly in view of the fact that the potential side effects impose an appreciable hazard.

There are currently no data bearing on the efficacy of immunosuppressive agents such as azathioprine in patients with acute glomerulonephritis, and the routine use of such agents cannot be recommended.

TONSILLECTOMY AND OTHER MEASURES

Although tonsillectomy has been said to have an important role in promoting recovery and in preventing exacerbations of the disease, there is no evidence that the procedure has any therapeutic value. Controlled observations indicate that the speed of healing and the frequency of recovery are the same whether or not the tonsils are removed [123]. In fact, the only demonstrable effects of tonsillectomy on the kidney are undesirable; surgery is frequently followed by a marked intensification of hematuria, cylindruria, and proteinuria. Such exacerbations usually last for only a few days but may persist in some cases for as long as one or two weeks [123]. From these observations, it follows that there is no specific indication for tonsillectomy in children with acute glomerulonephritis. If operation is deemed necessary on other grounds, it should be deferred until a later date.

A variety of other therapeutic methods have been tried over the past 50 years. These have included starvation diets, decapsulation of the kidney, antihistamine therapy, and deep diathermy. None of these measures have proved efficacious, and they have no place in modern therapy.

URINARY TRACT INFECTIONS

The urinary tract infection that occasionally occurs as a complication of acute glomerulonephritis should be treated promptly, with due regard in choice of drug and dose to the degree of renal insufficiency [147–151, 238]. Treatment should be continued for three to four weeks. After cessation of therapy, the patient should be followed at regular intervals by means of quantitative bacteriologic studies of the urine to detect recurrences that may occur in the absence of symptoms.

ACUTE RENAL FAILURE

Oliguric patients with acute glomerulonephritis should be treated in a fashion similar to those with other types of intrinsic acute renal failure. The principles of conservative treatment can be briefly summarized as follows. To prevent overhydration, fluid intake should be restricted to the net insensible water loss (approximately 500 ml. daily in adults) plus an amount equal to the volume of urine and of other fluid losses (sweat, diarrhea, and vomitus). The most sensitive guide to the accuracy of the fluid-replacement program is the careful daily measurement of body weight. During the period of oliguria the patient should lose about half a pound daily.

To avoid the risk of potassium intoxication and cardiac arrest every effort should be made to prevent a marked rise in serum potassium concentration. Potassium should not be given by either the oral or the parenteral route. The release of potassium from cells should be minimized by the provision of at least 150 gm. of glucose daily. If, despite these measures, the serum potassium concentration rises above 6 mEq. per liter, extrarenal depletion of potassium should be promoted by the use of an osmotic cathartic, such as sorbitol, in conjunction with an ion-exchange resin. When severe hyperkalemia is present, or when there is electrocardiographic evidence of impending cardiac standstill, measures must be employed that will produce a more rapid fall in serum potassium concentration than can be achieved by the above methods. The rapid infusion of a sodium bicarbonate solution or of hypertonic glucose with insulin will usually effect a prompt reduction in serum potassium concentration by promoting the transfer of potassium from the extracellular fluid into cells. In acidotic patients, sodium bicarbonate therapy is likely to be a particularly effective means of achieving this goal [237].

In the patient with severe renal insufficiency, dialysis should be used promptly and frequently to avoid the unfavorable clinical consequences of azotemia. This procedure will, of course, also successfully control hyper-

kalemia and other electrolyte disturbances and can be used to correct overhydration if it becomes a significant problem.

References

1. Addis, T. *Glomerular Nephritis. Diagnosis and Treatment.* New York: The Macmillan Company, 1949.

2. Akerrén, Y., and Lindgren, M. Investigation concerning early rising in acute haemorrhagic nephritis. *Acta Med. Scand.* 151: 419, 1955.

3. Albert, M. S., Leeming, J. M., and Scaglione, P. R. Acute glomerulonephritis without abnormality of the urine. *J. Pediat.* 68:525, 1966.

4. Albert, R. E., Smith, W. W., and Eichna, L. W. Hemodynamic changes associated with fluid retention induced in noncardiac subjects by corticotropin (ACTH) and cortisone; comparison with the hemodynamic changes of congestive heart failure. *Circulation* 12:1047, 1955.

5. Aldrich, C. A. Nephritis in children; prognosis and differential diagnosis. *Amer. J. Dis. Child.* 41:766, 1931.

6. Alper, C. A., and Rosen, F. S. Studies of the in vivo behavior of human C'3 in normal subjects and patients. *J. Clin. Invest.* 46: 2021, 1967.

7. Alyea, E. P., and Parish, H. H., Jr. Renal response to exercise — urinary findings. *J.A.M.A.* 167:807, 1958.

8. Anderson, A., and Kolff, W. J. Artificial kidney in the treatment of uremia associated with acute glomerulonephritis (with a note on regional heparinization). *Ann. Intern. Med.* 51:476, 1957.

9. Anthony, B. F., Chapman, S. S., Kaplan, E. L., Quie, P. G., and Wannamaker, L. W. Epidemic acute nephritis with reappearance of type-49 streptococcus. *Lancet* 2:787, 1967.

10. Anthony, B. F., Perlman, L. V., and Wannamaker, L. W. Skin infections and acute nephritis in American Indian children. *Pediatrics* 39:263, 1967.

11. Arnold, O. H., and Bock, K. D. The prob-

lem of postnephritic hypertension. *German Med. Monthly* 3:175, 1958.

12. Ash, R., Rubin, M. I., and Rapoport, M. Electrocardiographic variations in acute glomerulonephritis. *Amer. J. Dis. Child.* 67: 106, 1944.

13. Baehr, G. Renal complications of endocarditis. *Trans. Ass. Amer. Physicians* 46: 87, 1931.

14. Baehr, G., and Lande, H. Glomerulonephritis as a complication of subacute streptococcus endocarditis. *J.A.M.A.* 75:789, 1920.

15. Bain, R. C., Edwards, J. E., Scheifley, C. H., and Geraci, J. E. Right-sided bacterial endocarditis and endarteritis. *Amer. J. Med.* 24:98, 1958.

16. Barker, P. S. A clinical study of subacute bacterial infection confined to the right side of the heart or the pulmonary artery. *Amer. Heart J.* 37:1054, 1949.

17. Bell, E. T. Glomerular lesions associated with endocarditis. *Amer. J. Path.* 8:639, 1932.

18. Bengtsson, E., and Birke, G. Complications in penicillin-treated acute throat infections caused by β-haemolytic streptococci and among carriers of haemolytic streptococci. *Acta Med. Scand.* 143:120, 1952.

19. Berg, K. J., and Ritland, S. The long-term prognosis of acute glomerulonephritis: A follow-up study. *Acta Med. Scand.* 181:13, 1967.

20. Berlyne, G. M., and De C. Baker, S. B. Acute anuric glomerulonephritis. *Quart. J. Med.* 33:105, 1964.

21. Berman, L. B., and Schreiner, G. E. Clinical and histologic spectrum of the nephrotic syndrome. *Amer. J. Med.* 24:249, 1958.

22. Berman, L. B., and Vogelsang, P. Poststreptococcal glomerulonephritis without

proteinuria. *New Eng. J. Med.* 268:1275, 1963.

23. Bernstein, S. H., and Stillerman, M. A study of the association of group A streptococci with acute glomerulonephritis. *Ann. Intern. Med.* 52:1026, 1960.

24. Blackman, S. S., and Rake, G. Acute pneumococcal nephritis. *Bull. Johns Hopkins Hosp.* 51:217, 1932.

25. Blount, J. G. Bacterial endocarditis. *Amer. J. Med.* 38:909, 1965.

26. Blumberg, R. W., and Feldman, D. B. Observations on acute glomerulonephritis associated with impetigo. *J. Pediat.* 60:677, 1962.

27. Bodian, M., Black, J. A., Kobayashi, N., Lake, B. D., and Shuler, S. E. Recurrent haematuria in childhood. *Quart. J. Med.* 34:359, 1965.

28. Bone, M., Braude, A. I., and Kleinman, H. Complement-fixing antibody response to M protein of nephritogenic streptococci in glomerulonephritis. *J. Lab. Clin. Med.* 50:705, 1957.

29. Boswell, D. C., and Eknoyan, G. Acute glomerulonephritis in the aged. *Geriatrics* 23:73, 1968.

30. Boyarsky, S., Burnett, J. M., and Barker, W. H. Renal failure in embolic glomerulonephritis as a complication of subacute bacterial endocarditis. *Bull. Johns Hopkins Hosp.* 84:207, 1949.

31. Boyle, H. H., Aldrich, C. A., Frank, A., and Borowsky, S. The Addis count in children following clinical recovery from postinfectious nephritis. *J.A.M.A.* 108:1496, 1937.

32. Bradley, S. E., Bradley, G. P., Tyson, C. J., Curry, J. J., and Blake, W. D. Renal function in renal disease. *Amer. J. Med.* 9:766, 1950.

33. Breese, B. B., Disney, F. A., and Talpey, W. B. The prevention of type specific immunity to streptococcal infections due to the therapeutic use of penicillin: Occurrence of second attacks due to the same type of group A hemolytic streptococci. *Amer. J. Dis. Child.* 100:353, 1960.

34. Briggs, A. P., Fowell, D. M., Hamilton, W. F., Remington, J. W., Wheeler, N. C.,

and Winslow, J. A. Renal and circulatory factors in the edema formation of congestive heart failure. *J. Clin. Invest.* 27:810, 1948.

35. Brod, J. Acute diffuse glomerulonephritis. *Amer. J. Med.* 7:317, 1949.

36. Brun, C., Gormsen, H., Hilden, T., Iverson, P., and Raaschou, F. Kidney biopsy in acute glomerulonephritis. *Acta Med. Scand.* 160:155, 1958.

37. Bull, G. M., Joekes, A. M., and Lowe, K. G. Renal function studies in acute tubular necrosis. *Clin. Sci.* 9:379, 1950.

38. Bunn, P. A., and Cook, E. T. Treatment of subacute bacterial endocarditis. *Ann. Intern. Med.* 41:487, 1954.

39. Burke, F. G., and Ross, S. Acute glomerulonephritis: A review of ninety cases. *J. Pediat.* 30:157, 1947.

40. Burnett, C. H., Greer, M. A., Burrows, B. A., Sisson, J. H., Relman, A. S., Weinstein, L. A., and Colburn, C. G. The effects of cortisone on the course of acute glomerulonephritis: Report of a case. *New Eng. J. Med.* 243:1028, 1950.

41. Cardozo, E. L. Hydremia in acute nephritis. *Acta Med. Scand.* 125:333, 1946.

42. Cargill, W. H., and Hickam, J. B. The oxygen consumption of the normal and the diseased human kidney. *J. Clin. Invest.* 28:526, 1949.

43. Cates, J. E., and Christie, R. V. Subacute bacterial endocarditis. A review of 442 patients treated in 14 centres appointed by the Penicillin Trials Committee of the Medical Research Council. *Quart. J. Med.* 20:93, 1951.

44. Chaplin, H., and Mollison, P. L. Red cell life-span in nephritis and in hepatic cirrhosis. *Clin. Sci.* 12:351, 1953.

45. Christian, H. A. The kidneys in subacute *Streptococcus viridans* endocarditis. *J. Mt. Sinai Hosp.* 8:427, 440, 1941.

46. Cohen, J. A., and Levitt, M. F. Acute glomerulonephritis with few urinary abnormalities: Report of two cases proved by renal biopsy. *New Eng. J. Med.* 268:749, 1963.

47. Combined Staff Clinics. Acute diffuse glomerulonephritis. *Amer. J. Med.* 7:382, 1949.

48. Corcoran, A. C., Taylor, R. D., and Page,

I. H.   Functional patterns in renal disease. *Ann. Intern. Med.* 28:560, 1948.

49. Cullhed, I., Juhlin, I., Werner, I., and Laurell, G.   Type-specific antibodies in acute glomerulonephritis. *Acta Med. Scand.* 165: 17, 1959.

50. Daikos, G., and Weinstein, L.   Streptococcal bacteriostatic antibody in patients treated with penicillin. *Proc. Soc. Exp. Biol. Med.* 78:160, 1951.

51. Danowski, T. S., and Mateer, F. M.   Therapy of acute and chronic glomerulonephritis. *J. Chronic Dis.* 5:122, 1957.

52. Davies, C. E.   Heart failure in acute nephritis. *Quart. J. Med.* 20:163, 1951.

53. Davis, J. H., and Faber, H. K.   The prognosis in acute glomerulonephritis in children. *J. Pediat.* 27:453, 1945.

54. Davis, J. O., Urquhart, J., Higgins, J. T., Jr., Johnston, C. I., and Brown, T. C.   Effects of deoxycorticosterone acetate in unilaterally nephrectomized dogs with renal artery constriction. *Endocrinology* 78:316, 1966.

55. DeFazio, V., Christensen, R. C., Regan, T. J., Baer, L. J., Morita, Y., and Hellems, H. K.   Circulatory changes in acute glomerulonephritis. *Circulation* 20:190, 1959.

56. Denny, F. W., Jr., Perry, W. D., and Wannamaker, L. W.   Type-specific streptococcal antibody. *J. Clin. Invest.* 36:1092, 1957.

57. Derow, H.   The diagnostic value of serial measurements of albuminuria in ambulatory patients. *New Eng. J. Med.* 227:827, 1942.

58. Derow, H.   Management of acute glomerulonephritis. *New Eng. J. Med.* 249:144, 1953.

59. Dillon, H. C., Jr.   Pyoderma and nephritis. *Ann. Rev. Med.* 18:207, 1967.

59a. Dixon, F. J.   The pathogenesis of glomerulonephritis. *Amer. J. Med.* 44:493, 1968.

60. Dodge, W. F., Daeschner, C. W., Jr., Brennan, J. C., Rosenberg, H. S., Travis, L. B., and Hopps, H. C.   Percutaneous renal biopsy in children: II. Acute glomerulonephritis, chronic glomerulonephritis, and nephritis of anaphylactoid purpura. *Pediatrics* 30:297, 1962.

61. Dodge, W. F., Spargo, B. H., and Travis, L. B.   Occurrence of acute glomerulonephritis in sibling contacts of children with sporadic acute glomerulonephritis. *Pediatrics* 40:1029, 1967.

62. Dunn, M. J.   Acute glomerulonephritis with normal results from urinalyses: A report of two cases and comments on four additional cases with atypical findings from urinalyses. *J.A.M.A.* 201:933, 1967.

63. Earle, D. P., and Seegal, D.   Natural history of glomerulonephritis. *J. Chronic Dis.* 5:3, 1957.

64. Earle, D. P., and Jennings, R. B.   Studies of poststreptococcal nephritis and other glomerular diseases. *Ann. Intern. Med.* 51: 851, 1959.

65. Earle, D. P., Taggart, J. V., and Shannon, J. A.   Glomerulonephritis: A survey of the functional organization of the kidney in various stages of diffuse glomerulonephritis. *J. Clin. Invest.* 23:119, 1944.

66. Earle, D. P., Farber, S. J., Alexander, J. D., and Pellegrino, E. D.   Renal function and electrolyte metabolism in acute glomerulonephritis. *J. Clin. Invest.* 30:421, 1951.

67. Earley, L. E., and Friedler, R. M.   The effects of combined renal vasodilatation and pressor agents on renal hemodynamics and the tubular reabsorption of sodium. *J. Clin. Invest.* 45:542, 1966.

68. Edelmann, C. M., Jr., Greifer, I., and Barnett, H. L.   The nature of kidney disease in children who fail to recover from apparent acute glomerulonephritis. *J. Pediat.* 64:879, 1964.

69. Editorial.   Dietary protein in acute nephritis. *Brit. Med. J.* 2:423, 1955.

70. Eichna, L. W.   Circulatory congestion and heart failure. The George E. Brown Memorial Lecture. *Circulation* 22:864, 1960.

71. Eichna, L. W., Farber, S. J., Berger, A. R., Earle, D. P., Rader, B., Pellegrino, E., Albert, R. E., Alexander, J. D., Taube, H., and Youngwirth, S.   The interrelationships of the cardiovascular, renal and electrolyte effects of intravenous digoxin in congestive heart failure. *J. Clin. Invest.* 30:1250, 1951.

72. Eisenberg, S.   Blood volume in patients with acute glomerulonephritis as deter-

mined by radioactive chromium tagged red cells. *Amer. J. Med.* 27:241, 1959.

73. Ellenberg, S. L., and Martin, A. T. Acute nephritis simultaneously affecting three siblings. *Arch. Pediat.* 57:38, 1940.

74. Ellis, A. Natural history of Bright's disease: Clinical, histological and experimental observations. *Lancet* 1:34, 72, 1942.

75. Emerson, C. P. The pathogenesis of anemia in acute glomerulonephritis: Estimations of blood production and blood destruction in a case receiving massive transfusions. *Blood* 3:363, 1948.

76. Ernstene, A. C., and Robb, G. P. Familial epidemic of acute diffuse glomerulonephritis: Relation to pathogenesis of disease. *J.A.M.A.* 97:1382, 1931.

77. Etteldorf, J. N., Smith, J. D., and Johnson, C. The effect of reserpine and its combination with hydralazine on blood pressure and renal hemodynamics during the hypertensive phase of acute nephritis in children. *J. Pediat.* 48:129, 1956.

78. Etteldorf, J. N., Smith, J. D., Tharp, C. P., and Tuttle, A. H. Hydralazine in nephritic and normal children with renal hemodynamic studies. *Amer. J. Dis. Child.* 89:451, 1955.

79. Faith, G. C., and Trump, B. F. The glomerular capillary wall in human kidney disease: Acute glomerulonephritis, systemic lupus erythematosus, and preeclampsia-eclampsia. Comparative electron microscopic observations and a review. *Lab. Invest.* 15:1682, 1966.

80. Farber, S. J. Physiologic aspects of glomerulonephritis. *J. Chronic Dis.* 5:87, 1957.

81. Farnsworth, E. B. Studies on the Influence of Adrenocorticotrophin in Acute Nephritis, in Simple Nephrosis and in Nephrosis with Azotemia. In Mote, J. R. (Ed.), *Proceedings of the First Clinical ACTH Conference.* Philadelphia: Blakiston, 1950. Pp. 297–317.

82. Farquhar, M. G., Vernier, R. L., and Good, R. A. An electron microscope study of the glomerulus in nephrosis, glomerulonephritis, and lupus erythematosus. *J. Exp. Med.* 106:649, 1957.

83. Farr, L. E., and Smadel, J. E. The effect of dietary protein on the course of nephrotoxic nephritis in rats. *J. Exp. Med.* 70:615, 1939.

84. Feldman, J. D., Mardiney, M. R., and Shuler, S. E. Immunology and morphology of acute poststreptococcal glomerulonephritis. *Lab. Invest.* 15:283, 1966.

85. Ferris, T. F., Gorden, P., Kashgarian, M., and Epstein, F. H. Recurrent hematuria and focal nephritis. *New Eng. J. Med.* 276:770, 1967.

86. Fischel, E. E. Immune reactions in human glomerulonephritis. *J. Chron. Dis.* 5:34, 1957.

87. Fischel, E. E., and Gajdusek, D. C. Serum complement in acute glomerulonephritis and other renal diseases. *Amer. J. Med.* 12:190, 1952.

88. Fishberg, A. M., and Oppenheimer, B. S. The differentiation and significance of certain ophthalmoscopic pictures in hypertensive diseases. *Arch. Intern. Med.* 46:901, 1930.

89. Fison, T. N. Acute glomerulonephritis in infancy. *Arch. Dis. Child.* 31:101, 1956.

90. Fleisher, D. S., Voci, G., Garfunkel, J., Purugganan, H., Kirkpatrick, J., Jr., Wells, C. R., and McElfresh, A. E. Hemodynamic findings in acute glomerulonephritis. *J. Pediat.* 69:1054, 1966.

91. Fleming, J. An epidemic of acute nephritis. *Lancet* 1:763, 1949.

92. Flood, F. B. Albuminuria and hematuria in boxers. *J.A.M.A.* 171:1678, 1959.

93. Friedberg, C. K. Congestive heart failure of renal origin: Pathogenesis and treatment in four cases of carbon tetrachloride nephrosis. *Amer. J. Med.* 9:164, 1950.

94. Friedberg, C. K., Goldman, H. M., and Field, L. E. Study of bacterial endocarditis: Comparisons in ninety-five cases. *Arch. Intern. Med.* (Chicago) 107:6, 1961.

95. Frisk, A., and Klackenberg, G. A study of the onset and prognosis of nephritis in children. *Acta Paediat.* 33:349, 1946.

96. Gachet, F. S. Course and prognosis of hemorrhagic nephritis in children. *Amer. J. Dis. Child.* 61:1175, 1941.

97. Gardner, K. D., Jr. "Athletic pseudonephritis" — alteration of urine sediment by

athletic competition. *J.A.M.A.* 161:1613, 1956.

98. George, J. T., McDonald, J. C., Payne, D. J., and Slade, D. A.   Nephritis in North Yorkshire. *Brit. Med. J.* 2:1381, 1958.

99. Goldring, W.   Studies of the kidney in acute infection: III. Observations with the urine sediment count (Addis) and the urea clearance test in lobar pneumonia. *J. Clin. Invest.* 10:355, 1931.

100. Goldsmith, H. J., Cowan, M. A., and Gooder, E.   Familial outbreak of acute glomerulonephritis due to Griffith Type-1 streptococcus. *Lancet* 2:674, 1958.

101. Goorno, W., Ashworth, C. T., and Carter, N. W.   Acute glomerulonephritis with absence of abnormal urinary findings. Diagnosis by light and electron microscopy. *Ann. Intern. Med.* 66:345, 1967.

102. Gore, I., and Saphir, O.   Myocarditis associated with acute and subacute glomerulonephritis. *Amer. Heart J.* 36:390, 1948.

103. Gorlin, R., Favour, C. B., and Emery, F. J.   Long-term follow-up study of penicillin-treated subacute bacterial endocarditis. *New Eng. J. Med.* 242:995, 1950.

104. Gotoff, S. P., Fellers, F. X., Vawter, G. F., Janeway, C. A., and Rosen, F. S.   The beta$_{1C}$ globulin in childhood nephrotic syndrome: Laboratory diagnosis of progressive glomerulonephritis. *New Eng. J. Med.* 273:524, 1965.

105. Grishman, E., and Churg, J.   Acute glomerulonephritis: A histopathologic study by means of thin sections. *Amer. J. Path.* 33:993, 1957.

106. Guild, H. G.   The prognosis of acute glomerular nephritis in childhood. *Bull. Johns Hopkins Hosp.* 48:193, 1931.

107. Harrington, J. T., and Senior, B.   Recovery following 36 days of oliguria in a child with acute glomerulonephritis. *Amer. J. Dis. Child.* 115:611, 1968.

108. Harris, L. D., and McNeil, J. H.   Recurrent focal glomerulitis; a case report with renal biopsy. *Ann. Intern. Med.* 49:679, 1958.

109. Harrison, C. V., Loughridge, L. W., and Milne, M. D.   Acute oliguric renal failure

in acute glomerulonephritis and polyarteritis nodosa. *Quart. J. Med.* 33:39, 1964.

110. Hayman, J. M., Jr., and Martin, J. W., Jr.   Acute nephritis: Review of 77 cases. *Amer. J. Med. Sci.* 200:505, 1940.

111. Hebert, H. J.   Acute glomerulonephritis in childhood: A study of the late prognosis of twenty-seven cases. *J. Pediat.* 40:549, 1952.

112. Heller, B. I., and Jacobson, W. E.   Renal hemodynamics in heart disease. *Amer. Heart J.* 39:188, 1950.

113. Herdson, P. B., Jennings, R. B., and Earle, D. P.   Glomerular fine structure in poststreptococcal acute glomerulonephritis. *Arch. Path.* (Chicago) 81:117, 1966.

114. Heymann, W., and Wilson, S. G. F.   Hyperlipemia in early stages of acute glomerular nephritis. *J. Clin. Invest.* 38:186, 1959.

115. Heymann, W., Rothenberg, R. A., Gilkey, C., and Lewis, M.   Difference in color of hematuria in the nephrotic syndrome and glomerulonephritis. *Pediatrics* 21:375, 1958.

116. Hilden, T.   Diodrast clearance in acute nephritis. *Acta Med. Scand.* 116:1, 1943–44.

117. Hill, L. W.   Studies in the nephritis of children: Clinical considerations of classification, etiology, prognosis and treatment. *Amer. J. Dis. Child.* 17:270, 1919.

118. Hirschfelder, A. D.   Clinical manifestations of high and low plasma magnesium: Dangers of epsom salt purgation in nephritis. *J.A.M.A.* 102:1138, 1934.

119. Hoyer, J. R., Michael, A. F., Fish, A. J., and Good, R. A.   Acute poststreptococcal glomerulonephritis presenting as hypertensive encephalopathy with minimal urinary abnormalities. *Pediatrics* 39:412, 1967.

120. Hughes, W. M., Moyer, J. H., and Daeschner, C. W.   Parenteral reserpine in treatment of hypertensive emergencies. *A.M.A. Arch. Intern. Med.* 95:563, 1955.

121. Hughes, W. T., Steigman, A. J., and De-Long, H. F.   Some implications of fatal nephritis associated with mumps. *Amer. J. Dis. Child.* 111:297, 1966.

122. Hutt, M. S. R., Pinniger, J. L., and de Wardener, H. E.   The relationship between the clinical and the histological features of acute glomerular nephritis: Based

on a study of renal biopsy material. *Quart. J. Med.* 27:265, 1958.

123. Illingworth, R. S. Tonsillectomy and nephritis of childhood. *Lancet* 2:1013, 1939.

124. Illingworth, R. S., Philpott, M. G., and Rendle-Short, J. A controlled investigation of the effect of diet on acute nephritis. *Arch. Dis. Child.* 29:551, 1954.

125. Iseri, L. T., and Mader, I. J. The effect of ACTH on acute glomerulonephritis. *J. Lab. Clin. Med.* 42:821, 1953.

126. James, R. F. Prognosis of nephritis in childhood. *J.A.M.A.* 76:505, 1921.

127. Jennings, R. B., and Earle, D. P. Poststreptococcal glomerulonephritis: Histopathologic and clinical studies of the acute, subacute and early chronic latent phases. *J. Clin. Invest.* 40:1525, 1961.

128. Jensen, M. M. Viruses and kidney disease. *Amer. J. Med.* 43:897, 1967.

129. Jones, A. M., Herring, R., Langley, F. A., and Oleesky, S. Penicillin treatment of subacute bacterial endocarditis. *Brit. Heart J.* 9:38, 1947.

130. Joseph, M. C., and Polani, P. E. The effect of bed rest on acute hemorrhagic nephritis in children. *Guy Hosp. Rep.* 107: 500, 1958.

131. Kaipainen, W. J., and Seppälä, K. Endocarditis lenta: A review of 118 patients treated during the ten-year period 1945 to 1954. *Acta Med. Scand.* 155:71, 1956.

132. Kallen, R. J., Zaltzman, S., Coe, F. L., and Metcoff, J. Hemodialysis in children: Technique, kinetic aspects related to varying body size, and application to salicylate intoxication, acute renal failure and some other disorders. *Medicine* 45:1, 1966.

133. Kassirer, J. P., and Schwartz, W. B. Acute glomerulonephritis. *New Eng. J. Med.* 265:686, 736, 1961.

134. Kaye, M. The anemia associated with renal disease. *J. Lab. Clin. Med.* 52:83, 1958.

135. Keefer, C. S. Subacute bacterial endocarditis: Active cases without bacteremia. *Ann. Intern. Med.* 11:714, 1937.

136. Kelly, D. K., and Winn, J. F. Renal lesions produced by group A, type 12, streptococci. *Science* 127:1337, 1958.

137. Kempe, C. H., Olmsted, R. W., and Curnen, E. C. Outbreak of acute nephritis in adolescent schoolboys. *Pediatrics* 8:393, 1951.

138. Kerr, A., Jr. Rheumatic activity in bacterial endocarditis — antistreptolysin measurements. *Ann. Allerg.* 11:73, 1953.

139. Kiil, F., Aukland, K., and Refsum, H. E. Renal sodium transport and oxygen consumption. *Amer. J. Physiol.* 201:511, 1961.

140. Kilbourne, E. D., and Loge, J. P. The comparative effects of continuous and intermittent penicillin therapy on the formation of antistreptolysin in hemolytic streptococcal pharyngitis. *J. Clin. Invest.* 27:418, 1948.

141. Kilpatrick, L. G. Susceptibility to acute nephritis. *Brit. Med. J.* 1:222, 1945.

142. Kimmelstiel, P., Kim, O. J., and Beres, J. Studies on renal biopsy specimens, with the aid of the electron microscope: II. Glomerulonephritis and glomerulonephrosis. *Amer. J. Clin. Path.* 38:280, 1962.

143. Kirkpatrick, J. A., Jr., and Fleisher, D. S. The roentgen appearance of the chest in acute glomerulonephritis in children. *J. Pediat.* 64:492, 1964.

144. Kleinman, H. Epidemic acute glomerulonephritis at Red Lake. *Minn. Med.* 37:479, 1954.

145. Kobayashi, O., Wada, H., and Moriuchi, M. Needle renal biopsy of acute glomerulonephritis in children. *Acta Med. Biol.* 7: 241, 1960.

146. Koffler, D., and Paronetto, F. Immunofluorescent localization of immunoglobulins, complements, and fibrinogen in human diseases: II. Acute, subacute, and chronic glomerulonephritis. *J. Clin. Invest.* 44:1665, 1965.

147. Kunin, C. M. A guide to use of antibiotics in patients with renal disease. A table of recommended doses and factors governing serum levels. *Ann. Intern. Med.* 67:151, 1967.

148. Kunin, C. M., and Finland, M. Persistence of antibiotics in blood of patients with acute renal failure: III. Penicillin, streptomycin, erythromycin and kanamycin. *J. Clin. Invest.* 38:1509, 1959.

149. Kunin, C. M., and Finland, M. Restric-

tions imposed on antibiotic therapy by renal failure. *Arch. Intern. Med.* 104:1030, 1959.

150. Kunin, C. M., Glazko, A. J., and Finland, M. Persistence of antibiotics in blood of patients with acute renal failure: II. Chloramphenicol and its metabolic products in the blood of patients with severe renal disease of hepatic cirrhosis. *J. Clin. Invest.* 38:1498, 1959.

151. Kunin, C. M., Rees, S. B., Merrill, J. P., and Finland, M. Persistence of antibiotics in blood of patients with acute renal failure: I. Tetracycline and chlortetracycline. *J. Clin. Invest.* 38:1487, 1959.

152. Kushner, D. S., Armstrong, S. H., Dubin, A., Szanto, P. B., Markowitz, A., Maduros, B. P., Levine, J. M., River, G. L., Gynn, T. N., and Pendros, J. P. Acute glomerulonephritis in the adult. *Medicine* (Balt.) 40:203, 1961.

153. Kuttner, A. G., and Lenert, T. F. The occurrence of bacteriostatic properties in the blood of patients after recovery from streptococcal pharyngitis. *J. Clin. Invest.* 23:151, 1944.

154. LaDue, J. S. The role of congestive heart failure in the production of the edema of acute glomerulonephritis. *Ann. Intern. Med.* 20:405, 1944.

155. LaDue, J. S., and Ashman, R. Electrocardiographic changes in acute glomerulonephritis. *Amer. Heart J.* 31:685, 1946.

156. Lancefield, R. C. Persistence of type-specific antibodies in man following infection with group A streptococci. *J. Exp. Med.* 110:271, 1959.

157. Lange, K., Wasserman, E., and Slobody, L. B. The significance of serum complement levels for the diagnosis and prognosis of acute and subacute glomerulonephritis and lupus erythematosus disseminatus. *Ann. Intern. Med.* 53:636, 1960.

158. Lassen, N. A., Munck, O., and Thaysen, J. H. Oxygen consumption and sodium reabsorption in the kidney. *Acta Physiol. Scand.* 51:371, 1961.

159. Lawrence, J. R., Pollak, V. E., Pirani, C. L., and Kark, R. M. Histologic and clinical evidence of post-streptococcal glomerulonephritis in patients with the nephrotic syndrome. *Medicine* (Balt.) 42:1, 1963.

160. Lee, H. A., Stirling, G., and Sharpstone, P. Acute glomerulonephritis in middle-aged and elderly patients. *Brit. Med. J.* 2:1361, 1966.

161. Lemieux, G., Cuvelier, A. A., and Lefebvre, R. The clinical spectrum of renal insufficiency during acute glomerulonephritis in the adult. *Canad. Med. Ass. J.* 96:1129, 1967.

162. Levinsky, N. G. Nonaldosterone influences on renal sodium transport. *Ann. N.Y. Acad. Sci.* 139:295, 1966.

163. Levy, I. J. Cardiac response in acute diffuse glomerulonephritis. *Amer. Heart J.* 5:277, 1930.

164. Libman, E., and Friedberg, C. K. In Christian, H. A. (Ed.), *Subacute Bacterial Endocarditis* (2d ed.). New York: Oxford University Press, 1948.

165. Lieberman, E., and Donnell, G. N. Recovery of children with acute glomerulonephritis. *Amer. J. Dis. Child.* 109:398, 1965.

166. Loeb, E. N., Lyttle, J. D., Seegal, D., and Jost, E. L. On the permanence of recovery in acute glomerulonephritis. *J. Clin. Invest.* 17:623, 1938.

167. Loge, J. P., Lange, R. D., and Moore, C. V. Characterization of the anemia associated with chronic renal insufficiency. *Amer. J. Med.* 24:4, 1958.

168. Longcope, W. T. Studies of the variations in the antistreptolysin titer of blood serum from patients with hemorrhagic nephritis: II. Observations on patients suffering from streptococcal infections, rheumatic fever and acute and chronic hemorrhagic nephritis. *J. Clin. Invest.* 15:277, 1936.

169. Longcope, W. T. Some observations on the course and outcome of hemorrhagic nephritis. *Internat. Clin.* 1:1, 1938.

170. Longcope, W. T., O'Brien, D. P., McGuire, J., Hansen, O. C., and Denny, E. R. Relationship of acute infections to glomerular nephritis. *J. Clin. Invest.* 5:7, 1928.

171. Lyttle, J. D. The treatment of acute glomerulonephritis in children. *Bull. N.Y. Acad. Med.* 14:212, 1938.

172. Lyttle, J. D., and Rosenberg, L. The prognosis of acute nephritis in childhood. *Amer. J. Dis. Child.* 38:1052, 1929.

173. Lyttle, J. D., Seegal, D., Loeb, E. N., and Jost, E. L. The serum antistreptolysin

titer in acute glomerulonephritis. *J. Clin. Invest.* 17:631, 1938.

174. McCarty, M. (Ed.). The Antibody Response to Streptococcal Infections. In *Streptococcal Infections*. New York: Columbia University Press, 1954. Pp. 130–142.

175. McCluskey, R. T., and Baldwin, D. S. Natural history of acute glomerulonephritis. *Amer. J. Med.* 35:213, 1963.

176. McCrory, W. W., and Rapoport, M. Effects of hydrazinophthalazine (Apresoline®) on blood pressure and renal function in children with acute nephritis. *Pediatrics* 12:29, 1953.

177. McCrory, W. W., and Shibuya, M. Acute glomerulonephritis in childhood: Long-term follow-up. *New York J. Med.* 68:2416, 1968.

178. McCrory, W. W., Fleisher, D. S., and Sohn, W. B. Effects of early ambulation on the course of nephritis in children. *Pediatrics* 24:395, 1959.

179. McCullough, G. C., Coffee, J. Y., Trice, P. A., Stone, J. J., and Crandall, H. L. Acute glomerulonephritis: Impetigo as an etiological factor. A review of 124 cases at Lloyd Noland Hospital, Fairfield, Ala. *J. Pediat.* 38:346, 1951.

180. Manser, R. W. E., and Wilson, M. M. Epidemic of hemolytic streptococcal (group A) infection associated with considerable incidence of acute nephritis. *Med. J. Aust.* 2:339, 1952.

181. Martino, J. A., and Earley, L. E. Demonstration of a role of physical factors as determinants of the natriuretic response to volume expansion. *J. Clin. Invest.* 46:1963, 1967.

182. Martino, J. A., and Earley, L. E. Relationship between intrarenal hydrostatic pressure and hemodynamically induced changes in sodium excretion. *Circ. Res.* 23:371, 1968.

183. Master, A. M., Jaffe, H. L., and Dack, S. The heart in acute nephritis. *Arch. Intern. Med.* 60:1016, 1937.

184. Matthew, H., and Gilchrist, A. R. Subacute bacterial endocarditis and its treatment with penicillin. Session 128, Tr. Med.-Chir. Soc. Edinburgh, pp. 25–48, 1948–49; in *Edinb. Med. J.* 1949.

185. Merrill, A. J. Edema and decreased renal

blood flow in patients with chronic congestive heart failure: Evidence of "forward failure" as the primary cause of edema. *J. Clin. Invest.* 25:389, 1946.

186. Merrill, J. P. The use of the artificial kidney in the treatment of glomerulonephritis. *J. Chronic Dis.* 5:138, 1957.

187. Michael, A. F., Jr., Drummond, K. N., Good, R. A., and Vernier, R. L. Acute poststreptococcal glomerulonephritis: Immune deposit disease. *J. Clin. Invest.* 45:237, 1966.

188. Minkowitz, S., Wenk, R., Friedman, E., Yuceoglu, A., and Berkovich, S. Acute glomerulonephritis associated with varicella infection. *Amer. J. Med.* 44:489, 1968.

189. Mortensen, V. Treatment of acute glomerulonephritis with high protein diet. *Acta Med. Scand.* 129:321, 1947.

190. Movat, H. Z., Steiner, J. W., and Huhn, D. The fine structure of the glomerulus in acute glomerulonephritis. *Lab. Invest.* 11:117, 1962.

191. Murphy, F. D., and Peters, B. J. Treatment of acute nephritis: The immediate results and the outcome ten years later in eighty-nine cases. *J.A.M.A.* 118:183, 1942.

192. Murphy, F. D., and Rastetter, J. W. Acute glomerulonephritis with special reference to the course and prognosis: Study of 150 cases. *J.A.M.A.* 111:668, 1938.

193. Murphy, F. D., Grill, J., and Moxon, G. F. Acute diffuse glomerular nephritis: Study of 94 cases with special consideration of stages of transition into chronic form. *Arch. Intern. Med.* 54:483, 1934.

194. Murphy, T. R., and Murphy, F. D. The heart in acute glomerulonephritis. *Ann. Intern. Med.* 41:510, 1954.

195. Muth, R. G. Diuretic response to furosemide in the presence of renal insufficiency. *J.A.M.A.* 195:190, 1966.

196. Muth, R. G. Diuretic properties of furosemide in renal disease. *Ann. Intern. Med.* 69:249, 1968.

197. Neale, A. V. Kidneys in pneumococcal infections. *Brit. Med. J.* 2:891, 1928.

198. Nesson, H. R., and Robbins, S. L. Glomerulonephritis in older age groups. *Arch. Intern. Med.* 105:23, 1960.

199. Neustein, H. B., and Davis, W. Acute glo-

merulonephritis: A light and electron microscopy study of eight serial biopsies. *Amer. J. Clin. Path.* 44:613, 1965.

200. Newman, W., Torres, J. M., and Guck, J. K. Bacterial endocarditis: Analysis of 52 cases. *Amer. J. Med.* 16:535, 1954.

201. Osman, A. A., Close, H. G., and Carter, H. Studies in Bright's disease: Observations on aetiology of scarlatinal nephritis. *Guy. Hosp. Rep.* 83:360, 1933.

202. Parrish, A. E., Rubenstein, N. H., and Howe, J. S. Correlation between renal function and histology. *Amer. J. Med. Sci.* 229:632, 1955.

203. Perlman, L. V., Herdman, R. C., Kleinman, H., and Vernier, R. L. Poststreptococcal glomerulonephritis: A ten-year follow-up of an epidemic. *J.A.M.A.* 194:175, 1965.

204. Peters, J. P. Edema of acute nephritis. *Amer. J. Med.* 14:448, 1953.

205. Pillsbury, P. L., and Fiese, M. J. Subacute bacterial endocarditis: Follow-up study of thirty patients treated with penicillin. *A.M.A. Arch. Intern. Med.* 85:675, 1950.

206. Pittinos, G. E., Craig, J. D., and DeSanctis, A. G. The prognosis of acute hemorrhagic nephritis in childhood. *J.A.M.A.* 117:1855, 1941.

207. Pleydell, M. J., and Hall-Turner, W. J. An outbreak of nephritis in Northamptonshire. *Brit. Med. J.* 2:1382, 1958.

208. Poon-King, T., Mohammed, I., Cox, R., Potter, E. V., Simon, N. M., Siegel, A. C., and Earle, D. P. Recurrent epidemic nephritis in South Trinidad. *New Eng. J. Med.* 277:728, 1967.

209. Potter, E. V. Type 12 streptococci and acute glomerulonephritis: I. Presence and recall of type-specific streptococcal antibodies in patients with healed acute glomerulonephritis. *J. Lab. Clin. Med.* 65:40, 1965.

210. Potter, E. V., Moran, A. F., Poon-King, T., and Earle, D. P. Characteristics of beta hemolytic streptococci associated with acute glomerulonephritis in Trinidad, West Indies. *J. Lab. Clin. Med.* 71:126, 1968.

211. Potter, E. V., Siegel, A. C., Simon, N. M., McAninch, J., Earle, D. P., Poon-King, T., Mohammed, I., and Abidh, S. Streptococ-

cal infections and epidemic acute glomerulo nephritis in South Trinidad. *J. Pediat.* 72 871, 1968.

212. Proger, S. Acute hemorrhagic nephritis with "heart failure": Presentation of case with hypothesis as to mechanism. *Bull. New Eng. Med. Center* 3:108, 1941.

212a. Rabinovich, S., Evans, J., Smith, I. M., and January, L. E. A long-term view of bacterial endocarditis: 337 cases 1924 to 1963. *Ann. Intern. Med.* 63:185, 1965.

213. Rake, G. Nephritis in pneumococcal infections. *Guy Hosp. Rep.* 83:430, 1933.

214. Ramberg, R. The prognosis for acute nephritis. *Acta Med. Scand.* 127:396, 1947.

215. Rammelkamp, C. H., Jr. Glomerulonephritis. Frank Billings Lecture. *Proc. Inst. Med. Chicago* 19:371, 1953.

216. Rammelkamp, C. H., and Weaver, R. S. Acute glomerulonephritis: The significance of the variations in the incidence of the disease. *J. Clin. Invest.* 32:345, 1953.

217. Rammelkamp, C. H., Wannamaker, L. W., and Denny, F. W. The epidemiology and prevention of rheumatic fever. *Bull. N.Y. Acad. Med.* 28:321, 1952.

218. Rammelkamp, C. H., Stetson, C. A., Krause, R. M., Perry, W. D., and Kohen, R. J. Epidemic nephritis. *Trans. Ass. Amer. Physicians* 67:276, 1954.

219. Randall, R. E., Jr., Cohen, M. D., Spray, C. C., Jr., and Rossmeisl, E. C. Hypermagnesemia in renal failure: Etiology and toxic manifestations. *Ann. Intern. Med.* 61:73, 1964.

220. Rapoport, M., Rubin, M. I., and Waltz, A. D. The influence of sulfanilamide therapy upon the course of acute glomerulonephritis in children. *Amer. J. Med. Sci.* 211:307, 1946.

221. Reed, R. W. An epidemic of acute nephritis. *Canad. Med. Ass. J.* 68:448, 1953.

222. Reimann, H. A. Nephropathy and viroses. *Postgrad. Med. J.* 44:853, 1968.

223. Reinstein, C. R. Epidemic nephritis at Red Lake, Minnesota. *J. Pediat.* 47:25, 1955.

223a. Retan, J. W., and Dillon, H. C., Jr. Furosemide in the treatment of acute poststreptococcal glomerulonephritis. *Southern Med. J.* 62:157, 1969.

224. Richards, D. W., Jr.   Dynamics of congestive heart failure. *Amer. J. Med.* 6:772, 1949.

225. Richter, A. B.   Prognosis in acute glomerular nephritis. *Ann. Intern. Med.* 9:1057, 1935.

226. Robinson, M. J., and Ruedy, J.   Sequelae of bacterial endocarditis. *Amer. J. Med.* 32:922, 1962.

227. Roscoe, M. H.   Biochemical and hematological changes in type 1 and type 2 nephritis. *Quart. J. Med.* 19:161, 1950.

228. Rosenblatt, P., and Lowe, L.   Healed subacute bacterial endocarditis. *Arch. Intern. Med.* 76:1, 1945.

229. Ross, J. H.   Recurrent focal nephritis. *Quart. J. Med.* 29:391, 1960.

230. Rubin, M. I., and Rapoport, M.   Cardiac complications of acute hemorrhagic nephritis. *Amer. J. Dis. Child.* 55:244, 1938.

231. Rubin, M. I., Rapoport, M., and Waltz, A. D.   A comparison of routine urinalysis, Addis count, and blood sedimentation rate as criteria in acute glomerulonephritis. *J. Pediat.* 20:32, 1942.

232. Rudebeck, J.   Clinical and prognostic aspects of acute glomerulonephritis. *Acta Med. Scand.* Suppl. 173:1–184, 1946.

233. Samiy, A. H., Field, R. A., and Merrill, J. P.   Acute glomerulonephritis in elderly patients: Report of seven cases over sixty years of age. *Ann. Intern. Med.* 54:603, 1961.

234. Sapir, D. G., Yardley, J. H., and Walker, W. G.   Acute glomerulonephritis in older patients. *Johns Hopkins Med. J.* 123:145, 1968.

235. Saslaw, M. S., and Streitfeld, M. M.   Glomerulonephritis in Miami, Florida. Studies on types 12, 4, and Red Lake group A beta-hemolytic streptococci isolated over a three-year period (1953–1955). *Amer. J. Dis. Child.* 91:555, 1956.

236. Schreiner, G. E., Marc-Aurele, J., Talamas, A., and Mostofi, F. K.   Anuria in acute glomerulonephritis. *Clin. Res.* 8:233, 1960.

237. Schwartz, W. B.   Fluid, Electrolyte and Acid-Base Balance. In Beeson, P. B., and McDermott, W. (Eds.), *Cecil-Loeb Textbook of Medicine* (12th ed.). Philadelphia: Saunders, 1967. Pp. 753–774.

238. Schwartz, W. B., and Kassirer, J. P.   Medical management of chronic renal failure. *Amer. J. Med.* 44:786, 1968.

239. Schwartz, W. B., and Kassirer, J. P.   Unpublished data, 1970.

240. Seabury, J. H.   Subacute bacterial endocarditis: Experiences during past decade. *Arch. Intern. Med.* 79:1, 1947.

241. Seegal, D.   Acute glomerulonephritis following pneumococcic lobar pneumonia: Analysis of 7 cases. *Arch. Intern. Med.* 56:912, 1935.

242. Seegal, D., and Earle, D. P.   A consideration of certain biological differences between glomerulonephritis and rheumatic fever. *Amer. J. Med. Sci.* 201:528, 1941.

243. Seegal, D., Seegal, B. C., and Jost, E. L.   A comparative study of the geographic distribution of rheumatic fever, scarlet fever and acute glomerulonephritis in North America. *Amer. J. Med. Sci.* 190:383, 1935.

244. Seegal, D., Lyttle, J. D., Loeb, E. N., Jost, E. L., and Davis, G.   On the exacerbation in chronic glomerulonephritis. *J. Clin. Invest.* 19:569, 1940.

245. Siegel, A. C., Johnson, E. E., and Stollerman, G. H.   Controlled studies of streptococcal pharyngitis in a pediatric population: 2. Behavior of the type-specific immune response. *New Eng. J. Med.* 265:566, 1961.

246. Singer, D. B., Hill, L. L., Rosenberg, H. S., Marshall, J., and Swenson, R.   Recurrent hematuria in childhood. *New Eng. J. Med.* 279:7, 1968.

247. Spain, D. M., and King, D. W.   The effect of penicillin on the renal lesions of subacute bacterial endocarditis. *Ann. Intern. Med.* 36:1086, 1952.

248. Stead, E. A., Jr., Warren, J. V., and Brannon, E. S.   Cardiac output in congestive heart failure: An analysis of the reasons for lack of close correlation between the symptoms of heart failure and the resting cardiac output. *Amer. Heart J.* 35:529, 1948.

249. Stetson, C. A., Rammelkamp, C. H., Krause, R. M., Kohen, R. J., and Perry, W. D.   Epidemic acute nephritis: Studies on etiology, natural history and prevention. *Medicine* (Balt.) 34:431, 1955.

250. Strauss, M. B., and Raisz, L. G.   *Clinical*

Management of Renal Failure. Springfield (Ill.): Thomas, 1956.

251. Strunk, S. W., Hammond, W. S., and Benditt, E. P.   The resolution of acute glomerulonephritis. An electron microscopic study of four sequential biopsies. *Lab. Invest.* 13: 401, 1964.

252. Thorn, G. W., Merrill, J. P., Smith, S., III, Roche, M., and Frawley, T. F.   Clinical studies with ACTH and cortisone in renal disease. *Arch. Intern. Med.* 86:319, 1950.

253. Tudor, R. B.   Acute glomerulonephritis occurring in three children in the same family. *Amer. J. Dis. Child.* 66:528, 1943.

254. Tumulty, P. A., and Harvey, A. M.   Experiences in the management of subacute bacterial endocarditis treated with penicillin. *Amer. J. Med.* 4:37, 1948.

255. Uwaydah, M. M., and Weinberg, A. N.   Bacterial endocarditis — a changing pattern. *New Eng. J. Med.* 273:1231, 1965.

256. Verel, D., Turnbull, A., Tudhope, G. R., and Ross, J. H.   Anaemia in Bright's disease. *Quart. J. Med.* 28:491, 1959.

257. Villarreal, H., and Sokoloff, L.   The occurrence of renal insufficiency in the subacute bacterial endocarditis. *Amer. J. Med. Sci.* 220:655, 1950.

258. Vogler, W. R., Dorney, E. R., and Bridges, H. A.   Bacterial endocarditis: A review of 148 cases. *Amer. J. Med.* 32:910, 1962.

259. Wagener, H. P.   Retinopathy in glomerulonephritis. *Amer. J. Med. Sci.* 209:257, 1945.

260. Wahrer, C. F.   An epidemic of hemorrhagic nephritis following scarlet fever. *J.A.M.A.* 51:1410, 1908.

261. Warren, J. V., and Stead, E. A., Jr.   The protein content of edema fluid in patients with acute glomerulonephritis. *Amer. J. Med. Sci.* 208:618, 1944.

262. Watt, M. F., Howe, J. S., and Parrish, A. E.   Renal tubular changes in acute glomerulonephritis. *Arch. Intern. Med.* 103:690, 1959.

263. Weinstein, L., and Tsao, C. C. L.   Effect of types of treatment on development of antistreptolysin in patients with scarlet fever. *Proc. Soc. Exp. Biol. Med.* 63:449, 1946.

264. Weinstein, L., Bachrach, L., and Boyer, N. H.   Observations on the development of rheumatic fever and glomerulonephritis in cases of scarlet fever treated with penicillin. *New Eng. J. Med.* 242:1002, 1950.

265. Welty, J. W.   Febrile albuminuria. *Amer. J. Med. Sci.* 194:70, 1937.

266. Wertheim, A. R., Lyttle, J. D., Loeb, E. N., Earle, D. P., Jr., Seegal, B. C., and Seegal, D.   The association of type-specific hemolytic streptococci with acute glomerulonephritis. The Presbyterian and Babies Hospitals, New York, N.Y., in the years 1936–1942. *J. Clin. Invest.* 32:359, 1953.

267. West, C. D., Winter, S., Forristal, J., McConville, J. M., and Davis, N. C.   Evidence for in vivo breakdown of $\beta_1 C$ globulin in hypocomplementemic glomerulonephritis. *J. Clin. Invest.* 46:539, 1967.

268. West, C. D., Northway, J. D., and Davis, N. C.   Serum levels of beta$_{1C}$ globulin, a complement component, in the nephritides, lipoid nephrosis, and other conditions. *J. Clin. Invest.* 43:1507, 1964.

269. White, R. H. R.   "Silent" nephritis: A study based on renal biopsies. *Guy Hosp. Rep.* 113:190, 1964.

270. Whitehill, M. R., Longcope, W. T., and Williams, R. D.   The occurrence and significance of myocardial failure in acute hemorrhagic nephritis. *Bull. Johns Hopkins Hosp.* 64:83, 1939.

271. Williams, R. D.   Electrocardiographic changes in acute hemorrhagic nephritis. *Bull. Johns Hopkins Hosp.* 65:434, 1939.

272. Wilson, S. G. F., and Heymann, W.   Acute glomerulonephritis with the nephrotic syndrome. *Pediatrics* 23:874, 1959.

273. Winkenwerder, W. L., McLeod, N., and Baker, M.   Infection and hemorrhagic nephritis. *Arch. Intern. Med.* 56:297, 1935.

274. Yuceoglu, A. M., Berkovich, S., and Minkowitz, S.   Acute glomerulonephritis as a complication of varicella. *J.A.M.A.* 202:879, 1967.

275. Yuceoglu, A. M., Berkovich, S., and Minkowitz, S.   Acute glomerulonephritis associated with ECHO virus type 9 infection. *J. Pediat.* 69:603, 1966.

14

Focal Glomerulonephritis

R. H. Heptinstall

One of the main causes of confusion in present-day medicine is the lack of a precise terminology, and for this reason focal glomerulonephritis must be clearly defined. To some, it is a term used to denote that only a portion of a given glomerulus is affected [12], but in this chapter it is regarded as a form of glomerulonephritis in which only a certain number of glomeruli are affected, the remainder being normal. It is singular, however, that the change within a given glomerulus is almost always confined to one or two lobules of the tuft, the term *local* being used to describe this type of involvement.

Focal glomerulonephritis is a histological diagnosis, although certain clinical syndromes are frequently associated with the lesion as defined. It may be seen in several systemic diseases, such as systemic lupus erythematosus (SLE) and polyarteritis nodosa, and it is one of the commoner lesions seen in Schönlein-Henoch syndrome. Not all patients with this renal lesion, however, have these systemic diseases, and a number of different clinical pictures may be seen. These include recurrent attacks of hematuria, nephrotic syndrome, and the chance finding of protein in the urine. Be-

cause of the diverse settings in which focal glomerulonephritis may be encountered, it must be clearly understood that there are likely to be different etiologic factors and different pathogenetic mechanisms at work.

Historical

Löhlein [46], in 1910, described a focal involvement of the glomeruli in patients with subacute bacterial endocarditis. He called this embolic nonsuppurative focal nephritis, but as a rule it is now simply referred to as focal embolic nephritis. In this condition there are red blood cells in the urine, and renal insufficiency does not commonly occur. Histologically, certain of the glomeruli show localized areas of necrosis, while others show localized solidified or hyaline areas. Until recent years this was the only well-established form of focal glomerular disease with a definite clinical counterpart, and even today is apparently regarded by many as the only form of focal glomerulonephritis.

Volhard and Fahr [74] appreciated that focal nephritis could occur, and in their 1914 monograph they described three main forms: (1) focal glomerulonephritis, which could be acute or chronic; (2) interstitial nephritis; and (3) embolic focal nephritis. The first form, focal glomerulonephritis, presented clinically in the acute stage with hematuria and usually occurred in association with an infection. Tonsillitis or scarlatina were the infections most commonly encountered, and it was noticed that the hematuria occurred at the height of the infection rather than after a latent period of several days, a feature that characterizes the more generally recognized diffuse post-streptococcal form of glomerulonephritis. There was no rise in blood pressure — an important distinguishing feature from the diffuse forms — and edema was rare. Nitrogen retention did not occur except as part of a severe infection. The urine contained small quantities of albumin, and red and white blood cells and hyaline casts appeared in the urinary sediment. The prognosis in general was excellent. Hematuria often disappeared permanently after a few days, but occasionally it persisted for months or years. Subsequent acute infective attacks frequently caused a reappearance of the hematuria, and transient hematuria sometimes followed such procedures as tonsillectomy. In certain patients with this clinical picture the disease passed into a chronic stage with persistent hematuria. Difficulties were encountered, however, in distinguishing between this chronic stage of focal glomerulonephritis and the less severe forms of chronic diffuse glomerulonephritis. In the majority of cases renal function was not impaired, but some patients showed persistence of blood and albumin in the urine and some lability of the blood pressure. In considering these observations of Volhard and Fahr [74] it is interesting to note that they called attention to the earlier work of Scheidemandel [66], who discussed the significance and importance of bacteriologic examination of the urine, and described how recurrences of infection, such as tonsillitis, caused an increased

excretion of red blood cells and bacteria (usually streptococci) in the urine of patients with this hemorrhagic form of nephritis. Moreover, Scheidemandel noted that removal of the tonsils could also produce hematuria in these patients.

In 1926, Baehr [6] described a form of hemorrhagic nephritis that occurred mainly in young adults. In this condition, hematuria accompanied by albuminuria was the chief abnormality. The illness could be recurrent or persistent, the interval between attacks in the recurrent form being variable and extending from days to years. A sore throat usually preceded the attacks by one or two days. The persistent form tended to have a more insidious onset, the patient seldom being conscious of a sore throat. Subjective symptoms were completely absent, and the more chronic cases persisted for many months. Hematuria was a constant finding, and albuminuria, from a trace to a cloud, was always present. Red-cell, granular, and hyaline casts were also observed. The urinary concentrating ability was unimpaired, and in neither form was there edema or hypertension. Baehr [6] considered that the pathologic lesions were probably not unlike those described by Löhlein [46] in focal embolic nephritis. In a previous paper Baehr [5] claimed to have shown that the damaged loops in the affected glomeruli in focal embolic nephritis often contained bacterial emboli, but he thought that the focal glomerular lesions of the benign hemorrhagic form of nephritis need not necessarily be produced in the same way. He referred to two cases in which he had seen such glomerular changes in the absence of endocarditis.

Fishberg [27] discussed focal nephritis and described how, during the course of various infections, hematuria, albuminuria, and casts appeared in the urine without edema or hypertension. He chose to call the condition focal nephritis rather than focal glomerulonephritis because he considered that independent glomerular, tubular, and interstitial changes occurred, although any one of these might predominate in a given case. He believed that the renal lesions were caused by a direct invasion by microorganisms, and as evidence for this he cited the demonstration of the causative organism in the tissues. The various infective conditions with which focal nephritis was associated were streptococcal infections of the throat, skin, and uterus; pneumonia; typhoid fever; malaria; and relapsing fever. Pathologically there were hemorrhages into the glomerular capsular space, with foci of endothelial proliferation, increase in leukocytes, and swelling of capillary walls in the glomerular tuft. Only a certain number of glomeruli were affected, and lesions were usually confined to a portion of the affected tuft. Sometimes focal necrosis of tubules was present, and scattered collections of lymphocytes were found in the interstitium. It is difficult to judge from Fishberg's [27] account how constantly these various clinical and pathologic correlations were confirmed at autopsy, or with what degree of severity the glomeruli were affected.

A general review on the concept of focal nephritis was made by Payne and Illingworth [54] in 1940. Their object was to decide whether anything was to be gained by distinguishing between focal and diffuse glomerular nephritis. Their main conclusion was that focal glomerular nephritis was not a distinct clinical entity.

In 1942 Ellis [24] devised a new classification of glomerulonephritis, separating it into two types. Type 1 was characterized by an acute onset with hematuria, hypertension, edema, and mild nitrogen retention, usually following an upper-respiratory-tract infection after an interval of several days. The great majority of patients recovered completely, but others died from renal failure in the early stages; some progressed into a chronic stage, death ultimately occurring with the patient in chronic renal failure and having a raised blood pressure. Type 2 began insidiously with a nephrotic syndrome and was associated with a

poor prognosis. In addition, Ellis [24] described a small group of patients who presented with hematuria but who did not have hypertension and edema such as that found in type 1. The hematuria occurred at the height of an infection, which was usually tonsillitis or otitis media. The prognosis was good, and recovery took place as soon as the infection cleared. Occasionally there were repeated attacks of hematuria related to a recurrence of infection, which again was usually tonsillitis or otitis media. The prognosis was good, and recovery took place as soon as the infection cleared. The recurrences in 11 out of 35 patients with this benign condition were considered to be acute focal nephritis. Although in general the prognosis was good, two of the patients showed persistent albuminuria, and after many years the blood pressure rose and death occurred in uremia. Ellis [24] kept these 35 cases separate from type 1 glomerulonephritis.

It was not until the advent of the renal biopsy, however, that the concept of focal glomerular involvement was solidified. Bates et al. [7] performed renal biopsies in a group of 10 young men who presented with hematuria and proteinuria, but usually without hypertension and edema. The renal manifestations appeared within 5 days of a sore throat, which on both immunologic and clinical grounds was not caused by group A hemolytic streptococci. Microscopic hematuria persisted, but proteinuria disappeared in at least eight of the patients during a six-month period of observation. The biopsies showed that the majority of the glomeruli were normal, but that occasional ones showed epithelial crescents or hyalinization. Red blood cells were present in capsular spaces and tubular lumina, suggesting that glomerular damage had occurred. These authors suggested that their findings were consistent with a focal type of lesion.

In 1959 Heptinstall and Joekes [36] published an account of 13 patients with a focal type of glomerular lesion, and by 1961 they [37] had collected a total of 31 cases. The diagnosis was made on renal biopsy, the histologic picture showing a form of glomerulonephritis that affected only a certain number of glomeruli, the others being normal in appearance. The clinical picture was not constant: while some patients had systemic lupus erythematosus, presumed polyarteritis nodosa, or Schönlein-Henoch syndrome, others had varied clinical findings which are described in a later section. Subsequent publications have amply confirmed the existence of focal glomerulonephritis, and reference will be made to these at appropriate places in this chapter.

Diseases or Syndromes in Which Focal Glomerulonephritis May Be Found

Before the days of the renal biopsy it had been appreciated that focal glomerulonephritis could occur as part of various generalized diseases, and these impressions have been amply confirmed by the renal biopsy. The more important of these generalized diseases are considered.

FOCAL EMBOLIC GLOMERULONEPHRITIS

This condition has been well described by several authors [5, 9, 46] as the renal lesion that may complicate subacute bacterial endocarditis, the causative organism in the great majority of cases being the *Streptococcus viridans*.

Clinically, there is very little to suggest renal disease apart from hematuria. This may either be so slight that it is found only on examination of the urinary sediment or be so great that it leads to discoloration of the urine. In the latter instance it is much more likely that the hematuria has its origin in an infarct of the kidney rather than through leakage of red cells across affected glomeruli. Renal insufficiency does not commonly occur, but in

some cases it may; it is then usually associated with a more widespread pathologic lesion.

Most of the information on the pathologic changes in this particular type of kidney disease comes from autopsy studies. The kidneys are smooth and swollen, with numerous petechial hemorrhages on the subcapsular surface and gross infarcts in a substantial number of cases. This type of kidney is frequently referred to as the flea-bitten kidney. Histologically most of the glomeruli are normal, but some show changes consisting of eosinophilic areas confined to single lobules in the capillary tufts. These areas of intracapillary thrombosis, sometimes with necrosis of the adjacent capillary walls, may be accompanied by proliferation of cells in the nearby tuft capillaries, or by increase in number of cells lining Bowman's capsule leading to epithelial-crescent formation. This is usually referred to as the acute type of lesion. In addition, however, and frequently in the same case, there is a more quiescent-looking lesion in the glomeruli. This lesion consists of a solidification at the periphery of a lobule of a glomerular tuft, usually with adherence to Bowman's capsule. Baehr [5] traced the evolution of the first (acute) lesion into the second, which he regarded as the healed phase. Bell [10] disagreed and considered the two types of lesions as independent of each other. On the basis of serial biopsies of focal glomerulonephritis in situations outside endocarditis, I would agree with Baehr on this point. Focal glomerular lesions similar to those found in bacterial endocarditis have been described in fungal endocarditis, the organism in the four recorded cases being of the *Candida* species [61].

The pathogenesis of the lesion has not finally been resolved. On the basis of having noticed streptococci in an embolus that had become impacted in an artery in the kidney, thereby causing infarction, Löhlein [46] suggested that the glomerular lesions were caused by bacterial emboli. Baehr [5] supported this concept and claimed to have seen bacterial emboli in glomeruli in 5 out of 25 cases. On the other hand, Longcope [47], Jungmann [39], and Allen [2] considered the glomerular lesions to be of allergic origin. I have observed in autopsy cases of subacute bacterial endocarditis that the glomerular lesions occur in groups, frequently around the periphery of infarcts. The effects of interference with the blood supply to glomeruli in such positions as the edges of infarcts has not been generally appreciated, but all the changes of focal glomerulonephritis may be simulated. It is therefore conceivable that many of the glomerular lesions are explicable on an embolic basis, although not in the sense envisaged by Löhlein [46] and Baehr [5].

Certain authors have been impressed with the degree of diffuse involvement of glomeruli in subacute bacterial endocarditis — for example, Bell [9] reported a frequency of diffuse hypercellularity of the glomeruli of over 60 per cent and Christian [16] of over 80 per cent of cases. In my own experience the frequency has been much smaller, being of the order of 17 per cent.

POLYARTERITIS (PERIARTERITIS) NODOSA

Certain patients with polyarteritis nodosa have a renal lesion in which many glomeruli show necrotizing changes in the tufts, sometimes associated with localized proliferation of the cells in the tuft and occasionally of the cells lining Bowman's capsule. Other glomeruli within the same kidney may show fibrous lesions, probably representing a healed phase of the necrotizing form; other glomeruli may appear to be completely normal. Such cases were described [19] as microscopic periarteritis or polyarteritis to distinguish them from the classic form in which the glomeruli are not affected in this way, and show merely the consequences of ischemia brought about by occlusive lesions of the segmental and arcuate arteries. The renal lesions encountered in microscopic polyarteritis are considerably more widespread than in the other forms of focal glomerulonephritis, and the degree of involvement becomes so great that renal failure is

the usual cause of death. This is seen in particular in Wegener's syndrome [77], a variant of polyarteritis. In spite of widespread glomerular involvement, many glomeruli may be spared, the changes in affected glomeruli being of a characteristically localized type.

SYSTEMIC LUPUS ERYTHEMATOSUS (SLE)

The early renal lesion of SLE has been well demonstrated by the percutaneous renal biopsy. Up to recent times the renal lesion of SLE appeared to be more or less diffuse because only the end stage was seen in autopsy material. Muehrcke et al. [49] have shown the focal and local involvement of the glomeruli by the biopsy method, and two of our original cases [36] showed an essentially focal and local involvement. It should be repeated that the term *local* describes the change within an affected glomerulus and signifies that only a portion of the glomerulus is involved. Because of the similarity of the words focal and local, and the difficulty certain people encounter in distinguishing between them, the term *segmental* has been suggested as an alternative for local. I take no violent objection to this, although it is highly questionable whether established nomenclature should be altered for the benefit of those with feeble memories. The early change in SLE consists of peripherally located areas of cellular proliferation in certain glomeruli, often associated with karyorrhexis of nuclei and necrosis of the affected lobule of the tuft. The localized or segmental involvement of glomeruli is very often apparent even in cases where virtually all of the glomeruli are affected in the later stages. Systemic lupus erythematosus is described elsewhere in this volume and no more will be said at this stage.

SCHÖNLEIN-HENOCH SYNDROME

In this condition there is a combination of a skin eruption and pains in the joints and abdomen. It is not unusual to encounter hematuria associated with proteinuria in such cases. The frequency of renal involvement varies considerably from one investigation to another, and in a review of several series I have found a range of 14.0 to 63.4 per cent [35]. The ultimate outcome likewise exhibits great variance, and in several series the frequency of residual damage to the kidney varied from 6 to 38 per cent [35]. The scatter is undoubtedly explained by the different criteria used for assessing damage; the high figure of 38 per cent found by Wedgwood and Klaus [76] was based merely on the persistence of red blood cells and casts in the urine. Gairdner's [28] paper did much to give a sinister prognosis for patients with renal involvement in this syndrome, 4 out of his 11 patients being left with chronic nephritis or persistent proteinuria and hematuria.

The best-known renal lesion in the Schönlein-Henoch syndrome is a rapidly progressing glomerulonephritis that is characterized by widespread glomerular change with crescent formation; this course is comparatively rare. Little information about the milder forms was available until the renal biopsy came into use, but several series of biopsy studies in children have now appeared. The most commonly described lesion is that of a focal glomerulonephritis. Vernier et al. [73] have described 11 renal biopsies in children and one in an adult patient, commenting on the segmental (local) nature of the lesion in scattered glomeruli. The individual lesions consisted of endothelial hypercellularity associated with accumulation of amorphous PAS-positive material. Focal capillary thrombi were also described. Bergstrand et al. [13] described similar lesions in children, and in two patients in whom a repeat biopsy was performed two years later, there was no progression of the lesion.

The largest series to date is that of Kobayashi et al. [40], who described the findings in 74 biopsies on 54 children. They again commented on the focal nature of the glomerular involvement. One of their cases, described in detail, started out as a focal glomerulonephritis in which only 5 out of 11 glomeruli showed changes. A biopsy taken three months later showed many glomeruli in the process of hyalinization, while a third biopsy 20 months after the onset of illness showed that 5 of the 6 glomeruli in the biopsy were completely hyalinized. These authors also described a case in which, at autopsy after a two-year illness, the characteristic alterations of chronic glomerulonephritis were present, with large numbers of glomeruli being completely sclerosed. It is unfortunate that they did not report on the initial biopsy of this patient. However, their study does indicate that a certain number of patients with renal involvement in Schönlein-Henoch syndrome may progress to a chronic stage with obliteration of large numbers of glomeruli.

Information on the renal picture of this syndrome in older patients is scarce. However, I have had the opportunity of studying biopsies from six adult patients, and of these, four showed a focal form of glomerulonephritis. Daeschner et al. [18] demonstrated focal glomerular changes in 6 out of 10 children with Schönlein-Henoch syndrome and coexistent hematuria and proteinuria. They went on to comment that no normal glomeruli were seen in these six cases, so clearly they were referring to widespread localized glomerular lesions rather than focal glomerulonephritis. In the single case with a repeat biopsy there was no change over a 13-month period. They described a further case with advanced focal glomerular lesions, presumably advanced local lesions, which showed progressive glomerular changes in a repeat biopsy six months later.

Bouissou et al. [15] described diffuse proliferative glomerular changes, and in a later paper Vernier and his co-workers [71] described a more widespread renal lesion characterized by proliferation of mesangial cells, which they called diffuse proliferative glomerulonephritis. The kidneys in certain of their patients showed more severe diffuse lesions with crescent formation, while others showed scarring and hyalinization of glomeruli; in one patient in the latter group renal transplantation was required. Bodian et al. [14], while describing focal and local lesions in this syndrome, also described patients with more widespread lesions with all the glomeruli showing involvement of all the tuft, or with all the glomeruli showing the localized type of lesions within the tuft.

It is of considerable interest that many patients with Schönlein-Henoch syndrome also have a concomitant nephrotic syndrome. The renal lesion here has also been described as a focal glomerulonephritis. As in other cases of the nephrotic syndrome with a histologic picture of focal glomerulonephritis, I have been impressed by the absence of necrotizing lesions in the glomeruli. The nephrotic syndrome may also accompany the severe, rapidly progressing azotemic form with widespread glomerular involvement.

Electron microscopy of the renal lesion in Schönlein-Henoch syndrome [25, 40, 53, 59, 71] reveals endothelial hyperplasia, laying down of basement membrane-like material in the glomeruli, and localized fusion of foot processes. Irregular masses of electron-dense deposits were described in a subendothelial position in the glomerular tuft by Kobayashi et al. [40] and Urizar et al. [71]. The latter authors also described a splitting of the lamina densa into layers by these deposits and commented on the increased numbers of mesangial cells as well as increase in mesangial material. It is not clear from their description whether the mesangial changes were found in those with the focal involvement or whether it was confined to those with diffuse lesions. Subepithelial electron-dense deposits (humps) were not seen. These authors [40, 71] were particularly impressed with the presence of platelets and fibrin in the capillary lumina, suggesting that intravascular coagulation may play a role in producing the lesions. In the cases associated with a nephrotic syndrome, fusion of the foot processes of the tuft epithelial cells has been described.

Immunofluorescent studies are sparse, and those described refer to the more widespread lesion. Bodian et al. [14] described positive fluorescence to antihuman globulin in one case out of three tested; the histologic diagnosis of this case was generalized diffuse glomerulonephritis. Urizar et al. [71] described positive fluorescence to immunoglobulins and beta$_{1c}$ globulin occurring in a focal and local distribution in one patient with a focal and local histologic lesion. They commented on the mesangial distribution of fluorescence in the patients with more widespread glomerular involvement. Lange [43], however, has studied a 7-year-old girl with Schönlein-Henoch syndrome in whom renal biopsy showed some glomeruli to be affected whereas others appeared to be normal in the routine histological preparation. The frozen-section studies with immunofluorescent technics revealed all glomeruli as showing a granular fluorescence to IgG and beta$_{1c}$ globulin. Although it cannot be stated with certainty, these observations strongly suggest that the glomeruli that appeared normal by conventional microscopy did in fact contain immune complexes.

LUNG HEMORRHAGE AND GLOMERULONEPHRITIS (SO-CALLED GOODPASTURE'S SYNDROME)

Increasing numbers of cases of the syndrome characterized by hemoptysis and renal failure are being described. This condition is found most commonly in young men, although no age group is exempt, and a certain number of cases have been recorded in women. The first symptom is usually hemoptysis, and this is usually of small amount and repeated at intervals of varying duration. Anemia is a common feature and is frequently out of proportion to the amount of blood expectorated. Dyspnea is another common feature. These patients usually pursue a rapidly progressive downhill course, with death occurring in renal failure several months later.

In the early stages the changes in the urine are usually slight, consisting of abnormalities in the spun-down deposit. Protein is sometimes present, but usually only in small amounts. In cases that have been biopsied at this early stage, a focal form of glomerulonephritis has been described [11, 22, 36, 38, 63]. However, the character of the renal involvement rapidly changes to that of a very florid diffuse glomerulonephritis with widespread crescent formation. Several cases are now on record in which serial biopsies have shown this rapid transformation from a focal to a diffuse form of glomerular involvement. Rusby and Wilson [63] described a 20-year-old man who had various episodes of spitting up blood, and dyspnea. On examination he was found to be anemic and mildly hypertensive, with protein, red cells, and granular casts in the urine. On admission a renal biopsy showed 3 out of 12 glomeruli to have localized areas of cellular proliferation, irregular thickening of basement membranes, adhesions to Bowman's capsule, and localized proliferation of epithelial cells. A second biopsy taken 6 weeks later showed all 22 glomeruli to be severely disorganized, with partial or complete necrosis of the tufts, capsular adhesions, and crescent formation. This same severe involvement was seen in a third biopsy one month after this, and in the kidneys at autopsy three months later. This man died within six months of admission with a remarkable transformation from a focal to a diffuse glomerular nephritis over a period of 6 weeks. Johnson and McGovern [38] have also described a case with a rapid transformation from a focal type to a diffuse type of lesion over a period of four weeks. Benoit et al. [11] described their experience with a 19-year-old man who presented with hemoptysis, exertional dyspnea, and urinary changes suggesting renal involvement. The initial biopsy showed a mild focal glomerulonephritis, only 1 in 16 glomeruli showing small localized changes, the other glomeruli being normal in appearance. Two months later a second biopsy showed a still largely focal picture, but there appeared to be a mild nuclear increase in many glomeruli. The patient pursued a hectic azotemic course and died nine weeks after the second biopsy.

The kidney at autopsy showed widespread glomerular involvement, crescent formation, and proliferative and sclerosing changes in the tufts.

It should not be assumed, however, that all cases of lung hemorrhage with glomerulonephritis pursue this rapidly progressive course following an original diagnosis of a focal glomerulonephritis. For example, a 20-year-old man (Case 13 of our original publication [36]) with an 8-month history of coughing up blood was found to have red blood cells and protein in the urine, together with a severe degree of anemia and elevation of blood pressure. Renal biopsy revealed a focal glomerulonephritis, half of the 30 glomeruli showing involvement (i.e., localized areas of proliferation). A second biopsy 13 months later showed changes in some one-third of the 22 glomeruli present, but proliferative activity appeared to be much decreased and localized solidification more apparent. Six years after the initial presentation he was well, although with some residual proteinuria [75]. A similar type of case was described by Crosnier et al. [17] in which a renal biopsy in a 48-year-old man showed a local or segmental change in many glomeruli. A biopsy one year later showed substantially the same changes. This patient, however, had some residual renal impairment. Duncan et al. [22] have also described the case of a 21-year-old woman who showed only a trace of albumin and occasional red cells in the urine, 20 months after a biopsy which showed one-third of the glomeruli to be affected. Other cases with a more favorable course are reviewed by Duncan et al. [22].

Apart from being yet another example of the various conditions that can be attended by a focal glomerulonephritis, this particular syndrome is of undue interest because it demonstrates the way in which a focal form of glomerulonephritis can be transformed into a more diffuse one. It is apparent that this behavior is in contrast to the usual situation in Schönlein-Henoch syndrome.

The etiology and pathogenesis of lung purpura and glomerulonephritis are poorly understood, to say the least, largely because of a paucity of information about the early stages when the lesion in the kidney is still focal. Benoit et al. [11] commented that certain cases followed in the wake of epidemics of influenza, thereby suggesting a viral etiology. In this respect it is worthy of note that Duncan et al. [22] demonstrated virus-like particles in glomerular endothelial and epithelial cells on electron microscopy.

Fluorescent-antibody studies have shown a linear pattern of immunoglobulins along the basement membranes of the glomeruli [8, 22, 45, 65, 69], and Lerner et al. [45] have presented evidence to demonstrate the presence of antiglomerular basement membrane (anti-GBM) antibodies in affected kidneys. This evidence was based on several observations. First, a linear fluorescence was obtained in glomerular capillaries when sections were treated with antibody to IgG and beta$_{1C}$ globulin; this is the pattern of distribution of heterologous anti-GBM antibodies localized in vivo in nephrotoxic serum nephritis and of autologous anti-GBM antibodies in the autoimmune version of this disease. Second, eluates from kidneys with so-called Goodpasture's disease fix strongly to sections of normal human kidney in vitro, and furthermore, the eluates rapidly produce severe glomerulonephritis when injected into monkeys, establishing the pathogenicity of the antibodies.

Kroe and Pitcock [42] found gamma globulin in areas of lobular glomerular sclerosis and along capillary basement membranes in a single case. The distribution along the basement membranes in their illustration is focal instead of the regular linear pattern regarded as indicating the pattern of anti-GBM antibodies.

All these studies on the demonstration of antibodies to glomerular basement membrane have been carried out on advanced cases, but Vernier [72] has shown that this same linear fluorescence is present at an early stage. In a 21-year-old woman with hemoptysis and red blood cells in the urine, biopsy revealed some glomeruli to have localized areas of cellular proliferation, whereas others had a normal appearance. Immunofluorescent studies revealed that all glomeruli had a linear fluorescence to IgG, showing that immunoglobulins were diffusely present at a relatively early stage.

There is a close antigenic similarity between the lung and the kidney, and it is tempting to suggest a common immunologic mechanism to be operative in the so-called Goodpasture's disease. Fluorescent-antibody studies carried out on the lung at autopsy in such patients have shown differing results. On the one hand, Scheer and Grossman [65] and Duncan et al. [22] failed to demonstrate immunoglobulins in the lung capillaries, whereas on the other Sturgill and Westervelt [69], Kroe and Pitcock [42], and Beirne et al. [8] demonstrated them in the alveolar septa.

HEREDITARY NEPHRITIS (ALPORT'S SYNDROME)

Hereditary nephritis is a condition in which one or several members of a family are subject to recurrent bouts of hematuria precipitated by infections or more rarely by certain items in the diet. Proteinuria is present in variable quantities, and in some patients there may be an actual nephrotic syndrome. Some patients may also have an associated nerve deafness. In time, progressive renal failure occurs in the majority of patients affected; it is interesting that male subjects fare worse than females, some of whom may live to old age.

This condition, well described by Guthrie [33] and later by Alport [3], is inherited as an autosomal dominant [51], and several large pedigrees have now been recorded [50, 51, 55, 56, 79]. It is described more fully in Chapter 37 and is mentioned here only because in the early stages it is characterized by focal glomerular involvement.

The glomerular changes vary from case to case; in some there are proliferative changes in the glomerular tuft, and crescents may be seen. In others, rather bland eosinophilic areas appear in the glomeruli; with the passage of time more glomeruli are affected and individual glomeruli become more severely involved until virtually all are affected.

The pathogenesis of the lesion is not understood, and immunofluorescence studies are sparse. Spear et al. [68] have recorded the absence of IgG in four biopsies and one nephrectomy specimen, which may indicate that the pathogenesis is different from other forms of glomerulonephritis.

RECURRENT HEMATURIA

The condition of recurrent hematuria, in which a patient has repeated attacks of hematuria, is worthy of separate mention because of the way in which focal glomerulonephritis or focal glomerulitis has been repeatedly observed. Reference has already been made to this condition (page 464) and to the way in which Baehr [6] speculated that the pathological picture might be a focal form of glomerular disease. It is important that one not confuse this condition with the more serious condition of hereditary nephritis just described. Recurrent hematuria may be found in children [4, 14, 48, 62], young adults [1, 5, 26, 57], and exceptionally in persons over the age of 40 years [57]. The patient usually seeks advice because of dark urine and frequently gives a history of an upper-respiratory-tract infection immediately preceding the attack. The latter is in marked contrast to poststreptococcal acute glomerulonephritis in which there is a latent interval between the infective episode and onset of symptoms. It is also a feature of the patients with recurrent hematuria that evidence of streptococcal etiology is usually lacking [4, 7, 26, 48, 57, 62]. McConville et al. [48] have shown that the serum beta$_{1c}$ globulin (component of complement) levels are normal, in contrast to the usual low levels found in poststreptococcal glomerulonephritis. Intervals of weeks or months may separate the recurrent attacks of hematuria; in one of Ross's [62] cases no less than 12 separate episodes had taken place. Episodes of hematuria may be precipitated by factors other than infection, such as tonsillectomy [6, 66], dental extractions [62], exercise [57], and inoculation against typhoid fever. Alexander [1] has described recurrence caused by influenza A virus.

Proteinuria is frequently inconspicuous in the first few attacks, but it may become persistent after several episodes. Microscopic hematuria may be found in the urine in the interval between the overt attacks [14, 62]. The blood pressure is usually not raised during the attacks, another feature that distinguishes it from poststreptococcal glomerulonephritis. There is commonly no nitrogen retention, although this may occur as a transient phenomenon. Edema is usually absent and venous pressure is not elevated. In general the prognosis is excellent with no progressive impairment of renal function [4, 6, 20, 26, 57, 74], but death occurred in renal failure in 2 of the 11 cases of recurrent hematuria described by Ellis [24].

An interesting feature emerged from the studies of Ayoub and Vernier [4] and McConville et al. [48]. In the former, it was found that of 17 children with multiple episodes of gross hematuria, 7 gave a family history of nephritis or hematuria. The mothers of three patients had an unexplained history of hematuria, and another patient's mother had acute nephritis. A sister of one, and a brother of another, had hematuria; in both instances the siblings had their attacks at the same time. The niece of the final patient was described as having nephritis. In the series of McConville et al. [48] there was a family history in only 2 out of 17 children with recurrent hematuria. However, when the urine of family members was tested for blood by a chemical method, a familial incidence was found in 10 cases. These two series are of interest because of the similarity of presentation to the condition of hereditary nephritis, a condition with a sinister prognosis, particularly in the male. However, deafness — a common accompaniment of hereditary nephritis — was specifically sought in these two series and was absent in all patients; it was also absent in those relatives who were tested. In addition, the renal biopsies in the series of Ayoub and Vernier [4] either were normal or showed only minimal focal glomerulonephritis. Those in the series of McConville et al. [48] showed little more than equivocal glomerular hypercellularity, except in one patient who was considered to have nephritis in an indeterminant stage. It was specifically mentioned that there was no difference between those with and those without the familial association. Foam cells — a feature of hereditary nephritis — were apparently absent in both series. The subsequent clinical courses were benign in all cases in both series. Singer et al. [67] have recorded a similar family history of hematuria in patients with recurrent hematuria.

Many of these patients with recurrent hematuria have a focal glomerulonephritis or focal glomerulitis on biopsy [4, 14, 26, 57, 62, 67]. On the other hand, more diffuse proliferative glomerular lesions have been recorded [14, 26, 57, 70], while no abnormalities at all have been described in certain biopsies [4, 26, 34, 48, 57, 67]. I have seen several cases over the last several years with no demonstrable histologic abnormalities in the glomeruli by light microscopy. It is important to record the technic by which glomeruli are deemed normal, because Singer et al. [67], using electron microscopy, have demonstrated electron-dense deposits on both the epithelial and the endothelial aspects of the lamina densa in patients with no abnormality by light microscopy.

There are unfortunately insufficient cases in which serial biopsies have been performed to state with certainty the natural history of the renal lesion. In his paper on recurrent focal nephritis, Ross [62] described how he studied the old records of nine patients who had been considered to have had recurrent focal nephritis. Unfortunately biopsies were not performed on these patients, but autopsy records were available on two who had died in uremia. One had developed hypertension after four years of recurrent episodes of hematuria, with no hypertension, edema, or impairment of renal function during these attacks. Death occurred in uremia two years after the development of hypertension, and at autopsy the glomeruli were reduced in numbers in the contracted kidneys; those glomeruli that survived showed proliferative and necrotic lesions in the tufts with crescent formation. In the other patient a nephrotic syndrome developed after two years of repeated attacks of hematuria, death occurring in uremia seven years later. Hypertension and renal failure developed four years before death. The kidneys at autopsy were contracted, and the majority of glomeruli were seen to be reduced to fibrohyaline discs surrounded by dense interstitial fibrosis. The surviving glomeruli showed capillary basement membrane thickening with "intercapillary" hyalinization.

Electron microscopy has revealed electron-dense material in a subendothelial position [44, 67], and an increase in basement membrane-like material in the denser areas [44]. Subepithelial deposits of electron-dense material have also been recorded in biopsies from patients with recurrent hematuria, where the biopsy shows no change or localized proliferative lesions in glomeruli [67] by light microscopy. If subepithelial deposits can be regarded as specific for poststreptococcal glomerulonephritis, then we may be provided with some clue as to the etiology of some cases of recurrent hematuria. At this particular time, however, it may be wrong to assume that subepithelial deposits (humps) are specific for poststreptococcal glomerulonephritis. There are few reports of immunofluorescent studies, but Bodian et al. [14] commented on the fact that those cases with focal and local

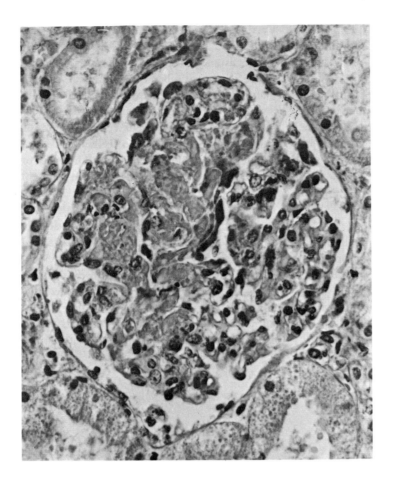

Figure 14-2. Glomerulus with extensive necrosis in part of tuft. From a patient with microscopic form of polyarteritis in which many glomeruli were normal. Hematoxylin and eosin. ×450.

that they represent the scars of healed acute lesions. Occasionally entire glomeruli may be solidified. Certain types of lesions seem to predominate in certain clinical states — for example, necroses in the glomerular tufts are the predominant changes in polyarteritis.

Tubular changes are inconstant and usually amount to little more than focal loss or atrophy. Tubular changes are greater in those cases with more extensive glomerular involvement. Small collections of chronic inflammatory cells and small areas of fibrosis may be seen in the interstitium. Vascular changes are not conspicuous. Culture of renal tissue, in our own experience, has invariably been sterile. Electron microscopy and immunofluorescence microscopy have been described

earlier in the chapter under the various settings in which focal glomerulonephritis is found.

Clinical Features

Focal glomerulonephritis, being a histologic entity, may be found in many different clinical settings. The clinical pictures of such entities as systemic lupus erythematosus and polyarteritis are described in other parts of this book, while brief accounts of the clinical side of the Schönlein-Henoch syndrome, lung hemorrhage and glomerulonephritis, and recurrent hematuria are given with the general account of these conditions earlier in this chap-

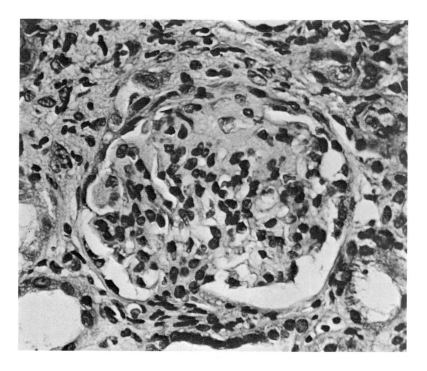

Figure 14-3. Glomerulus showing older solidified area adherent to Bowman's capsule from a case of Schönlein-Henoch syndrome with focal glomerulonephritis. Hematoxylin and eosin. ×450.

ter. Certain general points, however, need stressing, as do the features of patients who have histologic focal glomerulonephritis outside specific systemic diseases.

The clinical presentations may be extremely varied, ranging from the chance finding of proteinuria to a severe acute illness — possibly with generalized signs and symptoms. In some cases there may be an acute illness in which evidence of renal involvement is associated with monoarthritis or polyarthritis, with erythematosus skin lesions, with anemia, and in certain instances with colicky intestinal pain. The associated symptoms can occur individually or in combination.

In many patients there is no clear-cut association of an infection — and in particular, a streptococcal infection — and the histologic finding of focal glomerulonephritis. In patients in whom either a sore throat, some local septic infection, or pneumonia occurs, there

is no clear interval of time between the onset of infection and evidence of renal involvement. In some cases of recurrent hematuria the episode has been closely related to a sore throat; in others, the hematuria may follow exertion or occur for no apparent reason.

There is usually a good inverse correlation between the degree of histologic damage and the tendency for the clinical parameters to improve. In some patients with recurrent attacks there has been complete remission after each episode, but in a few instances, although remission occurred after the earlier episodes, renal involvement persisted after the later ones.

When focal glomerulonephritis is recognized by renal biopsy at an early stage, it is important to remember that there is no evidence that a single disease process is involved. Also, any attempt to build up a "clinical syndrome" which will enable the diagnosis to be made without histologic confirmation is unjustified.

The *nephrotic syndrome* may be present, and the clinical findings are similar to those in the nephrotic syndrome with other pathologic pictures. West et al. [78] noted gross hematuria in some of their nephrotic patients with focal glomerulonephritis; these patients have normal serum complement levels, and only a small proportion of them have an elevated ASO titer. With regard to the prognosis in the nephrotic syndrome, our own experience has been good [37], as has been the experience of West et al. [78]. As recorded previously (page 474), however, Goldman et al. [32] noted that the response to treatment was less favorable than in the nephrotic syndrome with other pathologic pictures.

Skin rashes are common, and in patients with the Schönlein-Henoch syndrome, typical purpuric spots and ecchymoses are found. In some other patients without specific systemic disease there have been erythematosus rashes at the outset of the illness; these are usually confined to the skin and dorsa of the feet, and consist of irritating circular erythematous patches, with a darker center up to a centimeter in diameter. The rash fades after several days, leaving a brown discoloration for two or three weeks.

Joint pains are common features, even in patients without the Schönlein-Henoch syndrome and the other specific systemic diseases. Most commonly one or two joints, such as the ankle, knee, or wrist, are affected at the outset, but occasionally a fleeting polyarthritic picture resembling rheumatic fever is seen. The acute joint symptoms usually disappear after several weeks but show a tendency to recur in those with a recurrent renal picture.

Gastrointestinal symptoms have occasionally been seen in patients other than those with the Schönlein-Henoch syndrome. Colicky abdominal pain has been the usual complaint, with occult blood in the stool in some.

Edema is variable and is usually related to the urinary protein loss and the level of albumin in the serum. *Hypertension* is fairly common and is usually of a modest degree; it is most frequent when glomerular involvement is extensive. It may be fleeting, but in some patients it persists indefinitely. In our experience, it has been singular that even in the presence of hypertension and edema in the early stages of the disease, there has been no elevation in the venous pressure. This is in marked contrast to the situation in acute post-streptococcal glomerulonephritis.

Urinary changes are in no way characteristic. There may be gross proteinuria or frank hematuria, or there may be nothing more than a trivial increase in the excretion of formed elements. The urinary abnormalities tend to disappear more rapidly in patients with the least severe renal involvement, although it is not uncommon for some urinary abnormality, usually proteinuria, to disappear very slowly after a single episode of focal glomerulonephritis. Proteinuria in some patients has persisted for several years with no evidence of new episodes or of deterioration of renal function.

Renal function varies, but in most patients there is neither nitrogen retention nor significant renal functional impairment at any stage of a single episode of focal glomerulonephritis. A certain number of patients, however, show a transient reduction in renal function, and in some there are severely elevated blood urea nitrogen levels. Renal functional impairment is very short-lived, in most instances with full recovery in three weeks, but in some there is full recovery after several months of impairment. Transient nitrogen retention may occur with successive attacks in patients who have recurrent hematuria. A minority of patients develop persistent nitrogen retention.

Other laboratory investigations may show abnormalities. Anemia is sometimes noted, and the erythrocyte sedimentation rate is usually moderately raised. High sedimentation rates may be found when there is a disturbance of the plasma protein pattern. Low serum albumin concentration, elevation of the alpha-2 globulin level, and raised serum cholesterol levels may be found in patients with the nephrotic syndrome. Serum electrolyte abnormalities have been found only when there is severe renal functional disturbance. Laboratory evidence of previous group A streptococcal infections is almost invariably lacking.

Treatment

With the considerable variation in the degree of renal involvement and different circumstances in which focal glomerulonephritis may be encountered, assessment of the effects of therapy is extremely difficult. The treatment of the specific conditions in which focal glomerulonephritis may be found, such as systemic lupus erythematosus, polyarteritis, and so forth, is described in the appropriate chapters. In other cases certain points need emphasizing.

In patients with recurrent hematuria, tonsillectomy has proved of value. There is also some evidence to show that blood transfusion may occasionally lead to an extension of the renal lesion.

Hypertension, often present in the early stages of focal glomerulonephritis, may continue indefinitely. It frequently responds satisfactorily to reserpine, although other antihypertensive drugs may be needed and may have to be used indefinitely. Because hypertension may be difficult to control later on in the illness, there is an absolute indication for its treatment at an early stage. However, when it is difficult to differentiate the clinical picture from that of acute diffuse poststreptococcal glomerulonephritis, in which the blood pressure will fall rapidly and spontaneously, it is justifiable to wait two or three weeks before initiating treatment.

In lung hemorrhage with nephritis (so-called Goodpasture's syndrome) energetic treatment with steroids and possibly immunosuppressive drugs is necessary. With few exceptions the prognosis is extremely poor, and intractable progression to renal failure is the usual story.

Steroid therapy is usually efficacious in those patients with the nephrotic syndrome associated with focal glomerulonephritis. However, Goldman et al. [32] found that the response to steroids and other forms of treatment (including azathioprine) was disappointing.

Etiology and Pathogenesis

The diverse settings in which focal glomerulonephritis may be found make it unlikely that there are common etiologic agents and pathogenetic mechanisms. An example of this is provided by the apparently different pathogenetic mechanisms of two conditions which initially show a focal glomerulonephritis — namely, systemic lupus erythematosus and the so-called Goodpasture's syndrome. There is growing evidence to show that systemic lupus erythematosus is an example of immune-complex disease with deoxyribonucleic acid being the antigen [41]; on the other hand, it appears that the so-called Goodpasture's syndrome, at least in its later stages, is an example of disease caused by antibodies to glomerular basement membrane [21, 45].

Immunologic mechanisms undoubtedly play some role in certain cases, for, even excluding such conditions as SLE and polyarteritis, many of the patients give a history of skin rashes, joint pains, and other features consistent with this explanation. In Schönlein-Henoch syndrome there is some evidence for an immune mechanism. As reported on page 469, a granular fluorescent pattern has been noted by Lange [43] at an early stage in the disease, and Bodian et al. [14] described fluorescence to gamma globulin in one of their three cases in which this technic was used. The pattern of involvement was not stated. Urizar et al. [71] were impressed with the mesangial pattern of fluorescence for gamma globulin and complement in their cases of Schönlein-Henoch syndrome. They were of the opinion that, although the nephritis of anaphylactoid purpura may have an immune pathogenesis, the mechanism may differ significantly from that of other forms of renal disease.

In recurrent hematuria specific infections do not appear to play any constant role, and this is true in particular of group A streptococcal infections. Such a background has been assiduously sought and found to be lacking by several investigators [7, 26]. A virus etiology has been suspected in certain series [1, 4, 7], but this is by no means certain. It is a singular fact, however, that many patients with recurrent hematuria have their attacks concomitantly with, or shortly after, nonspecific upper-respiratory-tract infections. Bodian et al. [14] have studied the immunofluorescent picture in recurrent hematuria and in those cases with focal glomerulonephritis found that immunoglobulins were present in glomeruli that were not abnormal by conventional histologic technics, and were distributed diffusely in those glomeruli that were affected in a localized or segmental way.

In the so-called Goodpasture's syndrome reference has been made to the thoughts about a possible viral background (page 471) and on the likelihood of the renal lesion being brought about by antiglomerular basement membrane antibodies (page 471).

In the nonspecific groups, several studies have been carried out on serum complement levels, in particular in patients with hematuria and focal glomerulonephritis and in those with the nephrotic syndrome associated with focal glomerulonephritis. In their original study of acute nephritis not associated with group A streptococcal infection (see page 465) Bates et al. [7] found decreased serum complement levels suggesting that some antigen-antibody mechanism was at work, although the possibility of participation of group A streptococci had been virtually eliminated. On the other hand, West et al. [78] measured beta$_{1c}$ globulin in the serum, as a measure of complement activity, in a group of patients with focal glomerulonephritis associated with a nephrotic syndrome and hematuria; they found that the levels were not decreased. Rapoport et al. [58] studied a group of patients with hematuria or proteinuria, or both, in the absence of systemic disease who showed features different from those seen in poststreptococcal glomerulonephritis. On biopsy, focal proliferative glomerulonephritis was found in over half, and in these — as in those with no specific glomerular changes on biopsy — the serum beta$_{1c}$ globulin was normal or elevated. The exact significance of the normal complement levels in these two series is not altogether clear, but it is in contrast to the decreased levels that are found in poststreptococcal glomerulonephritis, and might suggest a different operative mechanism for the patients with focal glomerulonephritis.

In the nonspecific groups there are very few studies in which immunofluorescent technics have been applied to tissue sections of biopsies with focal glomerulonephritis. Earle and Jennings [23] depict a glomerulus from a patient with focal glomerulitis who did not have polyarteritis, SLE, or evidence of streptococcal infection. Localized fluorescence to gamma globulin and beta$_{1c}$ globulin was found, and in addition, fibrin was deposited focally. The exact significance of the localized areas of gamma globulin and beta$_{1c}$ globulin is not clear, and it must not be readily assumed that this constitutes proof of an antigen-antibody reaction; such a picture could come about as a pooling of protein in an area of injury.

Irrespective of the circumstances in which focal glomerulonephritis may be found, the way in which certain glomeruli may be involved, with others showing no change, is intriguing and at the present time entirely unexplained. The way in which the glomeruli can be "protected" by narrowing of the renal artery in diffuse proliferative glomerulonephritis in man [52], in immune-complex disease experimentally [30], and in nephrotoxic nephritis experimentally [64] indicates the importance of hemodynamic factors. While it is probable that the perfusion pressure of the juxtamedullary glomeruli is greater than of the glomeruli further out in the cortex, it is unlikely that such differences by themselves could be the sole explanation for focal glomerulonephritis in man. Such an explanation would be dependent on a demonstration that the juxtamedullary glomeruli are those selectively involved in focal glomerulonephritis; so far as I am aware there is no proof that this is the case, although as mentioned earlier, Rich [60] showed a greater vulnerability to sclerosis of these particular glomeruli in lipoid nephrosis.

Dosage effects also could be postulated as an explanation for the focal distribution of lesions. That is, if a greater dose of soluble complexes or antiglomerular basement membrane antibody were delivered to certain glomeruli, these would be more likely to show reactive changes than others. The demonstration of immunoglobulins in histologically unaffected glomeruli in Schönlein-Henoch syndrome [43], so-called Goodpasture's syndrome [72], and recurrent hematuria [14] suggests that additional local factors are necessary before injury takes place.

Germuth et al. [31] have shown the profound effects of cortisone on the genesis of the glomerular lesion in experimental serum sickness nephritis. Briefly, it was shown that cortisone inhibited the development of glomerulonephritis by impeding the transit of immune complexes from the circulation across the walls of the glomerular loops. Germuth [29] has informed me that when subinhibitory doses of cortisone are administered, a focal glomerulonephritis with localized or segmental histologic changes in the affected glomeruli is produced. This experimental production of a focal glomerulonephritis is unique and may provide valuable clues to the problem of why certain glomeruli, and not others, are affected in focal glomerulonephritis.

While none of the above explanations by itself can explain the focal distribution of glomerular lesions, it is conceivable that combinations of such factors might be operative. More information on the intrarenal circulation is needed before this question can be finally resolved.

References

1. Alexander, E. A. Recurrent hemorrhagic nephritis with exacerbation related to influenza A. *Ann. Intern. Med.* 62:1022, 1965.

2. Allen, A. C. *The Kidney. Medical and Surgical Diseases* (2d ed.). New York: Grune & Stratton, 1962. P. 203.

3. Alport, A. C. Hereditary familial congenital haemorrhagic nephritis. *Brit. Med. J.* 1: 504, 1927.

4. Ayoub, E. M., and Vernier, R. L. Benign recurrent hematuria. *Amer. J. Dis. Child.* 109:217, 1965.

5. Baehr, G. Glomerular lesions of subacute bacterial endocarditis. *J. Exp. Med.* 15:330, 1912.

6. Baehr, G. A benign and curable form of hemorrhagic nephritis. *J.A.M.A.* 86:1001, 1926.

7. Bates, R. C., Jennings, R. B., and Earle, D. P. Acute nephritis unrelated to group A hemolytic streptococcus infection: Report of ten cases. *Amer. J. Med.* 23:510, 1957.

8. Beirne, G. J., Octaviano, G. N., Kopp, W. L., and Burns, R. O. Immunohistology of the lung in Goodpasture's syndrome. *Ann. Intern. Med.* 69:1207, 1968.

9. Bell, E. T. Glomerular lesions associated with endocarditis. *Amer. J. Path.* 8:639, 1932.

10. Bell, E. T. *Renal Diseases* (2d ed.). Philadelphia: Lea & Febiger, 1950.

11. Benoit, F. L., Rulon, D. B., Theil, G. B., Doolan, P. D., and Watten, R. H. Goodpasture's syndrome: A clinicopathologic entity. *Amer. J. Med.* 37:424, 1964.

12. Berger, J., and de Montera, H. Les glomérulo-néphrites focales nécrotiques chroniques. *J. Urol. Nephrol.* (Paris) 70:122, 1964.

13. Bergstrand, A., Bergstrand, C. G., and Bucht, H. Kidney lesions associated with anaphylactoid purpura in children. *Acta Paediat.* 49:57, 1960.

14. Bodian, M., Black, J. A., Kobayashi, N., Lake, B. D., and Shuler, S. E. Recurrent haematuria in childhood. *Quart. J. Med.* 34:359, 1965.

15. Bouissou, H., Dupont, H.-G., and Régnier, Cl. L'atteinte rénale au cours du syndrome de Schönlein-Henoch. Étude clinique. Étude histologique par ponction biopsie du rein. *Arch. Franc. Pediat.* 16:890, 1959.

16. Christian, H. A. The kidneys in subacute streptococcus viridans endocarditis. *J. Mount Sinai Hosp. N.Y.* 8:427, 1941–1942.

17. Crosnier, J., Mery, J-Ph., de Montera, H., Zaltzman, S., and Rueff, B. Sur un syndrome associant une glomérulite segmentaire nécrotique et une pneumopathie hémoptoïque avec alvéolite hémorragique. *J. Urol. Nephrol.* (Paris) 68:569, 1962.

18. Daeschner, C. W., Jr., Dodge, W. F., Travis, L. B., and Hopps, H. C. Observations on the renal lesion of anaphylactoid purpura–nephritis. *Amer. J. Dis. Child.* 102:496, 1961.

19. Davson, J., Ball, J., and Platt, R. The kidney in periarteritis nodosa. *Quart. J. Med.* 17:175, 1948.

20. Davson, J., and Platt, R. A clinical and pathological study of renal disease: I. Nephritis. *Quart. J. Med.* 18:149, 1949.

21. Dixon, F. J. The pathogenesis of glomerulonephritis. *Amer. J. Med.* 44:493, 1968.

22. Duncan, D. A., Drummond, K. N., Michael, A. F., and Vernier, R. L. Pulmonary hemorrhage and glomerulonephritis: Report of six cases and study of the renal lesion by the fluorescent antibody technique and electron microscopy. *Ann. Intern. Med.* 62:920, 1965.

23. Earle, D. P., and Jennings, R. B. Glomerulonephritis. In Becker, E. L. (Ed.), *Proceedings Third International Congress of Nephrology.* Basel: Karger, 1967. P. 51.

24. Ellis, A. Natural history of Bright's disease: Clinical, histological and experimental observations. *Lancet* 1:1, 1942.

25. Falls, W. F., Jr., Ford, K. L., Ashworth, C. T., and Carter, N. W. Renal vasculitis in a nonfatal case of Henoch-Schönlein purpura. *Ann. Intern. Med.* 64:1276, 1966.

26. Ferris, T. F., Gorden, P., Kashgarian, M., and Epstein, F. H. Recurrent hematuria and focal nephritis. *New Eng. J. Med.* 276:770, 1967.

27. Fishberg, A. M. *Hypertension and Nephritis* (5th ed.). Philadelphia: Lea & Febiger, 1954.

28. Gairdner, D. Schönlein-Henoch syndrome (anaphylactoid purpura). *Quart. J. Med.* 17:95, 1948.

29. Germuth, F. G., Jr. Personal communication, 1969.

30. Germuth, F. G., Jr., Kelemen, W. A., and Pollack, A. D. Immune complex disease: II. The role of circulatory dynamics and glomerular filtration in the development of experimental glomerulonephritis. *Johns Hopkins Med. J.* 120:252, 1967.

31. Germuth, F. G., Jr., Valdes, A. J., Senterfit, L. B., and Pollack, A. D. A unique influence of cortisone on the transit of specific macromolecules across vascular walls in immune complex disease. *Johns Hopkins Med. J.* 122:137, 1968.

32. Goldman, R., Costa, C., Tinglof, B., and Wilkerson, J. Focal glomerulonephritis and the nephrotic syndrome. Presented as free communication at Third International Congress of Nephrology, Washington, D.C., 1966.

33. Guthrie, L. G. "Idiopathic" or congenital, hereditary and family haematuria. *Lancet* 1:1243, 1902.

34. Hamburger, J. Discussion. In Wolstenholme, G. E. W., and Cameron, M. P. (Eds.), *Ciba Foundation Symposium on*

Renal Biopsy. Boston: Little, Brown, 1961. P. 216.

35. Heptinstall, R. H. *Pathology of the Kidney.* Boston: Little, Brown, 1966.

36. Heptinstall, R. H., and Joekes, A. M. Focal glomerulonephritis: A study based on renal biopsies. *Quart. J. Med.* 28:329, 1959.

37. Heptinstall, R. H., and Joekes, A. M. Focal Glomerulonephritis. In Wolstenholme, G. E. W., and Cameron, M. P. (Eds.), *Ciba Foundation Symposium on Renal Biopsy.* Boston: Little, Brown, 1961. P. 194.

38. Johnson, J. R., and McGovern, V. J. Goodpasture's syndrome and Wegener's granulomatosis. *Aust. Ann. Med.* 11:250, 1962.

39. Jungmann, P. Ueber chronische Streptokokkeninfektionen. *Deutsch. Med. Wschr.* 50:71, 1924.

40. Kobayashi, O., Wada, H., Kanasawa, M., and Kamiyama, T. The anaphylactoid purpura-nephritis in childhood. *Acta Med. Biol.* (Niigata) 13:181, 1965.

41. Koffler, D., and Kunkel, H. G. Mechanisms of renal injury in systemic lupus erythematosus. *Amer. J. Med.* 45:165, 1968.

42. Kroe, D. J., and Pitcock, J. A. Goodpasture's syndrome: An immunofluorescent study of the pulmonary and renal lesions. *Southern Med. J.* 61:183, 1968.

43. Lange, K. Personal communication, 1969.

44. Lannigan, R., and Insley, J. Light and electron microscope appearances in renal biopsy material from cases of recurrent haematuria in children. *J. Clin. Path.* 18:178, 1965.

45. Lerner, R. A., Glassock, R. J., and Dixon, F. J. The role of antiglomerular basement membrane antibody in the pathogenesis of human glomerulonephritis. *J. Exp. Med.* 126:989, 1967.

46. Löhlein, M. Ueber hämorrhagische Nierenaffektionen bei chronischer ulzeröser Endokarditis. (Embolische nichteiterige Herdnephritis.) *Med. Klin. Berl.* 6:375, 1910.

47. Longcope, W. T. The susceptibility of man to foreign proteins. *Amer. J. Med. Sci.* 152:625, 1916.

48. McConville, J. M., West, C. D., and McAdams, A. J. Familial and nonfamilial benign hematuria. *J. Pediat.* 69:207, 1966.

49. Muehrcke, R. C., Kark, R. M., Pirani, C. L., and Pollak, V. E. Lupus nephritis: A clinical and pathologic study based on renal biopsies. *Medicine* (Balt.) 36:1, 1957.

50. Mulrow, P. J., Aron, A. M., Gathman, G. E., Yesner, R., and Lubs, H. A. Hereditary nephritis: Report of a kindred. *Amer. J. Med.* 35:737, 1963.

51. Opitz, J. Hereditary Hematuria. In Metcoff, J. (Ed.), *Hereditary, Developmental, and Immunologic Aspects of Kidney Disease.* Evanston, Ill.: Northwestern University Press for National Kidney Disease Foundation, 1962. P. 3.

52. Palmer, J. M., Eversole, S. L., and Stamey, T. A. Unilateral glomerulonephritis: Virtual absence of nephritis in a kidney with partial occlusion of the main renal artery. *Amer. J. Med.* 40:816, 1966.

53. Panner, B. Nephritis of Schönlein-Henoch syndrome: Electron microscopic study of the glomerular lesion in an adult. *Arch. Path.* (Chicago) 74:230, 1962.

54. Payne, W. W., and Illingworth, R. S. Acute nephritis in childhood, with special reference to the diagnosis of focal nephritis. *Quart. J. Med.* 9:37, 1940.

55. Perkoff, G. T., Nugent, C. A., Jr., Dolowitz, D. A., Stephens, F. E., Carnes, W. H., and Tyler, F. H. A follow-up study of hereditary chronic nephritis. *A.M.A. Arch. Intern. Med.* 102:733, 1958.

56. Perkoff, G. T., Stephens, F. E., Dolowitz, D. A., and Tyler, F. H. A clinical study of hereditary interstitial pyelonephritis. *A.M.A. Arch. Intern. Med.* 88:191, 1951.

57. Pryor, J. S., and Joekes, A. M. Recurrent Haematuria. In Vostál, J., and Richet, G. (Eds.), *Proceedings of the Second International Congress of Nephrology.* Amsterdam: Excerpta Med., 1964. P. 804.

58. Rapoport, A., Saiphoo, C., deVeber, G., Ranking, G. N., and McClean, C. R. Focal proliferative glomerulonephritis — a cause of hematuria. Presented at American Society of Nephrology Meeting, Los Angeles, 1967.

59. Régnier, Cl., and Bouissou, H. Apport de la microscopie électronique dans les néphropathies du syndrome de Schönlein-Hénoch. *Arch. Franc. Pediat.* 17:384, 1960.

60. Rich, A. R. A hitherto undescribed vulner-

ability of the juxtamedullary glomeruli in lipoid nephrosis. *Bull. Johns Hopkins Hosp.* 100:173, 1957.

61. Roberts, W. C., and Rabson, A. S. Focal glomerular lesions in fungal endocarditis. *Ann. Intern. Med.* 56:610, 1962.

62. Ross, J. H. Recurrent focal nephritis. *Quart. J. Med.* 29:391, 1960.

63. Rusby, N. L., and Wilson, C. Lung purpura with nephritis. *Quart. J. Med.* 29:501, 1960.

64. Sarre, H., and Wirtz, H. Geschwindigkeit und Ort der Antigen-Antikörper-Reaktion bei der experimentellen Nephritis. *Deutsch. Arch. Klin. Med.* 189:1, 1942.

65. Scheer, R. L., and Grossman, M. A. Immune aspects of the glomerulonephritis associated with pulmonary hemorrhage. *Ann. Intern. Med.* 60:1009, 1964.

66. Scheidemandel, E. Ueber die Bedeutung der bakteriologischen Harnuntersuchung für die Diagnose und Therapie (speziell der akuten Nephritis). *Munchen. Med. Wschr.* 60:1722, 1778, 1913.

67. Singer, D. B., Hill, L. L., Rosenberg, H. S., Marshall, J., and Swenson, R. Recurrent hematuria in childhood. *New Eng. J. Med.* 279:7, 1968.

68. Spear, G. S., Whitworth, J. M., and Konigsmark, B. W. Hereditary nephritis with nerve deafness: Immunofluorescent studies on the kidney. Presented at Fourth International Congress of Nephrology. Stockholm, 1969.

69. Sturgill, B. C., and Westervelt, F. B. Immunofluorescence studies in a case of Goodpasture's syndrome. *J.A.M.A.* 194:172, 1965.

70. Travis, L. B., Daeschner, C. W., Dodge, W. F., Hopps, H. C., and Rosenberg, H. S. "Idiopathic" hematuria. *J. Pediat.* 60:24, 1962.

71. Urizar, R. E., Michael, A., Sisson, S., and Vernier, R. L. Anaphylactoid purpura: II. Immunofluorescent and electron microscopic studies of the glomerular lesions. *Lab. Invest.* 19:437, 1968.

72. Vernier, R. L. Personal communication, 1969.

73. Vernier, R. L., Worthen, H. G., Peterson, R. D., Colle, E., and Good, R. A. Anaphylactoid purpura: I. Pathology of the skin and kidney and frequency of streptococcal infection. *Pediatrics* 27:181, 1961.

74. Volhard, F., and Fahr, T. *Die Brightsche Nierenkrankheit.* Berlin: Springer, 1914.

75. Walker, J. M., and Joekes, A. M. Survival after haemoptysis and nephritis. *Lancet* 2:1199, 1963.

76. Wedgwood, R. J. P., and Klaus, M. H. Anaphylactoid purpura (Schönlein-Henoch syndrome): Long-term follow up with special reference to renal involvement. *Pediatrics* 16:196, 1955.

77. Wegener, F. Über eine eigenartige rhinogene Granulomatose mit besonderer Beteiligung des Arteriensystems und der Nieren. *Beitr. Path. Anat.* 102:36, 1939.

78. West, C. D., McAdams, A. J., and Northway, J. D. Focal glomerulonephritis in children. *J. Pediat.* 73:184, 1968.

79. Whalen, R. E., Huang, S., Peschel, E., and McIntosh, H. D. Hereditary nephropathy, deafness and renal foam cells. *Amer. J. Med.* 31:171, 1961.

15

nical Aspects of Chronic Glomerulonephritis

Arnold S. Relman

concerned mainly with the
tural history of chronic glo-
n the eight years that have
first edition of this book,
s happened to change our
reas. There has been much
about the immunologic
esis, and advances continue
treatment of chronic renal
pics are discussed in other
lected, therefore, not to
rmat of this chapter and
a few new paragraphs

ne glomerulonephritis as
tity, for there are still
erstanding of the clinical
mena usually grouped
1. For the purposes of
define the subject rather

nonspecifically as a renal disease (or diseases)
characterized by morphologic and sometimes
functional evidence of primary and relatively
diffuse involvement of the glomeruli. Excluded from consideration are other, more or
less well-defined clinical and histologic entities
which may also primarily affect the glomeruli,
such as intercapillary glomerulosclerosis and
systemic lupus erythematosus.

In Chapter 13 on acute glomerulonephritis
the discussion was devoted mainly to what
appears to be a fairly specific disorder etiologically related in some way to beta-hemolytic streptococcal infection. The present
chapter deals with glomerulonephritis as a
subacute or chronic disease, the pathogenesis
of which is often uncertain and the classification difficult. As will be elaborated, there is
considerable doubt whether all such cases begin as acute poststreptococcal glomerulonephritis. Designations such as type 1 and type 2
nephritis, membranous nephritis, and lipoid
nephrosis are often used to suggest the possibly
diverse etiologies of the more chronic mani-

festations of glomerulonephritis. The following discussion includes all these types of renal disease and attempts to summarize such evidence as is relevant to the question of their interrelationship. However, no detailed consideration is given to so-called lipoid nephrosis or to the general subject of nephrotic syndrome, because these are treated at length in Chapter 16.

Incidence

It seems safe to say that subacute and chronic glomerulonephritis, as defined here, are second in frequency only to pyelonephritis as a cause of serious renal disease.* The autopsy records of the Massachusetts Memorial Hospitals during the interval 1950–1957 reveal an approximately 1 per cent incidence of subacute and chronic glomerulonephritis [41]. Similar estimates of frequency in autopsy material have been reported from widely separated places, the figure ranging from 0.5 to 1.5 per cent [7, 42, 53]. In the Boston City Hospital and in the Massachusetts Memorial Hospitals it was estimated from review of the clinical and autopsy records that in approximately three-quarters of the cases of glomerulonephritis the renal lesion contributed significantly to the cause of death [41, 42]. By contrast, the autopsy incidence of acute and chronic pyelonephritis at these two hospitals is approximately 10 to 20 per cent, but the pyelonephritic lesion was judged to be a major factor in causing death in only about one-third of these cases [41, 42]. As a cause of renal failure, therefore, pyelonephritis is probably several times more common than glomerulonephritis. For example, in a study of 147 deaths due to uremia in Copenhagen, Raaschou [45] found that 58 per cent were caused by chronic pyelonephritis and 23 per cent by glomerulonephritis, sub-

acute or chronic in the great ma stances.

My own clinical experience, w that chronic pyelonephritis is a three times as frequent as subacu glomerulonephritis, is in substan with the autopsy data just cit there are no definitive publishe relative clinical incidence of the of chronic renal disease. Comp ing from biased selection of m uncertainties involved in the terms and the application of dia would in any event make suc to interpret.

For unknown reasons, ma affected by glomeruloneph quently than females, most ing a male preponderance clinical as well as autopsy ex

Vital statistics from the U Great Britain seem to indi reduction in the death ra nephritis" from 1950 to 1964. significant rise in deaths fr the kidney" [31]. Althougl represent changing diagnc is reason to believe that ch phritis may well have dec perhaps because of advanc streptococcal infections. A the incidence of rheumatic same explanation.

Excluding those with majority of patients with glomerulonephritis first r after the age of 10. Table apparent onset in a comb of subacute and chroni seen from 1950–1961 by setts Memorial Hospital Schwartz at the New pital.† The data in the

---

* The most common renal *lesion* found at autopsy is benign nephrosclerosis, but this is of little or no clinical significance in the great majority of cases.

† I am indebted to Dr. W mission to include his case Dr. Jacob Lemann, Jr., ass

chronic glomerulonephritis could also be distinguished on histologic grounds. He stated that patients dying of type 1 subacute glomerulonephritis almost always are found to have considerable proliferation of endothelial and epithelial elements in the glomeruli and usually show a characteristic proliferation of the parietal epithelium of the capsule in the form of so-called crescents. In type 1 glomerulonephritis of longer duration, crescent formation is not as common, but the characteristic feature of endothelial and epithelial proliferation is still apparent; there is also a varying degree of fibrosis, contraction, and disappearance of glomeruli. In contrast to this description, the histologic findings in type 2 glomerulonephritis, according to Ellis, are chiefly characterized by lobulation of tufts, a minimal degree of proliferation, generalized thickening of basement membranes, and deposition of a hyalin-like material in intercapillary spaces. Glomeruli usually remain enlarged, and marked contraction of the kidney is unusual.

In the years since Ellis's contribution, there have been many clinical and pathologic studies attempting to classify chronic glomerulonephritis and to define the relationship of the latter to acute poststreptococcal nephritis [11–14, 19, 22, 26, 27, 34, 44, 48–50]. The weight of evidence supports Ellis's view that there is more than one pathogenetic mechanism responsible for chronic nephritis and that those cases due to poststreptococcal disease constitute only a part of the whole spectrum. Type-specific antibodies against nephritogenic streptococci are often absent in patients with chronic glomerulonephritis [50]. As these antibodies are usually detectable for months or years after known poststreptococcal acute glomerulonephritis, this finding suggests a nonstreptococcal etiology for many chronic cases. Careful prospective studies of acute poststreptococcal nephritis with serial biopsies have revealed that proliferation of endothelial and axial mesangial cells in the glomerulus appears to be the characteristic lesion

of this disease, at least during the acute and early chronic stages [28]. These histologic criteria are probably not completely specific, but if they are applied to biopsy material obtained from adults with chronic glomerulonephritis, it becomes apparent that many cases are not due to poststreptococcal disease [11, 26, 27, 34, 44].

Further support for the Ellis hypothesis is provided by a study of the incidence of the nephrotic syndrome in the two types of chronic nephritis. In the MMH-NECH series *none* of the 16 patients with known acute glomerulonephritis developed the nephrotic syndrome, whereas 47 of the remaining 92 patients went through a nephrotic phase. Although there is no doubt that a sustained nephrotic syndrome does occasionally occur in chronic poststreptococcal nephritis, the general experience has been that the great majority of cases of nephrotic syndrome due to chronic nephritis in adults occur in persons without past history or immunologic evidence of acute glomerulonephritis. Renal biopsies from large groups of patients with the nephrotic syndrome agree with this view, inasmuch as they demonstrate proliferative glomerular changes in no more than a third of cases [26, 34, 48].

On the other hand, the sharp morphologic distinction Ellis tried to draw is not supported by the new information available from kidney biopsies. It is the general experience that extensive capsular proliferation, with widespread crescent formation and necrosis of glomeruli, is almost always associated with an acute onset and a rapidly progressive or subacute course. Less extensive proliferation, especially that involving endothelium and mesangium, may or may not be associated with an acute onset. There is also agreement that most cases with minimal "membranous" changes, or with almost no glomerular abnormalities detectable by light microscopy, have an insidious onset and follow a course characteristic of type 2 nephritis. In between these extremes, however, there are many cases in which proliferative and "membranous" changes occur together. In some of these the clinical picture fits type 1 and in others type 2 [26, 27].

No discussion of the pathogenesis and classification of chronic glomerulonephritis would be complete without some consideration of so-called *lipoid nephrosis*. This disorder, as well as other causes of the *nephrotic syndrome,* is discussed in more detail in Chapter 16, but it is also necessary to mention it here, however briefly, because of its intimate relation to type 2 nephritis. As Ellis pointed out [21], lipoid nephrosis in childhood and type 2 nephritis in adults have many clinical features in common which seem to set them apart from type 1 nephritis. Both disorders begin insidiously, without relation to streptococcal or other respiratory infections. Proteinuria, hypoalbuminemia, and edema are relatively more marked, and microscopic hematuria less marked, in these two diseases than in acute or chronic type 1 nephritis. As noted previously, a true nephrotic syndrome is unusual in the chronic stages of type 1 nephritis.

Striking similarities between childhood nephrosis and type 2 nephritis in adults are also seen when the histologic lesions in each are compared. In both instances there may be a wide spectrum of lesions, ranging from barely perceptible changes in the basement membrane to the fully developed picture of so-called membranous nephritis, which includes a variable degree of endothelial proliferation. As already noted, some cases of type 1 and type 2 nephritis may be histologically indistinguishable, but both childhood nephrosis and type 2 nephritis in adults share the common feature of rarely showing the extensive degree of epithelial and capsular proliferation and adhesion characteristic of many of the cases of type 1 nephritis. In addition, extensive leukocytic infiltration and necrosis of glomeruli are almost never found in either childhood nephrosis or type 2 nephritis, although they are common in severe cases of type 1 nephritis.

Indeed, the only obvious and significant distinctions between childhood nephrosis and type 2 nephritis in adults seem to be the greater frequency of endothelial proliferation and thickened basement membranes early in the course of the latter disorder, and the correspondingly poorer prognosis in the adult disease. Childhood nephrosis heals spontaneously in roughly a third to a half of all cases [5, 6, 18], and it usually responds to treatment with adrenal steroids. While there are no definitive data on the frequency of spontaneous remission in all forms of the adult disease, approximately one-fifth of adults with nephrotic syndrome due to type 2 nephritis will ultimately heal spontaneously and another 10 or 20 per cent will respond well to steroid therapy [38]. That this difference in prognosis between children and adults with nephrotic syndrome may not be a sharp one is suggested by the data of Barnett and Eder [6], who point out that there appears to be a steady and progressively unfavorable change in prognosis with increasing age. Those children with nephrosis who do not heal develop signs of progressive renal damage and follow a course that is quite indistinguishable from the natural history of progressive type 2 nephritis in adults. Although follow-up studies of patients with lipoid nephrosis show that in most cases the minimal glomerular lesions in this disorder do not progress [44], there is clear evidence that occasionally progressive sclerosis and even proliferative changes may develop and lead to progressive renal insufficiency [25].

The similarities between childhood nephrosis and type 2 nephritis suggest a common etiology. This, in turn, supports the concept of at least two different types of chronic glomerulonephritis, for there are many reasons for believing that in children nephrosis is a pathologic entity distinct from poststreptococcal glomerulonephritis [5, 6, 16, 54]. However, in the absence of information about the fundamental nature of the underlying processes, none of the present arguments can be considered decisive.

The recent application of immunofluorescent staining technics to the study of renal biopsy material has led to renewed interest in the role of immune mechanisms and to an effort to classify clinical renal diseases on this basis [15, 16, 32]. In acute and chronic poststreptococcal glomerulonephritis, deposits of material are found along the subepithelial surface of the basement membrane, which stain for immunoglobulin G (IgG), complement, and fibrin. In acute cases, there is also some evidence that antigenic components of nephritogenic streptococci are also localized in these deposits [2]. This has led to the view that poststreptococcal glomerulonephritis is caused by the deposition of antigen-antibody complexes along the glomerular basement membrane [15]. In patients with the nephrotic syndrome who have minimal glomerular lesions there are usually no deposits of globulin to be found [16], but in those who have thickened basement membranes or proliferative changes, varying degrees and patterns of immunofluorescent staining may be observed [16, 32]. A similar variation in immune staining patterns has been found in patients with chronic glomerulonephritis of uncertain etiology [32]. The significance of these findings, and the nosological value of the immunofluorescent technic remain to be determined.

Symptoms and Signs

Chronic glomerulonephritis usually begins quietly and insidiously. It may first be discovered when a random or routine urinalysis leads to the chance disclosure of *proteinuria*. Not infrequently peripheral *edema* is the first manifestation; sometimes this is minimal in degree and only transient in duration. In other instances there may be progressive and fairly rapid development of a full-blown *nephrotic syndrome* with massive generalized edema. Approximately one-half of all patients with chronic glomerulonephritis develop the nephrotic syndrome sometime during the course of the disease. Thus, Bloom and Seegal [8] found that 27 of 50 consecutive autopsied cases had a nephrotic phase, while the nephrotic syndrome developed in 47 of the 108 patients in the MMH-NECH series even though many were still living and had been followed for only relatively short periods.

In some patients the presence of chronic glomerulonephritis is first discovered because of the development of *hypertension*. This sign appears sooner or later in the majority of cases, but usually not until renal insufficiency has become well established. In general, therefore, the presence of hypertension indicates a relatively advanced stage of the disease, although in a few instances blood pressure may be elevated relatively early, long before significant renal impairment is detectable. The hypertension may be of any degree of severity; 5 patients in the MMH-NECH series had papilledema or a diastolic pressure greater than 130 mm. Hg, or both.

Finally, there are occasional instances in which the patient is apparently totally oblivious of his disease until the final stages have been reached. In such cases weakness, anorexia or nausea, unusual pallor, fatigue, pruritus, hemorrhagic phenomena, or other symptoms and signs of *uremia* may be the first manifestations of the disease.

Laboratory Findings

The cardinal laboratory finding in chronic glomerulonephritis and the sine qua non for the diagnosis is *proteinuria*. In the latent stages of the disease the rate of protein excretion may be only slightly greater than normal and therefore its presence may be overlooked, particularly if the urine is dilute (see Chapter 3). In almost all adult cases, however, the 24-hour excretion of protein will exceed 100 mg. per day, even in the latent and relatively inactive stages of the disease. When the nephritis is more active, protein excretion is considerably higher, and in the nephrotic syndrome it may be as large as 20 or 30 gm. per day. It is a moot question whether truly intermittent proteinuria ever occurs in well-established chronic glomerulonephritis, but it is known that the severity of the proteinuria may vary considerably with activity and posture.

As emphasized by Addis [1], the excretion of red cells as well as of leukocytes and epithelial cells in the *urinary sediment* is always increased in chronic nephritis although the absolute and relative amounts of these elements may vary. In general, the degree of *hematuria* is a reflection of the activity of the inflammatory process in the glomeruli. Acute exacerbations are characterized by a marked increase in hematuria, which may even become gross. Large numbers of *leukocytes* and *renal epithelial cells* may also be a sign of the activity of the inflammatory process, but usually they are not as numerous as red blood cells. When proteinuria is severe, as in the nephrotic syndrome, the sediment also contains *oval fat bodies* (i.e., renal epithelial cells which have undergone fatty degeneration) as well as variable quantities of droplets and particles of fatty debris.

The number of *casts* in the sediment is almost always increased. *Hyaline* and *granular casts* are usually predominant, but the relative number as well as the nature of other types of casts will depend upon the stage, severity, and activity of the disease. *Red blood cell casts* usually mean active glomerulitis, and are particularly noticeable during acute exacerbations and in progressive subacute disease. They are frequently present during other phases, but they may be rare or absent during the latent stage. *Fatty casts* are particularly characteristic of the nephrotic syndrome, regardless of cause, and are found only when proteinuria is marked. Very broad, granular, or waxy casts (*renal failure casts*) are seen in large numbers in the end stages of nephritis, after renal insufficiency is well developed.

It cannot be too strongly emphasized that a careful qualitative examination of the urinary sediment will virtually always reveal abnormalities in patients with chronic glomerulonephritis, irrespective of stage or severity. Although the pattern of the formed elements in the sediment may not be of specific diagnostic value, it is of considerable help in establishing the presence of some type of renal disease, in the estimation of its severity and activity, and in providing useful clues to the nature of the disease.

A negative qualitative test for protein on a reasonably concentrated urine specimen (i.e., specific gravity greater than 1.020) and a normal sediment examination virtually rule out the possibility of chronic glomerulonephritis.

Many other laboratory abnormalities may also be found in patients with chronic glomerulonephritis, but these are the nonspecific results of renal failure or of hypertensive vascular disease, and therefore will not be detailed here. The clinical and laboratory features of uremia are discussed in Chapter 6.

Early in the course of chronic nephritis, specific physiologic measurements indicate that glomerular filtration rate is relatively more reduced than is tubular secretory capacity, but in the advanced stages this preponderance of glomerular damage disappears [20]. However, as is pointed out in Chapter 3 (see Fig. 3-13), the usual clinical tests of renal function fail to reveal any distinctive pattern. To follow the course of the renal damage, endogenous creatinine clearances are probably the most useful clinical measurement; this function appears to give an approximately accurate estimate of the severity of the histologic lesions [10]. Recent work [47] suggests that endogenous creatinine clearance, as well as the ability to concentrate and acidify the urine, is better correlated with the degree of tubular damage than with the extent of glomerular involvement.

Prognosis and Natural History

The extreme variability in the natural history of chronic glomerulonephritis makes accurate prognosis at the onset of the disease frequently impossible. There is a wide spectrum of possibilities. At one extreme are those patients with *subacute glomerulonephritis* whose disease remains continuously active from the start and who die of hypertension and uremia within six months to two years. At the other extreme are those more fortunate patients in whom the disease seems to remain indefinitely suspended in a latent or inactive stage. In such cases minimal proteinuria and cylindruria are the only manifestations of glomerulonephritis, and there may be no detectable progression of renal damage for periods of up to 30 or 40 years. Indeed, in some patients it is a moot question whether it would not be more accurate to say that the disease has healed, although leaving some minimal residual glomerular damage.

The average patient with type 1 chronic glomerulonephritis passes from the acute stage into a latent or inactive phase within the first few months of the illness. The latent phase lasts for a variable period of months to many years before the first definite signs of renal functional impairment appear. The disease then enters its final phase, characterized by progressively rapid deterioration of renal function and the appearance of hypertensive vascular disease. This phase usually lasts only a few years. At any time during the inactive or preterminal phases of the type 1 disease, *acute exacerbations* may occur (see below). In rare instances the nephrotic syndrome may appear, following which the disease may return to its latent stage or progress rapidly into the preterminal azotemic phase.

In type 2 nephritis there is usually no latent stage as such, since profuse proteinuria and edema are common even at the beginning, and signs of renal damage appear soon thereafter. In general, after a period of several years during which edema may be continuous or intermittent, progressive renal insufficiency ensues. In a significant minority of patients with type 2 nephritis, however, there is no gross edema and the phase of asymptomatic proteinuria slowly merges into a stage of progressive renal failure and hypertension.

As noted in Chapter 13, the initial severity of an attack of acute glomerulonephritis does not predict the subsequent course; on the other hand, the persistence of azotemia, hypertension, and edema beyond the first several weeks is an unfavorable sign, and indicates the likelihood of a progressive subacute course. Regardless of hypertension or evidence of functional impairment, if continuous proteinuria is still present at the end of a year, it is very probable that the disease has become chronic and will persist indefinitely. Nevertheless, occasional patients who have shown proteinuria for years will ultimately heal completely and lose all evidences of renal disease [1, 23, 30, 40]. Delayed healing of this sort never occurs, however, once sustained azotemia or hypertension has become established.

In the MMH-NECH series, as of 1961, 31 patients had been followed until death. The average known duration of their disease was approximately 7½ years, with a range of 1 to 38 years. All but five had died within 10 years of the first manifestation of their disease. On the other hand, of the 77 patients in the series still alive in 1961, 7 were known to have had their disease for more than 25 years.

Azotemia may develop within the first year or two, or it may be delayed for several decades, but once it appears it tends to increase progressively, and the outlook for survival becomes shortened. In the MMH-NECH series there were a few patients whose disease seemed to be remaining stationary over periods of two to nine years despite modest elevations of BUN or creatinine concentration. In general though, these values rise rapidly in the course of a few years, and the majority of patients do not survive more than five years after the blood nitrogen level has first become increased. Addis stated that 90 per cent of his patients who developed renal insufficiency died within six years of the initial onset of their disease, and none survived more than 12 years [1]. These gloomy statistics should not obscure the fact that it is not uncommon to see patients without renal insufficiency alive and well even after two or three decades.

Another serious prognostic sign is the appearance of sustained diastolic *hypertension*. In general, significant hypertension does not occur until after some degree of renal insufficiency has appeared. When hypertensive vascular disease is severe, the progress of the renal damage is undoubtedly accelerated. Patients with azotemia and papilledema or diastolic blood pressure levels above 120 mm. Hg have a particularly grave outlook and are usually near the terminal phase of their disease.

Severe persistent *edema* also carries a relatively poor prognosis, at least in adults. As already noted, the nephrotic syndrome usually occurs in the patients with type 2 nephritis whose disease has begun insidiously without known antecedent acute glomerulonephritis. In most instances the edematous phase remits before the development of advanced azotemia, although it is not unusual for azotemia to begin before the nephrotic phase has cleared. On the average, the nephrotic phase lasts about two years and rarely, if ever, recurs. Sometimes adults with the nephrotic syndrome will heal completely and apparently permanently, either spontaneously or under therapy with steroids (see Chapter 16). Such

remissions rarely occur after hypertension and azotemia have become established. These statements are not true of childhood nephrosis. Relapses following temporary remissions are quite common in children, and the permanent cure rate is substantially higher than in adults.

All of the above statements about survival apply to patients treated by conventional means. In recent years, the widespread application of chronic hemodialysis and renal homotransplantation has significantly prolonged the survival of patients beyond the point at which their own kidneys would have been able to support life.

ACUTE EXACERBATIONS

Acute exacerbations [51] are defined as sudden, usually transient, increases in the manifestations of glomerulonephritic activity, resembling an acute attack of glomerulonephritis. They are characterized by marked hematuria, increase in proteinuria and cylindruria, and often transient hypertension, edema and decrease in renal function. Such episodes occur only in a small percentage of patients with chronic glomerulonephritis, almost always among those with the type 1 disease, and may occur several times in the same patient. They seem to occur mainly in children. Exacerbations are usually preceded by an upper-respiratory-tract infection, the majority of which are due to group A hemolytic streptococci. The reduction in renal function which sometimes accompanies these episodes is usually transient, and there is no good evidence that they often contribute significantly to the ultimate progression of the disease. Occasionally, however, a progressive and rapidly fatal downhill course may be initiated by an exacerbation. The differential diagnosis between initial attacks of acute glomerulonephritis and acute exacerbations of chronic type 1 glomerulonephritis has been discussed in Chapter 13.

PREGNANCY

In the latent stage of chronic glomerulonephritis, when renal function and blood pressure are normal and proteinuria and cylindruria are the only manifestations of the disease, pregnancy does not appear to have any significant deleterious effect on the course of the disease [55]. Although there may be a slightly higher incidence of preeclampsia (as manifested by increased proteinuria, edema, and hypertension), fetal survival and long-term prognosis of the maternal disease do not seem to be affected [24, 29]. On the other hand, the hazards of pregnancy are significantly increased and fetal mortality is enhanced if the patient has moderate or marked hypertension at the time she becomes pregnant. Serious difficulties are the rule if any degree of azotemia is present.

Azotemic women with chronic glomerulonephritis are often infertile, but if they should become pregnant their renal disease is usually exacerbated, and a spontaneous abortion is to be expected. The more significant the azotemia, the poorer is the fetal prognosis [29]. For these reasons, pregnancy is strongly contraindicated in chronic glomerulonephritis once azotemia has appeared.

Differential Diagnosis

Persistent proteinuria and the finding of abnormal formed elements in the urinary sediment are the minimal criteria necessary to establish the possibility of chronic glomerulonephritis, but they cannot by themselves distinguish between glomerulonephritis and all the other diseases that may produce diffuse renal involvement and glomerular damage. Obviously, a clear-cut history of acute glomerulonephritis in the past is of great value in establishing the diagnosis. Renal biopsy, of course, usually can provide a definitive diagnosis of glomerulonephritis, provided that an adequate specimen of tissue is obtained.

However, an accurate differential diagnosis can be made without a biopsy in the great majority of cases if due consideration is given to history, physical examination, urine analysis, and a few of the commonly employed laboratory and x-ray studies. In the following paragraphs a few of these diagnostic points are discussed in relation to the renal diseases most likely to be confused with chronic glomerulonephritis.

ARTERIOLAR NEPHROSCLEROSIS

If it can be clearly established that proteinuria has *preceded* the onset of hypertension, the diagnosis of primary hypertensive disease of the kidney is unlikely. Conversely, a history of long-standing hypertension prior to any signs of renal damage is a strong argument against chronic glomerulonephritis and in favor of arteriolar nephrosclerosis. Generally the hypertensive vascular disease is relatively more severe than the renal impairment in nephrosclerosis, whereas in glomerulonephritis the renal impairment tends to outstrip the hypertensive vascular disease during most of the course of the illness. Except when hypertension is very severe or "malignant," nephrosclerosis usually causes minimal or only intermittent proteinuria. Persistent hematuria and the excretion of red-cell casts occur but rarely in benign nephrosclerosis. Occasionally in benign nephrosclerosis "renal epistaxis" occurs, due probably to rupture of a small vessel in the epithelial lining of the urinary tract. Under these circumstances transient gross or microscopic hematuria appears, but there are usually no red-cell casts.

Renal failure due to malignant nephrosclerosis can in most cases be distinguished from glomerulonephritis with secondary hypertensive disease if the following points are considered. Uremia usually develops fairly rapidly in malignant nephrosclerosis, but relatively slowly in chronic glomerulonephritis. Therefore, anemia, skin pigmentation, and malnutrition are more prominent in nephritis than in nephrosclerosis. For the same reason, bone disease is much more apt to occur in glomerulonephritis than in malignant nephrosclerosis. Contraction of the kidneys is also more common and more severe in glomerulonephritis, and when the renal shadows in an x-ray reveal both kidneys to be markedly reduced in size, this diagnosis is to be preferred. Finally, the urinary sediment often contains many red cells and red-cell casts in malignant nephrosclerosis; in terminal glomerulonephritis, on the other hand, the characteristic casts are the broad, waxy, and granular types, and hematuria is less prominent.

CHRONIC PYELONEPHRITIS

There are a number of characteristic features of this ubiquitous renal disease which serve to distinguish it from chronic glomerulonephritis. In contrast to glomerulonephritis, chronic pyelonephritis often causes hypertension without azotemia, or azotemia without hypertension; the first situation occurs in nonobstructive pyelonephritis, while the second is found usually in obstructive pyelonephritis. Pyelonephritis never, by itself, causes the nephrotic syndrome. Edema is uncommon, and when it occurs it is usually due to congestive heart failure or some other recognizable extrarenal mechanism.

One of the most reliable differential points is that pyelonephritis is often asymmetrical or even unilateral. Furthermore, pyelonephritis usually produces characteristic anatomic changes in the calyces, pelves, or ureters [9, 46]. Therefore, *pyelography* is of the greatest value in differentiating pyelonephritis from glomerulonephritis. Any difference in kidney size, or any abnormality in the visible collecting system, favors the diagnosis of pyelonephritis. X-ray evidence of stones or nephrocalcinosis also tends to indicate pyelonephritis

rather than glomerulonephritis, but it should be noted that a few instances of nephrocalcinosis (mainly cortical in distribution) have been observed in association with chronic glomerulonephritis [4].

Except in acute exacerbations, or when there is severe secondary hypertensive vascular disease, the formed elements of the urinary sediment in chronic pyelonephritis are relatively scanty. There is usually a perceptible increase in white blood cells on qualitative examination, but red cells and casts are few.* The few casts found in the sediment in uncomplicated pyelonephritis consist mainly of cellular and coarsely granular types; this is in sharp contrast to chronic glomerulonephritis, in which hyaline, finely granular, and sometimes waxy casts usually are more numerous. Another distinguishing feature of the urine is that proteinuria is scanty, intermittent, or sometimes even absent in chronic pyelonephritis, compared with the persistent and more marked proteinuria of glomerulonephritis. When severe secondary hypertensive disease is superimposed on chronic pyelonephritis many of these characteristics are altered, for now the urine may resemble that seen in malignant nephrosclerosis. Thus, proteinuria, hematuria, and cylindruria may become profuse, and virtually all sorts of casts will appear. In the terminal uremic stages of chronic pyelonephritis, broad, granular, and waxy casts occur, but in the absence of severe hypertensive vascular disease the sediment will usually still be distinguishable from that of advanced glomerulonephritis because of the relative increase in white cells and the scanty proteinuria.

Symptoms, signs, or bacteriologic evidence

---

* It should be borne in mind that there are occasional exceptions to this rule. Microscopic, and even gross, hematuria may occur in chronic pyelonephritis. This hematuria differs from that seen in active glomerulonephritis in that it is not accompanied by heavy proteinuria or the excretion of red-cell casts.

of active infection of the urinary tract, if present, are of course very important in recognizing pyelonephritis, but it must be remembered that active bacterial infection is often absent in chronic pyelonephritis [46].

Glomerular and tubular functional impairment generally advance together in chronic glomerulonephritis, but in pyelonephritis it is not unusual to find evidences of tubular defects without accompanying azotemia. Furthermore, since the pyelonephritic process primarily involves interstitium and tubules, these tubular defects are apt to be more severe in pyelonephritis than in glomerulonephritis. Therefore, hyperchloremic acidosis, severe salt-wasting defects, renal osteomalacia, and other primary tubular disorders occur in pyelonephritis but are rare in glomerulonephritis.

Finally, it is not uncommon to find pyelonephritis as a complication of glomerulonephritis. In the MMH-NECH series, histologically proved acute or chronic pyelonephritis was superimposed on the chronic glomerulonephritis in 23 per cent of the cases. One can only speculate on the factors responsible for this association, but whatever the cause, it should be obvious that the diagnoses of pyelonephritis and glomerulonephritis should not be considered as mutually exclusive.

"LIPOID NEPHROSIS"

As discussed under *Pathogenesis and Classification,* it is impossible to draw a clear distinction between this disorder and type 2 nephritis. Nevertheless, some would still wish to reserve the term *lipoid nephrosis* for those cases of nephrotic syndrome of insidious and apparently idiopathic onset in which the glomerular lesions are limited to changes in the epithelial foot processes revealed only by electron microscopy. Routine examination by light microscopy usually is normal. Hypertension, azotemia, and hematuria (considered in this view to be "nephritic" rather than

"nephrotic" manifestations) are minimal or absent.

LUPUS NEPHRITIS

Renal involvement in systemic lupus erythematosus may produce a clinical and histologic picture which closely resembles chronic glomerulonephritis [39]. Lupus nephritis often results in the nephrotic syndrome. Differentiation depends chiefly on the recognition of other manifestations of lupus, such as rash, arthritis, fever, leukopenia, and hypergammaglobulinemia. The demonstration of LE cells is of great help in the diagnosis. Sometimes renal biopsy will reveal focal "wire-loop" lesions in the glomeruli, but more often the findings are less specific, and indicative only of a diffuse membranoproliferative glomerulonephritis [39].

INTERCAPILLARY GLOMERULOSCLEROSIS

The renal manifestations of this disease are very much like those of type 2 nephritis. The clinical distinction depends chiefly on the presence of diabetes mellitus and the characteristic microaneurysms and punctate hemorrhages in the fundi. It is a fairly safe assumption that any diabetic patient with the nephrotic syndrome has intercapillary glomerulosclerosis, but it must be remembered that diabetic patients are not immune to glomerulonephritis or to any of the other causes of heavy proteinuria. I have seen several cases of the nephrotic syndrome in young diabetic patients which proved on biopsy to be due to chronic membranous glomerulonephritis rather than to diabetic nephropathy.

AMYLOID KIDNEY

Primary systemic amyloidosis involving the kidney, as well as secondary amyloidosis, can produce a clinical syndrome of microscopic hematuria, proteinuria, and cylindruria, often associated with hypertension and progressive renal insufficiency which may at times be confused with chronic glomerulonephritis. Sometimes renal insufficiency progresses without the development of hypertension until the terminal stages of the disease, and this characteristic should suggest the possibility of amyloidosis. With the primary type, renal disease may be the only clinical manifestation of the amyloidosis, but often the systemic nature of the disease is revealed by the involvement of skeletal or cardiac muscle or by the development of macroglossia. In the secondary type, renal involvement almost always is associated with hepatomegaly or splenomegaly and the clinical picture may be overshadowed by the primary inciting disease. With either type of amyloidosis, hyperglobulinemia will often suggest the diagnosis. When amyloid is due to multiple myeloma, the presence of myeloma cells in the bone marrow, severe anemia, and the characteristic myeloma protein in the plasma or urine are of diagnostic value. In the last analysis, however, many cases of amyloidosis of the kidney cannot be diagnosed antemortem without the aid of renal biopsy.

PERIARTERITIS NODOSA AND
DIFFUSE VASCULITIS

Occasionally renal involvement in these diseases will result in a clinical picture almost indistinguishable from a subacute or chronic active glomerulonephritis. The differential diagnosis depends mainly on the evidences of extrarenal disease and sometimes may be aided by the finding of leukocytosis, eosinophilia, or anemia out of proportion to the severity of the azotemia. The renal lesions may be indistinguishable from those of acute or subacute proliferative glomerulonephritis, and renal biopsy is often less helpful than is biopsy of the skin and muscle.

BENIGN PROTEINURIA

Occasionally the finding of proteinuria, and sometimes hematuria and cylindruria, in patients who have postural or other functional causes will lead to the erroneous diagnosis of chronic nephritis. The diagnosis and significance of postural and other types of benign proteinuria have been discussed in detail in Chapter 3. Suffice it to say here that proteinuria in established chronic glomerulonephritis, although it may vary considerably in severity under the influence of position, activity, and many other physiologic factors, is almost always a continuous phenomenon. The demonstration of truly intermittent proteinuria, therefore, makes chronic glomerulonephritis unlikely, but it does not rule out many other types of renal disease. Intermittency of protein excretion may occur as a phase in the healing of acute glomerulonephritis, but it may also be the prelude to persistent proteinuria and the development of various types of chronic progressive renal disease. The prudent physician will consequently reserve final judgment about intermittent proteinuria until he has had adequate opportunity to follow such cases over a prolonged period.

Treatment

There is no known therapy that will significantly change the natural history of chronic glomerulonephritis once it has developed. Rational approaches to treatment are restricted to relieving symptoms, preventing complications, and thereby attempting to prolong life. The management of the nephrotic syndrome in chronic glomerulonephritis is not fundamentally different from its management (see Chapter 16) in any other renal disorder. Similarly, there is nothing unique about the uremic syndrome as it occurs in chronic glomerulonephritis. (See Chapter 6 for the treatment of this syndrome with all its manifold complications, including hypertension.) The following comments refer, therefore, chiefly to the latent and inactive stages of chronic glomerulonephritis.

There is no rational basis for restricting *activity* in the inactive phase of the disease as long as the patient feels able to carry on.

However, in view of the fact that intense physical exertion is known to produce transient renal ischemia as well as hematuria, proteinuria, and cylindruria, it seems wise to advise patients to avoid such activity.

Addis [1] and his students contended that moderate restriction of protein in the *diet* was beneficial because it reduced the "work" of the kidney in the excretion of urea. This concept has fallen out of favor in recent years, and most students of renal disease would agree that no special dietary restrictions of any sort are indicated in the latent, uncomplicated stage of glomerulonephritis. At the present time most physiologists would doubt the existence of any simple, direct relation between protein intake and the chemical work of the kidney. It has been shown that the oxygen consumption of the kidney is closely related to the rate of sodium transport [33], which would indicate that the latter function is far more important in determining renal "work" than is the excretion of urea. Regardless of theoretical considerations, however, there is no convincing evidence that a normal, unrestricted protein intake has any deleterious effect on the kidney. Much more harm is likely to be done by too rigid insistence on dietary restrictions. When edema, hypertension, congestive heart failure, or uremia appears, the manipulation of diet may be of value. This is discussed in Chapters 6 and 16.

Because of the known relation between streptococcal infections and acute exacerbations of type 1 nephritis, some students of the disease advocate routine prophylactic use of *penicillin*. Such therapy is undoubtedly of value in reducing the incidence of streptococcal infections, but its effect on the underlying chronic nephritic process is entirely unknown. Since the disease appears to progress in the great majority of cases without acute exacerbations and without any evidence of continuing or recurrent respiratory infection, the value of routine prophylactic antibacterial treatment is dubious. It is my current practice to restrict the use of such therapy to those few patients with chronic nephritis who have had a past history of recurrent streptococcal infections or who seem to be particularly prone to upper-respiratory-tract disease.

Adrenal steroids have been used in the treatment of the nephrotic syndrome in chronic nephritis; this is discussed in Chapter 16. There is no evidence that these agents have any favorable effect on the course of chronic nephritis *without* the nephrotic syndrome, and the numerous complications that may attend their use make such treatment of dubious value [3]. Recent evidence suggesting that immune processes are involved in the pathogenesis of chronic glomerulonephritis [15], and the availability of new agents that inhibit cell-mediated immune responses, have led to increased interest in the possible value of *immunosuppressive therapy*. Several investigators have treated relatively small groups of patients with a combination of an adrenal steroid (usually prednisone) and an immunosuppressive drug such as azathioprine or mercaptopurine. Although there have been some encouraging results in individual cases, there is as yet no solid basis on which to draw definite conclusions about this type of therapy [37, 52]. Carefully controlled studies will be required to determine whether the risks attending the inevitable suppression of bone marrow that is produced by these drugs are justified by their long-term therapeutic effects.

Appendix

THE "MMH-NECH SERIES"

This group of 108 patients with subacute or chronic glomerulonephritis was selected from the records of the Renal Clinics of the Massachusetts Memorial Hospitals or the Pratt Clinic–New England Center Hospital on the basis of the following criteria:

Histologic Diagnosis (48 patients). In 24

cases the diagnosis was made from renal biopsy, and in 24 from autopsy.

Clinical Diagnosis. All patients in the series had persistent proteinuria and cylindruria for at least one year. In addition, they had at least one of the following criteria: (1) definite clinical history of acute glomerulonephritis; (2) nephrotic syndrome at some time in the course, with adequate clinical evidence to exclude intercapillary glomerulosclerosis and systemic lupus erythematosus; (3) red blood cell casts in the urinary sediment, without evidence of any other diffuse vascular disease which might have produced a glomerulitis.

There were 63 males (58 per cent) and 45 females (42 per cent). Thirty-one patients had already died; the other 77 were still being followed at the time these observations were completed in 1961.

References

1. Addis, T. *Glomerular Nephritis. Diagnosis and Treatment.* New York: Macmillan, 1948.
2. Andres, G. A., Accinni, L., Hsu, K. C., Zabriskie, J. B., and Seegal, B. C. Electron microscopic studies of human glomerulonephritis with ferritin-conjugated antibody: Localization of antigen-antibody complexes in glomerular structures of patients with acute glomerulonephritis. *J. Exp. Med.* 123: 399, 1966.
3. Armstrong, S. H., Jr., and Kushner, D. S. Current status of steroid therapy in chronic glomerulonephritis in the adult. *Amer. J. Med.* 29:377, 1960.
4. Arons, W. L., Christensen, W. R., and Sosman, M. C. Nephrocalcinosis visible by x-ray associated with chronic glomerulonephritis. *Ann. Intern. Med.* 42:260, 1955.
5. Barness, L. A., Moll, G. H., and Janeway, C. A. Nephrotic syndrome: I. Natural history of the disease. *Pediatrics* 5:486, 1950.
6. Barnett, H. L., and Eder, H. A. The nephrotic syndrome. *J. Chron. Dis.* 5:108, 1957.
7. Bell, E. T. *Renal Disease* (2d ed.). Philadelphia: Lea & Febiger, 1950.
8. Bloom, W. L., and Seegal, D. The nephrotic phase: Its frequency of occurrence and its differential diagnostic value in determining the nature of the renal lesion in 120 patients who died of renal failure. *Ann. Intern. Med.* 25:15, 1946.
9. Brod, J. Chronic pyelonephritis. *Lancet* 1: 973, 1956.
10. Brod, J., and Benesova, D. A comparative study of functional and morphological renal changes in glomerulonephritis. *Acta Med. Scand.* 157:23, 1957.
11. Chase, W. H., and Price, J. D. E. Glomerulonephritis: A review based on 52 renal biopsies. *Canad. Med. Ass. J.* 94:105, 1966.
12. Churg, J., Grishman, E., Goldstein, M. H., Yunis, S. L., and Porush, J. G. Idiopathic nephrotic syndrome in adults: A study and classification based on renal biopsies. *New Eng. J. Med.* 272:165, 1965.
13. Clark, N. S. Nephritis in childhood: A clinical assessment of the Ellis classification. *Arch. Dis. Child.* 31:12, 1956.
14. Davson, J., and Platt, R. A clinical and pathological study of renal disease: I. Nephritis. *Quart. J. Med.* 18:149, 1949.
15. Dixon, F. J. The pathogenesis of glomerulonephritis (Editorial). *Amer. J. Med.* 44:493, 1968.
16. Drummond, K. N., Michael, A. F., Good, R. A., and Vernier, R. L. The nephrotic syndrome of childhood: Immunologic, clinical and pathologic correlations. *J. Clin. Invest.* 45:620, 1966.
17. Eales, L. The nephrotic syndrome: Aetiological considerations. *South African J. Lab. Clin. Med.* 1:135, 1955.
18. Eales, L. Resolution of the nephrotic syndrome. *South African J. Lab. Clin. Med.* 2: 179, 1956.
19. Earle, D. P., Jr., and Jennings, R. B. Studies on poststreptococcal nephritis and other glomerular diseases. *Ann. Intern. Med.* 51:851, 1959.
20. Earle, D. P., Jr., Taggart, J. V., and Shannon,

J. A. Glomerulonephritis: A survey of the functional organization of the kidney in various stages of diffuse glomerulonephritis. *J. Clin. Invest.* 23:119, 1944.

21. Ellis, A. Natural history of Bright's disease: Clinical, histological and experimental observations. *Lancet* 1:72, 1942.

22. Enticknap, J. B., and Joiner, C. L. Bright's disease: An attempt at a statistical assessment of the classification proposed by Ellis. *Brit. Med. J.* 1:1016, 1953.

23. Fishberg, A. M. *Hypertension and Nephritis* (5th ed.). Philadelphia: Lea & Febiger, 1954.

24. Hamilton, H. F. H. Nephritis in pregnancy: A follow-up study. *J. Obstet. Gynaec. Brit. Emp.* 59:25, 1952.

25. Hayslett, J. P., Krassner, L. S., Bensch, K. G., Kashgarian, M., and Epstein, F. H. Progression of "lipoid nephrosis" to renal insufficiency. *New Eng. J. Med.* 281:181, 1969.

26. Heptinstall, R. H. *Pathology of the Kidney.* Boston: Little, Brown, 1966.

27. Hutt, M. S. R., and Sommers, S. C. A clinicopathologic analysis of biopsy specimens in persistent glomerulonephritis. *Amer. J. Path.* 43:459, 1963.

28. Jennings, R. B., and Earle, D. P. Post-streptococcal glomerulonephritis: Histopathologic and clinical studies of the acute, subsiding acute and early chronic latent phases. *J. Clin. Invest.* 40:1525, 1961.

29. Kaplan, A. L., Smith, J. P., and Tillman, A. J. B. Healed acute and chronic nephritis in pregnancy. *Amer. J. Obstet. Gynec.* 83:1519, 1962.

30. Keith, N. M., and Odel, H. M. Outlook for patients with glomerulonephritis. *J.A.M.A.* 153:1240, 1953.

31. Kessner, D. M., and Florey, C. Du V. Mortality trends for acute and chronic nephritis and infections of the kidney. *Lancet* 2:979, 1967.

32. Lange, K., Treser, G., Sagel, I., Ty, A., and Wasserman, E. Routine immunohistology in renal diseases. *Ann. Intern. Med.* 64:25, 1966.

33. Lassen, U. V., and Thaysen, J. H. Correlation between sodium transport and oxygen consumption in isolated renal tissue. *Biochim. Biophys. Acta* 47:616, 1961.

34. Lawrence, J. R., Pollak, V. E., Pirani, C. L., Kark, R. M. Histologic and clinical evidence of post-streptococcal glomerulonephritis in patients with the nephrotic syndrome. *Medicine* 42:1, 1963.

35. Longcope, W. T. The pathogenesis of glomerular nephritis. *Bull. Johns Hopkins Hosp.* 45:335, 1929.

36. Longcope, W. T. Some observations on the course and outcome of hemorrhagic nephritis. *New Int. Clin.* 1:1, 1938.

37. Michael, A. F., Vernier, R. L., Drummond, K. N., Levitt, J. I., Herdman, R. C., Fish, A. J., and Good, R. A. Immunosuppressive therapy of chronic renal disease. *New Eng. J. Med.* 276:817, 1967.

38. Miller, R. B., Harrington, J. T., Ramos, C. P., Relman, A. S., and Schwartz, W. B. Long-term results of steroid therapy in adults with idiopathic nephrotic syndrome. *Amer. J. Med.* 46:919, 1969.

39. Muehrcke, R. C., Kark, R. M., Pirani, C. L., and Pollak, V. E. *Lupus Nephritis.* Baltimore: Williams & Wilkins, 1957.

40. Murphy, F. D., and Schulz, E. G. Natural history of glomerular nephritis: A report of patients treated from ten to twenty-five years after the acute stage. *A.M.A. Arch. Intern. Med.* 98: 783, 1956.

41. Nesson, H. R., and Relman, A. S. Unpublished observations.

42. Nesson, H. R., and Robbins, S. L. Glomerulonephritis in older age groups. *Arch. Intern. Med.* (Chicago) 105:23, 1960.

43. Perlman, L. V., Herdman, R. C., Kleinman, H., and Vernier, R. L. Poststreptococcal glomerulonephritis: A ten-year follow-up of an epidemic. *J.A.M.A.* 194:175, 1965.

44. Pollak, V. E., Rosen, S., Pirani, C. L., Muehrcke, R. C., and Kark, R. M. Natural history of lipoid nephrosis and of membranous glomerulonephritis. *Ann. Intern. Med.* 69:1171, 1968.

45. Raaschou, R. *Studies of Chronic Pyelonephritis.* Copenhagen: Ejnar Munksgaard, 1948.

46. Relman, A. S. Some Clinical Aspects of Chronic Pyelonephritis. In Quinn, E. L., and

Kass, E. H. (Eds.), *Biology of Pyelonephritis*. (Henry Ford Hospital International Symposium.) Boston: Little, Brown, 1960. Chap. 25.

47. Ridson, R. A., Sloper, J. C., and de Wardener, H. E. Relationship between renal function and histological changes found in renal-biopsy specimens from patients with persistent glomerular nephritis. *Lancet* 2:7564, 1968.

48. Robson, J. S. The Nephrotic Syndrome. In Black, D. A. K. (Ed.), *Renal Disease* (2d ed.). Philadelphia: F. A. Davis, 1967. Chap. 11.

49. Roscoe, M. H. Biochemical and haematological changes in type 1 and type 2 nephritis. *Quart. J. Med.* 19:161, 1950.

50. Schmidt, W. C., and Rammelkamp, C. H., Jr. Etiology and pathogenesis of glomerulonephritis. *Advances Intern. Med.* 9:181, 1958.

51. Seegal, D., Lyttle, J. D., Loeb, E. N., Jost, E. L., and Davis, G. On the exacerbation in chronic glomerulonephritis. *J. Clin. Invest.* 19:569, 1940.

52. Urizar, R. E., Tinglof, B., McIntosh, R., Litman, N., Barnett, E., Wilkerson, J., Smith, F., Jr., and Vernier, R. L. Immunosuppressive therapy of proliferative glomerulonephritis in children. *Amer. J. Dis. Child.* 118:411, 1969.

53. Uys, C. J. The pathology of renal disease in the Bantu on the Witwatersrand: Glomerulonephritis. *South African J. Lab. Clin. Med.* 2:232, 1956.

54. Vernier, R. L., Farquhar, M. G., Brunson, J. G., and Good, R. A. Chronic renal disease in children: Correlation of clinical findings with morphologic characteristics seen by light and electron microscopy. *A.M.A. J. Dis. Child.* 96:306, 1958.

55. Werko, L., and Bucht, H. Glomerular filtration rate and renal blood flow in patients with chronic diffuse glomerulonephritis during pregnancy. *Acta Med. Scand.* 153:177, 1956.

16

The Nephrotic Syndrome

George E. Schreiner

Definition

The nephrotic syndrome has been classically defined as a clinical entity characterized by massive proteinuria, edema, hypoproteinemia, lipidemia, and lipiduria. Nephrosis has not, in recent years, been regarded as a disease in itself, since it may have multiple causes and may occur as a complication of well-defined morbid disorders. In addition, the diagnostician has had to face the perplexing fact that most of the "cardinal features" of the nephrotic syndrome are secondary rather than essential to the pathologic process. Edema results from interplay of renal, hormonal, dietary, and hemodynamic factors. Hypoproteinemia is the resultant of absorption, renal and gastrointestinal loss, and hepatic synthesis. Continued experience in treating patients with the nephrotic syndrome has impressed me with the variability of these cardinal features and has led me to prefer the following description:

The nephrotic syndrome is a clinical entity having multiple causes and characterized by increased glomerular membrane permeability that is manifested in massive proteinuria and

the excretion of fat bodies. There is a variable tendency toward edema, hypoproteinemia, and hyperlipemia. Protein excretion rates are usually in excess of 3.5 gm. per 24 hours per 1.73 square meters of body surface area in the *absence* of *depressed* glomerular filtration rates.

The present review includes data from 183 patients with the nephrotic syndrome thus defined, who were studied in the Renal and Electrolyte Division (now Division of Nephrology) of Georgetown University Hospital between 1952 and 1960. Of these patients, 92 were male, 68 Caucasian.

Etiology

In the past two decades concepts of the nephrotic syndrome have been enormously broadened by the realization that it can be produced by a wide variety of inciting agents and seen as part of the clinical spectrum in a number of systemic diseases [56, 345, 682]. A reasonable classification of the causes of the nephrotic syndrome is presented in the following list.

Causes of the Nephrotic
Syndrome

1. Glomerular disease
   Minimal change
   Idiopathic membranous [151, 345]
   Proliferative — acute
              — subacute
              — chronic
   Lobular [593]
2. Metabolic diseases
   Diffuse and nodular diabetic glomeru-
      losclerosis [210, 386, 534, 544, 564, 565]
   Amyloidosis [97, 107, 209, 412, 479, 511,
      512, 578, 618, 718]
   Multiple myeloma [640]
   Myxedema [236]
3. Systemic diseases [453]
   a. Collagen vascular disease
      Systemic lupus erythematosus [50,
         75, 88, 137, 305, 333, 450, 469, 626]
      Periarteritis [591]
      Goodpasture's syndrome [67]
      Dermatomyositis
      Central pontine myelinolysis [426]
      Takayasu disease (Table 16-1)
      Erythema multiforme
   b. Malignant diseases
      Hodgkin's disease [79, 448]
      Lymphocytic leukemia [79]
      Adult carcinomas [98, 336, 401,
         491]
4. Circulatory diseases
   Sickle cell anemia [56, 57, 162]
   Spherocytosis [436]
   Renal artery stenosis [517]
   Renal vein thrombosis [15, 26, 40, 65, 85,
      110, 111, 122, 124, 130, 150, 180, 181,
      190, 247, 297, 327, 344, 411, 456, 465,
      507, 524, 575, 650, 671]
   Pulmonary artery thrombosis [407, 455,
      657, 681]
   Inferior vena cava stenosis or thrombo-
      sis [222, 402]
   Constrictive pericarditis [65, 518]
   Congestive heart failure [298, 516, 640]

Tricuspid valvular insufficiency [345]
Pheochromocytoma [558]
5. Nephrotoxins
   Organic mercurial diuretics [90, 108,
      125, 480, 543, 598]
   Ammoniated mercury ointment [48,
      620, 673]
   Inorganic mercury [37, 86, 710]
   Bismuth [47]
   Gold [80, 675, 695]
6. Allergens and drugs
   Pollen [260]
   Bee stings [345, 584]
   Poison oak, poison ivy, and "purified"
      rhus toxin [583]
   Trimethadione and paramethadione
      [33, 185, 284, 286, 303, 483, 570, 662,
      703, 722]
   Insect repellents [302]
   Snake bites [12, 645]
   Probenecid [602, 628]
   Penicillamine [183, 323, 346, 606, 646]
   Miscellaneous allergens and serum ther-
      apy, e.g., wool, "cold pills," globulin,
      and poliomyelitis vaccine
7. Diseases due to infection
   Cytomegalic inclusion disease [721]
   Syphilis [36, 164, 304, 471]
   Malaria [10, 53, 328, 362–365]
   Typhus
   Chronic jejunoileitis [354]
   Tuberculosis [72, 388]
   Subacute bacterial endocarditis [345]
   Herpes zoster
   Miscellaneous bacteremia [63, 649, 672]
8. Congenital nephrotic syndrome [253, 358]
9. Hereditofamilial nephritis [147, 173, 208,
   215, 246, 252, 359, 516, 679, 680]
10. Miscellaneous causes
   Pregnancy [197, 278, 281, 525, 529, 608]
   Transplantation [267, 380, 462]
   Cyclic recurrence [585]
   Intestinal lymphangiectasia [128]

   The cause, as inferred from the clinical history of the patient, does not always correlate

exactly with the histologic classifications, as shown in Table 16-1. Nephrotic syndromes that bear a temporal relationship to streptococcal infections account for the widest variety of glomerular lesions. In some patients with minimal-change disease and deposits of antigen-antibody complexes within the basement membrane, such as occurs in lupus erythema-

Table 16-1. Summary of the Clinical History and the Interpretation of the Histologic Characteristics in 183 Patients with the Nephrotic Syndrome[a]

Clinical History	Acute Glomerulonephritis	Subacute Glomerulonephritis	Chronic Glomerulonephritis	Membranous Glomerulonephritis	Diabetic Glomerulosclerosis	Amyloidosis	Unknown	Total
β streptococcus	9	5	14	8	0	0	0	36
Diabetes mellitus			1	2	34			37
Collagen-vascular								
Lupus erythematosus			11					11
Other				1				1
Pregnancy				4				4
Nephrotoxins								
Mercury				1				1
Ammoniated mercury				1				1
Paint remover containing mercury				1				1
Hydroquinone				1				1
Intramuscular gold salts				1				1
Nephroallergens								
Herpes zoster				1				1
Insect bite				1				1
"Cold pill"				1				1
"Cold shot"				1				1
Rhus				1				1
Suppurative disease								
Chronic ulcerative colitis						1		1
Hodgkin's disease						1		1
Tuberculosis						1		1
Miscellaneous								
Varicella				1				1
Poliomyelitis vaccine				1				1
Sickle cell disease				2				2
Gamma globulin	1							1
Takayasu syndrome							1	1
Unknown	8	4	28	31	0	3	1	75
Totals	18	9	54	60	34	6	2	183

[a] The vertical listing represents the clinical setting in which the disease developed. The horizontal headings represent the diagnostic interpretations, which were based on biopsy, autopsy, or unequivocal clinical course.

tosus, the histologic picture on light microscopy may appear to be perfectly normal, and
lesions can be demonstrated only by the newer
electron microscopic or immunofluorescent
methods.

The general relationships between onset of
the nephrotic syndrome due to specific causes
and the age of the patient are shown in Figure
16-1. The nephrotic syndrome occurs in the
early stages of infancy, all the way through to
the very elderly. I have seen several patients in
their seventies, and one at age 92 was recently
reported [192]. In our own clinical experience,
acute glomerulonephritis was seen predominantly in persons under 45 years of age, chronic
proliferative and idiopathic membranous glomerulonephritis extended through all age
groups, systemic lupus erythematosus was
largely a disease of young females, while diffuse diabetic glomerulosclerosis and amyloidosis were seen in the middle and older age
groups. The nephrotic syndrome has been reported in premature neonates [147]. Parker

and Piel [516] reported data concerning five
nephrotic infants under the age of seven
months. Worthen et al. [721] had 12 patients
under one year of age, and there are other reports of an infantile type of nephrotic syndrome [215, 241, 246, 437]. In the neonatal or
congenital forms of nephrotic syndrome, the
prognosis appears to be particularly guarded.
Perhaps for this reason it is rare to have a patient with childhood nephrosis or nephritis develop a second acute disease in later childhood
or adult life, but this has occasionally been reported in the nephrotic syndrome due to allergens and in the classic cyclic nephrotic syndrome, as well as rarely in glomerulonephritis
[25].

Perhaps the most confusing aspect of discussions on the nephrotic syndrome is the tendency to combine clinical and pathologic
terms. If this admixing is done on the basis of
biopsy experience, the presentations may be
reasonably accurate. But there is reason to
assume that the diagnosis in most of the pub-

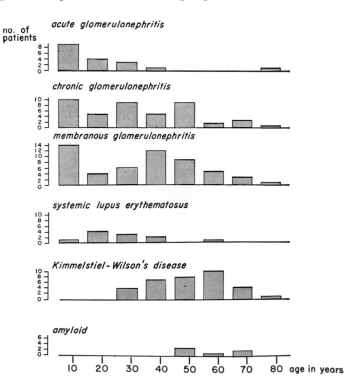

Figure 16-1. Age at onset in relation to the specific nature of the
nephrotic syndrome.

lished series to date was based on some clinical prejudice (e.g., protein and red cells equal glomerulonephritis, acute or subacute; protein and no red cells equal membranous glomerulonephritis). We have found these clinical methods to be reliable in about two-thirds of the cases, and believe that tabulations based on them should be approached with skepticism.

In Table 16-2 are summarized our final diagnoses in 183 patients. The 111 in the first column are histologically proved, and hence quite reliable. The 72 in the second column were classified according to the best of clinical criteria but are still suspect. The diagnosis in patients with lupus erythematosus and diabetes mellitus is apt to be fairly accurate. It can be seen that the classic forms of proliferative glomerulonephritis are a common cause of the nephrotic syndrome.

Table 16-2. Final Diagnoses in 183 Patients with the Nephrotic Syndrome[a]

Diagnosis	Histologically Proved	Not Histologically Proved	Total
Acute glomerulo-nephritis	7	11	18
Subacute glomerulo-nephritis	3	6	9
Chronic glomerulo-nephritis	26	18	44
Membranous glomerulonephritis	41	19	60
Amyloidosis	6	0	6
Diabetic glomerulo-sclerosis	19	15	34
Systemic lupus erythematosus	8	3	11
Takayasu syndrome	1	0	1
Totals	111	72	183

[a] Diagnoses not histologically proved were based on typical clinical course, studies of renal function, urinary sediment, etc., but are still subject to doubt. Proliferative glomerulonephritis appears to be a frequent cause of the nephrotic syndrome.

Nature of the Lesion

Volhard and Fahr [683], in 1914, linked clinical nephrotic syndrome to primary degenerative tubular disease without notable changes in the glomerulus. With a gradual return to emphasis on the primacy of glomerular rather than tubular lesions, the very survival of the term *nephrosis* has raised an etymologic storm. The resulting proliferation of terminology must leave the nonrenal scholar wondering how we communicate. The nomenclature in this chapter may appear arbitrary — and is — but we have found that it is also intelligible.

GROSS PATHOLOGY

The kidneys in the nephrotic syndrome are classically larger than normal and have a swollen appearance, both on radiographic and gross examination. The internal swelling may be reflected radiographically by a narrowing of the infundibula (Fig. 16-2). A smooth, pale-yellow surface is characteristic of the "pure" type. On cut sections, yellow cortices stand in relief from pale pyramids. Hemorrhagic glomeruli are seen only in the mixed type.

MICROSCOPIC PATHOLOGY

The filtering unit of the kidney, the glomerulus, is composed of an incoming or afferent arteriole, an outgoing or efferent arteriole, and coils of specialized capillaries hung from a mesangium. The capillaries extend into a space outlined by Bowman's capsule, which is made of attenuated epithelial cells.

The filtering membrane of the glomerular capsule consists of three basic structures:

1. The cytoplasm of the endothelial cell lining the capillary is thickened locally at the endothelial cell nucleus, but spreads out thinly in a signet-ring fashion to the periphery of the cell, forming a layer of 0.1 micron or less in thickness. On electron microscopy, the nucleus is surrounded by mitochondria, Gol-

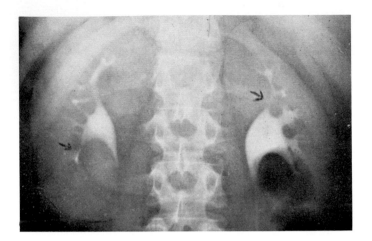

Figure 16-2. Intravenous pyelogram on a patient with the nephrotic syndrome. The kidneys appear large and edematous, and interval swelling is reflected radiographically by narrowing of the infundibula (*arrows*). It is this characteristic that makes nephrotic kidneys easier to biopsy than kidneys with other types of organic disease. The nephrotic kidney is "soft" to the biopsy needle, and excellent samples are usually obtained.

gi's apparatus, endoplasmic reticulum with ribonucleoprotein granules, and granules free in the cytoplasm. Fenestrations may be seen at the thinned-out portions of the endothelial cell.

2. A basement membrane is a hydrated gel, containing mucopolysaccharides and mucoprotein; its true cross-sectional thickness measures up to 3500A in adults, but is thinner in children. On electron microscopy it is composed of a central lamina densa with a lamina rara externa and a lamina rara interna on either side. On light microscopy the basement membrane is best demonstrated by aniline blue–orange G, periodic acid–Schiff (PAS), and the periodic acid–silver methenamine stains. The basement membrane has a constant metabolic turnover rate which may be enhanced by disease or injury. Fractions of its protein may be found in the urine, and the substance is regarded as foreign material by animals, in whom, as shown by Lerner and Dixon [405], it has produced renal lesions. The basement membrane itself appears to be the prime barrier to filtration, determining the molecular size of solutes filtered.

3. The epithelial cell or podocyte has numerous ribonucleoprotein granules both free and in the endoplasmic reticulum; mitochondria, fine fibrils, and vesicles may also be present. The foot processes are attached to the luminal side of the capillary basement membrane at intervals that are 200A to 500A apart in true linear sections. The areas between form epithelial slits bridged by a thin line, the "slit membrane." In animals injected with large electron-dense molecules such as human myeloperoxidase, these accumulate at the epithelial side of the basement membrane and appear to clog up the epithelial slits. They do not pass into Bowman's space, whereas small molecules traverse the slit membrane freely and enter the glomerular filtrate in Bowman's space. The podocytes may have vesicles that change in size in response to water diuresis. For further details on the fine anatomy of the kidney, refer to Chapter 1 in the excellent text on renal pathology by Heptinstall [275] and to Chapter 1 in this volume.

Renal biopsy has contributed importantly to our improved understanding of the pathology in the nephrotic patient. Very little autopsy material is available for study of the mild or early lesions. Sequential examination, correlation of structure and function, and experimental manipulation have been possible only since the development of percutaneous biopsy. In addition, freshly fixed material yields far superior slides even in routinely stained specimens (Fig. 16-3).

The most common histologic findings in the glomeruli of nephrotic patients are:

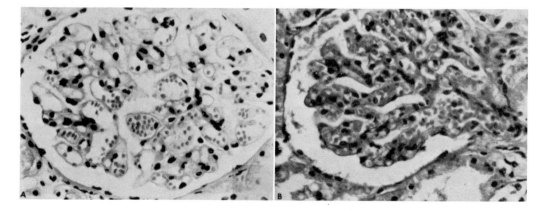

Figure 16-3. A. Normal glomerulus as seen on thin section from renal biopsy specimen of a young man studied for orthostatic proteinuria. Hematoxylin and eosin. ×402. B. Normal glomerulus from autopsy on a patient who died from unrelated causes. Hematoxylin and eosin. ×450.

Minimal Change or Lipoid Nephrosis. This change is also called "no change," "nil disease," "glomerular epithelial disease," or "foot process disease." It is a frequent lesion in children, and when the biopsy is performed early in the clinical course, the glomeruli are frequently read as normal on the routine pathologic specimen. Table 16-3 indicates the frequency of "minimal change" in six series of patients with nephrotic syndrome.

Table 16-3. Frequency of "Minimal Change" in Series of Patients with Nephrotic Syndrome

Series	Total No. of Cases	No. of Cases with Minimal Change	Fre-quen-cy (%)
Heptinstall	70	17	24
Bjørneboe	8	2	25
Kark	98	11	12
Blainey	29	6	20
Earle & Jennings	29	8	27
Habib	127	35	28
Total		79	
Weighted mean			24

When examined with great care, there is little change on light microscopy, except for dilated capillary loops and a general thick appearance of the tufts [248]. On higher magnification edema and swelling of the endothelial cytoplasm may sometimes be seen. On electron microscopy the earliest changes have been noted in the foot processes of the podocytes, which contain more vacuoles than normal and, in the presence of massive proteinuria, may appear fragmented. The basement membrane may appear slightly thickened and of abnormal texture. Where thickened, the endothelial side is irregular and appears attached to the cytoplasm of the endothelial cell which may have cytoplasmic extensions into it. Small droplets are seen in the endothelial cytoplasm. These changes have been demonstrated to be reversible in association with adrenal steroid therapy [193]. The tubules may show fine vacuolization from fat which may stain with oil red-O or be refractile on polarized light (Fig. 16-4). Hyaline-droplet formation occurs in the cells, and casts are seen in some tubular lumina. The interstitial tissue may show edema.

Classically, patients with this lesion have only proteinuria and lipiduria and do not have hematuria, red cell casts, diminished re-

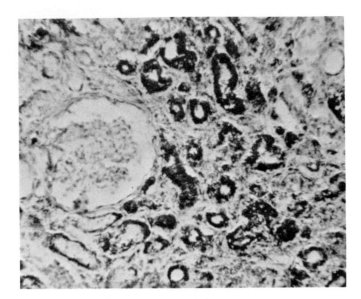

Figure 16-4. Oil red-O stain showing intratubular cell fat deposition in the kidney of a woman who had four separate nephrotic episodes coinciding with four of her five pregnancies. Routine stains revealed no tubular changes or vacuole formation. (Stain courtesy of Dr. Albert Cannon.)

nal clearances, or azotemia. Some degree of cellular proliferation is noted, most often in the early stage of the mixed type. Epithelial cell changes may be aggravated by intravenous administration of albumin.

Idiopathic Membranous Glomerulonephritis. This change consists in regular thickening in a diffuse manner of capillary loops in the glomerulus. It occurs classically without an increase in cells or proliferation of the epithelial elements of Bowman's capsule. In more advanced cases, there is a condensation of tufts and hyaline solidification of the glomerulus. The membrane thickening is usually eosinophilic and refractile, and is well demonstrated with PAS stain or methenamine–silver, which shows a silver-positive inner line from which silver-positive projections extend outward. The hyaline material stains green with Masson's trichrome stain. On electron microscopy the thickening of the basement membrane can be resolved even further. An irregular accumulation of electron-dense material between the lamina densa and the fused foot processes is a constant feature [22, 186, 248, 475]. Deposits are not homogenous, are often flecked with darker granular elements, and are separated by light "moth-eaten" zones. These al-

ternating areas may give a "spiked" appearance.

Basement membrane defects up to 1000A have been reported in human beings with nephrotic syndrome [637], but this has not been confirmed. Membranous glomerulonephritis has been demonstrated to develop in as short a time as 10 days in a human homotransplant [380]. Similar deposits of electron-dense material have been noted in acute glomerulonephritis and in variants of systemic lupus erythematosus with the nephrotic syndrome as well as in other colagen diseases. Fluorescent-antibody studies have shown the presence of gamma globulin in the thickened capillary basement membranes in this condition [453].

Mixed Membranoproliferative Glomerulonephritis. This histologic change is also called Ellis type 1 [151] or Longcope type A glomerulonephritis, proliferative glomerulonephritis with nephrotic component, and nephritic nephrosis. This is the classic lesion seen in the nephritic nephrotic patient who has proteinuria, hematuria, and diminished renal clearances. It was found in 21 of our 45 cases [57], and by Fiaschi [184] in eight out of nine children and 16 out of 20 adults. McCluskey and

Baldwin [438] found a nephrotic syndrome in 10 out of 25 cases of poststreptococcal acute glomerulonephritis. Actually, the lesion may be seen in all forms of proliferative glomerulonephritis — acute, subacute, and chronic — which are described in detail elsewhere in this volume. In addition to the membranous changes, there may be an inflammatory lesion with an increase in epithelial, mesangial, and endothelial cells. There may also be an accumulation of leukocytes, swelling of endothelial and epithelial cytoplasm, and a functional narrowing of the capillary lumen. In the typical subacute lesions, there is a piling up of the thin epithelial layer forming Bowman's capsule, with formation of epithelial crescents. In the more chronic form, hyalinization appears. In any one glomerulus either endothelial or epithelial cell proliferation may predominate, but usually both are present to some degree. There is every reason to believe that these are poststreptococcal in origin, and some of them have been reasonably well documented serologically and bacteriologically to follow an episode of streptococcal infection.

Lobular Glomerulonephritis. Habib et al. [248] described this picture in 15 out of 108 nephrotic patients. The entity begins with the lesion limited to the glomerular lobule and progressively develops into a simplification of the capillary structure by a decrease in the number of loops and a coalescence around a fibrohyaline stalk which is eosinophilic and PAS positive. When this material accumulates, it bears a striking resemblance to some nodular lesions of intercapillary glomerulosclerosis, but it occurs in nondiabetic patients [275].

Some cases of the lobular disease are related to poststreptococcal glomerulonephritis. The reasons why the nephrotic syndrome should develop in association with this particular form is not known.

Glomerulosclerosis. This is a gradual reduction in the number of cells of the glomerulus, both epithelial and endothelial, by progressive atrophy. There may be pyknosis of nuclei, thin, atypically staining cytoplasm, dilatation of capillary loops, aneurysm formation at the base, and a general simplification of the glomerular architecture, with some lobules devoid of capillaries.

Glomerular Involvement in Other Diseases. A number of systemic diseases affect the basement membrane and in addition produce lesions that may be characteristic of a specific pathologic entity. Lupus erythematosus may present with any of the membranoproliferative changes and may have the more characteristic addition of verrucous capillaritis with piling up of endothelial and basement membrane and focal areas of fibrinoid necrosis. Infiltration with amyloid may produce a basement membrane which is much thickened and rather loosely spongy in appearance. Intercapillary glomerulosclerosis may present with a diffuse, hard, gel-like infiltration of the basement membrane or discrete collections in the typical concentric nodules.

Foam Cells in the Glomerulus. In some forms of chronic membranous glomerulonephritis, a suggestion of vacuolization may be seen in the PAS-positive material at a magnification of 1200 to 3000 times. Occasionally, large foam cells may be seen within the glomerulus (Fig. 16-5). Their role is unknown.

Hyalinization. Reduction of portions or all of the glomerular tuft to a hyalinized ball may occur in the progression of any of the above lesions. At this point the glomerulus becomes virtually acellular and ischemic.

Kimmelstiel has recently done one of the few quantitative studies of lipoid nephrosis (personal communication). Twenty cases were studied independently by blind review of conventional light microscopy, electron microscopy, clinical data, and by quantitative analysis of light microscopy sections. When arranged according to ascending size of mesangium (as percentage of total glomerular area), it was found that the mesangial area and number of mesangial nuclei (as percent-

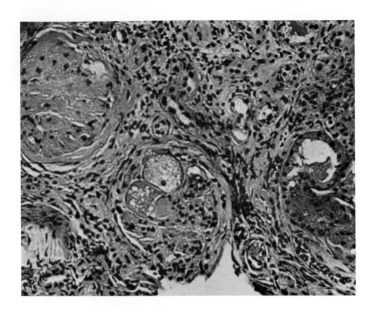

Figure 16-5. Photomicrograph of a renal biopsy specimen from a Chinese male with chronic glomerulonephritis and the nephrotic syndrome. The glomerulus in the lower midcenter shows a fatty sclerosis with foam cells. Hematoxylin and eosin. Enlarged from ×100.

age of total) of each individual glomerulus was considerably lower than the average values of glomeruli in cases of postacute, focal glomerulonephritis, including such glomeruli of the latter series that were "normal" by conventional microscopy.

In 11 of these 20 instances of lipoid nephrosis the highest values were significantly lower than the lowest values of any individual glomerulus in the series of focal glomerulonephritis. Also, all 11 cases met the criteria of conventional microscopy, electron microscopy, and clinical data presently recognized as indicative of "lipoid nephrosis." Of the remaining nine cases the size of mesangium or number of mesangial cells (or both) slightly exceeded the lowest value found in microscopy sections of glomerulonephritis. Three cases had been reevaluated as glomerulonephritis, three were listed as questionable glomerulonephritis, and one was found to have membranous changes by electron microscopy. Only two cases met the requirements for lipoid nephrosis by all other criteria. In the majority of these cases (six) the duration of illness was one year or less. Reevaluation of this group is therefore indicated. This fourfold blind study, which in-

cluded quantification of camera lucida drawings, confirms the noninflammatory nature of the glomerular lesions in idiopathic glomerulonephrosis (nonmembranous). Conspicuous on electron microscopy were numerous dense fibrillary deposits in the mesangium, which rapidly disappeared after one month's duration of the illness.

GEORGETOWN UNIVERSITY HOSPITAL
EXPERIENCE WITH RENAL BIOPSY
IN THE NEPHROTIC SYNDROME

In our series of 183, 100 biopsy attempts were made in 95 patients. Two of the successful biopsies were performed as open procedures in the operating room. Six attempts yielded inadequate tissue samples. In 68 instances the biopsy interpretation supported the clinical diagnosis made at the time of the patient's admission. There was disagreement between the clinical and the histologic diagnosis in 21 instances. Five of these involved the distinction between amyloidosis and glomerulonephritis; five, differentiation of diabetic glomerulosclerosis from glomerulonephritis; and one, differentiation of amyloidosis from diabetic glomerulosclerosis. In the remaining patients the discrepancy was between various stages of glomerulonephritis. Thus a 94 per cent diagnostic accuracy was obtained by renal biopsy. Diagnostic security without additional information was gained in 68 cases. In many of these cases, diagnostic security was of more than academic significance. It enabled us to pursue planned therapeutic regimens with conviction and enthusiasm, sometimes in the face of complications or difficulties. From the remaining successful procedures, also, information having a direct bearing on the planning of therapy was obtained.

The problem of sampling always enters into the interpretation of renal biopsy material. Many pathologists are unwilling to make interpretations of biopsy material because of the possibility that the sample may not be characteristic. Our experiences proved that this is not a practical problem in diseases producing the nephrotic syndrome, since most of them are diffuse. The interpretation is, of course, more reliable if the number of glomeruli in the biopsy specimen is large. In 18 patients (approximately 10 per cent of our entire series) sections were available both from percutaneous renal biopsy and from postmortem examination. The biopsy specimens contained 2 to 41 glomeruli per section. In no instance was there a disagreement in histologic interpretation between the biopsy and subsequent autopsy.

Immunologic Considerations

Most investigators regard the nephrotic syndrome as a sensitivity disease produced by a poorly understood antigen-antibody complex occurring in the patient's kidneys. Those who regard all primary nephrosis (excluding groups 2 through 10 in the etiologic classification on page 504) as being a variant of acute glomerulonephritis place much stress on antecedent beta-hemolytic streptococcal infection. Other investigators, among them most

pediatricians, regard primary "nephrosis" (lipoid nephrosis) as a separate disease entity clinically distinguishable from glomerulonephritis [224].

Both schools of thought currently are inclined to accept an immunologic basis for the disease in at least some patients with the idiopathic nephrotic syndrome [136]. In one attempted "immunodissection" of 35 children with the nephrotic syndrome, 22 showed no deposition of IgG and β_1C globulin and responded to steroid therapy. Of the remaining 13 patients seven had focal depositions and six showed marked deposition together with extensive pathologic alterations. None responded to steroid therapy. The positive lines of evidence for immunologic pathogenesis in the nephrotic syndrome may be summarized as follows:

1. Extrarenal allergic manifestations and other sensitivity diseases have a higher than normal frequency in patients with the nephrotic syndrome [193].

2. There is a higher than expected frequency of multiple allergies in the families and forebears of patients with nephrosis [680].

3. Eosinophilia may occur during activity and recede during remission [390].

4. Serum complement is low in the nephrotic syndrome, rises in spontaneous remission or successful treatment, and falls again in relapse [29, 152, 187–189, 299, 390, 391–395, 397, 398]. Complement abnormalities have been found in unusual forms of the nephrotic syndrome, including that due to malaria [494, 632]. In 15 Nigerian nephrotic children, Allison et al. [10] found immune complexes along the epithelial side of the glomerular membrane. Antibody eluted from the kidney of one patient gave precipitates with a preparation of *Plasmodium malariae* antigens, but none with *P. falciparum* or normal kidney antigens. Specific components of complements such as C′3A have received particular attention in patients with glomerulonephritis [631].

5. Experimental nephrosis may be pro-

duced by nephrotoxic serum containing anti-kidney antibodies in the rabbit [432, 433], rat [432, 622, 625], and dog [493].

6. Antikidney antibody in experimental nephrosis is located in the globulin fraction of the serum [622].

7. Experimental nephrosis has been produced by iso- and autoimmunization by intraperitoneal injection of rat kidney protein mixed with Freund's adjuvant [287, 290, 318].

8. Adrenal corticosteroids increase the incidence and nitrogen mustards prevent the occurrence of autoimmune experimental disease [318].

9. The antibody to rat kidney antigen is species-specific [318].

10. Glomerulonephritis has been reported to have been induced in sheep by direct, intramuscular and subcutaneous injection of human glomerular basement membranes in Freund's adjuvant [318].

11. Nephrotoxic serum exhibits glomerular localization by radioisotopic labeling technics [531].

12. Fluorescein-labeled antiserum, prepared against the immunoproteins IgG and β_1C globulin, and also against human complement, fibrinogen, and other serum components of hypersensitivity lesions, concentrates on the basement membrane of glomeruli in patients with the nephrotic syndrome due to poststreptococcal glomerulonephritis [460], disseminated lupus erythematosus [136], in experimental nephrotoxic serum nephritis [254], antigen-antibody complex nephritis [132], and the autoimmune experimental model of Heymann [285, 504]. Positive immunofluorescent staining occurs in beaded form in streptococcal disease, in a "lumpy, bumpy" distribution in lupus and other immune-complex diseases, and in linear form where antiglomerular basement membrane antibodies are involved (e.g., Goodpasture's syndrome). The immunofluorescent staining in idiopathic membranous glomerulonephri-tis seems to be much more frequent in adult morphologic material [195, 396a, 453, 455]. It is more frequent in adults with idiopathic nephrotic syndrome than in the childhood variety [136]. Intensive studies of complement fractions and immunoglobulin fractions, with the use of immunoelectrophoresis and immunofluorescent staining, have been applied in a number of clinical situations involving the nephrotic syndrome [347, 378, 396a, 439, 467], including such unusual forms as the nephrotic syndrome accompanying renal vein thrombosis [650] and malaria [632].

13. Circulating human antikidney autoantibodies have been detected by the tanned red cell hemagglutination test [414, 415], and by immunofluorescent technics. Antibodies directed against the glomerular basement membrane (anti-GBM) have been most consistently found in Goodpasture's syndrome and in subacute or rapidly progressive glomerulonephritis. These antibodies may be found in the serum in patients who have had kidneys removed preparatory to transplantation. This material has even been eluted from glomeruli in the elegant experiments of Dixon and his colleagues [132].

Proof that experimental nephrosis is an autoimmune disease lies in the ability to transfer it from a diseased to a healthy animal. Intravenous injection of serum, ascites, and spleen emulsion, and intraperitoneal transplant of spleen emulsion, has failed to transfer the disease to recipients [318]. However, an exciting experiment has been reported in which experimental nephrosis was transferred by the transplant of lymph nodes into a paired animal rendered susceptible to tissue transplantation by previous injection of spleen cells during the neonatal period [280]. Membranous glomerulonephritis has been demonstrated in human renal homografts within 10 [380] and 21 [462] days after grafting. Perhaps the most convincing evidence for an active immunologic factor is the demonstrated transmission of periarteritis and subacute glomerulonephritis to human renal transplants [317].

Search for recent or current exposure to beta-hemolytic streptococcal infections was carried out in 108 of our 183 patients. Cultural growth of an organism, an initial ASO titer of 1:320, or a twofold rise in ASO titer on serial examination was considered presumptive laboratory evidence. Of 108 patients, 11 had histories and laboratory test results suggesting recent streptococcal infections, 13 had evidence from the history alone, and 16 had laboratory evidence alone. Thus, recent beta-streptococcal infection, by history or laboratory evidence, was seen in 27 per cent of our nephrotic patients. The positive cases were predominantly in persons with proliferative glomerulonephritis. However, a streptococcal encounter was demonstrated in 14 per cent of those with purely membranous glomerulonephritis (excluding preeclampsia and sickle cell disease). It has recently been reported [400, 587] that substantial quantities of ASO protein were excreted in the urine of 10 out of 15 nephrotic children with low serum ASO titers (0 to 50 Todd units). Five children with the nephrotic syndrome had no ASO protein in the urine, but 10 had quantities ranging from 480 to 150,000 units per 24 hours. It is our impression that with more diligent testing by present methods, recognition of potential urinary losses or the development of more sensitive technics [586, 587], one would probably increase the proportion of patients with the nephrotic syndrome in whom infection with beta-hemolytic streptococci could be established.

It is also apparent that any statistics on streptococcal causality must take into consideration a meticulous classification of the nephrotic syndrome. Thus, evidence of streptococcal infection was found in 56 per cent (15) of patients with acute proliferative glomerulonephritis, 55 per cent (9) of those with

subacute glomerulonephritis, and 32 per cent (44) of those with chronic glomerulonephritis in our series of 183 patients with the nephrotic syndrome.

Pathologic Physiology

MEMBRANE PERMEABILITY

The causes of the nephrotic syndrome in human patients apparently are multiple and disparate. Regardless of the cause, the common denominator appears to be an abnormality in protein and fat metabolism. I believe that the initiating event in pathogenesis is increased glomerular basement membrane permeability. In our series of 183 nephrotic patients protein losses in the urine ranged from 0.05 to 35 gm. per day, with a mean of 7.3 gm. per day. Quantitative protein excretion alone, when measured in a large variety of renal diseases, has a generally bimodal distribution. The vast majority of patients with diseases such as nephrosclerosis, hypertension, and chronic glomerulonephritis have protein excretion rates below 2 gm., whereas the majority of those with diseases producing nephrotic syndrome have excretion rates above 3 to 4 gm. per 24 hours consistently when measured in the presence of a reasonably good filtration rate. Figure 16-6 indicates the suitability of using the quantitative protein excretion to differentiate between nephrotic and nonnephrotic phases of common renal diseases. Occasionally, massive proteinuria may lead to discovery of unexpected glomerular lesions, as in the three cases of vesicoureteral reflux reported by Pillay et al. [523].

Three explanations have been offered for proteinuria in the nephrotic syndrome: (1) abnormal circulating proteins are present which can pass through a normal glomerulus while leaving normal plasma proteins behind; (2) glomerular permeability is increased for normal plasma proteins; and (3) in the nor-

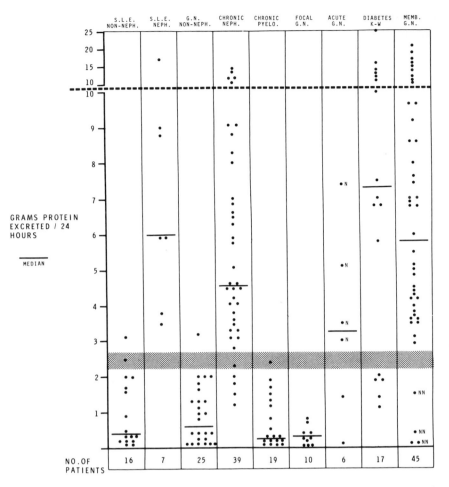

Figure 16-6. Daily protein excretion in patients with frequently encountered renal diseases with and without the nephrotic syndrome. Black lines are the mean of the group. Note dearth of points in shaded area reflecting the bimodal distribution pattern. Most nonnephrotic (NN) patients with organic renal disease excrete less than 2.0 gm. per day. Most nephrotic (N) patients excrete over 3.0 gm. per day.

mal kidney, plasma proteins are filtered and then reabsorbed. In the nephrotic syndrome tubular reabsorption is decreased. Thus, normally filtered proteins escape in the urine.

The first theory is, of course, valid for multiple myeloma (Fig. 16-7), in which Bence Jones proteinuria, massive in quantity, is related to the formation of a protein that has a smaller-than-normal molecular size. This concept has been applied to the nephrotic syndrome [4, 101, 419, 423, 424]. However, the evidence at present is in favor of immuno-

chemical [219] and electrophoretic [196, 648] identity between the urine and serum proteins in both nephrotic and normal subjects.

The third theory of proteinuria gained its strength from the detection of significant concentrations of protein in a fraction of micropuncture specimens [684], and from the fact that all the specimens could contain up to 30 to 40 mg. per 100 ml. of protein undetected by the biochemical methods employed. Normal subjects given human serum albumin may develop proteinuria [690], and tubular transport

Figure 16-7. Renal biopsy specimen from a young male with multiple myeloma and albuminuria in the nephrotic range. Original clinical diagnosis was glomerulonephritis. Hematoxylin and eosin. ×160.

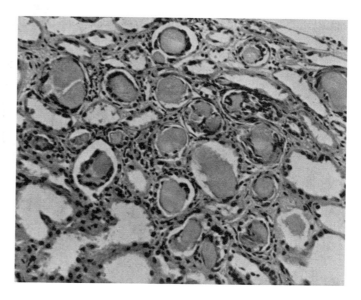

of proteins has been suggested by experiments with protein labels and by associated metabolic experiments [149, 227, 609, 610]. For the rat, the rate of tubular reabsorption has been estimated at 5 mg. per hour.

The tubular rejection theory cannot adequately explain the amounts of proteinuria encountered clinically in the nephrotic syndrome. We therefore lean toward the second theory, *increased glomerular permeability,* as the primary explanation of nephrotic proteinuria. Studies with graded dextran [76, 685] have set the average glomerular "screen" at a molecular weight of 5000 or less, with fewer than 1 in 10,000 pores permeable to compounds of molecular weights in the range of beta globulin. The approximate molecular weights of standard plasma proteins are:

Beta lipoprotein	1,300,000
Alpha-2 globulin	300,000
Alpha-1 globulin	200,000
Gamma globulin	160,000–320,000
Beta globulin	90,000
Albumin	69,000
Hemoglobin	68,000
Alpha-1 mucoprotein	44,000

GLOMERULAR PERMEABILITY INDEX

The 24-hour excretion of protein measured in terms of grams varies with the accuracy of the urine collection, the technical accuracy of the protein determination in urine, the size of the subject, and the filtered load of protein. The filtered load would normally be calculated by the following expression:

$$P_{ALB} \times GFR$$

where P_{ALB} is the plasma albumin and GFR, the glomerular filtration rate. However, the propriety of using albumin filtered load as a concept rests on the degree of selectivity in the glomerular permeability. If it is a highly selective proteinuria with albumin as the major urinary protein, the calculation becomes more valid, although the clearance will be a minimal rather than a true clearance, since the completeness of albumin filtration is unknown in relation to the chemically measured fraction. In the case of unselective proteinuria with larger protein molecules represented in the urine, the plasma albumin is not the sole moiety to be considered, nor can one use the total protein excreted. However, for practical clinical purposes P_{ALB} can be considered in the calculation of the filtered load and albumin clearance calculated as a minimum value from urine and blood. By this method glomerular permeability may be studied in the living patient [593, 595]. One simply divides the rate of albumin excretion (milligrams per minute) by the serum albumin concentration (milligrams per milliliter) and a value for albumin clearance (C_{ALB}) is obtained:

$$\frac{UV_{ALB}}{P_{ALB}} = C_{ALB}$$

This value may then be corrected to a standard surface area of 1.73 square meters.

If the albumin clearance (C_{ALB}) is divided by the creatinine clearance (C_{CR}) or some suitable estimate of the glomerular filtration rate, similarly connected, the permeability index (PI) may be obtained. For example:

$$\frac{C_{ALB}}{C_{CR}} \times 10^3 \quad or \quad \frac{C_{TP}}{C_{CR}} \times 10^3$$
$$= PI \text{ (permeability index)}$$

Since clearances are conventionally corrected to 1.73 M^2 standard surface area, the calculation takes care of the variability between different-sized individuals, as well as variations in the serum albumin concentration. Division by the filtration rate encompasses the other component of the filtered-load formula, and, therefore, all variables are in the expression except the technical ones of collection and analytical determination. Glomerular permeability index thus becomes a more physiologic expression than quantitative measurement of proteinuria. We have calculated the permeability index ($C_{ALB}/C_{CR} \times 10^3$) in 29 nephrotic patients (Table 16-4).

The left side of Figure 16-8 shows the permeability indices of individual patients plotted to indicate the frequency pattern. The median value is 3. On the right side, the permeability indices are plotted against the serum cholesterol taken at the same time. There appears to be a more linear relationship between the

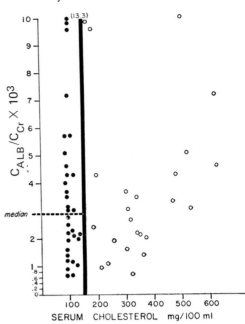

Figure 16-8. Glomerular permeability index in the nephrotic syndrome.

permeability index and the serum cholesterol than between the quantitative absolute amounts of protein excreted and the serum cholesterol, or between the serum albumin concentration and the serum cholesterol (Fig. 16-9).

McCrory et al. [442], in a study of 20 nephrotic children, found a statistically significant correlation between a low permeability measurement and a good response to cortical steroid therapy.

CONCEPT OF SELECTIVITY

Hardwicke and Squire [261] have found that the differential globulin clearance of alpha-1 mucoprotein is equal to 124 per cent of the albumin clearance, and that the beta globulin clearance is 29 per cent, the gamma globulin clearance 27 per cent, and the alpha-2 globulin clearance 13 per cent of the albumin clearance. They have developed a concept, a mathematical expression, for selectivity which is defined as the slope of the line relating the logarithm of the relative renal clearance of

Figure 16-9. Scattergram showing relationship of the serum albumin to cholesterol in 174 patients.

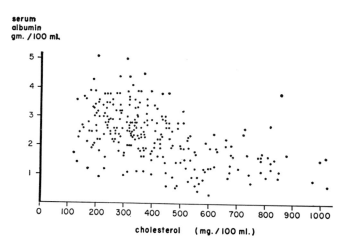

protein to the logarithm of their molecular weights. The formulation for a two-protein system is

$$Kg = \frac{\text{Log } C_1 - C_2}{\text{Log } X_1 - X_2},$$

where C_1 and C_2 represent the relative clearances of two proteins — for example, transferrin and alpha-2 macroglobulin — and X_1 and X_2 represent the molecular weights of the two proteins. In this system, a steep slope means the excretion of small amounts of a high-molecular-weight protein, or a selective proteinuria; whereas a flat slope means the excretion of large amounts of high-molecular-weight protein, or unselective proteinuria. Robson [62] has calculated the selectivity constant in 60 patients with the nephrotic syndrome of varying causes (Fig. 16-10). Minimal-lesion glomerulonephritis possessed the highest value of selectivity and did not overlap values for membranous or mixed membranous and proliferative glomerulonephritis.

With infusions of dextran or concentrated albumin, an increase in the glomerular permeability index may occur, which may be due to vascular distention associated with an increase in plasma volume. This phenomenon has been studied by Wasserman and Mayerson [689], who found the concentration of albumin in lymph plasma increased following sudden expansion with dextran. Lauson et al. [399] demonstrated a decline in permeability index in children treated with ACTH. There is some relationship between proteinuria and filtering surface. Very high protein excretion rates are rarely seen in chronic disease.

Farquhar et al. [170, 172], utilizing electron microscopy and ferritin as a marker in the glomeruli of rats with aminonucleoside nephrosis, have demonstrated that the basement membrane functions principally as the filtration area and may be permeated by small amounts of protein subsequently removed by the podocytes or epithelial cells. Loss of foot processes and the formation of vacuoles and hyaline droplets are the visible signs of increased epithelial activity marshaled by the increased passage of protein through a defective basement membrane. Penetration of ferritin molecules is deeper in the nephrotic basement membrane [172]. Membrane defects ranging from a few hundred to a thousand Angström units have been reported in human nephrosis [637]. Membranous changes are reversed by steroid therapy, especially in children. Subsidence of proteinuria along with reversal of the lesion affords an excellent example of the correlation between basement membrane structure and glomerular permeability as the major mechanism for nephrotic proteinuria.

Table 16-4. Glomerular Permeability in the Nephrotic Syndrome

Name	Date	Age (yr.), Race, & Sex[a]	Diag-nosis[b]	BUN (mg./ 100 ml.)	P_CR (mg./ 100 ml.)	Protein (gm./ day)	Protein (mg./ min.)	Serum Albu-min (mg./ ml.)	C_ALB (ml./ min.)	C_CR (ml./ min.)	C_ALB/ C_CR × 10³	Serum Choles-terol (mg./ 100 ml.)	Remarks
LO'S	3-22-57	45WF	A	10	1.05	6.0	4.17	10	.417	73	5.7	450	Before prednisone
	7-31-57			17		2.5	1.74	18	.097	126	.8	550	After prednisone
	1-17-58			16	2.15	5.4	3.75	19	.197	88	2.2	530	
	4-30-58			21		6.9	4.8	18	.267	20	14.8	516	After I.V. albumin
	9-21-58			19	.55	11.4	7.9	15	.527	103	5.1	516	
	4- 3-59			20	1.1	7.9	5.5	28	.196	49	4.0	512	
PM	8-10-59	46WF	B	14	.7	3.98	2.76	18	.153	110	1.4	360	
SZ	7-21-59	5WF	C		.8	10.68	7.42	27	.275	38	7.2	612	
CP	7-13-59	42WF		27	1.14	12.7	8.82	27	.327	71	4.60	632	
NA	7- 2-59	43WF	D	40	1.9	6.0	4.17	24	.174	40	4.35	194	
LD	4-16-57	23CM	D	20	1.0	8.4	5.83	34	.171	150	1.14	532	
SL	4-13-56	4WF	C	23	1.1	3.3	2.3	8	.288	50	5.7	580	
BA	6- 6-57	29WF	E	25	1.0	7.6	5.28	24	.22	87	2.5	404	
HB	9-27-59	18WM	B	26	1.0	5.2	3.61	17	.212	134	1.6	300	
JL	8- 2-59	28WM	D	40	1.1	7.3	5.07	16	.317	130	2.4	370	
AN	7-29-59	47WM	B	20	.94	6.7	4.65	16	.291	135	2.16	348	
MP	6-10-59	29CM	F	13	1.2	4.1	2.85	44	.065	90	.7	320	
PK	6- 4-59	37WM	G	24	1.1	5.7	3.96	33	.120	104	1.15	236	
EC	5-13-59	6WM	C	13	0.8	7.9	5.5	33	.167	60	2.78	315	

CP	5- 7-59	45WF	B	40	1.7	9.6	6.67	29	.230	65	3.54	330
CB	5-29-59	6WM	B		.8	7.6	5.28	33	.160	86	1.86	252
JM	3-19-59	66WM	H	36	2.2	5.04	3.5	32	.109	36	3.03	301
JS	1-12-59	34WF	D		1.0	16.0	11.1	42	.264	87	3.03	525
HP	7-23-58	51WF	B	15	.94	3.9	2.7	31	.087	94	.9	206
JW	12-19-58	10WM	C		.98	6.25	4.34	29	.150	67	2.24	166
TMcG	9-25-58	37WM	H	26	4.8	6.7	4.65	40	.116	32	3.62	300
CC	7- 8-58	41WM	D	18	1.4	9.1	6.32	25	.253	80	3.16	470
WC	6-12-58	45WM	H	43	3.0	12.7	8.82	20	.441	33	13.4	500
PM	3-25-58	29WM	D	172	13.4	2.9	2.01	34	.059	6	9.8	180
AD	4-11-58	34CF	B	16	.85	3.9	2.71	30	.090	84	1.07	680
MF	3- 7-58	23WF	I	20	1.0	7.2	5.0	39	.128	64	2.0	366
WP	11-10-57	71WM	B		1.0	8.8	6.12	18	.339	80	4.24	480
AC	9-24-57	1½WF	D	12	0.75	4.8	3.33	29	.115	12	9.6	176
EM	9-24-57	36WM	D	45	3.1	4.1	2.85	35	.081	39	2.1	340

[a] W: White, C: colored.

[b] A: Amyloidosis
B: Membranous glomerulonephritis
C: Mixed type glomerulonephritis
D: Chronic glomerulonephritis
E: Pregnancy
F: Subacute glomerulonephritis
G: Acute glomerulonephritis, cause unknown
H: Chronic lobular glomerulonephritis
I: Collagen disease

SOURCE: Reprinted from Schreiner [593].

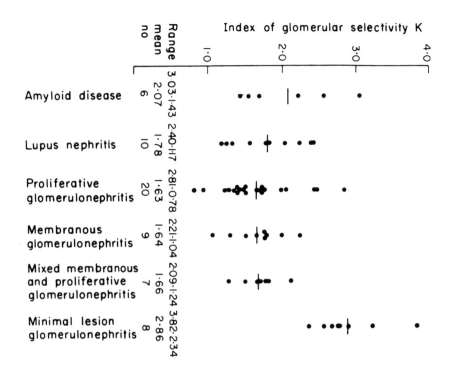

Figure 16-10. Glomerular selectivity (K) in 60 patients with the nephrotic syndrome due to a variety of causes. Minimal-lesion glomerulonephritis possesses the highest value of selectivity and does not overlap the values for membranous or mixed membranous and proliferative glomerulonephritis. A small number of patients with proliferative glomerulonephritis, lupus nephritis, and amyloid disease also have highly selective proteinuria. (From Black [62]. Reproduced by permission.)

THE FATE OF FILTERED PROTEIN

What happens to large molecules that progress through the filtration slits and how large are the molecules that can do so? The main possibilities for the fate of filtered protein are: disposal within the glomerular capsule (the mesangium is thought to be the active organ of disposition); reabsorption, modification, or addition to filtered protein by the action of renal tubular cells; excretion in the urine as soluble protein; and gel or cast formation. In the laboratory animal this has been studied by Graham and Karnovsky [235] using markers of varying molecular weight (Table 16-5). The smaller horseradish peroxidase, when injected into the test animal, rapidly appeared in Bowman's space; however, the larger molecular weight, human myeloperoxidase, tended to concentrate at the epithelial margin of the basement membrane, and appeared to clog up the filtration slits (Fig. 16-11).

The thickened mesangium seen in patients with poststreptococcal glomerulonephritis and lupus nephritis (Fig. 16-12) may represent the disposition process for the proteins of larger molecular weight, which are seen in the unselective proteinuria in these diseases. Indeed, the pathologic picture seen in renal biopsies may be less a function of the rate of deposition of these proteins than it is a resultant of the rate of deposition related to the rate of removal. This probably accounts for the finding of thickened mesangium that persists for a year or more after apparent healing of an

Figure 16-11. Myeloperoxidase (MPO). (From Graham and Karnovsky [235]. Reproduced by permission.)

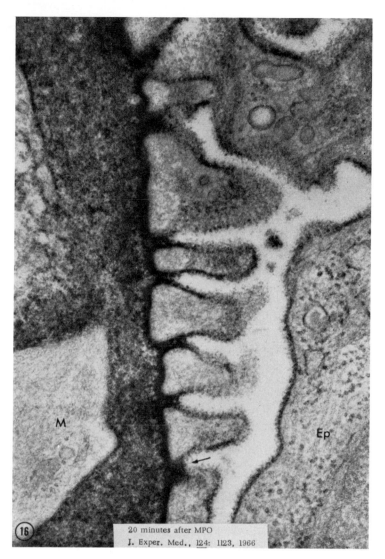

20 minutes after MPO
J. Exper. Med., 124: 1123, 1966

acute attack of poststreptococcal glomerulonephritis.

PROTEIN METABOLISM

Hypoproteinemia is one of the hallmarks of the nephrotic syndrome. In the older literature, a decrease in chemically determined total protein or in albumin concentration was considered an essential diagnostic feature; the severity of the decrease of albumin was described many years ago [156]. Information on serum proteins has been refined by the widespread application of paper electrophoresis, acrylamide gel separation, immunochemistry, and other modern methods of separation, to serum and urine obtained from patients with the nephrotic syndrome and related diseases. The classic pattern described in the literature [219, 226, 239, 258, 260, 335, 371, 416, 514, 577, 648] involves low albumin; normal or low alpha-1 globulin; a relative and often absolute increase of alpha-2 globulin, beta globulin, and fibrinogen; and a decrease in gamma globulin. Bernstein et al. [59] studied

Table 16-5. Molecular Weight and Glomerular Clearance Data for Some Representative Substances

Substance	Molecular Weight	Glomerular Clearance (creatinine = 1)
Ferritin	462,000[a]	—[b]
Myeloperoxidase	160,000–180,000	—[b]
7S gamma globulin	160,000	—[b]
Plasma albumin	69,000	<0.01
Hemoglobin	68,000	0.03–0.1
Egg albumin	43,500	0.22
Horseradish peroxidase	40,000	—[b]
Bence Jones protein	22,000–44,000	—[b]
Myoglobin	17,000	0.75
Inulin	5,500	>0.97

[a] Value represents the molecular weight of the protein portion of the molecule.
[b] Glomerular clearance data unavailable for these substances.
SOURCE: Graham and Karnovsky [235].

electrophoretic patterns on normal subjects and patients with poststreptococcal glomerulonephritis and the nephrotic syndrome. The results are summarized in Table 16-6.

By grouping the alpha-2 and gamma globulin values together, Bernstein et al. were able to obtain a high degree of discrimination between glomerulonephritis and the nephrotic syndrome in the group which contained both children and adults, as shown in Figure 16-13. The only clinical conditions with serum protein patterns resembling that of the idiopathic nephrotic syndrome are protein-losing enteropathy and thermal burns [35, 312]. Acrylamide gel separations suggest that the elevated alpha-2 globulin may be partially accounted for by a particular alpha-2 macroglobulin. There is yet no satisfactory explanation for such hyperglobulinemia. Kluthe et al. [371] reported normal absolute catabolic rates for alpha-2 macroglobulin turnover in nephrotic patients and from their data inferred a normal rate of alpha-2 macroglobulin synthesis. They therefore ascribed the elevation of alpha-2 macroglobulin to selective retention of the high-molecular-weight protein by the kidney and diminution of plasma volume, giving it a further apparent increase in concentration. Immunochemical methods have shown that urinary albumin and other proteins are identical with serum proteins. Immunofluorescent staining with fluorescent-labeled antibodies, in our own laboratory [582], have identified the following serum proteins as localized on the granules inside hyaline casts excreted in patients with the nephrotic syndrome: albumin, alpha acid glycoprotein and alpha-2 lipoprotein, beta globulin, ceruloplasmin, alpha-2 macroglobulin, complement β_1C and β_1A,

Table 16-6. Electrophoretic Protein Fractions in Normal Subjects and Patients with Nephrotic Syndrome

Condition of Subjects	Total Protein (gm./100 ml.)	Albumin (gm./100 ml.)	Alpha-2 Globulin (gm./100 ml.)	Gamma Globulin (gm./100 ml.)	$\overline{N}$
Normal subjects	7.20 (±0.42)[a]	4.20 (±0.43)	0.74 (±0.11)	1.02 (±0.23)	58
Nephrotic syndrome	4.84 (±0.94)	1.92 (±0.83)	1.66 (±0.51)	0.40 (±0.16)	25
Poststreptococcal glomerulonephritis	6.60 (±0.55)	3.06 (±0.53)	1.08 (±0.20)	1.51 (±0.34)	25

[a] Standard deviation.
SOURCE: From Bernstein [59]; reproduced by permission.

Figure 16-12. Renal glomerulus from kidney of patient with lupus nephritis. The thickened mesangium may represent the disposition process for the larger molecular weight proteins. Silver methenamine. ×325, before 15% reduction.

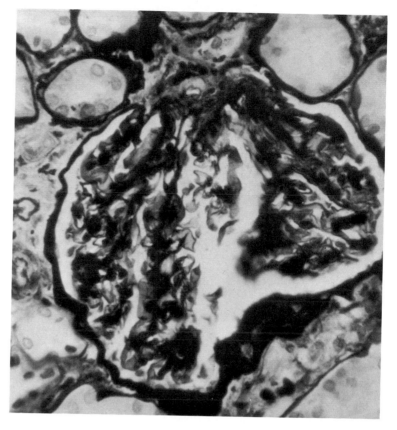

transferrin, fibrinogen, beta lipoprotein, IgA and IgG, and IgM.

Unfortunately, many electrophoretic studies have been done on patients whose nephrotic syndrome was not identified histologically or even from a proved clinical pattern. In our own clinical material, serum electrophoretic patterns in 49 nephrotic patients were examined (Fig. 16-14) and can be grouped into four major diagnostic categories:

1. *Glomerulonephritis.* Acute and chronic glomerulonephritis of nonlupus origin had similar protein patterns. Albumin was subnormal, alpha-1 globulin was normal or slightly elevated, alpha-2 globulin was distinctly elevated, beta globulin varied but showed no significant trend, gamma globulin was rarely elevated and frequently depressed.

2. *Systemic Lupus Erythematosus.* The same pattern as in glomerulonephritis was noted, except that gamma globulin was slightly to moderately elevated in four out of eight patients examined.

3. *Intercapillary Glomerulosclerosis.* All patients had low albumin and high alpha-1 globulin. Alpha-2 globulin was elevated in half, and beta globulin tended to be increased. Three out of four patients had increased gamma globulin levels.

4. *Amyloidosis.* Alpha-1 globulin was normal, alpha-2 globulin was elevated in 80 per cent of patients, and beta and gamma globulin showed no deviations [211].

It has thus been our experience that while deviations in electrophoretic pattern may be more characteristic in some etiologic categories, they are not sufficiently definitive to be really useful in determining the cause of the

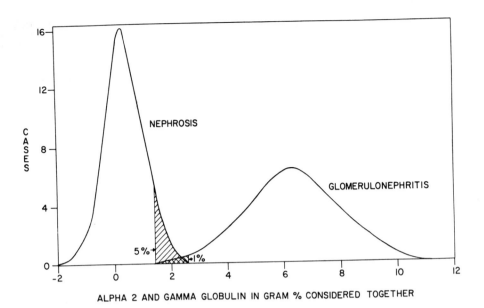

Figure 16-13. Distribution of alpha 2 and gamma globulin levels when considered together in the differentiation of nephrosis from nephritis (discriminant function analysis). (From Bernstein et al. [59]. Reproduced by permission.)

nephrotic syndrome. They may, however, be able to discriminate between idiopathic nephrotic syndrome and glomerulonephritis.

The most obvious explanation for both hypoproteinemia in general and hypoalbumin-

emia in particular is the absolute loss of proteins in the urine. Other possible mechanisms could be either increased turnover of plasma proteins (catabolism) or decreased synthesis. The rate of synthesis in turn is prob-

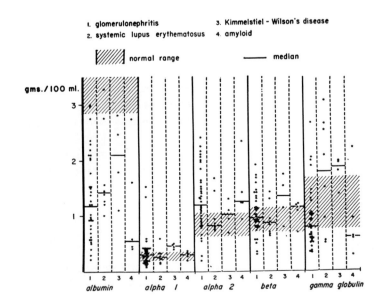

Figure 16-14. Findings in electrophoretic studies of serum proteins in 49 nephrotic patients.

ably affected by dietary factors, the quantitative stress which urinary losses put on the mechanism of synthesis, specific metabolic consequences of the disease process, unknown absorptive defects in the gastrointestinal tract, a possible role for the kidney in the degradation of albumin [349, 350], or albumin "leak" in the intestinal tract [329]. Evidence for the latter hypothesis has been difficult to obtain. The nephrotic syndrome has, of course, been associated with intestinal lymphangiectasia [128], in which case there is an unequivocal protein-losing enteropathy. Jensen et al. [104] studied protein loss by means of albumin labeled with radioactive chromium (^{51}Cr). Out of 13 patients examined, four had a slight increase in fecal ^{51}Cr output, but in the remaining nine, the excretion was normal. Contrary results have been reported by others [334, 372, 427, 499, 500]; however, most of these studies have employed less reliable iodine labeling of the albumin under study.

There have been many important experimental studies on protein metabolism in nephrotic patients [134, 220, 332, 340, 356, 636, 653]. In general, urinary losses represent the primary defect. In the case of selective proteinuria [94, 95, 261], concepts of albumin metabolism are simplified since there is an immunochemical identity between serum and urinary albumin and direct albumin clearances may be calculated or, as we have previously seen, related to the glomerular filtration rate as a permeability index.

In the case of nonselective proteinuria, turnover times and clearance rates are much less precise because of difficulties in the chemical determinations of larger fractions and because changes may occur in permeability due to alterations in the disease state, in hemodynamics, in posture, methodology, and treatment [5, 259, 315, 316]. In simplified physiologic terms a urinary loss of protein initiates reduction in the size of the protein pool. There is often increased fractional catabolism in relation to pool size, and synthesis

may be normal or slightly increased, but in general it is not sufficiently increased to compensate for the loss and the increase in fractional catabolism. Immobilization of the patient and rigid dietary intake in the course of these metabolic studies may, in some cases, have affected the outcome. Quantitative data for assessing the practical impact of qualitative and quantitative factors in nutritional protein intake, the effect of exercise, the possible contribution of absorptive effects from the renal tubule or absorptive defects from an edematous gastrointestinal tract are, in general, not available in existing metabolic studies. We have observed clinically at least three patients who have excreted more than 12 gm. of protein a day for periods longer than six months without a lowering of serum albumin below normal levels. They were muscular persons with high protein intakes who engaged in heavy physical activity. At the other end of the spectrum, I have seen sedentary, elderly women with a marked decline in serum albumin consequent to the excretion of less than 5 gm. of protein daily. Exercise and dietary intake apparently can elevate protein synthesis even when urinary losses are substantial. Observations of positive nitrogen balance on high intake form a rational basis for the use of high-protein diets in the management of the nephrotic syndrome [345].

In addition to albumin metabolism, there have been several detailed studies on the metabolism of other serum proteins — for example, gamma-A and gamma-M immunoglobulins [467], gamma-B globulin [13], serum haptoglobin [706], thyroxine-binding globulin [482], and fibrinogen metabolism and fibrinolysis [658, 688]. Complement and gamma globulin levels, in particular, may be affected by the nature of the initial underlying disease (e.g., malaria) [494], by elevation of ASO titers in disease secondary to streptococcal infections, and by superimposed bacterial infections such as pyelonephritis which occurs in a significant number of nephrotic syndromes and which has been rarely documented in the reported investigations.

LIPID METABOLISM

Lipiduria was included in our definition as an essential feature of the nephrotic syndrome. The observation of fat bodies in the urine was made early on in the study of nephrosis and probably accounted for its original designation as "lipoid" nephrosis by Munk [481] and in the description of the syndrome by Volhard and Fahr [683]. The term *lipoid nephrosis* has, in fact, recently been revived by Heptinstall [275]. An enormous literature has accumulated on the relationship of lipid metabolism in the nephrotic syndrome. The general chemistry of lipids and lipoproteins has been

adequately reviewed by Eder [141], Oncley [508], and others [44, 232, 370, 445, 611].

Incidence of Abnormal Lipidemia in Nephrosis. Clinically the best-studied plasma lipids are cholesterol, cholesterol esters, phospholipids, and triglycerides. Fatty acids may also be included. Plasma lipids are generally insoluble in water and yet may be present in clear solution in the plasma in relatively high concentrations which readily enter into chemical reactions. This solubilization is achieved by close association with proteins and polypeptides in complexes that are generally classified under the term *lipoproteins*. On the other hand, high concentrations of neutral fats or triglycerides impart a characteristic creamy, turbid appearance to serum, generally de-

Table 16-7.   Concentrations of Alpha and Beta Lipoproteins of Human Plasma

Investigators and Subjects	Mean Concentration (mg./100 ml.)				Per Cent Total	
	Cholesterol		Lipoprotein		Plasma	Proteins
	Alpha	Beta	Alpha	Beta	Alpha	Beta
Cohn et al.[a]						
Men & women	50	126	310	360	4.4	5.0
Pearsall and Chanutin[b]						
Men, 20–30 years	35	131	0	375	3.0	5.1
Lever et al.[c]						
Men, 18–40 years	56	154	345	440	4.8	6.2
Russ et al.[d]						
Men, 18–35 years	50	147	310	420	3.9	5.3
45–65 years	55	184	345	525	4.4	6.6
Women, 18–35 years	64	123	400	350	5.1	4.4
45–65 years	59	193	370	550	4.7	7.1
Swahn[e]						
Men & women	47	126	294	360	4.3	5.0
Barclay et al.[f]						
Women, 20–30 years	70	140	430	400	5.5	5.1

[a] Cohn, E. J., Strong, L. E., Hughes, W. L., Jr., Mulford, D. J., Ashworth, J. N., Melin, M., and Taylor, H. L. *J. Amer. Chem. Soc.* 68:459, 1946.
[b] Pearsall, H. H., and Chanutin, A. *Amer. J. Med.* 7:297, 1949.
[c] Lever, W. F., Gurd, F. R. N., Uroma, E., Brown, R. K., Barnes, B. A., Schmid, K., and Schultz, E. L. *J. Clin. Invest.* 30:99, 1951.
[d] Russ, E. M., Eder, H. A., and Barr, D. P. *Amer. J. Med.* 11:468, 1951.
[e] Swahn, B. *Scand. J. Clin. Lab. Invest.* 5: No. 6, 1953.
[f] Barclay, M., Cogin, G. E., Escher, G. C., Kaufman, R., Kidder, E. D., and Petermann, M. L. *Cancer* 8:253, 1955.
SOURCE: From Oncley [508].

scribed as lactescence. In many patients the nephrotic syndrome has been diagnosed by the simple clinical observation of lactescence in a tube of clotted blood. However, lactescence is also observed in diabetic acidosis, familial hyperlipemia, and acute pancreatitis [7, 8].

Table 16-7 lists the composition and properties of the major lipoproteins of human plasma. Alpha and beta lipoproteins are distinct from each other with respect to molecular weight, density, size, viscosity, solubility and composition of their protein fractions, and content of cholesterol, cholesterol ester, phospholipid, and other constituents [207, 508]. Lipoproteins have also been classified according to their density as determined by relative rates of flotation when serum is ultracentrifuged. They may be simply classified as (1) lipoproteins of very low density (less than 1.019 Sf 10–200), which include chylomicrons; (2) lipoproteins of low density (1.019 to 1.063

Sf 1–10), which include most of the beta lipoproteins; and (3) lipoproteins of high density (1.063 to 1.21), which include the lipoproteins that migrate with alpha-1 globulin.

Table 16-8 shows the typical changes in lipid and lipoprotein fractions in the serum of patients with the nephrotic syndrome. These patients are classified into three groups according to whether their serum was clear, slightly creamy, or very creamy. Thus, the serum of patients with the nephrotic syndrome is characterized by great increase of all lipid constituents, with both quantitative and qualitative alterations in lipoproteins.

In severe cases the major serum lipids are transported in a form that has greater solubility and electrophoretic mobility than the beta lipoprotein of normal serum. Similar increases in low-density beta lipoproteins with normal or occasionally decreased alpha lipoproteins have also been reported by Gitlin

Table 16-8. Lipids and Lipoprotein Fractions in Serum of Patients with Nephrosis

Patients and Ages (yr.)	Serum						Albumin (gm./ 100 ml.)	Lipoprotein Fraction (Density)		
	TC	FC	PL	TG	TC/TG			1.019 TC	1.019– 1.063 TC	1.063– 1.21 TC
	(mg./100 ml.)					Appearance		(mg./100 ml.)		
Normal	180	45	225	100	1.8	Clear	4.0	25	100	50
SS-29	1522	435	942	3210	0.5	Very creamy	0.8	1247	98	46
LG-22	1234	349	785	2440	0.5		0.6	1023	78	21
WT-10	715	235	636	2387	0.3		0.5	624	63	19
JH-2½	677	200	620	3920	0.2		0.6	609	52	16
OH-41	588	149	497	570	1.0	Slightly creamy	1.1	326	229	46
RS-3½	682	154	562	390	1.7		0.6	234	333	54
FF-30	471	125	419	400	1.2		0.8	208	201	47
EW-50	857	251	691	480	1.8		0.9	210	604	57
SS-31	379	91	399	197	1.9	Clear	2.5	23	219	68
AR-4	586	124	479	120	4.9		2.0	60	382	85
DP-3	703	166	514	174	4.0		0.9	48	541	97
MH-5	678	181	499	169	4.0		1.2	64	520	49

TC = total cholesterol, FC = free cholesterol, PL = phospholipids, TG = triglycerides.

SOURCE: From Baxter [42]; reproduced by permission.

[217, 218] and others [495, 496]. It has long been known that intravenous injection of heparin could produce rapid clearing of serum lactescence in some metabolic states. Recently the clearing factor has been identified as a heparin-activated lipoprotein lipase [377]. This substance has been administered by a number of investigators of the nephrotic syndrome without notable success. Nikkila et al. [495, 496] assigned the failure of clearing to a deficiency of acceptor protein, and believe that albumin is an essential component of the lipidemia-clearing process. Some years ago we tried a series of daily injections of high concentrations of depoheparin in adult nephrotic patients. There were no detectable changes in any clinical signs, although a few patients had an apparent improvement in the ultracentrifugation pattern and in the severity of gross lactescence.

Rodbell [563] has employed interesting technics for the characterization of individual proteins by chemical marking of the terminal amino groups, and has found variations in the protein fractions associated with particular classes of lipoproteins. Those amino acids associated primarily with lipoproteins are serine, threonine, and aspartic acid. In the Sf 0–8 and Sf 3–17 classes, which contain a very large cholesterol component, glutamic acid containing protein appears.

Mechanism of Lipidemia. There are many fundamental questions concerning the mechanism of lipidemia in the nephrotic syndrome in which experimental data are conflicting. Some of the major ones are: (1) Is lipidemia due to hypoalbuminemia? (2) Is it due to a deficiency in clearing factor such as the lipoprotein lipase which has been implicated as an explanation for familial hyperlipemia? (3) Is it due to an abnormality in the absorption of lipids from the gastrointestinal tract? (4) Is it due to excess or unbinding or enhancement of some lipid-mobilizing hormone such as that which has been described by Seifter et al. [607]? (5) Is it due to some metabolic

block in the interconversion of one lipoprotein to another? (6) Is it due to an increase in lipid synthesis which runs parallel to the stimulation of protein synthesis secondary to massive proteinuria? (7) Are plasma lipids actually synthesized in the diseased kidney? (8) Are metabolic consequences of nephrosis such as lipidemia due to the same antigen-antibody reaction which affects the kidney but in this instance also affects an extrarenal (e.g., liver) site of lipid synthesis?

Friedman et al. [202, 203, 572, 574] have done extensive studies on the mechanism of nephrotic hyperlipemia in laboratory animals. They have taken a particularly strong stand favoring the causal role of hypoalbuminemia, having demonstrated that hyperlipemia may be aggravated by dietary sources but is primarily of endogenous origin. If urinary loss of albumin was prevented by ureteral ligation prior to the administration of nephrotoxic serum, no rise in the serum cholesterol or lipids appeared even though their animals developed other features of the nephrotic syndrome [573].

Heymann and his co-workers have also done extensive studies on this subject [282, 283, 288, 289, 293, 294]. They found no correlation between the severity of hypoalbuminemia and hyperlipemia in nephrotic rats. The development of hyperlipemia preceded rather than succeeded the hypoalbuminemia; intraperitoneal administration of nonprotein-containing rat urine decreased hyperlipemia in nephrotic rats; subtotal hepatectomy inhibited the development of hyperlipemia; and the severity of hyperlipemia was related to the amount of nephrotic kidney tissue present. Their data have led them to discount the causal role of hypoproteinemia in nephrotic hyperlipemia [293]. Moreover, they have demonstrated transient hyperlipemia in the early stages of acute glomerulonephritis in children [296].

A third possible explanation for hyperlipemia has been presented by Marsh and

Drabkin [428]. With the use of ^{14}C acetate labeling they demonstrated a decreased rate of synthesis of fatty acids and cholesterol despite an elevated content of cholesterol in the blood, liver, and kidney of nephrotic rats. They therefore postulated that the hyperlipemia was a mobilization phenomenon which supplied fat for energy.

With respect to the lipidemia of human nephrosis, it seems clear that there is no unifying hypothesis that is consistent with all the observations to date. The data of Baxter and his colleagues [42] show that a reasonable correlation exists between decreased serum albumin and elevated levels of lipid, although almost all clinical observers can find exceptions to this correlation. In Figure 16-9 (page 519), serum albumin concentration is plotted against serum cholesterol concentration for 174 nephrotic patients. The paucity of patients in the right upper quadrant emphasizes the relatively rare occurrence of a markedly elevated cholesterol in the presence of normal serum albumin. There are, however, many instances of low levels of cholesterol in the presence of hypoalbuminemia. It is well known that other clinical entities, marked by protein deficiency (nutritional deficit, kwashiorkor, cirrhosis, idiopathic hypoproteinemia), may not have associated hyperlipemia. Lupus nephritis [345, 478] has been singled out as one cause of the nephrotic syndrome often characterized by a normal or low serum cholesterol. This is equally true of the nephrotic syndrome in acute glomerulonephritis, as is shown in Figure 16-15. It is also well known that inadequate dietary intake such as may be seen with severe anorexia, nausea, vomiting, and diarrhea may be associated with lowered cholesterol levels. When the nephrotic syndrome occurs late in the course of chronic glomerulonephritis and early uremia supervenes, the cholesterol concentration in serum often falls. We have also noted that the

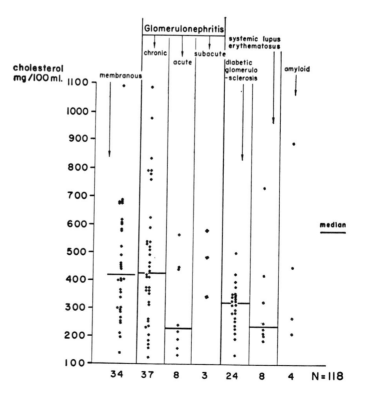

Figure 16-15. Relationship of the serum cholesterol to specific causes of the nephrotic syndrome in 118 nephrotic patients.

acute onset of salt retention and edema may artificially lower the cholesterol, so that patients with rapidly accumulating edema or acute congestive heart failure may have, when first seen, borderline or even normal concentrations. This decrease is presumably due to rapid expansion of circulating plasma volume. Cholesterol and the large molecules of lipoprotein seem to occupy an essentially intravascular position and do not appear in large concentrations in pleural effusions or ascites. When diuresis ensues, such patients [594, 597] may develop elevation of the cholesterol to abnormally high levels in the nonedematous state. This phenomenon has been reproduced in essential or familial hyperlipemia by the administration of DOCA and salt to reduce cholesterol concentrations, followed by diuretic therapy which restores them.

When quantitative urinary losses of protein are plotted against elevated levels of cholesterol, there is no significant correlation. However, when losses are expressed in terms of $C_{ALB}/C_{CR} \times 10^3$ (Fig. 16-8, page 518), there appears to be a more direct correlation. We have occasionally observed nephrotic-nephritic patients who became anuric. One such patient maintained an elevated serum cholesterol (352–460 mg. per 100 ml.) during two months of virtually complete anuria when urinary protein losses were impossible and serum albumin rose from 1.2 to 3.3 gm. per 100 ml. Other investigators have also failed to find a correlation between the "lipidogram" of infants and the further course of the nephrotic syndrome [309, 311].

In experimental nucleoside nephrosis in rats, Hoak et al. [301] noted a significant positive correlation between the amount of proteinuria and the serum cholesterol level in nephrotic animals and a significant negative correlation between blood urea nitrogen (BUN) and both the serum cholesterol and the serum triglyceride. Thus, the serum cholesterol increased progressively with proteinuria and declined with azotemia. Significantly low cholesterol

levels have been described in clinical uremia [598]. These investigators also found that hypophysectomy in rats prevented the usual rise in serum cholesterol and triglyceride. It is known that cholesterol synthesis in the liver is enhanced in rats having aminonucleoside nephrosis [231, 348], and that a depression of cholesterol synthesis has been found in liver slices taken from hypophysectomized rats [217]. Clofibrate, an inhibitor of cholesterol synthesis, may cause a decrease in serum cholesterol and triglyceride concentrations both in normal rats and in rats made nephrotic by injections of aminonucleoside [300].

In summary, it appears that elevation of triglycerides and high-density lipoproteins is the primary abnormality in the nephrotic syndrome. There appears to be an inability to carry out the proper rate of interconversion from large to small lipoprotein fractions. Whether this represents a deficiency of a specific carrier substance is unknown, but albumin seems to have a major role as an acceptor in the transport chain required for interconversion. In the presence of low serum albumin, less marked limitations in the rate of the interconversion process may be uncovered. These interconversions may even be due to changes in the protein fraction. At any rate, hyperlipemia is sometimes improved by albumin or dextran administration or by any therapeutic effort that produces a decrease in glomerular permeability and a resulting rise in serum albumin.

EDEMA

Edema is an expansion of fluid volume of the interstitial space which has progressed to the point at which it is evident on physical examination. This edema shifts with position owing to the effects of gravity; it is best to examine the soft tissues of the periorbital space in the morning or after the patient has been in the horizontal position and to examine the medial surface of the ankle after sitting or standing. Edema has generally been accepted as a cardinal feature of the nephrotic syndrome. The presence of clinical edema, however, is not necessary for the diagnosis of nephrotic syndrome. Edema was seen in about three-fourths of our nephrotic patients at the time they were referred to us by their primary physician. It is present, however transiently, in almost all nephrotic patients *at some period* of the clinical course. Edema is unquestionably the sign that is most important to the patient, and usually the one that brings him to the doctor; it therefore tends to dominate the clinical picture. Preoccupation with edema, however, must never become an obstacle to accurate diagnosis, and should not be used as an absolute guide to therapy or prognosis in the nephrotic syndrome.

Edema should be regarded as a secondary manifestation. Its comings and goings may often be related to events extrinsic to the fundamental pathologic process. Isonatremic edema, for example, may depend on salt intake, posture and position of the patient, tissue turgor, presence and severity of heart or liver disease, quantity of parenteral fluid administered, and a host of other factors. The tide of hyponatremic edema may rise and fall with excess ingestion of fluid, metabolic water production, vagaries of the thirst mechanism, and excessive ADH secretion. What, then, are the essential physiologic steps in the accumulation of nephrotic edema?

Figure 16-15a presents what is perhaps the currently most acceptable scheme for the pathogenesis of nephrotic edema. A central role is assigned to the albumin deficit, which is largely due to increased glomerular permeability. As seen in the section on *Protein Metabolism,* intestinal loss and impaired synthesis may also play a role [73, 77]. However, there is little positive evidence for a generalized increase in the permeability of peripheral capillaries. In fact, the protein content of nephrotic edema, pleural effusions, and ascites is extremely low. Squire et al. [638–640] have pointed out that there is a direct relationship

between serum albumin and colloid osmotic pressure in the serum of patients with the nephrotic syndrome. A serum albumin of 2 gm. per 100 ml. corresponds to a colloid osmotic pressure just under 20 cm. of water and a serum albumin of 1 gm. per 100 ml. to a colloid osmotic pressure of just under 10 cm. of water. For clinical purposes, therefore, one can translate the serum albumin concentration into colloid osmotic pressure in the majority of adult nephrotic patients. Substantial edema was seen by these investigators whenever the serum albumin fell below 1.6 gm. per 100 ml. (16 cm. of water). Such correlations are generally less reliable in children.

In our observations on 150 nephrotic patients, 36 had no edema, three had periorbital edema only, 50 had lower leg edema, 35 had leg plus sacral edema, and 26 had generalized anasarca with fluid accumulation in serous cavities. The relationship between the serum albumin concentration and the edema in these patients is graphically expressed in Figure 16-16. With the exception of the three patients who had only periorbital edema, there was a reasonable correlation between the concentration of serum albumin and the severity of edema on admission to the hospital. Four patients, however, with serum albumin concentrations of less than 2 gm. per 100 ml. had no edema. Two of these were at or below the critical level drawn by Squire et al. [640]. Metcoff [458] infused hypertonic sodium into nephrotic children and found that the excretion of a sodium load was impaired during the accumulation of edema, but was otherwise normal. Sodium retention was accompanied by excessive excretion of potassium. In many instances this may be due to renal hemodynamic factors [32, 74]. Wesson [697], who emphasizes the primacy of glomerular filtration rate, found that at the time of diuresis the filtration rate was measurably increased in 85 to 90 per cent of more than 30 experiments cited. Albumin deficit, theoretically, should cause a contraction in effective plasma volume, a re-

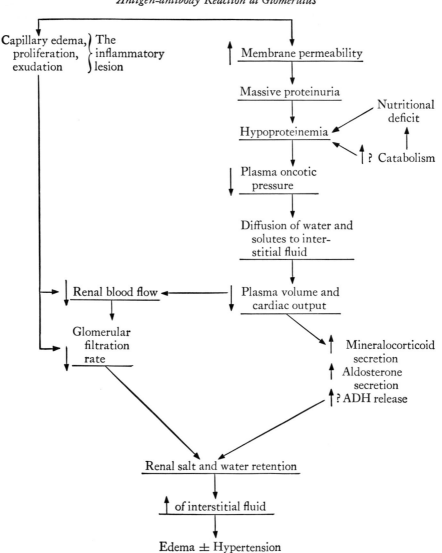

Figure 16-15a. The currently most acceptable scheme for the pathogenesis of nephrotic edema.

duction in glomerular filtration rate, increased fractional reabsorption of filtrate in the proximal tubule, and activation of the renin-angiotensin system to increase the aldosterone secretory rate [6, 39, 118, 320].

A reduction of circulating plasma volume in the range of 20 to 30 per cent was, in fact, reported by early investigators of the nephrotic syndrome [639], and has been reconfirmed with more modern methods. Yamauchi and Hopper [725] found that the blood volume was normal or reduced in 90 per cent of a group of patients with the nephrotic syndrome. Garnett and Webber [207] found

Figure 16-16. Relation between edema and serum albumin concentration in 150 nephrotic patients.

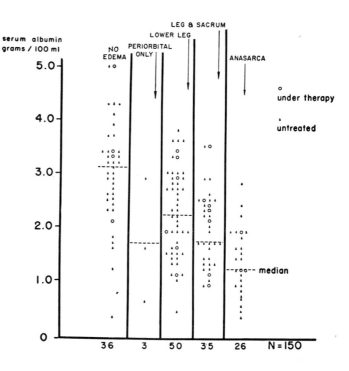

measured blood volume to be normal or reduced in all except 1 of 14 nephrotic patients studied. Volumes continued to fall by a liter or more during diuretic treatment, a highly significant finding since it represents a sequential change and is independent of the normal value chosen for "predicted" blood volume. Further falls of effective volume may occur with upright posture, and six patients developed postural hypotension or fainted on standing. Fawcett and Wynn [177] ascribed hypotension to hypovolemia. Hypovolemic shock is known to complicate the nephrotic syndrome in children [181], and one sudden death has been reported [250]. Eisenberg [148] measured the blood volume in 15 edematous subjects with the nephrotic syndrome. In 9 of the 15 subjects the venous hematocrit was decreased, and in each of these patients the red cell mass was significantly reduced, indicating a true anemia. There was no consistent change in blood volume when these patients had become edema-free following treatment.

In the majority of patients with the ne-

phrotic syndrome treated with diuretics, the serum albumin concentration, and hence the colloid oncotic pressure, remains low even when the patients are no longer edematous. In the absence of edema, interstitial pressure is negligible, and therefore, the capillary hydrostatic pressure must be low. This has been ascribed to a preferential constriction of precapillary vessels by Garnett and Webber [207] and by Oberg [502]. The existence of normal or supernormal glomerular filtration rates in some untreated nephrotic patients (particularly children) has made many investigators unwilling to accept renal hemodynamic changes as the only explanation for salt retention and a rise in glomerular filtration rate as the sole mechanism of diuresis [142, 155, 506].

Luetscher [419, 421] discovered in the urine of a nephrotic child a substance trophic for renal tubules and capable of producing potent sodium retention and potassium excretion. This substance was subsequently identified as aldosterone, and is extensively discussed elsewhere in this volume. The urine of nephrotic patients may have a high aldosterone content during sodium accumulation. The aldosterone level falls when spontaneous diuresis due to improvement in the nephrotic state occurs or when diuresis is induced by infusions of colloid-containing solutions or treatment with ACTH or with steroids. It may increase during further effective plasma volume depletion when prolonged treatment with diuretics is used. Potassium depletion from such therapy represents an additional danger, and one should caution against the prolonged use of diuretics in the nephrotic syndrome. Hypovolemia acts as a potent stimulator for aldosterone production, presumably through the now well-defined renin-angiotensin system (discussed elsewhere). More recently there has been great investigational interest in the so-called "third factor" which may be produced by volume expansion.

These mechanisms can provide an adequate physiologic explanation for the occurrence and subsidence of edema in the vast majority of nephrotic patients. They are the coarse adjustments of the renal mechanisms of salt and water homeostasis. From time to time exceptional patients may be observed who do not have hypoalbuminemia, do not have plasma volume contraction, or who do not have mineralocorticoid excess. Such exceptions should be meticulously recorded by all investigators of this disease, since a detailed study of them may lead to a better insight into the "fine" adjustment involved in salt and water homeostasis.

HYPERTENSION

Elevation of the blood pressure is not generally considered an essential feature of the nephrotic syndrome, and most reports fail to mention it among the clinical signs. Hypertension in relation to renal insufficiency and renal failure has been reviewed [598]. Obviously, the incidence of hypertension is meaningless in the nephrotic syndrome unless a series of cases is subdivided into individual etiologic groups. For example, all patients classified by Squire et al. [640] as having acute and subacute nephritis were hypertensive. Of the 10 patients they classified as having "uncomplicated" nephrotic syndrome, 4 had initial diastolic blood pressures of 90 mm. Hg or above, and 4 showed final diastolic pressures of 100 mm. Hg or above.

In our own clinical material, multiple hospital blood pressure recordings were available for 140 nephrotic patients. If we define hypertension as a diastolic pressure above 90 mm. Hg in persons over age 12, and above 70 mm. Hg in persons under age 12, and if we further exclude all blood pressure readings taken on patients under medication which might affect blood pressure (e.g., adrenal corticosteroids, antihypertensive drugs, chlorothiazide type diuretics), as many as 90 of the 140 patients were hypertensive. Of the patients with membranous glomerulonephritis, 21 out of 44 were hypertensive (Table 16-9).

Table 16-9. Incidence of Hypertension in the Nephrotic Syndrome

(Excluding blood pressure recordings taken during significant medications.)

Disease Category	Number of Patients
Membranous glomerulonephritis	21 of 44
Acute glomerulonephritis	8 of 11
Subacute glomerulonephritis	6 of 8
Chronic glomerulonephritis	28 of 39
Amyloidosis	0 of 2
Intercapillary glomerulosclerosis	21 of 28
Systemic lupus erythematosus	6 of 9

Pollak et al. [527] studied 21 patients each in the histologically differentiated categories of lipoid nephrosis and membranous glomerulonephritis. The diastolic blood pressure exceeded 90 mm. Hg in seven patients (or one-third of each group) and 100 mm. Hg in a patient with membranous glomerulonephritis.

Hypertension has also been noted in a pediatric series [308].

In our opinion, the incidence of hypertension in the nephrotic syndrome has been largely understated in the clinical literature because of two circumstances. Firstly, most observations on patients with the nephrotic syndrome have been accumulated in children, in whom blood pressures are less reliable and the boundaries of normal less definitely established than in adults. Secondly, contraction of plasma volume makes it difficult to achieve hypertensive blood pressure levels even when a tendency toward hypertension exists. In our series of nephrotic patients, which has a preponderance of adults, hypertension was present in more than half the patients even when we excluded readings taken during medications which might conceivably have affected blood pressures. If one adds to such series the many normotensive patients who become hypertensive when they are either repleted with albumin or treated with ACTH or adrenocortical steroids, it becomes apparent that hypertension is both more frequent and more important in the nephrotic syndrome than has previously been recognized. Furthermore, when one recalls that it was in the urine of a patient with the nephrotic syndrome that aldosterone was first recognized and that recent information points to a stimulation of the renin-angiotensin-aldosterone system in this disease, the relationship between hypertension and the nephrotic syndrome would seem to merit more attention from researchers. Occasionally in my clinical experience I have seen severe hypertension and even encephalopathy in a nephrotic patient after treatment with steroids. These sequelae suggest that a previous tendency toward severe hypertension was ameliorated by hypovolemia, much as essential hypertension may be ameliorated by prolonged salt and protein restriction [104] or the use of diuretics [594, 597]. This type of secondary rise in blood pressure is now the most common cause of encephalopathy in our

nephrotic-nephritic patients. It may be seen in a particularly malignant form in patients with disseminated lupus erythematosus.

THYROID FUNCTION

It is an old observation that nephrotic patients have lowered basal metabolic rates. These deviations were exaggerated in the older literature by the failure to distinguish between nonedematous and edematous weight in the calculations. However, the combination of a low basal metabolic rate (BMR) and lipidemia understandably led to the assumption that nephrotic patients have a metabolic disturbance related to hypothyroidism, and also led to the employment of thyroid medication in treatment [157]. Peters and Man [520] later observed that although the serum protein-bound iodine (PBI) level was reduced in nephrotic patients, exogenous thyroid administration failed to elevate it. This subject was extensively investigated by Recant and Riggs [539]. In a series of 16 patients with active nephrotic syndrome, largely adults and ranging in age from 9 to 62, the mean BMR was subnormal in 15 even when calculated on the basis of edema-free weight. The serum protein-bound iodine was below 3 micrograms per 100 ml. in 13, borderline (i.e., 3 to 3.4 micrograms per 100 ml.) in 2, and "normal" (3.5 to 7 micrograms per 100 ml.) in only 1 patient. The mean PBI in the 16 patients was 2.2 micrograms per 100 ml. However, the uptake of radioactive iodine by the thyroid gland was normal or above normal. There was a definite rise in the serum protein-bound iodine in response to thyrotropic hormone.

As a result of the work of Recant and Riggs, several hypotheses can be presented regarding thyroid metabolism in the nephrotic syndrome:

1. *There is a specific thyroid gland abnormality in the nephrotic syndrome.* There is no real support for this concept. With few exceptions [717] the thyroid gland in nephrotic patients is clinically and histologically normal

and appears to respond normally to exogenous thyroid-stimulating hormones [539].

2. *There is abnormal loss of thyroid hormone in the urine.* Peters and Man [520] observed losses ranging from 16 to 48 micrograms per day. Recant measured 36 micrograms per day as the greatest loss of PBI in four nephrotic patients. With intravenously administered thyroxine, urinary losses in 48 hours represented 6 to 7 per cent of the dose [539]. Recant and Riggs tend to discount thyroid hormone loss as a significant physiologic feature. Rasmussen [536], however, in a later study, measured the metabolic fate of ^{131}I-labeled thyroxine and found the half-time shorter than normal, with significant loss of iodine in urine and feces. The urinary iodine was in the form of both thyroxine and diiodotyrosine. He calculated that 25 to 30 per cent of the secreted thyroxine entering the circulation was lost in the nephrotic urine. He would thus assign a greater role to urinary losses than that indicated by Recant and Riggs.

3. *Thyroid function and supply of hormone to the tissues may be normal, but the low PBI is due to a change in concentration or binding capacity of the plasma proteins in nephrotic patients.* This would relate the low PBI to hypoalbuminemia or preempting of binding sites (or both). This explanation implies that a lower plasma binding would enable the peripheral tissues to take up relatively more from a lower concentration and would thus permit the transport and delivery of a normal supply of thyroid hormone to tissues despite a decreased concentration of hormone in the bloodstream. As a corollary, certain patients may have thyroid hyperactivity to compensate for urinary hormonal loss. Recant and Riggs favor this latter theory. Rasmussen, on the other hand, seems to feel that the low PBI is a result of at least four factors: (1) significant loss of organic iodide in the urine; (2) proportionately greater loss in the feces; (3) dilution of organic iodide in the circulating fluid because of an expanded extra-cellular fluid volume in edematous patients; and (4) inability of the pituitary-thyroid axis to augment thyroxine in the face of an apparent deficiency.

This problem was studied by Kalant et al. [342] in experimental nephrosis in rats. Their animals were apparently able to maintain normal oxygen consumption and PBI. However, they had an impaired response to exogenously administered hormones. Considerable thyroxine was lost with proteinuria. There was also a decreased response to triiodothyronine in the absence of sufficient urinary loss to explain it. Freinkel et al. [198] found that circulating thyroxine is distributed among plasma proteins according to their relative binding affinities for this material and is principally associated with a fraction having electrophoretic mobility between the alpha-1 and alpha-2 globulins. They examined a nephrotic urine which had a PBI of 8.6 micrograms per 100 ml. with a total iodine of 15.4 micrograms per 100 ml. and an albumin concentration of 2 gm. per 100 ml. Recant [537] reported an abnormality in thyroxine binding in the serum of nephrotic patients which has also been described by Robbins et al. [560]. Further studies by these investigators [561] indicate that the serum proteins which interact with thyroxine are normal from a physical standpoint. The urine in one nephrotic patient was found to contain thyroxine in combination chiefly with thyroid-binding protein. Excess thyroxine added to this urine became associated with albumin.

Since many of these investigations are highly technical and confusing to the average reader, we shall provide a summary which attempts to present a unified although perhaps oversimplified explanation of thyroid function in the nephrotic syndrome.

We have seen that there are considerable variations in glomerular permeability in patients with different types of the nephrotic syndrome, and even in patients at different stages of the same disorder. It is perhaps unfortunate that many investigators of the more esoteric aspects of protein binding have failed to relate their data either to the proved cause of the nephrotic syndrome or, preferably, to the glomerular permeability as reflected by the microscopic changes in biopsy, the calculation of the permeability coefficient, or the distribution of proteins in the urine. It seems reasonable that the amount of thyroxine-binding protein (alpha-1 to alpha-2 globulin or prealbumin) should vary with glomerular permeability. If a deficiency should develop, presumably secreted thyroxine might bind proportionately more to albumin or to other proteins. It is also reasonable that this compensation might be affected by the biologic spectrum of changes in serum proteins seen in patients with the nephrotic syndrome. If the net result of these compensations is a net loss of PBI, this represents the first step in a stimulus to the thyroid gland in the nephrotic patient. Some patients apparently respond by increased thyroid activity. Others do not. Failure to respond is presumably due to failure of the pituitary-thyroid axis since exogenous stimulation is possible. Pituitary failure may, in turn, be related to protein deficit since similar alterations in response occur among patients with partial hypopituitarism or with hypogonadism, and among patients maintained for a long time on a rice diet. The nephrotic rat is able to compensate by increasing his rate of iodine uptake and thyroxine secretion to restore a normal PBI and oxygen consumption. The human nephrotic patient rarely achieves this degree of compensation. Both humans and laboratory animals may have some problems in peripheral utilization, but the stimulus to thyroid hyperfunction may well be initiated by protein loss.

Some Speculation. The predominant considerations thus far have been concerned with the physiologic phenomena, and very little attention has been directed to the regulation of these phenomena. The essential question is, why does the patient with the nephrotic syndrome apparently fail in some way to respond to excessive urinary protein losses of thyroxine? Is it because his protein metabolism is essentially anabolic, with a normal or supernormal rate of albumin synthesis? Is it a direct effect of the antigen-antibody reaction on the pituitary-thyroid axis, or is the problem fundamentally one of heat balance? Most nephrotic patients sweat poorly and their edematous surface layer may act as an insulating blanket minimizing heat loss and the demand for caloric expenditure, which is further decreased in most cases by immoblization or bed rest. Since furry animals do not depend on skin for heat loss, perhaps their ability to compensate for urinary thyroxine losses is made possible by the added condition of a normal heat loss, a physiologic mechanism that is denied to the edematous, nephrotic patient.

AMINOACIDURIA AND TUBULAR DYSFUNCTION

There have been scattered reports of aminoaciduria in the course of untreated nephrotic syndrome in children. This subject has been reviewed by Hooft and Herpal [307]. The diverse reports may be grouped into three categories:

1. Reports of no significant increase in urinary excretion of free amino acids [34].

2. Reports of hyperaminoaciduria only under special conditions such as treatment with high-protein diet [64, 640], administration of protein hydrolysates [463], treatment with ACTH [567], and the presence of intercurrent infections such as infectious hepatitis [307].

3. Reports of particular patterns of aminoaciduria in particular nephrotic patients. Woolf and Giles [720] found hyperaminoaciduria in 25 out of 28 children with uncomplicated nephrotic syndrome. The patterns of amino acid excretion seem to fall into groups. H pattern is characterized by compounds no longer containing α-amino nitrogen (e.g., ethanolamine, β-aminoisobutyric acid, taurine) and somewhat lesser quantities of tyro-

sine, leucine, and valine. R type contains amino acids which may be found in blood but rarely in normal urine. These are chiefly proline, leucine and isoleucine, valine, and alanine. Hooft and Herpal [307] analyzed 58 urine samples from 10 nephrotic patients who had been followed closely, and 25 urine samples from 12 other nephrotic patients who were followed occasionally. In the active stage, before treatment, either a normal aminoaciduria or a characteristic kind conforming to the R pattern was found. Only one patient, and this was during the course of infectious hepatitis, showed hyperaminoaciduria resembling the H pattern [720].

In a few patients the R pattern was found independently of any therapy and was interpreted to indicate a tubular dysfunction. It may occur in combination with renal glycosuria and decreased phosphate reabsorption. The clinical course of patients showing hyperaminoaciduria with the R pattern differed from that of patients with uncomplicated "lipoid" nephrosis. One patient developed a complete de Toni-Fanconi syndrome and two others showed unresponsiveness to ACTH with progressive development of further tubular dysfunction. Defects in tubular function were also noted by Stanbury and Macaulay [641], who made observations on a nephrotic child with aminoaciduria, glycosuria, polyuria, tubular acidosis, and potassium depletion. Similar experiences have been reported by others [307, 663, 667]. We have seen one child with cystinosis and edema with hyperlipemia. It is not clear in many of these cases whether the tubular dysfunction resulted from persistent proteinuria or whether the tubular dysfunction and the proteinuria resulted from the same original insult. Simultaneous injury to both tubule and glomerulus is understandable, especially in the case of those nephrotic syndromes which are due to nephrotoxic injury. Quantitative studies of amino acid excretion have been carried out in this country by Shreeve et al. [619] and in Japan by Sumida

[652]. Great caution must be observed in the handling and preservation of urine specimens containing plasma proteins, since artifactual breakdown of protein moieties may be mistaken for aminoaciduria.

In studying tubular syndromes in nephrotic patients, it is of critical importance to use untreated cases, since some of the immunosuppressive drugs used in treatment have been thought to produce acquired tubular dysfunction [91]. We have reported one patient with acquired renal tubular acidosis and later nephrotic syndrome following renal homotransplantation with multiple rejection episodes that were reversed by large doses of steroids and immunosuppressive agents [431].

PHYSIOLOGIC ABERRATIONS IN THE
NEPHROTIC SYNDROME

Clinical investigation of patients with the nephrotic syndrome has proved to be a rich source of increased understanding in many areas of pathologic physiology. Besides those that have already been mentioned in a specific context, the recent literature reports hypomagnesemia [374, 375], hypocalcemia [338], increased catecholamine excretion [505], alteration of blood fibrinolytic activity [384], factor IX deficiency [256], transferrin deficiency [270], increased urinary excretion of iron [117], abnormalities in urinary lactic dehydrogenase, alkaline phosphatase, and lysozyme [223], and TAMe esterase activity [381].

Experimental Nephrosis

Transient syndromes in animals bearing a clinical and laboratory resemblance to the nephrotic syndrome in humans have now been produced in a wide array of species by a remarkable variety of technics. Some of these syndromes have appeared to involve primarily an immune mechanism, others a direct nephrotoxicity, and still others varying combinations of the two. Interpretations drawn from experimental nephrotic syndromes have been criticized on the ground that marked biologic differences in the disease are produced as one goes from species to species with the same basic method, or from method to method with the same species. Few investigators would claim that they have an absolute analogue of human nephrotic disease in laboratory animals; yet modern understanding of the clinical nephrotic syndrome has been enormously enriched by the contributions of investigators working with experimental nephrosis. This has been accomplished largely by providing conceptual models or by testing the validity of various suggested mechanisms for the pathogenesis of the nephrotic syndrome. Some of the attempts to produce experimental glomeru-

lonephritis are summarized in Table 16-10. Our account of the development of experimental nephrosis is limited to a brief description of the major types.

AVIAN ANTISERUM NEPHROSIS

This has also been called the delayed or biphasic type. The classic experiment uses anti-rabbit-kidney duck serum, which characteristically has produced a nephrotic syndrome in rabbits after a latent period of four to five days, although Seegal [605] described certain high titer duck anti-rat-kidney serum and duck anti-rat-lung serum made with Freund's adjuvant [200] which are capable of producing an immediate onset of disease.

The mechanism of avian nephritis has usu-

Table 16-10. Experimental Nephritis-Nephrosis

Investigator	Reference[a]	Donor Species	Antibody-producing Species	Recipient Species	Interval of Injection to Onset
Lindeman	481	Rabbit	Guinea pig	Rabbit	Immediate
Masugi	532	Rat	Rabbit	Rat	Immediate
Smadel	772–775	Rat	Rabbit	Rat	Immediate
Seegal	753	Rat[b]	Rabbit	Rat	Immediate
Heymann	365, 366, 382	Rat	Rabbit	Rat	Immediate
Steblay	481	Dog	Rabbit	Dog	Immediate
Stickler	481	Dog	Rabbit	Dog	Immediate
Mellors	481	Rabbit	Goat	Rabbit	Immediate
Steblay	799	Human	None	Sheep	Unknown
Masugi	533, 534	Rabbit	Duck	Rabbit	5+ days
Fouts	266	Dog	Chicken	Dog	5+ days
Kay	437	Rabbit	Duck	Rabbit	4+ days
Lange	471, 480, 481	Rabbit	Duck	Rabbit	4+ days
Lange	481	Rat	Duck	Rat	3+ days
Stavitsky	481	Rat	Duck	Rat	3+ days (some immediate)
Lange	481	Rabbit	Chicken	Rabbit	4+ days
Seegal	754	Rabbit[c]	Duck	Rabbit	Variable, sometimes immediate

[a] Reference numbers are found in *Diseases of the Kidney* (1st edition), pages 411–444. Boston: Little, Brown, 1963.
[b] Placenta rather than kidney.
[c] Freund's adjuvant [200].

ally been explained by the following scheme: (1) Rabbit kidney acts as an antigen when injected into a duck. (2) The duck forms antibody against rabbit kidney which is localized in the globulin fraction. (3) Reinjection of duck globulin into the rabbit produces a harmless combination of rabbit kidney antigen and duck globulin antibody which localizes on the kidney. (4) The rabbit regards duck globulin as a foreign protein. (5) The rabbit makes antibody against it. (6) The combination of rabbit antiglobulin and previous antigen-antibody complex reaches a high titer within three to five days and in the presence of serum complement produces nephritis.

Kay [351] has demonstrated that prior injection of duck serum into the rabbit eliminates the latent period. Seegal's data suggest that dosage of antibody may play a role since some ducks provided pools of antisera which elicited an immediate nephrotic syndrome [605].

MAMMALIAN NEPHROTOXIC
ANTISERUM NEPHROSIS

This type has also been termed immediate, monophasic, direct, passive transfer, and rat-type. Masugi [432] injected rat kidney into rabbits and produced a serum containing potent anti-rat-kidney antibodies capable of producing glomerular changes in as little time as four hours. This technic was thoroughly explored by Smadel and Farr [622–624] but was originally considered to be an analogue of diffuse glomerulonephritis. Later workers [249, 629] observed thickening of the capillary basement membrane after multiple injections of antiserum, and this technic has subsequently been used as a model for the nephrotic syndrome [292]. As noted in Table 16-10, a similar experimental syndrome has been produced using other species systems, including various combinations of rabbit, guinea pig, rat, dog, and goat. It has also been developed with other tissues, such as placenta.

The generally accepted mechanism has the following scheme: (1) A specific protein in the kidney of species A (e.g., rat) when injected into species B (e.g., rabbit) acts as an antigen. The antibodies may be fortified by using numerous immunizing injections. (2) When the serum from the rabbit is given to a rat, immediate disease is produced. (3) Complement falls sharply for less than 24 hours, suggesting a direct antigen-antibody reaction between the affected organ (glomerulus) and the antiorgan antibody.

The initial lesion of nephrotoxic serum nephritis best fits the concept of passive transfer of antibodies. Pfeiffer [521], Stavitsky et al. [643], and Lange [389] have demonstrated rapid drops in serum complement shortly after the injection of potent antibody-containing serum, and Lange and Wenk [398] have done experiments perfusing rat kidney with blood of constant complement level. With the addition of nephrotoxic serum, most or all of the complement is removed on one passage through the kidney. Ehrich and his colleagues [143–146] have shown that the clinical experimental disease as well as the histologic picture can be graded in proportion to the dose of nephrotoxic serum used, so that a spectrum may be achieved ranging from mild proteinuria with transitory edema to the more classic, severe syndrome of hypoproteinemia, hyperlipemia, and azotemia. Basement membrane thickening was seen within 1 to 1½ days.

Seegal [605] has developed an extremely potent nephrotoxic antiserum by prolonged immunization lasting three to four months when the organs were incorporated in Freund's adjuvant and five to six months using saline suspensions. Potent sera could be obtained by immunization with kidney, placenta, or lung, but anti-rat-brain serum and anti-rat-serum serum failed to localize in glomeruli. Anti-rat-aorta serum could localize in the glomeruli to some extent but failed to produce disease. There was a variation in the pattern of response to the injection of all other nephrotoxic sera. In some animals an immediate onset of a nephrotic syndrome occurred,

be accomplished with the rat's own kidney.

The mechanism of antigen-antibody interaction as a basis for autoimmune mechanism has been reviewed by Najjar [485–490]. When an antibody molecule reacts with an antigen molecule, a change in surface configuration of the two parts is produced in the resulting complex. This change may give rise to new antigen sites involving either antigen surface, antibody surface, or their adjoining surfaces. Specific antibody would then form against the new antigen sites on the complex. Where antibodies so formed react with their respective sites, a still newer complex is formed, with further alteration of surface, which can provide additional antigen sites. In like manner further complexes are subsequently formed. This process might well be self-perpetuating and continue as long as antigen is present. Theoretically, it should stop when antigen disappears from the organism or when no further alteration in surface configuration is obtained.

Najjar and Robinson [489] report experimental data to support this concept. It may be summarized as follows: (1) It is possible to absorb exhaustively a sample of rabbit antiserum to a given antibody-antigen complex yet leave behind antibodies that react only with free antigen. (2) It is possible to fractionate antisera and obtain fractions that react only with antibody-antigen complex. (3) Rabbits injected with rabbit antibody-antigen complex prepared from other immunized rabbits show in some animals antibodies that do not react with antigen but react only with complex. (4) It is possible in a large complex to aggregate many more antibody molecules on an antigen of smaller size than could possibly be accommodated because of steric hindrance.

This concept therefore implies that an antibody molecule normally considered familiar and nonantigenic to an organism may in the same animal, as a consequence of altered configuration caused by union with antigen, be rendered unfamiliar, foreign, and thereby antigenic. The production of possible disease by

such a mechanism involves the variables of dose, localization, solubility, and time, and perhaps one of the problems in the transfer of autoimmune disease from animal to animal has been failure to use the proper antibody or allow sufficient time for secondary antibody formation to occur. A recent experiment by Hess et al. [280] which demonstrated the transfer of experimental nephrosis by the transplant of lymph nodes from animals whose somatic antigen "memory" development was previously altered by the injection of spleen cells may represent a major link between our understanding of experimental nephrosis and our present concepts of human nephrotic syndrome as a continuing autoimmune disease involving antibody-antigen reaction. Grupe [243] has presented an in vitro demonstration of cellular sensitivity in experimental autoimmune nephrosis in rats. Much recent interest and investigative effort has been expanded on a genetically transmittable autoimmune disease in NZB mice. The nephrotic syndrome is one of the autoimmune and immunoproliferative diseases that occur in the NZB/BL mice in hybrids [452].

OTHER FORMS OF EXPERIMENTAL NEPHRITIS

Fisher et al. [190] have explored experimental renal vein constriction in relationship to the renal lesions observed in human renal vein thrombosis producing the nephrotic syndrome. Exudative, proliferative, and necrotizing lesions of glomeruli have been produced by a variety of experimental procedures. Many of these are really reactions to foreign protein such as may be obtained by injecting bovine gamma globulin or horse serum into rabbits [144, 264, 599], rabbit anticollagen serum into rats [576], or human basement membrane into sheep [644]. These syndromes, if fulminating, may be characterized by heavy proteinuria but rarely produce a condition resembling the human nephrotic syndrome. If anything, they are probably better models for collagen vascular disease. Similarly, "diffusion chamber nephritis" [159, 357] and experimental nephritis using type 12 beta-hemolytic streptococcal polypeptide in monkeys are probably better models for acute poststreptococcal nephritis than for the nephrotic syndrome.

Clinical Features of the Nephrotic Syndrome

As seen in the sections on *Etiology* and *Incidence,* the nephrotic syndrome is a rare disease with an extraordinary list of etiologies and occurring in varied clinical settings which can easily overshadow it. It is unusual, therefore, for a physician in a single lifetime to be able to study the nephrotic syndrome in the broad context of its many ramifications. The history, physical examination, and laboratory findings of patients with the nephrotic syndrome must always be considered in relation to both the underlying disease and the abnormalities due to the nephrotic syndrome itself. At one end of the spectrum a patient may present, for example, with all manifestations of disseminated lupus erythematosus, while her nephrotic syndrome remains solely a laboratory diagnosis and may go undetected unless she is subjected to the necessary blood and urine examinations. On the other hand, a patient may present only with the nephrotic syndrome, due to some obscure cause, such as wool allergy or inunction of a mercury-containing ointment. In such instances, the manifestations of the underlying disease may be so subtle as to be clinically undetectable, and the clinical findings are then wholly attributable to the nephrotic syndrome.

The most frequent item in the histories of nephrotic patients is edema. It is often quite subtle, and may be localized to the periorbital, scrotal, or abdominal wall or pedal areas. Its onset may be almost impossible to date. Many patients have related that, in retrospect, their edema had been accumulating for weeks or months. The patient shown in Figure 16-17

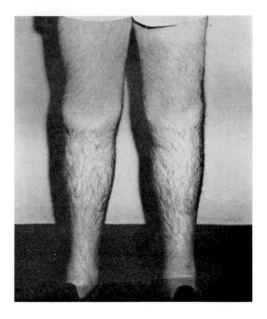

Figure 16-17. Hydrarthrosis and asymmetrical nephrotic edema.

failed to note the hydrarthrosis and leg edema for a period of six months. Edema may be cyclic, aggravated by excessive periods of salt intake or by premenstrual factors. Intermittent mediastinal widening has been noted on x-ray films in nephrotic patients. The lateral roentgenogram may be valuable [221]. Nephrotic edema may simulate cardiac compression [81] and produce skin pallor, falsely suggestive of anemia. In children, orbital edema may impair vision. The patient may also complain of severe anorexia, lassitude, or bizarre headaches, or may present with anxiety, depression, or other psychologic symptoms. Labial swelling in young girls and scrotal edema in young boys will be rarely mentioned by mothers unless specific searching questions are asked. On physical examination, findings due to the nephrotic syndrome consist of edema in any part of the body, wet retinal sheen on funduscopic examination, and skin pallor. Muehrcke [476] has reemphasized the paired white lines in the fingernails which have for a long time been known as a sign of

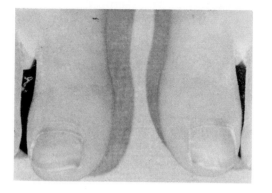

Figure 16-18. Paired parallel white lines in the nails of the great toes of a young girl with the nephrotic syndrome and hypoalbuminemia.

chronic hypoalbuminemia. Figures 16-18 and 16-19 illustrate some of the nail changes that may be seen in nephrotic patients. We have made a point of watching the fingernails and toenails of all our nephrotic patients, and have found a rather wide range of fingernail abnormalities. The major ones are a broad white band occupying the lower two-thirds of the nail bed or occasionally the entire nail bed, a whitening of the normally pink part of the nail with associated pinking of the normally white half-moon, and paired white lines which are seen best when viewed in an oblique light. These appear to be most often due to the blanching out of selective areas of the hemoglobin-filled capillaries of the nail bed, presumably by localized bands of edema. In occasional patients, however, the white bands appear to be imbedded in the nail itself. In patients with advanced disease, signs of fluid in the chest may be detected by physical or x-ray examination, and in children ascites and umbilical herniation are not uncommon.

Nephrotic children are known to have a markedly increased susceptibility to infection, and bacterial sepsis may occur [708]. Many

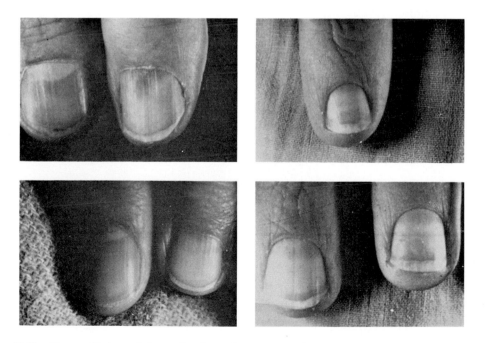

Figure 16-19. Fingernail signs of the nephrotic syndrome. *Upper left*: Normal nail on left. Patient's nail on right. The semilune of the patient is red and soft. The nail bed is white. *Lower left*: Normal nail on left. Note the broad white band on patient's nail. *Upper right*: Parallel white lines and red semilune. *Lower right*: Broad white band combined with single horizontal thin white line.

clinicians make a conscious attempt to isolate nephrotic patients from exposure to infected persons in public places, and to minimize the extent and frequency of hospitalization or to use reverse isolation procedures when available. In patients on corticosteroids and immunosuppressive agents, a wide variety of bacterial yeast and fungal infections have been seen. A fatal case of strongyloidiasis has been reported [114].

Nephrotic "crisis" consists clinically of fever, leukocytosis, prostration, a sudden change in affect, abdominal pain, vomiting, distention, and constipation. This may be confused with an abdominal disorder requiring surgery. In the preantibiotic area, such crises were usually due to pneumococcal peritonitis and were associated with hypoaminoacidemia [176]. In recent years, we have also seen such episodes from staphylococcal enterocolitis, from enteritis secondary to antibiotics, and from localized collections of edema. Eruptive xanthomas may be seen in nephrotic patients with lipidemia [140, 201].

LABORATORY DIAGNOSIS

A listing of the laboratory features in the nephrotic syndrome should distinguish those due to the underlying disease from those due to the nephrotic syndrome per se. The former are considered under the specific diseases discussed elsewhere in this volume. The blood abnormalities most commonly found in the nephrotic syndrome are gross lactescence in serum, marked elevation of the sedimentation rate, elevation of the serum cholesterol, which may occasionally exceed 1000 mg. per 100 ml., and elevation of cholesterol esters, triglycerides, phospholipids, and low-density lipoproteins on ultracentrifugation. The serum albumin level is generally decreased. Urine abnormalities include persistent proteinuria, which is occasionally increased by erect posture, by intravenous infusions of fluid and albumin, and by steroid administration. As seen in Figure 16-6, there is a bimodal distribution of protein excretion in patients with a wide variety of frequently encountered renal disease when the glomerular filtration rates are reasonably normal. Patients with the nephrotic syndrome are characterized as excreting in excess of 3 gm. of protein per 24 hours per 1.73 square meters of body-surface area (Fig. 16-20). A history of excessive foaming and stickiness of urine may be helpful in dating the onset of massive proteinuria. Most character-

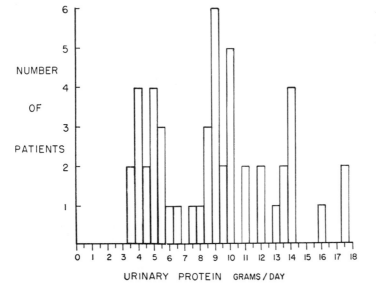

Figure 16-20. Quantitative excretion of protein in a group of nephrotic patients.

istic urinary findings, however, are detected only on careful microscopic observation of freshly voided urine.

URINARY SEDIMENT IN THE NEPHROTIC SYNDROME

The value of careful microscopic examination of the urinary sediment cannot be overestimated in both the diagnosis and the management of the nephrotic syndrome. This is the simplest and least expensive form of laboratory examination, is carried out with no discomfort to the patient, and is constantly available for repeated examinations. In many causes of the nephrotic syndrome, sedimentary changes may occur early, before obvious clinical and chemical signs of the syndrome develop, and may persist after chemical abnormalities have improved. In fact, we have followed some patients during an interval of apparent remission between exacerbations and have found the persistence of abnormalities in the urinary sediment (especially fat bodies) to be the only objective manifestation of a continuing disease process.

Because of the marked proteinuria, the sediment is usually characterized by a profusion of casts. In discussing these, we prefer the following descriptive classification [592]:

Classification of Urinary Sediment Contents

A. Urinary casts
  1. Plain casts
    a. Pure hyaline (transudation believed to be a protein gel)
    b. Hyaline-granular (matrix is Tamm-Horsfall; granules are serum proteins)
    c. Waxy (both Tamm-Horsfall and albumin diffuse in matrix)
  2. Plain cast with inclusions: Red blood cells, white blood cells, renotubular cells, doubly refractile fat bodies, bacteria, fat, bile-stain granules, etc.
  3. Epithelial (desquamation): Fresh, granular, fatty, broad, and gouty
  4. Casts of unusual composition: Bence Jones, myoglobin, globin, and amyloid
  5. Pseudocasts: Packed urates, red blood cells, white blood cells, mucus threads, sperm, and artifacts

B. Other formed elements in the urine
  1. Cells originating in the blood: Red blood cells, white blood cells, lymphocytes, histiocytes, plasma cells, etc.
  2. Erythropoietic cells (extramedullary erythropoiesis)
  3. Cells originating in the kidney: Renal tubular cells, foam cells, etc.
  4. Neoplastic cells: Especially lymphoma, carcinoma, mycosis fungoides, etc.
  5. Cells from the lower urinary tract: Transitional-squamous
  6. Cellular inclusions: Cytomegalic, rosette, LE cell
  7. Bacteria, mycelia, yeast, and parasites such as Trypanosoma
  8. Crystals
  9. Sperm
  10. Other

The most important characteristic of the urinary sediment of the nephrotic patient is the presence of lipoid material. This may be present in any of the following forms:

1. Degenerative fatty vacuoles in the fragmented cytoplasm of desquamated renal epithelial cells.

2. Coalescent droplets of neutral fat which appear to be deposited in the cytoplasm of epithelial cells and in casts and stain red with Sudan or oil red-O (Fig. 16-21).

3. Neutral fat droplets in the urine (Fig. 16-22).

4. Oval fat bodies which have a yellow or

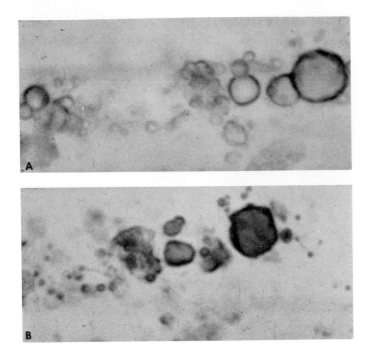

Figure 16-21. A. Fat droplets within a hyaline cast in nephrotic urine. B. The same cast with the droplets stained with Sudan III. ×860.

black appearance on reduced light and may occur singly or in aggregates.

5. Birefringent and/or anisotropic crystals called doubly refractile fat bodies (DRFB), which are crystals of cholesterol esters (Figs. 16-23, 16-24).

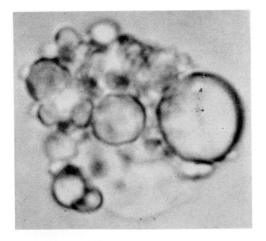

Figure 16-22. Neutral fat droplets in the urine from a nephrotic patient.

Degenerative fatty vacuolation may occur as a postmortem change, but fat bodies and DRFB's represent vital deposits formed during the cell's life. They must therefore represent an abnormality of fat storage or transport, or possibly they are evidence for an extrahepatic site of cholesterol synthesis. Munk [481] is generally credited with having made the first observation on the diagnostic importance of refractile fat bodies in the nephrotic syndrome, and the observation has subsequently been confirmed by many others [206, 403, 532, 544, 569, 589, 592, 686]. Doubly refractile fat bodies have recently been found useful in the study of nephrotic syndrome among Filipinos [120].

Anisotropism, or the exhibition of different physical properties when tested along axes of different directions, is a property of many crystals, and the sporadic finding of an isolated fat body should not be overinterpreted. For example, many forms of lubricating jelly commonly used for catheterization and some forms of uric acid crystals are doubly refractile.

Several points of technic are worth noting. The ideal equipment is a polarizing microscope or Nicol prisms which include a polarizer and analyzer. Less expensive polarizing films are available [589] but are of poor optical quality. Some of these films contain optical artifacts, and should not be left in place during the conventional microscopic examination, but should be inserted into the visual field only when the polaroids are to be crossed (Fig. 16-23). In examinations with a standard monocular microscope, we use an intact ocular to scan sediments, pick out epithelial cells, fat bodies, granular casts, etc., at a magnification of 50 to 200; we then swing a filter holder containing a polarizing film into the condenser and employ a separate ocular in which a film has been permanently installed. The light source should be fairly bright. The classic "Maltese cross" appearance of doubly refractile fat bodies will be apparent only if they are in sharp focus, and one should keep focusing up and down with the fine adjustments during the examination. In ordinary light the DRFB's have bright achromatic Maltese crosses with dark crossed lines which rotate when the stage is rotated. With the insertion of a red quartz filter, the cross lines may be optically stained a bluish-green against the red background. When viewed in unpolarized light, casts containing fat bodies may be easily mistaken for granular casts.

DRFB's frequently exist as one large crystal surrounded by small satellite crystals (Fig. 16-24). They may occur free in urine but are more typically seen in the cytoplasm of degenerating or intact renal epithelial cells. It is said that the lipoprotein-polysaccharide com-

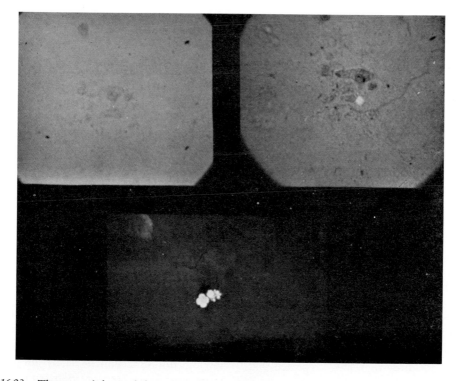

Figure 16-23. The upper left panel shows a renal epithelial cell under reduced light. In the upper right panel, the light source is partially polarized, delineating the nucleus and the anisotropic crystal. In the lower panel the Maltese cross appearance is typical of doubly refractile fat bodies.

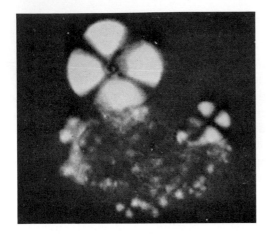

Figure 16-24. Doubly refractile fat body and satellite crystals.

plex which forms the infiltrative material in Kimmelstiel-Wilson disease contains birefringent crystals when thin frozen sections are observed under polarized light. We have noted prominence of free DRFB's, as distinguished from those in epithelial cells, in the urine of patients with known Kimmelstiel-Wilson disease and with less than "nephrotic" amounts of proteinuria. It is possible that in this situation the DRFB's may be coming from a source other than renal epithelial cells. DRFB's have been seen in patients with a nephrotic syndrome due to membranous glomerulonephritis, chronic glomerulonephritis, amyloidosis, syphilis, lupus erythematosus, leptospirosis, renal vein thrombosis, and in the Kimmelstiel-Wilson syndrome with or without a nephrotic syndrome. They have also been seen in the healing stage of acute renal insufficiency, and rarely in patients with severe arteriosclerosis in whom epithelial cells are desquamating as a consequence of nephrosclerosis. They may also be seen in gout, but are difficult to distinguish from the doubly refractile forms of uric acid crystals.

Quinn and Zimmerman [532] reported that oval fat bodies exhibiting anisotropism usually coexist with others which do not. Visible evidence of anisotropism depends upon the orientation of each crystal in the light field. They believed that anisotropic fat bodies were clearly indicative of renal parenchymal disease. Walz and James [687] examined 3633 urine specimens and found DRFB's 23 times in the urine from 22 patients with a wide variety of medical diseases. Fat bodies were not consistently present in repeated examinations of urine from any one patient. It is probably not wise to assign significance to the DRFB's when the urine might contain uric acid crystals or an unknown foreign material, or when the presence of an isolated Maltese cross is a sporadic and inconsistent finding.

In our own laboratory, a search for doubly refractile fat bodies was carried out on fresh urine from 152 nephrotic patients. On initial examination all but 17 had significant oval fat bodies or DRFB's in their urine. In our earlier series of 45 patients [56] with nephrosis proved by tissue study, all urine examinations were done personally by the investigators, and DRFB's were found in every instance. It is probable that the real incidence of DRFB's depends to a considerable extent on the interest, persistence, and skill with which they are sought.

There have been attempts in the past to relate the presence of DRFB's to the degree of hyperlipemia. Figure 16-25 demonstrates no difference in the median value of the serum cholesterol in the presence or absence of fat bodies in the urine. Normal urinary fat (less than 11 mg. per liter) has been found in a small number (12 patients) of diabetic patients [78]. Urine fat is elevated in acute alcoholism, but has not been well studied in the various etiologies of the nephrotic syndrome.

In patients who have a membranoproliferative disease, the urinary sediment may also reflect glomerular damage. The severity of the damage may be graded according to the following findings, which reflect progressively more severe degrees of glomerulitis: (1) a small number of red cells; (2) many red cells; (3) hyaline casts with red cell inclusions (Fig.

Figure 16-25. Scattergram showing the relation of serum cholesterol to the presence or absence of fat bodies in the urine. Most nephrotic patients had fat bodies, but the median serum cholesterol did not differ in the group with fat bodies absent.

16-26); (4) blood casts; and (5) blood casts with fibrin strands. When an exudative lesion is present, there may also be leukocytes, and rarely leukocyte casts. When these are associated with bacteriuria, they are frequently due to a superimposed bacterial pyelonephritis seen as a complication of the nephrotic syndrome. In patients with chronic glomerulonephritis, dilatation of distal tubules and collecting ducts may lead to the passage of large, broad (renal failure) casts. Either hyaline or granular casts which have remained in situ for a long time may take on a highly refractile or waxy appearance.

Figure 16-26. Red cells, free and included in a hyaline cast, from the urine of a 10-year-old girl with membranoproliferative glomerulonephritis and a clinical nephrotic syndrome.

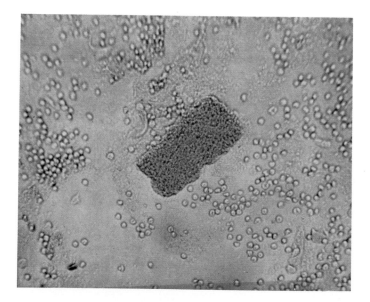

Patients with the nephrotic syndrome secondary to collagen disease tend to have a greater spread in the stage of involvement among the glomeruli which leads to alterations in the urinary sediment which include almost all those alluded to earlier. Such sediment is often referred to as a "telescoped" urinary sediment [592] (Table 16-11), and may rarely be found in selected cases of chronic glomerulonephritis when the nephrotic syndrome has been superimposed on the late renal failure stage of the nephritis [590]. More frequently, however, telescoped urinary sediment is found in systemic lupus erythematosus and other collagen diseases, as listed in Table 16-11. We have also seen it in the nephritis associated with subacute bacterial endocarditis.

Special Forms of Nephrotic Syndrome

HEREDOFAMILIAL, INFANTILE, AND CONGENITAL NEPHROSIS

Hereditary transmission with a more than chance occurrence in particular families has long been recognized in certain cases of pyelonephritis, interstitial nephritis, glomerulonephritis, and a number of renal tubular disorders. True hereditary chronic nephritis (congenital hereditary hematuria [205], Alport's syndrome [11], hereditary familial congenital hemorrhagic nephritis) is a term used for the familial association of a nephropathy together with varied combinations of other abnormalities, such as nerve deafness, polyneuropathy, and ocular defects (especially cataracts, spherophakia, and anterior lenticonus) [519]. The nephrotic syndrome, on the other hand, has been rare in multiple siblings and has generally not been listed in classifications of heredofamilial diseases. There have been increasing reports, however, of the occurrence of the nephrotic syndrome in two or more siblings [11, 32, 117, 165, 205, 212, 244, 252, 257, 262, 314, 343, 373, 446, 447, 497, 509, 519, 530, 679, 696]. Not all of these reports, however, have adequately differentiated between hereditary, congenital, and infantile nephrotic syndromes. A workable classification of the neonatal nephrotic syndromes follows:

1. Nephrotic stage of hereditary chronic nephritis (Alport's syndrome)
2. Familial nephrosis
3. Congenital nephrosis [358]
   a. Microcystic disease
   b. Congenital membranous glomerulonephritis
   c. Congenital syphilis
   d. Renal vein thrombosis
   e. Cytomegalic inclusion disease [723]
   f. Other diseases
   g. Malaria [632]
4. Infantile nephrosis

Table 16-11.   Urinary Findings in the Separate Stages of Glomerulonephritis

Acute	Nephrotic Syndrome	Chronic
Red cells	Massive albuminuria	Decreased albuminuria
Hyaline casts with red cell inclusions	Hyaline casts	Pigmented granular casts
	Cellular casts, vacuoles	Waxy casts
Blood casts	Oval fat bodies	Broad, renal failure casts
Positive benzidine test	Doubly refractile fat bodies	

Telescoped in

1. Collagen kidney — periarteritis, lupus erythematosus, progressive systemic sclerosis (scleroderma), angiitis.
2. Focal necrotizing glomerulonephritis (subacute bacterial endocarditis).
3. Rare cases in which exacerbation of chronic glomerulonephritis follows nephrotic syndrome.

The nephrotic syndrome may occur in patients with hereditary chronic nephritis with or without any of the other features associated with Alport's syndrome. Several such cases have already been reported [373, 509, 562]. It is a rarity, however, occurring in less than 1 per cent of patients with the disease. The nephrotic syndrome is then superimposed much as any syndrome may be superimposed on any stage of glomerulonephritis. In familial nephrosis the syndrome is simply seen in two or more siblings without other features of hereditary chronic nephritis. In the case of congenital nephrosis, the syndrome may be secondary to an insult in utero [244], or to other known specific causes or congenital diseases, such as congenital syphilis [164, 528]. Infantile nephrosis is simply the nephrotic syndrome occurring in the first year of life [215, 314, 343, 446, 516, 721]. The patient reported by Grupe et al. [244] was particularly interesting since the patient had an abnormality of external genitalia, suggesting a maturation arrest at about seven weeks' gestation. There is a possibility that the nephrotic syndrome originated with the same insult. The patient also developed an iron-deficiency anemia, which is more frequent in the very young nephrotic patient [117].

Vernier et al. [679] have reported detailed studies on four children with familial nephrosis. It was diagnosed in two of the children at the age of 4 months and in one at the age of 5½ years; the other child exhibited proteinuria in the first urine voided after delivery. There was a strong family history of multiple allergies, and the mother had had scarlet fever and had developed hypertension, edema, and albuminuria during the last trimester of each of her four pregnancies. Transplacental circulation of an antikidney antibody and autoimmunization against some product of the placenta were among the mechanisms considered, but no antibodies specific for glomeruli could be detected in maternal serum by a fluorescent tagging technic.

Experimental nephrosis has been produced by injection of rabbit antidog placental serum [192, 604]. The familial form of nephrosis is generally more severe, begins at an earlier age, is more resistant to treatment, and carries a poorer prognosis than the sporadic disease. In the case of specific causes of congenital nephrosis, such as malaria or syphilis, the underlying disease should, of course, be fully treated.

PROLIFERATIVE GLOMERULONEPHRITIS

Proliferative glomerulonephritis is one of the prominent lesions encountered in nephrotic patients. In children it may be the result of streptococcal infection. It differs from the more usual acute hemorrhagic glomerulonephritis in having a membranous component which leads to protein loss and the nephrotic syndrome.

Clinically the diagnosis of acute proliferative glomerulonephritis is based upon the presence of hematuria and blood casts, early azotemia which diminishes on healing, and acute elevation of the blood pressure. Confirmation is obtained by renal biopsy.

Some investigators think that steroids should be withheld from patients with proved proliferative glomerulonephritis. This conviction is based on the observation that steroid therapy fails to alter the clinical course of hemorrhagic glomerulonephritis and that the prognosis of children with proliferative disease is less favorable than those with minimal change or lipoid nephrosis, and also less favorable than some varieties of membranous glomerulonephritis. The well-controlled multistation study of the British Medical Research Council suggests that steroid therapy is of no avail in patients with proliferative glomerulonephritis.

In our series, 18 patients, or approximately 10 per cent of the total, were found to have acute proliferative glomerulonephritis. Histologic confirmation was obtained in seven. Age at the time of diagnosis ranged from 2 to 76 years (median, 13). Twelve of the 18 patients received corticosteroids, with six achieving a group 3 to 4 response, and three entering upon complete remission.* Four had a group 1 response and two showed no response, one of these dying within a month. Among the six patients who did not receive early steroid therapy, there were no complete remissions; one patient made a group 3 response, three a group 1, and two a group 0 response, with one death.

Long-term follow-up (mean, 33 months; median, 16 months) has been possible with seven patients having acute proliferative glomerulonephritis. All but one of these were treated with steroids initially. Four of the seven progressed to complete remission without subsequent steroids. Three who remain on steroid treatment continue to have a group 3 response.

Except for the two deaths from proliferative glomerulonephritis, which occurred in each case with a BUN greater than 200 mg. per 100 ml., there was no firm correlation of therapeutic response with either maximal BUN or maximal proteinuria. However, of the six patients making a group 3 to 4 (favorable) response, five had maximal proteinuria of less than 5 gm. per 24 hours, while five of eight patients making a less satisfactory response had proteinuria greater than 5 gm. per 24 hours. Five patients with a satisfactory response were under 4 years of age, and all of the patients who have achieved a long-term complete remission were less than 4 years old at the onset of the disease. There was only one patient under age 4 with an unsatisfactory response. From this small group, it appears that the age at onset has an important bearing in the prognosis of acute membranoproliferative glomerulonephritis.

AMYLOIDOSIS

Amyloidosis, which is discussed in greater detail in Chapter 21, is characterized by the variable local and general deposition of an un-

known intercellular substance related to protein metabolism. Since it may be distributed irregularly through various organs, a wide spectrum of clinical findings is produced. Both course and prognosis are uncertain. Except in the case of amyloidosis secondary to a known suppurative process, there is no specific form of therapy.

Although there are many mixed or overlapping cases, a useful working classification of amyloidosis may be formulated as follows:

1. *Primary or "atypical" amyloidosis.* The material stains metachromatically and is irregularly distributed. The heart, tongue, skin, and gastrointestinal tracts are favorite sites.

2. *Secondary or "typical" amyloidosis.* This form is associated with known predisposing diseases such as long-standing suppuration, ulcerative colitis, rheumatoid arthritis, lymphoma, and familial Mediterranean fever [109]. Favorite sites are the kidneys, thyroid gland, liver, spleen, and adrenal glands.

3. *Amyloidosis which is a complication of multiple myeloma.* Amyloidosis occurs in 5 to 10 per cent of myeloma patients.

4. *Tumor-forming amyloidosis.* The predominant sites are the larynx, trachea, mediastinum, bronchi, heart, and skin. This form of amyloidosis occurs preponderantly in males.

The theories of the pathogenesis of amyloidosis include disturbances in general or local protein metabolism, an antigen-antibody reaction with precipitation in tissues, a primary abnormality resembling neoplasia in the reticuloendothelial system, a direct relationship to hyperglobulinemia with amyloid as a possible intermediary and abnormal form of gamma globulin, and the concept that amyloidosis may be a degenerative disease that promotes the formation of pathologic ground substance. Hallen and Rudin [251] have recently studied 51 cases of pericollagenous amyloidosis.

* The grouping of responses is explained on page 581.

Experimental amyloidosis has been produced in rabbits by injection of pus from caries, sodium caseinate, rabbit globulin, and ribonucleotide, and by high cholesterol feeding. It has been produced in mice by eggs, milk, and cheese, and by injection of Friedländer's bacillus; in ducks by methyl cholanthrene; and in all these animals by injection of staphylococci, pseudomonas, and endotoxin. It is also observed in horses that are given repetitive injections and used as donors for diphtheria antitoxin.

Giles and Calkins [216] have studied the differential staining properties of secondary amyloid and have noted that it is eosinophilic with hematoxylin and eosin, anachromatic with methyl violet, has an affinity for Congo red, is periodic acid–Schiff positive, stains yellow with Verhoeff's and van Gieson's elastic tissue stain, and is negative to Schultz's stain, Sudan III, Baker's acid hematin stain for phospholipids and Feulgen's stain for deoxyribonucleic acid. Amyloid also stains dark brown with iodine, blue with iodine and sulfuric acid, red with crystal violet, red with gentian violet, and violet with methyl violet. Some forms of amyloid also exhibit autofluorescence. It appears from histochemical studies that amyloid infiltrates are protein-polysaccharide complexes of varying compositions. In the glomerulus on electron microscopy, they give a foamy appearance and both electron and polarization microscopy suggest deposition in a fiber pattern with a periodicity of about 100A.

Renal involvement occurs in about three-quarters of patients with secondary amyloidosis, in a third of patients with multiple myeloma, and in a quarter of those with the primary form. The reported incidence in secondary amyloidosis has been as high as 93 per cent. In a rather large series reported by Rukavina et al. [578], renal involvement was present in 27 per cent of 154 cases of primary systemic amyloidosis.

Although chronic suppuration is the classic background, secondary amyloidosis has been described in connection with a rather formidable number of conditions. A partial list would include tuberculosis, empyema, bronchiectasis, lung abscess, osteomyelitis, syphilis, actinomycosis, ulcerative colitis, regional enteritis [686], dysentery, subacute bacterial endocarditis, pemphigus, malaria, leprosy, rheumatic fever, paranasal sinusitus, rheumatoid arthritis, familial Mediterranean fever [109], diabetes mellitus, gout, thermal burns, cirrhosis, Hodgkin's disease, leukemia, and carcinoma of the bronchus and stomach. In suppurative diseases in which the gamma globulin concentration has been distinctly elevated due to infection, there may be a sharp decrease in the serum gamma globulin concentration coinciding with the development of amyloidosis. This is probably due to a decreased synthesis of complete immunoglobulins, a view which is supported by the coincident excretion of excessive quantities of low molecular weight and light-chain fragments of the Bence Jones type in the urine of patients with secondary amyloidosis.

It has generally been taught that hypertension and renal failure are relatively rare in amyloidosis as distinct from other forms of renal disease. Impaired renal tubular reabsorption of bicarbonate has been reported in renal amyloidosis [604]. In Bell's series there was a 17 per cent incidence of hypertension in 40 patients without uremia and a 50 per cent incidence in 20 patients with uremia. Zuckerbrod and his colleagues [728] extracted 347 cases of secondary amyloidosis from the literature and added 39 of their own. In this series of 386 patients, 138 had renal insufficiency — an incidence of about 36 per cent. About one-fifth of the patients in Zuckerbrod's own group had hypertension, and the other investigators reported incidences varying from 4 to 35 per cent. Death due to progressive hypotension has been reported [97].

Primary systemic amyloidosis is a much rarer disease than the secondary type and only infrequently has produced an overt nephrotic syndrome. Muehrcke et al. [479], in 1955, reported only 10 cases of nephrotic syndrome due to primary amyloidosis in the English literature. Rukavina et al. [578] reviewed 154 cases and found evidence for renal involvement in 42 (27.2 per cent) with an age range from 15 to 78 years (mean, 44 years).

The common complaints in primary amyloidosis are weakness, easy fatigability, and weight loss, with albuminuria in persons with renal involvement. Almost any other constellation of symptoms may be seen in an individual case, depending on the pattern of organ involvement. A number of cases have been reported in which the diagnosis was finally made as a result of curiosity concerning eye symptoms. Specific findings have been diplopia, sudden blindness, inability to keep the eyes open, blurring of vision, and progressive visual defects. One of the earliest ocular signs is the occurrence of perivascular retinal deposits, which appear to form first around the wall of the capillaries, then about arteries, and later on the surface of cells. Opacities of the vitreous may also be seen. Both peripheral and central neurologic findings are common.

A familial form of primary amyloidosis was first described by Ostertag [512]. In the family studied by Rukavina et al. [578] about half the patients had an abnormal or poorly resolved alpha-2 globulin demonstrated by free electrophoresis. Similar protein patterns were found in 13 unaffected members of the family who were younger. Nephrotic syndrome with amyloidosis due to familial Mediterranean fever has also been reported and could be responsible for amyloidosis in multiple siblings [109].

In our own series, six patients with histologically proved amyloidosis were seen. Three cases were secondary to chronic ulcerative colitis, Hodgkin's sarcoma, and tuberculosis. Three other patients had no apparent antecedent disease, and these cases were considered instances of primary amyloidosis producing the nephrotic syndrome (Fig. 16-27). The mean age at the time of the diagnosis, which was unsuspected until the advent of the nephrotic syndrome, was 50 years. Duration of survival after diagnosis ranged from one month to four years. Chemical changes in amyloidosis are, in general, either confusing or noncontributory; there is therefore no substitute for a tissue diagnosis. In patients who have albuminuria or the frank nephrotic syndrome, the tissue of choice is, of course, that obtained by renal biopsy [429, 596].

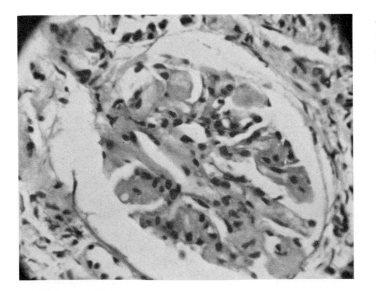

Figure 16-27. Glomerulus from a renal biopsy on a patient with nephrotic syndrome due to amyloidosis.

The importance of serial examination is emphasized by Muehrcke et al. [479] and has been amply confirmed in our own series. One patient treated with steroids at an early stage of her disease had a sharp rise in endogenous creatinine clearance and PSP excretion. This was apparently due to a nonspecific effect of the steroids in expanding extracellular fluid volume, although a sharp drop in the permeability index was demonstrated at the same time. Renal biopsy revealed a progression of the glomerular lesion. A year later a second trial of corticosteroids produced a precipitous fall in glomerular filtration rate from 88 to 20 ml. per minute. After steroids were discontinued, the C_{CR} rose to 77 ml. per minute. Later a nonspecific rise in endogenous creatinine clearance occurred shortly after an intravenous infusion of albumin. The chemical data are summarized in Table 16-12. In four other patients with amyloid disease proved by tissue diagnosis, edema was refractory to therapy, an uncommon event in cases of the nephrotic syndrome of other etiology. The serum proteins in the amyloid patients showed a consistent decrease in albumin, alpha-1 glob-

ulin was normal, alpha-2 globulin was elevated in four out of five, and beta and gamma globulin showed no striking deviation. Figure 16-28 shows macroglossia in a patient who had the nephrotic syndrome and myxedema from thyroid infiltration by primary amyloid.

DIABETIC GLOMERULOSCLEROSIS

Other names for this disease are intercapillary glomerulosclerosis, Kimmelstiel-Wilson syndrome, diabetic nephropathy, and Kimmelstiel-Wilson glomerulonephropathy.

Although albuminuria in diabetic patients has been noted for centuries, a reasonably firm association between diabetic nephropathy and the nephrotic syndrome was not established until 1936, when Kimmelstiel and Wilson [367] described concentric hyaline masses in glomerular lobules of elderly diabetic patients. Despite the prevalence of the edema of congestive heart failure in this type of patient, they were adroit enough to describe the edema in the patients of their own series as nephrotic. Clinicians interested in diabetes seized upon this new entity and created the concept of "Kimmelstiel-Wilson syndrome."

Table 16-12. Physiologic Measurements in a 45-Year-Old White Female with Primary Amyloidosis and the Nephrotic Syndrome

Date	BUN Cr (mg./100 ml.)		Protein Excretion (gm./ day)	(mg./ min.)	Serum Albumin (mg./ ml.)	C_{ALB}	C_{CR}	Permeability Index[a]	Serum Cholesterol (mg./ 100 ml.)	Remarks
3-22-57	10	1.05	6.0	4.17	10	0.417	73	5.7	450	Before prednisone
7-31-57	17		2.5	1.74	18	0.097	126	0.8	550	After prednisone
1-17-58	16	2.15	5.4	3.75	19	0.197	88	2.2	530	
4-30-58	21		6.9	4.8	18	0.267	20	14.8	516	
9-21-58	19	0.55	11.4	7.9	15	0.527	103	5.1	516	After intravenous albumin
4-3-59	20	1.1	7.9	5.5	28	0.196	49	4.0	512	

[a] $C_{ALB}/C_{CR} \times 10^3$.

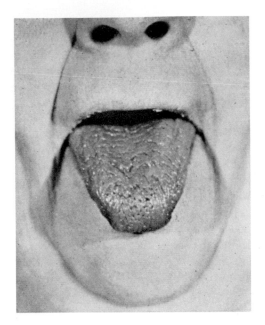

Figure 16-28. Macroglossia in a woman with primary amyloidosis, nephrotic syndrome, and myxedema (a rare complication).

The basic criteria are long-standing diabetes, hypertension, significant albuminuria, and edema. Rogers and his colleagues [564, 565] reviewed these criteria in relation to the structural lesion in 100 consecutive cases, and found that 32 per cent of the patients who met the criteria of the clinical syndrome did not have the histologic correlate. Conversely, in 57 patients who had the lesion at autopsy, it had not been diagnosed during life. This led many subsequent observers to conclude either that the criteria were incomplete or that the nodular lesion originally described was not, in fact, the structural correlate of the nephrotic syndrome. In our view, both criticisms appear to be valid. It has more recently been found that nodular glomerulosclerosis is usually, if not always, accompanied by the diffuse lesion and that the nephrotic syndrome may occur with the diffuse lesion in the absence of the nodular lesion. Gellman et al. [210] correlated the clinical findings with those of renal biopsy. They found that the increasing severity

of diffuse diabetic glomerulosclerosis was closely associated with increases in diastolic blood pressure, proteinuria, serum urea nitrogen, and serum creatinine levels, and with decreases in serum albumin concentration and urea and creatinine clearances. It was also associated with increased frequency of ketosis, retinopathy, edema, and the nephrotic syndrome. They suggested that "the abnormalities associated with the presence of nodular glomerulosclerosis are in fact caused by the diffuse glomerulosclerosis which invariably accompanies the nodular lesion."

It is also apparent that the original clinical criteria [158] for Kimmelstiel-Wilson syndrome are both too general and too limited. More exact criteria for diabetic nephrotic syndrome are:

1. A history or the proved presence of diabetes mellitus
2. Quantitative protein excretion in the nephrotic range
3. Variable diastolic hypertension
4. Variable edema of the nephrotic type
5. Hypoalbuminemia
6. Hyperlipemia, especially hypercholesterolemia and an abnormal pattern of serum lipids
7. Doubly refractile fat bodies in the urine, preferably "free"
8. Reduction in renal function
9. Retinal microaneurysms
10. Elevated alpha-2 globulin with normal alpha-1 and gamma globulin

No counterpart of the Boston City Hospital [564, 565] study has been published using modern clinical criteria. It is our own and the general experience [210], however, that a satisfactory renal biopsy in patients selected by the above clinical criteria shows diffuse glomerulosclerosis in almost 100 per cent. Since the numerous names for this disease have led to confused thinking, it is preferable to use the term "diabetic nephrotic syndrome" for the clinical entity meeting these new criteria and the term "diffuse diabetic glomerulosclerosis" for the pathologic entity now believed to be its clinical correlate.

In addition to the semantic problem, understanding of the nephrotic syndrome in diabetes has been complicated by vague descriptions of the pathology and by the usual occurrence of multiple pathologic entities in the biopsy and autopsy sections of diabetic patients. The following diagnostic terms are the most satisfactory for reporting the pathology revealed by renal biopsies in these patients:

Intercapillary glomerulosclerosis
    Diffuse — Nodular
Nephrosclerosis
    Mild — Moderate — Severe
Pyelonephritis
    Acute — Focal — Chronic — Interstitial
Papillitis
    Acute — Necrotizing — Healed
Fatty nephrosis
Glycogen nephrosis

To formulate a reasonably complete descriptive diagnosis from renal biopsies on diabetic patients, one must carefully examine the glomeruli for eosinophilic thickening between the capillary loops (diffuse glomerulosclerosis; Figs. 16-29, 16-30), concentric nodular infiltration (nodular diabetic glomerulosclerosis; Fig. 16-31), atrophied fibrosis, and hyalinization of the glomerular tuft (ischemic glomerulosclerosis). Other changes include exudative lesions, capillary aneurysms, adhesions within Bowman's capsule, periglomerular fibrosis, foam cells, and fat in blood vessels [66, 84, 263]. One also may find medial thickening (mild nephrosclerosis), medial and intimal thickening with early collateral formation (moderate nephrosclerosis), and gross thickening, hyalinization, PAS-staining deposits, and thickened collateral vessels (marked nephrosclerosis). Siperstein [621] has found thickening of capillary membranes in muscle in diabetic homozygotes without carbohydrate intolerance. In the interstitial tissue, one must search for fibrocytic proliferations, edema, cellular infiltrates composed of mononuclear and polymorphonuclear cells (both focal and diffuse), necrosis, and hemorrhage. In the tubules, one should search for atrophy, dilatation, fat deposits, necrosis, reactive hyperplasia, peritubular hyaline cuffing, vacuolization (the

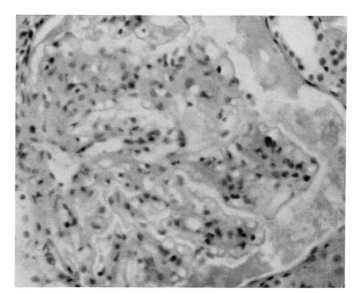

Figure 16-29. Diffuse diabetic glomerulosclerosis in an elderly diabetic with the nephrotic syndrome who had not been receiving insulin. Hematoxylin and eosin. ×400.

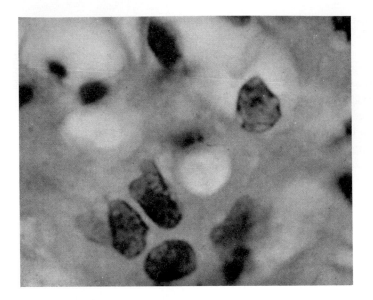

Figure 16-30. High power view of severe thickening of the capillary wall in a patient with diffuse diabetic glomerulosclerosis and nephrotic syndrome. Note the slightly foamy appearance. Hematoxylin and eosin. ×1800.

Armanni-Ebstein lesion), and intraluminal casts.

These findings may be summarized in descriptive terms as follows:

Glomeruli
  Eosinophilic thickening between capillary loops
  Nodular infiltration
  Glomerulosclerosis

Blood vessels
  Mild nephrosclerosis: medial thickening
  Moderate nephrosclerosis: medial and intimal thickening; early collaterals
  Marked nephrosclerosis: hyalinization; PAS-positive deposits; thickened collaterals
Interstitium
  Fibrocytic proliferation
  Edema

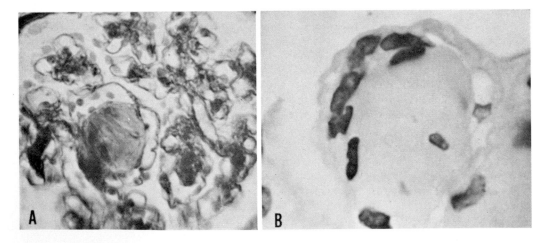

Figure 16-31. A. Nodular lesion in diabetic glomerulosclerosis. PAS. ×430. B. High power view of a single nodule showing displacement of endothelial cell nuclei. Hematoxylin and eosin. ×1800.

Cellular infiltrate — mono- and polynuclear,
    focal and diffuse
Necrosis and hemorrhage
Tubule
    Atrophy
    Vacuolization
    Fat deposits — exfoliative; doubly refractile
        fat bodies
    Necrosis

Using these criteria in examining both autopsy and biopsy material from diabetic patients over the past 20 years, we have found
that diabetic patients referred for evaluation of
a renal disorder because of suspicious findings
rarely if ever present with an isolated pathologic lesion. Rather, we have observed, in decreasing order of frequency, nephrosclerosis,
pyelonephritis, diabetic glomerulosclerosis,
fatty nephrosis, glycogen nephrosis, and papillitis. Papillary necrosis is an extreme complication of diabetic microvascular disease in the
kidney. The need for separation of the lesions
and estimation of the relative responsibility for
the patient's disorder consitutes one of the major indications for renal biopsy. Indeed, diabetic patients comprise about 15 per cent of our
entire renal biopsy series, which is now in
excess of 600 patients. An incomplete review
of this series includes 38 patients with proved
diabetes. In this group we found arteriolar
nephrosclerosis in 87 per cent, pyelonephritis
in 74 per cent, diffuse diabetic glomerulosclerosis in 37 per cent, and nodular diabetic glomerulosclerosis in 29 per cent.

Gellman and his co-workers [210], in the
largest renal biopsy series yet published, have
studied 53 diabetic patients who had at least
one renal biopsy. Eight had more than one
biopsy and nine were examined at autopsy.
Diffuse diabetic glomerulosclerosis was found
in 75 per cent, nodular diabetic glomerulosclerosis in 48 per cent, vascular lesions in 83 per
cent, interstitial fibrosis in 82 per cent, round
cell infiltration in 50 per cent, and 26 per cent
of these patients had clinical features of the

nephrotic syndrome. There is increasing
interest in studying the site of early deposition
of the infiltrate in diabetic glomeruli employing electron microscopy [54, 55, 171].

In our total series of 183 patients with the
nephrotic syndrome, 37 (20 per cent) had
diabetes mellitus documented by the history or
glucose tolerance studies. Three of these were
shown by renal biopsy to have pure membranous or chronic sclerosing glomerulonephritis.
The diagnosis in the remaining 34 was diabetic nephrotic syndrome on the basis of clinical and laboratory findings. In 20 of these
cases, the diagnosis was proved by histologic
evidence obtained through biopsy or postmortem examination, with the finding of diffuse
diabetic glomerulosclerosis. The mean age of
these patients at the onset of the nephrotic syndrome was 46.8 years (range, 26 to 72 years)
and the mean duration of known diabetes preceding the onset of nephrotic syndrome was
11.8 years (range, 1 to 30 years). Twenty-seven
of these patients have been available for follow-up study. Eighteen died after an average
survival of 3.3 years (range, 3 months to 12
years) from the onset of the nephrotic syndrome. For the nine patients still living
(1962), the mean survival time is 19 months
and the longest 6 years. Adequate blood pressure recordings for 28 of the diabetic patients
when they were not receiving antihypertensive
therapy showed diastolic hypertension in 21.*

Patients with diabetic nephrotic syndrome
have been treated with close regulation of the
diabetes mellitus, control of congestive heart
failure with early digitalization, mild sodium
restriction and diuretics when indicated, and
restriction of saturated fats in the diet. Diabetic
nephrotic syndrome has been considered a
contraindication to steroid therapy. Sexual
disturbances are more frequent in the diabetic
than in other nephrotic patients [322].

---

* Criteria: Over age 12, diastolic blood pressure greater
than 90 mm. Hg on multiple readings. Under age 12,
diastolic pressure greater than 70 mm. Hg on multiple
readings.

Comment. There is an open debate as to whether the nodular lesion of diabetic glomerulosclerosis is specific for diabetes or has been aggravated by insulin therapy, as suggested by Robbins [561] and by a study at the Boston City Hospital [319] in which all kidney sections from 42 diabetic patients autopsied prior to the introduction of insulin were reviewed, with the finding of only one case of nodular glomerulosclerosis.

There have been scattered reports in the past of intercapillary glomerulosclerosis in nondiabetic patients, although it is possible to quibble about the criteria for the absence of diabetes in specific cases as well as the criteria for the description of intercapillary glomerulosclerosis. In an examination of this subject [534], lesions resembling those of the Kimmelstiel-Wilson syndrome were found in 12 of 20 cases of necrotizing pancreatitis (also found in chronic pancreatitis [612]), 6 of 33 cases of alcoholic fatty infiltration of the liver, and 4 of 23 cases of alcoholic portal cirrhosis. The lesions were believed to be caused by embolization of mixtures of fat and lysed red cells. Most were of the exudative type [534].

Gellman and his colleagues [210] stated that "in 600 renal biopsy specimens and numerous autopsies, we have never seen nodular glomerulosclerosis in any disease other than diabetes mellitus." Proponents of this point of view have criticized reported cases on the ground that the criteria employed to exclude diabetes were inadequate; yet they themselves have related glomerulosclerosis to the duration of the diabetes. In the Gellman series the duration of the diabetes was 13.0 ± 6.9 years in 41 patients with diffuse diabetic glomerulosclerosis and 13.5 ± 6.3 years in 28 patients with nodular diabetic glomerulosclerosis. Indeed, it is possible that the use of the glucose tolerance test may serve to include patients who really do not have diabetes.

We have noted [598] that a very high proportion of uremic patients have diabetic-type glucose tolerance curves. Since many patients with diabetic nephropathy are presented for study during a stage of the disease when renal failure has already supervened, it is quite possible that truly nondiabetic patients with uremic hyperglycemia have been *falsely included* in studied series of "diabetic" nephropathy. Up to the present time, we have observed four patients with classic nodular glomerulosclerosis who have never overtly been clinically diabetic. In two of these cases, we were fortunate enough to obtain biopsies at an early stage of renal functional impairment, when glucose tolerance tests were normal. The renal biopsy specimen from one of these patients is shown in Figure 16-32. We therefore keep open the possibility of nondiabetic nodular glomerulosclerosis while acknowledging that it must, indeed, be rare [263].

SYSTEMIC LUPUS ERYTHEMATOSUS

Systemic lupus erythematosus (SLE) is a "collagen vascular" disease of unknown cause which is occurring or being diagnosed with increasing frequency in recent years. The disease occurs at all ages, but most often between 15 and 40, and there is a female preponderance of about 4:1. Physicians interested in anthropography have emphasized the typical occurrence of SLE in red-haired young women with a tendency to freckling or an inability to tan. However, many cases have been reported among Negroes and in persons of divergent types of skin. The disease occasionally occurs in families and in twins. A set of three-year-old identical twins has recently been reported in which one became nephrotic and the other nephritic [410]. Its general renal and systemic manifestations are considered elsewhere in this volume (page 838). The essential histologic features are "veruccal capillaritis" (focal thickening), focal hematoxylin bodies, hyaline thrombi, and advanced "wire-looping." Representative lesions are shown in Figure 16-33. Marked wire-looping is seen in Figure 16-34. Current pathologic technics have demon-

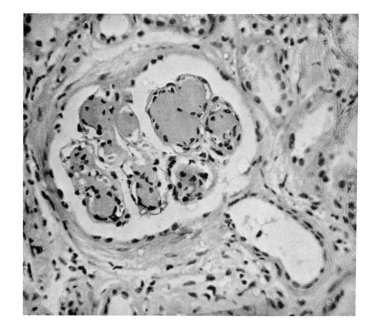

Figure 16-32. Nodular lesions in a nondiabetic nephrotic, uremic patient. Hematoxylin and eosin. ×140.

documen
Muehrck
tologic e
per cent
abnorma
incidence
markably
drome in
lier study
seven rep
phrotic sy
cases from

They a
hibited al
drome e
cases hav
nate tern
namic der
oped in th
patients
olemia at
We there
pseudo-ne
SLE is on
drome,
absence or
blood lipi
would the
drome, an
Presbyteri
[627], of
20 had bo
tients who
use of go
arthritis-li
tive LE tes
question r
really pat
rheumatoi
tivity to g
patient wi

The pos
for lupus
fluorescent
tion of gar
endothelia

strated many patients in whom light microscopy of the kidney is essentially negative, but in whom electron-dense antigen-antibody "complexes" and complement may be demonstrable on electron microscopy within the basement membranes. By immunofluorescent microscopy, immune globulins or complements may be seen deposited in the same areas (Fig. 16-35).

It is difficult to state the true incidence of renal involvement in SLE. Many of the larger series have been obtained from review of charts or by investigators whose orientation was not directed particularly to the kidney. In

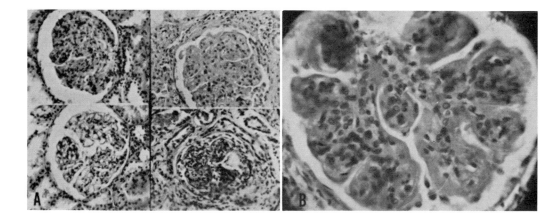

Figure 16-33. A. The range of glomerular lesions in four patients with lupus nephritis. Hematoxylin and eosin. ×136. B. Classic lobulation, homogeneous thickening, veruccal capillaritis, fibrinoid degeneration, and wire-loop thickening in the glomerulus of a young girl with systemic lupus erythematosus. She had a rapidly deteriorating clinical course and died within six months. Hematoxylin and eosin. ×400

There were two males and nine females. The mean duration of symptoms attributable to SLE was 2.7 years. At the time of onset of the nephrotic syndrome, the mean age was 34.4 years (range, 8.6 to 60 years). All 11 patients were treated with corticosteroids equivalent to 100 to 300 mg. of cortisone per day. In addition, four patients received nitrogen mustard after an unsatisfactory response to steroid therapy. We have seen a few patients become oliguric on high steroid therapy and recover on withdrawal. Both pericardial effusion [27] and retroperitoneal fibrosis [413] have been seen as special features of SLE in nephrotic syndrome. We have seen in a patient with Sjøgren's syndrome [87] a combination of keratoconjunctivitis sicca (sicca syndrome), xerostomia, and rheumatoid arthritis. Other renal effects reported are hyposthenuria [339], the Fanconi syndrome [615], and renal tubular acidosis [443, 472, 659, 711]. In the patients of Talal et al. [660] glomeruli were normal and free of immunoglobulin in those with renal tubular acidosis, but the glomeruli contained large amounts of IgM and a component of complement in the patients with glomerulonephritis. Hyperglobulinemic purpura occurred frequently in the patients with Sjøgren's syndrome and renal disease; the authors suggest that the three features of sicca syndrome, nonthrombocytopenic purpura, and renal tubular acidosis may constitute a clinical triad [660].

Treatment. Holman [305] has emphasized the importance of sustained high doses of steroids over long periods in patients with mild or moderate lupus nephritis. At the Rockefeller Institute, 40 to 50 mg. of prednisone are continued for two to seven months in SLE patients with renal involvement. At this dosage level arthritis, fever, pleuritic pain, and rash usually improve or disappear within a few days. Blood abnormalities change toward normal only after two weeks to a month or more of treatment. Hematuria is likely to persist for a minimum of two months. High doses of steroids are continued until proteinuria diminishes. The steroid is then slowly withdrawn, and the patients are maintained on antimalarial drugs. Of 38 patients so treated, 31 have returned to normal activity, five have died, and two have retained significant renal abnormalities. There have been 10 relapses within a period of 3½ years. Harvey has noted a death rate of about 10 per cent per year after the initial high mortality (13 per cent in three months) seen in hospitalized patients [88].

We have adopted a general approach similar to that of the Rockefeller group in recent years. The results are not reflected in our overall series, since many of these patients were studied before newer steroids were available and a significant number were specifically referred to us because of renal involvement not responding to massive steroid dosage. Among the 11 nephrotic SLE patients, a group 3 or 4 response was seen in three. In the remainder, proteinuria remained virtually unchanged although edema was usually controlled. We have noted particularly that some patients may achieve total remissions with steroids and that others are steroid-resistant but respond to nitrogen mustard. Two Negro females have achieved complete remissions of the nephrotic syndrome without developing renal failure.

In summary, systemic lupus erythematosus is responsible for a significant percentage of adult nephrotic syndromes. The nephrotic syndrome occurs in about one-third of lupus patients presenting with renal complaints. Disregarding the peripheral manifestations of SLE, features of lupus nephrotic syndrome are all typical except for decreased occurrence of hypercholesterolemia, and increased frequency of telescoped urinary sediments and severe hypertension. All patients with the nephrotic syndrome due to SLE should be given a prolonged course of corticosteroids in high dosage. Some patients will apparently worsen on this regimen, and oliguria has been seen. Those who fail to improve should probably be given a course of nitrogen mustard, 6-mercaptopurine, heparin, or other immunosuppressive agents.

CYCLIC NEPHROTIC SYNDROME

A number of frank allergies have been noted as causes of the nephrotic syndrome. Poison oak, bee stings, pollen [260], dust, and serum used in therapy have been among the allergens cited in review articles [345]. Insect bites, injections to minimize the incidence of respiratory infections, and poison ivy have been recorded in our own series. Rytand [583] studied the nephrotic syndrome in seven patients sensitive to poison oak. It is curious that subsequent recurrence of the nephrotic syndrome in demonstrably sensitive persons is extremely rare. Physicians with broad experience, however, can usually recall a case or two of recurrent nephrotic syndrome in allergic patients. Addis [4] has recorded at least three instances of patients with recurrent syndromes. Rytand and Cox [583] presented a detailed report of a patient who had at least six and possibly eight separate episodes of the nephrotic syndrome. Proteinuria was absent during remissions. They also reviewed the literature of what they call the "polycyclic nephrotic syndrome." Among these patients, two episodes started in December and January and the remainder in April to June. Allergic phenomena were prominent in the past history and in the acute episodes. Four relapses were related to infections or hay fever.

Nephrotic syndrome in pregnancy might well be included in the category of cyclic syndrome. We have one patient with chronic membranous glomerulonephritis and cyclic edema related to menses.

We have had occasion to discuss an interesting case of cyclic disease with Dr. Ethan A. H. Sims, and the following history is included with the permission of Dr. Sims, Dr. R. J. Reveillaud, and Dr. John W. Heisse.

Case History. A 24-year-old white farmer had a completely normal medical examination early in 1955. In June of that year, he had a severe respiratory infection with asthmatic manifestations and the onset of a severe nephrotic syndrome accompanied by accumulation of 20 pounds of edema. The blood pressure rose to 130/90. There were 8 per cent eosinophils on the blood film, a sedimentation rate of 20 mm. per hour, hypoalbuminemia of 1 gm. per 100 ml., hypercholesterolemia of 782 mg. per 100 ml., and massive proteinuria with two to three white blood cells per high power field and two to three granular casts. Inulin clearances were 97, 62, and 42 ml. per minute in successive clearance periods. PAH clearances were 697, 680, and 499 ml. per minute.

The patient responded to adrenocorticosteroid therapy with decreasing clinical manifestations of the nephrotic syndrome. The albuminuria disappeared by December, 1955. He was continued on steroid therapy and developed Cushingoid features. By February, 1956 the endogenous creatinine clearance was 128 ml. per minute. In July, 1956 he again developed respiratory infection, mild edema, hypoalbuminemia, and proteinuria of 3.9 gm. per day which cleared rapidly. In 1957 the patient remained symptom-free, and steroids were discontinued. In the summer of 1958, during the haying season, he noted the onset of burning of the eyes and sneezing while in a particular pasture in which his father had developed a skin rash. The allergic manifestations cleared, but albuminuria and edema supervened, and he gained 6½ pounds in weight. This episode was treated at once with 100 mg. of prednisone daily, and promptly subsided. In the latter part of the subsequent summers of 1959, 1960, and 1961 symptoms of hay fever developed, followed each time by recurrence of proteinuria and, at times, by mild edema. The patient monitored his proteinuria at home, and each episode was treated with steroids.

The pasture associated with the allergic reactions contained mainly timothy grass in addition to an undue amount of molds. Skin tests showed strong sensitivity to mill dust, but not to molds. There was no reaction to ragweed through 1958, but thereafter sensitivity developed to this as well as to most grasses. Complement-fixation tests for anti-renal antibodies in 1960 and 1962 were negative. Desensitization with mixed antigens was begun in the summer of 1959 and continued through the years to the time of writing (1970). In the winter of 1959 there was transient proteinuria associated with a respiratory infection, and in 1962 a relapse with edema and proteinuria of as much as 3 to 6 gm. per day. At this time an open renal biopsy showed increased glomerular cellularity with occasional neutrophils, but without eosinophilia. By electron microscopy there was slight to moderate thickening of portions of the basement membrane of glomerular capillaries and of Bowman's capsule. The endothelial and epithelial cells showed changes consistent with proteinuria. The patient has continued the regimen of desensitization to the present (1970), and coincidentally has had no further proteinuria and has been asymptomatic. In 1966 the BUN and cholesterol were normal and serum creatinine was 0.9 mg. per 100 ml. Figure 16-36 is a diagram of the clinical course of this patient. The scale of reference of prednisone therapy totals 100 mg. per day.

Rytand has taken the view that the glomerular lesion may persist during clinical remissions in some patients with the nephrotic syndrome and that cyclic nephrosis is probably not an exception to the observation that proliferative glomerulonephritis does not recur once it is healed. There is need for continued close observation of cases of cyclic nephrotic syndrome, and particularly for serial renal biopsies during the stages of remission and exacerbation. The management of such patients presents a rare challenge to the clinician interested in renal disease.

NEPHROSIS OF PREGNANCY

Wegner [693] called attention to the occurrence of the nephrotic syndrome with pregnancy and cited a frequency of 0.028 per cent. Others, such as Dieckmann and Eastman, have been quoted [529] as citing frequency of nephrosis in pregnancy consistently less than 0.1 per cent. Tillman [668] reported a frequency of between 0.025 and 0.050 per cent. Sporadic case reports of the nephrotic syndrome in pregnancy have appeared in the medical litera-

ture [197, 272, 278, 281, 492, 503, 529, 608]. A cause-and-effect relationship is difficult to assign when the syndrome occurs as a single episode during a pregnancy. There is no doubt that many types of organic renal disease may be coincidental with a pregnancy. These, combined with the known hemodynamic changes of the gravid state, may result in a slightly more florid clinical and laboratory picture.

Nephrosis of pregnancy is of importance to the obstetrician because its clinical features may appear for the first time during pregnancy. The syndrome may be mistaken for preeclampsia. Underlying renal disease may have an adverse effect on the pregnancy. Nephrotic patients have an increase of susceptibility to infections and thromboembolic disease. Severe proteinuria may affect pregnancy tests [360].

We have encountered in pregnant women classic acute poststreptococcal glomerulonephritis associated with hypertension and heavy proteinuria. We have also seen the nephrotic phase of chronic glomerulonephritis in pregnant women, and rarely diabetic intercapillary glomerulosclerosis. Moreover, there are a number of diseases which are aggravated by pregnancy in which the glomerular permeability may rise. This has been our experience particularly with systemic lupus erythematosus and renal involvement.

It has been pointed out [345, 525] that some patients with preeclampsia may have focal vascular lesions in the glomeruli and the small arterioles which may lead to increased proteinuria. We have had some experience in studying glomerular permeability and renal biopsies in patients with preeclampsia and have found that quantitative protein excretion often rises at the very end of pregnancy. In one or two instances it advanced into the nephrotic range a day or two before delivery. It is possible that if the gestation period had been longer, these particular individuals might have gone on to a full-fledged nephrotic syndrome. In general, however, obstetricians have made the

Figure 16-36. Clinical course of a patient with severe cyclic nephrosis from 1955 through 1962.

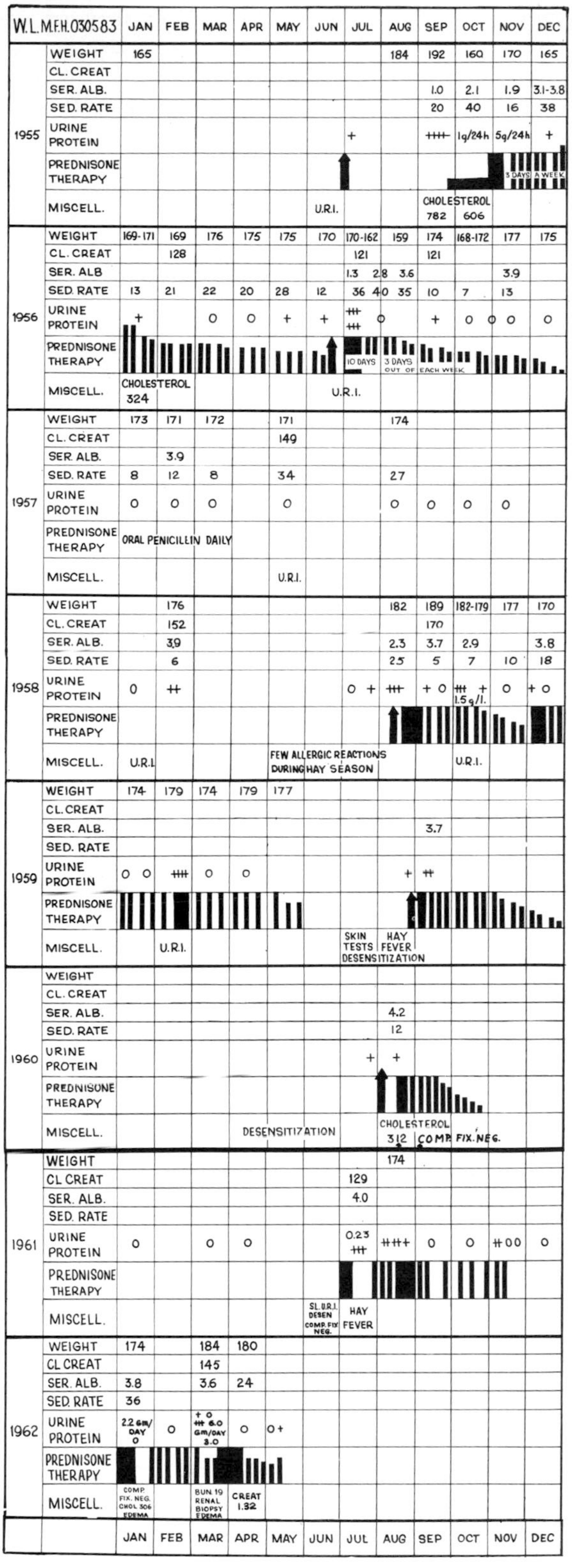

W.L.M.F.H.030583		JAN	FEB	MAR	APR	MAY	JUN	JUL	AUG	SEP	OCT	NOV	DEC
1955	WEIGHT	165							184	192	160	170	165
	CL. CREAT												
	SER. ALB.									1.0	2.1	1.9	3.1-3.8
	SED. RATE									20	40	16	38
	URINE PROTEIN						+			++++	1g/24h	5g/24h	+
	PREDNISONE THERAPY												5 DAYS A WEEK
	MISCELL.						U.R.I.			CHOLESTEROL 782	606		
1956	WEIGHT	169-171	169	176	175	175	170	170-162	159	174	168-172	177	175
	CL. CREAT		128					121		121			
	SER. ALB							1.3	2.8 3.6			3.9	
	SED. RATE	13	21	22	20	28	12	36 40	35	10	7	13	
	URINE PROTEIN	+		0	0	+	+	+++ +++	0	+	0	0 0	0
	PREDNISONE THERAPY							10 DAYS	3 DAYS OUT OF EACH WEEK				
	MISCELL.	CHOLESTEROL 324					U.R.I.						
1957	WEIGHT	173	171	172		171			174				
	CL. CREAT				149								
	SER. ALB.		3.9										
	SED. RATE	8	12	8		34			27				
	URINE PROTEIN	0	0	0		0			0	0	0	0	
	PREDNISONE THERAPY	ORAL PENICILLIN DAILY											
	MISCELL.						U.R.I.						
1958	WEIGHT		176						182	189	182-179	177	170
	CL. CREAT		152							170			
	SER. ALB.		3.9						2.3	3.7	2.9		3.8
	SED. RATE		6						25	5	7	10	18
	URINE PROTEIN	0	++					0 +	+++	+ 0	+++ 1.5g/l.	0	+ 0
	PREDNISONE THERAPY												
	MISCELL.	U.R.I.				FEW ALLERGIC REACTIONS DURING HAY SEASON					U.R.I.		
1959	WEIGHT	174	179	174	179	177							
	CL. CREAT												
	SER. ALB.									3.7			
	SED. RATE												
	URINE PROTEIN	0 0	+++	0	0				+	++			
	PREDNISONE THERAPY												
	MISCELL.		U.R.I.				SKIN TESTS DESENSITIZATION	HAY FEVER					
1960	WEIGHT												
	CL. CREAT												
	SER. ALB.									4.2			
	SED. RATE									12			
	URINE PROTEIN							+	+				
	PREDNISONE THERAPY												
	MISCELL.					DESENSITIZATION				CHOLESTEROL 312	COMP. FIX. NEG.		
1961	WEIGHT								174				
	CL CREAT							129					
	SER. ALB.							4.0					
	SED. RATE												
	URINE PROTEIN	0		0	0			0.23 +++	++++	0	0	++ 0 0	0
	PREDNISONE THERAPY												
	MISCELL.						SL. U.R.I. DESEN COMP FIX NEG.	HAY FEVER					
1962	WEIGHT	174		184	180								
	CL CREAT			145									
	SER. ALB.	3.8		3.6	24								
	SED. RATE	36											
	URINE PROTEIN	2.2 gm/DAY 0	0	+ 0 ++ 8.0 gm/DAY 3.0	0	0 +							
	PREDNISONE THERAPY												
	MISCELL.	COMP. FIX. NEG. CHOL. 506 EDEMA		BUN 19 RENAL BIOPSY EDEMA	CREAT 1.32								
		JAN	FEB	MAR	APR	MAY	JUN	JUL	AUG	SEP	OCT	NOV	DEC

diagnosis of nephrotic syndrome in pregnancy only when edema, massive proteinuria, hypo-albuminemia, and hypercholesterolemia have been present with a normal blood pressure. When hypertension coexists, most obstetricians would be inclined to classify such patients as having either preeclampsia or organic renal disease.

Finnerty [186] followed some 15 nephrotic patients who throughout pregnancy were maintained on corticosteroids, chlorothiazide, and supplemental potassium. Their course was favorable, with no superimposed toxemia. He reported four patients with what appeared to be toxemia of pregnancy in the last trimester who developed massive edema and albuminuria during the first two weeks after delivery. No explanation is at hand.

The term *nephrotic syndrome of pregnancy* should probably be reserved for cyclic nephrotic syndromes recurring with pregnancy and regressing after delivery and thus suggesting a sensitivity response to some product of the pregnancy itself. The mechanism might be analogous to that described above for cyclic nephrotic syndrome. Presumably this could represent a form of hyperimmunization, perhaps to a minor blood type of the fetus (with subsequent introduction of fetal cells into the maternal circulation) or to an abnormal protein in the placenta, or to some other product of pregnancy. Since separate recurrences of the nephrotic syndrome are rather rare, recurrences would at least serve to separate the true nephrotic syndrome of pregnancy from the coincidental disorders which may occur in the pregnant woman. In a case of deteriorating renal function, early delivery may be desirable, and in a case of recurrent nephrotic syndrome, the patient should, of course, be counseled against repeated pregnancies [493].

A rather striking example of cyclic nephrotic syndrome in pregnancy is illustrated in the following case history:

Case History. FIRST ADMISSON TO GEORGETOWN UNIVERSITY HOSPITAL. B. A., a 28-year-old white female, was admitted to Georgetown University Hospital on June 4, 1957, with the following history:

1947. Near the end of her first pregnancy, ankle swelling and a sudden increase in weight occurred, to a total gain of 55 pounds. Albuminuria, without hypertension, was noted by the obstetrician. There was normal term delivery of an infant weighing 6 pounds, 13 ounces.

1948. In her second pregnancy, at the fifth month, sudden edema again occurred, accompanied by intense albuminuria. Edema involved the legs and upper thighs. At the six-week checkup after this and the first delivery, albumin was absent from the urine. No particular studies were made.

1950. In her third pregnancy, there was slight swelling, localized to the ankles. She was not told of albuminuria, and the total weight gain in this pregnancy was 18 pounds (from 117 to 135 pounds).

1956. In her fourth pregnancy, marked edema leading to anasarca was noted in the fifth month (weight, 156 pounds). By the eighth month, pitting edema had spread above the level of the umbilicus and was accompanied by marked albuminuria. The patient was admitted to a community hospital, unable to walk and with such massive edema of the perineum that her obstetrician had grave fears about the mechanical problems involved in the delivery. We saw her in a single consultation when she was in critical condition with massive anasarca, and confirmed the presence of massive albuminuria, hypercholesterolemia, and doubly refractile fat bodies in the urine. She was treated with large doses of intravenous salt-poor albumin and acetazolamide, which promoted a diuresis during which she lost 22 pounds. Following this she went into normal labor and delivered an infant weighing 6 pounds, 7 ounces. She continued to have albuminuria and some edema and was treated with infusions of albumin periodically. Other symptoms included slight back pain, increasing nervousness, occasional substernal pain, one episode of sharp, hot pain in the interphalangeal joints of the third and fourth fingers of both hands, accompanied by swelling of the fingers, a single attack suggestive of hyperventilation syndrome, periods of crying spells and depression, and consciousness of the heart beat.

PAST HISTORY. Relevant past history included a tonsillectomy at age 6, an appendectomy at age 12, severe sore throat between the first and second pregnancies followed in 1 week by severe bilateral back pain which was diagnosed as pleurisy, and poor teeth, with many removed because of infection and replaced by a full upper plate. Administration of a sulfonamide drug once produced dizziness and a possible allergic reaction.

FAMILY HISTORY. The patient's father died at age 65 and had an unknown type of arthritis and heart trouble. Her mother died at age 66 with a heart attack and had a goiter. Two brothers and one sister were born dead. A maternal aunt had hypertension, and a daughter has urticaria.

HOSPITAL COURSE. During the first admission the patient had a limited ability to concentrate the urine (specific gravity of 1.011 to 1.013), 20 to 30 red cells and 2 to 4 white blood cells per high power field, 50 per cent glitter cells, occasional bacteria, doubly refractile fat bodies, oval fat bodies, oxalate crystals, and urate crystals. Some of the urine sample had many yeast cells. Quantitative protein excretion was 7.6 gm. per 24 hours. The Addis count revealed 107,000,000 red blood cells, 6,000,000 white blood cells, and 5,000,000 casts per 24 hours. The endogenous creatinine clearance in three determinations was 82, 104, and 103 ml. per minute per 1.73 square meters of body surface area with a plasma creati-

nine of 1.0 mg. per 100 ml. Phenolsulfonphthalein excretion was 30 per cent in 15 minutes, 15 per cent in 30 minutes, and 17 per cent in 60 minutes. There was no Bromsulphalein retention. The serologic findings were negative. There were gram-negative rods on stain of the urine, and a culture grew *Escherichia coli*. The hematocrit was 41 volumes per 100 ml., hemoglobin 12.8 gm. per 100 ml., white count 5700 per cubic millimeter, with 51 per cent segmented forms, 1 per cent band form, 40 per cent small lymphocytes, 6 per cent monocytes, and 2 per cent eosinophils. The results of serologic and LE cell preparations were normal. The cholesterol was 404 mg. per 100 ml., the total protein 4.4 gm. per 100 ml., with an albumin of 2.4 and a globulin of 2.0 gm. per 100 ml. The BUN was 25 mg. per 100 ml. Coagulation studies showed normal reactions.

A renal biopsy on June 10, 1957 (Fig. 16-37), showed some diffuse interstitial fibrosis with mononuclear infiltrate. There were foci of infiltration with polymorphonuclear cells. The glomeruli showed diffuse membranous thickening with proliferation. An area of fibrinoid necrosis was seen in one glomerulus.

The histologic diagnosis was subacute to chronic membranoproliferative glomerulonephritis. The patient was discharged with the diagnosis of nephrotic syndrome, cause undetermined —

Figure 16-37. Asymmetrical glomerular lesion in a renal biopsy specimen from a woman who had recurrent nephrotic syndrome associated with each pregnancy. Hematoxylin and eosin. ×215.

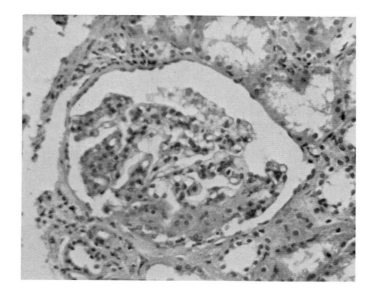

possibly due to chronic glomerulonephritis, with some clinical features suggestive of systemic lupus erythematosus and pyelonephritis secondary to nephrotic syndrome. Chloramphenicol was the only medication ordered.

SECOND ADMISSION TO GEORGETOWN UNIVERSITY HOSPITAL. The patient entered the hospital on August 25, 1958, in the eighth month of her fifth pregnancy, with swelling of the legs and ankles of three to four months' duration. She had had persistent albuminuria between her fourth and fifth pregnancies and had a continued elevation of cholesterol. There was no hypertension at any time. At about the third month of this fifth pregnancy severe edema was noted. With chlorothiazide therapy she was able to walk until she experienced a sharp rise in body weight accompanied by a rise in the serum cholesterol. The edema progressed despite salt restriction and diuretics, and she was admitted for study and a second renal biopsy.

PHYSICAL FINDINGS. The findings were: blood pressure 122/70, pulse 80, respiration 20, a grade 3 systolic murmur at the apical area and left sternal border, fetus in the ROA position, and 4+ pitting edema to the knees.

LABORATORY STUDIES. These studies revealed 2+ to 4+ proteinuria, quantitatively 6.4 and 7.3 gm. per 24 hours. On urinalysis there were hyaline, granular, and white cell casts, 1 to 3 red cells, 3 to 4 white cells, per high power field, renal epithelial cells, mixed casts with fatty material, oval fat bodies, doubly refractile fat bodies, and renal tubular cell casts. The serum protein was 4.8 gm. per 100 ml., with an albumin of 1.6 and a globulin of 3.2 gm. per 100 ml. The uric acid was 7.8 mg. per 100 ml., cholesterol 636 mg. per 100 ml., and esters 342 mg. per 100 ml. The test for cryoglobulin was positive.

COURSE. A second renal biopsy was attempted, but revealed only perirenal fat, capsule, and a small area of renal tubules without glomeruli. The patient was placed on prednisone, 40 mg. per day, chlorothiazide, and salt restriction. She lost 2½ pounds of edema and was discharged on August 30 from the hospital. Discharge diagnoses included chronic glomerulonephritis, possibly lupus in origin; hypersensitivity reaction aggravated by pregnancy; the nephrotic syndrome; nephrocalcinosis; and cryoglobulinemia.

INTERVAL COURSE. The patient had an un-eventful delivery on October 4, 1958, with subsequent diminution of edema but persistent hypertension and proteinuria. Delivery was at another hospital. Following this a tubal ligation was performed, and she was discharged home, where persistent bilateral lower abdominal pain and fever, headache, and lethargy were treated by her private physician. She proved to be anemic and was hospitalized elsewhere. She was found to have a hematocrit of 17 per cent, a BUN of 100 mg. per 100 ml., and thrombocytopenia. She passed a large bloody clot from the vagina, received a blood transfusion and some unknown injections, and was transferred back to Georgetown University Hospital on October 23, 1958.

THIRD ADMISSION TO GEORGETOWN UNIVERSITY HOSPITAL. When admitted to the hospital, the patient had a blood pressure of 170/90 and appeared pale and considerably more ill than on previous admissions. The hematocrit was 17.5 volumes per 100 ml., the hemoglobin 5.5 gm. per 100 ml., the platelet count 148,000 per cubic millimeter, the bleeding time 9 minutes, with >20 petechiae in a 2.5 cm. diameter ring on tourniquet test, a 2.9 per cent reticulocyte count, and a normal prothrombin time. It was believed that she had underestimated uterine bleeding and that the fall in hematocrit from 37 to 17 volumes per 100 ml. represented primarily acute blood loss. The stools were consistently guaiac-positive, and she had repeated emeses. The urinary sediment was unchanged, BUN 122 mg. per 100 ml., quantitative protein excretion 1.7 gm. per 24 hours, and the urine culture was positive, with a high colony count of paracolon, escherichia, and enterococci. The patient was given transfusions, digitalis, and antibiotics, and developed virtually all clinical manifestations of the uremic syndrome.

She was maintained by five hemodialyses during four weeks, with a stormy course including muscle twitching, pericardial friction rub, intermittent hematemesis, pulmonary rales, epigastric pain, dyspnea and lethargy, pleural effusion, ascites, peripheral edema, and episodes of coma. The chemical changes on the five dialyses are summarized in Table 16-14. Serum calcium determinations ranged between 9 and 9.5 mg. per 100 ml.

She was sent home for Christmas with her

Table 16-14. Chemical Changes in Patient B. A. on Five Hemodialyses

Dialyses	BUN	Creatinine	Uric Acid	Phosphorus	Na	K	Cl	CO$_2$
	(mg./100 ml.)				(mEq./L.)			(mM/L.)
November 4, 1958								
Before dialysis	315	14.0	12.5	22.8	135	4.7	100	8.6
After dialysis	113	6.8	5.2	9.1	143	4.4	108	19.2
November 13, 1958								
Before dialysis	205	12.0	6.7	7.1	131	3.9	116	14.5
After dialysis	83	5.9	3.5	4.4	135	3.9	108	23
December 1, 1958								
Before dialysis	91	13.8	13.8	—	128	5.1	98	22.4
After dialysis	48	6.8	6.2	—	142	4.0	102	24.5
December 12, 1958								
Before dialysis	99	6.2	12.5	10.9	130	6.5	89.3	18.6
After dialysis	40	7	7.2	7	133	4.9	102	20.4
December 22, 1958								
Before dialysis	93	13.2	11.2	9.7	134	5.1	91	19
After dialysis	53	8	7.8	6.5	136	4.2	93	24.8

family. She was moderately confused, exhibited compulsive water drinking, gained 10 pounds in three days, and was readmitted in pulmonary edema. The BUN was 154 mg. per 100 ml., and she was given an emergency ultrafiltration dialysis against 300 mm. Hg filtration pressure and an elevated bath glucose concentration varying from 600 to 800 mg. per 100 ml. She was dialyzed for six hours on the twin coil artificial kidney with a net loss of 7 pounds and improvement in pulmonary edema, but complained of loss of vision at the end of the dialysis; she escaped the restraints and pulled out her arterial cannula, with subsequent marked loss of whole blood. This was immediately replaced, and she demonstrated no circulatory problems as a result of the blood loss. She was given supportive treatment. Prednisone was reinstituted. However, she remained oliguric, and died on January 5, 1959.

At autopsy the heart was not enlarged but microscopically showed uremic pericarditis, pericardial fat necrosis, myocardial hypertrophy, focal myocarditis, and moderate coronary sclerosis. The lungs showed chronic pleuritis and pulmonary edema. There was ascites, and the liver weighed 1900 gm. and showed serous hepatitis and chronic passive congestion. The kidneys weighed 100 gm. each and showed subacute lobular glomerulone-phritis with arteriolar nephrosclerosis. The ovaries showed corpus albicans and multiple follicular cysts. There were no other organ changes. The vessels of the spleen were examined for systemic lupus erythematosus, but this was not seen.

FINAL DIAGNOSES. (1) Nephrotic syndrome with unusual deposition of fat in the glomeruli and tubules (Fig. 16-4). (2) Subacute lobular glomerulonephritis. (3) Nephrosclerosis. (4) Uremic syndrome including pericarditis, pneumonitis, pleural effusion, and a chronic passive congestion of multiple organs.

COMMENT. The patient is believed to represent a unique entity of cyclic nephrotic syndrome, probably produced by hyperimmune response related to some product of pregnancy. Certain features of her clinical course — notably, the single episode of joint pain and substernal pain — suggested systemic lupus erythematosus, but no pathologic or hematologic confirmation was possible. The nature of the sensitizing agent as a product of pregnancy was not identified.

SICKLE CELL DISEASE

Sickle cell anemia is included in our classification of the causes of the nephrotic syndrome (see page 504). Two of the patients referred [56] were, to our knowledge, the first reported examples of persons with a nephrotic syndrome occurring in sickle cell disease. Additional reports have appeared from other centers [30, 656]. Mostofi et al. [474] described in detail the pathologic lesions in kidneys removed for unilateral hematuria in sickle cell disease. There were stasis of sickled red cells in small vessels, and hemorrhages in the interstitium, tubules, and pelvis. Glomerular damage was conspicuously absent. Subsequently Bernstein and Whitten [58] studied kidney sections from 15 patients with sickle cell disease. Alterations in the pyramids were compounded of edema, telangiectasia, fibrous scarring, and obliteration of tubular elements. Enlargement, vascular dilatation, and increased vascularity of juxtamedullary glomeruli were noted in older children, and in the oldest patients there appeared to be progressive ischemia and fibrosis leading to glomerular obliteration. Renal failure developed in one of their patients. Berman and Tublin [57] have also reported physiologic studies on a third patient with the nephrotic syndrome. This 9-year-old boy with sickle cell disease had multiple glomerular lesions with pyelonephritis, a vasopressin-resistant concentrating defect [352], and gross hematuria. Administration of corticotropin had no significant effect. Focal asymmetrical glomerular hyalinization, which appears to originate in the region of the arteriole, has been described in all three reported cases (Fig. 16-38).

In summary, the nephrotic syndrome and sickle cell disease appears to be a new and real entity in which glomerular lesions are developed as a result of vascular dilatation and fibrosis presumably secondary to recurrent ischemia.

VASCULAR THROMBOSES

As indicated in the section on *Etiology*, renal vein thrombosis is now a well-recognized cause of the nephrotic syndrome [15, 26, 40, 65, 85, 122, 124, 130, 150, 172, 181, 247, 297, 327, 344, 407, 456, 465, 526, 671]. The nephrotic syndrome has also been reported after thrombosis of the aorta [681], the renal artery [517], and the pulmonary arteries [407]. Conversely, thromboembolism of the pulmonary artery has been noted as a complication of nephrosis [657]. The appearance of a very high concentration of protein in the urine may be quite sudden in this special form of nephrosis. The

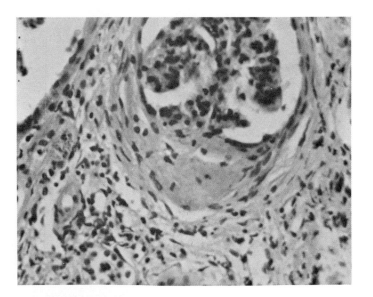

Figure 16-38. Focal glomerular fibrosis in region of afferent arteriole seen in a renal biopsy specimen from a 39-year-old man with the nephrotic syndrome and sickle cell anemia. Hematoxylin and eosin. ×300.

kidneys rapidly increase in size, and venography of the inferior vena cava shows absence of flow from one or both renal veins and roughening of the vena cava at the orifices of the renal vein. Renal venograms may also be helpful; the hippurate renogram is usually abnormal. Pathologic changes include thickening of the basement membrane, prominent margination of polymorphonuclear leukocytes in capillaries, marked interstitial edema, and on electron microscopy deposits of osmiophilic protein materials, both within and on either side of the basement membrane. Kowal et al. [379] reviewed the literature and found that 41 of 65 adults with renal vein thrombosis had a fatal termination within two months of onset and another 10 died within two years. Only 14 survived, and almost all had persistent proteinuria. Pollak et al. [526] reported complete clinical recovery after treating a patient with 75 to 100 mg. of heparin intravenously every four hours. The coagulation time was kept in excess of 30 minutes. Michon et al. [461] also reported improvement after infusion of large amounts of heparin into a patient with severe acute neonatal renal vein thrombosis.

MALIGNANCY NEPHROSIS

From an enormous outpouring of individual case reports and small studies, the problem of malignancy nephrosis has just recently emerged as an important special form of the nephrotic syndrome. The relationship is important in three major ways:

1. The nephrotic syndrome and other hypersensitivity or autoimmune manifestations may be an *early clue* to the diagnosis of malignancy. It may be clinically manifest months or even years before the cancer is diagnosable.

2. Malignancy or its catabolic products may initiate autoantibodies to produce the nephrotic syndrome and provide an important clue to pathogenesis.

3. Since immunosuppressive drugs are being used with increasing frequency in chronic states associated with the nephrotic syndrome, and since immunosuppression may defeat one of the body's defenses against neoplasia, a late-appearing malignancy in a treated patient may very well be a complication of treatment.

In addition to these considerations, a number of patients undergoing renal homotransplantation and treatment with immunosuppressive drugs and antilymphocytic serum have developed malignancy and, particularly, lymphomas. In some cases these were apparently transplanted with the kidney, and in others the relationship is not clear. Some patients undergoing chronic repeated rejection reactions in the long-term survival group from cadaveric homotransplantations have also developed the nephrotic syndrome. The interrelationship between these two occurrences is not as yet clearly delineated.

The autoimmune syndromes have recently been reviewed by Greenberg et al. [237]. They include manifestations resembling dermatomyositis [23, 99, 115, 234], chronic lymphocytic thyroiditis [99], systemic lupus erythematosus [138], and other collagen diseases [82].

It has been traditionally taught that the major association between malignancy and nephrosis lies in the secondary development of amyloidosis [112, 366, 542, 617, 716] (see section on *Amyloidosis*). There has also been an association between malignancy and renal vein thrombosis [129, 264, 444], and occasionally both causes [501]. Lee et al. [401] have reported 11 adult patients representing 10.9 per cent of their adult nephrotic series of 101 patients through the decade from 1953 to 1962 in whom cancer developed or was found at a closely related time (0 to 14 months) in the course of their nephrotic syndrome. This is well above the expected frequency of cancer, and there was no predominance of a specific tumor. In addition, causal associations have been suggested by others [98, 336, 491]. An association between the nephrotic syndrome and other forms of malignancy, including nephroblastoma, has been noted [105, 133, 425, 729].

There have been at least four cases reported in which chronic lymphocytic leukemia or Hodgkin's disease was clearly associated with the nephrotic syndrome, where the renal histology was studied [79, 464, 603]. An additional three patients with Hodgkin's disease clinically associated with the nephrotic syndrome, but without renal histology, have also been reported [566, 630, 661]. Since the kidney is infiltrated by the primary disease process in 30 to 60 per cent of patients with Hodgkin's disease, malignant lymphomas, and leukemia, other reported incidences seem curiously low. Three of the four best cases reported had control of both their primary disease and their nephrotic syndrome by nitrogen mustard, chlorambucil, and radiation therapy, respectively. Tapie [661] described a man with Hodgkin's disease, unilateral neck lymphadenopathy, edema, and proteinuria. The neck nodes were excised, and six months later there was neither edema nor proteinuria.

In NZB/B1 mice an association between membranous glomerulonephritis and malignant lymphoma has been observed. In these interesting animals a membranous glomerulonephritis, nephrotic syndrome, Coombs-positive, autoimmune hemolytic anemia, and malignant lymphomas developed spontaneously [61, 306]. The most common causes of death are membranous glomerulonephritis and lymphoid neoplasms [306]. Cyclophosphamide has been used in this model [580, 581]. Cyclophosphamide, in a dose of 1.8 mg. per mouse per week, decreased the frequency of severe renal disease from 100 to 6.7 per cent. Cessation of cyclophosphamide at one year is not associated with a return of the kidney disease. Treatment initiated at 150 days of age seemed particularly effective, and no mice so

treated showed evidence of renal change. Although kidney disease was suppressed, antinuclear antibodies were not completely suppressed. Transiently positive tests for antinuclear factor and for latex-detected antinuclear antibodies were found. When short-term therapy was used the frequency of proteinuria rose on cessation of cyclophosphamide, and short-term treatment resulted in earlier and more extensive rise in proteinuria than did long-term therapy. Russell and Hicks [580] have suggested that cyclophosphamide has its greatest effect when given during the initial stages of the kidney disease. They employ the clonal theory as an explanation. Treatment given to mice before 150 days must allow pathogenic clones to be repopulated, whereas when given after the age of 150 days, the treatment is insufficient to wipe out all aberrant cells. These cells produced nephritis in some fraction of the mice.

Opposing theoretical views have been presented by Lewis, Dixon, and others. Lewis et al. [408] observed autoimmune complications in 18 of 100 patients with lymphocytic leukemia or lymphosarcoma. In five the complications occurred shortly after irradiation or the use of alkylating agents. One must face the possibility that immunosuppressive agents can also cause an increase in antibody synthesis and serve as a trigger mechanism. Dixon has emphasized, in the pathogenesis of renal lesions, the important quantitative relations between the amount of antigen and the amount of antibody present in producing complex depositions. Some of this difference may be resolved by the contrast between short-term and long-term therapy in the mouse model. The patients reported by Brodovsky et al. [79], however, seem to clearly establish a relationship between the nephrotic syndrome and Hodgkin's disease, for their patients became nephrotic before any antitumor therapy had been given and both the hematologic and renal diseases improved pari passu.

GOODPASTURE'S SYNDROME

Goodpasture's syndrome, an interesting variant of glomerulonephritis, is featured by hemoptysis, pulmonary hemosiderosis, and hematuria [51, 230, 579, 642, 691]. On light microscopy there is usually an acute or subacute proliferative glomerulonephritis with rapid progression, and there are fairly specific basement membrane changes by electron microscopy and linear deposits of immunoglobulin by fluorescent techniques. Occasionally immunofluorescence has also been demonstrated in the basement membrane of alveoli. The majority of patients die of uremia within two years. Features of the nephrotic syndrome have been reported in a number of cases, but have been overshadowed by progressive renal failure [113, 121, 213, 409]. Bloom et al. [67] have recently reported on five patients with Goodpasture's syndrome complicated by typical nephrotic syndrome, accompanied by profound anemia, changes in the optic fundi, transient coagulation defects in one patient, and episodes of major venous thrombosis. In one patient on corticosteroid therapy a dramatic clinical improvement occurred, but in three others there was no effect [67].

Treatment and Prognosis

Any disease which affects people of all ages, is found prominently in children, produces striking cosmetic changes (as shown in Figure 16-39), persists for periods stretching out into years, is fatal in a disturbing percentage of cases, and is etiologically puzzling can be expected to have been treated by almost everything available and with every possible variation in deployment and combination. The nephrotic syndrome is such a disease. Barnes et al. [28] list 64 methods of treatment used in Boston between 1926 and 1948. Since then, more specific forms of therapy have emerged which are based on the nature of the lesion.

Evaluation has been difficult for the following reasons:

1. The syndrome may have a vague onset, varied causes, and protean clinical manifestations.

2. The natural history of many forms of the nephrotic syndrome is characterized by spontaneous remissions and exacerbations.

3. One-third of young clinical investigators in America change their addresses every year, whereas continuity of observation is desirable when a disease extends over many years.

4. Too few studies proceed on the basis of crisp definitions. Treatment groups may mix up adults and children, minimal change and proliferative changes, and systemic diseases. These series make no attempt to ascertain the etiology by modern methods. It is fair to note, however, that from the long list of causes seen

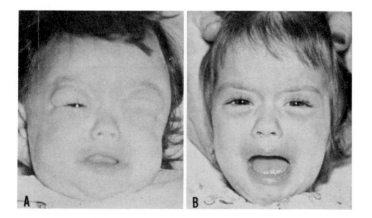

Figure 16-39. A. Marked periorbital edema progressing to the point of blindness in a 15-month-old girl with acute glomerulonephritis and the nephrotic syndrome. B. Same patient eight days later after diuresis brought her weight down from 29 to 19 pounds.

in the section on *Etiology,* it is quite possible to mistakenly assign a cause.

5. In a few well-established series the criteria for definition of classification have been rendered obsolete by newer diagnostic technics, such as electron microscopy and immunofluorescence.

6. New drugs are introduced into therapy before those already available have been completely evaluated. Too many clinicians automatically assume that each new steroid or antibiotic is superior to its predecessor. Furthermore, it has become fashionable for the clinician to attempt to associate himself with a new "method" of treating the nephrotic syndrome. Corticosteroid therapy, for example, has not only been given by a widely varying number of agents, but in the most imaginative ways — for example, intravenously; orally; daily in divided doses; daily in single doses; alternate daily in divided doses; alternate daily in single doses; intermittently; three days on, four off; four on, three off; and sliding scale.

Skeptical critics may conclude that nothing scientific has been learned concerning the effect of any particular treatment on the patient's longevity or ultimate mortality of the nephrotic syndrome. Riley and his associates [546, 555] are to be commended, however, for their attempt to compile an evaluation of the efficacy of steroid treatment. (The reader is referred especially to references 553 and 555 for the compilation of these data.) Numerous references to the problem of treatment are contained also in all the proceedings of the twelve annual Conferences on the Nephrotic Syndrome, sponsored by the National Kidney Foundation. More recently, cooperative studies, such as that reported by Cameron [93] and the control trial sponsored by the Medical Research Council of Great Britain [568], and other cooperative series have approached the therapeutic evaluation in a more scientific way [29].

GENERAL PRINCIPLES

General principles of therapy may be summarized as follows:

1. A diagnosis revealing the cause of the syndrome should be established whenever possible before therapy based on the nature of the lesion is begun.

2. As many physiologic factors as possible should be studied before treatment is started. Of particular significance are those that define the degree of glomerular permeability, the selectivity of the proteinuria, the presence of renal tubular syndromes, etc.

3. The pathology of the lesion should be established with the application of modern methods to biopsy and autopsy material. At this time it seems important to separate minimal change in the disease from membranous glomerulonephritis, and both of these from proliferative glomerulonephritis and systemic disease. It also seems important to establish the presence or absence of inflammatory elements in the glomerulus by electron microscopy, to note whether deposits are present subendothelially, in the membrane, or in a subepithelial position, and to know by immunofluorescence what proteins are deposited on the glomerular basement membrane and whether in linear or "lumpy-bumpy" fashion, or whether "humps" or evidence of streptococcal etiology are present.

4. Treatment should be started as early as possible consistent with accurate diagnosis. This makes early referral from pediatrician or general physician imperative.

5. Initial therapy should be continued long enough to determine reliably the degree of the patient's response.

6. The response should be clearly described.

7. The patient and his family should be prepared for continued studies for at least five to ten years.

8. Patients who make a partial response should receive continued therapy, and relapses

should be treated with multiple courses of therapy.

9. The prognosis should be expressed in terms of clearly defined categories related to the advance of the disorder.

A corollary of the first principle is that in the absence of a classic clinical picture for a disease of known cause most patients require renal biopsy before treatment is begun. This procedure is particularly important in the adult. Nothing is gained by including a patient with amyloid nephrosis in the statistics of a series of patients with membranous glomerulonephritis. In our series, a 94 per cent diagnostic accuracy was obtained through the use of renal biopsy, which was attempted 100 times in 183 patients. There was disagreement between clinical and histologic diagnoses in 21 patients. In virtually all patients who had had renal biopsies and who have come to autopsy, the light microscopy diagnosis has been substantiated. However, recently we have seen a significant number of patients with normal glomeruli or minimal change on light microscopy, but distinct abnormalities on either electron microscopy or immunofluorescent microscopy, or both.

THERAPEUTIC CLASSIFICATIONS

In treating any chronic condition, especially one subject to remissions or exacerbations, it is imperative to have a clearly established classification of therapeutic results based on accessible objective methods. Since presenting this in the last edition, we have received a large number of reprints and letters testifying to the utility of the following therapeutic classification which may be used for series of patients treated with corticosteroids, immunosuppressive agents, combinations of these, or new drugs to be developed in the future. The classification may be used for the initial therapeutic response to the initial therapy (e.g., three weeks of steroids), or it can also be used as a categorized patient group during chronic therapy, or for a follow-up study.

Group 4 Response: Complete remission with clearing of all features of the nephrotic syndrome (e.g., reduction of proteinuria to less than 90 mg. per day, restoration of serum albumin to normal, loss of all signs and symptoms).

Group 3 Response: Substantial but incomplete, as evidenced by marked decrease

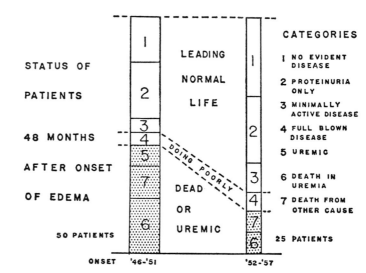

Figure 16-40. Status of patients at Babies' Hospital four years after onset of nephritis. Height of each column represents 100 per cent. (From Riley [553]; reproduced by permission.)

in proteinuria (e.g., less than 2 gm. per day), increase in serum albumin nearly to normal levels (e.g., more than 3.0 gm. per 100 ml.), decrease in hypercholesterolemia (e.g., to less than 300 mg. per 100 ml.), and a loss of nephrotic signs and symptoms.

Group 2 Response: Quantitative lessening of proteinuria (e.g., from 12 to 6 gm. per day, but not below the "nephrotic range"). Serum albumin concentration does not rise to normal; many clinical features of the nephrotic syndrome, including edema, may show improvement.

Group 1 Response: Control of edema alone, with no significant change in proteinuria, serum proteins, or lipids.

Group 0 Response: Failure to improve significantly in any critical respect, or death during the initial therapeutic trial.

Figure 16-40 depicts the graphic presentation originally used by Riley [553].

PROGNOSIS IN CHILDREN

It is generally stated in the older literature that 50 per cent of nephrotic children will be dead within five years after the onset of the disease. There has been considerable discussion in many of the published proceedings of the Conferences on the Nephrotic Syndrome, relative to the interpretation of published data, on whether or not this mortality has been substantially affected by the introduction of steroids. Riley and his co-workers [553, 555] initiated a cooperative study in an attempt to evaluate this question. Survival figures for 872 children are shown in Figure 16-41. These figures indicate that 75 per cent of children with recent onset of nephrosis can expect to be alive four years after the onset of their disease, whereas only about 60 per cent of their counterparts in the presteroid era could expect to live four years. The children were under 12 years of age and were seen within six months of onset of their disease, and the cases were selected from 1500 reports by 18 different physicians throughout the United States.

Information on the prognosis can also be gathered from figures presented by other investigators. Todd [669] reported that one-

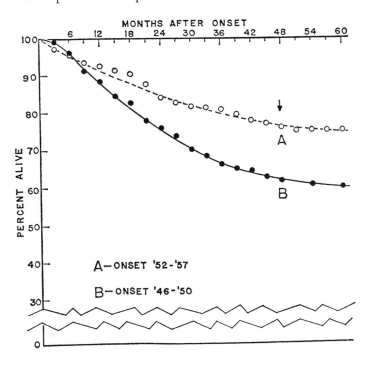

Figure 16-41. Survival curves of children with nephrosis whose disease began in the years indicated. Group A — based on 554 cases; Group B — based on 318 cases. (From Riley [553]; reproduced by permission.)

third of 32 children died during an eight-year follow-up period from 1948 to 1955. Barnes et al. [28] reported recovery in 50 per cent of 208 patients seen from 2 to 23 years after onset of nephrosis. Schwartz et al. [600, 601] reported recovery in 45 per cent of 40 patients studied up to 20 years. Farr [174, 175] reported recovery in 28 per cent of 36 patients. Rapoport et al. [535] reported complete remission in 44 per cent of 40 patients studied between 1949 and 1952. Cameron [93], in a study of 400 nephrotic patients, found that the major difference between children and adults was the much greater frequency of minimal-change lesions in children, and the near absence of glomerular disease secondary to systemic disorders. There was little difference in treatment response which was not related to the minimal-change lesion. This lesion was the only histologic appearance regularly associated with complete response to corticosteroid therapy within eight weeks. Highly selective differential protein clearances were strongly associated with response to steroids, but this depended on the relationship between this type of protein clearance and the minimal-change lesion. In the age group of from one to five, the absence of purpura, hypertension, hematuria, and a highly selective pattern of urinary protein clearance provide a very good indication that the minimal-change lesion is present in the kidneys. Sharpstone et al. [613] suggest that over 80 per cent of children with primary glomerular disease and 30 per cent of similar adults have the minimal-change lesion on renal biopsy. Adult patients with the minimal-change lesion seem to follow a relapsing course less often than similar children. For details of other individual studies, the reader is referred to the following references [19, 20, 368, 369, 498, 633, 634, 647, 707].

Specific Therapy

Since the nephrotic syndrome is complex in its pathologic physiology and symptomatology, there are logically a number of different therapeutic measures which may be directed toward specific aspects of the pathologic physiology. Some of these methods of treatment may be carried on simultaneously, but we shall discuss them in terms of the specific goals of the treatment regimen, under the following headings:

1. Treatment based on the nature of the lesion.
2. Treatment determined by the altered physiology and its immediate consequences.
3. Treatment to eliminate the more indirect consequences or the complications of the nephrotic syndrome.
4. Long-term treatment and management considering the whole patient and his environment.

TREATMENT BASED ON THE NATURE OF THE LESION

Assuming that the fundamental pathologic physiology of the nephrotic syndrome is increased permeability of the basement membrane, probably due to a structural or metabolic alteration, it is important to seek therapeutic measures in relationship to some considered pathogenesis. From the widely varied list of the etiologic classification of nephrotic syndrome, it is apparent that injury to the basement membrane may occur by chemical means, by antibodies directed against the membrane, or by the deposition of antigen-antibody complexes which may also contain complement and other immune components. It is important to note that these can be deposited to some extent without apparent injury, but injury seems more prominent when white cell margination and inflammatory reaction ensues. Drugs specifically directed toward the nature of the lesion most effectively have been those known to have some immunosuppressive effect, some anti-inflammatory effect, or some combination of both. The major successful regimens have included corticosteroids in various forms and immunosuppressive drugs with varying actions.

Adrenal Corticotropic Hormone and Adrenal Cortical Steroids. Ever since Farnsworth [498, 501] noted that a diuresis might be achieved in the nephrotic syndrome by the use of ACTH [499], many investigators have studied the effect of specific treatment regimens on other features of the syndrome. Most of these regimens attempt to alter the natural history of the nephrotic syndrome. Therapeutic variations have included successive trials of ACTH, cortisone, hydrocortisone, prednisone, triamcinolone, decamethazone, and each new steroid as it has become available from the chemists. Suggested dosages have ranged from the very small to the very large, but in recent years there has been a tendency toward increased dosage. Exact dosage regimens have been calculated on weight, body surface area, age, previous response, and the presence or absence of anasarca. Investigators have recommended that the initial course of treatment should extend to seven, ten, fourteen, sixteen days, three weeks, a month, two months. Other studies have given the corticosteroid intravenously, orally daily in divided doses, daily single dose at noon, alternate-day dosages, intermittent therapy of three days on and four days off, or four days on and three days off, or sliding scale, with a tapering dose from Monday to Saturday of each week. Some have recommended that steroids should be continued in constant high dosage until there has been a demonstrable change in some critical feature of the nephrotic syndrome, others that it be continued until proteinuria has disappeared. Criteria for the time to stop the initial course and the time to continue steroids vary. Most investigators agree that for patients who do not have a total remission, some form of long-term program should be instituted. Readers desiring more detailed historical information may glean it from the following references [2, 17, 18, 31, 46, 49, 94, 100, 116, 118, 119, 123, 139, 167, 224, 228, 271, 295, 310, 331, 341, 361, 396, 420, 430, 441, 457, 459, 473, 522, 535, 546–556].

Our current regimen — which is undergoing continued evolution — is outlined as follows. After making the specific diagnosis of the nephrotic syndrome and its cause, treatment is begun by administering prednisone, 60 mg. a day in divided doses for large or massively edematous individuals, 40 mg. a day for smaller or nonedematous individuals. Equivalent doses of other adrenocortical steroids may be used. In edematous individuals making a group 0 response, these large doses are continued uninterruptedly for 21 days, and a withdrawal diuresis is then attempted, often in association with one of the diuretic regimens outlined below. In patients making a group 1 response, treatment is continued for three weeks, and a decision is made as to whether to try a higher dosage or proceed to a combination of corticosteroid and immunosuppressive therapy. With a group 3 response in the first two weeks, intensive therapy is continued until the partial response has reached a plateau. The patient then receives alternate-day therapy with a single dose given at noon. With a group 4 response at any point in the program, the patient is immediately changed to alternate-day therapy, with a single dose given at noon for a period of two months, and is then gradually tapered off steroids under observation. We have only one patient who failed to respond at the 60 mg. dosage level and then showed a clear-cut response at a higher dosage level. This has been the experience of other investigators also [45]. We do have, however, patients who responded to nitrogen mustard or other immunosuppressive therapy after failure with steroids.

RESULTS OF STEROID THERAPY. In our series of 183 patients, 60 had renal disorders diagnosed as membranous glomerulonephritis. In four instances it was related to pregnancy, and in two to sickle cell disease. Of the remaining

54 patients, 22 were treated with some regimen of adrenocortical steroids and have been available for satisfactory follow-up study. Of these, 15 showed a group 3 to 4 response, five showed a group 1 to 2 response, and two had no response and were dead within one month. One patient failed to respond to steroids alone but has maintained a good response for 18 months since receiving nitrogen mustard.

During the first few days of steroid administration, there may be a nonspecific rise in glomerular filtration rate with a transient increase in proteinuria before the definitive effect on the basement membrane obtains. This phenomenon is shown in Figure 16-42, which depicts the course of an exacerbation of nephrosis in a 10-year-old girl. Note the rise and fall of proteinuria on steroid therapy and the return of proteinuria after withdrawal of the drug.

Out of our total series, adequate follow-up data are currently available on 132 patients.

The status of treatment response in all the specific diagnostic categories is summarized in Tables 16-15 to 16-19.

Cameron [93] has reported on a group of 400 nephrotic patients. Unfortunately, qualitative studies of the urine were used to assess effectiveness, and an occasional positive finding was regarded as protein-free on "stick" methods; however, response was assessed as loss of proteinuria by the end of three weeks, and would probably correspond roughly to a combination of our grade 3 and 4 responses. Ninety per cent of the 77 children with minimal-change lesions responded, as did 77 per cent of the adults. A highly selective pattern of differential protein clearances ($C_{IgG}/C_{transferrin}$ of less than 0.1) was associated with a response to corticosteroids, but the association was dependent on a correlation with the minimal-change lesion. This suggests that a response to steroids within eight weeks, coupled with a selective proteinuria, is a very

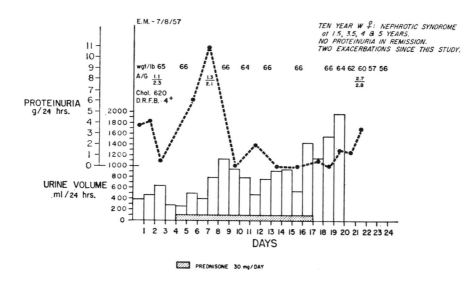

Figure 16-42. A typical pattern of proteinuria during exacerbation of nephrosis in a 10-year-old girl. Initial proteinuria of 4 gm. per day fell on bed rest. With steroid therapy there was an early, nonspecific rise, then a decline to protein-free urines on the tenth day. A short subsequent rise coincided with a respiratory infection passing through the pediatric ward. Following this, diminished proteinuria continued until discontinuation of the drugs, when there was a prompt exacerbation. The patient lost 9 pounds of edema, blood chemistries have been restored to normal, and a group 4 response has been obtained. Focal membranoproliferative disease was present on later biopsy.

Table 16-15. Course of Nephrotic Syndrome due to Membranous Glomerulonephritis[a]

Therapy	Number of Patients	Response Group		
		4	3	2–0
Initial evaluation				
Corticosteroid	29	9	8	12
Corticosteroid + nitrogen mustard	3	0	2	1
No corticosteroid	22	4	0	18
Total	54	13	10	31
Late evaluation				
Corticosteroid[b]	13	7	6	0
Corticosteroid + nitrogen mustard	2	0	2	0
No corticosteroid	20	3	1	16
Total	35	10	9	16[c]

[a] Diagnosed at that time by light microscopy only. Some patients' lesions would now be described as "minimal change." These were predominantly in adults.
[b] Includes those who had at any time received corticosteroids.
[c] Short-term follow-up only.

Table 16-16. Course of Nephrotic Syndrome due to Acute Glomerulonephritis

Therapy	Number of Patients	Response Group		
		4	3	2–0
Initial evaluation				
Corticosteroid	13	3	3	7[a]
No corticosteroid	6	0	1	5[b]
Total	19	3	4	12
Late evaluation				
Corticosteroid	5	4	1	0
Corticosteroid + nitrogen mustard	1	0	1	0
No corticosteroid	1	0	1	0
Total	7	4	3	0

[a] Includes 2 deaths.
[b] Includes 1 death.

Table 16-17. Course of Nephrotic Syndrome due to Subacute Glomerulonephritis

Therapy	Number of Patients	Response Group		
		4	3	2–0
Initial evaluation				
Corticosteroid	6	0	1	5
Corticosteroid + nitrogen mustard	1	0	1	0
No corticosteroid	2	0	0	2
Total	9	0	2	7
Late evaluation				
Corticosteroid	5	1	2	2[a]
Corticosteroid + nitrogen mustard	0	0	0	0
No corticosteroid	0	0	0	0
Total	5	1	2	2

[a] Both patients have died.

Table 16-18. Course of Nephrotic Syndrome due to Chronic Glomerulonephritis

Therapy	Number of Patients	Response Group		
		4	3	2–0
Corticosteroid	14	5	2	7
No corticosteroid	17	2	2	13
Total	31	7	4	20

Table 16-19. Course of Nephrotic Syndrome due to Systemic Lupus Erythematosus

Therapy	Number of Patients	Response Group		
		4	3	2–0
Corticosteroid	5	1	1	3
Corticosteroid + nitrogen mustard	4	0	1	3
Total	9	1	2	6

good indication that the minimal-change lesion is present or predominant. Selectivity alone is an inadequate criterion on which to base this diagnosis, since patients with amyloidosis and lupus nephritis sometimes show selectivity, especially when their lesions are relatively mild. However, a selectivity index of less than 0.1 makes the existence of minimal change very likely, and one of 0.3 makes such a possibility remote. The presence of the minimal-change lesion can be established definitively only by renal biopsy. In the study sponsored by the British Medical Research Council, the lesions of a group of 125 patients were classified as minimal-change (31 cases), membranous (19 cases), or proliferative (75 cases), although there were some discrepancies because of individual pathologists looking at the same material differently. This is undoubtedly a problem in many other series, but is less candidly stated. Sixty-four persons were kept as controls and 61 received prednisone in a range of 20 to 30 mg. Patients with minimal-change lesions showed an earlier improvement compared to controls in respect to proteinuria, hypoprotcinemia, and edema. There is also the suggestion that renal function may be maintained at a higher level in these patients given steroids. However, in the first two years the number of patients dying from renal failure and the number of those maintained on dialysis was similar in both steroid and control groups. In patients with glomerulonephritis the risks of steroids seem to outweigh the possible benefits. Patients in the high-risk groups seem to be those of more advanced age with higher blood pressure. The trial suggested that steroids should not be used for long periods of time in patients who do not show clinical remission.

COMPLICATIONS OF STEROID THERAPY.   All the usual complications of corticosteroid therapy [313] may be seen in our patients. The most bothersome are: *expansion of the extracellular fluid volume* with initial increase in edema; *rise in blood pressure,* occasionally precipitat-

ing encephalopathy in the patients with acute and subacute glomerulonephritis; all the clinical features of *Cushing's syndrome,* including moon face, buffalo hump, striae, acne, and muscle wasting; and marked *behavioral changes,* including agitated depression, euphoria, paranoia, and excessive stimulation. The most dangerous of these is agitated depression. (One patient in our series escaped from a mental institution and committed suicide while on steroids and reserpine for severe nephrotic syndrome, chronic glomerulonephritis, and hypertension.) In addition, we have observed retardation of growth, a delay or absence of pubescence, osteoporosis, induction of abnormal carbohydrate intolerance, and gastritis. Steroid-induced leukocytosis may be misconstrued as an infection; the mean leukocyte count on 30 mg. of prednisone per day is about 14,000 cells per cubic millimeter [191].

The added salt retention induced by steroid therapy can be minimized by the employment of salt restriction, administration of large doses of potassium supplements, and the judicious use of diuretic therapy (avoiding mercurial diuretics), and by a transition to alternate-day or intermittent therapy at an early stage when the patient is making a group 3 or group 4 response or showing severe side effects of the steroid. It is remarkable that we have not encountered peptic ulceration as a complication of steroid therapy in the nephrotic syndrome, since in many other diseases, such as rheumatoid arthritis, there has been a variable but rather high frequency of peptic ulceration among patients undergoing long-term steroid therapy [654]. This observation, if confirmed by others, might warrant study by those interested in peptic ulceration.

The deep philosophic implications of a decision to pursue treatment of the nephrotic syndrome with steroids at the risk of inducing Cushing's disease have been reviewed by Armstrong [17]. Variations in the Cushingoid response to corticotropin given intramuscularly have been ascribed to tissue edema in nephrotic patients. However, biologic variations in disposal of exogenous hormone must be considered analogous to the experience described by Howard and Migeon [313] of a patient with myxedema who developed Cushing's syndrome while taking 25 mg. of cortisone per day.

Among the frequently encountered hormonal effects are moon facies, hypertension, muscular cramps and wasting, ecchymosis, epigastric distress, hirsutism (especially in brunette children), voracious appetite, flushes, acne, headache, osteoporosis, behavioral changes, and frank psychosis. Arthralgia, muscle wasting, and even toxic dermatitis [69] have been reported as complications of steroid therapy which may, at times, be worse than the disease being treated [434, 576, 674]. Alternate-day corticosteroid therapy can minimize effects on growth hormone and on adrenocortical responsiveness [1, 430, 724]. However, stress responsiveness may be diminished. Children who have marked suppression of growth hormone and impaired growth at the time of the prepubertal spurt have been shifted to ACTH temporarily. This procedure may allow normal growth to continue while still maintaining the patient in remission.

Immunosuppressive Therapy. Since the early trial of nitrogen mustard in the nephrotic syndrome by Chasis et al. [102, 103], a wide variety of drugs have become available for immunosuppression. Their pharmacologic action permits the following simple classification.

1. *Alkylating agents.* The principal drugs are nitrogen mustard, cyclophosphamide (Cytoxan), and busulfan (Myleran). These interact directly with protein and DNA molecules, causing their denaturation. They act on nucleoprotein and affect the cell nucleus disproportionately. They have also been termed radiomimetic agents because of their similarity to the effects of irradiation.

2. *The purine antagonists.* The principal drugs are 6-mercaptopurine, 6-thioguanine, and azathioprine (Imuran). These act by blocking the interconversion of nucleotides, especially the conversion of inosinic acid to adenylic acid. This leads to widespread effects on subcellular structures, especially the synthesis of nucleic acids. Azathioprine also binds sulfhydryl groups.

3. *The halogenated pyrimidines or pyrimidine-antagonists.* The principal drugs are 5-fluorouracil (FUDR) and 5-bromodeoxyuridine (BUDR). These are specifically incorporated into DNA with the result that an abnormal DNA is synthesized, which cannot support mitosis. Cell multiplication slows and may halt.

4. *Folic acid antagonists.* The principal drug is amethopterin. These drugs, which are largely folic acid analogues, block the action of dihydrofolic reductase required to convert folic acid to folinic acid. Folinic acid is required in transmethylation and the metabolism of one-carbon fragments. This transmethylation is important in the biosynthesis of purine, pyrimidines, and some amino acids. Folinic acid malnutrition renders the cell unable to build nucleic acid and proteins.

5. *Inhibitors of messenger RNA.* The principal drug is a polypeptide antibiotic, actinomycin D, which has been used principally in homograft rejection.

CLINICAL EXPERIENCE WITH IMMUNOSUPPRESSIVE DRUGS. Chasis et al. [102, 103] administered nitrogen mustard (HN-2) to eight patients with glomerulonephritis and a nephrotic component. The rationale of this trial was based on the knowledge that HN-2 could prevent the development of experimentally induced Shwartzman phenomenon, Arthus reaction, and glomerulonephritis. The 24-hour quantitative protein excretion showed a significant reduction in 25 out of 28 courses. Six out of 16 courses resulted in marked diureses of from 10 to 40 pounds, and in three patients there was complete disappearance of the edema. The duration of the response was generally 3 to 13 days, although in three patients repeated induction of temporary changes was followed by permanent improvement in the disease. This was accompanied in many cases by a measured increase in glomerular filtration rate.

These interesting results were generally submerged in the deluge of clinical reports which followed the introduction of corticotropin and, subsequently, steroids into clinical therapeutics. However, there have been scattered reports of the use of nitrogen mustard either alone, following the demonstration of refractoriness to steroids, or in combinations with corticotropin or steroid therapy [355, 406, 661a, 702]. Taylor [661b] treated 22 nephrotic patients (0.1 mg. per kilogram on each of 4 successive days) and followed them for three to five years after treatment. Nine showed apparent complete recovery, seven were unchanged, and six died during the follow-up period. In general, the patients who did poorly had more significant hematuria and possibly greater glomerular involvement. The mean pretreatment urea clearance among the patients who recovered was 71 per cent of normal, among the unchanged group 69 per cent, and among those who died 42 per cent. Startzman reported seven patients in remission (in a group of patients who had been previously treated but had relapsed) when they received a combined course consisting of ACTH, 10 mg. every six hours intramuscularly for 10 days, with nitrogen mustard at a dosage of 0.1 mg. per kilogram intravenously on the last four days. Among clinicians employing this therapy, the vote for combined therapy continued to grow [96, 238, 355, 406, 704, 705, 714, 719, 727]. West [702], who reported cessation of albuminuria in 14 of 16 patients treated with combined steroids and nitrogen mustard, expressed a strong opinion that combined therapy induced remission with a greater frequency than either agent used alone. Many clinicians have emphasized that steroid hormones should be given for a prolonged period

before embarking on nitrogen mustard therapy. Nitrogen mustard has also found widespread use in the therapy of disseminated lupus erythematosus with nephritis, with and without the nephrotic syndrome. Nitrogen mustard has been reported to alter wound healing without impairing fibroblastic proliferation [166].

With the advent of the purine antagonists, particularly 6-mercaptopurine, 6-thioguanine, and azathioprine, many clinical trials have been reported using these agents in varying dose levels, for varying periods following or combined with varying levels of steroid administration for varying periods. The results of these studies, as one might expect, have been variable. They have been further confused by the fact that in many large series the histologic basis for the nephrotic syndrome has not been established. In most of the older series, even when renal biopsies have been done, the newer technics of electron microscopy and immunofluorescent microscopy have not been used to establish an immunologic basis for the nephrotic syndrome being treated. In the many patients with early forms of mesangial thickening, lobular glomerulonephritis, and membranous glomerulonephritis without significant deposition of immunoglobulin or complement, immunosuppressive therapy is probably destined to have little or no effect. However, undoubtedly immunosuppressive drugs have some effect in the patient with the steroid-resistant nephrotic syndrome. For example, Shearn [614] administered 14 courses of 6-mercaptopurine to 10 patients with nephrotic syndromes of diverse etiology. In each patient the nephrotic syndrome had proved to be steroid resistant, failing to respond to 60 mg. or more of prednisone daily for a minimum of three weeks. With 6-mercaptopurine therapy a clinical remission, evidenced by marked decrease in proteinuria, loss of edema, and rise in serum albumin, occurred in half the patients. Toxic side effects were observed in virtually all.

When classified according to the therapeutic classification of Schreiner, the results could be summarized in Table 16-20.

Table 16-20. Response of the Nephrotic Syndrome to 6-Mercaptopurine

Diagnosis	Number of Patients	Response Group		
		4	3	2–0
Lipoid nephritis	3	1[a]	1	1
Membranous glomerulonephritis	2			2
Systemic lupus erythematosus	4		2	2
Henoch-Schönlein purpura	1		1	

[a] Subsequently relapsed to group 0.

Grupe and Heymann [245] administered azathioprine, cyclophosphamide, or chlorambucil to 16 children with idiopathic nephrotic syndrome; six with lupus, two with chronic glomerulonephritis; and one with anaphylactoid purpura and the nephrotic syndrome. The treatment was initiated because of either an unremitting course or serious side effects from steroid therapy. Of the 25 children, seven entered complete remission and five experienced incomplete remission. No improvement occurred in the seven courses in which the cytotoxic drug was administered alone. Lagrue et al. [382, 383] reported improvement in about 50 per cent of patients with steroid-resistant nephrotic syndrome following the use of an alkylating agent. Goodman et al. [229], using 6-thioguanine alone, had no response in four patients with steroid-resistant nephrotic syndrome. Three of these patients were subsequently given combined therapy — that is, 6-thioguanine and prednisone; there was one response. Adams et al. [3] treated 19 adults with 2 to 14 months of azathioprine. They reported improvement in two out of seven patients with proliferative glomerulone-

phritis, two out of two with minimal-change nephrotic syndrome, one out of one with focal glomerulonephritis, and three out of four with lupus nephritis.

In an international cooperative study,* which was prospective and double blind, the role of azathioprine was evaluated in children with the nephrotic syndrome who either failed to respond to adrenocorticosteroid therapy or relapsed as often as twice in a six-month period and were considered likely to develop steroid toxicity. In this series of nearly 200 previously untreated patients, 19 per cent were nonresponders and 24 per cent were frequent relapsers. On renal biopsy, frequent relapsers and other patients who responded to steroid therapy had, in almost every case, only minimal pathologic changes. However, a few nonresponders also had minimal changes. Almost all of the steroid-resistant patients had either focal glomerular lesions or proliferative changes. Of a total of 29 patients failing to respond, 2 responded on placebos, 2 on azathioprine, and proteinuria persisted in the rest. In 33 frequent relapsers, the occurrence of relapses was not significantly different in patients treated with azathioprine from that in patients given placebos. From their observations, these investigators concluded that they had failed to demonstrate the usefulness of azathioprine in *children* with the nephrotic syndrome.

The exact mechanism of action of immunosuppressive agents on the nephrotic syndrome is not known. While they do diminish the antibody response to known antigens, most of these agents also have an anti-inflammatory action [321], and it is possible that their salutary effect on the nephrotic syndrome could be either a direct effect on the basement membrane or an anti-inflammatory effect, rather than their fundamental action as immunosuppressive agents [655].

For more than a decade, we have followed

* International Study of Kidney Disease in Children, New York, 1969.

the practice (outlined in the section on *Steroids*) of treating nephrotic patients with an initial added course of steroids for a minimum of three to four weeks, and then treating them in accordance with our therapeutic classification. Patients who give grade 3 to 4 responses are not treated with immunosuppressive agents, whereas those with grade 0 to 2 responses are first treated with very high doses of prednisone, often in the range of 100 to 120 mg. per day. The duration of this therapy is usually determined by the patient, since virtually all will develop steroid toxicity evidenced by frank Cushingoid features, hypertension, hyperglycemia, beginning striae, or psychosis. In all these years, only one patient who failed to respond to 60 mg. of prednisone daily subsequently responded to 120 mg. per day, continued for several months. In the series of Goodman and Baxter no patient responded to 120 mg. who had failed to respond to 60 mg. of prednisone. Following this kind of clear-cut demonstration of steroid unresponsiveness, patients who continue to fall in the therapeutic classification of grades 0, 1, and 2 have over the years, in phases, been treated with nitrogen mustard in a dose of 0.4 mg. per kilogram in two divided doses on successive nights after the administration of a sedative or an antiemetic, or azathioprine, 2.5 to 3.5 mg. per kilogram per day, or cyclophosphamide, 1.5 to 2.5 mg. per kilogram per day. These are initial doses, and the patients must be monitored carefully for leukopenia, thrombocytopenia, or a drop in reticulocyte count. Biologic tolerance varies considerably, and dosage may have to be adjusted upward or downward, depending on progress of the disease weighed against the toxic effects of the drugs.

Looked at in overview, we are still not sure about the long-term value of these drugs. Trials do seem justified in the unrelenting cases that have a poor prognosis. Our results have been best in the patients with nephrotic syndrome due to lupus erythematosus and in

patients with atypical forms of early membranous disease which may very well be conceptually a form of lupus. An occasional patient with idiopathic nephrotic syndrome may have a partial response, and a still smaller number of patients may actually depend on the use of the immunosuppressive agent for maintenance of a remission. A typical example of this last group is illustrated in Figure 16-43.

Two unique experiences in this series are worth noting. One patient with severe nephrotic syndrome and high glomerular permeability was a metabolic cripple, with wasting and anasarca and no response to long trials of massive steroids, diuretics, and parenteral albumin. At one point during a long course of azathioprine severe leukopenia developed, and while leukopenic, he acquired a hospital-based staphylococcal infection with pneumonia and septicemia. During the course of the severe life-threatening septicemia, he experienced a period of profound hypotension, and acute tubular necrosis developed. After therapy with antibiotics and hemodialysis, he had a classic diuretic phase, and following this the nephrotic syndrome remitted and has remained in remission for several years, with gradually improving renal function and complete reversal of all symptoms. Another patient who proved resistant to long courses of both high-dose steroids and immunosuppressives remained nephrotic for several years after withdrawal from all forms of therapy. Following a laparotomy, he sustained a subdiaphragmatic abscess with severe infections from multiple organisms and septicemia. After recovery from this severe infection, the status of the nephrotic syndrome as well as the glomerular filtration rate improved for the first time in many years.

CYCLOPHOSPHAMIDE. There has been a recent upsurge in interest in an alkylating agent, cyclophosphamide [160, 242, 698], which more closely resembles nitrogen mustard in action than its temporal successor, the

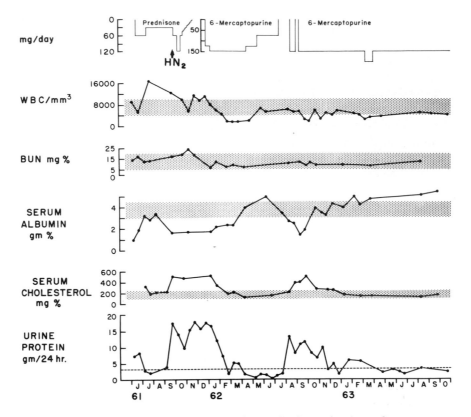

Figure 16-43. Combined steroid-immunosuppressive therapy in the nephrotic syndrome.

purine antagonist azathioprine. Cyclophosphamide can be given by mouth in long courses, and it is presumably inert in tissues and is activated only by the presence of certain enzymes found within the cells. West et al. [700] gave cyclophosphamide to four steroid-resistant patients with lipoid nephrosis and induced a long-term remission in all four. In eight courses in seven patients with frequent recurrences of the nephrotic syndrome, the durations of remissions were significantly lengthened, and in four courses in four patients with persistent residual proteinuria, one course of cyclophosphamide led to disappearance of the proteinuria. Cyclophosphamide did not affect the development of aminonucleoside nephrosis in rats. It was reported

from the same clinic [699] that cyclophosphamide produced an elevation of β_1C-globulin levels to normal range and a reduction of proteinuria in one out of four patients with persistent hypocomplementemic glomerulonephritis. There seemed to be no clear correlation between serum β_1C-globulin level and progression of the nephritis [701]. Drummond et al. [135] treated 12 nephrotic children with minimal-lesion or foot-process type of nephrotic syndrome. Five were proved steroid dependent with frequent relapses. Seven were proved steroid resistant after at least one month of daily steroid therapy. Cyclophosphamide was given for periods up to one year in a dosage of 75 mg. per 1.73 square meters of body surface area per day. The steroid-dependent patients responded within 15 days with clearing of the proteinuria and had no relapses for a follow-up period of one year. In the steroid-resistant group, the response was slower (over three to four months), but all patients became well, without proteinuria for a mean follow-up period of over two years. The successful use of cyclophosphamide in trimethadione-induced nephrosis has also been reported [498]. Etteldorf et al. [161] used a much higher dose of cyclophosphamide and found that in the patients who responded the urine became protein free within 14 days. In the report of West et al. [700], the beneficial effects were usually seen in 30 to 50 days, and in that of Grupe and Heymann [245], one patient began to respond after one month and continued to improve for a period of six months.

The principal complication of cyclophosphamide therapy is alopecia, which occurs in one-third to one-half of the patients and is probably dose dependent. It is usually reversible. Bone marrow suppression and other side effects of radiomimetic agents may be seen. Hemorrhagic cystitis and fatal postvaricella pneumococcal sepsis have been reported [161, 588]. Cyclophosphamide has been used in the treatment of kidney disease in NZB and NZW F1 mice in a dosage of 1.8 mg. per week; a significant prolongation of life span was obtained — that is, 77 per cent of the treated mice were alive 100 days longer than the maximum life expectancy of the untreated controls. Only two out of 43 treated mice died of kidney disease, and microscopic studies showed that the disease process was halted by cyclophosphamide treatment [581].

Therapeutic Subclassification. As a result of our experience and review of the literature, we believe that it is very useful to treat patients with adequate doses of steroids as outlined above, and then use our therapeutic classification. On the basis of such a trial or additional exposure to higher doses of steroids

(or both), the patients should then be subclassified as follows:

1. *Steroid responsive.* Patient sustains a grade 3 or 4 response for more than six months after course of steroid therapy.
2. *Steroid dependent.* Patient sustains a grade 3 or 4 response, but relapses when steroids are substantially reduced or omitted. (Patient who moves downward in classification within six months after intensive course or who requires ongoing steroid medication at same level in order to maintain therapeutic classification is probably steroid dependent.)
3. *Steroid resistant.* Patient maintains a grade 0, 1, or 2 therapeutic response in spite of prolonged trial with steroids at high dosage.

One should probably try immunosuppressive therapy in steroid-responsive or steroid-dependent cases only when there is clear evidence of steroid toxicity to a degree that the clinician is unable to maintain the patient in his previously established therapeutic classification. The usual reasons are accelerating hypertension, hyperglycemia, serious personality and behavioral changes, frank psychosis, recurrent infections, rare gastrointestinal problems, and serious adverse cosmetic effects from the Cushingoid syndrome, especially bothersome in young ladies. When a carefully administered program of immunosuppressive drugs is used in these steroid-responsive and steroid-dependent groups, the clinician can confidently expect good results in the vast majority of cases. In our experience three-quarters or more of such patients will experience additional beneficial effects from the immunosuppressive agent or at least a substitutive effect — that is, the immunosuppressive agent will replace whatever benefit that particular patient has received from high toxic doses of steroids. This seems to be a very practical positive role for immunosuppressive drugs. We have seen many patients with severe adverse reactions from steroids alone, or severe toxic effects from immunosuppressive agents alone, who were easily managed, with little toxicity, by a combination of modest steroid administration and a careful immunosuppressive regimen.

When one undertakes, however, to treat a group of *proved* steroid-resistant nephrotic patients, the results will be very much poorer. Only a small percentage of these patients (e.g., Figure 16-44) will have a clear-cut therapeutic response to immunosuppressive therapy if one carefully excludes from the series, by renal biopsy with electron microscopy and immu-

nofluorescence, those patients who represent lupus or a "forme fruste" syndrome resembling lupus with deposits of immune complexes within the basement membrane. Of these, even a smaller percentage can be demonstrated to be immunosuppressive dependent — that is, to have exacerbations on withdrawl of the drug and responses on readministration. Until some reliable way is found to identify these patients in advance, it will probably be open season on philosophical discussion as to whether one is justified in exposing a large number of persons to the toxic effects of immunosuppressive drugs in order to find the relatively small percentage of patients who really need them. The justification for immu-

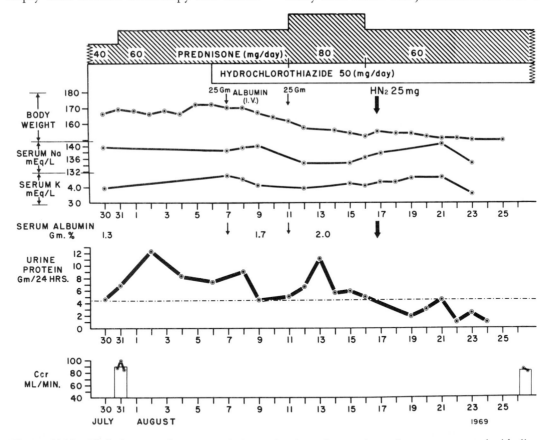

Figure. 16-44. Clinical course of patient with the nephrotic syndrome whose edema was managed with diuretics and intravenous albumin infusions, but whose glomerular permeability was unaffected by either 40, 60, or 80 mg. per day of prednisone. A remission was induced with 25 mg. of nitrogen mustard (HN2), and proteinuria dropped below the nephrotic range, with restoration of serum albumin.

nosuppressive therapy seems to be less in young children than in adults.

SIDE EFFECTS OF IMMUNOSUPPRESSIVE THERAPY. Major side effects of immunosuppressive therapy are, of course, bone marrow depression, with a fall in the reticulocyte count as an early finding, followed by thrombocytopenia, leukopenia, and occasionally aplastic anemia. Other toxic manifestations are nausea, vomiting, vague gastrointestinal complaints, anemia, cataracts [635], pituitary-adrenal suppression [533], and secondary infections. Infections are apt to be of the so-called opportunistic type, including unusual bacteria such as pseudomonas, klebsiella, or common coagulase-negative staphylococci, rare fungi, yeasts, and molds. In our long experience with these agents in the treatment of nephrotic syndrome, lupus erythematosus, and in cadaver homotransplantation, we have encountered *Candida albicans,* Nocardia, Aspergillus, and the protozoan pneumocystis carinii. Others have reported *Coccidioides immitis* and *Cryptococcus neoformans.* Unusual behavior of skin infections, particularly disseminated herpes simplex, herpes zoster, cytomegalovirus, varicella, measles, and histoplasmosis, has been noted [515]. One fatal case of herpes simplex and three contributing to fatality have been reported in one transplant series [468]. A fatal case of measles in a nephrotic child has been reported [449].

We know of several women, both in nephrotic and in transplant series, who have normally conceived and carried a normal fetus to term while being maintained on immunosuppressive therapy. In the Swiss-Webster mouse, azathioprine did not appear to affect either male or female fertility or the estrous cycle [571]; the bone marrow, however, was more susceptible in the fetus than in the mother. Skeletal anomalies, cleft palate, and decrease in thymic size were noted in the fetus when the drug was administered during the embryonic period of development. It would be well, therefore, to monitor carefully any pregnancy that occurs in the course of immunosuppressive treatment.

A number of patients with repeated rejection reactions following cadaveric renal homotransplantation have developed basement membrane thickening on renal biopsy and proteinuria in the nephrotic range. Curiously enough, many of these patients will respond to either an increase in steroids or the addition of immunosuppressive agents, or an increase in both of these modalities of treatment, if they have been maintained at low level dosages for maintenance of their transplant. Our longest survivor (four years, four months) has a steroid-dependent nephrotic syndrome which can be reversed only by going to high-dose intermittent therapy, and which relapses regularly when the steroid level is reduced.

Some concern has been voiced regarding the permanent effects of immunosuppressive drugs. Hersh et al. [277] studied 16 patients who were stimulated with three antigens during and after intensive five-day courses of 6-mercaptopurine and methotrexate. There was marked inhibition of the primary antibody response to the antigen given 24 hours after the start of therapy. All patients responded to a different antigen given 24 hours after the last dose of the five-day course. The median titers of antibodies were lower in the patients than in the control subjects. The third antigen, given 72 hours after the end of therapy, elicited a normal response. Thus, short-term intensive chemotherapy appears to be a potent inhibitor of the antibody response, but its effect ceased within 24 hours after the end of therapy.

Heparin. Because of the demonstrated relationship between small-vessel coagulation and experimental glomerulonephritis [676–678] and because of the ease with which fibrin deposition may be seen on light, electron, and immunofluorescent microscopy in patients with chronic proliferative glomerulonephritis, a number of investigators have recently employed large doses of heparin in the management of this disease. Kincaid-Smith and others have shown demonstrable improvement in both glomerular permeability and renal function in patients with proliferative disease which may also have a membranous component. Cade et al. [92] recently studied 18 patients with biopsy-proved chronic proliferative glomerulonephritis treated with daily injections of depo heparin. Eight showed significant improvement in endogenous creatinine clearance, Addis count, protein permeability index, and renal biopsy. Of carefully followed eight control patients, six demonstrated progressive diminution of renal function and four died in renal failure.

In adult glomerulonephritis, the lymphatic drainage by thoracic duct fistula may produce favorable effects in many cases. The main effect is disappearance of immunosuppressive resistance. A complete recovery (3 out of 11 cases) or improvement (4 out of 11 cases) has been found after 4 to 12 months in previously azathioprine-resistant patients. After thoracic duct fistula, patients with some azathioprine-resistant glomerulonephritis may respond favorably to azathioprine [70].

TREATMENT DETERMINED BY THE
ALTERED PHYSIOLOGY AND ITS
IMMEDIATE CONSEQUENCES

Diuretics. Much of the older literature on the nephrotic syndrome reflects preoccupation with the problem of edema. This preoccupation has often interfered with efforts to discover the cause of the syndrome when making the diagnosis, and changes in the edema have been misinterpreted as changes in the natural history of the disease process. For this reason, we emphasize the secondary role of edema, dependent as it is on dietary intake of salt, exercise, posture, aldosterone production, and the state of renal function. Thus, a patient with chronic glomerulonephritis and the nephrotic syndrome may get rid of his edema because of a change in diet, bed rest, transition into the nonedematous phase with reduc-

tion in filtration rate, or because of a diuresis in response to some therapeutic regimen. Nevertheless, edema is the most common manifestation that brings the patient to the physician. It is unsightly, it is obvious, and it may be uncomfortable (Fig. 16-39; page 579). It looms large in the patient's mind, and successful management of the edema may promote a satisfactory doctor-patient relationship. The most direct means of managing the edema is diuretic therapy [597].

The patient with nephrosis reacts in a physiologic manner to manipulation of the large number of mechanisms that alter urine flow. These mechanisms are summarized in the accompanying classification.

Classification of Diureses*

Osmotic Diuresis. Increase in urine volume due to the presentation of more solute and water to the distal nephron. Major methods:

1. Raising the plasma concentration of physiologic substances and therefore their filtered load (e.g., urea, intravenous hypertonic saline; glucose or fructose)
2. Administering osmotically important foreign substances or nonreabsorbable solute (e.g., mannitol; sucrose; sulfate)
3. Blockade of tubular reabsorption of physiologic substances (e.g., glucose by phlorizin; NaCl by saluretic agents; $NaHCO_3$ by carbonic anhydrase inhibitors)

Filtration Diuresis. Increase in urine volume due to the elevation of glomerular filtration rate. Methods are:

1. Raising the cardiac output and renal blood flow (e.g., digitalis in congestive heart failure; hydralazine in hypertension; extracellular expansion, corticosteroids, albumin, dextran; horizontal posture in syncope and severe heart failure)

* From Schreiner [594].

2. Raising the hydrostatic pressure (e.g., transfusion or plasma expanders in hypovolemic shock; pressors in vasodilatation; posture in orthostatic hypotension)
3. Inducing vasodilatation (e.g., xanthine diuretics)

Water Diuresis. Increase in urine volume due to a reduction in distal water reabsorption. Methods are:

1. Impaired production of ADH (diabetes insipidus; hypnosis; conditioned reflex)
2. Physiologic suppression of ADH (hydration; alcohol)
3. Impaired tubular response to ADH (nephrogenic diabetes insipidus; postrelease of obstruction; periureteral fibrosis; nephrocalcinosis; potassium depletion; chronic pyelonephritis. No drug is as yet available to manipulate this function.)

Perhaps the most important element in the clinical evaluation of diuretics is an accurate estimation of renal function in the patient. If one uses an agent that blocks sodium reabsorption in the nephron, the magnitude of the response is limited by the total load of sodium. This, of course, is the product of the sodium concentration of plasma water and the glomerular filtration rate. Since the concentration of serum sodium usually varies less than 10 per cent, the important reductions in filtered sodium load come from severe reductions in the glomerular filtration rate. One should therefore attempt to classify patients according to their filtration rates and corresponding filtered sodium loads. Azotemic patients, or those with marked reduction in filtration rate, will have impaired response to any diuretic regimen.

Another conditioning factor is the sodium, potassium, and water content of the patient's diet. Patients with organic renal disease are likely to have unusual dietary habits and may have substantial losses of electrolytes from vomiting and diarrhea. Other factors are

posture and the degree of physical activity. A continued horizontal position, as in bed rest in the hospital, may produce spontaneous diuresis in the nephrotic syndrome without measurable change in renal function. The patient's protein metabolism is also important. There is a correlation between hypoalbuminemia and the severity of clinical edema. There is an even greater correlation between serum albumin concentration in adults and the ability to attain diuresis with diuretics alone. In general, it is extremely difficult to achieve satisfactory diuresis and a clearing of edema with the usual doses of the common diuretic agents when the serum albumin is less than 1.5 gm. per 100 ml., although obviously this is not a clinical rule without exceptions. The role of steroid therapy should also be considered, since the salt-retaining effect of adrenal steroids varies, both with the drug employed and with the patient. Lastly, there are unknown factors that may preclude a diuresis even when all known physiologic factors favor a good effect.

The first really valuable agents in the control of nephrotic edema were the thiazide diuretics, which block the reabsorption of sodium [597]. Figure 16-45 depicts the renal response to intravenous chlorothiazide. In the first three columns are shown responses of a young girl with nephrotic syndrome due to disseminated lupus erythematosus. The first two 60-minute clearance periods represent controls taken in the basal state and those following the dashed line are the results after rapid administration of intravenous chlorothiazide in the dosage indicated. Column I shows the response in the untreated stage, column II the response after elevation of serum albumin by administration of concentrated albumin solution over a period of days, and column III the response after 19 days of intramuscular ACTH gel in a dosage of 40 units twice a day.

Noteworthy is the fact that this patient reacted to steroid therapy and the use of di-

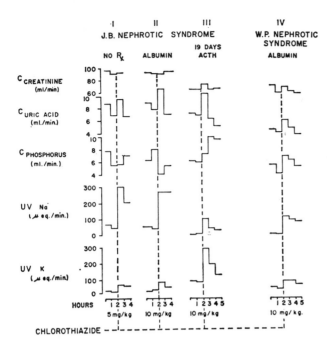

Figure 16-45. Renal response to intravenous chlorothiazide in the nephrotic syndrome. See text.

uretics with a distinct fall in endogenous creatinine clearance. This seriously modified the sodium diuresis, which was approximately the same in the first two studies. Although a higher dosage was administered in the albumin studies, these data corroborate the maximal dose response phenomenon which has been observed with chlorothiazide. There is no rationale for increasing the dose of chlorothiazide in nonresponding patients. The clearance of phosphorus generally declined except after ACTH therapy, when there was an appreciable rise.

The most significant change appeared in potassium excretion, which increased after chlorothiazide administration but was massive after corticosteroid therapy. It seems reasonable to suppose that the sodium-for-potassium ion exchange in the distal nephron site is enhanced by endogenous or exogenous levels of corticosteroid. Thus, the delivery of large amounts of sodium by an effective diuretic agent might provide enough sodium for a massive potassium exchange and produce rapid potassium depletion of the organism.

We have observed several nephrotic patients on steroid therapy who excreted only potassium with their chloruresis. In such patients, reduction of dose or the addition of dietary or pharmacologic supplements of potassium is vital, in order to prevent the metabolic and renal effects of intracellular potassium depletion as well as the increased susceptibility to pyelonephritis which has been noted experimentally in the kaliopenic state.

Column IV depicts the results of a study in a patient with an extremely low serum albumin concentration who had previously shown no measurable response to chlorothiazide. There was a significant elevation of sodium excretion following artificial elevation of the serum albumin concentration by intravenous albumin infusion. Judicious use of chlorothiazide diuretics and potassium supplements may enable a physician to obtain very significant weight losses and reduction of both edema and hypertension (see Table 16-21).

Other complications of thiazide diuretic therapy are increased serum uric acid with occasional precipitation of a gouty syndrome,

Table 16-21. Chlorothiazide in Nephrosis: Electrolyte Balance Studies

Diagnosis	Renal Function[a]	Sodium (mEq./24 hours)			Sodium Balance (mEq.)	Weight Loss (pounds)	Duration of Treatment (days)
		Dietary Intake	Control Excretion	Treatment Excretion			
Etiology unknown	BUN 9	8	17	118	−329	−3	3
Lupus nephritis	BUN 35	17	55	424	−2848	−46	7
Membranous glomerulonephritis	C_{CR} 150	17	0	82	−131	−½	2
Chronic glomerulonephritis	BUN 30	8	17	106	−293	−6½	3
Membranous glomerulonephritis	BUN 27	17	0	64	−94	−3½	2
Subacute glomerulonephritis	BUN 35	8	4	13	−16	−½	3
Renal amyloidosis	C_{CR} 75	8	0	5		−2	3
Chronic glomerulonephritis	BUN 105	17	45	76		−6	6
Membranous glomerulonephritis	C_{CR} 102	8	71	191		−20	6

[a] Blood urea nitrogen (BUN) given in milligrams per 100 ml.; creatinine clearance (C_{CR}) in milliliters per minute.
SOURCE: From Schreiner [594].

and further elevations of azotemia, which may reflect fluid loss or be an indirect manifestation of uric acid nephrotoxicity or pyelonephritis secondary to hypokalemia. We have previously documented alterations in renal function which may occur as a result of long-term salt depletion with a rice diet [330].

Similar effects may be seen after the long-term administration of potent diuretic agents, which may also produce the effect in a much shorter time than dietary factors. Table 16-22 presents the renal hemodynamic changes seen in the major types of salt depletion.

If the response to chlorothiazide diuretics

Table 16-22. Renal Effects of Depletion Regimens

Regimen	Blood Pressure	Plasma Flow	Filtration Rate	Filtration Fraction
Acute hypovolemia Blood removal Limb congestion Quiet standing	↓	↓	↓	↑
Chronic hypovolemia Rice diet Marked sodium restriction Chronic use of resins	↓	Little changed	↓	↓
Prolonged diuretic therapy	↓	Unchanged	↓	↓

is suboptimal, they may be reinforced by the addition of carbonic anhydrase inhibitors, xanthine diuretics such as aminophylline, or an osmotic diuretic agent such as mannitol. In patients with urinary electrolyte findings that suggest hyperaldosteronism (low sodium excretion, high potassium excretion) the short-term use of aldosterone antagonists, such as the spirolactones or triamcinolone, may be beneficial. They are also helpful in reversing the hypokalemia of prolonged therapy with diuretics and steroids. In patients with diminished glomerular filtration rates, however, these agents must be used very carefully, since they can rapidly reverse the potassium loss and lead to significant and even dangerous degrees of hyperkalemia [276].

More recently, the development of more potent diuretics, such as ethacrynic acid [324] and furosemide, enable the delivery to the urine of much higher percentages of the filtered sodium load. These agents, of course, have side effects that include deafness from large intravenous doses of ethacrynic acid and effects on uric acid excretion leading to hyperuricemia, and on carbohydrate metabolism [659]. Figure 16-46 represents a metabolic study done on a nephrotic patient given ethacrynic acid [426]. With the addition of these potent diuretics to our armamentarium, resistant edema in the nephrotic syndrome has become such a clinical rarity that it is almost a curiosity. We no longer receive requests for consultations for refractory edema, but we do get them for the side effects of prolonged or too vigorous diuretic therapy.

It is my personal view that mercurial diuretics should never be used in the nephrotic syndrome. To date we have observed six cases of acute tubular necrosis secondary to the administration of organic mercurial diuretics, and several instances where a nephrotic syndrome occurred after the prolonged use of oral mercurial diuretics or cutaneous exposure to mercury [48].

Albumin Replacement. A considerable body of clinical experience indicates that albumin replacement has a salutary effect in nephrotic patients who have significant hypoalbuminemia. In the presteroid era, administration of intravenous albumin or serum was often followed by diuresis [14, 263], and in some cases there was an apparent improvement in well-being and amelioration of the progress of the disease, which may or may not have been coincidental. Even with modern therapy, one still encounters clinical situations in which the nephrotic patient appears to regress acutely. This may occur after immunization procedures, nonspecific exposure to allergens, respiratory infection, or even with physical exertion and simple fatigue. Infusion of salt-poor albumin may be of considerable value in transient exacerbations during steroid therapy. Adult patients with a serum albumin concentration under 2 gm. per 100 ml. are often unable to achieve diuresis in response to appropriate procedures. Acute elevation of serum albumin in such persons may be accompanied by a diuresis as a direct result of plasma expansion or may improve the filtered load of sodium to such a degree that even though no great diuresis is achieved from albumin alone, the patient becomes susceptible to the effects of tubular blocking agents such as the thiazide diuretics.

It is not difficult to explain these phenomena theoretically as resulting from an increase in intravascular volume and in the filtered load of sodium. However, one wonders how the patient with nephrosis differs from patients with congenital analbuminemia or hypoalbuminemia due to losses in the gastrointestinal tract which have been described in Germany and in the United States. The latter patients, who may have little or no measurable serum albumin, do not seem to have massive edema. In fact, they appear to get along quite well.

From the beginning of any exogenous albumin infusion there is progressive distur-

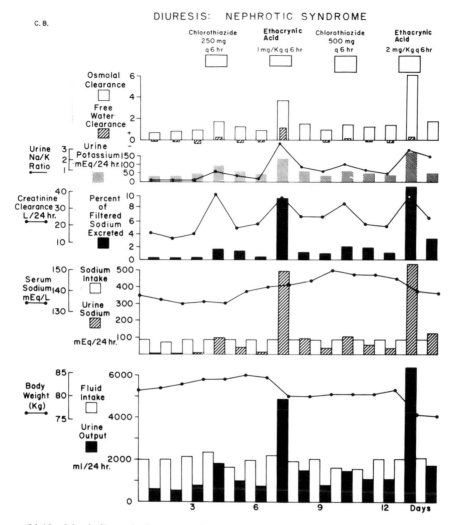

Figure 16-46. Metabolic study done on nephrotic patient during administration of ethacrynic acid.

bance of capillary membrane equilibrium all over the body. This is seen grossly from increases in thoracic and hepatic lymph and increased protein losses through the kidney, but physiologically it must be visualized as occurring throughout the capillary bed. Armstrong [16] has characterized the responses as "iso-osmotic" and "isometric." Chinard et al. [106] studied serial changes in plasma volume following intravenous administration of albumin to nephrotic patients. The change in plasma volume per gram of albumin re-tained was less than that predictable by an iso-osmotic response, thus suggesting an increase in capillary hydrostatic pressure. The estimated decrease in interstitial fluid pressure was in the order of 1.3 mm. Hg for net shifts of water approaching 1 liter.

Luetscher and his colleagues [418, 422] also studied the treatment of the nephrotic syndrome with concentrated albumin and were able to render 5 of 13 patients edema free after administration of 50 gm. a day for a period of four to six days. They noted very large increases of plasma volume in some patients, and increased venous pressure and dyspnea in patients whose vital capacity was reduced by infusion, which suggests that doses larger than 50 to 75 gm. a day should be given with great caution. In patients with large losses of the administered protein, efficiency of albumin replacement was poor. At the end of treatment a fairly constant proportion of the administered albumin could not be found in urine or plasma. At the end of two weeks, all the nitrogen injected as albumin could be accounted for as excess albumin and nonprotein nitrogen in the urine. The proportion of their patients who responded with a diuresis and the variations in the relationship between the rise in serum albumin and the diuretic results were in general agreement with reports of Janeway [326] and Thorn [665].

In my own experience, the patients with massive proteinuria, in general, have made the less dramatic responses to intravenous albumin, and patients who have failed to achieve a diuresis have been, in general, the ones who have shown the poorest elevations of serum albumin in response to an infusion. In the steroid era we have used calculated albumin retention as a good clinical index of permeability under the stress of plasma volume expansion. If one has a good control period of measured protein excretion on standard diet and activity, and administers the albumin rapidly during the first four to six hours of a 24-hour collection, the percentage of retention can be calculated on a 24- to 48-hour basis by subtracting from the protein excretion the mean control value and expressing the difference as a percentage of the amount administered. Patients whose glomerular permeability is diminishing with steroids and those who will go on to a full diuresis and a more favorable response will often excrete as little as 10 to 20 per cent of the administered albumin. Patients who ex-

crete more than half of the administered albumin will usually continue to be therapeutic problems.

Orloff et al. [510] reexamined carefully the sequence in albumin diuresis and found that the osmotic efficiency in the body was reasonably close to the osmotic efficiency of albumin by in vitro measurements. They measured no significant shifts in the electrolytes within the body or changes of endogenous creatinine clearance. Albumin first induced diuresis of water, and only when this resulted in an increased serum sodium concentration was salt excretion significantly augmented.

Other Oncotic Agents. The expense of continued albumin administration and its unavailability in many parts of the world has led to continued exploration of all types of plasma substitutes [131, 233, 387, 404] in patients with hypovolemia due to the nephrotic syndrome. These have included plasma, gum acacia, globin, polyvinyl pyrrolidone, and the whole gamut of plasma expanders.

As a striking example, the availability of dextran [68, 240] led logically to its use in oligemic subjects [255] and in those with the nephrotic syndrome [325, 466]. James et al. [325] found that the intravenous infusion of 12 per cent (hyperoncotic) dextran initiated a water diuresis followed often by a natriuresis and removal of edema fluid. Transient hypertension was the most common complication. Diuresis was associated with marked increase in plasma volume and with increased effective renal plasma flow in seven patients. Maximal diuresis could be transiently inhibited by intravenous injection of vasopressin (Pitressin). Observations during the dextran infusion in four children suggested that glomerular membrane permeability for albumin may increase further during dextran infusion and appears to be independent of that for water.

There are fewer indications for massive

use of oncotic agents in patients with the nephrotic syndrome since the introduction of therapy which is based on the nature of the lesion. However, in patients who first come under medical care with extensive anasarca or strategic, life-threatening serous effusions, oncotic agents have a place in reducing the morbidity from edema during the two to three weeks necessary to ascertain the efficacy of specific therapy. For transient episodes of increased glomerular permeability during maintenance of steroid therapy, the judicious use of albumin or other oncotic agents may contribute materially to the comfort and well-being of the patient.

TREATMENT TO ELIMINATE THE MORE
INDIRECT CONSEQUENCES OR COMPLICATIONS
OF THE NEPHROTIC SYNDROME

Infection. There is an old clinical observation that patients with the nephrotic syndrome may have increased susceptibility to intercurrent bacterial infections. In the pre-antibiotic era, the term *nephrotic crisis* was applied to acute attacks in children, and occasionally in adults, which were characterized by abrupt onset with high temperatures (105 to 106°F.), often with a chill, and accompanied by generalized abdominal pain, rigidity, nausea, vomiting, prostration, and marked leukocytosis (20,000 to 40,000 cells per cubic millimeter). In some cases an organism, usually a pneumococcus, would be found in the blood or peritoneal fluid; in others, no organism could be cultured. The attacks recurred many times. Metabolic studies indicated a markedly negative nitrogen balance preceding by several days the onset of the crisis, and low plasma amino acid nitrogen has been observed during attacks, rising promptly with their cessation [174, 176, 601].

In addition to pneumococcal and, rarely, streptococcal peritonitis, confluent broncho-pneumonia, bacteremia, pleurisy, pericarditis, and erysipelas may also be seen. The naso-

pharynx should be cultured frequently since it is the focus of the carrier state for pathogenic microorganisms in nephrotic children.

The mechanism for increased susceptibility to infection is not completely known. It has been ascribed to protein deficiency, to low complement levels, and to gamma globulin deficit, which may be seen as a result of marked glomerular porosity.

In recent years, the availability of antibiotics has markedly decreased the danger of those infectious complications which used to represent a major cause of death in nephrotic children. It is our custom to culture the throat and nasopharynx of all children with nephrosis appearing in the hospital, to isolate them from known pneumococcal, streptococcal, and staphylococcal infections insofar as is possible, and to treat with oral penicillin those patients with positive cultures. When the carrier state has been identified in the family or in immediate contacts, we treat the children prophylactically. It is helpful, during the acute stages, to keep these children out of school or social situations involving contact with infection.

Infection has sometimes been used therapeutically in the nephrotic syndrome. Diuresis has been reported in about four out of five patients with anasarca who developed intercurrent measles [547], and has also occurred after other viral diseases, such as dengue fever [547] and hepatitis [52]. The once common practice of deliberately exposing children with nephrosis to measles on the hospital wards has been abandoned since the advent of steroids and the occurrence of a number of untoward complications.

Infections of all types have likewise produced acute exacerbation during a remission. This has been observed especially after the common cold, nasopharyngitis, and streptococcal pharyngitis. We observed a patient whose original nephrotic syndrome occurred after a bout of herpes zoster. He had made a group 4 response (remission), but had an exacerbation after siblings developed chickenpox, a virus closely related to the herpes zoster which produced his original nephrotic syndrome.

We do not advocate the long-term prophylactic use of penicillin. This is reserved for family or school epidemics, in which oral penicillin, 250 mg. three times a day for two to three weeks, is generally desirable.

Hypertension. Hypertension is a formidable problem in the management of the nephrotic syndrome. It has, however, become much more tractable under modern diuretic therapy. Hypertension is seen in its most severe state in the setting of florid disease, edema, and steroid therapy. Very high diastolic blood pressures can be reduced in the majority of nephrotic patients by elimination of the edema with diuretic therapy. In the case of accelerated hypertension, ethacrynic acid or furosemide have been very helpful. In the remainder of patients, the blood pressures are usually manageable by mild antihypertensive drugs, such as the rauwolfia alkaloids. In patients with azotemia, alphamethyldopa is often the most effective drug. Rarely have we had to use ganglionic blockade with drugs such as guanethidine (Ismelin). An occasional patient responds well to high doses of spironolactone, and a very high percentage of patients with azotemia and severe accelerated hypertension, when they respond to nothing else, will respond transiently at least to intravenously administered diazoxide [692].

Nutritional Problems. The most severe nutritional problems revolve, of course, about the loss of serum albumin or specifically identifiable globulin fractions. Reams have been written about the dietary management of the nephrotic syndrome. There are very few good data to suggest that one can "force" albumin synthesis by diets excessively high in protein, although the converse seems true, that protein wasting would be more cata-

strophic with dietary deficiency. It is therefore our practice to allow patients an unrestricted diet, in general, but to encourage a protein intake of 2 gm. per kilogram per day if they have moderately reduced or normal glomerular filtration rates. A protein intake of 1 gm. per kilogram per day is recommended when there is a marked reduction of filtration rate; and 0.5 gm. of protein per kilogram per day when there is more severe reduction in filtration rate which is accompanied by a serum urea nitrogen level in excess of 60 mg. per 100 ml. It is not unusual for nephrotic patients to have gamma globulin concentrations on serum electrophoresis which are less than 20 to 30 per cent of normal. Indeed, these have been offered as one of the explanations for the frequency of intercurrent infection. In patients plagued with boils or recurrent infection and a persistent low gamma globulin, the administration of exogenous gamma globulin may be occasionally rewarded with a lessening of infectious complications. If a nephrotic patient has acquired unusual appetite fads as a result of his disease or steroid therapy, or if his diet is not adequate in vitamin-containing foods, it is advisable to place the patient on maintenance vitamin therapy during his active disease.

Pyelonephritis. When closely following the urinary sediment in patients with nephrosis, one is impressed by the transient occurrence of pyuria, especially in children. It is important to investigate the causes of this pyuria and not to remain preoccupied with the nephrotic syndrome alone. We have found in a number of children with transient pyuria urethral obstruction, contracture of the bladder neck, and other anomalies leading to lower urinary tract infection. We have also been impressed, in reviewing biopsy material, by a rather significant incidence of focal leukocytic infiltrations in the interstitial areas of kidneys in patients who have not had symptoms of an infection. Other patients have had both symptomatic clinical and histologic evidence of pyelonephritis. We believe that the association of pyelonephritis and the nephrotic syndrome is probably conditioned by a general susceptibility to infection and by the local factor of intrarenal obstruction which may occur in large edematous kidneys. In fact, the unusual narrowing of the infundibula seen on the intravenous pyelogram of nephrotic patients is evidence of pressure on the collecting system by edematous pyramids (Fig. 16-2).

There have been a number of correlative studies indicating a high frequency of bladder-neck obstruction or anomalies of the lower urinary tract in children with the nephrotic syndrome. Whether this simply reflects a greater diagnostic exposure to these children who are generally in good medical centers, or whether there is a truly elevated correlation is not clear. In some series the yield of anomalies of the urinary tract is sufficiently high to justify further diagnostic studies in nephrotic children during the recovery phase.

Growth Retardation and Decalcification of Bone. There have now been abundant reports that prolonged steroid therapy can induce significant growth retardation in young children [205, 385] and may also produce possible complications of osteoporosis [376] and urinary lithiasis. Most such children will accelerate and resume their previous growth curve after cessation of steroid therapy. In some, however, cessation of steroid therapy leads to exacerbation of the nephrotic syndrome. Under these circumstances, we have resorted, particularly during the pubertal growth spurt, either to a period of ACTH administration during which growth is usually resumed [204] or to a single–dose alternate-day regimen with the entire day's steroid dose being given at noon. This technic has enabled some patients to grow while controlling their steroid-dependent nephrotic syndrome. A third possible maneuver is to substitute immunosuppressive agents and re-

duce the steroid dose to very low levels. Theoretically, if severe retardation of growth continues in spite of these measures, the child should probably be studied with one of the newer technics for measuring the quantitative growth-hormone response, and if found quantitatively deficient, growth may be inducible by daily injections of a synthetic growth hormone.

TREATMENT AND MANAGEMENT, CONSIDERING THE WHOLE PATIENT AND HIS ENVIRONMENT

A successful blending of scientific background and the art of medicine is a desideratum in approaching any ill patient. No clinical situation imposes a greater challenge in this regard than the long-term management of the patient with nephrosis through remissions and exacerbations, complications and vicissitudes. A successful conclusion requires constant attention to detail, patience, and an unusual degree of educational activity on the part of the physician.

To tell the upset mother of a nephrotic child, "This is just a little kidney swelling. A few days of this new miracle drug and we will have her all cured," is hazardous. It is our policy to sit down initially with the patient or parent and explain the necessity of facing up to the fact that this is a potentially chronic disease which is characterized by remissions and exacerbations, and which will require a long medical follow-up therapy and evaluation and a great amount of patience and cooperation from the patient and his family. We never speak of a cure in this disease, any more than we would to a diabetic patient, since exacerbations have occurred after remissions of longer than five years. We point out that this disease will affect constantly their day-to-day living, but we emphasize that it is possible to adapt successfully and happily to the situation and that we will make the regimen no more formidable than is necessary for the immediate medical situation. We indicate in general terms the prognosis we can offer on the basis of urine examination, clearance data, and renal biopsies, and we permit patient and family to hope that an early group 3 or group 4 response will prove to be a good omen for the long-term prognosis.

Diet. Protein is regulated in accordance with the principles outlined in our discussion of nutritional problems (see page 604). We recommend only small amounts of salt in the diet. We do not impose any further dietary restrictions on the average patient, because small accumulations of edema are much more easily managed with modern diuretic therapy.

Activity. This remains a highly controversial point. We advocate restricted activity during the acute phase and for several months after it. Initial hospitalization for one to two months is a great educational help to this end. Patients with group 3 to group 4 responses are then allowed normal activity. For those with a group 0 response, we prescribe absolute bed rest; and for those with group 1 to group 2 responses, modified bed rest, with bathroom privileges, permission to get up for meals, and so forth. We warn all children against excessive fatigue or long periods of standing. There are some nephrotic patients who regularly experience exacerbations after colds or respiratory infections. We suggest that they avoid overt exposure in theaters, department stores, and large crowds during the respiratory-virus season. It is important not to make psychologic cripples or neurasthenic individuals out of patients with the nephrotic syndrome. Gentle exercise combined with a high protein intake is probably the best stimulus to albumin synthesis.

Immunization. We have personally encountered clear-cut exacerbations of the nephrotic syndrome in patients who have been in long remissions who received smallpox vaccination or immunizations against tetanus, typhoid, and influenza. Because the nephrotic syndrome is considered a hyperimmune disease, and because of this experience after innoculations, we recommend that patients with the nephrotic syndrome avoid all immunizations and skin testing for allergies during the period of active disease. When investigating a patient with polycyclic nephrotic syndrome due to pollen, it may be necessary to try to find the specific nephroallergen in order to initiate desensitization procedures.

Surgery. This question comes up most often in connection with tonsillectomy in children. It is our general policy to avoid surgical stress as much as possible during a period of active disease. Existence of an active state may be judged from residual clinical laboratory findings and elevation of the sedimentation rate. In patients who have very bad tonsils which are considered a focus of infection and who have not responded to other therapeutic measures, a tonsillectomy may well be tried.

Travel. We do not recommend long travel in the upright position. Many of our patients are able to tolerate family excursions well when a back seat bed is prepared and they are allowed to travel horizontally.

Sunburn. Sunburn has been known to precede an exacerbation of lupus nephritis, the transplant reaction, and acute and subacute glomerulonephritis. We therefore recommend that sunburn be avoided in patients in the active stage of nephrosis.

Allergic Experience. Nephrotic patients known to be allergic to poison oak, poison ivy, etc., are cautioned to avoid exposure at all times, and especially when their disease is active. Since desensitization has been known to produce the nephrotic syndrome, it is not recommended in these patients. The interesting problems of cyclic nephrotic syndrome related to pollen have already been discussed.

Sedation. For patients rendered hyperexcitable by administration of steroids, small doses of phenobarbital have proved most effective. Antihistamines may also be employed for their sedative properties.

School. It is our policy to remove nephrotic children from school at the time of their attack. If this occurs in the fall or winter, arrangements are made for a visiting teacher to instruct the child at home, since he will be on steroid therapy for a minimum of two and a half months. We do not return child patients to school until the following year. If the disease remains extremely active for more than one year and the child has obtained what appears to be maximum benefit from bed rest, steroids, and other therapeutic media, it is our practice to send him back to school in an attempt to avoid a psychologically crippling situation.

Acknowledgments

From the Department of Medicine and the Division of Nephrology, Georgetown University School of Medicine, Washington, D.C.

Supported in part by the John A. Hartford Foundation Inc., the Georgetown University Kidney Research Fund, and TO1 HE 05256-09.

We wish to acknowledge the assistance of our Editorial Assistant, Miss Joan P. Ryan, in the preparation of this chapter.

References

1. Ackerman, G. L., and Nolsn, C. M. Adrenocortical responsiveness after alternate-day corticosteroid therapy. *New Eng. J. Med.* 278:405, 1968.

2. Adams, D. A., Gold, E. M., and Gonick, H. C. Adrenocortical function during intermittent corticosteroid therapy. *Ann. Intern. Med.* 64:542, 1966.

3. Adams, D. A., Gordon, A., and Maxwell, M. H. Azathiozone treatment in immunologic renal disease. *J.A.M.A.* 199:459, 1967.

4. Addis, T. Renal degenerations due to protein reabsorption by the kidney. *Stanford Med. Bull.* 31:67, 1945.

5. Afonso, E. Evaluation of renal filter selectivity by quantitative immunoelectrophoresis. *Clin. Chim. Acta* 17:239, 1967.

6. Aida, M., Maebashi, M., and Yoshinaga, K. Estimation of plasma renin and renin-substrate in various diseases in man. *Tohoku J. Exp. Med.* 87:35, 1965.

7. Albrink, M. J. Lactescence of serum following episodes of acute alcoholism and its probable relationship to acute pancreatitis. *Amer. J. Med.* 23:26, 1957.

8. Albrink, M. J., Man, E. B., and Peters, J. P. The relation of neutral fat to lactescence of serum. *J. Clin. Invest.* 34:26, 1955.

9. Aldrich, C. A., Stokes, J., Jr., Killingsworth, W. P., and McGuiness, A. C. Concentrated human blood serum as a diuretic in the treatment of nephrosis. *J.A.M.A.* 111:129, 1938.

10. Allison, A. C., Houba, V., Hendrickse, R. G., de Petris, S., Edington, G. M., and Adenihi, A. Immune complexes in the nephrotic syndrome of African children. *Lancet* 1:1232, 1969.

11. Alport, A. C. Hereditary familial congenital haemorrhagic nephritis. *Brit. Med. J.* 1:504, 1927.

12. Amorin, M. F., and Mello, R. F. Intermediate nephron nephrosis from snake poisoning in man. *Amer. J. Path.* 30:479, 1954.

13. Andersen, S. B., Jarnum, S., and Jensen, H. Metabolism of gamma-G-globulin in the nephrotic syndrome in adults. *Scand. J. Clin. Lab. Invest.* 21:42, 1968.

14. Andersen, S. B., and Ward, P. S. Diagnostic significance of hypogammaglobulinemia. *Acta Med. Scand.* 180:253, 1966.

15. Annotations. Nephrosis and renal-vein thrombosis. *Lancet* 2:1932, 1956.

16. Armstrong, S. H. Mechanisms of action of serum albumin therapy in internal medicine. *Amer. J. Med.* 4:390, 1948.

17. Armstrong, S. H., and Kushner, D. S. Current status of steroid therapy in chronic glomerulonephritis in the adult. *Amer. J. Med.* 29:377, 1960.

18. Arneil, G. C. Age Incidence of Nephrosis in Britain and Scotland. In Metcoff, J. (Ed.), *Proceedings of the Eighth Annual Conference on the Nephrotic Syndrome.* New York: National Nephrosis Foundation, 1956. P. 123.

19. Arneil, G. C. Management of the nephrotic syndrome. *Arch. Dis. Child.* 43:257, 1968.

20. Arneil, G. C., and Lam, C. N. Long-term assessment of steroid therapy in childhood nephrosis. *Lancet* 2:819, 1966.

21. Arneil, G. C., and Wilson, H. E. ACTH in nephrosis. *Arch. Dis. Child.* 28:372, 1953.

22. Arnold, J. D., and Spargo, B. Clinical use of the percutaneous renal biopsy. *Circulation* 19:609, 1959.

23. Arundell, F. D., Wilkinson, R. D., and Haserick, J. R. Dermatomyositis and malignant neoplasms in adults: A survey of 20 years' experience. *Arch. Derm.* (Chicago) 82:772, 1960.

24. Azoury, F. J., and Gum, O. B. Antinuclear factors in nephrotic syndrome secondary to systemic lupus erythematosus and in leprosy. *Amer. J. Med. Sci.* 253:661, 1967.

25. Ballard, H. S., and Eisinger, R. P. Childhood nephrosis followed by acute glomerulonephritis in adulthood. *Brit. Med. J.* 1:477, 1967.

26. Balsløv, J. T. Nephrotic syndrome with bilateral thrombosis of renal veins in two cardiac patients. *Ugeskr. Laeg.* 121:197, 1959.

27. Banerjea, J. C., and Mukherjee, S. K. Pericardial effusion with nephrotic syndrome in systemic lupus erythematosus: A case report with review of literature. *Indian Heart J.* 19:358, 1967.

28. Barnes, L. A., Moll, G. H., and Janeway, C. A. Nephrotic syndrome: Natural history of the disease. *Pediatrics* 5:486, 1950.

29. Barnett, H. L. In discussion on Lange, K., and Wenk, E. J. Investigations into the site of complement loss in acute human and experimental glomerulonephritis and the nephrotic syndrome. *A.M.A. Amer. J. Dis. Child.* 88:639, 1954.

30. Barnett, H. L. Clinicopathological conference. Albert Einstein College of Medicine, Bronx, New York. *J. Pediat.* 73:936, 1968.

31. Barnett, H. L., Forman, C. M., McNamara, H., and McCrary, W. W. Effect of adrenocorticotrophic hormone on children with nephrotic syndrome: II. Physiologic observations on discrete kidney functions and plasma volume. *J. Clin. Invest.* 30:227, 1951.

32. Barnett, H. L., Forman, C. W., and Lauson, H. D. The Nephrotic Syndrome in Children. In Levine, S. Z., and others (Eds.), *Advances in Pediatric*, Vol. 5. Chicago: Year Book Publishers, 1952. P. 53.

33. Barnett, H. L., Simons, D. J., and Wells, R. E. Nephrotic syndrome occurring during Tridione therapy. *Amer. J. Med.* 4:760, 1948.

34. Barow, R., and Hartmann, F. Die Ausscheidung freier Aminosäuren im Urin bei Gesunden, Leber- und Nephrosekranken. *Deutsch. Arch. Klin. Med.* 203:260, 1956.

35. Barr, S. Serum and plasma proteins in thermally injured patients treated with plasma, its admixture with albumin or serum alone. *Ann. Surg.* 161:112, 1965.

36. Barr, J. H., Cole, H. N., Driver, J. R., DeLeas, R., Miller, M., and Strauss, L. G. Acute syphilitic nephrosis successfully treated with penicillin. *J.A.M.A.* 131:741, 1946.

37. Barrett, F. R. Determination of mercury inurine with results in cases of pink disease. *Med. J. Aust.* 2:411, 1955.

38. Bartlett, P., and Bossart, J. F. Effects of the potent nephrotogenic aminonucleoside of puromycin on phospholipid metabolism in rat kidney cortex subcellular fractions. *Henry Ford Hosp. Med. J.* 16:137, 1968.

39. Bartter, F. C. *The Clinical Use of Aldos-*

88. Bunim, J. J., Harvey, A. M., Bollet, A. J., Hilbish, T. F., Van Scott, E., Sokoloff, L., and Brecher, G. Systemic lupus erythematosus. *Circulation.* 14:125, 1956.

89. Burke, E. C. Survival in a group of steroid-treated nephrotic children; preliminary report. *Proc. Staff Meet. Mayo Clin.* 33:12, 1958.

90. Burston, J., Darmady, E. M., and Stranack, F. Nephrosis due to mercurial diuretics. *Brit. Med. J.* 1:1277, 1958.

91. Butler, H. E., Jr., Morgan, J. M., and Smythe, C. M. Mercaptopurine and acquired tublar dysfunction in adult nephrosis. *Arch. Intern. Med.* (Chicago) 116:853, 1965.

92. Cade, J. R., de Quesada, A. M., Shires, D. L., Levin, D. M., Hackett, R. L., Spooner, G. R., Schlein, E. M., Pickering, M. J., and Holcomb, A. The effect of long-term high dose heparin treatment on the course of chronic proliferative glomerulonephritis. *Nephron,* 8:67, 1971.

93. Cameron, J. S. Histology, protein clearances, and response to treatment in the nephrotic syndrome. *Brit. Med. J.* 4:352, 1968.

94. Cameron, J. S. The clinical significance of glomerular permeability studies. *Proc. Roy. Soc. Med.* 59:512, 1966.

95. Cameron, J. S., and Blandford, G. The simple assessment of selectivity in heavy proteinuria. *Lancet* 2:242, 1966.

96. Campbell, R. A., and Jacinto, E. Y. Combined immunosuppressive therapy in steroid-resistant, chronic glomerular diseases of childhood. *J. Lancet* 87:149, 1967.

97. Campbell, T. N., and Goldman, R. Primary amyloidosis with death due to progressive hypotension. *Calif. Med.* 104:208, 1966.

98. Castleman, B. Case records of the Massachusetts General Hospital. Case 29—1963 *New Eng. J. Med.* 268:943, 1963.

99. Chamberlain, M. J., and Whittaker, S. R. Hashimoto's disease, dermatomyositis, and ovarian carcinoma. *Lancet* 1:1398, 1963.

100. Charlton, D., Latner, A. L., Platt, J. W., Smart, G. A., Thompson, R. B., and Walker, W. The nephrotic syndrome: Observations of the effects of ACTH in 40 patients. *Acta Med. Scand.* 161:33, 1958.

101. Charlwood, P. A. Sedimentation and diffusion of human albumins: II. Nephrotic human albumins at a low concentration. *Biochem. J.* 52:279, 1952.

102. Chasis, H., Goldring, W., and Baldwin, D. S. Effect of febrile plasma, typhoid vaccine and nitrogen mustard on renal manifestations of human glomerulonephritis. *Proc. Soc. Exp. Biol. Med.* 71:565, 1949.

103. Chasis, H., Goldring, W., and Baldwin, D. S. The effects of nitrogen mustard on renal manifestations of human glomerulonephritis. (Abstract.) *J. Clin. Invest.* 29:804, 1950.

104. Chasis, H., Goldring, W., Breed, E. S., Schreiner, G. E., and Bolomey, A. A. Salt and protein restriction: Effects on blood pressure and renal hemodynamics in hypertensive patients. *J.A.M.A.* 142:711, 1950.

105. Chassagnon, C., and Robillard, J. Syndrome néphrotique révélateur d'un cancer bronchique. *Lyon Med.* 213:1063, 1965.

106. Chinard, F. P., Lauson, H. D., Eder, H. A. and Greif, R. L. Plasma volume changes following administration of albumin to patients with the nephrotic syndrome. *J. Clin. Invest.* 33:629, 1954.

107. Christian, H. A. Nephrosis syndrome associated with idiopathic amyloidosis. *Med. Clin. N. Amer.* 15:805, 1932.

108. Christiansen, W. E. Nephrotic syndrome after use of mercurial diuretics. *Ugeskr. Laeg.* 121:200, 1959.

109. Clancy, R. L., and Stiel, J. N. Familial Mediterranean fever with amyloidosis. *Med. J. Aust.* 1:495, 1968.

110. Cohn, L. H., Lee, J., and Hopper, J. The treatment of bilateral renal vein thrombosis and nephrotic syndrome. *Surgery* 64:387, 1968.

111. Coon, W. W., and Willis, P. W. Thrombosis of axillary and subclavian veins. *Arch. Surg.* (Chicago) 94:657, 1967.

112. Cornig, H. J. Une forme nouvelle de la maladie de Hodgkin: Lymphogranulomatose maligne à type de Néphrose Lipoidique, Thèse de Paris 1939, No. 517. Cited by Tapie, J., Laporte, J., and Ricalens, S. U. C. Syndrome néphrotique au cours de la mala-

die de Hodgkin-Sternberg. *Presse Med.* 65: 287, 1957.

113. Cruickshank, J. G., and Parker, R. A. Pulmonary haemosiderosis with severe renal lesions. *Thorax* 16:22, 1961.

114. Cruz, T., Reboucas, G., and Rocha, H. Fatal strongyloidiasis in patients receiving corticosteroids. *New Eng. J. Med.* 275:1093, 1966.

115. Curtis, A. C., Heckaman, J. H., and Wheeler, A. H. Study of the autoimmune reaction in dermatomyositis. *J.A.M.A.* 178: 571, 1961.

116. Daeschner, C. W., Dodge, W. F., and Hill, L. L. Management of the nephrotic syndrome with particular reference to the use of triamcinolene. *J. Pediat.* 56:48, 1960.

117. Dagg, J. H., Smith, J. A., and Goldberg, A. Urinary excretion of iron. *Clin. Sci.* 30:495, 1966.

118. Danowski, T. S., Mateer, F. M., and Puntereri, A. J. ACTH or adrenocortical steroid therapy of proteinuria in adolescents and in adults. *Amer. J. Med. Sci.* 237:545, 1959.

119. Dawdle, E., and Saunder, S. J. Acute effect of hydrocortisone sodium succinate on the proteinuria of the nephrotic syndrome. *S. Afr. J. Lab. Clin. Med.* 3:39, 1957.

120. Daysog, A., Jr., and Campos, P. C. The nephrotic syndrome among Filipinos: Clinical and histologic studies with special reference to doubly refractile fat bodies in the urine. *J. Philipp. Med. Ass.* 42:779, 1966.

121. De Gowin, R. L., Ida, Y., and Evans, R. H. Nephritis and lung hemorrhage. *Arch. Intern. Med.* (Chicago) 111:16, 1963.

122. Deparis, M., Auguier, L., Canivet, J., Levillain, R., and Lissac, J. Thrombose des veines rénales et néphrose lipoidique. *Presse Med.* 62:1363, 1954.

123. Derow, H. A. The nephrotic syndrome. *New Eng. J. Med.* 258:77, 1958.

124. Derow, H. A., Schlesinger, M. J., and Savitz, H. A. Chronic progressive occlusion of inferior vena cava and renal and portal veins, with clinical picture of nephrotic syndrome: Report of a case with review of literature. *Arch. Intern. Med.* 63:626, 1939.

125. Derow, H. A., and Wolff, L. Oral administration of mercupurin tablets in am-

bulatory patients with chronic congestive heart failure. *Amer. J. Med.* 3:693, 1947.

126. Derr, R. F., Alexander, C. S., and Nagasawa, H. T. Metabolism of puromycin aminonucleoside in the normal "pre-nephrotic" and nephrotic rat. *Proc. Soc. Exp. Biol. Med.* 125:248, 1967.

127. Derr, R. F., Loechler, D. K., and Alexander, C. S. Inhibition of aminonucleoside nephrosis in rats: IV. Prevention by N6-methyladenosine. *J. Lab. Clin. Med.* 72:363, 1968.

128. De Sousa, J. S., Guerreiro, O., and Cunha, A. Association of nephrotic syndrome with intestinal lymphangiectasia. *Arch. Dis. Child.* 43:245, 1968.

129. Deleted in proof.

130. DeSwiet, J., and Wells, A. L. Nephrotic syndrome associated with renal venous thrombosis and bronchial carcinoma. *Brit. Med. J.* 2:1341, 1957.

131. Dick, M. W., Warweg, E., and Andersch, M. Acacia in the treatment of nephrosis. *J.A.M.A.* 105:654, 1935.

132. Dixon, F. J., Feldman, J. D., and Vasquez, J. J. Experimental glomerulonephritis. The pathogenesis of a laboratory model resembling the spectrum of human glomerulonephritis. *J. Exp. Med.* 113:899, 1961.

133. Domart, A., Hazard, J., and Modal, J. Syndrome nephrotique apparement primitif associe a un corticosurrenalome malin. *Bull. Soc. Med. Hop. Paris* 116:1161, 1965.

134. Drabkin, D. L., and Marsh, J. B. Metabolic channeling in experimental nephrosis: I. Protein and carbohydrate metabolism. *J. Biol. Chem.* 212:623, 1955.

135. Drummond, K. N., Hillman, D. A., Marchessault, J. H. V., and Feldman, W. Cyclophosphamide in the nephrotic syndrome of childhood: Its use in two groups of patients defined by clinical, light microscopic, and immunopathologic findings. *Canad. Med. Ass. J.* 98:524, 1968.

136. Drummond, K. N., Michael, A. F., Good, R. A., and Vernier, R. L. The nephrotic syndrome of childhood: Immunologic, clinical, and pathologic correlations. *J. Clin. Invest.* 45:620, 1966.

137. Dubois, E. L. Systemic lupus erythematosus: Recent advances in its diagnosis and treatment. *Ann. Intern. Med.* 45:163, 1956.

138. Dubois, E. L. (Ed.) *Lupus Erythematosus: A Review of the Current Status of Discoid and Systemic Lupus Erythematosus and Their Variants.* New York: Blakiston Div., McGraw-Hill, 1966. P. 479.

139. Dunn, J. S. Nephrosis or nephritis? *J. Path. Bact.* 39:1, 1934.

140. Durand, P., and DeToni, E. Ricercho clinico-sperimentali sulla patogenesi e terapia delle sindromi nefrosiche. *Minerva Pediat.* 5:717, 1953.

141. Eder, H. A. The lipoproteins of human serum. *Amer. J. Med.* 23:269, 1957.

142. Eder, H. A., Lauson, H. D., Chinard, F. P., Greif, R. L., Cotzia, G. C., and Van Slyke, D. D. A study of the mechanisms of edema formation in patients with the nephrotic syndrome. *J. Clin. Invest.* 33:636, 1954.

143. Ehrich, W. E. Glomerular nephritis and lipoid nephrosis: Identities and mechanisms. *J. Chron. Dis.* 5:14, 1957.

144. Ehrich, W. E., Forman, C. W., and Seifer, J. Diffuse glomerular nephritis and lipid nephrosis: Correlation of clinical, morphological and experimental observations. *A.M.A. Arch. Path.* 54:463, 1952.

145. Ehrich, W. E., and Piel, C. Morphologic Differentiation of Nephritis and Nephrosis in the Rat and the Therapeutic Effects of Anticoagulants and Proteolytic Enzymes. In Metcoff, J. (Ed.), *Proceedings of the Fifth Annual Conference on the Nephrotic Syndrome.* New York: National Nephrosis Foundation, 1953. P. 117.

146. Ehrich, W. E., Sharma, G. P., Rajou, R. A., Bhamarapravati, N., and Seifter, J. Identity of renal lesion in rats treated with antikidney serum. *Fed. Proc.* 15:514, 1956.

147. Eiben, R. M., Kleinerman, J., and Cline, J. C. Nephrotic syndrome in a neonatal premature infant. *J. Pediat.* 44:195, 1954.

148. Eisenberg, S. Blood volume in persons with the nephrotic syndrome. *Amer. J. Med. Sci.* 255:320, 1968.

149. Eliasch, H., Sellers, A. L., Rosenfeld, S., and Marmouston, J. Protein metabolism in the mammalian kidney. *J. Exp. Med.* 101:129, 1955.

150. Elliott, T. A., Gattman, G. B., Billings, E. R., and Ivy, J. H. Thrombosis of the inferior vena cava and the nephrotic syndrome. *J. Indiana Med. Assoc.* 52:976, 1959.

151. Ellis, A. Natural history of Bright's disease. *Lancet* 1:1, 34, 72, 1942.

152. Ellis, H. A., and Walton, K. W. Variations in serum complement in the nephrotic syndrome and other forms of renal disease. *Immunology* 1:234, 1958.

153. Ellis, J. T. Glomerular lesions and the nephrotic syndrome in rabbits given saccharated iron intravenously, with special reference to the part played by intracapillary precipitates in the pathogenesis of lesions. *J. Exp. Med.* 103:127, 1956.

154. Ellis, J. T. Glomerular lesions in rabbits with experimentally induced proteinuria as disclosed by electron microscopy. (Abstract.) *Amer. J. Path.* 34:559, 1958.

155. Emerson, K., Jr., and Dole, V. P. Diodrast and inulin clearances in nephrotic children with supernormal urea clearances. *J. Clin. Invest.* 22:447, 1943.

156. Epstein, A. A. The nature and treatment of chronic parenchymatous nephritis (nephrosis). *J.A.M.A.* 79:444, 1917.

157. Epstein, A. A. Thyroid therapy and thyroid tolerance in chronic nephrosis. *J.A.M.A.* 87:913, 1926.

158. Epstein, F. H., and Zuta, V. J. Clinical correlates of the Kimmelstiel-Wilson lesion. *New Eng. J. Med.* 254:896, 1956.

159. Eschenbrenner, A. B. The Diffusion Chamber Technique in the Study of Nephritogenic Bacteria. In Metcoff, J. (Ed.), *Proceedings of the Eleventh Annual Conference on the Nephrotic Syndrome.* New York: National Kidney Disease Foundation, 1959. P. 77.

160. Etteldorf, J. N. Cyclophosphamide therapy for nephrosis. *J. Pediat.* 73:641, 1968.

161. Etteldorf, J. N., Roy, S., 3rd, and Summitt, R. L. Cyclophosphamide in the treatment of idiopathic lipoid nephrosis. *J. Pediat.* 70:758, 1967.

162. Evans, P. V., and Symmes, A. T. Bone marrow infarction with fat embolism and nephrosis in sickle cell disease. *J. Indiana Med. Ass.* 50:1101, 1957.

163. Fahr, T. Pathologische Anatomie des morbus Brightii. In Henke, F., and Lubarsch, O. (Eds.), *Handbuch der speziellen pathologischen Anatomie und Histologie.* Berlin: Springer-Verlag, 1925. Vol. 6, p. 156.

164. Falls, W. F., Jr., Ford, K. L., and Ashworth, C. T. The nephrotic syndrome in secondary syphilis: Report of a case with renal biopsy findings. *Ann. Intern. Med.* 63:1047, 1965.

165. Fanconi, G., Kousmine, C., and Frischknecht, W. Die konstitutionelle Bereitschaft zum Nephrosesyndrom. *Helvet. Paediat. Acta* 6:199, 1951.

166. Farhat, S. M., Amer, N. S., Weeks, B. S., and Musselman, M. M. Effect of mechlorethamine hydrochloride (nitrogen mustard) on healing of abdominal wounds. *Arch. Surg.* 76:749, 1958.

167. Farnsworth, E. B. Acute and subacute glomerulonephritis modified by adrenocorticotropin. *Proc. Soc. Exp. Biol. Med.* 74: 57, 1950.

168. Farnsworth, E. B. Studies on the Influence of Adrenocorticotrophin in Acute Nephritis, in Simple Nephrosis and in Nephrosis with Azotemia. In Mote, J. R. (Ed.), *Proceedings of the Second Clinical ACTH Conference.* New York: Blakiston, 1951. Vol. 1, p. 297.

169. Farnsworth, E. B. Studies on adrenocortical function in relation to the nephrotic syndrome. *J. Clin. Endocr.* 13:1169, 1953.

170. Farquhar, M. G. Electron Microscopic Studies on the Renal Glomerulus in the Nephrotic Syndrome. In Moyer, J. H., and Fuchs, M. (Eds.), *Edema, Mechanisms and Management.* Philadelphia: Saunders, 1960. P. 497.

171. Farquhar, M. G., Hopper, J., and Moon, H. D. Diabetic glomerulosclerosis: Electron and light microscopic studies. *Amer. J. Path.* 35:721, 1959.

172. Farquhar, M. G., and Palade, G. E. Segregation of ferritin in glomerular protein absorption droplets. *J. Biophys. Biochem. Cytol.* 7:297, 1960.

173. Farquhar, M. G., Vernier, R. L., and Good, R. A. Studies on familial nephrosis: II. Glomerular changes noted with the electron microscope. *Amer. J. Path.* 33:791, 1957.

174. Farr, L. E. Nephrosis. *Advances Intern. Med.* 1:225, 1942.

175. Farr, L. E. Abstract of discussion of Schwartz, H., Kohn, J. L., and Weiner, S. B. Lipid nephrosis: Observations over a period of 20 years. *Amer. J. Dis. Child.* 65:362, 1943.

176. Farr, L. E., and MacFayden, D. A. Hypoamino-acidemia in children with nephrotic crises. *Amer. J. Dis. Child.* 59:782, 1940.

177. Fawcett, J. K., and Wynn, V. Effects of posture on plasma volume and some blood constituents. *J. Clin. Path.* 13:304, 1960.

178. Feigelson, E. B., Drake, J. W., and Recant, L. Protein metabolism in experimental nephrosis. (Abstract.) *J. Lab. Clin. Med.* 48:806, 1956.

179. Feigelson, E. B., Drake, J. W., and Recant, L. Experimental amino-nucleoside nephrosis in rats. *J. Lab. Clin. Med.* 50:437, 1957.

180. Fein, R. L., Chait, A., and Leviton, A. Renal vein thrombectomy for the treatment of renal vein thrombosis associated with the nephrotic syndrome. *J. Urol.* 99:1, 1968.

181. Feinerman, B., Burke, E. C., and Bahn, R. C. The nephrotic syndrome associated with renal vein thrombosis; report of a case in an infant. *J. Pediat.* 51:389, 1957.

182. Feldman, J. D., and Fisher, E. R. Renal lesions of aminonucleoside nephrosis as revealed by electron microscopy. *Lab. Invest.* 8:371, 1959.

183. Felts, J. H., King, J. S., and Boyce, W. H. Nephrotic syndrome after treatment with D-penicillamine. *Lancet* 1:53, 1968.

184. Fiaschi, E., Andres, G., Giacomelli, F., and Naccarato, R. Renal histopathology in the para-nephritic nephrotic syndrome: Optical and electron microscopic studies of kidney biopsies. *Sci. Med. Ital.* (Eng.) 7:639, 1959.

185. Finkel, K. C., and Israel, S. Paradione nephrosis. *J. Lancet* 79:243, 1959.

186. Finnerty, F. Edema: Mechanisms and

Management. In Moyer, J., and Fuchs, M. (Eds.), *A Hahnemann Symposium on Salt and Water Retention*. Philadelphia: Saunders, 1960. P. 481.

187. Fischel, E. E., and Gajdusek, D. C. Serum complement in acute glomerulonephritis and other renal diseases. *Amer. J. Med.* 12: 190, 1952.

188. Fisher, E. R., and Gruhn, J. Aminonucleoside nephrosis in rats. *A.M.A. Arch. Path.* 65:545, 1958.

189. Fisher, E. R., and Gruhn, J. Aminonucleoside nephrosis. *Arch. Path.* (Chicago) 71: 129, 1961.

190. Fisher, E. R., Sharkey, D., and Pardo, V. Experimental renal vein constriction: Its relation to renal lesions observed in human renal vein thrombosis and the nephrotic syndrome. *Lab. Invest.* 18:689, 1968.

191. Floyd, M., Muckle, T. J., and Kerr, D. N. S. Prednisone-induced leucocytosis in nephrotic syndrome. *Lancet* 1:1192, 1969.

192. Flynn, V. J., and Roland, A. S. Nephrotic syndrome in a 92-year-old woman. *Geriatrics* 22:119, 1967.

193. Folli, G., Pollak, V. E., Reid, R. T., Pirani, C. L., and Kark, R. M. Electromicroscopic studies of reversible glomerular lesions in the adult nephrotic syndrome. *Ann. Intern. Med.* 49:775, 1958.

194. Franz, H. E., and Franz, M. Influence of aminonucleoside on the pyridine nucleotide concentration of the rat kidney. *Nature* (London) 206:947, 1965.

195. Freedman, P., Peters, J. K., and Kark, R. M. Localization of gamma-globulin in the diseased kidney. *Arch. Intern. Med.* (Chicago) 105:524, 1960.

196. Freeman, T., and Joekes, A. M. Nephrotic proteinuria: A tubular lesion? *Acta Med. Scand.* 157:43, 1957.

197. Freidell, H. V., and Zener, F. B. The nephrotic syndrome in pregnancy: A case report. *Amer. J. Obstet. Gynec.* 79:154, 1960.

198. Freinkel, W., Ingbor, S. H., and Dowling, J. T. The influence of extracellular thyroxine-binding protein upon the accumulation of thyroxine by tissue slices. *J. Clin. Invest.* 36:25, 1957.

199. Frenk, S., Antonowicz, I., Craig, J. M., and Metcoff, J. Experimental nephrotic syndrome induced in rats by aminonucleoside: Renal lesions and body electrolyte composition. *Proc. Soc. Exp. Biol. Med.* 89:424, 1955.

200. Freund, J., Lipton, M. M., and Thompson, G. E. Aspermatogenesis in the guinea pig induced by testicular tissue and adjuvants. *J. Exp. Med.* 97:711, 1953.

201. Friedman, R., Nelson, W. E., Stritzler, C., and Roxby, J. B., Jr. Xanthoma eruptive secondary to lipid nephrosis. *Arch. Derm. Syph.* 60:828, 1947.

202. Friedman, M., Rosenman, R. H., and Byers, S. O. The role of exogenous lipids in the hyperlipemia and hypercholesterolemia of nephrotic rats. *J. Clin. Invest.* 33:1103, 1954.

203. Friedman, M., Rosenman, R. H., and Byers, S. O. Lipid and cholesterol content of hepatic lymph in experimental nephrosis. *Amer. J. Physiol.* 190:180, 1957.

204. Friedman, M., and Stimmer, L. Effect of corticotrophin on growth hormone secretion in response to insulin-induced hypoglycemia in children. *Lancet* 2:944, 1966.

205. Friedman, M., and Strang, L. B. Effect of long-term corticosteroids and corticotrophin on the growth of children. *Lancet* 2:569, 1966.

206. Fuller, R. H. Lipoids in the kidney. *Arch. Path.* 32:556, 1941.

207. Garnett, E. S., and Webber, C. E. Changes in blood-volume produced by treatment in the nephrotic syndrome. *Lancet* 2:798, 1967.

208. Gautier, P., and Miville, D. Syndrome de néphrose lipoidique congénitale. *Rev. Med. Suisse Rom.* 62:740, 1942.

209. Geer, J. C., Strong, J. P., McGill, H. C., and Muslow, I. Electron microscopic observations on the localization of amyloid in the kidney in secondary amyloidosis. *Lab. Invest.* 7: 554, 1958.

210. Gellman, D. D., Pirani, C. L., Soothill, J. F., Muehrcke, R. M., and Kark, R. M. Diabetic nephropathy: A clinical and pathologic study based on renal biopsies. *Medicine* (Balt.) 38:321, 1959.

211. Ghai, C. L., Chugh, K. S., and Kumar, S. Electrophoretic pattern of serum proteins in secondary renal amyloidosis with nephrotic

syndrome. *J. Ass. Physicians India* 14:141, 1966.

212. Ghosal, S. P., and NagChandhuri, J. Nephrotic syndrome in children: A survey of 45 cases. *Indian J. Pediat.* 25:637, 1958.

213. Ghose, R. R. Goodpasture's syndrome. *Brit. Med. J.* 1:262, 1962.

214. Giebisch, G. Electrical potential measurements on single nephrons of Necturus. *J. Cell. Comp. Physiol.* 51:221, 1958.

215. Giles, H. M., Pugh, R. C., Darmady, E. M., Stranack, F., and Woolf, L. I. The nephrotic syndrome in early infancy: A report of three cases. *Arch. Dis. Child.* 32:167, 1957.

216. Giles, R. B., and Calkins, E. Studies of the composition of secondary amyloid. *J. Clin. Invest.* 34:1476, 1955.

217. Gitlin, D., and Cornwell, D. Plasma lipoprotein metabolism in normal individuals and in children with nephrotic syndrome. *J. Clin. Invest.* 35:706, 1956.

218. Gitlin, D., Cornwell, D. G., Nakasato, D., Oncley, J. L., Hughes, W. L., Jr., and Janeway, C. A. Studies on the metabolism of plasma proteins in the nephrotic syndrome: II. The lipoproteins. *J. Clin. Invest.* 37:172, 1958.

219. Gitlin, D., and Janeway, C. A. An immunochemical study of the albumins of serum, urine, ascitic fluid and edema fluid in the nephrotic syndrome. *J. Clin. Invest.* 31:223, 1952.

220. Gitlin, D., Janeway, C. A., and Farr, L. E. Studies on metabolism of plasma proteins in nephrotic syndrome: I. Albumin, γ-globulin, and iron-binding globulin. *J. Clin. Invest.* 35:44, 1956.

221. Gleason, D. C., and Steiner, R. E. The lateral roentgenogram in pulmonary edema. *Amer. J. Roentgen.* 98:279, 1966.

222. Goldberg, H. S. Nephrotic syndrome with inferior vena cava stenosis. *Arch. Intern. Med.* (Chicago) 120:94, 1967.

223. Goldberg, W. M., Chakrabarti, S., Filipich, R. Urinary lactic dehydrogenase, alkaline phosphatase, and lysozyme studies in renal disease. *Canad. Med. Ass. J.* 94:126, 1966.

224. Goldring, W., Chasis, H., Merrill, J. P., Riley, D. M., and Schreiner, G. E. Glomerulonephritis and pyelonephritis. *Bull. N.Y. Acad. Med.* 36:662, 1960.

225. Goodman, H. Attempted Characterization of Nephrotoxic Serum Antigen. In Metcoff, J. (Ed.), *Proceedings of the Seventh Annual Conference on the Nephrotic Syndrome.* New York: National Nephrosis Foundation, 1955. P. 12.

226. Goodman, H. (Ed.). *Proceedings of the Twelfth Annual Conference on the Nephrotic Syndrome.* National Kidney Disease Foundation, 1961. P. 245.

227. Goodman, H., Sellers, A. L., Smith, S., and Marmorston, J. Endocrine influences on proteinuria in the rat. *Proc. Soc. Exp. Biol. Med.* 77:725, 1951.

228. Goodman, H. C., and Baxter, J. H. The nephrotic syndrome; clinical observations on therapy with prednisone and other steroids *J.A.M.A.* 165:1798, 1957.

229. Goodman, H. C., Wolff, S. M., and Carpenter, R. R. Current studies on the effect of anti-metabolites in nephrosis, other non-neoplastic diseases, and experimental animals. *Ann. Intern. Med.* 59:388, 1963.

230. Goodpasture, E. W. The significance of certain pulmonary lesions in relation to the etiology of influenza. *Amer. J. Med. Sci.* 158:863, 1919.

231. Goodrich, I., and Harmes, W. S. Synthesis of endogenous cholesterol in experimental nephrosis. *Metabolism* 13:141, 1964.

232. Gordon, R. S., Jr. Interaction between oleate and lipo proteins of human serum. *J. Clin. Invest.* 34:477, 1955.

233. Goudsmit, A., Jr., Binger, M. W., and Power, M. H. Acacia in the treatment of nephrotic syndrome: Influence of acacia, injected intravenously, on concentration of proteins and on colloid osmotic pressure of the serum. *Arch. Intern. Med.* 68:701, 1941.

234. Grace, J. T., Jr., and Dao, T. L. Dermatomyositis in cancer: A possible etiological mechanism. *Cancer* 12:648, 1959.

235. Graham, R. C., Jr., and Karnovsky, M. J. Glomerular permeability: Ultrastructural cytochemical studies using peroxidases as protein tracers. *J. Exp. Med.* 124:1123, 1966.

236. Green, W. L. Guidelines for the treatment

of myxedema. *Med. Clin. N. Amer.* 52:431, 1968.

237. Greenberg, E., Divertie, M. B., and Woolner, L. B. A review of unusual systemic manifestations associated with carcinoma. *Amer. J. Med.* 36:106, 1964.

238. Greenman, L., Weigand, F. A., and Danowski, T. S. Therapy of the nephrotic syndrome. *Amer. J. Dis. Child.* 89:169, 1955.

239. Grieble, H. G., Courcon, J., and Grabar, P. The immunochemical heterogeneity of proteins and glycoproteins in normal human urine. *J. Lab. Clin. Med.* 66:216, 1965.

240. Gronwall, A., and Ingelman, B. Dextran as a substitute for plasma. *Nature* 45:155, 1945.

241. Gruenwald, P., and Popper, H. The histogenesis and physiology of the renal glomerulus in early postnatal life: Histological examinations. *J. Urol.* 43:452, 1940.

242. Grunberg, J. Cyclophosphamide therapy for nephrosis. *J. Pediat.* 73:641, 1968.

243. Grupe, W. E. An in vitro demonstration of cellular sensitivity in experimental autoimmune nephrosis in rats. *Proc. Soc. Exp. Biol. Med.* 127:1217, 1968.

244. Grupe, W. E., Cuppage, F. E., and Heymann, W. Congenital nephrotic syndrome with interstitial nephritis. *Amer. J. Dis. Child.* 111:482, 1966.

245. Grupe, W. E., and Heymann, W. Cytotoxic drugs in steroid-resistant renal disease. *Amer. J. Dis. Child.* 112:448, 1966.

246. Gruskay, F. L., and Turcino, A. Nephrosis in a newborn infant. A syndrome difficult to explain by existing theories of etiology. *A.M.A. Amer. J. Dis. Child.* 94:107, 1957.

247. Guillemin, P., Larcan, A., and Bessot, M. Nephrotic syndrome and thrombosis of vena cava. *Rev. Med. Nancy* 84:249, 1959.

248. Habib, R., Michielsen, P., de Montera, E., Hinglais, N., Galle, P., and Hamburger, J. Clinical Microscopic and Electron Microscopic Data in the Nephrotic Syndrome of Unknown Origin. In Wolstenholme, G. E. W., and Cameron, M. P. (Eds.), *Ciba Foundation Symposium on Renal Biopsy.* Boston: Little, Brown, 1961. P. 70.

249. Hackel, D. B., Portfolio, A. G., and Kinney, T. D. Experimental nephrotoxic nephritis in the rat treated with ACTH or cortisone. *Proc. Soc. Exp. Biol. Med.* 74:458, 1950.

250. Hagge, W. W., Burke, E. C., and Stickler, G. B. Sudden death in the nephrotic syndrome: Salt depletion as a probable mechanism. *Clin. Pediat.* 6:524, 1967.

251. Hallen, J., and Rudin, R. Peri-collagenous amyloidosis: A study of 51 cases. *Acta Med. Scand.* 179:483, 1966.

252. Hallman, N., and Hjelt, L. Congenital nephrotic syndrome. *J. Paediat.* 55:152, 1959.

253. Hallman, N., Norio, R., and Kouvalainen, K. Main features of the congenital nephrotic syndrome. *Acta Paediat. Scand.* Suppl. 172:75, 1967.

254. Hammer, D. K., and Dixon, F. J. Experimental glomerulonephritis: II. Immunologic events in the pathogenesis of nephrotoxic serum nephritis in rats. *J. Exp. Med.* 117:1019, 1963.

255. Hammarsten, J. F., Heller, B. I., and Ebert, R. V. The effects of dextrans in normovolemic and oligemic subjects. *J. Clin. Invest.* 32:340, 1953.

256. Handley, D. A., and Lawrence, J. R. Factor-IX deficiency in the nephrotic syndrome. *Lancet* 1:1079, 1967.

257. Hansen, M. F., and Coye, R. D. Congenital nephrosis with renal arteriolar hypertrophy. *Amer. J. Dis. Child.* 102:28, 1961.

258. Hardwicke, J. Serum and urinary protein changes in the nephrotic syndrome. *Proc. Roy. Soc. Med.* 47:834, 1954.

259. Hardwicke, J. Estimation of renal permeability to protein on sephadex G 200. *Clin. Chim. Acta* 12:89, 1965.

260. Hardwicke, J., Soothill, J. F., Squire, J. R., and Holti, G. Nephrotic syndrome with pollen hypersensitivity. *Lancet* 1:500, 1959.

261. Hardwicke, J., and Squire, J. R. The relationship between plasma albumin concentration and protein excretion in patients with proteinuria. *Clin. Sci.* 14:509, 1955.

262. Harkin, J. C., and Recant, L. The earliest lesion in aminonucleoside nephrosis; an electron microscopic study. (Abstract.) *Amer. J. Path.* 34:559, 1958.

263. Harrington, A. R., Hare, H. G., and Chambers, W. N. Nodular glomerulosclerosis

suspected during life in a patient without demonstrable diabetes mellitus. *New Eng. J. Med.* 275:206, 1966.

264. Harrison, C. V., Milne, M. D., and Steiner, R. E. Clinical aspects of renal vein thrombosis. *Quart. J. Med.* 25:285, 1956.

265. Hartman, M. E. Some metabolic and structural characteristics of experimental nephrosis. *Amer. Heart J.* 58:483, 1959.

266. Harvey, A. M., Shulman, L. E., Tumulty, P. A., Couley, C. L., and Schoenrich, E. H. Systemic lupus erythematosus: Review of the literature and clinical analysis of 138 cases. *Medicine* (Balt.) 33:291, 1954.

267. Hawn, C. V., Hume, D. M., Merrill, J. P., and Miller, B. F. Pathologic changes in eight human renal transplants. *Fed. Proc.* 12:391, 1953.

268. Hawn, C. V., and Janeway, C. A. Histological and serological sequences in experimental hypersensitivity. *J. Exp. Med.* 85:571, 1947.

269. Heidorn, G. H. The effect of corticotrophin (ACTH) on ammonia production in the nephrotic syndrome. *Amer. J. Med. Sci.* 231:644, 1956.

270. Heilmeyer, L., Merker, H., and Wetzel, H. P. Transferrin deficiency associated with nephrotic syndrome. *German Med. Monthly* 11:219, 1966.

271. Hellman, L., Zumoff, B., Minsky, A., Kretchmer, N., and Kramer, B. Treatment of the nephrotic syndrome with triamcinolone. *Pediatrics* 28:686, 1959.

272. Hellman, L. M., and Johnson, W. L. Nephrotic syndrome. *Amer. J. Obstet. Gynec.* 97:719, 1967.

273. Hendel, J. P. Lipoid nephrosis; a review. *Ugeskr. Laeg.* 121:185, 1959.

274. Henes, E., Jr. The prognostic value of cholesterinemia in chronic nephritis. *Arch. Intern. Med.* 25:411, 1920.

275. Heptinstall, R. H. *Pathology of the Kidney.* Boston: Little, Brown, 1966. P. 836.

275a. Herbert, H. J. Acute glomerulonephritis in childhood: A study of the late prognosis of twenty-seven cases. *J. Pediat.* 40:549, 1952.

276. Herman, E., and Rado, J. Fatal hyperkalemic paralysis associated with spironolactone: Observation on a patient with severe renal disease and refractory edema. *Arch. Neurol.* (Chicago) 15:74, 1966.

277. Hersh, E. M., Carbone, P. P., and Freireich, E. J. Recovery of immune responsiveness after drug suppression in man. *J. Lab. Clin. Med.* 67:566, 1966.

278. Hervé, R. Lipoid nephrosis and pregnancy. *Rev. Franc. Gynec. Obstet.* 51:170, 1956.

279. Herxheimer, G. Über hyaline Glomeruli der Neugeborenen und Säuglinge. *Frankfurt. Ztschr. Path.* 2:138, 1909.

280. Hess, E. V., Ashworth, C. I., and Ziff, M. Transfer of autoimmune nephrosis in rats by means of lymph node cells. *Clin. Res.* 9:48, 1961.

281. Hewitt, L. F. Urine proteins in nephrosis, pregnancy, and myelomatosis. *Lancet* 1:66, 1929.

282. Hewmann, W., and Clark, E. C. Pathogenesis of nephrotic hyperlipemia. *Amer. J. Dis. Child.* 70:74, 1945.

283. Heymann, W. Pathogenesis of Nephrotic Hyperlipemia. In Metcoff, J. (Ed.), *Proceedings of the Eighth Annual Conference on the Nephrotic Syndrome.* New York: National Nephrosis Foundation, 1956. P. 95.

284. Heymann, W. Trimethadione (Tridione) nephrosis. *Pediatrics* 22:614, 1958.

285. Heymann, W. (Ed.). *Proceedings of the Fifteenth Annual Conference on the Kidney.* New York: National Kidney Foundation, 1964. P. 217.

286. Heymann, W. Nephrotic syndrome after use of trimethadione and paramethadione in petit mal. *J.A.M.A.* 202:127, 1967.

287. Heymann, W., Gilkey, C., and Salehar, M. Antigenic property of the renal cortex. *Proc. Soc. Exp. Biol. Med.* 73:385, 1950.

288. Heymann, W., and Hackel, D. B. Role of liver in pathogenesis of experimental nephrotic hyperlipemia. *Metabolism* 4:258, 1955.

289. Heymann, W., and Hackel, D. B. Effect of ethionine on blood and depot lipids in experimental nephrotic hyperlipemia. *Proc. Soc. Exp. Biol.* 92:41, 1956.

290. Heymann, W., Hackel, D. B., Harwood, S., Wilson, S. G., and Hunter, J. L. Produc-

tion of nephrotic syndrome in rats by Freund's adjuvants and rat kidney suspensions. *Proc. Soc. Exp. Biol. Med.* 100:660, 1959.

291. Heymann, W., Kmetec, E. P., and Wilson, S. G. Experimental autoimmune renal disease in rats. *Ann. N.Y. Acad. Sci.* 124:310, 1965.

292. Heymann, W., and Lund, H. Z. Nephrotic syndrome in rats. *Pediatrics* 7:691, 1951.

293. Heymann, W., Matthews, L. W., Bergman, A. B., and Nash, G. Studies on the causal role of hypoalbuminemia in experimental nephrosis. *J. Clin. Invest.* 37:808, 1958.

294. Heymann, W., Matthews, L. W., Lemm, J., Olynyk, P., Salehar, M., and Gilkey, C. Fat metabolism in nephrotic hyperlipemia. *Metabolism* 3:27, 1954.

295. Heymann, W., Spector, S., Matthews, L. W., and Shapiro, D. J. Treatment of the nephrotic syndrome with corticotropin (ACTH) and cortison: A 4½-year survey of results with short-term courses. *A.M.A. Amer. J. Dis. Child.* 90:22, 1955.

296. Heymann, W., and Wilson, S. G. F. Hyperlipemia in early stages of acute glomerular nephritis. *J. Clin. Invest.* 38:186, 1954.

297. Hilden, T., and Nielsen, O. E. Renal vein thrombosis with nephrotic syndrome. *Nord. Med.* 62:1108, 1959.

298. Hilton, P. J., Jones, N. F., and Tighe, J. R. Nephrotic syndrome with heart disease: A reappraisal. *Brit. Med. J.* 3:584, 1968.

299. Himmel, A., Markiewicz, K., and Szydlowski, A. Serum complement level in patients with the nephrotic syndrome. *Polish Med. J.* 5:734, 1966.

300. Hoak, J. C., Connor, W. E. Armstrong, M. L., and Warner, E. D. Effect of clofibrate on serum and hepatic lipids in nephrotic rats. *Lab. Invest.* 19:370, 1968.

301. Hoak, J. C., Connor, W. E., and Stone, D. B. Effect of hypophysectomy on serum lipids in aminonucleoside nephrosis. *Proc. Soc. Exp. Biol. Med.* 122:588, 1966.

302. Hoehn, D. Nephrosis probably due to excessive use of "Sta-way" insect repellent. *J.A.M.A.* 128:513, 1945.

303. Höfle, K. H., and Schoop, W. Acute nephrotic syndrome caused by mesantoin

treatment. *Deutsch. Med. Wschr.* 84:837, 1959.

304. Holman, D. V., and Makovsky, I. H. Acute syphilitic nephrosis treated with penicillin. *New York J. Med.* 46:520, 1946.

305. Holman, H. Systemic lupus erythematosus. *J. Pediat.* 56:109, 1960.

306. Holmes, M. C., and Burnett, F. M. The natural history of autoimmune disease in NZB mice. *Ann. Intern. Med.* 59:265, 1963.

307. Hooft, C., and Herpal, J. Aminoaciduria in the course of lipoid nephrosis in children: The influence of ACTH. *Acta Paediat.* 48:135, 1959.

308. Hooft, C., and Van Acker, K. J. The natural history of the idiopathic nephrotic syndrome in children. *Ann. Paediat.* (Basel) 207:1, 1966.

309. Hooft, C., and Vandenberghen, C. Lipoid nephrosis. *Ann. Paediat.* 185:212, 1955.

310. Hooft, C., Vandenberghen, C., and Eeckels, R. Results of the treatment of lipoid nephrosis with ACTH. *Acta Paediat. Belg.* 11:123, 1957.

311. Hooft, C., Vandenberghen, C., and Van Belle, M. Les lipoproteines dans la néphrose lipoidique de l'enfant. *Rev. Belg. Path.* 24:155, 1956.

312. Housley, J. Alpha-2 macroglobulin levels in disease in man. *J. Clin. Path.* 21:27, 1968.

313. Howard, J. E., and Migeon, C. J. Cushing's syndrome produced by normal replacement doses of cortisone in a patient with defective mechanism for steroid degradation. *Amer. J. Med. Sci.* 235:387, 1958.

314. Hoyer, J. R., Michael, A. F., Jr., and Good, R. A. The nephrotic syndrome of infancy: Clinical, morphologic, and immunologic studies of four infants. *Pediatrics* 40:233, 1967.

315. Huang, F., Hutton, L., and Kalant, N. Molecular sieving by glomerular basement membrane. *Nature* (London) 216:87, 1967.

316. Hulme, B., and Hardwicke, J. Human glomerular permeability to macromolecules in health and disease. *Clin. Sci.* 34:515, 1968.

317. Hume, D. M., Merrill, J. P., Miller, B. F., and Thorn, G. W. Experience with renal homotransplantation in humans: Report of nine cases. *J. Clin. Invest.* 34:327, 1955.

318. Hunter, J. Auto-immune Nephrotic Disease in Rats. In Metcoff, J. (Ed.), *Proceedings of the Eleventh Annual Conference on the Nephrotic Syndrome*. New York: National Kidney Disease Foundation, 1959. P. 148.

319. Hyman, H. T., Hurwitz, D., Robbing, S. L., MacDonald, R. A., and Freinkel, M. Personal communication, 1962.

320. Imai, M., and Sokabe, H. Plasma renin and angiotensinogen levels in pathological states associated with oedema. *Arch. Dis. Child.* 43:475, 1968.

321. Immunosuppressive or anti-inflammatory. *Brit. Med. J.* 1:650, 1967.

322. Irisawa, S., Shirai, M., and Matsushita, S. Sexual disturbances in diabetes. *Tohoku J. Exp. Med.* 88:311, 1966.

323. Jaffe, I. A., Treser, G., and Suzuki, Y. Nephropathy induced by D-penicillamine. *Ann. Intern. Med.* 69:549, 1968.

324. James, J. A. Ethacrynic acid in edematous states in children. *J. Pediat.* 71:881, 1967.

325. James, J., Gordillo, G., and Metcoff, J. Effects of infusion of hyperoncotic dextran in children with the nephrotic syndrome. *J. Clin. Invest.* 33:1346, 1954.

326. Janeway, C. A., Gibson, S. T. Woodruff, L. M., Heyl, J. T., Bailey, O. T., and Newhauser, L. R. Chemical, clinical and immunologic studies on the products of human plasma fractionation: VII. Concentrated human serum albumin. *J. Clin. Invest.* 23:465, 1944.

327. Janower, M. L. Nephrotic syndrome secondary to renal vein thrombosis: The value of inferior vena cavography. *Amer. J. Roentgen.* 95:330, 1965.

328. Jelliffe, E. F. The prevalence of plasmodium malariae in a Baganda community in Uganda. *Trop. Geogr. Med.* 19:15, 1967.

329. Jensen, H., and Jarnum, S. Investigations on gastrointestinal protein loss in the nephrotic syndrome. *Nuclearmedizin* 211:6, 1967.

330. Jensen, H., Jarnum, S., and Hart Hansen, J. P. Gastrointestinal protein loss and intestinal function in the nephrotic syndrome. *Nephron* 3:209, 1966.

331. Jensen, H., and Jensen, E. Steroid treatment of the nephrotic syndrome in adults. *Acta Med. Scand.* 182:741, 1967.

332. Jensen, H., Rossing, N., and Andersen, S. B. Albumin metabolism in the nephrotic syndrome in adults. *Clin. Sci.* 33:445, 1967.

333. Jessar, R. A., Lamont-Havers, R. W., and Ragan, C. A. Natural history of lupus erythematosus disseminatus. *Ann. Intern. Med.* 38:717, 1953.

334. Jimenez Diaz, C., Linazasoro, J. M., and Rios, M. S. The elimination of seroalbumin by feces in nephrosis. *Bull. Inst. Med Res. Univ. Madrid* 14:105, 1963.

335. Joachim, G. R., Cameron, J. S., Schwartz M., and Becker, E. L. Selectivity of protein excretion in patients with the nephrotic syndrome. *J. Clin. Invest.* 43:2332, 1964.

336. Johnson, J. R., and Reader, R. Prognosis in the nephrotic syndrome; a study with particular reference to the adult and older child. *Aust. Ann. Med.* 8:200, 1959.

337. Johnston, C. C., and Podsiadly, C. J. Oxidative enzyme content of kidneys from normal and aminonucleoside-nephrotic rats. *Proc. Soc. Exp. Biol. Med.* 124:988, 1967.

338. Jones, J. H., Peters, D. K., and Morgan, D. B. Observations on calcium metabolism in the nephrotic syndrome. *Quart. J. Med.* 36:301, 1967.

339. Kahn, M., Merritt, A. D., Wool, M. J., and Orloff, J. Renal concentrating defect in Sjögren's syndrome. *Ann. Intern. Med.* 56:883, 1962.

340. Kaitz, A. L. Albumin metabolism in nephrotic adults. *J. Lab. Clin. Med.* 53:186, 1959.

341. Kalant, N., Missra, R. P., Manley, R. St. J., and Wilson, J. Glomerular basement membrane in experimental nephrosis: X-ray defraction and electrophoretic studies. *Nephron* 3:167, 1966.

342. Kalant, N., McIntyre, W. C., and Wilausky, D. L. Thyroid function in experimental nephrotic syndrome. *Endocrinology* 64:333, 1959.

343. Kanasawa, M. Idiopathic nephrotic syndrome of childhood: A light-microscopic study of the histologic spectrum as revealed by renal biopsies. *Acta Med. Biol.* (Niigata) 14:217, 1967.

344. Kaplan, B. M., Newman, J. S., Kaplan, E., Baker, L. A., and Lee, J. M. Bilateral renal vein thrombosis and the nephrotic syndrome. *Ann. Intern. Med.* 45:505, 1956.

345. Kark, R. M., Pirani, C. L., Pollak, V. E., Muehrcke, R. C., and Blainey, J. D. The nephrotic syndrome in adults: A common disorder with many causes. *Ann. Intern. Med.* 49:751, 1958.

346. Karp, M., Lurie, M., and Yonis, Z. Nephrotic syndrome in the course of treatment of Wilson's disease with DL-penicillamine. *Arch. Dis. Child.* 41:684, 1967.

347. Kasukawa, R., Anthone, R., and Abeyounis, C. J. Studies on the serology of renal diseases: II. Unusual antibodies in glomerulonephritis sera. *Int. Arch. Allerg.* 32:563, 1967.

348. Kattermann, R., Reutter, W., and Decker, K. Über die cholesterinsynthese bei der aminonucleosid-nephrise der ratte. *Klin. Wschr.* 43:393, 1965.

349. Katz, J., Rosenfeld, S., and Sellers, A. L. Role of the kidney in plasma albumin catabolism. *Amer. J. Physiol.* 198:814, 1960.

350. Katz, J., Sellers, A. L., and Bunores, G. The effect of nephrectomy on the plasma albumin catabolism in experimental nephrosis. *J. Lab. Clin. Med.* 63:680, 1964.

351. Kay, C. F. Mechanism by which experimental nephritis is produced in rabbits injected with nephrotoxic duck serum. *J. Exp. Med.* 72:559, 1940.

352. Keitel, H. G., Thompson, D., and Itano, H. A. Hyposthenuria in sickle cell anemia; a reversible renal defect. *J. Clin. Invest.* 35:998, 1956.

353. Keitel, H. G., Goodman, H. C., Havel, R. J., Fordon, R. S., and Baxter, J. H. Nephrotic syndrome in congenital quartan malaria. *J.A.M.A.* 161:520, 1956.

354. Keith, N. M., and Daugherty, G. W. The occurrence of nephrosis with chronic jejuno-ileitis. *Proc. Staff Meet. Mayo Clin.* 33:391, 1958.

355. Kelley, V. C., and Panos, T. C. Nephrotic syndrome in children: Clinical response to nitrogen mustard therapy. *J. Pediat.* 41:505, 1952.

356. Kelley, V. C., Ziegler, M. R., Doeden, D., and McQuarrie, I. Labelled methionine as an indicator of protein formation in children with lipoid nephrosis. *Proc. Soc. Exp. Biol. Med.* 75:153, 1950.

357. Kelly, D. K., and Winn, J. F. Renal lesions produced by group A, type 12, streptococci. *Science* 127:1337, 1958.

358. Kendall-Smith, I. M., Pullon, D. H., and Tomlinson, B. E. Congenital nephrotic syndrome in Maori siblings. *New Zeal. Med. J.* 68:156, 1968.

359. Kerenyi, N., and Balogh, K. Kongenitale Glomerulosklerose. *Frankfurt. Ztschr. Path.* 67:359, 1956.

360. Kew, M. C., Seftel, H. C., and Bloomberg, B. M. Pregnancy tests and proteinuria. *Lancet* 1:902, 1967.

361. Khandelwal, M. K. Steroid therapy in nephrotic syndrome in relation to nephrobiopsy. *Indian Pediat.* 4:393, 1967.

362. Kibukamusoke, J. W. Malaria prophylaxis and immunosuppressant therapy in management of nephrotic syndrome associated with quartan malaria. *Arch. Dis. Child.* 43:598, 1968.

363. Kibukamusoke, J. W. The nephrotic syndrome in Lagos, Nigeria. *W. Afr. Med. J.* 15:213, 1966.

364. Kibukamusoke, J. W., and Hutt, M. S. R. Histological features of the nephrotic syndrome associated with quartan malaria. *J. Clin. Path.* 20:117, 1967.

365. Kibukamusoke, J. W., Hutt, M. S. R., and Wilks, N. E. The nephrotic syndrome in Uganda and its association with quartan malaria. *Quart. J. Med.* 36:393, 1967.

366. Kimball, K. G. Amyloidosis in association with neoplastic disease: Report of an unusual case and clinicopathological experience at Memorial Center for Cancer and Allied Diseases during eleven years (1948–1958). *Ann. Intern. Med.* 55:958, 1961.

367. Kimmelstiel, P., and Wilson, C. Intercapillary lesions in glomeruli of kidney. *Amer. J. Path.* 12:83, 1936.

368. Kinoshita, Y., Kosokabe, K., and Yokoyama, Y. Relationship between histologic findings and effects of glucocorticoid

therapy on the nephrotic syndrome. *Acta Med. Biol.* (Niigata) 13:79, 1965.

369. Kinoshita, Y., Mikami, A., and Ichinose, M. Steroid nephropathy: A case of renal disease showing similar changes of lipoid nephrosis modified by steroid treatment. *Acta Med. Biol.* (Niigata) 14:51, 1966.

370. Klahr, S., Tripathy, K., and Bolanos, O. Qualitative and quantitative analysis of urinary lipids in the nephrotic syndrome. *J. Clin. Invest.* 46:1475, 1967.

371. Kluthe, R., Hagemann, U., and Klein, N. The turnover of alpha-2 macroglobulins in the nephrotic syndrome. *Vox Sang* (Basel) 12:308, 1967.

372. Kluthe, R., Liem, H. H., Nussle, D., and Barandun, S. Intestinal plasma protein loss (protein diarrhea) in the nephrotic syndrome. *Klin. Wschr.* 41:15, 1963.

373. Knepshield, J. H., Roberts, P. L., Davis, C. J., and Moser, R. H. Hereditary chronic nephritis complicated by nephrotic syndrome. *Arch. Intern. Med.* (Chicago) 122:156, 1968.

374. Kobayashi, A. Hypomagnesaemia in nephrosis. *Lancet* 1:748, 1968.

375. Kobayashi, A. Serum magnesium level in idiopathic nephrotic syndrome. *Paediat. Univ. Tokyo* 15:12, 1968.

376. Kobayashi, O., Wada, H., and Utsumi, J. Urinary lithiasis in children treated with adrenocorticosteroid hormone. *Acta Med. Biol.* (Niigata) 15:91, 1967.

377. Korn, E. D. Clearing factor, a heparin-activated lipoprotein lipase. *J. Biol. Chem.* 215:1, 1955.

378. Kouvalainen, K. Immunoglobulins in pediatric disorders: An immunoelectrophoretic study. *Ann. Paediat. Fenn.* 12:83, 1966.

379. Kowal, J., Figur, A., and Hitzig, W. M. Renal vein thrombosis in the nephrotic syndrome with complete remission. *J. Mt. Sinai Hosp. N.Y.* 30:47, 1963.

380. Krieg, A. F., Bolande, R. P., Holden, W. D., Hubay, C. A., and Persky, L. Membranous glomerulonephritis occurring in a human renal homograft. *Amer. J. Clin. Path.* 34:155, 1960.

381. Kumagai, N., Abe, K., and Mouri, T. TAMe esterase activity in human plasma

under normal and pathological conditions. *Tohoku J. Exp. Med.* 95:121, 1968.

382. Lagrue, G., Bariéty, J., and Kérautem, Y. de Résultats de la chimothérapie prolongée au cours de certains syndromes néphrotiques. *J. Urol. Nephrol.* 70:156, 1964.

383. Lagrue, G., Bariéty, J., and Milliez, P. Moutards azotées et antimétabolites dans le traitement des syndromes néphrotiques et de certaines néphropathies glomérulaires. *Actualités Néphrologiques* 1:219, 1964.

384. Laha, P. N., and Agarwal, R. C. Blood fibrinolytic activity in acute glomerulonephritis and nephrotic syndrome. *J. Ass. Physicians India* 15:151, 1967.

385. Lam, C. N., and Arneil, G. C. Long-term dwarfing effects of corticosteroid treatment for childhood nephrosis. *Arch. Dis. Child* (Chicago) 43:589, 1968.

386. Lambie, A. T., and MacFarlane, A. A. A clinico-pathologic study of diabetic glomerulosclerosis. *Quart. J. Med.* 24:125, 1955.

387. Landis, E. M. Observations on acacia therapy in nephrosis. *J.A.M.A.* 109:2030, 1937.

388. Landouzy, L., and Bernard, L. La néphrite parenchymateuse chronique des tuberculeux. *Presse Med.* 9:121, 1901.

389. Lange, K. Complement Components in Human Nephritis and Nephrosis. In Metcoff, J. (Ed.), *Proceedings of the Sixth Annual Conference on the Nephrotic Syndrome.* New York: National Nephrosis Foundation, 1954. P. 77.

390. Lange, K. The immunologic basis of glomerulonephritis and the nephrotic syndrome. *New York J. Med.* 57:2095, 1957.

391. Lange, K., Craig, F., Oberman, J., Slobody, L., Ogur, G., and LoCasto, F. Changes in serum complement during the course and treatment of glomerulonephritis. *A.M.A. Arch. Intern. Med.* 88:433, 1951.

392. Lange, K., Slobody, L., Craig, F., Ogur, G., Oberman, J., and LoCasto, F. The influence of ACTH and nitrogen mustard therapy on serum complement of patients in the nephrotic stage. *Bull. N.Y. Med. Coll.* 14:90, 1951.

393. Lange, K., Slobody, L. B., and Strang, R. H. Serum complement levels as a guide for

diagnosis and therapy of the nephrotic syndrome. *J. Clin. Invest.* 32:581, 1953.

394. Lange, K., Slobody, L. B., and Strang, R. H. Prolonged intermittent ACTH and cortisone therapy in the nephrotic syndrome: Immunologic basis and results. *Pediatrics* 15:156, 1955.

395. Lange, K., Slobody, L. B., and Wenk, E. J. Experimental glomerulonephritis: Relation of antibody titer, complement levels, and clinical course with and without therapy. *A.M.A. Amer. J. Dis. Child.* 92:474, 1956.

396. Lange, K., Strang, R., Slobody, L. B., and Wenk, E. J. The treatment of the nephrotic syndrome with steroids in children and adults. *A.M.A. Arch. Intern. Med.* 99:760, 1957.

396a. Lange, K., Treser, G., Sagel, I., Ty, A., and Wasserman, E. Routine immunohistology in renal diseases. *Ann. Intern. Med.* 64:25, 1966.

397. Lange, K., and Wenk, E. J. Complement components in the sera and urine of patients with severe proteinurias. *Amer. J. Med. Sci.* 228:448, 1954.

398. Lange, K., and Wenk, E. J. Investigations into the site of complement loss in experimental glomerulonephritis. *Amer. J. Med. Sci.* 228:454, 1954.

399. Lauson, H. D., Forman, C. W., McNamara, H., Mattar, G., and Barnett, H. L. The effect of corticotrophin (ACTH) on glomerular permeability to albumin in children with the nephrotic syndrome. *J. Clin. Invest.* 33:657, 1954.

400. Lazerson, J., Goldin, M., Grossman, A., and Mandel, E. E. Urinary antistreptolysin O in children with nephrosis. *Clin. Res.* 8:288, 1960.

401. Lee, J. C., Yamauchi, H., and Hopper, J., Jr. The association of cancer and the nephrotic syndrome. *Ann. Intern. Med.* 64:41, 1966.

402. Leiter, E. Inferior vena-caval thrombosis in malignant renal lesions. *J.A.M.A.* 198:1167, 1966.

403. Leiter, L. Nephrosis. *Medicine* (Balt.) 10:135, 1931.

404. Lepore, M. J. Acacia therapy in nephrotic edema. *Ann. Intern. Med.* 11:285, 1937.

405. Lerner, R. A., and Dixon, F. J. The induction of acute glomerulonephritis in rabbits with soluble antigens isolated from normal homologous and autologous urine. *J. Immunol.* 100:1277, 1968.

406. Lestina, F. A., Freeman, S., and Wilson, H. Treatment of the nephrotic syndrome with nitrogen mustard and ACTH. *J. Lab. Clin. Med.* 42:918, 1953.

407. Levin, S. E., Zamit, R., and Schmaman, A. Thrombosis of the pulmonary arteries and the nephrotic syndrome. *Brit. Med. J.* 1:153, 1967.

408. Lewis, F. B., Schwartz, R. F., and Dameshek, W. X-radiation and alkylating agents as possible trigger mechanisms in the autoimmune complications of malignant lymphoproliferative diseases. *Clin. Exp. Immun.* 1:3, 1966.

409. Lexow, P., and Sigstad, H. Glomerulonephritis with initial lung purpura. *Acta Med. Scand.* 168:405, 1960.

410. Lieberman, E., Heuser, E., and Hanson, V. Identical 3-year-old twins with disseminated lupus erythematosus: One with nephrosis and one with nephritis. *Arthritis Rheum.* 11:22, 1968.

411. Lindenbaum, J., and Scheidt, S. S. Chylous ascites and the nephrotic syndrome: Report of a case, associated with renal vein thrombosis. *Amer. J. Med.* 44:830, 1968.

412. Lindsay, S. Primary systemic amyloidosis with nephrosis. *Amer. J. Med.* 4:765, 1948.

413. Lipman, R. L., Johnson, B., and Berg, G. Idiopathic retroperitoneal fibrosis and probable systemic lupus erythematosus. *J.A.M.A.* 196:1022, 1966.

414. Liu, C. Search for Anti-kidney Antibodies in Patients. In Metcoff, J. (Ed.), *Proceedings of the Ninth Annual Conference on the Nephrotic Syndrome.* New York: National Nephrosis Foundation, 1957. P. 74.

415. Liu, C. T., and McCrory, W. W. Autoantibodies in human glomerulonephritis and nephrotic syndrome. *J. Immunol.* 81:492, 1958.

416. Lubran, M. Paper electrophoresis. J.A.M.A. 197:360, 1966.

417. Luetscher, J. A., Jr. Electrophoretic analysis of plasma and urinary proteins. *J. Clin. Invest.* 19:313, 1940.

418. Luetscher, J. A., Jr. The effect of a single injection of concentrated human serum albumin on circulating proteins and proteinuria in nephrosis. *J. Clin. Invest.* 23:365, 1944.

419. Luetscher, J. A., Jr. The Nephrotic Syndrome. In *Transactions of the Fifth Conference on Renal Function.* New York: Josiah Macy, Jr. Foundation, 1953.

420. Luetscher, J. A., Jr., Deming, Q. B., Harvey, J., Lew, W., and Pool, L. J. Treatment of nephrosis with cortisone. *J. Clin. Invest.* 29: 1576, 1950.

421. Luetscher, J. A., Jr., Dowdy, A., Harvey, J., Neher, R., and Wettstein, A. Isolation of crystalline aldosterone from urine of a child with the nephrotic syndrome. *J. Biol. Chem.* 217:505, 1955.

422. Luetscher, J. A., Jr., Hall, A. D., and Kremer, V. L. Treatment of nephrosis with concentrated human serum albumin: II. Effects on renal function and on excretion of water and some electrolytes. *J. Clin. Invest.* 29:896, 1950.

423. Luetscher, J. A., Jr., and Mubrew, P. J. The nephrotic syndrome. *DM* August 3, 1956.

424. Luetscher, J. A., Jr., Piel, C. F., and Curtis, R. H. The nephrotic syndrome. *J. Chron. Dis.* 1:442, 1955.

425. Lumeng, J., and Moran, J. F. Carotid body tumor associated with mild membranous glomerulonephritis. *Ann. Intern. Med.* 65: 1266, 1966.

426. Maher, J. F., and Schreiner, G. E. Studies on ethacrynic acid in patients with refractory edema. *Ann. Intern. Med.* 62:15, 1965.

427. Marchal, C. *Les Gastro-Enteropathies Exsudatives Chez L'enfant.* Nancy: Georges Thomas, 1965.

428. Marsh, J. B., and Drabkin, D. L. Metabolic channeling in experimental nephrosis: II. Lipid metabolism. *J. Biol. Chem.* 212:633, 1955.

429. Martin, J. H., Brown, A. L., Jr., and Daugherty, G. W. Renal amyloidosis: A biopsy study. *Amer. J. Med. Sci.* 251:129, 1966.

430. Martin, M. M., Gaboardi, F., and Podolsky, S. Intermittent steroid therapy: Its effect on hypothalamic-pituitary-adrenal function and the response of plasma growth hormone and insulin to stimulation. *New Eng. J. Med.* 279:273, 1968.

431. Massry, S. G., Preuss, H. G., Maher, J. F., and Schreiner, G. E. Studies on the mechanism of renal tubular acidosis occurring after cadaver kidney homotransplantation. *Amer. J. Med.* 42:284, 1967.

432. Masugi, M. Über das Wesen der spezifischen Veränderungen der Wiev und der Leber durch das Nephrotoxin bzw. das Hepatotoxin: zugleich ein Beitrag zur Pathogenese der Glomerulonephritis und der eklamptischen Lebererkrankung. *Beitr. Path. Anat.* 91:82, 1933.

433. Masugi, M., and Sato, Y. Über die allergische Gewebsreaktion der Niere, zugleich ein experimenteller Beitrag zur Pathogenese der diffusen Glomerulonephritis und der periarteritis nodosa. *Virchow. Arch. Path. Anat.* 293:615, 1934.

434. Mathur, K. S., and Srivastava, S. C. Total complication with prednisolone therapy in nephrotic syndrome — with a case report. *J. Indian Med. Ass.* 33:414, 1959.

435. Mathur, K. S., Wahal, P. K., and Singh, K. K. Aminonucleoside nephropathy: An experimental study. *J. Ass. Physicians India* 16:1, 1968.

436. Matsuda, I., Shida, N., Takase, A., and Sasaki, K. Nephrotic syndrome and spherocytosis. *Lancet* 2:1204, 1969.

437. Maxwell, M. H. The nephrotic syndrome in adults. *Postgrad. Med.* 23:427, 1958.

438. McCluskey, R. T., and Baldwin, D. S. Natural history of acute glomerulonephritis. *Amer. J. Med.* 35:213, 1963.

439. McCluskey, R. T., Vassalli, P., Gallo, G., and Baldwin, D. S. An immunofluorescent study of pathogenic mechanisms in glomerular diseases. *New Eng. J. Med.* 274:695, 1966.

440. McCormick, W. F., and Danneel, C. M. Central pontine myelinolysis. *Arch. Intern. Med.* (Chicago) 119:444, 1967.

441. McCrory, W. W., and Macaulay, D. Recent advances in the management of renal disease in children (Part I). *Pediatrics* 19: 481, 1957.

442. McCrory, W. W., Rapoport, M., and Fleisher, D. S. Estimation of severity of the nephrotic syndrome in childhood as a guide to therapy and prognosis. *Pediatrics* 23:861, 1959.

443. McCurdy, D. K., Cornwald, G. C., III, and Deprante, V. J. Hyperglobulinemic renal tubular acidosis. *Ann. Intern. Med.* 67:110, 1967.

444. McDonald, J. R. The prognostic significance of thrombosis of the renal vein secondary to malignant neoplasms of the kidney. *Proc. Mayo Clin.* 18:289, 1943.

445. McKenzie, I. F., and Nestel, P. J. Studies on the turnover of triglyceride and esterified cholesterol in subjects with the nephrotic syndrome. *J. Clin. Invest.* 47:1685, 1968.

446. McLean, R. H., and Herdman, R. Childhood nephrosis: The influence of infection on therapy. *J. Pediat.* 71:579, 1967.

447. Meadow, S. R. Congenital nephrotic syndrome. *Develop. Med. Child. Neurol.* 9: 500, 1967.

448. Meadow, S. R., and Shite, R. H. Steroids and nephrotic syndrome. *Brit. Med. J.* 2: 119, 1968.

449. Meadow, S. R., Weller, R. O., and Archibald, R. W. R. Fatal systemic measles in a child receiving cyclophosphamide for nephrotic syndrome. *Lancet* 2:876, 1969.

450. Meesen, H., and Litton, M. A. Morphology of the kidney in morbus caeruleus. *A.M.A. Arch. Path.* 56:480, 1953.

451. Mehta, S., Kumar, K. K., and Gupta, M. L. Hodgkin's disease with nephrotic syndrome and erythema multiforme. *J. Indian Med.* 48:279, 1967.

452. Mellors, R. C. Autoimmune and immunoproliferative disease of NZB/BL mice and hybrids. *Int. Rev. Exp. Path.* 5:217, 1966.

453. Mellors, R. C., and Ortega, L. G. Analytical pathology: III. New observations on pathogenesis of glomerulonephritis, lipid nephrosis, periarteritis nodosa, and secondary amyloidosis in man. *Amer. J. Path.* 32:455, 1956.

454. Mellors, R. C., Ortega, L. G., and Holman, H. R. Role of gamma globulins in pathogenesis of renal lesions in systemic lupus erythematosus and chronic membranous glomerulonephritis, with an observation on the lupus erythematous cell reaction. *J. Exp. Med.* 106:191, 1957.

455. Menon, I. S. Pulmonary artery thrombosis and the nephrotic syndrome. *Brit. Med. J.* 2:110, 1967.

456. Mériel, P., Galinier, F., Moreau, G., Bastide, G., Suc, J. M., and Bounhoure, J. P. Two new cases of renal vein thrombosis with nephrotic syndrome: Diagnostic value of association of cavography with renal biopsy puncture. *Bull. Soc. Med. Hop. Paris* 75: 109, 1959.

457. Merrill, A. J., and Mitchell, G. L. Continuous ACTH therapy of nephrotic syndrome in children. *J. Clin. Invest.* 32:589, 1953.

458. Metcoff, J., Nakasone, N., and Rance, C. P. On the role of the kidney during nephrotic edema: Potassium excretion and sodium retention. *J. Clin. Invest.* 33:665, 1954.

459. Metcoff, J., Rance, C. P., Kelsey, W. M., Nakasone, N., and Janeway, C. A. Adrenocorticotrophic hormone (ACTH) therapy of the nephrotic syndrome in children. *Pediatrics* 10:543, 1952.

460. Michael, A. F., Jr., Drummond, K. N., Good, R. A., and Vernier, R. Acute poststreptococcal glomerulonephritis: Immune deposit disease. *J. Clin. Invest.* 45:237, 1966.

461. Michon, L., Aubertin, D., Jagerschmidt, G., and Valleteau de Moulliac, G. Two cases of primary thrombosis of the renal vein in the new born: Cure of one of them by heparin perfusion. *Ann. Ped. Paris* 9:119, 1962.

462. Michon, L., Hamburger, J., Occonomos, N., Deliniatte, P., Richet, G., Vaysse, J., and Antoine, B. Une tentative de transplantation rénale chez l'homme; aspects médicaux et biologiques. *Presse Med.* 61:1419, 1953.

463. Milhand, G., and Courvoissier, B. Appreciation du métabolism des acides amines par la chromatographie sur papier. *Helv. Med. Acta* 18:475, 1951.

464. Miller, D. G. The association of immune disease and malignant lymphoma. *Ann. Intern. Med.* 66:507, 1967.

465. Miller, G., Hoyt, J. C., and Pollock, B. E. Bilateral renal vein thrombosis and the ne-

phrotic syndrome. *Amer. J. Med.* 17:856, 1954.

466. Mollison, A. W., and Rennie, J. B. Treatment of renal oedema with dextran. *Brit. Med. J.* 1:893, 1954.

467. Momma, K. Immunochemical semiquantitative estimation of gamma-M and gamma-A immunoglobulins in healthy and diseased children: 2. Immunoglobulin levels in nephrotic syndrome, exudative enteropathy, acute leukemia, and malignant tumors. *Acta Paediat. Jap.* 7:13, 1965.

468. Montgomerie, J. Z., Becroft, D. M. O., Croxson, M. C., Doak, P. B., and North, J. D. K. Herpes-simplex-virus infection after renal transplantation. *Lancet* 2:867, 1969.

469. Montgomery, H. Disseminated lupus erythematosus as a systemic disease. *Oxford Medicine* 4:41, 1949.

470. Montgomery, H., and McCreight, W. G. Disseminated lupus erythematosus. *Arch. Dermat. Syph.* 60:356, 1949.

471. Moore, J. E. *Modern Treatment of Syphilis.* Springfield, Ill.: Thomas, 1933. P. 213.

472. Morris, R. C., and Fuedenburg, H. H. Impaired renal acidification in patients with hypergamma globulinemia. *Medicine* (Balt.) 45:57, 1967.

473. Moser, R. H. Treatment of nephrotic syndrome. *Southwest Med.* 48:28, 1967.

474. Mostofi, F. K., Vorder Bruegge, C. F., and Diggs, L. W. Lesions in kidneys removed for unilateral hematuria in sickle-cell disease. *A.M.A. Arch. Path.* 63:336, 1957.

475. Movat, H. Z., and McGregor, D. D. The fine structure of the glomerulus in membranous glomerulonephritis (lipoid nephrosis) in adults. *Amer. J. Clin. Path.* 32:109, 1959.

476. Muehrcke, R. C. The finger-nails in chronic hypoalbuminaemia. A new physical sign. *Brit. Med. J.* 1:1327, 1956.

477. Muehrcke, R. C., Kark, R. M., Pirani, C. L., Pollak, V. E., and Steck, I. E. Histological and clinical evolution of lupus nephritis. *Ann. Rheum. Dis.* 14:371, 1955.

478. Muehrcke, R. C., Kark, R. M., Pirani, C. L., and Pollak, V. E. Lupus nephritis: Clinical and pathologic study based on renal biopsies. *Medicine* (Balt.) 36:1, 1957.

479. Muehrcke, R. C., Pirani, C. L., Pollak, V. E., and Kark, R. M. Primary renal amyloidosis with the nephrotic syndrome studied by serial biopsies of the kidney. *Guy. Hosp. Rep.* 104:295, 1955.

480. Munck, O., and Nissen, N. I. Development of nephrotic syndrome during treatment with mercurial diuretics. *Acta Med. Scand.* 153:307, 1956.

481. Munk, F. Klinische Diagnostik der degenerativen Nierenerkrankungen. *Ztschr. Klin. Med.* 78:1, 1913.

482. Musa, B. U., Seal, U. S., and Doe, R. P. Excretion of corticosteroid-binding globulin, thyroxine-binding globulin and total protein in adult males with nephrosis: Effects of sex hormones. *J. Clin. Endocr.* 27:768, 1967.

483. Nabarro, J. D. N., and Rosenheim, M. L. Nephrotic syndrome complicating Tridione therapy. *Lancet* 1:1091, 1952.

484. Nagasawa, H. T., Swingle, K. F., and Alexander, C. S. Metabolism of aminonucleoside-8-14C in the rat and guinea pig. *Biochem. Pharmacol.* 16:2211, 1967.

485. Najjar, V. A. The Mechanism of Antibody-Antigen Interaction as a Theoretical Basis of Auto-immune Mechanisms. In Metcoff, J. (Ed.), *Proceedings of the Eleventh Annual Conference on the Nephrotic Syndrome.* New York: National Kidney Disease Foundation, 1959. P. 98.

486. Najjar, V. A., and Fisher, J. Mechanism of antibody-antigen reaction. *Science* 122:1272, 1955.

487. Najjar, V. A., and Fisher, J. The mechanism of antibody-antigen reaction. *Biochem. Biophys. Acta* 20:158, 1956.

488. Najjar, V. A. Discussion. In Shaffer, J. H., et al. (Eds.), *Mechanisms of Hypersensitivity* (Henry Ford Hospital International Symposium). Boston: Little, Brown, 1959. P. 198.

489. Najjar, V. A., and Robinson, J. P. A Unified Concept of Immunologic Reactions and Allergic States. In Najjar, V. A. (Ed.), *Immunity and Virus Infection.* New York: John Wiley & Sons, 1959. P. 71.

490. Najjar, V. A., Sidbury, J. B., Jr., and Fisher, J. Further studies on the mechanism of

antibody-antigen reaction. *Biochem. Biophys. Acta* 26:114, 1947.

491. Nesson, H. R., Sproul, L. E., Jr., Relman, A. S., and Schwartz, W. B. Adrenal steroids in the treatment of idiopathic nephrotic syndrome in adults. *Ann. Intern. Med.* 58:268, 1963.

492. Nettles, J. B. The kidney in normal and abnormal pregnancy: Differential diagnosis. *Southern Med. J.* 59:295, 1966.

493. Nettles, J. B., and Flanigan, W. J. Counseling the pregnant patient with renal disease. *Clin. Obstet. Gynec.* 11:594, 1968.

494. Ngu, J. L., and Monekosso, G. L. Variation of serum complement levels in the nephrotic syndrome in Lagos, Nigeria. *J. Trop. Med. Hyg.* 71:252, 1968.

495. Nikkila, E., and Gräsbeck, R. Heparin in lipoid nephrosis. *Acta Med. Scand.* 150:39, 1954.

496. Nikkila, E., and Hashti, E. On the mechanism of the heparin induced lipemia clearing reaction. *Acta Chem. Scand.* 8:363, 1954.

497. Norio, R. Heredity in the congenital nephrotic syndrome: A genetic study of 57 Finnish families with a review of reported cases. *Ann. Paediat. Fenn.* 12(Suppl. 27):1, 1966.

498. Northway, J. D., and West, C. D. Successful therapy of trimethadione nephrosis with prednisone and cyclophosphamide. *J. Pediat.* 71:259, 1967.

499. Nusslé, D., Barandum, S., and Witschi, H. P. Pertes digestives de proteines et syndrome nephrotique. In Schwartz, M. O., and Vesin, P. (Eds.), *Plasma Proteins and Gastrointestinal Tract in Health and Disease.* Copenhagen: Munksgaard, 1962.

500. Nusslé, D., and Royer, P. Pertes digestives de proteines plasmatiques dans les syndromes nephrotiques de l'enfant. Etude avec la ^{131}I-albumin et de la ^{131}I-globuline. In Schwartz, M. O., and Vesin, P. (Eds.), *Protides of the Biological Fluids.* Amsterdam: Elsevier, 1964.

501. O'Beirn, S. Renal vein thrombosis in amyloidosis. *Irish J. Med. Sci.* 6:181, 1953.

502. Oberg, B. Effects of cardiovascular reflexes on the net capillary fluid transfer. *Acta Physiol. Scand.* 62(Suppl. 229):1, 1964.

503. Ojo, O. A., and Akinkugbe, O. O. The nephrotic syndrome in pregnancy. *J. Obstet. Gynaec. Brit. Comm.* 74:919, 1967.

504. Okuda, R., Kaplan, M. H., Cuppage, F. E., and Heymann, W. Deposition of autologous gamma globulin in kidneys of rats with nephrotic renal disease of various etiologies. *J. Lab. Clin. Med.* 66:204, 1965.

505. Oliver, W. J., Kelsch, R. C., and Chandler, J. P. Demonstration of increased catecholamine excretion in the nephrotic syndrome. *Proc. Soc. Exp. Biol. Med.* 125:1176, 1967.

506. Oliver, W. J., and Owings, C. L. Sodium excretion in the nephrotic syndrome: Relation to serum albumin concentration, glomerular filtration rate, and aldosterone excretion rate. *Amer. J. Dis. Child.* 113:352, 1967.

507. Omae, T., Masson, G. M., and Corcoran, A. C. Experimental production of nephrotic syndrome following renal vein constriction in rats. *Proc. Soc. Exp. Biol. Med.* 97:821, 1958.

508. Oncley, J. L. Physical Chemistry of Lipoproteins. In Metcoff, J. (Ed.), *Proceedings of the Seventh Annual Conference on the Nephrotic Syndrome.* New York: National Nephrosis Foundation, 1955. P. 68.

509. Opitz, J. Hereditary Hematuria. In Metcoff, J. (Ed.), *Hereditary, Developmental, and Immunologic Aspects of Kidney Disease.* Evanston, Ill.: Northwestern University Press, 1962. P. 3.

510. Orloff, J., Welt, L. G., and Stowe, L. The effects of concentrated salt-poor albumin on the metabolism and excretion of water and electrolytes in nephrosis and toxemia of pregnancy. *J. Clin. Invest.* 29:770, 1950.

511. Osman, A. A. Preliminary observations on treatment of nephritis with edema by means of large doses of alkalies. *Guy. Hosp. Rep.* 76:412, 1926.

512. Ostertag, B. Familial amyloidosis. *Ztschr. Menschl. Vererb.-Konstitutionslehre* 30:105, 1950.

513. Ozen, M. A., Sandalci, O., and Berker, F. Ethacrynic acid and carbohydrate metabolism. *Amer. J. Med. Sci.* 252:558, 1966.

514. Pande, S. R., Mehrota, T. N., and Gupta, S. C. Electrophoretic studies of the serum and urinary proteins in nephrotic syndrome. *Indian J. Med. Sci.* 21:800, 1967.

515. Park, R. K., Goltz, R. W., and Carey, T. B. Unusual cutaneous infections associated with immunosuppressive therapy. *Arch. Derm.* (Chicago) 95:345, 1967.

516. Parker, R. A., and Piel, C. F. The nephrotic syndrome in the first year of life. *Pediatrics* 25:967, 1960.

517. Pasternack, A., Eklund, J., and Krohn, K. Renal artery stenosis and the nephrotic syndrome. *Acta Med. Scand.* 181:265, 1967.

518. Pastor, B. H., and Cahn, M. Reversible nephrotic syndrome resulting from constrictive pericarditis. *New Eng. J. Med.* 262:872, 1960.

519. Perkoff, G. T. The hereditary renal diseases. *New Eng. J. Med.* 277:79, 251, 1967.

520. Peters, J. P., and Man, E. B. The relation of albumin to precipitable iodine of serum. *J. Clin. Invest.* 27:397, 1948.

521. Pfeiffer, E. F., Schoffling, K., and Bruch, H. E. Serumkomplement und Masugi-Nephritis der Ratte. *Verh. Deutsch. Ges. Inn. Med.* 59 Kongress, 1953.

522. Piel, C. F., and Williams, G. F. Long continued adrenal hormone therapy in childhood nephrosis. *J. Amer. Med. Wom. Ass.* 12:273, 1957.

523. Pillay, V. K. G., Schwartz, F. D., Battifora, H., Buenger, R. E., and Kark, R. M. Massive proteinuria associated with vesico-ureteral reflux. *Lancet* 2:1272, 1969.

524. Pollak, V., Kark, R. M., Pirani, C. L., Shafter, H. A., and Muehrcke, R. C. Renal vein thrombosis and the nephrotic syndrome. *Amer. J. Med.* 21:496, 1956.

525. Pollak, V., Pirani, C. L., Kark, R. M., Muehrcke, R. C., Freda, V. C., and Nettles, J. B. Reversible glomerular lesions in toxaemia of pregnancy. *Lancet* 2:59, 1956.

526. Pollak, V. E., Pirani, C. L., and Seskind, C. Bilateral renal vein thrombosis: Clinical and electron microscopic studies of a case with complete recovery after anticoagulant therapy. *Ann. Intern. Med.* 65:1056, 1966.

527. Pollak, V. E., Rosen, S., Pirani, C. L., Muehrcke, R. C., and Kark, R. M. Natural history of lipoid nephrosis and of membranous glomerulonephritis. *Ann. Intern. Med.* 69:1171, 1968.

528. Pollner, P. Nephrotic syndrome associated with congenital syphilis. *J.A.M.A.* 198:263, 1966.

529. Posner, A. C., Goldman, J. A., and Forester, G. U. Pregnancy complicated by nephrotic syndrome; a case report. *Amer. J. Obstet.* 74:651, 1957.

530. Prader, A. Lipoidnephrose bei eineiigen Zwillingen. *Helv. Paediat. Acta* 5:392, 1950.

531. Pressman, D., Korngold, L., and Heymann, W. Localizing properties of antirat-kidney serum prepared in ducks. *A.M.A. Arch. Path.* 55:347, 1953.

532. Quinn, J. R., and Zimmerman, H. J. Significance of oval fat bodies in urinary sediment. *Amer. J. Clin. Path.* 29:787, 1954.

533. Rabhan, N. B. Pituitary-adrenal suppression and Cushing's syndrome after intermittent dexamethasone therapy. *Ann. Intern. Med.* 69:1141, 1968.

534. Raphael, S. S., and Lynch, M. J. G. Kimmelstiel–Wilson glomerulonephropathy. *A.M.A. Arch. Path.* 65:420, 1958.

535. Rapoport, M., McCrory, W. W., and Sohn, W. Adrenal steroid therapy of the nephrotic syndrome; an analysis of treatment results in 70 children. *A.M.A. Amer. J. Dis. Child.* 90:631, 1955.

536. Rasmussen, H. Thyroxine metabolism in the nephrotic syndrome. *J. Clin. Invest.* 35:792, 1956.

537. Recant, L. Abnormality in thyroxine binding in nephrosis. *J. Clin. Invest.* 35:730, 1956.

538. Recant, L., Borowsky, B. A., and Kessner, D. M. Aminonucleoside glomerulonephritis: Morphologic and metabolic studies. (Abstract.) *J. Clin. Invest.* 37:924, 1958.

539. Recant, L., and Riggs, D. S. Thyroid function in nephrosis. *J. Clin. Invest.* 31:789, 1952.

540. Reimold, E. W., and Marks, J. F. Hypovolemic shock complicating the nephrotic syndrome in children. *J. Pediat.* 69:658, 1966.

541. Reyersbach, G. C., and Butler, A. M. Con-

genital hereditary hematuria. *New Eng. J. Med.* 251:377, 1954.

542. Richmond, J., Sherman, R. S., Diamond, H. D., and Craver, L. F. Renal lesions associated with malignant lymphomas. *Amer. J. Med.* 32:184, 1962.

543. Riddle, M., Gardner, F., Beswick, I., and Filshie, I. The nephrotic syndrome complicating mercurial diuretic therapy. *Brit. Med. J.* 1:1274, 1958.

544. Rifkin, H., Parker, J. G., Polin, E. B., Berkman, J. I., and Spiro, D. Diabetic glomerulosclerosis; clinical and pathologic observations with special reference to doubly refractile fatty cells and casts in the urine. *Medicine* (Balt.) 27:429, 1948.

545. Rijnberk, A. A nephrotic syndrome in the dog, treated with prednisone. *Zbl. Veterinaermed.* (A) 13:102, 1966.

546. Riley, C. M. The nephrotic syndrome; effect of adrenocorticotrophic hormone. *Pediatrics* 7:475, 1951.

547. Riley, C. M. The management of the nephrotic syndrome. *Bull. N.Y. Acad. Med.* 28:630, 1952.

548. Riley, C. M. Experimental Pathology and Immunochemistry. In Metcoff, J. (Ed.), *Proceedings of the Fourth Annual Conference on the Nephrotic Syndrome.* New York: National Nephrosis Foundation, 1952. P. 45.

549. Riley, C. M. *Nephrosis in Childhood.* New York: National Nephrosis Foundation, 1955.

550. Riley, C. M. Therapy of the Nephrotic Syndrome. In Metcoff, J. (Ed.), *Proceedings of the Sixth Annual Conference on the Nephrotic Syndrome.* New York: National Nephrosis Foundation, 1955. P. 227.

551. Riley, C. M. Therapy of the Nephrotic Syndrome, Clinical and Therapeutic Studies. In Metcoff, J. (Ed.), *Proceedings of the Seventh Annual Conference on the Nephrotic Syndrome.* New York: National Nephrosis Foundation, 1955. P. 199.

552. Riley, C. M. The use of corticotropin, cortisone and hydrocortisone in the nephrosis of childhood. *Ann. N.Y. Acad. Sci.* 61:430, 1955.

553. Riley, C. M. Statistical Evaluation of Survival of Nephrotic Children Treated with Steroids. In Metcoff, J. (Ed.), *Proceedings of the Tenth Annual Conference on the Nephrotic Syndrome.* New York: National Kidney Disease Foundation, 1958. P. 273.

554. Riley, C. M., and Davis, R. A. Childhood nephrosis. *Pediat. Clin. N. Amer.* 2:893, 1955.

555. Riley, C. M., Davis, R. A., Fertig, J. W., and Berger, A. P. Nephrosis of childhood: Statistical evaluation of the effect of adrenocortical-active therapy. *J. Chron. Dis.* 3:640, 1956.

556. Riley, C. M., and Scaglione, P. R. Current management of nephrosis: Statistical evaluation and a proposed approach to therapy. *Pediatrics* 23:561, 1959.

557. Rinehart, J. F., Farquhar, M. G., Jung, H. C., and Abul-Haj, S. K. The normal glomerulus and its basic reactions in disease. *Amer. J. Path.* 29:21, 1953.

558. Rizutto, V. J., Mazzara, J. T., and Grace, W. J. Pheochromocytoma with nephrotic syndrome. *Amer. J. Cardiol.* 16:342, 1965.

559. Robbins, J., Rall, J. E., and Petermann, M. L. Protein binding of thyroxine in normal and nephrotic serum. *J. Clin. Invest.* 33:959, 1954.

560. Robbins, J., Rall, J. E., and Petermann, M. L. Thyroxine binding by serum and urine proteins in nephrosis; qualitative aspects. *J. Clin. Invest.* 36:1333, 1957.

561. Robbins, S. L. *Textbook of Pathology.* Philadelphia: Saunders, 1957.

562. Robin, E. D., and Gardner, F. H. Hereditary factors in chronic Bright's disease — A study of two affected kindreds. *Trans. Ass. Amer. Physicians* 70:140, 1957.

563. Rodbell, M. The Interconversion of Lipoproteins. In Metcoff, J. (Ed.), *Proceedings of the Ninth Annual Conference on the Nephrotic Syndrome.* New York: National Nephrosis Foundation, 1957. P. 104.

564. Rogers, J., and Robbins, S. L. Intercapillary glomerulosclerosis; a clinical and pathological study: I. Specificity of the clinical syndrome. *Amer. J. Med.* 12:688, 1952.

565. Rogers, J., Robbins, S. L., and Jeghers, H. Intercapillary glomerulosclerosis; a clinical and pathological study: II. A clinical study

of 100 anatomically proven cases. *Amer. J. Med.* 12:692, 1952.

566. Rohmer, P., and Sacrez, R.   Un cas de néphrose lipoïdique au cour d'une maladie de Hodgkin. *Strasbourg Med.* 108:45, 1948.

567. Ronzoni, E., Roberts, E., Fronkel, S., and Ramasarma, G. B.   Influence of administration of ACTH on urinary amino acids. *Proc. Soc. Exp. Biol. Med.* 82:496, 1953.

568. Rose, G. A., and Black, D. A. K.   Controlled trial of steroids in the nephrotic syndrome. *Quart. J. Med.* 36:607, 1967.

569. Rosen, G. M., Carp, L., and Vernon, C. M.   Double refractile lipoid bodies in the urinary sediment of a patient with progressive scleroderma and calcinosis. *N.Y. J. Med.* 51: Part I, 1183, 1951.

570. Rosenblum, J., Sonnenschein, H., and Minsky, A. A.   Trimethadione (Tridione) nephrosis. *A.M.A. Amer. J. Dis. Child.* 97:790, 1959.

571. Rosenkrantz, J. G., Githens, J. H., and Cox, S. W.   Azathioprine (Imuran) and pregnancy. *Amer. J. Obstet. Gynec.* 97:387, 1967.

572. Rosenman, R. H., and Byers, S. O.   Study of possible causal role of lipoprotein lipase deficiency in nephrotic hyperlipemia. *J. Clin. Invest.* 38:1036, 1959.

573. Rosenman, R. H., Friedman, M., and Byers, S. O.   The causal role of plasma albumin deficiency in experimental nephrotic hyperlipemia and hypercholesterolemia. *J. Clin. Invest.* 35:522, 1956.

574. Rosenman, R. H., and Smith, M. K.   Relationship between concentrations of albumin and lipids in experimentally nephrotic rats. *Amer. J. Physiol.* 191:40, 1957.

575. Rosenmann, E., Pollak, V. E., and Pirani, C. L.   Renal vein thrombosis in the adult: Clinical and pathologic study based on renal biopsies. *Medicine* (Balt.) 47:269, 1968.

576. Ross, I. P., and Ross, J. H.   Nephrotic syndrome: Prednisone therapy with two deaths from cellulitis. *Lancet* 272:354, 1957.

577. Routh, J. I., Knapp, E. L., and Kobayashi, C. K.   Electrophoretic studies of plasma and urinary protein in children with lipoid nephrosis. *J. Pediat.* 33:688, 1948.

578. Rukavina, J. G., Block, W. D., Jackson, C. E., Falls, H. F., Carey, J. H., and Curtis, A.

C.   Primary systemic amyloidosis: A review and an experimental, genetic and clinical study of 29 cases with particular emphasis on the familiar form. *Medicine* (Balt.) 35:240, 1956.

579. Rusby, N. L., and Wilson, C.   Lung purpura with nephritis. *Quart. J. Med.* 29:501, 1960.

580. Russell, P. J., and Hicks, J. D.   Cyclophosphamide treatment of renal disease in (NZB and NZW) F1 hybrid mice. *Lancet* 1:440, 1968.

581. Russell, P. J., Hicks, J. D., and Burnet, F. M.   Cyclophosphamide treatment of kidney disease in (NZB and NZW) F1 mice. *Lancet* 1:1279, 1966.

582. Rutecki, G. J., Goldsmith, C. M., and Schreiner, G. E.   Characterization and pattern of distribution in urinary casts. (Abstract.) *Amer. Soc. Neph.* 2:57, 1968.

583. Rytand, D. A.   Fatal anuria, the nephrotic syndrome and glomerular nephritis as sequels of the dermatitis of poison oak. *Amer. J. Med.* 5:548, 1948.

584. Rytand, D. A.   Onset of the nephrotic syndrome during a reaction to bee sting. *Stanford Med. Bull.* 13:224, 1955.

585. Rytand, D. A., and Cox, A. J., Jr.   Polycyclic nephrotic syndrome. *Amer. J. Med.* 22:297, 1957.

586. Rytand, D. A., and Randall, E.   Titers of heterophile antibodies and antistreptolysin "O" in acute glomerular nephritis and in the nephrotic syndrome. *Amer. J. Med.* 8:524, 1950.

587. Rytand, D. A., Rantz, L. A., and Randall, E.   Antistreptolysin "O" in urine and serum of patients with the nephrotic syndrome. Proceedings of the Society for Clinical Investigation. *J. Clin. Invest.* 29:843, 1950.

588. Scheinman, J. I., and Stamler, F. W.   Cyclophosphamide and fatal varicella. *J. Pediat.* 74:117, 1969.

589. Schreiner, G. E.   3-D for diagnosis. *GP* 9: 70, 1954.

590. Schreiner, G. E.   Some observations on telescoped urinary sediments. *Ann. Intern. Med.* 42:826, 1955.

591. Schreiner, G. E.   The differential diagnosis

of acute and chronic glomerulonephritis. *J. Chron. Dis.* 5:45, 1957.

592. Schreiner, G. E. Identification and clinical significance of urinary casts. *A.M.A. Arch. Intern. Med.* 99:356, 1957.

593. Schreiner, G. E. The Glomerular Membrane in the Nephrotic Syndrome. In Moyer, L. H., and Fuchs, M. (Eds.), *Edema, Mechanisms and Management.* Philadelphia: Saunders, 1960. P. 485.

594. Schreiner, G. E. The Use of Diuretics in Edema of Renal Origin. In Moyer, J. H., and Fuchs, M. (Eds.), *Edema, Mechanisms and Management.* Philadelphia: Saunders, 1960. P. 540.

595. Schreiner, G. E. Glomerular permeability in the nephrotic syndrome. *Trans. Amer. Clin. Climat. Ass.* In press.

596. Schreiner, G. E., and Berman, L. B. Experience with 150 consecutive renal biopsies. *Southern Med. J.* 50:733, 1957.

597. Schreiner, G. E., and Bloomer, H. A. The effect of chlorothiazide on edema, cirrhosis, nephrosis, congestive heart failure and chronic renal insufficiency. *New Eng. J. Med.* 257:1016, 1957.

598. Schreiner, G. E., and Maher, J. F. *Uremia: The Biochemistry, Pathogenesis and Treatment.* Springfield, Ill.: Thomas, 1961.

599. Schwab, L., Moll, F. C., Hall, T., Brean, H., Kick, M., Hawn, C. V., and Janeway, C. A. Experimental hypersensitivity in the rabbit: Effect of inhibition of antibody formation by X-radiation and nitrogen mustards in histologic and serologic sequences and on behavior of serum complement following single large injections of serum proteins. *J. Exp. Med.* 91:505, 1950.

600. Schwartz, H., and Kohn, J. L. Studies of nephritis in child: I. Nephrosis. *Amer. J. Dis. Child.* 24:125, 1922.

601. Schwartz, H., Kohn, J. L., and Weiner, S. B. Lipid nephrosis: Observations over a period of 20 years. *Amer. J. Dis. Child.* 65:355, 1943.

602. Scott, J. T., and O'Brien, P. K. Probenecid, nephrotic syndrome, and renal failure. *Ann. Rheum. Dis.* 27:249, 1968.

603. Scott, R. B. Chronic lymphocytic leukemia. *Lancet* 1:1162, 1957.

604. Sebastian, A., McSherry, E., Ueki, I., and Morris, R. C., Jr. Renal amyloidosis, nephrotic syndrome, and impaired renal tubular reabsorption of bicarbonate. *Ann. Intern. Med.* 69:541, 1968.

605. Seegal, B. Localization of Rabbit and Duck Anti-kidney Antibodies. In Metcoff, J. (Ed.), *Proceedings of the Ninth Annual Conference on the Nephrotic Syndrome.* New York: National Nephrosis Foundation, 1957. P. 1.

605a. Seegal, B. C., Hasson, M. W., Gaynor, E. C., and Rothenberg, M. S. Glomerulonephritis produced in dogs by specific antisera: I. The course of the disease resulting from injection of rabbit antidog-placenta serum or rabbit antidog-kidney serum. *J. Exp. Med.* 102:789, 1955.

606. Seelig, M. S. Penicillamine and the nephrotic syndrome. *J.A.M.A.* 199:767, 1967.

607. Seifter, J., Baeder, D. H., Zarafontis, C. J. D., and Kalas, J. Hormonal control of permeability and mobilization of fat depots. *Ann. N.Y. Acad. Sci.* 72:1031, 1959.

608. Seftel, H. C., and Schewitz, L. J. The nephrotic syndrome in pregnancy. *J. Obstet. Gynaec. Brit. Emp.* 64:862, 1957.

609. Sellers, A. L. The mechanism and significance of protein excretion by the normal kidney. *A.M.A. Arch. Intern. Med.* 98:801, 1956.

610. Sellers, A. L., Griggs, N., Marmorston, J., and Goodman, H. C. Filtration and reabsorption of protein by the kidney. *J. Exp. Med.* 100:1, 1954.

611. Shafrir, E. Partition of unesterified fatty acids in normal and nephrotic syndrome serum and its effect on serum electrophoretic pattern. *J. Clin. Invest.* 37:1775, 1958.

612. Shapiro, F. L., and Smith, H. T. Diabetic glomerulosclerosis in a patient with chronic pancreatitis. *Arch. Intern. Med.* (Chicago) 117:795, 1966.

613. Sharpstone, P., Ogg, C. S., and Cameron, J. S. Nephrotic syndrome due to primary renal disease in adults: II. A controlled trial of prednisolone and azathioprine. *Brit. Med. J.* 2:535, 1969.

614. Shearn, M. A. Mercaptopurine in the treat-

ment of steroid-resistant nephrotic syndrome. *New Eng. J. Med.* 273:943, 1965.

615. Shearn, M. A., and Tu, W. H. Nephrogenic diabetes insipidus and other defects of renal tubular dysfunction in Sjøgren's syndrome. *Amer. J. Med.* 39:312, 1965.

616. Sherman, J. F., Taylor, D. J., and Bond, H. W. Puromycin: III. Toxicology and pharmacology. *Antibiotics Ann.* 1954–55. P. 757.

617. Sherman, M. J., Morales, J. B., Bayrd, E. D., and Schierman, W. D. Amyloid nephrosis secondary to Hodgkin's disease: Report of a case. *A.M.A. Arch. Intern. Med.* 95:618, 1955.

618. Sherman, M. J., Morales, J. B., Bayrd, E. B., and Schierman, W. D. Amyloid nephrosis secondary to Hodgkin's disease. *A.M.A. Arch. Intern. Med.* 95:618, 1955.

619. Shreeve, W. W., Hutchin, M. E., Harper, H. A., Miller, C. D., and Doolan, P. D. Excretion of amino acids in nephrosis. *Proc. Soc. Exp. Biol. Med.* 88:510, 1955.

620. Silverberg, D. S., McPhaul, J. T., and Hunt, J. C. Nephrotic syndrome with use of ammoniated mercury. *Arch. Intern. Med.* (Chicago) 125:81, 1967.

621. Siperstein, M. D., Unger, R. H., and Madison, L. L. Studies of muscle capillary basement membranes in normal subjects, diabetic, and prediabetic patients. *J. Clin. Invest.* 47:1973, 1968.

622. Smadel, J. E. Experimental nephritis in rats induced by injections of antikidney serum: I. Preparation and immunolgic studies of nephrotoxin. *J. Exp. Med.* 64:921, 1936.

623. Smadel, J. E. Experimental nephritis in rats induced by injections of anti-kidney serum: III. Pathological studies of the acute and chronic diseases. *J. Exp. Med.* 65:541, 1937.

624. Smadel, J. E., and Farr, L. E. Experimental nephritis in rats induced by injections of anti-kidney serum: II. Clinical and functional studies. *J. Exp. Med.* 65:527, 1937.

625. Smadel, J. E., and Swift, H. F. Experimental nephritis in rats induced by injection of anti-kidney serum: V. Chronic nephritis

of insidious development following apparent recovery from acute nephrotoxic nephritis. *J. Exp. Med.* 74:345, 1941.

626. Smith, J. F. The kidney in lupus erythematosus. *J. Bact. Path.* 70:41, 1955.

627. Snyder, A. Systemic lupus erythematosus. In "Combined Staff Clinic." *Amer. J. Med.* 28:416, 1960.

628. Sokol, A., Bashner, M. H., and Okun, R. Nephrotic syndrome caused by probenecid. *J.A.M.A.* 199:43, 1967.

629. Solomon, D. H., Gardella, J. W., Fanger, H., Dethier, F. M., and Ferrebee, J. W. Nephrotoxic nephritis in rats: Evidence for the glomerular origin of the kidney antigen. *J. Exp. Med.* 90:267, 1949.

630. Solsona Conillera, J. Linfogranulomatosis maligna: Forma monoganglionar Y nefrosica. *Med. Clin.* 20:37, 1953.

631. Soothill, J. F. Altered complement component C3A (beta-1C–beta-1A) in patients with glomerulonephritis. *Clin. Exp. Immun.* 2:83, 1967.

632. Soothill, J. F., and Hendricks, R. G. Some immunologic studies of the nephrotic syndrome of Nigerian children. *Lancet* 2:629, 1967.

633. Soyka, L. F. The nephrotic syndrome: Current concepts in diagnosis and therapy advantages of alternate day steroid regimen. *Clin. Pediat.* (Phila.) 6:77, 1967.

634. Soyka, L. F. Treatment of the nephrotic syndrome in childhood: Use of an alternate-day prednisone regimen. *Amer. J. Dis. Child.* 113:693, 1967.

635. Spaeth, G. L., and Von Sallmann, L. Corticosteroids and cataracts. *Int. Ophthal. Clin.* 6:915, 1966.

636. Spector, W. G. Labelled glycine in the nephrotic syndrome. *Clin. Sci.* 13:1, 1954.

637. Spiro, D. The structural basis of proteinuria in man; electron microscopic studies of renal biopsy specimens from patients with lipid nephrosis, amyloidosis, and subacute and chronic glomerulonephritis. *Amer. J. Path.* 35:47, 1959.

638. Squire, J. R. The nephrotic syndrome. *Brit. Med. J.* 2:1389, 1953.

639. Squire, J. R. The nephrotic syndrome. *Advances Intern. Med.* 7:201, 1956.

The Nephrotic Syndrome 633

640. Squire, J. R., Blainey, J. D., and Hardwicke, J. The nephrotic syndrome. *Brit. Med. Bull.* 13:43, 1957.

641. Stanbury, S. W., and Macaulay, D. Defects of renal tubular function in the nephrotic syndrome; observations on a nephrotic child with aminoaciduria, glycosuria, polyuria, tubular acidosis, and potassium depletion. *Quart. J. Med.* 26:7, 1957.

642. Stanton, M. C., and Tange, J. D. Goodpasture's syndrome. (Pulmonary haemorrhage associated with glomerulonephritis.) *Aust. Ann. Med.* 7:132, 1958.

643. Stavitsky, A. B., Hackel, D. B., and Heymann, W. Reduction of serum complement following in vivo tissue antigen-antibody reactions. *Proc. Soc. Exp. Biol. Med.* 85:593, 1954.

644. Steblay, R. W. Nephritis in sheep induced by direct injection of human kidney tissue and Freund's adjuvant. *Clin. Res.* 8:289, 1960.

645. Steinbeck, A. W. Nephrotic syndrome developing after snakebite. *Med. J. Aust.* 1:543, 1960.

646. Sternlieb, I. Penicillamine and the nephrotic syndrome. *J.A.M.A.* 198:1311, 1966.

647. Steroid treatment in the nephrotic syndrome in childhood. *Brit. Med. J.* 1:530, 1968.

648. Stickler, G. B., Burke, E. C., and McKenzie, B. F. Electrophoretic studies of the nephrotic syndrome in children: Preliminary report. *Proc. Staff Meet. Mayo Clin.* 29:555, 1954.

649. Stickler, G. B., Shin, M. H., and Burke, E. C. Diffuse glomerulonephritis associated with infected ventriculoatrial shunt. *New Eng. J. Med.* 279:1077, 1968.

650. Sturgill, B. C., and Rowe, C. T. Renal vein thrombosis and the nephrotic syndrome. *Arch. Intern. Med.* (Chicago) 120:708, 1967.

651. Surbek, K. E. A striking case of quartana nephrosis. *Trans. Roy. Soc. Trop. Med. Hyg.* 25:201, 1931.

652. Sumida, Y. Studies on the combined amino acids in human urine. *Hiroshima J. Med. Sci.* 16:231, 1967.

653. Sussman, H. C., Fowler, B., and Findley, T. Observations on the renal metabolism of protein in experimental and clinical nephrotic syndromes. *Metabolism* 17:336, 1968.

654. Svanborg, A. Studies on renal hyperlipemia. *Acta Med. Scand.* 141: Suppl. 264, 1951.

655. Swanson, M. A., and Schwartz, R. S. Immunosuppressive therapy. The relation between clinical response and immunologic competence. *New Eng. J. Med.* 277:163, 1967.

656. Sweeney, M. J., Dobbins, W. T., and Etteldorf, J. N. Renal disease with elements of the nephrotic syndrome associated with sickle cell anemia. *J. Pediat.* 60:32, 1962.

657. Symchych, P. S., and Perrin, E. V. Thrombosis of the main pulmonary artery in nephrosis: Thromboembolism as a complication of nephrosis. *Amer. J. Dis. Child.* 110:636, 1965.

658. Takeda, Y., and Chen, A. Y. Fibrinogen metabolism and distribution in patients with the nephrotic syndrome. *J. Lab. Clin. Med.* 70:678, 1967.

659. Talal, N. Sjøgren's syndrome. *Bull. Rheum. Dis.* 16:404, 1966.

660. Talal, N., Zisman, E., and Schur, P. H. Renal tubular acidosis, glomerulonephritis and immunologic factors in Sjøgren's syndrome. *Arthritis Rheum.* 11:774, 1968.

661. Tapie, J., Laporte, J., and Richalens, S. U. C. Syndrome néphrotique au cours de la maladie de Hodgkin-Sternberg. *Presse Med.* 65:287, 1957.

661a. Taylor, R. Therapy of the Nephrotic Syndrome. In Metcoff, J. (Ed.), *Proceedings of the Sixth Annual Conference on the Nephrotic Syndrome.* New York: National Nephrosis Foundation, 1954. P. 245.

661b. Taylor, R. D. Nephrotic syndrome: Treatment with ACTH and nitrogen mustard. *Med. Clin. N. Amer.* 39:995, 1955.

662. Tegelaers, W. H. H., and Tiddens, H. Nephrosis due to Tridione. *Maandschr. Kindergeneesk.* 20:23, 1952.

663. Tegelaers, W. H. H., and Tiddens, H. K. Nephrotic-glucosuric-aminoaciduric dwarfism and electrolyte metabolism. *Helv. Pediat. Acta* 10:269, 1955.

664. Terry, R., Hawkins, D. R., Church, F. H.,

and Whipple, G. W. Proteinuria related to hyperproteinemia in dogs following plasma given parenterally: A renal threshold for plasma proteins. *J. Exp. Med.* 87: 561, 1948.

665. Thorn, G. W., Armstrong, S. H., Jr., Davenport, V. D., Woodruff, L. M., and Tyler, F. H. Chemical, clinical and immunological studies on the products of human plasma fractionation: XXX. The use of salt-poor concentrated human serum albumin solution in the treatment of chronic Bright's disease. *J. Clin. Invest.* 24:802, 1945.

666. Thurau, K., Kramer, K., Deetjen, P., and Brechtelsbanes, H. Renal medullary blood flow and its relation to renal function. *Fed. Proc.* 19:360, 1960.

667. Tiddens, H. A. W. M. Het Renale Syndroom van De Toni met Dwerggroei. M.D. Thesis, Utrecht. Amsterdam: Diligentia, 1957.

668. Tillman, A. J. B. Toxemias of pregnancy: Their classification and management. *Med. Clin. N. Amer.* 35:677, 1951.

669. Todd, R. M. The natural history of nephrosis. *Arch. Dis. Child.* 32:99, 1957.

670. Tomkins, G. M., Chaikoff, I. L., and Bennett, L. L. Cholesterol synthesis by liver: II. Effect of hypophysectomy. *J. Biol. Chem.* 199:543, 1952.

671. Tublin, I. N. Renal vein thrombosis and the nephrotic syndrome in an adult: Report of a case and review of the literature. *Med. Ann. D.C.* 37:530, 1968.

672. Tully, J. G., Brown, M. S., and Sheagren, J. N. Septicemia due to mycoplasma hominis type 1. *New Eng. J. Med.* 273:648, 1965.

673. Turk, J. L., and Baker, H. Nephrotic syndrome due to ammoniated mercury. *Brit. J. Derm.* 80:623, 1968.

674. Valentine, G. H. Triamcinolone and intracranial hypertension: A side-effect? *Lancet* 1:892, 1959.

675. Vallery-Radot, P., Mauric, G., Wolfromm, R., and Guiot, G. Néphrose lipoidique secondaire à un traitement aurique. *Bull. Soc. Mem. Med. Hop. Paris* 58:96, 1942.

676. Vassalli, P., and McCluskey, R. T. Pathogenic role of fibrin deposition in immuno-logically indiced glomerulonephritis. *Ann. N.Y. Acad. Sci.* 116:1052, 1964.

677. Vassalli, P., and McCluskey, R. T. The pathogenic role of the coagulation process in rabbit masugi nephritis. *Amer. J. Path.* 45:653, 1964.

678. Vassalli, P., Simon, G., and Rouiller, G. Electron microscopic glomerular lesions resulting from intravascular fibrin formation. *Amer. J. Path.* 43:579, 1963.

679. Vernier, R. L., Brunson, J. G., and Good, R. A. Studies on familial nephrosis: I. Clinical and pathologic study of four cases in a single family. *A.M.A. Amer. J. Dis. Child.* 93:469, 1957.

680. Vernier, R. L., Farquhar, M. G., Brunson, J. G., and Good, R. A. Studies on familial nephrosis: Evidence for a unitarian concept. (Abstract.) *J. Clin. Invest.* 35:741. 1956.

681. Virabhak, N. K. Thrombosis of the aorta in a case of nephrotic syndrome. *J. Singapore Paediat. Soc.* 9:50, 1967.

682. Vivien, P., Gouffault, J., and Guillon, M. Peculiar etiological circumstances of the nephrotic syndrome in adults. *Bull. Soc. Mem. Med. Hop. Paris* 75:323, 1959.

683. Volhard, F., and Fahr, T. *Die Brightsche Nierenkrankheit.* Berlin: Springer-Verlag, 1914.

684. Walker, A. M., Bott, P. A., Oliver, J., and McDowell, M. C. The collection and analysis from single nephrons of the mammalian kidney. *Amer. J. Physiol.* 134:580, 1941.

685. Wallenius, G. Renal clearance of dextran as a measure of glomerular permeability. *Acta Soc. Med. Upsalien.* 59 (Suppl. 4):1, 1954.

686. Wallenstein, L., Serebro. H. A., and Calle, S. Chronic regional enteritis complicated by a nephrotic syndrome due to amyloidosis: Antemortem clinical study. *J.A.M.A.* 198:555, 1966.

687. Walz, D. V., and James, D. C. Significance of doubly refractile fat bodies in urinary sediment. *Amer. J. Clin. Path.* 25:598, 1955.

688. Wardle, E. N., and Taylor, G. Fibrin breakdown products and fibrinolysis in renal disease. *J. Clin. Path.* 21:140, 1968.

689. Wasserman, K., and Mayerson, H. S. The

permeability of capillaries to large molecules. *Amer. J. Med.* 19:154, 1955.

690. Waterhouse, C., and Holler, J. Metabolic studies on protein depleted patients receiving a large part of their nitrogen from human albumin administered intravenously. *J. Clin. Invest.* 27:560, 1948.

691. Wayne, D. J. Goodpasture's syndrome (pulmonary haemorrhage associated with glomerulonephritis). *Proc. Roy. Soc. Med.* 57:590, 1964.

692. Wegienka, L. C., Simpson, R. G., and Karam, J. H. Clinical experience with diazoxide. *Ann. N.Y. Acad. Sci.* 150:383, 1968.

693. Wegner, C. R. Nephrosis in pregnancy. *Amer. J. Obstet. Gynec.* 33:51, 1937.

694. Weinreb, M. S., Soules, H. K., and Wissler, R. W. Quantitative studies of acute nephrotoxic nephritis in rats. *Amer. J. Path.* 30:311, 1954.

695. Weissenbach, R. J., Martineau, J., Brocard, J., and Malinsky, A. Néphrose lipoïdique après chrysothérapie. *Bull. Mem. Soc. Med. Hop. Paris* 52:1076, 1936.

695a. Wermut, W. Paper electrophoresis of the proteins of cerebrospinal fluid in some renal diseases. *Pol. Med. J.* 5:62, 1966.

696. Werner, M. *Handbuch der Erbbiologie.* Berlin: Springer, 1942. P. 886.

697. Wesson, L. G. Glomerular and tubular factors in the renal excretion of sodium chloride. *Medicine* (Balt.) 36:281, 1957.

698. West, C. D. Cyclophosphamide therapy for nephrosis. *J. Pediat.* 73:641, 1968.

699. West, C. D., Holland, N. H., McConville, J. M., and McAdams, A. J. Immunosuppressive therapy in persistent hypocomplementemic glomerulonephritis and in lupus nephritis. *J. Pediat.* 67:1113, 1965.

700. West, C. D., Hong, R., and Holland, N. H. Effect of cyclophosphamide on lipoid nephrosis in the human and on aminonucleoside nephrosis in the rat. *J. Pediat.* 68:516, 1966.

701. West, C. D., and McAdams, A. J. Serum β_{1C} globulin levels in hypocomplementemic persistent glomerulonephritis: Variability unrelated to clinical course. *Nephron* 7:193, 1970.

702. West, D. C. Use of combined hormone and mechlorethamine (nitrogen mustard) therapy in lipoid nephrosis. *A.M.A. Amer. J. Dis. Child.* 95:498, 1958.

703. White, J. C. Nephrosis occurring during trimethadione therapy. *J.A.M.A.* 139:376, 1949.

704. White, R. H. Cytotoxic drug therapy in steroid-resistant glomerulonephritis. *Proc. Roy. Soc. Med.* 60:1164, 1967.

705. White, R. H., Cameron, J. S., and Trounce, J. R. Immunosuppressive therapy in steroid-resistant proliferative glomerulonephritis accompanied by the nephrotic syndrome. *Brit. Med. J.* 2:853, 1966.

706. Whittaker, M. Serum haptoglobin in the nephrotic syndrome: Other renal diseases and rheumatoid arthritis. *Amer. J. Clin. Path.* 50:454, 1968.

707. Wickes, I. G. Steroids and nephrotic syndrome. *Brit. Med. J.* 1:706, 1968.

708. Wilfert, C. M., and Katz, S. L. Etiology of bacterial sepsis in nephrotic children 1963–1967. *Pediatrics* 42:840, 1968.

709. Williams, K. S., and Ryan, T. J. Treatment of the nephrotic syndrome with concentrated serum albumin. *Lancet* 2:988, 1958.

710. Williams, N. E., and Bridge, H. G. The nephrotic syndrome after the application of mercury ointment. *Lancet* 2:602, 1958.

711. Wilson, I. D., Williams, R. C., Jr., and Tobian, L., Jr. Renal tubular acidosis: Three cases of immunoglobulin abnormalities in the patients and their kindreds. *Amer. J. Med.* 43:356, 1967.

712. Wilson, S., and Heymann, W. Work in Progress. In Metcoff, J. (Ed.), *Proceedings of the Ninth Annual Conference on the Nephrotic Syndrome.* New York: National Nephrosis Foundation, 1957. P. 213.

713. Wilson, S. G., Hackel, D. B., Horwood, S., Nash, G., and Heymann, W. Amino nucleoside nephrosis in rats. *Pediatrics* 21:963, 1958.

714. Wilson, S. G., and Heymann, W. Acute glomerulonephritis with the nephrotic syndrome. *Pediatrics* 23:874, 1959.

715. Wilson, S. G., Heymann, W., and Goldthwait, D. A. Studies on the mechanism of production of a nephrotic syndrome in

rats with a nucleoside. *Pediatrics* 25:228, 1960.

716. Winawer, S. J., and Feldman, S. M. Amyloid nephrosis in Hodgkin's disease. *A.M.A. Arch. Intern. Med.* 104:793, 1959.

717. Wolbach, S. B., and Blackfan, K. D. Clinical and pathological studies on so-called tubular nephritis (nephrosis). *Amer. J. Med. Sci.* 180:453, 1930.

718. Wolf, J., and Worker, B. Atypical amyloidosis and bone marrow plasmacytosis in a case of hypersensitivity to sulfonamides. *Amer. J. Med.* 16:746, 1954.

719. Wong, H. B. Treatment of childhood nephrotic syndrome with cytotoxic drugs. *J. Singapore Paediat. Soc.* 8:49, 1966.

720. Woolf, L. I., and Giles, H. M. Urinary excretion of aminoacids and sugar in the nephrotic syndrome: A chromatographic study. *Acta Paediat.* 45:489, 1956.

721. Worthen, H. G., Vernier, R. L., and Good, R. A. Infantile nephrosis: Clinical, biochemical and morphologic studies of the syndrome. *A.M.A. Amer. J. Dis. Child.* 98:731, 1959.

722. Wren, J. C., and Nutt, R. L. Nephrotic syndrome occurring during paramethadione therapy; report of case with clinical remission. *J.A.M.A.* 153:918, 1953.

723. Wright, A. D., Lowy, C., and Fraser, T. R. Serum-growth hormone and glucose intolerance in renal failure. *Lancet* 2:798, 1968.

724. Wright, W. T. Cell counts in urine. *A.M.A. Arch. Intern. Med.* 103:76, 1959.

725. Yamauchi, H., and Hopper, J., Jr. Hypovolemic shock and hypertension as a complication in the nephrotic syndrome. *Ann. Intern. Med.* 60:242, 1964.

726. Yoshida, T., Yamashita, F., and Metcoff, J. Metabolic basis of aminonucleoside nephrosis in rats: I. Inhibition of alpha-oxoglutarate oxidation by aminonucleoside. *J. Lab. Clin. Med.* 72:565, 1968.

727. Zosin, C., Manescu, N., and Schwarzkopf, A. Treatment of the nephrotic syndrome by an immunosuppressive medication. *Rom. Med. Rev.* 12:25, 1968.

728. Zuckerbrod, M., Rosenberg, B., and Kayden, H. J. Renal insufficiency and hypertension associated with secondary amyloidosis. *Amer. J. Med.* 21:227, 1956.

729. Zunin, C., and Soave, F. Association of nephrotic syndrome and nephroblastoma in siblings. *Ann. Pediat.* 203:29, 1964.

17

Acute Renal Failure

John P. Merrill

Acute failure of renal function is one of the most dramatic and important clinical problems with which the physician may be faced. Its importance stems in part from the fact that many patients with acute renal failure present the most severe clinical problems from which an individual may completely recover. Thus, both the severity and the reversibility of the situation demand attention.

Interest is stimulated also by our lack of ability to predict the onset of acute renal failure or to explain it when it does occur. It may follow major surgery, severe trauma or wounding, or it may be the sequel of hypotensive episodes mild enough to have gone unnoticed. It is a major problem in military medicine or in mass civilian catastrophes. In World War II, 40 per cent of one group of severely wounded patients developed acute post-traumatic renal insufficiency with a case fatality rate of 90 per cent among the severely oliguric [132]. Although in the conflict in Vietnam rapid evacuation of the wounded has reduced the incidence of acute renal failure, the mortality among those developing this complication has been about 50 per cent as it

has in the past. Acute renal failure was a frequent and grave complication of crushing injuries among the earthquake casualties at Agadir, Morocco [110]. In contrast, I have seen acute renal failure in a patient who walked into the hospital following the passage of a bloody stool at home.

Since it occurs so frequently in traumatized patients, the management of acute renal failure requires the skill not only of the nephrologist but of the physician well versed in general medicine and in surgical care. Optimally such care also requires considerable experience and common sense.

From the clinical standpoint it has seemed important to divide acute renal failure into three diagnostic categories: prerenal, renal, and postrenal. This division stresses the fact that only in the second category is there renal parenchymal damage adequate to cause in itself functional failure. By the same token it stresses the fact that prerenal and postrenal factors may be immediately remediable by specific procedures, whereas acute lesions of the renal parenchyma must heal spontaneously.

Obviously, prerenal factors such as hypotension, if severe or prolonged, may cause renal parenchymal damage, as may also postrenal factors such as obstruction of the lower urinary tract. However, since these two categories include situations in which the precipitating cause may be immediately remediable, it is convenient to include them in a separate category as "curable" renal failure. Damage to the kidney parenchyma, however, is not curable in the sense that the physician may specifically treat the lesion. The parenchymal lesion must heal by itself, and in this situation injudicious attempts to "force" the kidney to perform its urinary function may result in overhydration, pulmonary edema, and death. The stress laid upon this principle by Strauss [128] was undoubtedly responsible for the striking decrease in mortality in this syndrome in the past 20 years.

Treatable Causes of Renal Failure

Obstructive uropathy (calculi, etc.)
Pyelonephritis
Renal vascular disease
Renal allograft rejection reaction
Potassium depletion
Disorders of calcium metabolism
   Hyperparathyroidism
   Vitamin D intoxication
   Sarcoidosis
   "Milk-alkali" syndrome
Nephritis of bacterial endocarditis
"Lupus" nephritis
Methicillin "nephritis"
Membranous glomerulonephritis (nephrotic syndrome)
Gouty nephritis (?)
Myeloma kidney (?)
Circulatory insufficiency
   Water and electrolyte loss
   Whole blood or plasma loss
   Myocardial failure
   Vascular failure
Nephrotoxins
Intravascular hemolysis

The causes of acute renal failure are numerous and no real purpose is served by simply documenting the variety of clinical situations and toxins that have been reported to precipitate this syndrome. In general, two broad groups may be delineated. In the first are the many situations associated with vasomotor collapse and hypotension with resultant ischemia of renal tissue. The second is the group caused by the ingestion or inhalation of substances toxic to the renal parenchyma. The multiplicity of events included under the first heading, however, simply stresses our inability to pinpoint the causes of all cases. It is the experience of those who have dealt most with acute renal failure that 30 per cent or more of the cases cannot be attributed to any single causative agent [87, 136]. Two factors are probably responsible for this difficulty. The first is the fact that different patients, or even the same patient at a different time, may respond differently to the same insult. Secondly, it is the response of the renal vasculature which determines the renal lesion, and renal blood flow or perfusion is not always faithfully reflected by the status of the peripheral circulation.

Prerenal Failure

Inadequate maintenance of the circulation is frequently attended by renal ischemia. When this ischemia is severe enough to cause necrosis, organic lesions of the renal parenchyma occur. Decreases in renal blood flow and filtration rate of lesser degree may result in minimal or no renal parenchymal changes. They may, however, be associated with profound changes in urine volume and the excretion of solute which precede and mimic the consequences of lesions of the renal parenchyma. For want of a better term these nonparenchymal changes have been grouped under the heading *prerenal failure*.

The importance of this category lies in the

fact that such renal circulatory changes may be reversible before renal parenchymal damage occurs. The dependence of changes in the renal circulation upon changes in the general systemic circulation implies that prevention of cardiovascular insufficiency is a necessary component in the prophylaxis and treatment of acute renal failure. The extrarenal influences that modify renal function have been well studied — an exhaustive review of literature up to 1957 was published by Homer Smith [126] — and elsewhere in this volume they are discussed in relation to normal physiology. Therefore, in what follows they are described only insofar as an understanding of them is necessary for the diagnosis and treatment of prerenal failure.

The normal kidney receives some 20 to 25 per cent of the cardiac output. When the cardiac output decreases or when the blood or extracellular fluid volume is diminished by external loss or sequestration in the body, changes occur in the volume and concentration of the urine, the excretion of solute, and the renal circulation. These events have important consequences for the understanding of acute renal failure. Marked decreases in cardiac output, loss of blood, and dehydration are frequent precursors of acute renal failure. They may, however, result in modification of the volume and composition of the urine which may simulate changes secondary to destruction of renal parenchyma but which are completely reversible when the primary circulatory disorder has been corrected. With mild to moderate insults, urine volume may decrease and the urine become concentrated, possibly as the result of stimulation of secretion of the antidiuretic hormone. Experimental constriction of the renal artery with decreases in filtration rate which do not exceed 30 per cent cause marked decrease in urine volume with increase in urine concentration even in the absence of antidiuretic hormone [11]. Further decrease in filtration rate, however, then results in decreasing urine concentration

even in the presence of maximal antidiuretic hormone. In normal man, decreases in blood pressure following the use of ganglionic blocking agents may also result in decreased urine volume and increased urine concentration in the absence of antidiuretic hormone [60]. During acute and prolonged arterial hypotension marked redistribution of intrarenal blood flow occurs. The cortical flow fraction decreases from 80 per cent to about 10 per cent of total renal blood flow, while the corticomedullary fraction increases from 14 to 80 per cent. In initial stages this may be reversible, but the type of redistribution is also characteristic of persisting anuria [135]. These changes have their counterparts in clinical medicine under conditions of hypotension and blood loss. Teleologically, renal vasoconstriction under these circumstances may be thought of in terms of a shunt of blood from the kidney to more vital organs such as the brain. In this fashion, arterial pressure and central nervous system blood flow may be maintained at the expense of renal blood flow [69].

The effects of major surgical procedures, anesthesia, and trauma in stimulating secretion of antidiuretic hormone as well as causing a decrease in filtration rate and renal blood flow have been extensively studied [34, 101, 118]. Stimulation of antidiuretic hormone secretion following surgery or trauma would then result in increased urinary concentration with a decreased volume of urine, while decreases in filtration rate of more than 30 per cent might result similarly in decreased volume of urine and decreased concentration. The careful studies of Gullick and Raisz [49] have shown that renal concentrating ability may be markedly impaired during surgery and that this impairment may be transient, without evidence of frank renal parenchymal damage. In their studies, the impairment of concentrating ability was accompanied by parallel changes in filtration rate (creatinine clearance). Unfortunately, these authors give no data on the urine sediment, and renal biopsy was not done, so that it is not possible to exclude clinically insignificant degrees of parenchymal damage. Furthermore, as the authors themselves point out, the low protein intake and the tendency of these patients to retain water may both have contributed to the decrease in concentrating ability. It is quite possible, however, that their explanation is correct, since the fact remains that it is possible to impair concentrating ability by decreasing filtration rate in the absence of damage to the renal parenchyma. Furthermore, there is experimental evidence [101] which suggests that the renal blood flow must drop to less than 5 per cent before renal parenchymal damage (as evidenced by decreased extraction of para-aminohippuric acid) occurs.

Thus, under several circumstances, a decrease in urine volume and in solute excretion may occur which may mimic the oliguria of renal failure. Decreased excretion of urea may result in a rise of blood urea nitrogen, which may be accentuated by the increased protein breakdown attendant upon tissue necrosis or the accentuated catabolic response to surgery or trauma [89]. A decrease in the volume of urine and increase in its total solute concentration (osmolality) but with a decreased sodium concentration may be produced by constriction of the renal artery which is mild enough to produce little or no demonstrable drop in filtration rate [90]. These findings in a patient suggest prerenal failure without parenchymal damage.

Several authors have emphasized the value of the urinary sodium concentration and have suggested that the ability to produce urine with low sodium concentrations is inconsistent with the presence of continuing renal parenchymal damage. Conversely, they believe that in urines of low volume, sodium concentrations of 70 to 120 mEq. per liter presuppose renal damage [22, 47, 84]. In the studies of Gullick and Raisz, however, there was little correlation between urine sodium concentra-

tion and urine osmolality. It has also been suggested that the ratio of urinary sodium to potassium may be more accurate than sodium concentration alone in differentiating prerenal from renal failure. In one series of patients [84] with established acute renal failure, the ratio of urinary sodium to potassium was highest during the first few days of oliguria and fell steadily thereafter until the onset of diuresis. Exceptions to this, however, have been noted [99] in renal failure secondary to burns [47], diabetic coma [56], and transfusion reactions [98]. Furthermore, as suggested in the cases reported by Gullick and Raisz, the influence of previous hydration and of solute intake upon urine volume and concentration may also modify its significance. Oliguria can occur in individuals with normal renal function purely as a result of water restriction. Such individuals without impairment of renal function may elaborate only 400 ml. of urine per day with a specific gravity of 1.030 and an osmolality of 1200 mOsm per kilogram. Drastic restriction of dietary protein and sodium such as is common in management of the immediate postoperative period may so reduce the amount of solute (urea and sodium) which requires excretion that even further diminution of urine volume may occur [44]. Under such circumstances, persons with intact renal function may, in the absence of increased protein catabolism, excrete all their endogenous solute in a volume of 400 to 500 ml. per day with a urine specific gravity as low as 1.014 or 1.016.

On the other hand, the blood urea nitrogen level may rise as a result of increased protein catabolism or intake even in the presence of normal renal function. This fact was pointed out many years ago by Addis [2], who documented marked rises in blood urea nitrogen in normal young men whose protein intake was doubled. Since the adequacy of renal function is not reflected by the plasma level of urea alone but by its clearance, it has been suggested by Perlmutter et al. [99] that the ratio of urinary urea to plasma concentration may be of help in "differentiating the azotemia or oliguria of renal disease (U urea/ P urea < 10) from that of dehydration or that of inadequate blood flow." Since the accurate assessment of renal function by the clearance of substances excreted by glomerular filtration or tubular secretion depends upon adequate urine flow, these methods are of little value in borderline cases with marked oliguria. Significant glycosuria is rare in acute renal failure.

Postrenal Failure

The category of postrenal failure comprises only a small group of disorders. Nevertheless it is an important group because it is constituted largely of those cases in which urinary suppression is due to obstruction of the urinary tract, and in such cases it is imperative that the diagnosis be made at once so that relief of the specific obstruction may be effected. There are a number of diagnostic clues.

Total anuria is rare in acute renal failure due to parenchymal damage or to prerenal causes. Daily urine volumes of 75 to 300 ml. are the rule, although this may not be apparent when, in the absence of an inlying bladder catheter, complete emptying of the bladder is not obtained or when collection periods overlap. If, however, total anuria is truly present, the diagnosis is much more likely to be obstruction of the urinary tract, massive vascular accidents to the kidney, or acute glomerulonephritis. A history that is characteristic for obstructive uropathy is total anuria followed by 24 hours or more of polyuria and a sudden return to anuria. Although such a history is rarely obtained, it is important since it is diagnostic of obstruction, but it may be confusing to the inexperienced observer. Obstruction of a single ureter in the presence of two previously normal kidneys usually does not result in anuria. However, calculous disease of the kidney is frequently multiple, and if the contralateral kidney has previously been destroyed by obstruction or infection, sudden obstruction of the remaining kidney may give total anuria.

Renal colic or flank pain preceding anuria may be a valuable clue when present, but it is frequently absent in total obstruction. Pain in the costovertebral angle may be present with other forms of acute renal involvement. Edema of the ureters due to acute infection, particularly superimposed upon chronic disease, may be severe enough to cause obstruction of one or both ureters. Anuria following retrograde pyelography or catheterization of the ureters has been ascribed by Sirota and Narins [123] to edema and obstruction of the ureterovesical orifice rather than to "reflex" vasoconstriction secondary to manipulation of the ureters. However, temporary cessation of function of one kidney following the passage of a stone has recently been documented [95]. Prostatic hypertrophy may result in an apparent sudden onset of anuria. Here the diagnosis is made by a careful history of previous symptoms and the finding of a large distended bladder.

The use of ganglionic blocking agents which decrease bladder tone or of antihistaminics which act in much the same way may precipitate acute urinary retention in persons who have been previously compensated. Obstruction of the ureters due to the deposition of sulfonamide crystals is now rarely seen but may occur in patients receiving large doses of sulfadiazine under conditions of severe dehydration. The deposition of uric acid crystals may cause obstruction of the collecting system in dehydrated patients following the use of one of the uricosuric agents for the treatment of gout. The use of radiation or of the alkylating agents in the treatment of leukemia or

Hodgkin's disease may also result in precipitation of uric acid crystals in amounts sufficient to cause obstruction when alkalinization of the urine and adequate urine volume have not been maintained [62, 70, 111].

In chronic renal failure acute obstruction due to uric acid crystals is unusual because of the patient's inability to produce a concentrated urine. In such instances preexisting uric acid nephropathy due to the interstitial lesion or the vascular lesion, plus the superimposed dehydration, is a more likely cause. It has been reported that obstructive uropathy due to sulfonamide or uric acid crystals may respond to lavage of the renal pelves with warm bicarbonate solutions. Obstructive uropathy due to ligation of the ureters in the course of pelvic surgery or to retroperitoneal hematomas angulating and obstructing the ureter should also be ruled out when acute renal failure presents in individuals with previous pelvic surgery. This complication may occasionally be seen in patients on chronic anticoagulant therapy.

DIAGNOSIS

The diagnosis of obstructive uropathy can be made only by ascertaining the patency of the urinary tract. Since injudicious investigations of the upper urinary tract by bilateral catheterization of the ureters is unwise, careful consideration should be given to the diagnosis before undertaking this procedure. Frequently, however, it is impossible to rule it out without the help of cystoscopy. In such cases we have proceeded as follows:

A plain x-ray film of the abdomen is obtained. If two normal-sized or enlarged kidneys are visualized and the history is suggestive of obstructive uropathy, the ureter on one side only is carefully catheterized to the renal pelvis. No contrast material should be injected. If no urine is obtained from the normal-sized kidney, obstructive uropathy can be presumed not to be the basis of acute renal failure. If total anuria is due solely to obstruc-

tion, urine should be elaborated from a kidney of normal size regardless of the state of the contralateral kidney. Frequently, however, the perirenal fat line which outlines the kidney in the x-ray film may be obscured by edema and it is not possible adequately to visualize the renal mass. It should be remembered that occasionally when the ureter is edematous the catheter may act as a splint and while in place may allow adequate urine flow from the renal pelvis. When it is removed, obstruction may reoccur. For this reason, the ureteral catheter must be left in place until inflammation and edema have subsided and until adequate urine flow can be obtained without it. Occasionally following trauma to a solitary kidney, obstruction of the ureter by blood clot may result in acute renal failure. In at least one instance this markedly enlarged and traumatized kidney has been removed by the surgeon without regard for the significance of total anuria following damage to a single kidney.

Renal Failure

The most common and characteristic form of acute renal failure is that due to damage to renal parenchyma. The classic publication by Oliver et al. [92] gives a detailed description of this lesion based on preparations in which the entire nephron was separated by microdissection. Two main categories of lesion were described by Oliver and his associates, the ischemic and the nephrotoxic, with some overlap between them. With a few exceptions, this remains the major division.

The studies of Oliver et al. suggested that the parenchymal lesion produced by the ingestion or inhalation of a nephrotoxic agent was a uniform necrosis of the epithelium of the renal tubules down to, but not including, the basement membrane. With ischemia alone, the basement membrane might be fragmented and ruptured, with complete disintegration of the tubular structure and leakage of the tubular contents into the renal interstitium. This latter lesion the authors called tubulorrhexis. Lucké [78], who had described the ischemic lesion earlier, believed that it occurred largely in the distal portion of the nephron; he therefore named the syndrome resulting from the ischemic lesion "lower nephron nephrosis." The studies of Oliver et al., however, showed that this appellation was inappropriate since the lesion could and did occur in any part of the nephron. Oliver and others have emphasized the patchy nature of the lesion, pointing out that damaged areas were interspersed with areas in which tubular epithelium appeared quite normal. Grossly the kidneys were enlarged and swollen, with a tense capsule and parenchyma which bulged through the cut surface of the capsule. The cortex appeared pale and the medullary area congested, suggesting the presence of marked interstitial edema. Edema of the renal interstitium is frequently present in microscopic sections taken from postmortem material. Renal biopsies during life have been inconsistent in this regard, however. Some authors have found interstitial edema [57], while others have noted its absence [58].

The presence or absence of interstitial edema is a critical point upon which hinge many of the arguments about the etiology of the oliguria in acute renal failure. The studies of Oliver et al. revealed that healing of the lesion occurred with resorption of the interstitial edema and repair of the tubular epithelium. In the healing process, epithelial cells grew along the intact basement membrane to reestablish tubular integrity. Where disruption of the basement membrane had occurred, however, lack of a continuous supporting structure resulted in failure of reepithelialization of the tubular lining. In some instances growth of connective tissue into the tubular lumen through the rupture in the basement membrane also prevented the reestablishment of tubular integrity. Oliver et al. pointed out that the nephrotoxic lesion and

the ischemic lesion were not completely separable since in many of the kidneys damaged by nephrotoxins the lesions typical of ischemia might also occur.

Although in Oliver's studies the glomeruli were typically uninvolved, other authors studying both postmortem material and biopsy specimens [104, 119] have found glomerular involvement varying from hyalinization of glomeruli to periglomerular fibrosis. These changes were visualized by Price and Palmer [104] in both the ischemic and the nephrotoxic lesion and were present in individuals in whom biopsies were done months after apparent recovery from the episode of acute renal failure. In their follow-up material, tubular atrophy and interstitial fibrosis were also seen in the typical patchy distribution.

Since the blood supply to the renal tubules comes by way of the glomerulus, it seems reasonable that decrease in renal blood flow should first involve the postglomerular tissue, i.e., the tubules. Because the areas involved may alternate with uninvolved areas, recovery of a large degree of renal function may be possible even with total disruption of some of the affected nephrons. Involvement of the glomeruli in such a fashion as to produce hyalinization or periglomerular fibrosis is quite possible with severe and prolonged disruption . of blood supply to the nephron. Occlusion of nonischemic tubules by interstitial edema may also result in some degree of glomerular damage. When thrombosis of the afferent arteriole occurs (as in the lesion of postpartum cortical necrosis), the glomerulus becomes infarcted and destroyed, as does the entire nephron. Even in cortical necrosis, however, the patchy nature of the lesion may be consistent with survival of the patient [15] when resorption of edema and healing of the adjacent uninfarcted tissue takes place. When the vascular lesion is sufficiently severe so that all of the glomeruli are involved, the renal cortices are involved in a diffuse or symmetrical type of lesion in which the entire cortex is infarcted. This is "symmetrical cortical necrosis." The ultimate step in renal ischemia is, of course, obstruction of the renal artery, in which the entire kidney is infarcted. In this unified and perhaps over-simplified view, the entire spectrum of acute renal failure from prerenal failure to total infarction of the kidney is explicable upon the extent and duration of the renal ischemia.

NEPHROTOXIC RENAL FAILURE

The following toxins have been reported to cause acute renal failure:

Arsenic	Carbon tetrachloride
Bismuth	Chloroform
Cadmium	Methyl alcohol
Chromium	Phenol
Gold	Toluene
Lead	
Mercuric chloride	Mephenesin
Uranium	Phenurone
	Quinine
Phosphorus	Versene
Methicillin*	
Colistimethate	
Neomycin	(Di) Ethylene glycol
Polymyxin	Oxalic acid
Sulfonamides	
Cephaloridine	Potassium chlorate
Cantharides	
	Pesticides
Poisonous mushrooms	

Of these nephrotoxins, the most important are carbon tetrachloride, ethylene glycol, and mercuric chloride [30, 48, 74, 136]. The inhalation

---

* Methicillin and the sulfonamides may cause acute renal failure either through hypersensitivity to the drug or, less commonly with the sulfonamides, through obstruction due to crystal precipitation. Ethyl alcohol ingestion is also associated with acute renal failure, but its exact causative role is as yet unclear. Many of the pesticides contain phosphorus or arsenic or lead, and this may be the essential ingredient necessary for their nephrotoxicity.

of trichlorethylene has also been reported to cause acute renal failure. The diagnosis when any of these substances is the culprit may be unsuspected when the patient is first seen.

The presence of carbon tetrachloride in various solvents for the removal of grease may be unknown to the patient. Characteristically, the onset of oliguria following the inhalation of carbon tetrachloride may be insidious and may be apparent only two or even three days after actual exposure. The marked potentiation of its toxicity by the concomitant ingestion of alcohol is a well-established fact. Since exposure to the toxin may occur while the patient is inebriated, the history may be further confused. The presence of abdominal pain and jaundice may simulate an acute surgical condition. Because of the insidious onset of the renal failure, ingestion of salt and fluid may continue in the absence of their excretion, and some persons may present with a complaint of acute pulmonary edema. Red cells and even red-cell casts may be found in the urine of these patients, and the differential diagnosis between carbon tetrachloride intoxication and acute glomerulonephritis may be difficult.

Ethylene glycol, a constituent of antifreeze, may be ingested during alcoholic bouts or by mistake from unlabeled bottles. It is metabolized to oxalic acid, and crystals of calcium oxalate may be found in the kidney and in the brain. When large amounts are ingested, central nervous system manifestations and pulmonary symptoms may dominate the picture, and death from involvement of these systems may occur in the first few days. Or prolonged renal failure may result, with a degree of permanent renal damage greater than is seen in the pure ischemic lesion. One of our patients recovered after 31 days of marked oliguria, but had permanent and severe renal involvement due to the fibrosis of the interstitial lesions caused by the oxalate crystals as well as to the tubular degeneration.

The renal lesion produced by bichloride of

mercury is encountered chiefly in persons who have attempted suicide. For this reason, the history may be difficult to obtain, but the marked gastrointestinal symptoms and bleeding may be a clue to the diagnosis. The renal lesion occurs predominantly in the proximal tubule and recovery may take place if the lesions are not extensive. It has been my experience that permanent renal damage of a more severe nature is apt to follow acute renal failure due to bichloride of mercury poisoning. Renal calcification has been seen with some frequency in this syndrome. The use of Versene in the treatment of heavy metal poisoning may cause acute renal damage with failure [108].

MECHANISM OF ISCHEMIC
RENAL FAILURE

We know that the majority of cases of acute renal failure result from renal ischemia, but the complex mechanism by which this ischemia leads to renal damage is poorly understood. Where it has been measured in man, renal blood flow has been found to be decreased to 20 or 30 per cent of a normal value [22, 53]. Surprisingly, however, reduction of renal blood flow to these values is consistent with the elaboration of large volumes of urine in patients with chronic renal failure. It is on the discrepancy between this amount of renal blood flow and the virtual absence of urine formation in acute renal failure that the present controversy concerning the mechanism of oliguria hinges. It is of interest to return to the older work of Trueta and his associates [134] which was thought for many years to have little application to the problem of human renal failure. Trueta et al., working with rabbits, noticed that stimulation of the sciatic nerve and nerve endings in the splanchnic area caused a deviation in renal blood flow from the cortex to the medulla and suggested that bypassing of cortical glomeruli by diversion through the juxtamedullary glomeruli might explain the failure of urine formation in spite of continuation of some renal blood flow. An increase in the resistance of the cortical vasculature upon stimulation of nerves supplying this area was thought to account for the "bypassing" of cortical nephrons. Failure to perfuse these cortical nephrons would result in failure of urine formation in spite of considerable residual blood flow through the corticomedullary area.

Much support is available for the suggestion that the initiating factor in renal ischemia is an increase in renal vascular resistance [103, 118, 137], and evidence is available from dog experiments to support the role of nervous stimulation in producing this increase in renal resistance and decrease in renal blood flow. It has been shown [103] that renal damage following cross clamping of the abdominal aorta could be prevented by prior denervation of the kidney or ganglionic blockade. Other authors have similarly shown that renal vasoconstriction in the dog could be prevented by sectioning the spinal cord at the first lumbar segment and suggest that neurogenic stimuli at least initiate the fall in renal blood flow [131]. Although many observers have found decreases in renal blood flow with the stimulation of renal nerves [13, 129] and even through "venorenal reflexes" activated during manipulation of the renal pedicle, the inferior vena cava, and the femoral vessels [41, 42], the magnitude of the stimulation necessary to produce the ischemic lesion has not been defined. Recent work, however, indicates that mild renal nerve stimulation, which may not alter renal blood flow, decreases perfusion of the outer cortical peritubular capillaries and increases that of the outer medulla [102]. This sequence of events — i.e., medullary diversion of cortical blood, patchy cortical ischemia, and redistribution of blood to parts of the unaffected cortex — would be entirely consistent with the observations of many observers that renal blood flow continues, albeit at a markedly decreased rate [19, 22, 121].

As early as 1929 Richards [109], observing directly the kidney of the frog poisoned with mercury, reported that active filtration occurred in spite of the virtual absence of urine formation. In a more recent study Sims et al. [120], using a fluorescent dye to stain glomeruli in rats whose kidneys had been damaged by mercuric chloride, showed staining of many glomeruli under conditions of severe suppression of urine formation. The implication was that these glomeruli were continuing to function.

If it is agreed that renal blood flow and glomerular filtration continue at rates which in chronic renal failure should provide adequate volumes of urine, one is faced with the problem of accounting for the fate of the filtrate in the condition of acute renal failure with oliguria. Some observers hold that the filtrate disappears by nonselective back diffusion through damaged tubules whose structural integrity may be represented only by basement membrane. Attempts have been made to substantiate this suggestion by showing that molecules of different size and configuration normally cleared at the same rate may be cleared at different ratios in the various stages of acute renal failure [46, 80]. The evidence, however, is conflicting [22, 24]. Oliver's microdissections suggest that gross rents in the basement membrane might permit the back diffusion of filtrate, and occlusion of the tubule distal to the "leak" by casts might abet escape of the filtrate into the interstitium by this means. Edema secondary to ischemia and to leaks of this sort might account for the grossly swollen kidney seen at autopsy.

This sequence of events, however, still provides no explanation for continuing filtration and lack of urine formation. Some continuous means of removing filtrate from the renal interstitium even in the grossly edematous kidney must be postulated. The possibility that filtrate might be returned to the renal venous blood by way of the renal lymphatics has been raised by several authors [45, 125]. The only direct experiment on this of which I am aware was published only in abstract form by LeBrie and Meyerson [71]. In these experiments acute renal failure was induced by the subcutaneous injection of uranium nitrate. Renal capsular lymphatics were cannulated two to seven days after the injection, and lymph flow measured. The average flow was almost 15 times greater in the "nephrotic" animals than in the controls. Direct observations such as this are badly needed to investigate this logical hypothesis. It is possible to calculate indirectly that the difference between directly measured blood flows and urine volumes in acute renal failure may be accounted for by renal lymph flow [21].

Role of Interstitial Edema. A second controversial problem revolves around the role of edema in the production of acute renal failure. Edema in the kidney, as elsewhere in the body, results from ischemia and necrosis. Iversen and Brun [57] found interstitial edema in biopsy material obtained early in the course of acute renal failure. However, in view of the patchy nature of the lesion, it is not surprising that much other biopsy material, including my own specimens, has shown remarkably little abnormality early in the disorder.

De Wardener [29] found no striking increase in renal interstitial pressure by direct measurement in dogs with experimental acute renal failure; and the determination of the "wedged renal venous pressure" (analogous to the "wedged pulmonary capillary pressure") was interpreted as not indicating an increase in renal interstitial pressure in human acute renal failure by Brun et al. [18]. However, the validity of the technics is questionable, and there is a wide variance in the results of others investigating normal renal interstitial pressure.

Since the nephron population is believed to be heterogeneous rather than homogeneous [16], it is unlikely that interstitial edema would affect all nephrons equally. An increase in interstitial pressure might then decrease GFR in some nephrons before others and could well result in the observed patchy lesion. A rise in interstitial and intratubular pressure, whether or not accompanied by plugging with casts, would produce increased back pressure and thus a decrease in overall filtration rate. Similarly the effect of increased pressure on the peritubular capillaries would cause a decrease in renal blood flow. Further support is derived from the work of Hinshaw et al. [51], which suggests that the effective driving force for blood flow is the difference between the renal arterial and the tissue pressure. Thus, other things being equal, an increase in tissue pressure such as might occur with edema would diminish renal blood flow.

If renal edema were the cause of the oliguria, removal of the restricting capsule might be expected to bring about improvement. However, this has not proved to be the case [87]. Favorable results from this procedure reported earlier probably do not represent a cause-and-effect relationship, because "in a condition like acute anuria which is so dramatic for both patient and doctor, human patience with regard to desisting from interference seems to last about as long as the oliguric state of the disease [17].

The most significant additions to our knowledge of the pathophysiology of acute renal failure have come from carefully conceived experiments in animals. Micropuncture studies have systematically been applied by Oken and his associates to the pathophysiologic events leading to acute renal failure in laboratory animals [38, 91, 133, 140, 141]. These workers have shown that the oliguria and azotemia of both mercury-induced and hemoglobinuric acute renal failure in the rat is due to a primary decrease or cessation of glomerular filtration in individual nephrons. This abrupt attenuation of filtration was shown not to be the result of obstruction to urine outflow, as had been proposed, or to passive backflow of glomerular filtrate. Although there are data

discordant from these findings [5, 92], essentially the same conclusions have been reached by others using micropuncture methodology [7, 50, 114]. On critical evaluation, the experimental findings might be summarized as follows: Experimental acute renal failure is due primarily to a functional failure of glomerular filtration, presumably on the basis of afferent arteriolar constriction. This can and does occur in the absence of any sign of either obstruction or abnormal tubular permeability. (Most workers agree that the lesion is a patchy one and stress the role of the renin-angiotensin mechanism in effecting preglomerular constriction and decreased filtration rate.)

It is quite possible under certain experimental conditions, even in man, that back-diffusion of filtrate as well as obstruction of tubules by debris composed of necrotic tubular cells may contribute to the oliguria as a second note of phenomenon. Biber et al. [12] have reported a careful study of acute renal damage in rats secondary to injection of potassium dichromate and mercuric chloride. In these animals evidence from micropuncture studies was correlated with anatomic evidence from microdissection of the damaged nephrons. This group found evidence both for back-diffusion and for tubular obstruction and concluded that "it is apparent from the findings in the much simpler experimental situation, such as here described, that the phenomena of pathologic disturbances in the kidney do not have a cause but are rather the result of a constellation of factors which can vary in its constitution and in its effect." This seems a rational point of view, but in my opinion the bulk of the evidence would assign the *primary role* to failure of glomerular filtration, tubular ischemia, and tubular damage, the secondary result being back-diffusion of filtrate and obstruction of tubules in which filtration rate was lowered and tubular fluid flow decreased by the detritus of necrotic tubular cells. Further suggestive evidence for the primary role of renal hemodynamic change in the genesis

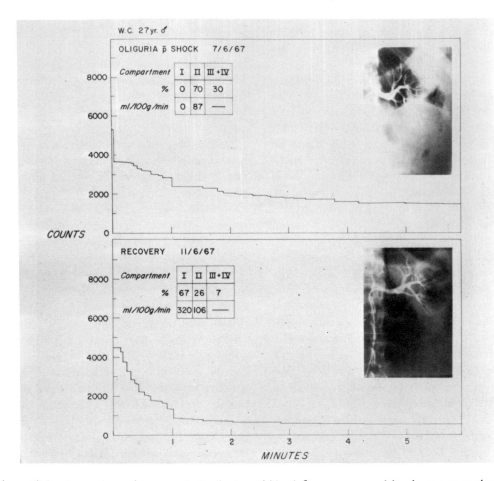

Figure 17-1. Comparison of intrarenal distribution of blood flow as measured by the xenon washout technique and selective renal arteriogram in a patient with oliguria following shock (left) and in a normal human subject given epinephrine directly into the renal artery (right). To be compared are the period during oliguria in the patient, and in the normal individual the period 10 seconds after epinephrine. It will be seen that in both instances blood flow to the cortical area (compartment I) is virtually absent. There is a relative increase in the flow through the corticomedullary area (compartment II). The angiogram shows virtual absence of the small cortical vessels both during epinephrine infusion and during the oliguric period. The control in the upper right-hand portion of the diagram shows normal distribution of blood flow with good filling of the cortical branches and in the lower left portion. Following recovery from oliguria, blood flow has returned to compartment I, and there is improved visualization of the smaller cortical vessels. The similarity between pharmacologically induced cortical vasoconstriction and that occurring following shock with resultant oliguria is striking [53].

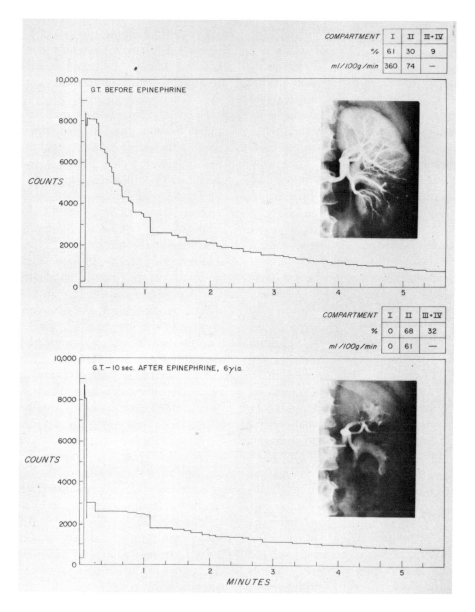

COMPARTMENT	I	II	III+IV
%	61	30	9
ml/100g/min	360	74	—

G.T. BEFORE EPINEPHRINE

COMPARTMENT	I	II	III+IV
%	0	68	32
ml/100g/min	0	61	—

G.T. — 10 sec. AFTER EPINEPHRINE, 6γi.a.

COUNTS

MINUTES

of acute renal failure in man is shown in Figure 17-1.

Although one might question whether such conclusions derived from experiments in the rat may be extrapolated to human disease, Hollenberg and his colleagues [53] have come to similar conclusions in a study of oliguric renal failure of different etiologies in 20 patients. Renal blood flow and its distribution was studied by the xenon washout technique and correlated with observations made by selective renal arteriography and by biopsy and autopsy material. In acute renal failure in five patients who had acute oliguric renal failure secondary to shock, trauma, sepsis, surgery, or nephrotoxins cortical blood flow was grossly decreased and angiography showed lack of filling of the vasculature distal of the arcuate and subarcuate arteries in the renal cortex. Total renal blood flow, however, was about one-third of normal. In contrast to the observations of Trueta, the transit time of the contrast medium through the kidney was prolonged. These results in man are consistent with the micropuncture results and suggest preferential renal cortical ischemia. Edema assessed by stretching and straightening of renal vessels and from renal size was present to a variable degree in 14 of the 20 oliguric cases studied. It was clearly absent in the others, however, and renal size correlated poorly with the degree of hemodynamic abnormality present. The kidney of one patient studied was 3 cm. shorter during the oliguric stage than during recovery. The emphasis on the hemodynamic contribution to acute renal failure from these human studies as well as from the micropuncture work suggests that "acute tubular necrosis" is inadequate as a descriptive term for the basic abnormality in acute renal failure.

DIFFERENTIAL DIAGNOSIS

The consequences and the management of renal failure per se are discussed elsewhere in this volume; hence, only those points specifically relevant to acute renal failure are dealt with here. The clinical course and its management are discussed together, so that therapeutic principles may be noted in context with the complications for which they are intended. The etiology of acute renal failure is so manifold and so poorly defined that little is to be gained by presenting a tabulation of all the factors which have been reported to be causative. However, a few pertinent observations can be made which may be useful from the clinical point of view.

The diagnosis of acute renal failure due to inhalation of *carbon tetrachloride* may be confused by the almost imperceptible onset of oliguria in this syndrome. The decrease in urine volume occurs gradually over a period of days, and because it may go unnoticed by the patient, the diagnosis of acute glomerulonephritis may be made. In addition, the association of abdominal pain, pulmonary edema, and hematuria with nausea and vomiting may further resemble nephritis. The presence of red blood cell casts is common both in acute glomerulonephritis and in carbon tetrachloride poisoning and rare in other forms of nephrotoxic lesions. Abdominal symptoms in both may frequently simulate an acute surgical emergency.

Acute renal failure following the use of distilled water as irrigating fluid during the *transurethral resection* of prostatic tissue was formerly a common problem. It is rarely seen today since the use of osmotically active nonelectrolytes in the irrigating fluid has been instituted.

Bichloride of mercury poisoning is frequently accompanied by severe bloody diarrhea and oral lesions. The reluctance of the patient to give a history of ingesting the toxin may further obscure the picture. Invasion of the bloodstream by *Clostridium welchii* in *septic abortions* characteristically produces hemoglobinemia with severe myalgia and high fever. Here again, denial by the patient of any attempts at instrumentation of the uterus is typical.

The intravenous injection of contrast material in the course of an *intravenous pyelogram* has occasionally been thought to be associated causally with acute renal failure. In my experience this has never been well documented, and frequently renal failure was already present at the time the dye was given. One exception to this, however, appears to be the presence of renal involvement by *multiple myeloma*. In this situation acute renal failure has been reliably reported to follow performance of an intravenous pyelogram [97]. Other authors, however, believe that intravenous pyelography per se is not hazardous but that deterioration of function is simply the result of the fluid restriction and dehydration preparatory to the procedure.

Renal medullary necrosis is secondary to acute overwhelming interstitial bacterial nephritis and occurs most frequently in elderly diabetic patients with preexisting urinary tract infections. It may occur, however, under any circumstances [68]. It has been reported in infants following replacement transfusion [79].

Although the so-called "ring sign," in which the medullary tip has been separated by calcification, may point to a preexisting acute inflammation, the roentgenologic diagnosis of the acute stage is not specific. Pathognomonic, but rarely seen, is the finding in the urine of the sloughed tip of a renal papilla. Excessive use of analgesics, notably phenacetin, may be associated with necrosis of renal papilla although this lesion does not usually present as acute renal failure unless severe infection is superimposed.

Paroxysmal myoglobinuria is occasionally associated with acute renal failure [107], and it has been reported in *sickle-cell crisis* [116]. *Acute glomerulonephritis, embolization* of the renal arteries, and *diffuse renal vasculitis* in polyarteritis and disseminated lupus erythematosus may all cause acute renal failure (see page 839) which may resemble that of tubular necrosis. The finding of red blood cell casts

suggests the former, as does the presence of total anuria, because total anuria for more than 48 hours is rare in tubular necrosis. When total anuria of more than two weeks is present, a renal biopsy should be made to ascertain the diagnosis, since glomerular involvement resulting in total anuria of more than two weeks rarely issues in recovery when it occurs in the adult. A history of total anuria with red-cell casts occurring after the administration of *sulfonamides* strongly suggests vasculitis. Steroid therapy has been of little help in these cases. Although the so-called *hepatorenal syndrome* is frequently only a chance association of hepatic and renal disease, renal hemodynamics may be disturbed specifically as a result of hepatic disease [94]. In any case, the association of severe liver disease with acute renal failure appears occasionally to be more than fortuitous, and in many instances the prognosis seems to be worse than in uncomplicated renal failure. Progressive renal failure in patients with cirrhosis of the liver may be due to a decrease in cortical blood flow; a marked and irregular renal vasoconstriction demonstrated by arteriography, which appears not to be present at autopsy, suggests that it is largely functional [35]. Acute hemorrhagic *pancreatitis* is frequently associated with acute renal failure. In large part this appears to be due to the shock frequently associated with pancreatitis, although the liberation of pancreatic enzymes into the circulating bloodstream has also been implicated.

Clinical Course and Treatment

Several extensive reviews of the clinical course and therapy of acute renal failure have appeared [17, 40, 86, 87, 130]. The authors are well agreed on most aspects of the clinical course and the principles of management. The discussion which follows summarizes their views.

The first concern of the physician must be

for the aspects of acute renal failure which may be specifically remediable. The diagnosis and management of obstructive lesions have already been discussed. Prompt and effective restoration of blood, plasma, and extracellular fluid volume must be accomplished whether or not renal parenchymal damage has already occurred. When electrolyte and water losses have progressed to the point of hypotension, blood volume expanders must be used to raise the blood pressure before the infusion of sodium salts and water can be effective.

Acute renal failure following a variety of insults may be manifest not by oliguria but by polyuria. Progressive azotemia may occur with volumes of urine greater than 1500 ml. per 24 hours [138]. The management of such patients is somewhat easier and their prognosis better than in the oliguric counterpart.

Occasionally doubt may exist as to whether the oliguria is prerenal or whether renal parenchymal damage has already occurred. The urine osmolality and the sodium-to-potassium ratio of the urine may be of some help in deciding the point. If, however, doubt exists, a therapeutic trial with intravenous fluid may be attempted. Hourly urine volumes must be carefully measured, and if there is no response to the infusion of 1500 ml. of the appropriate fluid, no attempts should be made to "force a diuresis" once the physician has assured himself that the volume of blood and extracellular fluid has been adequately repleted.

The prevention of acute renal failure by the infusion of mannitol following experimental clamping of the aorta [54, 103] has suggested the use of this substance to prevent tubular necrosis and oliguria after shock. The evidence indicates that, if given in time, it may prevent the clinical consequence of acute renal failure [9]. Twenty-five grams of mannitol in a 20 per cent solution should be given intravenously as a bolus. If the urine volume does not increase following this procedure, it is questionable whether larger doses will suc-

ceed; also, the infusion of excess amounts of mannitol which are not excreted may result in hyponatremia and acidosis. The intravenous administration of ethacrynic acid (50 to 100 mg.) or furosemide (40 to 80 mg.) appeared to be more effective than mannitol in this regard. Whether the increase in urine volume that results from any of these maneuvers actually "prevents" prolonged oliguria by "flushing out" nephrons is an unresolved question. In both the laboratory animal and man it must be remembered that dehydration, salt depletion, or intravascular volume deficits predispose to acute renal failure possibly through activation of the renin-angiotensin mechanism. The well-hydrated animal or patient with good urine volume is considerably less susceptible to acute renal failure following any precipitating cause than is his dehydrated, oliguric counterpart. This fact must be kept in mind in preparing patients for extensive surgery where preoperative fluid restriction is frequently practiced. Although oral intake must necessarily be restricted before operation, the patient should be well hydrated by the intravenous route.

Decapsulation of the kidney is of little value after acute renal failure has been present for several days. There also is some evidence, however, suggesting that decapsulation shortly after the initial insult may be of value in aborting the process that leads to renal failure [66]. The use of the adrenal steroids for their "anti-edema effect" has been of little value.

It has been suggested that the infusion of alkaline salts following an incompatible blood transfusion may prevent the precipitation of acid hematin in the tubules and abort incipient renal failure. It seems probable, however, that acute renal failure subsequent to incompatible transfusion depends more upon ischemia secondary to clumping of the red cells in the renal vasculature than it does upon the precipitation of acid hematin casts. In any case, if alkaline salts are to be of help, they must reach the tubular urine. They have little effect after the oliguria has occurred.

Of greater importance is the prophylaxis of oliguria following incompatible blood transfusions by the proper cross matching of blood. Antibodies against the weaker blood antigens such as Kell, Duffy, and Lewis may cause acute renal failure following the infusion of blood containing these antigens [43, 100]. "Delayed" renal failure has recently been reported some days following the infusion of Kell incompatible blood [52]. The use of albumin for cross matching is thus imperative for patients who have had previous transfusions. These antibodies cannot be detected by cross matching in saline. Specific therapy for the renal lesion following the ingestion or inhalation of nephrotoxins is usually of little avail. British anti-lewisite (BAL) should be administered in appropriate doses after the ingestion of bichloride of mercury, but it seems to be of little use once the renal lesion has actually developed. It should be remembered also that BAL in large doses may be nephrotoxic in itself [30].

Where adequate facilities exist the treatment of choice of acute renal failure is dialysis, either peritoneal dialysis or hemodialysis with the artificial kidney (see Chapter 10). These modalities should be utilized prophylactically — that is, to prevent the complications of uremia rather than to treat them after they have become manifest.

The course of acute renal failure is extremely variable and may be largely masked by the clinical course of the precipitating episode. It is frequently difficult to distinguish the signs and symptoms due to "uremia" from those of sepsis and anoxia in severely wounded individuals. It cannot be too strongly stressed that anoxia or hypercapnia may mimic in every regard the restlessness, irritability, and disorientation of uremia. Under these circumstances the provision of an adequate airway by

tracheostomy and the removal of secretions from the oropharynx may result in a marked improvement in what was thought to be the uremic syndrome. The marked increase in protein catabolism which accompanies trauma and surgical procedures accounts for the more rapid rise in the nonprotein nitrogen concentration, and may result in a striking increase in the incidence of potassium intoxication. Increased fat catabolism [130] contributes to the increase in body water. This relative increase in body water has been confirmed by a number of investigators [14, 37, 122]. The expansion of the extracellular fluid which has been documented in acute renal failure [37] may reflect in part this increase in "metabolic water" that frequently is aggravated by the injudicious administration of intravenous fluids. The hyponatremia that has been frequently reported may also result from excess water administration [130]. Acidosis and the toxic effect of "uremia" may impair transport systems that maintain the normal gradients for sodium and potassium between cell and extracellular fluid, and occasionally such impairment may result in intercompartmental shifts of sodium which contribute to hyponatremia [85]. It is possible to demonstrate by isotope-dilution technics that total body potassium may be low in the face of high serum levels. In the laboratory animal made anuric by ureteral ligation, muscle sodium and chloride concentrations have been found to be elevated [115]. The bulk of evidence in man, however, suggests that hyponatremia in acute renal failure is usually attributable to excess water administration. Edelman and his co-workers [33] found that in other abnormal clinical situations serum sodium concentrations were not a function of intercompartmental shift but of the relation of total exchangeable sodium, exchangeable potassium, and total body water. To some extent our inability to estimate accurately water requirements in acute renal failure may have been due to the fact that data for fluid replacement have been obtained from normal subjects. In addition, the criterion of surface area for the measurement of fluid requirement has recently been criticized.

For the clinician, the significance of these findings appears to be that water restriction should be even greater than that originally proposed by Strauss [128]. For the average 70 kg. adult, 300 to 400 ml. of water per day should be the basal requirement. To this should be added increments for gastrointestinal losses, increased respiratory rate, high fever, and profuse sweating. Daily measurements of the body weight appear to be the best gauge of adequate fluid replacement. A weight loss of 0.2 to 0.3 kg. per day should be effected. Failure to lose weight or weight gain in the face of inadequate caloric replacement can only mean excess fluid. In some instances this rate of weight loss may be slightly excessive. Since it is always easier to administer fluid to the dehydrated, anuric patient than it is to remove it from the overhydrated individual, it is a sound principle of therapy that some degree of weight loss should be maintained to avoid actual or incipient pulmonary edema.

The studies of Meroney [83] stress the value of the ratio of serum phosphate to nonprotein nitrogen in evaluating devitalization of muscle with cell damage and release of phosphate. However, Doolan et al. [32] were unable to confirm this, nor were they able to find that elevations of serum creatine out of proportion to those of creatinine were of any real use in predicting the presence of devitalized tissue. This is unfortunate, because devitalized tissue undoubtedly contributes to the mortality in acute renal failure. It is, however, probably unnecessary to utilize chemical means alone to detect this.

Unquestionably, the problem of acute spontaneous potassium intoxication is exaggerated by the presence of devitalized muscle and by undrained collections of blood and pus. Anything that contributes to protein breakdown

appears to accentuate this hazard. With the increased awareness of the principles of therapy of acute renal failure, acute potassium intoxication is less frequently seen than previously. In spite of the various factors that may influence its severity, the ultimate cause of death in potassium intoxication is cardiac arrhythmia [88]. Therefore, the use of the electrocardiogram is imperative in following patients with acute renal failure. The characteristic changes in the electrocardiographic pattern and the sequence of their development are shown in Figure 17-2. There is no direct correlation between the changes in the electrocardiogram and the level of the serum potassium. The complex that results in the disturbance of cardiac conduction appears to

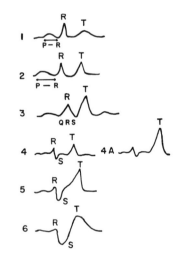

EKG IN POTASSIUM INTOXICATION

Figure 17-2. Sequential changes are shown beginning with peaking of the T wave, lengthening of the P-R interval, and a decrease in amplitude of the P wave. The T wave becomes higher and more pointed (2), the P-wave changes become more pronounced, and the QRS interval increases (3). A symmetrical or "tent-shaped" T wave (4) may have the same significance as a taller but asymmetric T wave (4A). The QRS interval increases, the S-T segment becomes nearly a continuous part of the ascending limb of the high pointed T wave (5), and these changes progress (6) to the so-called sine wave which precedes cardiac arrest.

depend upon the relation of intracellular-to-extracellular potassium, which may in turn be affected by the pH of body fluid and the intracellular-extracellular sodium ratio.

The emergency treatment of advanced potassium intoxication should be the infusion of hypertonic sodium bicarbonate. The antagonism of potassium ion by sodium and the beneficial effect of raising the serum pH are manifest in a few minutes. The benefit, however, is of relatively short duration, and this treatment should be reserved for patients in whom therapy cannot be postponed. The use of hypertonic sodium chloride solutions is somewhat less effective. Hypertonic calcium solutions may also be effective, although calcium in general is less effective therapy than sodium. The administration of hypertonic glucose solutions may also ameliorate electrocardiographic changes of potassium intoxication. This solution should be administered in the form of 25 or 30 per cent glucose with the addition of insulin in a ratio of 1 unit of insulin to 3 gm. of glucose. The beneficial changes are slower to appear than when electrolyte solutions are used, but their duration is somewhat longer. The removal of potassium by short-term peritoneal irrigation as described by Legrain and Merrill [72] in 1953 is an effective form of therapy for potassium intoxication. This technic has been employed with success in slightly modified form by other workers [31, 81], whose use of commercially prepared solutions has made it a more generally practicable form of therapy. The removal of potassium from body fluids by other methods is described elsewhere in this volume. The indications for and technics of dialysis are discussed in Chapter 10. Sodium polystyrene sulfonate* is a cation-exchange resin in the sodium cycle whose small mesh size makes it a practical means of therapy. The use of this resin in conjunction with D-sorbitol, a polyhydric alcohol which promotes diarrhea, has

* In the form of Kayexalate, Winthrop Laboratories, 90 Park Ave., New York, N.Y.

made resin therapy an extremely effective adjunct in the treatment of acute renal failure [39]. Unlike other forms of cathartics, sorbitol, if absorbed from the gastrointestinal tract, will be metabolized. The resin and sorbitol may also be given by enema. Administration of this resin by a rectal tube with a balloon to prevent its expulsion prolongs retention of the resin and allows removal of larger amounts of potassium from the large bowel. When the resin is given by mouth with sorbitol, the production of diarrhea not only causes effective passage of the resin through the gastrointestinal tract but promotes effective contact with intestinal secretions so that potassium may be removed.

Caloric Intake

The provision of nonprotein calories by the "forced" feeding of mixtures of fat and sugar [61] is now outmoded. The problems of administering such an intake to acutely ill, nauseated patients more than outweigh the possible benefits to be derived. The use of fat as an intravenous emulsion has been complicated by pyrogen reactions. Current preparations, however, are relatively pyrogen-free [26]. One must question the value of either oral or parenteral fat as a caloric supplement in acute renal failure since this disease is by and large a self-limited one. For this reason, body stores of fat usually suffice without the administration of exogenous fat supplements. One hundred grams or more of carbohydrate per day should be provided to prevent ketosis from fat catabolism and to reduce endogenous protein catabolism.

The route of administration of nonprotein calories constitutes a problem in acute renal failure. Since the volume of fluid may be limited, the oral route permits a more concentrated solution. In addition, it has the advantage of stimulating salivary flow and postponing drying and cracking of the lips which predispose to the oral lesions so frequently seen in uremia. I have found that small amounts of Karo syrup and ginger ale mixed in equal proportions and well iced are as well tolerated as any carbohydrate supplement.

In many instances nausea and vomiting or recent abdominal surgery contraindicate the ingestion of food or fluid. Therefore, parenteral supplements may be necessary. The hypertonic nature of this fluid either as solutions of glucose or as invert sugar necessitates the placing of a plastic catheter in veins whose caliber is large enough to prevent sclerosis by the hypertonic solution. Complications of this technic are clotting and infection. When such complications arise from catheters placed in the inferior vena cava, the resultant pulmonary emboli and abscesses may be lethal. Bansmer et al. [6] report a 46 per cent incidence of such complications. In another study Smits and Freedman [127] report that half the cases of staphylococcal sepsis in a seven-month period were directly attributable to the complications of venous cannulation. When utilized the site of insertion of the catheter should be treated daily with antibiotic ointment, and the catheter should be changed no less frequently than every 96 hours. The incidence of pulmonary emboli in catheters threaded into the brachial or axillary vein through the antecubital vessels is somewhat less, but infection remains a frequent complication here. It is to be noted, however, that the incidence of complications diminishes with the skill and experience of the physician who inserts the catheters.

Ethyl alcohol either by mouth or by vein also affords a good source of nonprotein calories. However, the specific pharmacologic effects of alcohol limit its general usefulness as a caloric source for patients with acute renal failure. In any case, the technic of providing a constant source of calories over a 24-hour period more than offsets the potential risk of venous catheterization, provided adequate precautions are utilized.

Attempts to minimize protein metabolism by the use of anabolic agents are widespread. In normal individuals on careful balance studies, it is possible to document the anabolic effects of testosterone derivatives. It is difficult accurately to assess their value in acutely ill patients, whose protein catabolism may be affected by many other factors. Since no toxic side effects have been demonstrated, however, it is my custom to use testosterone proprionate in doses of 50 mg. per day for a week or 10 days. The more slowly absorbed Depo-testosterone (100 mg. twice a week) may also be employed. Balance studies in a few patients whose anuria followed accidents of pregnancy [82] suggested that norethandrolone (Nilevar) has a significant effect in minimizing protein catabolism.

Cardiovascular System

Moderate degrees of hypertension may occur in acute renal failure, but frequently are accentuated by overhydration. Cardiac arrhythmias are a common complication. Patients with acute renal failure are particularly susceptible to the arrhythmias that accompany digitalis administration. For this reason, the intravenous administration of rapidly acting digitalis preparations may be extremely dangerous. A rise in serum potassium with the typical electrocardiographic changes may occur suddenly following the administration of rapidly acting digitalis preparations. In the laboratory animal with experimental uremia the production of acidosis with ammonium chloride markedly accentuates this sequence of events [117]. Even in the undigitalized patient, however, cardiac arrhythmias may occur, which appear to be due to sudden changes in concentration of electrolyte rather than to the absolute level of any one. A rapid rise in serum sodium or a decrease in serum potassium concentration effected by therapeutic maneuvers is most commonly responsible.

Supraventricular tachycardias, particularly paroxysmal atrial tachycardia and atrial fibrillation, are frequent. Ventricular premature contractions may occur even in undigitalized patients. The ventricular arrhythmias may account for sudden unexplained death in patients with acute renal failure. Fibrinous pericarditis with loud friction rubs and precordial pain occurs in some 18 per cent of patients with acute renal failure [139]. Pericarditis in the acute syndrome is perfectly compatible with spontaneous recovery. An occasional patient may show a striking and unexplained phenomenon mimicking in every way the sequelae of massive pulmonary embolus. Marked cyanosis, elevated venous pressure, dyspnea, and expiratory wheezes as well as the typical electrocardiographic criteria may be present. No pulmonary emboli, however, are found at autopsy. Electrocardiographic changes of subendocardial ischemia may be present. Both of these phenomena appear to be due to chemical abnormalities, since they may be reversed by dialysis with the artificial kidney [73].

Gastrointestinal Tract

The most common gastrointestinal complication of acute and chronic renal failure is nausea and vomiting. Either diarrhea or paralytic ileus may be present. The latter in combination with the marked leukocytosis which is so common may closely simulate the acute intraabdominal surgical condition. Bleeding from the gastrointestinal tract due to diffuse gastritis or even small gastric or duodenal ulcers is not uncommon. When the patient has been properly treated, particularly with dialysis, definitive surgery may be performed even in the face of continued oliguria.

Central Nervous System

The central nervous system manifestations of acute renal failure are many and varied. Decreased responsiveness may progress to frank coma. On the other hand, the patient may be wildly agitated and disoriented. The reflexes may be hyperactive or entirely flaccid, depending upon the chemical abnormalities or the way in which they have been modified by therapy. Hyperreflexia, twitching, and irritability are common. Unilateral pyramidal signs may be present and may change from day to day. The generalized hyperirritability has been attributed in the past to hypocalcemia. This appears to be rarely the cause, since the disorder partakes more closely of the nature of a generalized metabolic disturbance of the central nervous system and there appears to be no relation of the signs and symptoms to the levels of calcium in the serum or in the cerebrospinal fluid. Rarely if ever are these manifestations ameliorated by the intravenous infusion of calcium unless the previous administrations of alkaline solutions have produced tetany. Erratic flexor contractions of the extended hands (asterixis) may be seen which closely resemble "liver flap." Electroencephalographic studies show diffuse and gross abnormalities. The focal neurologic signs may change rapidly, and probably do not represent organic brain damage. It should be stressed again that such signs and symptoms may frequently represent anoxia secondary to an obstructed airway rather than the manifestations of uremia. No specific therapy for these disturbances is available, although the use of the anticonvulsant drugs such as diphenylhydantoin (Dilantin) and the avoidance of bright lights and noises may be beneficial. Prochlorperazine (Compazine), promazine hydrochloride (Sparine), or one of the short-acting barbiturates metabolized by the liver may be of value.

Infection

It is generally agreed that death in patients with acute renal failure is commonly not a direct consequence of the chemical abnormalities, but results from bacterial infection [4,

96, 136]. Acute renal failure frequently occurs in the setting of trauma or major surgery. Fresh wounds offer a convenient portal for infection, and prolonged immobility appears to enhance this proclivity. Impairment of wound healing as a result of severe uremia, malnutrition, and infection may result in wound dehiscence. Central nervous system depression and vomiting predispose the patient to the aspiration of stomach contents with a resultant chemical pneumonitis. The accumulation of secretions in the upper airway and inadequate respiratory movements are also predisposing factors. In all such patients the possible indications for tracheotomy must be carefully weighed.

The temptation to use "prophylactic" antibiotics in wounded, critically ill persons is almost irresistible. Unfortunately, however, the use of broad-spectrum antibiotics for this purpose predisposes to superinfection with antibiotic-resistant staphylococci [8, 112]. The uniform tendency toward leukocytosis in acute uremia and the frequent absence of fever in the face of infection make this diagnosis difficult. Infection, when present, should be treated promptly with antibiotics to which the organism cultured has been proved sensitive by in vitro studies. It must be kept in mind that certain antibiotics excreted primarily by the kidney may be effective in fractions of the doses ordinarily used. Severe toxic manifestations may result if this is not realized [63–65]. Streptomycin and kanamycin in particular are representative. A therapeutic blood level for these agents may be obtained for a period of 10 days with a single intramuscular dose of 1.5 gm.

Infection of the lower urinary tract is a common complication. The use of the inlying bladder catheter in patients with acute renal failure is a common practice. The quantity of urine elaborated is a hallmark of progress in these states, and it is only natural to attempt to gauge this from hour to hour by use of an inlying catheter. However, the indiscriminate use of such catheters predisposes to pyelonephritis [10]. Furthermore, in spite of the understandable impatience on the part of the physician, it is rarely of real prognostic benefit. Until the 24-hour urine volume in the diuretic stage is greater than 1000 ml., clearance of solute is minimal. Careful percussion of the bladder should reveal significant retention long before 1000 ml. has accumulated. Thus, for diagnostic purposes alone the inlying catheter is unnecessary. Awareness of the complications of the inlying catheter, however, has led to precautions in its management which have markedly decreased the bacterial complications of its presence [28].

Because of the hazards of infection, strict aseptic precautions should be observed, including scrubbing of the hands with an antiseptic solution and the use of gowns and masks. Although cumbersome, such precautions minimize the risk of contamination and make the attending personnel constantly aware of the problem of sepsis. No specific reason for the susceptibility of patients with acute renal failure to infection has been found. Phagocytosis and antibody production are apparently normal in such individuals [3]. Frequently, in spite of the best precautions and efforts to prevent environmental sepsis, such patients will become infected with the organisms of their own gastrointestinal flora and die of gram-negative pneumonia or septicemia. The administration of large amounts of intramuscular human gamma globulin (5 to 10 ml. daily) may be an effective adjunct.

Hematologic Considerations

Leukocytosis is the rule rather than the exception during acute renal failure. White blood cell counts of 20,000 per cubic millimeter or greater are not unusual. The peripheral bone marrow may be severely aplastic in acute renal anemia, but usually the erythroid-granulocyte ratio is slightly decreased or normal.

The anemia of renal failure is primarily due to lack of stimulation and proliferation of the erythroid elements of the bone marrow. Such patients show basal or subbasal erythropoiesis in the face of severe anemia. A blood smear is characteristically normochromic-normocytic with occasional burr forms or helmet cells [1]. Anemia in these individuals may result from dilution or from increased red cell destruction [76]. The hemoglobin value in each patient appears to stabilize at a point which represents a balance between hemolysis and red cell production. Transfusion of fresh packed red cells is the therapy of choice. Cardiac output appears not to be markedly affected until the normochromic, normocytic hematocrit has dropped below 25. In patients with acute renal failure, hematocrit levels above 30 obtained by transfusion tend to return rapidly to baseline levels. For practical purposes, therefore, the hematocrit should be maintained between 25 and 30. After the diuretic phase the anemia may persist for weeks after the return of the blood urea nitrogen to normal values. Reticulocytosis often reaching 10 to 20 per cent precedes the return of the hematocrit to normal. Bleeding defects and purpura are common during acute renal failure, but no single cause has been elicited. Multiple defects in hemostasis have been described, but no single defect appears to explain all of the bleeding abnormalities encountered [67, 75, 106]. However, it appears that a qualitative platelet defect, reversible by a dialysis, and manifested by impaired platelet adhesiveness and aggregation, is present in all uremic patients with obvious bleeding manifestations [23].

Diuresis

The onset of diuresis in acute renal failure is unpredictable. Increase in urine volume may begin within 48 hours after the onset of oliguria. On the other hand, I have seen one patient recover after 31 days of severe oliguria.

The urine volume usually increases in stepwise fashion. Rarely it increases from a volume of less than 300 ml. per day to greater than 1500 ml. in a 24-hour period. Sodium losses in the diuretic phase may be marked [55]. However, as renal function improves, urinary sodium losses may change in proportion to the status of body sodium stores. Frequently the marked loss of sodium during the diuretic period simply reflects the loss of previously acquired edema fluid. It is a mistake, therefore, to replace these losses simply on the basis of urinary measurements, since to do so is to perpetuate occult edema. Occasionally a patient who enters the diuretic phase critically ill may sustain sodium and water losses in the first two to three days which may endanger his state of hydration. However, if free access to water and sodium is allowed and the patient is conscious and capable of ingesting fluid, thirst and improving renal function will compensate for such losses. Hypokalemia may appear in the diuretic phase, with or without large urinary losses of potassium. Frequently this appears to be the "unmasking" of the stigmata of total body potassium depletion, which become apparent with the drop in serum potassium when acidosis is corrected. In the early part of the diuretic phase the urine may be markedly hypotonic to the plasma. Water is thus lost in excess of solute, and since urea clearance is not adequate to keep up with protein catabolism the urea concentration of the plasma may rise in the first few days in spite of improving renal function. Convulsions and central nervous system disturbances are not infrequently associated with this stage, particularly in the postpartum patient. They do not necessarily have a bad prognostic significance. However, in at least two instances prolonged psychiatric care has been required. Hypernatremia and hyperchloremia have been described as a complication of the diuretic phase [20]. These abnormalities have been variously thought to be associated with sulfonamide therapy and with central nervous system disturbances which in some way modify the tubular handling of sodium. In our opinion, they are more frequently the result of injudicious administration of hypertonic sodium solutions.

The prognosis for the renal lesion following acute renal failure is usually good. Some decrease in renal function may persist [36, 77], but this is rarely progressive or clinically significant. Inability to concentrate the urine and decreased maximal tubular excretory capacity for para-aminohippuric acid have been recorded as sequelae of the renal failure following

ing epidemic hemorrhagic fever [113]. Acute pyelonephritis may complicate the diuretic phase, and occasionally slowly progressive bacterial infection of the urinary tract may require treatment. One rare exception is worthy of notice. I have observed a patient in whom four renal biopsies over a period of six months of marked oliguria showed nothing but the lesions of tubular necrosis. When the kidneys were removed one year and a half after the onset of oliguria, diffuse interstitial fibrosis and atrophic glomeruli were the only significant lesions observed.

References

1. Adamson, J. W., Eschbach, J., and Finch, C. A. The kidney and erythropoiesis. *Amer. J. Med.* 44:725, 1968.
2. Addis, T. *Glomerular Nephritis*. New York: Macmillan, 1949.
3. Balch, H. H. The effect of severe battle injury and of post-traumatic renal failure on resistance to infection. *Ann. Surg.* 142:145, 1955.
4. Balch, H. H., Meroney, W. H., and Sako, Y. Observations on surgical care of patients with posttraumatic renal insufficiency. *Surg. Gynec. Obstet.* 100:439, 1955.
5. Bank, N., Mutz, B. F., and Ayndjian, H. S. The role of "leakage" of tubular fluid in anuria due to mercury poisoning. *J. Clin. Invest.* 46:695, 1967.
6. Bansmer, G., Keith, D., and Tesluk, H. Complications following use of indwelling catheters of inferior vena cava. *J.A.M.A.* 167:1606, 1958.
7. Barenberg, R. L., Solomon, S., Papper, S., and Anderson, R. Clearance and micropuncture study of renal function in mercuric chloride treated rats. *J. Lab. Clin. Med.* 72:473, 1968.
8. Barnes, J., Pace, W. J., Trump, T. S., and Ellison, E. H. Prophylactic postoperative antibiotics. *A.M.A. Arch. Surg.* 79:190, 1959.
9. Barry, K. G., Cohen, A., Knochel, J. P., Whelan, T. J., Jr., Beisel, W. R., Vargas, C. A., and LeBlanc, P. C., Jr. Mannitol infusion: II. The prevention of acute functional renal failure during resection of an aneurysm of the abdominal aorta. *New Eng. J. Med.* 264:967, 1961.
10. Beeson, P. B. The case against the catheter. *Amer. J. Med.* 24:1, 1958.
11. Berliner, R. W., and Davidson, D. G. Production of hypertonic urine in the absence of pituitary antidiuretic hormone. *J. Clin. Invest.* 36:14, 1957.
12. Biber, T. U. L., Mylle, M., Baines, A. D., Gottschalk, C. W., Oliver, J. R., and MacDowell, M. C. A study by micropuncture and microdissection of acute renal damage in rats. *Amer. J. Med.* 44:664, 1968.
13. Block, M. A., Wakim, K. G., and Mann, F. C. Circulation through kidney during stimulation of the renal nerves. *Amer. J. Physiol.* 169:659, 1952.
14. Bluemle, L. W., Jr., Potter, H. P., and Elkinton, J. R. Changes in body composition in acute renal failure. *J. Clin. Invest.* 35:1094, 1956.
15. Boucot, N. G., Guild, W. R., and Merrill, J. P. Bilateral renocortical necrosis with recovery. *New Eng. J. Med.* 257:416, 1957.
16. Bradley, S. E., Leifer, E., and Nickel, J. F. Distribution of Functional Activity Among the Nephron Population. In Lewis, A. A. G., and Wolstenholme, G. E. W. (Eds.), *Ciba Foundation Symposium on*

the Kidney. Boston: Little, Brown, 1954. P. 50.

17. Brun, C. *Acute Anuria*. Copenhagen: Ejnar Munksgaard, 1954.

18. Brun, C., Crone, C., Davidsen, H. G., Fabricius, J., Hansen, A. T., Lassen, N. A., and Munck, O. Renal interstitial pressure in normal and in anuric man: Based on wedged renal vein pressure. *Proc. Soc. Exp. Biol. Med.* 91:199, 1956.

19. Brun, C., Crone, C., Davidsen, H. G., Fabricius, J., Tybsaerg, H. A., Lassen, N., and Munck, O. Renal blood flow in anuric human subject determined by use of radioactive krypton 85. *Proc. Soc. Exp. Biol. Med.* 89:687, 1955.

20. Bull, G. Discussion, Acute renal failure. *Transactions of the Fifth Conference on Renal Function*. New York: Josiah Macy, Jr. Foundation, 1953. P. 129.

21. Bull, G. Personal communication, 1960.

22. Bull, G. M., Joekes, A. M., and Lowe, K. G. Renal function studies in acute tubular necrosis. *Clin. Sci.* 9:379, 1950.

23. Castaldi, P. A., Rosenberg, M. C., and Stewart, J. H. The bleeding disorders of uremia: A qualitative platelet defect. *Lancet* 2:66, 1966.

24. Chesley, L. C., and McCaw, W. H. A physiologic study of acute renal failure with follow-up observations. *Amer. J. Obstet. Gynec.* 62:1187, 1951.

25. Clark, J. K., Barker, H. G., and Crosley, A. P., Jr. Evidence against renal vascular shunts in a case of lower nephron nephrosis. *Amer. J. Med.* 9:268, 1950.

26. Conference on Intravenous Fat Emulsions. Final discussion and summary. *Metabolism* 6:823, 1957.

27. Conn, H. L., Jr., Wilds, L., and Helwig, J. Study of renal circulation, tubular function and morphology, and urinary volume and composition in dogs following mercury poisoning and transfusion of human blood. *J. Clin. Invest.* 33:732, 1954.

28. Desautels, R. E. Aseptic management of catheter drainage. *New Eng. J. Med.* 263:189, 1960.

29. de Wardener, H. E. Intrarenal pressure in experimental tubular necrosis. *Lancet* 1:580, 1955.

30. Doolan, P. D., Hess, W. C., and Kyle, L. H. Acute renal insufficiency due to bichloride of mercury. *New Eng. J. Med.* 249:273, 1953.

31. Doolan, P. D., Murphy, W. P., Wiggins, R. A., Carter, N. W., Cooper, W. C., Watten, R. H., and Alpen, E. L. An evaluation of intermittent peritoneal lavage. *Amer. J. Med.* 26:831, 1959.

32. Doolan, P. D., Theil, G. B., Wiggins, R. A., Lee, K. J., and Martinez, E. Acute renal insufficiency following aortic surgery. *Trans. Amer. Soc. Artif. Intern. Organs* 5:69, 1959.

33. Edelman, I. S., Leibman, J., O'Meara, M. P., and Birkenfeld, L. W. Interrelations between serum sodium concentration, serum osmolarity and total exchangeable sodium, total exchangeable potassium and total body water. *J. Clin. Invest.* 37:1236, 1958.

34. Eggleton, M. G., Richardson, K. C., Schild, H. C., and Winton, F. R. Renal damage due to crush injury and ischemia of the limbs of the anesthetized dog. *Quart. J. Exp. Physiol.* 32:89, 1943.

35. Epstein, M., Berk, D. P., Hollenberg, N. K., Adams, D. F., Chalmers, T. C., Abrams, H. L., and Merrill, J. P. Pathogenesis of the hepatorenal syndrome: The role of cortical ischemia. *Proceedings of the American Society of Nephrology*. (Abstract.) 2d Annual Meeting, 1968.

36. Finkenstaedt, J. T., and Merrill, J. P. Renal function after recovery from acute renal failure. *New Eng. J. Med.* 254:1023, 1956.

37. Finkenstaedt, J. T., O'Meara, M. P., and Merrill, J. P. Failure of equilibration of inulin in anuric subjects. *J. Clin. Invest.* 32:209, 1953.

38. Flanigan, W., and Oken, D. E. Renal micropuncture study of the development of anuria in the rat with mercury-induced acute renal failure. *J. Clin. Invest.* 44:449, 1965.

39. Flinn, R. B., Merrill, J. P., and Welzant, W. R. Treatment of the oliguric patient with a new sodium-exchange resin and sor-

bitol: A preliminary report. *New Eng. J. Med.* 264:111, 1960.

40. Franklin, S. S., and Merrill, J. P. Acute renal failure. *New Eng. J. Med.* 262:711, 1960.

41. Friedman, S. M., Radcliffe, R. W., Turpin, J. E. H., and Friedman, C. L. "Reflex" anuria in the dog. *Canad. J. Biochem. Physiol.* 34:158, 1956.

42. Friedman, S. M., Radcliffe, R. W., Turpin, J. E. H., and Friedman, C. L. Renal responses to remote surgical manipulations in the dog. *J. Int. Coll. Surg.* 25:744, 1956.

43. Fudenberg, H., and Allen, F. H., Jr. Transfusion reactions in the absence of demonstrable incompatibility. *New Eng. J. Med.* 256:1180, 1957.

44. Gamble, J. L. *Chemical Anatomy, Physiology, and Pathology of Extracellular Fluid.* Cambridge, Mass.: Harvard University Press, 1947.

45. Goodwin, W. E., and Kaufman, J. J. The renal lymphatics: I. Review of some of the pertinent literature. *Urol. Survey* 6:305, 1956.

46. Govaerts, P. The ratio of creatinine clearance to urea clearance in toxic nephropathies. *Stanford Med. Bull.* 6:71, 1848.

47. Graber, I. G., and Sevitt, S. Renal function in burned patients and its relationship to morphological changes. *J. Clin. Path.* 12:25, 1959.

48. Guild, W. R., Young, J. V., and Merrill, J. P. Anuria due to carbon tetrachloride intoxication. *Ann. Intern. Med.* 48:1221, 1958.

49. Gullick, H. D., and Raisz, L. G. Changes in renal concentrating ability associated with major surgical procedures. *New Eng. J. Med.* 262:1309, 1960.

50. Henry, L. N., Lane, C. E., and Kashgarian, M. Micropuncture studies of the pathophysiology of acute renal failure in the rat. *Lab. Invest.* 19:309, 1968.

51. Hinshaw, L. B., Day, S. B., and Carlson, C. H. Tissue pressure as a causal factor in the autoregulation of blood flow in the isolated perfused kidney. *Amer. J. Physiol.* 197:309, 1959.

52. Holland, P. V., and Wallerstein, R. O. De-layed hemolytic transfusion reaction with acute renal failure. *J.A.M.A.* 204:1007, 1968.

53. Hollenberg, N. K., Epstein, M., Rosen, S. M., Basch, R. I., Oken, D. E., and Merrill, J. P. Acute oliguric renal failure in man: Evidence for preferential renal cortical ischemia. *Medicine* (Balt.) 47:455, 1968.

54. Hostnik, W. J., Powers, S. R., Jr., Boba, A., and Stein, A. A. Observations on the effect of mannitol on the renal hemodynamics and O_2 tension in the urine and renal vein. *Surg. Forum* 10:872, 1960.

55. Hunter, R. B., and Muirhead, E. E. Prolonged renal salt wastage in lower acute renal insufficiency. *A.M.A. Arch Intern. Med.* 89:188, 1952.

56. Iseri, L. T., Batchelor, T. M., Boyle, A. J., and Mywers, G. B. Studies of fluid, electrolyte, and nitrogen balance in acute renal insufficiency. *A.M.A. Arch. Intern. Med.* 89:188, 1952.

57. Iversen, P., and Brun, C. Aspiration biopsy of the kidney. *Amer. J. Med.* 11:324, 1951.

58. Kark, R. M., Muehrcke, R. C., Pirani, C. L., and Pollak, V. E. The clinical value of renal biopsy. *Ann. Intern. Med.* 43:807, 1955.

59. King, L. R., Knoll, P. J., Hoy, J., and Margolin, E. G. Cerebrospinal and serum levels of Ca, Mg, P, and urea in uremia. *Clin. Res.* 8:288, 1960.

60. Kleeman, C. R., Maxwell, M. H., and Rockney, R. Production of hypertonic urine in humans in the probable absence of antidiuretic hormone. *Proc. Soc. Exp. Biol. Med.* 96:189, 1957.

61. Kolff, W. J. Treatment of uremia with forced high calorie-low protein diet. *Nutr. Rev.* 11:193, 1953.

62. Kravitz, S. C., Diamond, H. E., and Craver, L. F. Uremia complicating leukemia chemotherapy: Report of a case treated with triethylene melamine. *J.A.M.A.* 146:1595, 1951.

63. Kunin, C. M., Rees, S. B., Merrill, J. P., and Finland, M. Persistence of antibiotics in blood of patients with acute renal failure: I.

Tetracycline and chlortetracycline. *J. Clin. Invest.* 38:1487, 1959.

64. Kunin, C. M., Glazko, A. J., and Finland, M. Persistence of antibiotics in blood of patients with acute renal failure: II. Chloramphenicol and its metabolic products in the blood of patients with severe renal disease or hepatic cirrhosis. *J. Clin. Invest.* 38: 1498, 1959.

65. Kunin, C. M., and Finland, M. Persistence of antibiotics in blood of patients with acute renal failure: III. Penicillin, streptomycin, erythromycin and kanamycin. *J. Clin. Invest.* 38:1509, 1959.

66. Kuss, R., Legrain, M., Camey, M., Desarmenien, J., Mathe, G., Nedey, R., and Vourch, C. Homotransplantation rénale chez l'homme. *Mem. Acad. Chir.* (Paris) 87:183, 1961.

67. Larrain, C., and Adelson, E. Hemostatic defect of uremia: I. Clinical investigation of 3 patients with acute posttraumatic renal insufficiency. *Blood* 11:1059, 1956.

68. Lauler, D. P., Schreiner, G. E., and David, A. Renal medullary necrosis. *Amer. J. Med.* 29:132, 1960.

69. Lauson, H. D., Bradley, S. E., and Cournand, A. Renal circulation in shock. *J. Clin. Invest.* 23:381, 1944.

70. Lear, H., and Oppenheimer, G. D. Anuria following radiation therapy in leukemia. *J.A.M.A.* 143:806, 1950.

71. LeBrie, S. J., and Meyerson, H. S. Influence of uranium nitrate-induced nephrosis on flow and composition of renal lymph. *Physiologist* 3:102, 1960.

72. Legrain, M., and Merrill, J. P. Short-term continuous transperitoneal dialysis. *New Eng. J. Med.* 243:125, 1953.

73. Levine, H. D., Wanzer, S. H., and Merrill, J. P. Dialyzable currents of injury in potassium intoxication resembling acute myocardial infarction or pericarditis. *Circulation* 13:29, 1956.

74. Levy, R. I. Renal failure: Secondary to ethylene glycol intoxication. *J.A.M.A.* 173: 1210, 1960.

75. Lewis, J. H., Zucker, M. B., and Ferguson, J. H. Bleeding tendency in uremia. *Blood* 11:1073, 1956.

76. Loge, J. P., Lange, R. D., and Moore, C. V. Characterization of anemia associated with chronic renal insufficiency. *Amer. J. Med.* 24:4, 1958.

77. Lowe, K. G. Late prognosis in acute tubular necrosis: Interim follow-up report on 14 patients. *Lancet* 1:1086, 1952.

78. Lucké, B. Lower nephron nephrosis: The renal lesions of the crush syndrome, of burns, transfusion, and other conditions affecting the lower segments of the nephrons. *Milit. Surgeon* 99:371, 1946.

79. Marks, I. M. Renal medullary necrosis following exsanguination in infancy. *Lancet* 2:680, 1960.

80. Marshall, D., and Hoffman, W. S. The nature of the altered renal function in lower nephron nephrosis. *J. Lab. Clin. Med.* 34: 31, 1949.

81. Maxwell, M. H., Rockney, R. E., Kleeman, C. R., and Twiss, M. R. Peritoneal dialysis. *J.A.M.A.* 170:917, 1959.

82. McCracken, B. H., and Parsons, F. M. Use of Nilevar (17-ethyl-19-nortestosterone) to suppress protein catabolism in acute renal failure. *Lancet* 2:855, 1958.

83. Meroney, W. H. Phosphorus to nonprotein nitrogen ratio in plasma as index of muscle devitalization during oliguria. *Surg. Gynec. Obstet.* 100:309, 1955.

84. Meroney, W. H., and Rubini, M. E. Kidney function during acute tubular necrosis: Clinical studies and theory. *Metabolism* 8:1, 1959.

85. Merrill, J. P. Electrolyte changes in renal failure. *Metabolism* 5:419, 1956.

86. Merrill, J. P. Kidney disease: Acute renal failure. *Ann. Rev. Med.* 11:127, 1960.

87. Merrill, J. P. *The Treatment of Renal Failure.* New York: Grune & Stratton, 1955.

88. Merrill, J. P., Levine, H. D., Somerville, W., and Smith, S., III. Clinical recognition and treatment of acute potassium intoxication. *Ann. Intern. Med.* 33:797, 1950.

89. Moore, F. D., and Ball, M. R. *The Metabolic Response to Surgery.* Springfield, Ill.: Thomas, 1952.

90. Mueller, C. B., Surtshin, A., Carlin, M. R., and White, H. L. Glomerular and tubular

influences on sodium and water excretion. *Amer. J. Physiol.* 165:411, 1951.

91. Oken, D. E., Arce, M. L., and Wilson, D. R. Glycerol-induced hemoglobinuric acute renal failure in the rat: I. Micropuncture study of the development of oliguria. *J. Clin. Invest.* 45:724, 1966.

92. Oliver, J., MacDowell, M., and Tracy A. The pathogenesis of acute renal failure associated with traumatic and toxic injury: Renal ischemia, nephrotoxic damage and the ischemuric episode. *J. Clin. Invest.* 30:1307, 1951.

93. Pappenheimer, J. R., and Kinter, W. B. Hematocrit ratio of blood within mammalian kidney and its significance for renal hemodynamics. *Amer. J. Physiol.* 185:377, 1956.

94. Papper, S. The role of the kidney in Laennec's cirrhosis of the liver. *Medicine* (Balt.) 37:299, 1958.

95. Parker, R. M., Basch, R. I., and Harrison, J. H. Unilateral vasoconstrictive anuria. *Surg. Gynec. Obstet.* 127:66, 1968.

96. Parsons, F. M., and McCracken, B. H. Artificial kidney. *Brit. Med. J.* 1:740, 1959.

97. Perillie, P. E., and Conn, H. O. Acute renal failure after intravenous pyelography in plasma cell myeloma. *J.A.M.A.* 167:18, 1958.

98. Perlmutter, M. Unusual cases of acute tubular necrosis. *Ann. Intern. Med.* 47:81, 1957.

99. Perlmutter, M., Grossman, S. L., Rothberg, S., and Dobkin, G. Urine-serum urea nitrogen ration. (Simple test of renal function in acute azotemia oliguria.) *J.A.M.A.* 170:1533, 1959.

100. Peschel, E., McIntosh, H. D., Brown, I. W., Jr., Murdaugh, H. V. Acute tubular necrosis after transfusion reaction due to anti-Kell antibodies. *J.A.M.A.* 167:1736, 1958.

101. Phillips, R. A., Dole, V. P., Hamilton, P. B., Emerson, K., Jr., Archibald, R. M., and Van Slyke, D. D. Effects of acute hemorrhagic and chromatic shock on renal functioning of dogs. *Amer. J. Physiol.* 145:314, 1945.

102. Pomeranz, B. H., Birtch, A. G., and Barger, A. C. Neural control of intrarenal blood flow. *Amer. J. Physiol.* 215:1067, 1968.

103. Powers, S. R., Jr., Boba, A., and Stein, A. The mechanism and prevention of distal tubular necrosis following aneurysmectomy. *Surgery* 42:156, 1957.

104. Price, J. D. E., and Palmer, R. A. A functional and morphological follow-up of acute renal failure. *Arch. Intern. Med.* (Chicago) 105:114, 1960.

105. Quinton, W., Dillard, D., and Scribner, B. H. Cannulation of blood vessels for prolonged hemodialysis. *Trans. Amer. Soc. Artif. Intern. Organs* 6:104, 1960.

106. Rath, C. E., Mailliard, J. A., and Schreiner, G. E. Bleeding tendency in uremia. *New Eng. J. Med.* 257:808, 1957.

107. Reiner, L., Konikoff, N., Altschule, M. D., Dammin, G. J., and Merrill, J. P. Idiopathic paroxysmal myoglobinuria. Report of two cases and evaluation of the syndrome. *Arch. Intern. Med.* (Chicago) 97:537, 1956.

108. Reuber, M. D., and Bradley, J. E. Acute versenate nephrosis. *J.A.M.A.* 174:3, 1960.

109. Richards, A. N. Direct observations of change in function of the renal tubule caused by certain poisons. *Trans. Ass. Amer. Physicians* 44:64, 1929.

110. Richet, G., Alagille, D., and Fournier, E. L'erythroblastopénie aigue de l'anurie. *Presse Med.* 62:50, 1954.

111. Richmond, G. H., and Beardsley, G. D. Nitrogen mustard therapy complicated by acute renal failure due to uric acid crystallization. *Ann. Intern. Med.* 39:1327, 1953.

112. Rogers, D. E. The changing pattern of life-threatening microbial disease. *New Eng. J. Med.* 261:677, 1959.

113. Rubini, M. E. Renal residuals of acute epidemic hemorrhagic fever. *Arch. Intern. Med.* (Chicago) 106:378, 1960.

114. Ruiz-Guinazu, A., Coelho, J. B., and Paz, R. A. Methemoglobin-induced acute renal failure in the rat: In vivo observation, histology and micropuncture measurements of intratubular and postglomerular vascular pressures. *Nephron* 4:257, 1967.

115. Rush, B. F., Jr., and Randell, H. T. Postsurgical anuria: Experimental study of fluid

and electrolyte changes. *Surgery* 44:655, 1958.

116. Salisbury, P. F. Recovery from acute renal failure and acidosis in sickle-cell disease. *J.A.M.A.* 174:356, 1960.

117. Schafer, H. H., Witham, A. C., and Burns, J. H. Digitalis tolerance and effect of acetyl-strophanthidan upon serum potassium of dogs with acidosis and uremia. *Amer. Heart J.* 60:388, 1960.

118. Selkurt, E. E. Renal blood flow and renal clearance during hemorrhagic shock. *Amer. J. Physiol.* 145:699, 1946.

119. Sevitt, S. Pathogenesis of traumatic uraemia: Revised concept. *Lancet* 2:135, 1959.

120. Sims, E. A. H., Goldberg, H. I., Kelly, J. R., and Sisco, B. Glomerular profusion during acute renal insufficiency from mercury poisoning in rat. *J. Lab. Clin. Med.* 54:440, 1959.

121. Sirota, J. H. Carbon tetrachloride poisoning in man: I. The mechanisms of renal failure and recovery. *J. Clin. Invest.* 28:1412, 1949.

122. Sirota, J. H., and Kroop, I. G. Water and electrolyte disturbances in acute renal insufficiency. *Fed. Proc.* 10:126, 1951.

123. Sirota, J. H., and Narins, L. Acute urinary suppression after ureteral catheterization: The pathogenesis of "reflex anuria." *New Eng. J. Med.* 257:1111, 1957.

124. Smith, H. W. Note on the interpretation of clearance methods in the diseased kidney. *J. Clin. Invest.* 20:631, 1941.

125. Smith, H. W. *The Kidney: Structure and Function in Health and Disease.* New York: Oxford University Press, 1951.

126. Smith, H. W. Salt and water volume receptors: Exercise in physiologic apologetics. *Amer. J. Med.* 23:623, 1957.

127. Smits, H., and Freedman, L. R. Prolonged venous catheterization as a cause of sepsis. *New Eng. J. Med.* 276:1229, 1967.

128. Strauss, M. B. Acute renal insufficiency due to lower-nephron nephrosis. *New Eng. J. Med.* 239:693, 1948. Further data on lower-nephron and mercurial nephrosis. *Ibid.* 239:761, 1948.

129. Study, R. S., and Shipley, R. E. Comparison of direct with indirect renal blood flow,

extraction of insulin and Diodrast before and during acute renal nerve stimulation. *Amer. J. Physiol.* 163:442, 1950.

130. Swan, R. C., and Merrill, J. P. Clinical course of acute renal failure. *Medicine* (Balt.) 32:215, 1953.

131. Taylor, R. D., and Page, I. H. Origin of renal vasoconstriction in tourniquet shock. *Fed. Proc.* 8:155, 1949.

132. Teschan, P. E., Post, R. S., Smith, L. H., Jr., Abernathy, R. S., Davis, J. H., Gray, D. M., Howard, J. M., Johnson, K. E., Klopp, E., Mundy, R. L., O'Meara, M. P., and Rush, B. F., Jr. Post-traumatic renal insufficiency in military casualties. *Amer. J. Med.* 18:172, 1955.

133. Thiel, G., Wilson, D. R., Arce, M. L., and Oken, D. E. Glycerol induced hemoglobinuric acute renal failure in the rat: II. The experimental model, predisposing factors, and pathophysiologic features. *Nephron* 4:276, 1967.

134. Trueta, J., Barclay, A. E., Daniel, P. M., Franklin, K. J., and Prichard, M. M. L. *Studies of the Renal Circulation.* Oxford: Blackwell, 1947.

135. Truniger, B., Rosen, S. M., and Oken, D. E. Renale hämodynamik und hämorrhagische hypotension. *Klin. Wschr.* 44:857, 1966.

136. U.S. Army Surgical Research Unit. Proceedings, Study Group on Acute Renal Failure, Brooke Army Medical Center, Fort Sam Houston, Texas, Oct. 14–16, 1957. (Unpublished data.)

137. Van Slyke, D. D., Phillips, R. A., Hamilton, P. B., Archibald, R. M., Dole, V. P., and Emerson, K., Jr. Effect of shock on the kidney. *Trans. Ass. Amer. Physicians* 58:119, 1944.

138. Vertel, R. M., and Knochel, J. P. Nonoliguric acute renal failure. *J.A.M.A.* 200:598, 1967.

139. Wacker, W., and Merrill, J. P. Uremic pericarditis in acute and chronic renal failure. *J.A.M.A.* 156:764, 1954.

140. Wilson, D. R., Thiel, G., Arce, M. L., and Oken, D. E. Glycerol-induced hemoglobinuric acute renal failure in the rat: III. Micropuncture study of the effects of man-

nitol and isotonic saline on individual nephron function. *Nephron* 4:337, 1967.

141. Wilson, D. R., Thiel, G., Arce, M. L., and Oken, D. E. The role of the concentration mechanism in the development of acute renal failure: Micropuncture studies using diabetes insipidus rats. *Nephron* 6:128, 1969.

18

Urinary Tract Infection, Pyelonephritis, and Other Forms of Chronic Interstitial Nephritis

Lawrence R. Freedman

With the recognition of the importance of quantitative bacteriologic examination of the urine and the finding that large numbers of people are unaware of the presence of bacteria in their urine, culture of the urine has been utilized extensively in recent years and patients with urinary tract infections identified in ever increasing numbers. The parallel development of effective antimicrobial agents might have been anticipated to lead to the decline of urinary infections and pyelonephritis as serious clinical problems. Just the opposite has occurred. Interest in this area is steadily increasing, and the field abounds with controversy. The titles of a few papers exemplify some of the problems: "Asymptomatic Bacteriuria: A Therapeutic Enigma" [315], "Asymptomatic Bacteriuria, A Hypothetical Concept, Should Be Treated With Caution"

[220]. Perhaps even more to the point is the title of a recent symposium, "What Is Chronic Pyelonephritis?" [32].

These controversies may on the surface appear to be only semantic. I believe, however, that they indicate fundamental conceptual uncertainties which are frequently expressed in methods of patient care. It is common, for example, to encounter patients with serious urinary infections who are inadequately followed by their physicians. In contrast, other patients are treated for weeks or months with expensive and potentially toxic antimicrobial agents when the presumed infection did not exist at the outset. Particularly unfortunate is the subjugation of children to general anesthesia and potentially hazardous urologic diagnostic procedures without sufficient cause.

In order to deal with the issues that lie at

the heart of the controversies and remarkable differences in practice, it is necessary to begin by defining certain terms. *Chronic pyelonephritis* is kidney disease due to the immediate or late effects of bacterial infection in the renal substance and pelvocalyceal system. It can be suspected only when there is morphologic (radiologic) or functional evidence of renal disease and need not be associated with urinary tract infection at the time of study. On the other hand, *acute pyelonephritis* is either a pathologic lesion or a clinical symptom complex always associated with urinary tract infection which may, however, have no morphologic or functional components detectable by usual clinical technics. *Urinary tract infection* refers to the finding of bacteria in the bladder urine with or without clinical symptoms, with or without evidence of renal disease. Some authors use the term *bacteriuria* synonymously with urinary infections or restrict the term to the finding of bacteria in the urine of patients without pyuria or symptoms. Since there are no strict criteria for defining an abnormal number of white blood cells in the usual clinical examination of the urine and since eliciting a history of symptoms depends both on the patient's awareness of them and the physician's skill in detecting them, the broader term urinary tract infection will be employed to include all combinations of bacteriuria, pyuria, and symptoms of infection.

When one adheres to these definitions, it becomes apparent very soon that the majority of patients with urinary infections cannot be shown to have renal disease and the majority of patients with kidney disease morphologically resembling chronic pyelonephritis cannot be shown to have had their renal damage produced by the immediate or late effects of bacterial infection. It is necessary, therefore, to introduce another term, *chronic interstitial nephritis*, to designate those renal diseases with histologic findings resembling chronic pyelonephritis in which evidence of an etiologic

role for bacterial infection is lacking. Chronic interstitial nephritis which is believed due to bacterial infection becomes, in this scheme, just another way of saying chronic pyelonephritis. This system of classification is well established in Europe [127, 157].

The purpose of this discussion is to consider urinary infections, pyelonephritis, and other forms of chronic interstitial nephritis with emphasis on those concepts that provide a rational framework for patient management. At the outset, let us focus on the central area of debate, the relation between urinary infections and their potential for producing renal damage. Since the definition of the role of bacterial urinary infections in the production of chronic renal disease is intimately concerned with the problem of separating pyelonephritis from the larger group of morphologically similar interstitial nephritides, I shall begin with a description of chronic interstitial nephritis and a consideration of the various disorders capable of producing this type of renal disease.

Chronic Interstitial Nephritis

There is currently no way of accurately estimating the frequency or significance of chronic interstitial nephritis. It has become abundantly clear in the past five years, however, that there are many kinds of damage to the kidney which are expressed primarily as interstitial reactions. Interstitial changes, of course, are to some extent associated with all renal diseases. These changes are common in acute and chronic glomerulonephritis, diabetic kidneys with Kimmelstiel-Wilson nodular lesions, amyloidosis, and so forth. It is of considerable interest that decrease in a variety of renal functions correlates better with the amount of interstitial changes than with glomerular or vascular changes as seen in renal biopsy specimens [353]. In other disorders, interstitial changes represent the principal tissue reaction — for example, acute tubular necrosis, nephrocalcinosis, obstructive uropathy. In all these circumstances, however, characteristic lesions exist, permitting the application of a specific name which conveys morphologic if not pathogenetic distinction.

The issue becomes less clear when one turns to the lesions of nephrosclerosis. Here again, the kidney response is frequently interstitial, but the vascular lesion which is the presumed culprit not only may cause but may, following upon elevation of the blood pressure, be a result of the renal disease.

Confusion seems to have become the rule when one examines the use of the term chronic pyelonephritis, for here the tissue changes are also nonspecific, and it has been the custom to implicate bacterial infection in the pathogenesis of the lesion even when evidence of infection, at any time in the patient's life, was lacking. With such an open-ended set of diagnostic criteria it was no wonder that pyelonephritis became one of the most common causes of significant renal disease [5, 168, 267, 350]. The situation was still further complicated by the frequent superimposition of urinary tract infection and acute pyelonephritis in patients with other primary renal diseases as a result of infections resulting from indwelling catheters or diagnostic procedures involving instrumentation of the urinary tract [107].

This entire area is the subject of close scrutiny and careful investigation today. The clear identification of renal disease due to bacterial infection is of the utmost importance because these infections can be effectively combatted. Of equal importance, however, is the recognition that so many, perhaps the overwhelming majority, of the cases previously called nonobstructive pyelonephritis have other causes [15, 107].

Many of the interstitial nephritides are discussed in other chapters where they are identified by cause (e.g., obstructive uropathy) or by a unique morphologic feature (e.g., amyloidosis). In the future, when appropriate diagnostic technics are developed, all interstitial nephritides will have specific names. For the present, however, it is a convenient way of grouping renal diseases of unknown etiology with principally interstitial kidney changes, much as we use the term chronic glomerulonephritis for many renal diseases of unknown etiology with principally glomerular changes.

PATHOLOGY

The hallmark of chronic interstitial nephritis is cellular infiltration of the *interstitium* of the kidney, as a rule with lymphocytes and plasma cells (Fig. 18-1). Tubular atrophy and fibrosis are frequent, and foci of

Figure 18-1. Infiltration of plasma cells and lymphocytes between tubules and glomerular pericapsular fibrosis seen in chronic pyelonephritis.

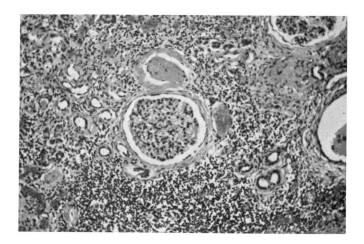

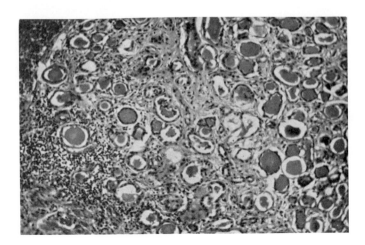

Figure 18-2. Typical colloid cast formation from a case of chronic pyelonephritis.

tubular dilatation and colloid cast formation may be prominent (Fig. 18-2). In some instances cast formation is so prominent as to give the appearance of thyroid tissue (Fig. 18-3). The scars may be separated by intervening zones of normal parenchyma or the scarring may be evenly distributed throughout the kidney. *Arteries and arterioles* located within scars may show medial hyaline change and intimal proliferation. Vessels in zones of normal kidney may be normal or similarly involved with hyaline and intimal changes. The level of blood pressure no doubt plays a significant role in the vascular changes in these otherwise normal zones of the kidney.

The state of the *glomeruli* is the most im-

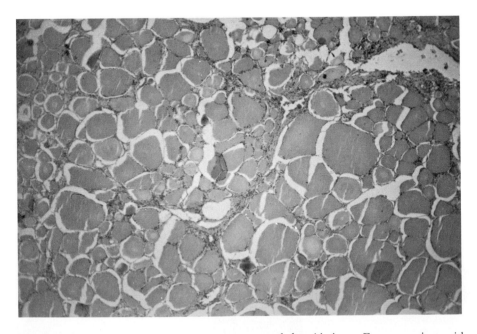

Figure 18-3. Colloid cast formation giving the appearance of thyroid tissue. From a patient with nephrosclerosis. No history of pyelonephritis. Urine cultures sterile.

portant finding distinguishing primary interstitial changes from those associated with primary glomerular disease. Although glomeruli within scars may be partially or completely hyalinized, glomeruli outside of these severely scarred zones are relatively normal (see Fig. 18-1) and, depending on the number of nephrons lost, hypertrophied. At autopsy, the extent to which normal renal architecture has been destroyed may be so great that the distinction between primary glomerular and interstitial disease is not possible. In addition, the alterative glomerulitis associated with severe hypertension and uremia may also render the separation of primary glomerular and interstitial diseases impossible [222]. Morphologically, these specimens are best referred to as *end-stage kidneys*. The nature of the process can be deduced only then if sufficiently distinctive clinical features were adequately documented during life.

The *renal papillae* are of much greater importance in the pathogenesis of renal parenchymal damage and functional change than their size suggests. Because a large number of nephron units occupying a considerable proportion of the surface of the kidney drain through papillae which are small in size and visible only when carefully searched for, changes in this zone may easily be overlooked and the role of papillary damage in the production of obvious cortical change not appreciated. Although the papillae may be affected with inflammatory changes to the same extent as the rest of the renal parenchyma, in other instances renal papillary necrosis or scarring is so prominent as to make it seem likely that damage localized to the renal papilla was responsible for the much more obvious widespread changes in the cortex.

Three special forms of severe renal papillary damage play a primary role in the production of severe interstitial nephritis: (1) acute papillary necrosis, (2) renal papillary sclerosis, and (3) medullary cystic change. *Acute papillary necrosis* is the form of injury which

until recently has received the greatest attention. This lesion consists of anemic infarction of the tip or central portions of the renal papillae. It has generally been considered to be a bilateral disease affecting most papillae, but in some patients the lesions occur in a single kidney or in one or two papillae [243]. The involved papillae may be separated from the remainder of the renal pyramid and may be found in the renal pelvis or excreted in the urine [250]. In some instances papillary fragments block the ureter, causing generalized hydronephrosis. Severe renal parenchymal infection usually accompanies acute papillary necrosis, and the possibility exists that infection plays a role in its pathogenesis. This view derives support from studies in rabbits where renal pedicle ligation for a short interval following the intravenous inoculation of *Escherichia coli* was associated with renal papillary necrosis and severe infection, whereas pedicle ligation or the intravenous inoculation of bacteria by themselves did not produce papillary necrosis or infection [117].

Severe *renal papillary sclerosis* may not be associated with evidence of renal infection but may, nevertheless, produce changes throughout the renal parenchyma typical of chronic interstitial nephritis [107]. The sclerotic process results in sharply demarcated acellular zones of papilla without evidence of surrounding inflammation (Fig. 18-4). To some extent these changes may be seen in kidneys from aged persons [217] and may be responsible for some of the cortical scar formation so common in kidneys from these patients.

Medullary cystic change is a lesion to which much attention has recently been directed. This subject has been carefully studied by Strauss and is considered in Chapter 36. For our purposes, the important point is that the cortical and medullary changes peripheral to cysts in the medulla are indistinguishable from chronic interstitial nephritis [107]. Indeed, many patients with severe renal salt wasting

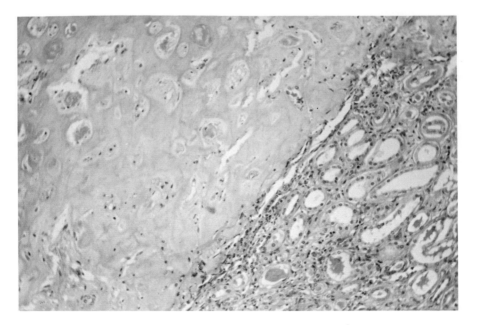

Figure 18-4. Severe papillary sclerosis in a patient with sickle hemoglobin and excessive consumption of analgesics. Urine cultures sterile. (Reprinted with permission from *Ann. Intern. Med.* [107].)

thought due to chronic pyelonephritis were later shown to have medullary cystic change accompanied by chronic interstitial nephritis without good evidence for a role of bacterial infection (Chapter 36).

It is of particular interest that the cortical projection of the interstitial changes accompanying papillary damage may be separated by zones of normal kidney (drained by uninvolved portions of papillae). The sharply demarcated interstitial changes produced by sterile papillary injury have been reproduced in animals (Fig. 18-5). In addition, cystic change throughout the kidney (resembling the infantile forms of polycystic kidney) has resulted from sterile papillary injury in the rabbit [101]. It appears, therefore, that papillary injury may result in focal tubular atrophy and chronic interstitial nephritis or cystic tubular change. The factors determining whether nephrons atrophy or dilate as a result of obstruction at the level of the renal papilla have not as yet been defined.

The *renal pelvis*, at autopsy, may be thickened and show changes of acute or chronic inflammation. Inflammation in this area is often the result of urinary tract infections, but because of the frequent superimposition of urinary infections in patients with other primary disorders, the presence of infection within the renal pelvis (or ureters or bladder) does not by any means establish infection as the cause of renal parenchymal disease.

The *gross appearance* of the kidney with interstitial damage will depend to a large extent on the nature of the underlying lesion. As a rule chronic renal insufficiency is associated with a considerable decrease in overall renal size to the extent that a single kidney will weigh less than 100 gm. The surface of the kidney may be finely or coarsely scarred and may have large deep scars separated by normal parenchyma. Although attention has been directed in the past to the significance of the shape of these large scars from the standpoint of pathogenesis, Heptinstall [172] does

Figure 18-5. Colloid cast formation (A) and glomerular pericapsular fibrosis (B) in the rabbit due to sterile mechanical injury to the renal medulla.

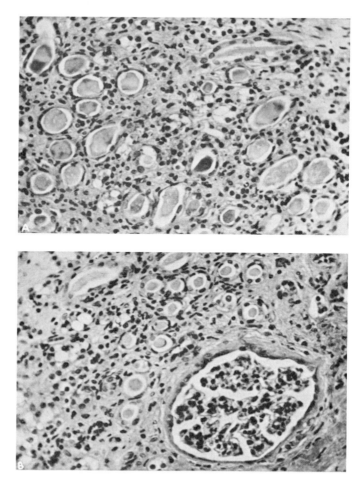

not find these distinctions useful. Asymmetrical involvement of the kidney has always been taken to favor infection as the causative agent, but it seems plausible that lesions of large or medium-sized arteries or asymmetrical papillary damage might result in a similar distribution of scarring.

PATHOGENESIS AND CLINICAL FEATURES

There are a great many injurious processes which produce significant interstitial changes in the kidney:

Obstruction [116, 166] (Chapter 27)
Nephrocalcinosis [261] (Chapter 24)
Potassium depletion [282] (Chapter 25)
Hyperuricemia [23a, 140, 369, 375] (Chapter 23)
Hypertension and renal vascular disease [232] (Chapter 20)
Diffuse intravascular coagulation [51]
Diabetes mellitus [329] (Chapter 22)
Congenital defects [69, 321]
Hereditary disorders [312] (Chapter 37)
Choline deficiency [18]
Immunologic reactions [369a, 370] (Chapters 11, 43)
X-irradiation [411] (Chapter 29)

Acute tubular necrosis [100, 106, 129]
  (Chapters 17, 30)
Sickle cell anemia [3, 107, 208, 289]
  (Chapter 33)
Hyperphosphatemia [184]
Leptospirosis [17]
Cystic disease of the renal medulla
  [107] (Chapter 36)
Sulfonamides [157, 172, 343]
Anticonvulsant drugs [157, 172]
Effects of aging [83, 214]
Lead and cadmium poisoning
  (see below)
Analgesic mixtures (see below)
"Balkan nephritis" (see below)
Bacterial infection (see below)

Almost one-third of the chapters in this book are devoted to detailed considerations of the renal diseases in which chronic interstitial change is a principal morphologic finding. It follows, therefore, that the clinical features and functional consequences of chronic interstitial nephritis can be understood only in relation to the particular disorder under consideration.

Certain *clinical features,* however, are common to those renal diseases with predominantly interstitial change. Most prominent is the absence of any symptom indicating the presence or the progression of renal disease. Frequently, patients will come to a physician for an unrelated complaint and be found to have hypertension, anemia, or some slight urinary abnormality. Much to the distress and surprise of the physician, the first determination of blood urea nitrogen may reveal it to be remarkably elevated, in the range of 100 to 200 mg. per 100 ml. These patients do not have episodes of ankle edema which bring patients with the nephrotic syndrome to a physician, and they do not have gross hematuria or periorbital edema which so often are the only clinical signs of acute glomerulonephritis. There may, of course, be prominent signs and symptoms of a variety of primary illnesses

which may underlie interstitial nephritis — for example, a history of renal colic, repeated episodes of pyelonephritis, diabetes mellitus, or severe hypertension.

There are three specific types of difficulties which, although not specific for interstitial nephritis, do serve to distinguish some patients with this type of renal disease: (1) increased urine production, (2) renal tubular acidosis, and (3) inability to conserve sodium. These problems have their origin in the disorders of renal tubular function resulting from damage to the papilla and interstitium of the kidney out of proportion to interference with renal blood flow and filtration at the glomerulus. *Increased urine production* resulting in polydypsia and polyuria (enuresis in children) is a consequence of inability normally to concentrate the urine. This condition is sometimes referred to as nephrogenic diabetes insipidus and is discussed in detail in Chapter 38. Interference with the mechanisms of *urinary acidification* may result in the syndrome of renal tubular acidosis producing symptoms related to potassium depletion (muscle weakness), urinary calcium loss (osteomalacia, renal stone, growth disturbances in children), or glycosuria and aminoaciduria (see Chapter 30). Finally, *inability to conserve sodium* (salt-losing nephritis) may lead to severe salt depletion with hypotension and vascular collapse much as one sees in Addison's disease (see Chapter 30).

The point to be emphasized here is that the most common alteration of renal function involves a proportionate loss of glomeruli and tubules and is not different from any other chronic renal disease. The unusual syndromes due to preponderant tubular dysfunction are, however, more common in interstitial nephritis than in glomerulonephritis, but these syndromes do not indicate the specific basis for the underlying disease process. A more detailed discussion of the medullary functional changes in relation to disease process is given in the section on *Chronic Pyelonephritis.*

LABORATORY FINDINGS

Examination of the Urine. Urinalysis may point to interstitial nephritis when abnormal elements are sparse, as is often the case when urinary concentrating power is diminished. On the other hand, there may be many casts and cellular elements, depending on the underlying process and whether or not infection is present. White-cell casts may be particularly helpful in calling attention to renal interstitial inflammation [15, 333]. Protein excretion is generally slight (less than 3.0 gm. per day) except when heart failure or very high blood pressure supervenes. There may be considerable proteinuria, of course, if interstitial nephritis should coexist with a glomerular lesion (amyloid, diabetes mellitus) promoting the filtration of protein.

Pyelography. The wide variety of patterns seen by excretory pyelography are described in other chapters according to underlying disorders. Aside from specific lesions such as obstruction, renal stone, and papillary necrosis, there seems to be considerable disagreement from one observer to the next as to the radiologic appearance of the kidney in different disease states. Based on the careful observations of Hodson [181], it is evident that interstitial nephritis is most commonly associated with irregularly spaced indentations of the outline of the kidney in association with papil-lary scarring, in contrast to chronic glomerulonephritis which is generally accompanied by symmetrical shrinkage of the kidney without papillary deformity. In practice, however, it is not uncommon to encounter patients to whose pyelogram the diagnosis pyelonephritis (caliectasis) is applied but who, when examined years later after many bouts of typical clinical acute pyelonephritis, are said to have normal kidneys on pyelography (Fig. 18-6). Conversely, patients with nonbacterial chronic interstitial nephritis (as far as could be determined) at autopsy may have symmetrical shrinkage of the kidney without papillary deformity by x-ray when examined during the course of the illness [107].

Although diagnostic criteria are not precise in the adult, Hodson and Wilson [182] have called particular attention to the pyelographic changes that occur in children with pyelonephritis (these will be considered later in this chapter). In general it can be stated that the uncertainties concerning the x-ray changes in kidney disease are only one facet of the general problem of correlating data across the disciplines of pediatrics, medicine, pathology, and radiology for diseases that extend over considerable time periods. These uncertainties are compounded by the obvious long list of possible causes of similar histopathologic and functional changes in the kidney.

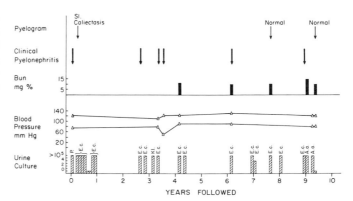

Figure 18-6. Clinical course of pyelonephritis in a married woman, age 21 when first seen. The urine cultures were positive virtually throughout 10-year period with six episodes of typical acute pyelonephritis. Blood pressure, blood urea nitrogen (BUN), and pyelogram have remained normal. P. = paracolon, E.c. = *E. coli,* Kl. = Klebsiella, A.a. = *Aerobacter aerogenes.*

Specific Forms of Chronic Interstitial Nephritis

ANALGESIC NEPHROPATHY AND RENAL PAPILLARY NECROSIS

Since the original suggestion by Spühler and Zollinger [382] relating excessive intake of analgesic mixtures (containing phenacetin, aspirin, caffeine, and often codeine) to chronic interstitial nephritis and renal papillary necrosis, evidence has continued to accumulate, leaving little doubt about the validity of the association [118, 128]. The excellent epidemiologic studies of Ulla Bengtsson [35] demonstrate clearly the increased frequency of analgesic abuse in women with interstitial nephritis, papillary necrosis, and urinary infection compared to those with interstitial nephritis and urinary infection alone. Bengtsson's subsequent report [36] and the careful work of Grimlund [141] go one step further to demonstrate the secondary nature of bacterial infection in the production of renal damage by these agents. The work of Gault et al. [122] and Dawborn et al. [79] substantiate these findings, and it seems possible now, after a number of equivocal efforts, to produce papillary necrosis with analgesic mixtures in animals using amounts of drugs comparable to those taken by patients [70, 99, 224].

Many questions concerning the nature of the agent(s) and the mechanisms involved remain unanswered. The difficulties in resolving these issues have been stated by Schreiner [356] and Gilman [124]. However, the original caution about accepting the existence of any causative relation between analgesics and interstitial nephritis seem to have been resolved [85c, 224a].

I am convinced that one of the main reasons relatively few patients with this association have been reported in the United States has to do with the effort necessary to obtain such a history. Grimlund [141] and Bengtsson

[36] have commented previously on the reluctance of many patients to admit to the ingestion of excessive quantities of analgesics. In my experience, a history of analgesic abuse is rarely volunteered. Many of these patients are neurotic, and when asked if they take any medicines, they usually reply in the negative. In the past year alone I have seen 10 patients with chronic renal disease who had been interviewed by a medical student, intern, resident, and frequently a fellow and private physician in whose notes no mention had been made of what was later found to be long-standing daily usage of analgesic compounds. Most patients do not consider nonprescription medications as drugs and therefore do not volunteer this information when asked if they are taking medications.

The difficulty in obtaining a history of analgesic abuse raises the question as to whether other forms of papillary necrosis may be related to drug toxicity. Other clinical states that have been implicated as predisposing to renal papillary necrosis include: severe bacterial interstitial nephritis [116, 133, 212], diabetes [243], urinary obstruction [364], sickle cell disease states [3, 208, 247a, 289], and chronic alcoholism [87, 259].

Harrow [160] has raised the possibility that obstruction might not be as significant a factor as previously believed and suggests that some ureteral obstructions considered primary might have been due to impacted papillary tissue — that is, a result of papillary necrosis perhaps due to analgesic excess. In this regard, I recently saw a chronic alcoholic patient with acute papillary necrosis who only after weeks of hospitalization with detailed questioning admitted to the excessive use of analgesics. Peptic disease may also be a consequence of this drug habit [79, 122, 302].

In a recent review of patients with chronic interstitial nephritis it was found that some patients with primary renal papillary disease have a variety of conditions predisposing to this disorder [107]. It is likely that there are many factors which, in combination, contribute to the production of renal papillary necrosis. This may, in part, explain why not all abusers of analgesics develop renal disease, but it may also point to a damaging role for quantities of analgesics not ordinarily considered toxic.

It is well known in man and has been shown in animals that papillary injury may serve as a nidus for renal stone formation [102, 330]. One wonders what role toxins may play in the general problem of renal stone. A recent report suggests that Worcestershire sauce, when taken in large quantities, may act in this fashion [292], and excessive analgesic intake has been documented in 27 per cent of one series of female stone formers [39]. The likelihood is that many agents will be discovered in the years to come, which, when passing through the renal medulla during the process of excretion into the urine, will achieve concentrations toxic to this zone of the kidney. It is not surprising that discovery of such agents should coincide with a period in our thinking about chronic renal disease which acknowledges our ignorance and reduces so many traditional terms to what they really are, hypotheses [217a].

Renal papillary necrosis is said to be found in 1 per cent of routine autopsies and in 3 to 7 per cent of autopsies of diabetic persons [243]. I suspect that this underestimates the true prevalence since frank papillary necrosis may be easily overlooked and there are no clear definitions for the classification of sclerotic lesions of the papilla which may not be frankly necrotic [66a].

Pathogenesis. The agent or agents responsible for analgesic nephropathy have not been identified, but vascular occlusion seems to be the lesion of importance. Small-vessel changes found in papillary necrosis in man have been carefully described by Lagergren and Ljungqvist [239] and point to papillary vascular insufficiency as the common denominator in urinary obstruction, diabetes mellitus, and analgesic abuse. Microscopic lesions of the vasa recta have also been described in experimental analgesic toxicity [224, 226a]. The excellent studies of Hill [178] in rats and rabbits suggest that the availability of collateral vascular channels to the renal papilla plays a significant role in determining its susceptibility to papillary necrosis. Papillary necrosis has been produced in animals by a variety of technics including anoxemia [129], toxins [243], dietary deficiency states [40], and by the intravenous administration of heterologous serum [142, 309].

Clinical Course. The clinical features of analgesic nephropathy are not distinctive. Women seem to abuse analgesics to a much greater extent than men do. The intake of various over-the-counter remedies appears to be so common that analgesic abuse should be suspected in any patient with renal disease or recurrent urinary tract infection. Psychoneurotic women, factory workers, and patients with headache are particularly prone to develop the habit.

As is the case with most types of chronic interstitial nephritis, prior to the development of renal insufficiency the patient is unaware of the progressive nature of his renal disease. When papillary damage ensues, it may take the form of fulminating illness or may progress so insidiously that the patient remains without symptoms until the stage of severe renal insufficiency develops [400a].

Acute papillary necrosis is almost uniformly associated with urinary tract infection and severe bacterial interstitial nephritis. The patients become seriously ill rapidly, and bacteremic shock may supervene. Other patients will present with severe acute pyelonephritis that will not respond satisfactorily to what would be expected to be effective antibiotic therapy. Kidney tenderness, signs of peritonitis, leukocytosis, and heavy pyuria may persist despite sterilization of the urine. Renal func-

urinary excretion of white cells is estimated quantitatively [188].

WHITE BLOOD CELL CASTS. Casts composed of polymorphonuclear leukocytes are commonly found during periods of active infection of the kidney, and represent good evidence of inflammation in renal parenchyma [333]. It is important, therefore, to carry out a painstaking examination of a fresh, acid urine specimen, since this may be one of the most reliable clues to diagnosis of chronic pyelonephritis. Unfortunately, white blood cell casts are sometimes found in other renal diseases and, therefore, cannot be considered pathognomonic of pyelonephritis.

HEMATURIA. Red blood cells are frequently found in small numbers in the urine of patients with pyelonephritis. Because they do not appear aggregated into tubular casts, it is thought that they originate in inflammatory foci distal to the renal parenchyma.

ALBUMINURIA. Massive proteinuria is uncommon in chronic pyelonephritis; the great majority of patients with this disease excrete less than 3 gm. of protein per day [229]. In the absence of congestive heart failure or malignant hypertension, excretion of more than 3 gm. per day argues against the diagnosis of chronic pyelonephritis as the main cause of renal disease.

EFFECT OF ENDOTOXIN ON URINE SEDIMENT. Pears and Houghton [311] and others [317] have described a sudden outpouring of leukocytes and nonsquamous epithelial cells in patients with pyelonephritis following intravenous injection of bacterial endotoxin. This phenomenon occurred within the first 30 minutes and was thought not to be related to changes in renal blood flow or body temperature. The effect was prevented by cortisone or aspirin and did not occur in normal patients. The phenomenon, while of interest, is not completely specific for pyelonephritis, since positive tests may be obtained also in patients with acute and chronic glomerulonephritis,

essential hypertension, and urethritis [93, 188, 284]. The test, as originally described, requires catheterization in the female and special technics of cell enumeration. Furthermore, endotoxin injection may be uncomfortable for the patient. Subsequent studies have demonstrated a similar increase in urinary excretion rate of white cells after the intravenous administration of prednisolone phosphate, and a measure of this urinary excretion rate can be obtained from the study of voided midstream urines, thus obviating the need for catheterization [206, 207, 253, 255]. These two modifications make it much easier to conduct the test and will undoubtedly permit more extensive inquiry into its usefulness.

Pyelography. The studies of Hodson and his colleagues [181, 182, 371] have focused attention on the occurrence of coarse scarring of the kidney in association with retraction of the corresponding papilla and dilatation of the calyces in children with urinary infections. As discussed earlier, these changes are of great clinical interest and offer the possibility of being able to document the development of renal disease as a consequence of infection. The remarkable aspect of Hodson's studies is the rarity of this change in adults, despite the common occurrence of acute symptomatic pyelonephritis. Indeed, careful study of the radiologic sequelae of acute pyelonephritis in adults by Little, McPherson, and de Wardener [257] have shown a decrease in overall kidney size in the affected kidney but no scarring in association with papillary deformity. The possibility exists that this decrease in size represents resolution of swelling present during the stage of acute inflammation.

It is still unsettled in my mind whether the changes described by Hodson have been shown to result from urinary tract infection in subjects with previously normal kidneys. In my own experience, I have not seen radiologic changes develop or progress in patients with urinary infections who did not have some other complicating lesion (e.g., analgesic excess or obstruction). Persky [313] has had a similar experience.

The lesions described by Hodson deserve continued study. Particularly important will be the results of correlations of clinical course with pathologic findings. The observations of Smith [374], providing the pathologic correlation of the x-ray findings of Hodson, were limited in number, were carried out in patients judged to have obstruction, and were rarely accompanied by clinical evidence of infection.

Renal Biopsy. Changes consistent with the diagnosis of chronic pyelonephritis are often demonstrated by percutaneous renal biopsy. This may support the clinical diagnosis, but cannot be relied upon as the sole evidence, because, as has already been pointed out, most or all of the histologic findings can be caused by other processes (see page 673). Conversely, the finding of normal renal tissue does not exclude a diagnosis of chronic pyelonephritis, because of the known patchy distribution [109, 169, 213, 221]. It must be borne in mind that needle aspiration provides a sample representing only about 1:10,000 of the total renal mass. Culture of biopsy tissue or of the needle is usually nonproductive in chronic pyelone-

phritis since in most cases bacteria are not found. Renal biopsy, therefore, has limited value as a clinical tool for the diagnosis of this disease.

Disturbance of Renal Function. MECHANISMS. The most direct effect of bacterial infection on renal function results from the destruction of nephrons. Although irreparable damage can occur at any level of the nephron, the tubular portion is apt to suffer to the greatest extent, since bacterial multiplication appears to begin in the medulla. In tissue sections, glomeruli are often seemingly untouched despite considerable adjacent inflammation (Fig. 18-9). The extensive inflammatory reaction, which may lead to scarring and other permanent alterations in the interstitial tissues, would be likely to interfere with tubular transport systems more than with glomerular filtration. It appears also that, because of their smaller total mass, medullary structures suffer proportionately greater injury from inflammation than cortical elements. This effect should be greater the more pointed the renal papilla. Furthermore, tubular functional abnormalities may vary with changes in the extent and character of the inflammatory exudate [27].

There are several mechanisms in pyelonephritis which could cause disturbance of renal

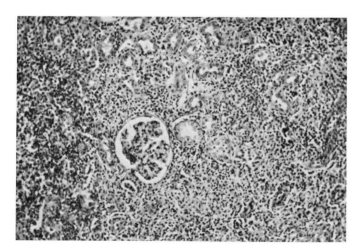

Figure 18-9. Preservation of glomerulus despite extensive acute inflammation in surrounding tissue. From a fatal case of postpartum acute pyelonephritis.

blood flow [52, 177, 183, 240]. The endotoxins of the gram-negative bacteria are known to have potent effects on small blood vessels. The elevated blood pressure so frequently associated with pyelonephritis may injure arterioles and small arteries, and the local effect of infection may affect blood vessels of all sizes. Kimmelstiel and Wilson [222] noted that a nonspecific type of glomerular scarring, sometimes resembling glomerulonephritis, is often a prominent finding in chronic pyelonephritis in the absence of uremia and hypertension. It may also be associated with proliferative endarteritis. These lesions seem to be unrelated to bacterial infection and offer a possible explanation for progressive deterioration of renal function despite the absence of infection.

Tissue necrosis resulting from infection or vascular changes predisposes to renal calcification and stone formation, processes which also may worsen the degree of renal insufficiency. The passage of concretions, necrotic tissue, or purulent debris can cause damage to the ureter, thereby interfering with the outflow of urine. This may in turn injure the kidney by its direct effect on renal function or by its tendency to increase further the kidney's susceptibility to infection. An additional means of injury in pyelonephritis is the possible nephrotoxic effect of antimicrobial drugs, such as sulfonamides, neomycin, or kanamycin [230, 425].

PATTERNS. Various abnormalities of renal function have been described in pyelonephritis in man [304, 328].

OVERALL REDUCTION IN FUNCTIONING MASS. This type of renal insufficiency is by far the most common result of pyelonephritis [229]. The manifestations are not distinctive and resemble those of any other disorder that results in chronic renal failure. The one feature which may suggest pyelonephritis or chronic interstitial nephritis is that the course of chronic renal insufficiency is unusually slow in progression. Addis [2] stated that "any prolonged uremic or suburemic state should in itself suggest the possibility of an inactive chronic pyelonephritis."

IMPAIRED ABILITY TO CONCENTRATE URINE. The concentrating ability of the kidney is believed to be largely a function of a countercurrent system located in the renal medulla. The ways by which pyelonephritis may damage this mechanism have already been described. It is of interest, therefore, that this defect, out of proportion to a decrease in glomerular filtration rate, is detected more frequently in patients with chronic pyelonephritis than in those with chronic glomerular nephritis [229]. Similar changes in maximal concentrating ability have been found in experimental pyelonephritis of rats [27, 131]. A decrease in maximal urinary concentration may be detected in renal insufficiency from other causes, because each surviving nephron must excrete an increased load of solute [55]. The significant point is that in pyelonephritis impairment in concentrating ability may be detected at a time when glomerular function is relatively normal [22, 386, 413]. The demonstration that ureteral obstruction also impairs renal concentrating ability may account for this functional abnormality in some patients with pyelonephritis [192, 326, 412].

OTHER ABNORMALITIES. A variety of other renal tubular disturbances have been described in patients thought to have chronic pyelonephritis and are considered in detail in other chapters. These include nephrogenic diabetes insipidus, sodium-losing nephritis, hyperchloremic acidosis, and potassium-losing nephritis. These disorders are rare and have been described in patients with various renal diseases. Although of great importance to the patient and of interest physiologically, their detection is of little value in establishing the nature of the underlying disease process.

Hypertension. The relationship of chronic pyelonephritis to hypertension is the subject of intense study and great controversy [85a].

There appears to be more than a chance association between the two conditions. The critical questions are:

1. Does pyelonephritis cause hypertension before renal insufficiency is evident, or only after renal insufficiency is evident?
2. Does pyelonephritis accelerate the course of essential hypertension?
3. Does hypertension increase susceptibility to pyelonephritis and urinary tract infection?

Some of the difficulties in attempting to answer these questions are related to lack of general agreement about basic terms such as hypertension, renal insufficiency, and chronic pyelonephritis.

The vascular lesions in the pyelonephritic kidney are discussed initially since, aside from generalized decrease in renal mass, it is these lesions that have led many workers to postulate a renal basis for hypertension. Weiss and Parker [406] studied the blood vessels in pyelonephritis in great detail. Their view, derived from the experimental studies of Goldblatt, was that narrowed vessels resulting from inflammation of the renal parenchyma were responsible for the development of hypertension, which, in turn, narrowed other renal vessels and aggravated the vascular process which initiated the cycle.

Kincaid-Smith [223] presented a somewhat different concept, based on the suggestion that narrowed vessels in pyelonephritic kidneys produced renal parenchymal changes called ischemic tubular atrophy. These areas were described as "showing small nephrons with glomerular crowding due to tubular atrophy. The atrophic tubules had small lumina lined by cuboidal epithelium." These atrophic tissue changes had previously been called incomplete infarcts by Fahr [92] and resemble the changes in Selye's [358] "endocrine kidney." Kincaid-Smith suggested that the vascular le-

sions described by Weiss and Parker may be found in pyelonephritis without hypertension and that it is the parenchymal lesion of ischemic tubular atrophy which is best correlated with high blood pressure. This lesion is not specific for pyelonephritis, however, since it is found in most cases of hypertension due to any type of renal disease as well as in essential and malignant hypertension not due to renal disease, and is most commonly associated with a marked decrease in renal mass [74, 226, 244]. The prevalence of ischemic tubular atrophy remains to be determined in cases of renal contraction where hypertension has not developed.

A similar tissue change is also characteristic of hydronephrosis. There is a sound explanation for this, since renal blood flow is diminished under the conditions of increased intrarenal pressure produced by obstruction to urine flow. If this lesion is the basic change associated with renal hypertension, it is surprising that high blood pressure is not more common in hydronephrosis [34], although recent studies suggest that age may be an important factor [368]. The interpretation of these lesions is further complicated by the demonstration by Heptinstall et al. [175] that ischemic tubular atrophy may result, in animals, from the parenchymal effects of infection alone without vascular occlusion demonstrable in tissue sections or by angiography.

The excellent angiographic studies of Hill [177] have fully confirmed Heptinstall's [172] view that organic vascular narrowing does not play a role in the production of the pyelonephritic scar. However, there is arterial vasoconstriction during the acute phase of infection which may well play a major role in the pathogenesis of the pyelonephritic lesion [52]. Indeed, short periods of vasoconstriction alone in animals may result in scarring of the kidney which is indistinguishable from the scars produced by infection [100, 106]. It is of interest to consider what role anoxemia may play in the events taking place in the kidney after transplantation.

Thus, a great deal has been learned about the sequence of events leading to the scars of pyelonephritis and the relation of these scars to vascular change, but pathologic studies have not been able to clarify the relation between hypertension and pyelonephritis.

The clinical relationship between pyelonephritis and hypertension is not better established. Isolated cases have been reported in which it is believed that unilateral pyelonephritis has produced hypertension in the absence of renal insufficiency [373]. It is also well established that renal insufficiency, whatever the cause, may be associated with hypertension. The point of contention relates to the role of pyelonephritis in the pathogenesis of what might be called "essential hypertension" prior to the development of renal insufficiency.

The frequency of hypertension in patients with pyelonephritis has been reported to range from 11.8 to 84.5 per cent, depending on methods of selection of patients, the criteria used for the diagnosis of hypertension and pyelonephritis, the ages of the patients, the presence of a family history of hypertension, and the stage and type (obstructive, atrophic, etc.) of renal disease [42, 56, 299]. One can find figures to support virtually any argument. Experimental studies have shown that hypertension can be produced and aggravated by pyelonephritis only when the infection is severe and widespread [174, 361].

In two studies evidence of histologic pyelonephritis has been found in 13.5 per cent [155] and in 51.5 per cent [379] of patients with essential hypertension. However, it is necessary to keep in mind the difficulties in making this diagnosis, particularly by biopsy, in the presence of hypertension [169]. The point to be emphasized in all these studies is that few of them have related pyelonephritis to bacterial infection. Not until this has been accomplished will it be possible to talk of the effects of pyelonephritis.

The findings of Sowry [380] and Kincaid-Smith et al. [226] are of particular interest in determining the relationship of pyelonephritis and hypertension. These workers noted that the incidence of a positive family history of hypertension in patients with pyelonephritis and high blood pressure was as high as it is in patients with essential hypertension. This is not true of patients with glomerular nephritis and hypertension, suggesting that patients with hypertension have an increased susceptibility to pyelonephritis. Experiments in animals support this viewpoint, since Woods [418, 419] and Shapiro [361, 362] have both shown that rats with hypertension due to administration of desoxycorticosterone have an increased susceptibility to pyelonephritis. Interestingly, rats with hypertension due to unilateral renal artery occlusion did not show this tendency [176].

In recent years a number of epidemiologic studies have focused particularly on the relation between urinary infection, chronic pyelonephritis, and hypertension. Kass and his associates [204, 279] were the first to find significantly higher mean blood pressure levels in women with urinary infections as compared with noninfected women. The findings were similar in a study of Japanese women [113] and were suggestive in three studies conducted in the United States [63, 238, 377]. Although the differences were small in all the studies and not statistically significant in the studies from the United States, all of them have demonstrated higher blood pressure values in bacteriuric women.

It is unlikely that the Japanese women had serious renal involvement since mean serum urea nitrogen levels were no different from those of controls [115]. On the other hand, the women with chronic pyelonephritis studied by Bengtsson [35] had very high levels of diastolic blood pressures even at a time when serum creatinine values were normal and, furthermore, family history data suggested that increased susceptibility to pyelonephritis did not alone explain the frequency of hypertension in subjects with pyelonephritis.

In summary, it appears that there are small increases in blood pressure in women with urinary infections and perhaps larger increases in women with pyelonephritis. There may be an increased susceptibility to pyelonephritis in subjects with hypertension, and pyelonephritis may be responsible for blood pressure elevation prior to the development of renal insufficiency. The relationship between pyelonephritis and hypertension is extraordinarily complex and is not likely to be easily resolved. Whatever the outcome in women, however, it must be emphasized that in none of the studies reported to date has a sufficient number of urinary infections in men been detected to suggest that urinary infections or pyelonephritis plays any significant role in the problem of hypertension in that sex. Even among women, the differences in blood pressure related to environment, race, and mode of living are not significantly influenced by eliminating subjects with urinary infections. *It seems clear, therefore, that although there is an intriguing and only partially defined relation between urinary infection, pyelonephritis, and blood pressure level, this relation does not appear to be important to the general problem of essential hypertension.*

Renal Stone. There is dispute as to the role of pyelonephritis and urinary tract infection in the formation of renal stone. Baker and Connelly [21] state:

There is no conclusive published evidence that infection, per se, is the etiological factor in human calculus disease. It is granted that recurrent pyelonephritis due to Gram-negative organisms thriving in an alkaline urine has considerably more than a chance association with calculi. The fact is that only a very small percentage of patients with acute or chronic pyelonephritis actually develop calculi, and approximately one-half of all patients with renal calculi have no infection.

On the other hand, Mortensen et al. [287] found chronic pyelonephritis to be the third most common cause of roentgenologically demonstrable nephrocalcinosis, accounting for 15.4 per cent of 91 cases. These data are difficult to interpret because of uncertainty regarding meaning of the terms pyelonephritis and urinary tract infection. In addition, one would have to define what was meant by renal stone. Anderson and McDonald [10] found microscopic renal calculi in all individuals over the age of 9.

Doubtless many factors can contribute to calcification within the genitourinary tract. Hellström [165] lists these:

1. A change in the solubility of stone-forming substances in the urine.
2. The occurrence in the urinary tract of, for example, epithelial defects, necroses or blood clots, which may serve as nidi for the stone-forming substances.
3. An obstacle to urinary flow, which prevents the excretion of the aforementioned stone nuclei, or of already formed minute concretions.

It is evident that urinary tract infection and pyelonephritis are capable of contributing to stone formation in all these categories.

Bacteria are well known to cause an increase in the pH of urine, thus making the common constituents of stones — that is, calcium phosphate and magnesium ammonium phosphate — markedly less soluble. In addition, any febrile or debilitating illness would increase urinary content of calcium salts.

Damage to the papilla produced by renal infection gives rise to foci which, under proper conditions of pH, etc., can become calcified [49, 102]. Randall [330] believed that the papillary damage due to pyelonephritis was the underlying lesion, which later became calcified, resulting in the formation of a plaque that could then break off and become a nidus for stone formation. That such plaques, however, are not the sole factor necessary for stone formation is illustrated by the study of Vermooten [402] in Africa. He found the frequency of Randall's plaque at autopsy in Africa to be as great as that in the Caucasian population in the United States; nevertheless, in Africa stone formation was extremely rare.

Stone formation within the urinary tract, by obstructing the flow of urine, undoubtedly increases susceptibility of the kidney to infection. The rates of infection in the presence of renal stone have varied from 47 per cent in some series [66] to 2 per cent in others [276]. A factor here is that instrumentation performed in diagnosis and treatment of stone is likely to introduce bacteria into the urinary tract, thus providing the ingredients for serious infection and renal damage.

A recent study by Braude and Siemienski [47] is of considerable interest in relating stone formation to urinary infection with L-forms of bacteria. These authors were able to detect bladder stone formation in rats in which Proteus L-forms had been injected into the urinary tract. The fascinating finding was that stones developed at a time when the bacterial L-forms could not be recovered from the urine and yet stone formation could be prevented by the administration of antibiotics.

Treatment. When a microorganism can be isolated from the urinary tract, it is evident that vigorous therapy should be administered. The particular antimicrobial agent should be selected according to in vitro sensitivity tests. This subject is considered in detail in the section devoted to urinary tract infection.

The management of renal disease due to infection is otherwise similar to the management of any irreversible renal disease. The guiding principle is to prevent continued destruction of nephrons. As pointed out previously, progressive renal damage may not be directly related to the agent which initiated disease. This concept is of particular importance in the management of patients with chronic pyelonephritis since their course, even

after the detection of renal insufficiency, is often slowly progressive. After a thorough search for evidence of reparable urinary obstruction, attention should be focused on preventing the introduction of bacteria into the urinary tract. Agents that are potentially nephrotoxic should be avoided, and meticulous care must be provided for minor illness such as colds or gastrointestinal upsets which might result in even transient dehydration. A detailed discussion of the care of patients with renal insufficiency is to be found elsewhere, and the principals of antibiotic therapy in the management of urinary infections are presented later in this chapter.

Urinary Tract Infection

In contrast to the difficulties encountered in the diagnosis of chronic pyelonephritis, the presence of urinary tract infection is established with a single simple laboratory test: urine culture. Nevertheless, much remains to be learned about the natural history of these infections.

Our attention will be focused on bacteriologic methods necessary for interpretation of urine cultures, significance of bacteriuria, natural history of urinary tract infection, and evaluation of therapy. Although the literature devoted to these problems is vast, much of it is difficult to evaluate, because of the use of qualitative bacteriologic technics. In addition, failure to recognize the role of instrumentation of the urinary tract in the initiation of infection and inadequate periods of follow-up after therapy have complicated interpretation.

MICROBIOLOGY

The Normal Urinary Tract. Observations on animals have demonstrated that the kidney, normally sterile, is a poor trap for bacteria. Approximately 1 in 10,000 microorganisms inoculated into the bloodstream lodge there [147]. Coliform bacteria, the most common pathogens to affect the urinary tract in man, are as a rule not able to establish infection in normal animal kidneys. Those bacteria that are arrested in the kidney slowly disappear without causing injury to the organ.

Bladder urine is normally sterile [423]. Bacteria are not excreted into the urine unless there is tissue infection. This is true even after the intravenous inoculation of those pathogens that produce infection in the normal kidney [116, 149].

In man, bacteria are normally present in the lower urethra, but they tend to diminish in frequency toward the bladder. The urethral mucosa appears to have some antibacterial effect, like that of the skin. In addition, this epithelial surface is frequently flushed toward the outside by urine flowing over it [179, 273, 385]. The predominance of urinary infections in females suggests that the male urethra might offer a greater barrier to bacteria than that of the female because it is longer and its meatus is relatively free from fecal contamination. In addition, Stamey et al. [384] and Gupta et al. [143] have demonstrated the antibacterial properties of prostatic fluid, a factor which may be of considerable significance in protecting the male from ascending urinary infections.

The Infecting Bacteria. The bacteria associated with urinary tract infection are a mixed group, most of which are constituents of the intestinal flora. The frequency with which different species have been isolated from the urine has varied somewhat, depending on the source of the patient population, the particular clinical problem under study, the bacteriologic technic, and the interpretation of the results [218].

The predominant cause of urinary tract infection is the coliform group of bacteria. These are found in at least 80 per cent of cases where infection has developed in the absence of obstruction, uninfluenced by antimicrobial treatment or urologic manipulation [104]. The remainder is comprised of several other groups: Proteus, Pseudomonas, Klebsiella, Aerobacter, Enterococcus, and Staphylococcus.

In patients who have acquired their infections in hospitals and have been treated by antimicrobial agents and by instrumentation of the urinary tract, the proportion of coliform isolations decreases considerably and infections due to enterococcus, proteus, Klebsiella, and pseudomonas bacteria assume greater importance [65, 218, 336]. One explanation is that mixed infections may be common, but are overlooked because a single species, usually the coliform, suppresses growth of another. When growth of the coliform is prevented by a chemotherapeutic agent, the less susceptible species is able to thrive and to be detected. In animals, however, it has been exceedingly difficult to produce pyelonephritis with two bacteria [341]. Pseudomonas infections are almost exclusively observed in patients who have been subjected to urethral instrumentation; the frequency with which this bacterial species is encountered in tap water and its resistance to many common sterilizing agents suggest iatrogenic infection. The circumstances under which klebsiella, aerobacter, proteus, or enterococcal infections develop in hospitals suggest transmission from person to person, via hands, catheters, bed pans, etc., analogous to the problem of "hospital staphylococcal" infections [218, 227, 272].

A small percentage of infections are caused by enterococci and staphylococci. In the older literature, staphylococci were reported as causing about 10 per cent of urinary infections. With the advent of quantitative bacteriologic technics, it has become apparent that staphylococcal urinary tract infection is comparatively rare. When such infections occur they are frequently associated with the hematogenous dissemination of bacteria such as is seen in osteomyelitis.

Although it is unusual for bacteria to produce infection in normal animal kidneys, certain strains are able to produce pyelonephritis with relative ease: enterococci [91, 130,

149], staphylococci [103, 116, 133, 136, 139], *E. coli* [420], Pseudomonas [132, 135, 137, 393], Proteus [403]. In other instances the slightest change in the animal host preventing the operation of normal defense mechanisms in the bladder can lead to prolonged bacteriuria [212].

Factors influencing nephropathogenicity of various bacteria have been studied experimentally [46, 58, 241, 322]. In man, some studies have shown certain types of bacteria to predominate in urinary infections [191, 215, 216, 390]. However, the general view is that the strains of bacteria recovered from the urine are representative of their distribution in the environment [215, 234, 236, 335, 399, 405].

Infections may also rarely be caused by *Bacillus anitratum,* Bacteroides, and various yeasts and fungi [94, 150, 156, 164, 203, 274]. Tubercle bacillus and gonococcal infections will not be considered here, since they present unique problems of pathogenesis, detection, and therapy and do not produce the type of pyelonephritis under discussion. Nevertheless, it is important to keep in mind the possibility of urinary tract tuberculosis as a cause of renal disease upon which common gram-negative infections may be superimposed. (See Chapter 40 for discussion of renal tuberculosis.)

Kidney tissue is an excellent host for viruses in the laboratory, and viruria is well known in many diseases. There has been scant evidence to implicate a virus etiology for urinary tract disease in man. Recent studies, however, suggest that there is a viral etiology for some cases of hemorrhagic cystitis in children [297]. To strengthen the potential role of viruses in urinary tract disease, Ginder [125] has convincingly produced an interstitial nephritis with adenovirus in the mouse and has demonstrated that infected animals have an increased susceptibility to *E. coli* pyelonephritis. It has also been observed that a variety of viruses survive satisfactorily in normal human urine [195].

PATHWAYS BY WHICH BACTERIA REACH THE KIDNEY

Controversy exists as to the pathways by which bacteria reach the kidney. Three main routes have been suggested: hematogenous, lymphatic, and urinary. Consideration of the available evidence leads to the conclusion that the hematogenous pathway, while possible, is probably not the common one [29]. Experimental and clinical evidence pointing to extraureteral lymphatic routes is scanty. There is, on the other hand, a wealth of clinical experience and substantial experimental evidence to indicate that the common pathway in pyelonephritis is the passage of bacteria from the bladder cavity to the kidney via the ureter.

It is sometimes possible to identify the means by which bacteria gain access to the bladder urine. Instrumentation of the urinary tract frequently precedes the onset of typical acute infection. It is presumed that bacteria are carried from the lower urethra to the bladder cavity by the catheter or cystoscope [148]. Large numbers of bacteria can make their way up the urethra and into the tissues of the upper urinary tract in animals [119]. The counterpart of this may be represented by fecal soiling of the urethral meatus in infants. Mechanical trauma to the female urethra during sexual intercourse seems to play a part in some instances, notably the infections that occur shortly after marriage. In children, bubble bath has been noted to be a factor of significance in some cases [24, 268].

Considerable attention has recently been directed to the role of urine as a culture medium in the pathogenesis of urinary infections [196, 289b, 389a, 405a]. Although it has long been known that the growth of bacteria in the urine was dependent on pH and osmolality [120, 190], it has only recently been emphasized that the first morning urine is not optimal for bacterial growth [19, 209]. Furthermore, urine from women appears better suited to support bacterial growth than that from men, and urine from pregnant women is better still [19]. In addition, as in the pleural and peritoneal cavities, bacteria in the bladder are not subject to surface phagocytosis encountered in body tissues, nor are they completely discharged from the bladder after micturition, since a film of urine coats the surface of the bladder, thereby supplying an inoculum for fresh supplies of urine entering from the ureter. Thus, there is a plausible explanation for the prolonged persistence of bacteria in urine and an intense curiosity about the mechanisms which permit most persons to maintain sterile bladder urine [86].

The ease with which bacteria are transported from the bladder cavity to the kidney is suggested by many clinical observations. For example, it is commonplace to obtain a history of symptoms of cystitis or urethritis preceding by hours or days the typical clinical picture of acute pyelonephritis. Instrumentation of the bladder is a well-known forerunner of pyelonephritis, undoubtedly related to contamination of urine and perhaps to the tissue trauma associated with instrumentation [210]. The importance of bacteriuria in the cause of pyelonephritis is clearly demonstrated by the studies of Kass [203] comparing the frequency of pyelonephritis in pregnant women, some of whom were treated for bacteriuria and some of whom were not. Pyelonephritis developed in as many as 40 to 50 per cent of those with untreated bacteriuria and in none whose urine cultures had been made sterile.

The facility of ascending infection has also been demonstrated in animals [8, 344]. Vivaldi et al. [403] inoculated bladder urine with an organism capable of producing infection in the normal kidney, and observed that division of the ureter markedly decreased the incidence of infection to that kidney. Studies of the ability of bacteria to rise against the flow of a stream have also supported the view that bacteria make their way to the kidney within the ureter [407].

Considerable emphasis has been placed on the role of ureteral reflux in facilitating the spread of bacteria from the bladder cavity to the kidney. It must be emphasized, however, that except for instances where there is total interruption of the urinary pathway, there is always a fluid connection between the kidney and the bladder [360]. In addition, observations on the character of normal flow down the ureter have shown that dye particles simultaneously ascend in the turbulence immediately adjacent to the ureteral wall [319].

The evidence seems convincing that most infecting bacteria reach the renal parenchyma by way of the urine, traveling in a direction opposite to its flow. *This important concept serves as the basis for the most promising means of preventing bacterial infection of the kidney, the elimination of bacteria from bladder urine.*

CLINICAL FACTORS INFLUENCING THE DEVELOPMENT OF URINARY TRACT INFECTIONS

Age, Race, and Sex. Surveys of large populations of school children and adults have demonstrated definite increasing rates of urinary infections with increasing age in both sexes (Fig. 18-10). Females with infections far outnumber males throughout all ages [281a]. In the study by Kunin et al. [236] of school children only two infections were found among nearly 8000 schoolboys between the ages of 5 and 19. In a survey in Japan no infections were found in 1200 adult males between the ages of 18 and 49 [113].

Although the preponderance of urinary infections in women has been recognized for some time, only recently has the magnitude of variation with age been appreciated. In addition, there is evidence that race (sickle hemoglobin [408]) and socioeconomic status also influence the rates for these infections [285, 398].

It has long been postulated that the shorter

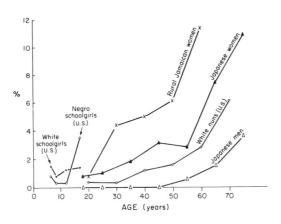

Figure 18-10. Prevalence of positive urine cultures. The data are from Miall et al. [279], Kunin et al. [236, 238], and Freedman et al. [113] and include surveys in which subject participation exceeded 80 per cent and the number of subjects in each age range exceeded 100.

female urethra is related to the higher rates of infection among women [76a]. However, the antibacterial properties of prostatic fluid may account for some of the resistence in men [143, 384], and the properties of urine as a culture medium may bear on this issue also [19].

Childbearing and sexual activity along with relaxation of the pelvic floor have usually been considered responsible for the increasing rates with age among women. Whereas this is substantiated to some extent by the lower rates of urinary infection in nuns, it is also evident that the effect of aging on susceptibility to infection is considerable even in women who do not bear children (Fig. 18-10) [238].

Pregnancy. The prevalence of urinary tract infections in pregnancy has varied widely in different studies depending on the bacteriologic methods employed and the character of the patient population. Bacteriuria has been detected in from 2 to 13 per cent of pregnant women, the rates being higher with increasing age, parity, frequency of sickle hemoglobin, and with lower socioeconomic status [198, 279, 295, 398, 408]. In general, positive urine cul-

tures are found in about 7 per cent of pregnant women. Although it has long been the clinical impression that pregnancy increases susceptibility to urinary infections [29] and experiments tend to support this view [12, 323a], it is not clear, considering all the factors to be controlled, whether urinary infections are more common during pregnancy than in similar groups of nonpregnant women. One must be particularly alert to stone presenting as pyelonephritis [159] and to pyelonephritis masquerading as toxemia of pregnancy [95].

It has been shown without question that among pregnant women with urinary infections, the rates of symptomatic pyelonephritis (40 to 50 per cent) are considerably lowered (5 to 10 per cent or less) by successful antibiotic treatment. The extent to which new infections arise in women with initially sterile urine cultures has varied among different studies, but new infections do occur, in some studies the number exceeding that detected at the initial prenatal visit. Thus, one cannot rely on a single urine culture, early in pregnancy, for the prevention of all cases of bacteriuria and pyelonephritis in pregnancy.

Considerable uncertainty exists concerning the significance of urinary tract infections in pregnancy. One of the most important clues relating bacteriuria to renal damage has been the demonstration of decreased urinary concentrating ability in pregnant women with urinary infections and a prompt increase in concentrating ability after sterilization of the urine [88, 197, 295, 295a, 296, 357]. Previous work in animals has suggested that changes in concentrating ability were related in part, at least, to inflammation or alterations in blood flow in the papilla [27]. It is also known, however, that large numbers of bacteria may persist in the pelvis of the animal kidney without producing renal damage [108]. Although it is not known whether concentrating defects can result from bacteria constantly bathing the renal papilla in the absence of renal damage, the possibility has certainly not been excluded.

In some series of pregnant women with urinary infections, pyelographic evidence of infection was common, particularly in women refractory to antibiotic treatment [225, 246]. On the other hand, using careful criteria to determine those pyelographic changes likely to have resulted from infection, high rates of acquired renal damage have not been observed [138].

Turning again to the evidence for functional renal damage, it should be emphasized that urinary infection by itself can produce changes in ureteral activity [392] and the superimposition of the hydronephrosis of pregnancy might result in the urinary concentrating difficulties due to obstruction alone [192, 326, 412]. Functional changes, therefore, may not be an unequivocal sign of renal damage due to destruction of the renal parenchyma by bacteria. Studies of antibody response have also been utilized as a measure of renal involvement in pregnant women with asymptomatic urinary infections, but the results cannot be considered conclusive [295]. Thus, functional, radiologic, and immunologic data suggest that urinary infections may damage the kidney during pregnancy. The relation remains unclear, however, since the functional changes are completely reversible, the radiologic changes may have preceded the infection, and the immunologic studies are indirect.

An association with toxemia of pregnancy was recognized many years ago, but the figures were based on unacceptable bacteriologic methods [314]. Recent studies have come up with all the possible results: no relation [82, 254], increased rates of toxemia in subjects with urinary infections [225, 389], and finally, decreased rates of toxemia in subjects with urinary infections [308]. Nevertheless, the subject is of great interest and probably of considerable significance to the general question of the cause of chronic interstitial nephritis. Weiss and Parker [406] noted the frequency with which toxemia was recorded in their patients with contracted kidneys, and the as-

sociation was commented on again recently in a study of chronic interstitial nephritis at autopsy [107]. The dangers of toxemia of pregnancy have been emphasized, and it will be no easy matter distinguishing the consequences of toxemia alone from those of toxemia and urinary infection. Part of the difficulty is establishing criteria for the diagnosis of toxemia of pregnancy.

Since Kass's initial studies, there has been intense interest in the relation between prematurity and urinary infections [26, 56a, 295, 352]. The subject is extraordinarily complex due to the many factors that can influence the birth weight. Most observers are agreed that whatever the effect of urinary infection in pregnancy on premature births, these infections could be responsible for only a small fraction of the large problem. Clearly, bacteriuria in pregnancy should be treated, with careful attention directed to the use of antibiotics which will not harm the fetus. It is possible, however, that the risk of urinary infections will be found to be greatest in women with preexisting renal disease [225, 246] or with the microangiopathy of diabetes [320].

A measure of the complexity of the issue can be seen by examining the effect of antibiotic therapy of urinary infections on prematurity. Many investigators have been able to "reduce" the rates of prematurity by successful antibacterial treatment. On the other hand, Elder and Kass [88] have data that suggest a beneficial effect of antibiotics in pregnancy even in patients without bacteriuria. This is of interest since antibiotics have also been recommended for the treatment of toxemia of pregnancy because of their effect on the intestinal bacterial flora [54]. The extensive literature concerned with urinary infections in pregnancy has been critically reviewed by Norden and Kass [295] and Beard and Roberts [26].

Urinary Obstruction. A frequent finding in patients with urinary tract infection and pyelonephritis is some type of lesion of the urinary tract impeding the outflow of urine. Lesions include neurogenic disorders, stricture, congenital valve, stone, or tumor. Although some have claimed that obstruction underlies all urinary tract infection, this does not seem to be the case. Careful urologic studies disclose a large group of patients in whom no extrarenal obstruction can be demonstrated. The reasons why renal susceptibility to infection is increased with urinary obstruction are given elsewhere in this discussion.

It is important to emphasize that obstruction above the level of the bladder is usually not associated with spontaneous infection. Observations in animals substantiate this. When ureteral obstruction is produced with meticulous attention to sterility at the time of operation, spontaneous infection does not occur [116]. This is an impressive finding since the susceptibility of the obstructed kidney to infection is considerably increased [147, 266, 322, 344]. Furthermore, even the increased susceptibility to infection produced by obstruction diminishes with the passage of time [112, 151].

These facts become critical when managing patients with obvious urinary obstruction who are not infected. One must weigh carefully the risk of introducing infection into a damaged urinary tract at the time of investigation or operation against the risk of doing nothing. As Bricker and Klahr point out (in Chapter 27), many obstructive lesions are compatible with good renal function and are not progressive. The introduction of bacteria into an obstructed urinary tract at the time of diagnostic or "therapeutic" manipulation may, however, lead to rapid and total destruction of the kidney.

Diabetes Mellitus. Diabetic patients are said to have very high rates of pyelonephritis as judged by autopsy diagnoses [90, 337]. It was of considerable interest, therefore, that surveys of urinary infection in patients with diabetes, when compared with subjects without diabetes, carefully matched for age and sex, have not shown differences between the groups [189, 305, 334]. In a survey of children with diabetes, the rates of urinary infection were comparable to those in nondiabetic children. Similarly, during pregnancy, diabetic women could not be found to have definitely increased rates of urinary infection [320]. Only in the study of Vejlsgaard [401] have diabetic women had significantly higher rates for urinary infection than nondiabetic women. This study is open to question, however, since the comparisons were made on the basis of a single clean-voided urine specimen. It might be anticipated that a single voided urine culture would be more likely to give false-positive results in diabetic than in nondiabetic women because of vulval irritation related to glycosuria.

Even if rates for urinary infection are not higher in diabetic patients, the possibility remains that pyelonephritis is more likely to result from urinary infection in diabetic than in nondiabetic subjects. Examination of autopsy series suggests, however, that it is not the altered metabolic state of diabetic patients but rather the severity of the renal disease that correlates best with the pathologic diagnosis of pyelonephritis [90]. Even this is unlikely, however, since autopsy evidence has, in general, not been adequate to determine the role of bacterial infection in the pathogenesis of interstitial scarring of the kidney. Raaschou [329] excluded diabetic persons from a study of pyelonephritis "because it is extremely difficult to separate the histologic pyelonephritis changes from the interstitial, inflammatory changes which appear as a consequence of the diabetic angiopathy." Thus, it cannot be stated whether the morphologic lesions of pyelonephritis are more common in diabetic as compared with nondiabetic persons, and convincing differences in the rates of urinary infections have not been found in the clinic.

Clinical evidence is incontrovertible, however, in assigning an important role in the production of metabolic disturbance to any infection in diabetes. In addition, diabetic subjects are especially liable to the serious, life-threatening complication of papillary necrosis [243, 337]. It is of the utmost importance, therefore, to take all measures to avoid unnecessary instrumentation of the urinary tract in diabetic patients and to eliminate or suppress bacterial growth in the urine.

Instrumentation of the Urinary Tract. Patients subjected to catheterization or other forms of urethral instrumentation risk infection and cannot be fully protected by prophylactic antimicrobial therapy [30]. Insufficient attention has been paid to these procedures as a cause of renal infection in many patients with unrelated renal diseases. This factor in urinary tract infection is the one most easily controlled by the physician. There is no longer justification for routine catheterization during parturition, and employment of an indwelling catheter as a standard procedure in the management of diabetic acidosis is to be condemned.

Patients with neurologic diseases, such as poliomyelitis and spinal cord injury, who have difficulty in control of micturition often develop pyelonephritis [65, 336, 394a]. These infections are undoubtedly favored by the introduction of bacteria into bladder urine due to the necessity for constant bladder drainage. Renal susceptibility to infection may also be increased by the obstruction of urine flow caused by nephrocalcinosis and urinary calculi which result from immobilization and demineralization of bone.

A great deal of experience has now been gained with the use of suprapubic needle aspiration of the bladder in lieu of urethral catheterization [20a, 271a, 346a, 385]. In addition, suprapubic drainage of bladder urine through a polyethylene catheter may be a useful procedure in postoperative states and in instances of transient inability to void in the male [155a]. The avoidance of urethral trauma and indwelling catheterization may significantly hasten recovery and decrease the risks

of initiating a urinary infection. It must be remembered that urine samples obtained directly from the bladder, particularly after forced hydration, are likely to have low numbers of bacteria (10^2 to 10^3) due to acute dilution even in the presence of significant infection. If the only type of culture carried out is that of a 1:1000 dilution of urine (as is the case in many hospitals), true infections may readily be overlooked.

CONTRIBUTIONS OF EXPERIMENTAL PATHOLOGY TO KNOWLEDGE OF FACTORS WHICH PREDISPOSE THE KIDNEY TO INFECTION

Role of Obstruction. The clinical observation that obstruction of urine flow is an important predisposing factor in pyelonephritis has received much support from animal experiments. Many workers have found that, whereas the normal kidney exhibits little susceptibility to coliform bacterial infection, the obstructed kidney is easy to infect [134, 147, 266].

The mechanisms by which interference with urine flow increases the susceptibility of the kidney to infection is still not clear. The phenomenon was first ascribed to increased trapping of circulating bacteria, or to interference with their excretion. Subsequent experiments have shown that neither of these factors can be responsible. "Stagnation of urine flow" is frequently cited as the responsible factor, the assumption being that urine not moving steadily toward the outside provides a medium in which bacteria can grow profusely, thus furthering a tendency to spread into the tissues of the urinary tract. This has been discussed in some detail elsewhere [112], and it is concluded that stagnation cannot be the sole factor in the initiation of infection; there must also be some secondary effect of the increased tissue pressure in the kidney [14], possibly on blood flow or on the biochemistry of the tissues.

As long ago as 1911, Brewer [53] showed that mechanical bruising of the renal parenchyma, in the absence of ureteral obstruction, increased the susceptibility of the kidney to coliform bacterial infection. Braude et al. [45] observed a similar effect from renal massage. De Navasquez [81] demonstrated susceptibility to coliform infection in rabbits which had sustained intrarenal scarring after recovery from staphylococcal pyelonephritis. The effect of all these procedures may be due to intrarenal obstruction of urine flow, not essentially different from obstruction at any lower level [110, 322, 340, 344].

Obstruction and consequent dilatation of the bladder has an important role in interfering with clearance of bacteria from the bladder urine. Distention of the bladder wall decreases blood flow to the bladder mucosa, thereby impairing the delivery of leukocytes and antibacterial serum factors [275], and the effect of residual urine on facilitating bacterial multiplication in the bladder cavity is well known clinically and experimentally [179]. It may be this effect of increasing bladder distention and provision of a constant source of "residual" urine which accounts for the adverse effects of water diuresis on host defense mechanism in the bladder of animals [108, 212].

Critical Importance of the Renal Medulla. The studies by Rocha et al. [344] revealed that infections which occurred within obstructed nephrons seemed to originate in the medullary portion of the kidney, since bacterial multiplication could be detected there before it was evident in the cortex. Further investigation of this finding, by direct inoculation of bacteria into different zones of the kidney, revealed that renal medullary tissue was far more susceptible to infection than cortical tissue [110]. Fewer than 10 coliform bacteria produced infection when injected into the medulla, whereas approximately 100,000 were required to infect the cortex. Studies with other bacteria have confirmed the exquisite sensitivity of the renal medulla to infection [103, 149].

The peculiarities of the renal medulla are further illustrated by the work of Paplanus [307], demonstrating that coliform bacteria which persist in the kidney for some hours or days after intravenous inoculation are located almost exclusively in the medulla. Rocha and Fekety [342] demonstrated that the inflammatory response was considerably delayed in the renal medulla as compared with the cortex providing a good basis for the facilitation of infection in this zone of the kidney.

Another explanation for the peculiar susceptibility of the medulla may be related to its role in ammonia production. This is suggested by studies showing that kidney homogenates interfere with the bactericidal action of blood serum on gram-negative bacteria [33]. The action was traced to inactivation of the fourth component of complement, a process which paralleled in vitro formation of ammonia by kidney tissue. Tests of this hypothesis in living animals showed that rats given an acid load, thus stimulated to excess ammonia production, developed typical acute pyelonephritis following intravenous injection of *E. coli.* The altered susceptibility could be nullified by the administration of alkali [111]. These studies were confirmed by Lyon and Tuttle [262], who went further and correlated infection with tissue ammonia content. Here, then, is susceptibility to infection on a biochemical basis, separate from any detectable morphologic abnormality of the kidney. Since the principal contribution of ammonia to urine occurs low in the nephron, these data are in accord with other findings regarding susceptibility of renal medullary tissue.

In studies of ascending renal infection in rats, particular attention has been directed to the initiation of infection in the fornices of the renal pelvis [8, 170]. This may be important in accounting for species differences in susceptibility to infection since there appear to be differences in the anatomy of the pelvic fornices among different animals [316].

Following the demonstration by Braude et al. [48] of bacterial variants in urine as a consequence of the action of antibiotics on bacterial cell walls, attention was immediately directed to the role of these cell-wall-deficient forms (spheroplasts, protoplasts, L-forms) in the pathogenesis of pyelonephritis. It was found that osmotically fragile bacterial forms could survive, revert to parent forms, and multiply in the hyperosmotic renal medulla but not in the cortex [4]. Variants that could not revert to parent forms have not been found to multiply or to produce renal lesions [415]. Variants have been identified in patients with urinary infections following antibiotic therapy and seem to be the form in which bacteria persist prior to reversion in some patients [144, 145]. Osmotically fragile forms have been detected indirectly by Eastridge and Farrar [84] and Guze and Kalmanson [152, 153] following penicillin treatment of enterococcal pyelonephritis in rats.

Since the survival of osmotically fragile bacterial variants depended on the conditions existing in the renal medulla, and since it was possible to lower the osmolality of the papilla by water diuresis, it appeared that a rational basis was provided for the time-honored clinical practice of forcing fluids in the treatment of pyelonephritis. Andriole and Epstein [11a, 11b, 13] demonstrated the beneficial effects of water diuresis on hematogenous pyelonephritis in rats, and Andriole [11] demonstrated the facilitation of the inflammatory response in the medulla by water diuresis. Mahoney and Persky [265] have shown similar benefits from water diuresis in a stone forming proteus infection.

In contrast to the above studies, the effect of chronic water diuresis on *E. coli* in the bladder urine is to facilitate bacterial multiplication [108]. Whereas as many as 10,000,000 *E. coli* placed in the bladder urine of man or normal animals are promptly cleared, as few as 10 multiply and persist for prolonged periods in animals undergoing water diuresis. Even though large numbers of bacteria are present in the renal pelvis under the conditions of these experiments, renal damage was not

found in rats. In mice, on the other hand, chronic bacteriuria in the presence of water diuresis led to severe pyelonephritis and papillary necrosis [212]. Thus, the effects of water diuresis in animals depend very much on the animal species tested, the microorganism employed, and the place at which it is introduced into the urinary tract. Despite traditional practice, the effects of water diuresis on pyelonephritis and urinary infections in man are not known.

The observations of Beeson and Rowley stimulated a search for other physiologic changes in the renal medulla or urine which might interfere with naturally occurring or acquired host defense mechanisms. Solutions of high osmolality and high urea concentration interfere with antigen-antibody combination, serum bactericidal systems, leukocyte sticking, phagocytosis, and bacterial multiplication [1, 25, 64, 68, 73, 186, 242, 281, 299]. Urine of low osmolality, on the other hand, makes certain microorganisms more susceptible to the action of antibiotics, but at the same time dilutes the concentration of antibiotic in the urine and in general provides a better medium for bacterial growth [301]. The effect of lowered urinary pH has a similar double effect in the urinary tract: Bacterial growth in the urine is inhibited [19, 209], but renal susceptibility to infection is increased [111]. The problem is further complicated by the effects of residual urine, frequency of voiding [179, 179a, 299a, 300], and the operation of an intrinsic bladder defense mechanism probably related to the availability of phagocytes [71, 98, 289a, 294a, 404].

It is apparent from these studies that it is no longer possible to consider the urinary tract as a single system when considering the pathogenesis of infection. Changes that favor bacterial multiplication in the urine may at the same time facilitate host defense mechanisms in the kidney and vice versa. Indeed, one cannot even think of the kidney as a single system because dramatic events occurring in the renal papilla may not significantly influence the environment of the renal cortex [11, 342]. When one adds the action of antibiotics to this complex system, there are the additional factors of urinary concentration and pH effect which must be considered [59, 201a, 301]. In addition, different microorganisms are influenced differently by changes in blood flow and physiologic environment, and animal species differences add still another dimension to the problem. It is necessary to conclude, at this time, that it is not clear from studies in animals whether forcing fluids works to the advantage or disadvantage of the patient with gram-negative urinary tract infection.

The studies of the effect of water diuresis in preventing clearance of E. coli from the bladder urine of animals point to the remarkably delicate balance between bacterial multiplication and host defense mechanisms as they operate in the bladder urine. The ability of a slight physiologic change such as water diuresis to bring about a 1,000,000-fold decrease in the efficiency of host defense mechanisms is a fact that may be useful in understanding phenomena that have been observed in the production and treatment of urinary infections in man.

The Role of Antibody. There has been speculation for many years concerning the role of antibody in the production of chronic pyelonephritis in man. Since it was so difficult to identify viable bacteria in kidney scars thought due to bacterial infection, it was suggested that perhaps inflammation persisted, causing progressive renal damage after bacteria had deposited their foreign antigens in the kidney [15a, 85b, 203a]. Studies in animals have demonstrated the persistence of antigen in the kidney damaged by bacterial infection at a time when viable bacteria could no longer be recovered [75, 347, 348]; renal damage, however, does not progress to involve portions of the kidney initially undamaged by infection. The significance of this antibody, which re-

cently has even been shown to be produced by antibody-forming cells in the kidney [245], is unknown.

Similarly, serum antibody has been shown to protect the animal kidney to some degree against hematogenous and ascending pyelonephritis [16, 97, 187, 349], but a role for these antibodies in human disease has not been identified [9, 60, 234, 295, 347, 414]. Furthermore, Kalmanson et al. [200, 201] were unable to correlate the different natural histories of pyelonephritis due to enterococci in rats and rabbits with the production of antibacterial antibody or with the enhancement of serum bactericidal properties.

Miscellaneous Factors in Susceptibility to Infection. Other kinds of injury increasing the susceptibility of the kidney to infection include hypertension and vascular disease [361, 418, 419], hypokalemia [421, 422], certain drugs (e.g., sulfonamide [343], analgesics [425]), and vascular obstruction [57, 129]. Possible explanations for these effects include damage to medullary nephrons (hypokalemia, sulfonamide) and alterations of blood flow (hypertension, renal vascular occlusion, analgesics). Whatever the ultimate explanation, it seems likely that several factors will eventually be recognized as favoring the initiation of infection in what we may now regard as the normal kidney.

Relation of Acute to Chronic Pyelonephritis. Studies of localized renal infections have provided an unusual opportunity to observe the evolution of pyelonephritis. The area involved is typically wedge-shaped, resembling the naturally occurring lesions of acute pyelonephritis in man. As this progresses through healing and fibrosis the area contracts, with only a linear scar remaining. The remarkable thing is that adjacent zones of renal tissue are not invaded by the infectious process [103, 110, 116, 344].

The evolution of the scarring process has been studied in detail by Heptinstall [172] and

Guze and his associates [52, 378], and the vascular changes in these lesions have been carefully documented by Hill [177, 178]. Despite the persistence of bacteria in some of these lesions for as long as a year, the long-term functional and morphologic changes do not seem to extend beyond the original zone of injury [52, 116, 131, 149, 363, 378]. Thus, chronic pyelonephritis in man may be conceived of as the end result of multiple circumscribed areas of infection.

PATHOLOGY OF ACUTE PYELONEPHRITIS

Acute pyelonephritis is characterized histologically by abscess formation in the renal parenchyma and the accumulation of polymorphonuclear leukocytes around and within tubules. Bacteria are often demonstrable in the foci of acute renal suppuration, and they are always present in large numbers in the urine. Glomeruli tend to be spared, and may remain as untouched islands within abscesses (see Fig. 18-9), though in severe lesions they too may be destroyed. Areas of infection are characteristically wedge-shaped, with the apex in the medulla. Because of this configuration, tissue destruction is invariably greater in the cortex than in the medulla [110]. Relative to its size, however, the inflammatory response would be expected to disturb the milieu of the medulla to a greater extent than that of the cortex [27, 116].

The distribution of the wedge-shaped areas of acute pyogenic infection is characteristically focal, sharply demarcated from areas of uninvolved parenchyma. In animals, where the progression of such lesions can be studied in detail, there is a notable lack of tendency to spread laterally. Only when there is ureteral obstruction, in animals or in man, is the entire kidney apt to be uniformly affected by acute pyogenic infection [110].

Polymorphonuclear leukocytic infiltration not associated with abscess formation occurs in many other kinds of renal injury. Such infiltration has been noted in man in association with drug toxicity, leukemia, acute glomerulonephritis, tubular necrosis, anoxemia, and ureteral obstruction (see Fig. 18-8) [5, 116, 172, 173, 306].

Evidence has accumulated from different laboratories indicating the presence of vascular spasm in the early stages of acute pyelonephritis [52, 172, 177]. It is of interest, in this regard, that short periods of vascular occlusion have been shown in animals to result in changes which very closely resemble those of chronic pyelonephritis [100, 129]. Vascular spasm may therefore be a significant factor in the pathogenesis of the pyelonephritic scar.

CLINICAL FEATURES OF URINARY TRACT INFECTION

Urinary tract infection may become clinically apparent in various ways. The fully developed features of *acute pyelonephritis* are characteristic. The patient is usually a woman between 15 and 40 years of age who complains of a sudden onset of fever, chills, flank pain, and frequent, burning urination. These symptoms often appear to be related to sexual intercourse or bladder catheterization. The patient may have noted cloudiness or a red discoloration of the urine. Sometimes the urine has a foul fishy odor. The pain of urination may be severe. The major finding on physical examination, in addition to fever, is tenderness of the kidney. This may be most marked anteriorly or posteriorly. Kidney pain is characteristically located in the lumbar region, although it may also be felt in the epigastrium, suggesting acute cholecystitis, or in one of the lower abdominal quadrants, thus making difficult the differentiation from acute appendicitis or diverticulitis.

There is often a polymorphonuclear leukocytosis, and urinalysis as a rule reveals an abundance of bacteria, polymorphonuclear leukocytes, clumps of white cells and white-cell casts. Red blood cells are often found during this stage of infection; sometimes the urine is grossly bloody. Hematuria usually disappears with the subsidence of the acute illness. The persistence of hematuria after the stage of acute infection should demand a search for evidence of other disease.

The development of abdominal pain in someone known to have bacilluria may present difficult problems of differential diagnosis. However, the finding of pyuria is as a rule sufficient to incriminate the urinary tract as the source of symptoms. Confusion may arise also in distinguishing pyelonephritis from glomerulonephritis. Abdominal pain is common in acute glomerulonephritis, and frequently the patient is seen after hematuria has subsided, when polymorphonuclear leukocytes may be the only abnormality of the urine sediment. Such patients may be thought to have bacterial infection of the kidney; however, repeatedly sterile urine cultures, profuse proteinuria and the ancillary signs of glomerulonephritis (hypertension, elevated streptococcal antibody titers, congestive heart failure, and azotemia with a normal phenolsulfonphthalein (PSP) excretion) are usually sufficient to distinguish the two diseases.

Azotemia does not result from uncomplicated acute pyelonephritis. Elevation of the blood urea nitrogen may, of course, occur in patients with underlying renal disease, obstruction, or circulatory collapse associated with gram-negative rod bacteremia. Hypertension, also, does not result from acute infections [229]. When acute pyelonephritis is associated with renal papillary necrosis, renal function may become severely compromised [243].

In contrast to the description just given, acute infection of the urinary tract may be accompanied by few signs and symptoms. The patients may complain only of back pain, or the symptoms of cystitis or urethritis, such as suprapubic pain, urgency and frequency of urination, and dysuria. Sometimes, particularly in children, the only complaint may be enuresis and incontinence of urine during the

day. In infants, the principal difficulty may be failure to thrive. Occasionally urine cultures will not reveal abnormalities during the first two or three days of symptoms — possibly because of walled-off infection of the kidney. Rarely, bacilluria appears only after the spontaneous disappearance of fever.

The onset and persistence of symptoms may vary considerably. In general, the acute illness lasts for only two to five days, then begins to subside. Along with the subsidence of symptoms there is a return of the white blood cell count to normal, and there may even be disappearance of white cells from the urine.

Even without therapy, the signs and symptoms of acute urinary tract infection frequently disappear promptly (Fig. 18-11). Despite complete relief of symptoms, bacteria continue to be found in the urine. It follows, therefore, that *alleviation of symptoms cannot be equated with bacteriologic cure.* Any agent directed against the infectious process must be evaluated by culture of the urine. This principle is most important, not only for proper evaluation of therapeutic agents but for the proper management of the patient. There is no substitute for urine culture in attempting to determine the presence or absence of urinary tract infection.

In the natural course of events the patient with symptomatic urinary tract infection, following the subsidence of symptoms, becomes a patient with asymptomatic bacteriuria. In the absence of therapy, and often despite therapy, asymptomatic bacteriuria has been observed to persist for years. The affected person may intermittently have acute flareups of signs and symptoms. On rare occasions bacteriuria may transiently disappear during asymptomatic periods only to return some months later, with or without symptoms (Fig. 18-12).

Although bacteriuria is common and the majority of patients may never develop significant kidney damage, there can be little question that some of these individuals develop serious renal disease. Evidence demon-

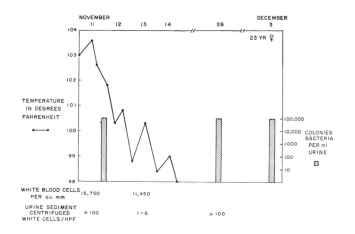

Figure 18-11. Clinical course of a case of *untreated* acute pyelonephritis. Flank pain and tenderness and dysuria had disappeared 72 hours after the patient's admission to the hospital. The patient remained without symptoms during the follow-up period despite repeated cultures showing large numbers of *Escherichia coli*.

strating the relationship between bacteriuria and chronic pyelonephritis is reviewed in the following section. It is not possible to anticipate which patients with bacteriuria will develop significant renal disease or how long this process might take. The conclusion seems inescapable that efforts should be made to eliminate bacteria from the urinary tract of any patient.

RELATIONSHIP BETWEEN BACTERIURIA AND PYELONEPHRITIS

Bacteriuria is found so commonly in hospital populations that its significance has been

questioned. As the preceding discussion has emphasized, the transport of bacteria from bladder urine to kidney is most likely the principal pathway by which the kidney becomes infected. In considering the meaning of bacteriuria, however, it is of equal importance to emphasize that large numbers of bacteria in the urine also result from kidney infection. A positive urine culture may be obtained for prolonged periods after the subsidence of the symptoms of acute pyelonephritis. The persistence of bacteriuria, therefore, even in the absence of symptoms, may indicate renal infection. That bacteriuria is an indica-

Figure 18-12. Clinical course of a patient treated for two episodes of acute pyelonephritis with prompt relief of symptoms each time. Bacteriuria persisted despite therapy. Subsequent disappearance and recurrence of bacteriuria occurred without change in asymptomatic state.

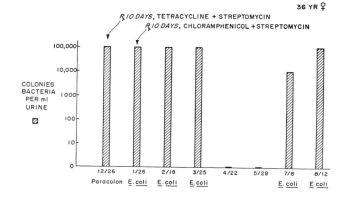

tion of renal infection in man has been suggested by autopsy studies [264] and by the detection of renal functional abnormalities in the clinic [88, 197, 296, 413]. Furthermore, in animals, the persistence of bacteria in the urine after acute pyelonephritis is practically always associated with bacteria in the renal parenchyma and with renal functional abnormalities [116]. In animals, cystitis and pyelitis have been shown to be a possible consequence of hematogenous pyelonephritis [43, 116, 136].

Bacteriuria may also be a reflection of acute bacterial infection of the kidney even in the absence of clinically recognizable symptoms. The detection of bacteriuria following renal biopsy supports this view [410].

Thus, the conclusion seems justified that the presence of bacteria in large numbers in the urine indicates (1) an increased risk of developing pyelonephritis, (2) persistent pyelonephritis, or (3) active new pyelonephritis.

There have been a considerable number of efforts to pinpoint the site of infection within the urinary tract by studies of white cell excretion [94, 119a, 206, 207, 253, 255, 284], antibody response [9, 60, 184a, 234, 295, 295a, 347, 414], "glitter" cells [388], renal concentrating ability [88, 197, 296, 357, 413], and ureteral catheterization [92a, 385, 400]. The purpose of these efforts is to be able to determine which patients have kidney involvement and to predict those who are likely to develop serious renal disease. The problem is complex, however, since patients have now been followed with urine cultures employing quantitative technics and have been observed to have repeated episodes of typical clinical acute pyelonephritis over a period of 10 years and yet have shown no evidence of renal damage as judged by intravenous pyelography, BUN, or blood pressure (see Fig. 18-6) [108a]. It is obviously going to take many years before it will be possible to determine those factors that promote the production of serious renal damage in patients with recurrent urinary in-

fections. *The important question is whether progressive serious renal damage ever occurs in subjects with recurrent or persistent urinary infections in the absence of diabetes mellitus, excessive analgesic ingestion, sickle hemoglobin, gross urinary obstruction, or other forms of underlying renal disease.*

DIAGNOSIS

Urinary tract infection can be diagnosed with certainty only when significant numbers of bacteria are detected in the urine. Catheterization is seldom necessary to secure a specimen for routine microscopic examination or bacteriologic study in men or women and carries with it the risk of introducing infection [148]. Clean-voided specimens for culture or microscopic examination can be obtained from female patients by a variety of technics [163]; generally they involve thorough cleansing of the vulva, as for catheterization, then the collection of a midstream sample in a wide-mouthed sterile vessel. Obviously this method may be unsatisfactory in the case of an unconscious or uncooperative patient, in the immediate postpartum period, etc.

Urine obtained by catheter, or as a clean-voided specimen, is liable to contamination by bacteria lying along the course of the urethra. Culture of such a specimen in liquid medium will yield luxuriant growth, and may thereby lead to a false impression of urinary infection [148]. To obviate this, some kind of quantitative estimate of the number of bacteria in urine must be made. The necessity for the use of such technics was appreciated in some clinics 25 years ago [331], but they have only recently been generally applied. The simplest procedure is to examine a stained film or unstained drop of freshly voided *uncentrifuged* urine [233]. If bacteria are found, it is fair to assume the presence of more than 10,000, probably more than 100,000, organisms per milliliter. This is more than would be expected from urethral contamination, and it indicates growth in the urine. Somewhat greater accuracy can be achieved by a quantitative cultural procedure. The simplest of these is to streak freshly voided uncentrifuged urine, collected on a calibrated bacteriologic loop, on the surface of an agar plate [163a, 163b]. Since this represents an inoculum of approximately 0.01 to 0.001 ml, the subsequent appearance of hundreds of colonies on the plate indicates infection. More accurate enumeration can be obtained by diluting the fresh specimen 1:1000, and making an agar pour plate containing 1 ml. of this dilution. Fewer than 1000 bacteria per milliliter of urine should be regarded as an insignificant number. Between 1000 and 10,000 per milliliter is of doubtful significance. A number of modifications of these simple quantitative technics have been described which may have advantages for specific field conditions [7a, 41, 67a, 82a, 82b, 146, 180, 260a, 298a, 320a, 325, 345, 354, 356b, 383]. An essential requisite for estimating the numbers of bacteria is that the test be set up before bacteria have an opportunity to multiply in the urine specimen. This means either immediate delivery to the bacteriology laboratory after collection, or storage of the specimen in a refrigerator until the test can be made. Refrigeration for 5 to 10 days or even longer does not significantly change the detectable number of bacteria [288].

Several additional precautions must be thoroughly kept in mind in examining clean-voided urine specimens. Antibacterial agents should not be employed in cleaning the periurethral area since they are effective in inhibiting bacterial growth, in the case of hexachlorophene (pHisoHex), in dilutions as high as 1:16,000. This material is also lytic for red cells in the urine at dilutions of 1:32,000, and when small amounts get into the urine, globules are formed which look like red blood cells under the microscope [67, 339]. It is also important to perform the microscopic exam-

ination for formed elements in the urine promptly since white blood cells may be lost in only a few hours depending on conditions of temperature, osmolality, and pH [395].

Several tests have been recommended as screening methods for the presence of bacteria in the urine. The principle of all these (Griess [196, 376], peroxidase [193], catalase [44]) is to indicate the presence of some product of bacterial metabolism or of inflammation. These may be useful for mass screening, but are too crude for individual examination, and are of little or no value in diagnosis of renal lesions resulting from preceding urinary tract infection.

Similarly, although many enzymes (LDH, alkaline phosphatase, beta-glucuronidase, lysozyme) are excreted in the urine in the presence of a variety of urinary tract diseases, none of the excretion patterns appear sufficiently specific to replace the need for urine culture and careful urinalysis in the management of patients with urinary tract infections [7, 23, 123, 199, 327, 338, 351].

PRINCIPLES OF THERAPY

Certain principles of therapy apply regardless of the particular agents employed in treatment. They are:

1. *Before antimicrobial therapy is begun, the presence of bacterial infection should be established.* Criteria for instituting therapy differ according to the nature of the clinical findings. In acute pyelonephritis a drop of uncentrifuged urine should show a profusion of microorganisms. If bacteria are not visible under these circumstances, one must question the diagnosis of acute urinary tract infection [258]. Unless there is particular reason to start treatment, antimicrobial treatment should be delayed until the etiologic agent is demonstrated by suitable cultural technics. If the patient has few or no generalized or local symptoms of urinary tract infection, a single urine culture, irrespective of the number of

bacteria found, is not a sufficient basis for the institution of therapy. There are so many potential sources of error inherent in the procedure that a culture should always be confirmed before administering drugs, which are usually expensive and never without some risk. Some possible sources of error in culturing the urine include: poor patient cooperation, contaminated containers, delay in delivery of the specimen to the laboratory, and laboratory error.

2. *Consideration must be given to the possible existence of urinary obstruction.* In patients with particularly severe systemic manifestations of infection, renal insufficiency, or symptoms suggesting renal colic it is important to obtain an intravenous pyelogram promptly to rule out the possibility of gross urinary obstruction. A similar radiologic study is indicated in men at the time of their first infection and in women if infections are recurrent.

3. *Therapy should be directed at eradicating bacteria from the tissues of the urinary tract if there are systemic signs of infection or kidney pain or tenderness.* There has been considerable discussion concerning the site of effectiveness of antibacterial agents in the urinary tract [38, 385, 400, 424]. It seems reasonable to use antibiotics that achieve effective levels in the tissues in the presence of signs and symptoms indicating tissue infection. In patients without symptoms or with symptoms referable to inflammation of the bladder and urethra, agents that act principally by achieving high urinary concentrations may be effective. Animal studies have demonstrated the ability to sterilize the urine without sterilizing the kidney following the administration of antibiotics [112, 251].

Certainly, many patients with evidence of tissue infection or with bacteria coming from the upper urinary tract may also be cured with agents which only achieve effective concentrations in the urine. This does not clarify the site of action of the drugs, however, since the usual prompt resolution of signs of pyelonephritis (see Fig. 18-11) may be associated with clearance of the tissue phase of infection leaving the patient with bacteriuria arising from the renal pelvis or within the bladder lumen.

In practice, therapy is often begun before the results of sensitivity testing are known. The particular antibiotics selected for use will depend very much on the patient's clinical condition. For example, if the patient is in shock and appears to be suffering from sepsis secondary to a gram-negative urinary infection, it may be necessary to administer kanamycin, colistimethate (Coly-micin), and ampicillin for the broadest possible emergency coverage. If, on the other hand, the patient is not seriously ill but has obvious tissue infection, such as acute pyelonephritis, a combination of tetracycline or ampicillin and streptomycin is likely to be effective. The choice of drugs would be different in this clinical situation if the infection were known to have developed after instrumentation of the urinary tract. In that case, kanamycin and Coly-micin would statistically be more likely to be effective.

For patients without symptoms or with lower urinary tract symptoms, one might decide to await the outcome of sensitivity testing. Lower urinary tract symptoms of urgency and dysuria can often be controlled for a day or two by having the patient drink 2 or 3 gm. of baking soda in a glass of water every 4 hours. Another approach which is useful is to have the patient take a sulfonamide, nitrofurantoin, or naladixic acid until the results of sensitivity tests are available. Since most hospital laboratories do not test the effectiveness of sulfonamides on media with controlled concentrations of para-aminobenzoic acid, it is necessary to culture a urine specimen after two or three days on therapy to determine the effectiveness of this class of drugs.

It is most important to appreciate that in the majority of instances patients with symptomatic urinary tract infections become asymptomatic in three or four days regardless of the therapy given (see Fig. 18-11). This is often not properly explained to patients with the result that they discontinue medication and do not return for follow-up examinations.

EFFECT OF THERAPY

It is evident from the foregoing discussion that any attempt to evaluate therapy in infections of the urinary tract must be based on the quantitative evaluation of the number of bacteria in the urine for a considerable time following the cessation of therapy. In addition, instrumentation of the tract must be avoided, if possible, during the follow-up period, so as to avoid reintroducing bacteria into the bladder urine.

Symptoms of acute urinary tract infection usually subside within a few days regardless of therapy. White cells in the urine also may decrease to very low numbers or disappear. Nevertheless, neither symptomatic response nor disappearance of pyuria can be taken as evidence that bacteriuria has been eliminated. On the other hand, the persistence of symptoms or pyuria with sterile urine cultures suggests either that there is other disease superimposed on urinary tract infection or that bacterial growth has only temporarily been inhibited by therapy.

Utilizing the aforementioned precautions, experience with a large series of patients has been that even in the absence of known urinary obstruction and with the use of antibiotics to which the infecting microorganism is sensitive in vitro (tetracycline or one of its derivatives, and streptomycin, in a dosage of 1 gm. each, daily for 10 days), long-term follow-up examination employing urine culture demonstrates that only about 50 per cent of patients treated with a single course of therapy remain free of infection [104]. Similar experiences have been reported by others [18a, 19a, 138, 225a, 246, 256, 270].

Treatment failure after vigorous antibiotic therapy may be due to (1) persistence of the original organism, (2) emergence of a second organism which had not been recognized initially, or (3) reinfection. Whether bacteria persist in the urinary tract or whether recurrent infection is the pattern depends to a considerable extent on the underlying pathology. For example, patients with renal stones are more likely to have a recurrence with their original organism. The young, newly married female, on the other hand, is more likely to become reinfected with different bacterial strains [104, 236, 249, 270, 396, 397, 400].

The critical aspect of treatment of urinary tract infections is long-term follow-up. It is desirable to obtain several follow-up cultures of the urine the first year after treatment. If the urine is not sterilized after two 10-day trials of an antibiotic to which the infecting bacteria are known to be sensitive, or if reinfection occurs two times, it is important to determine the blood urea nitrogen or serum creatinine level and to visualize the urinary tract by intravenous pyelography. If the intravenous pyelogram does not show evidence of urinary obstruction and if the bladder empties properly, there is no gross obstruction and clearly no urgent risk of destruction of renal parenchyma. At this point a decision must be made as to whether the patient should be given long-term suppressive antimicrobial therapy.

In patients with persistent urinary infections or frequent reinfections after short courses of therapy, it is as a rule possible to maintain the patient in an asymptomatic state with sterile urine by continuously administering small doses of a variety of antimicrobial agents [37, 116a, 303, 399a]. Useful agents include a short-acting sulfonamide, about 0.5 gm., two or three times a day or 1.0 gm. at bedtime; nitrofurantoin, 50 mg., two or three times a day or 100 mg. at bedtime; and nalidixic acid, 0.5 gm. twice a day or 1.0 gm. at bedtime. The dosages required will vary with different patients and with the problem under treatment. In young women with frequent recurrences, antimicrobials given at bedtime are usually sufficient to control the problem. In patients with staghorn calculi or nephrocalcinosis, antimicrobials given in the morning and at bedtime are usually necessary.

It is difficult to understand why such low doses of antibiotics should be effective in suppressing and preventing urinary infections. An explanation can perhaps be found by recalling the extremely delicate balance between bacteria and host defense mechanisms when bacteria are placed in the bladder. In animals, this balance can be tipped in favor of the bacteria so as to reduce the inoculum required by infection from 10,000,000 to 10 by merely subjecting the animals to water diuresis. Although it is not known what effect water diuresis has on bladder defense mechanisms in man, it is possible that the balance of forces within the bladder is similar to that demonstrated for animals. It may be that even low doses of antimicrobial drugs interfere with bacterial growth sufficiently to allow the normal host defense mechanisms to operate. Why these host defense mechanisms do not operate satisfactorily in patients with recurrent and persistent urinary infections is, in most instances, unknown.

The effect of antibiotic therapy on the ultimate course of urinary tract infections has not been determined. The principal problem here is that the natural history of these infections has not been documented well enough to determine if antibiotics, in the long run, have any effect at all. In a small series of untreated patients with urinary infections the rate of positive urine cultures four years later was no different from that in patients given a single 10-day course of therapy (about 50 per cent in each group) [114]. Similar experiences were reported by others [19a, 138, 389a]. However, there is no doubt that antimicrobial therapy frequently brings the signs and symptoms of inflammation to an abrupt end. Furthermore, a large number of patients are cured, and Kass's study showed that prolonged treatment during pregnancy sharply reduced the incidence of acute symptoms in patients with asymptomatic bacteriuria [352]. It is possible

that prevention of symptoms in this way forestalls additional renal injury, since successful treatment of bacteriuria is associated with improvement in renal function [88, 197, 295, 296, 357, 413]. This is not the full solution, however, since it is known that resistant bacteria not sensitive to the drugs used may appear, particularly in women during active sexual life. In addition, even after prolonged antimicrobial therapy, during which time the urine appears to be consistently sterile, discontinuation of treatment may be followed by the prompt return of bacteriuria [194]. Similarly, with agents that acidify the urine to a pH that inhibits bacterial multiplication, although the number of bacteria in the urine may be significantly lowered, thereby affording considerably relief of lower tract symptoms, return to a normal pH is likely to be accompanied by a return of bacteriuria to previous levels [205, 291]. Furthermore, experiments in animals have provided evidence that acidifying agents may increase the vulnerability of kidney tissue to bacterial infection [111], so that the number of bacteria in the urine may be reduced concomitantly with increasing susceptibility of the kidney to injury. The net result of this set of circumstances in man has not been determined.

Antibiotics highly effective against infections elsewhere may be ineffective in the urinary tract. As was discussed previously, the kidney is peculiar in affording bacteria an environment that theoretically interferes with the efficiency of a number of antimicrobial host factors — for example, the kidney produces ammonia which may inactivate complement locally; the elevated osmolality of the medulla is anticomplimentary and is an unfavorable medium for the proper function of polymorphonuclear leukocytes; and this same factor of osmolality might well inhibit the lysis of bacterial variants formed by the action of some antibiotics and normal serum. Also, since the kidney is essential in regulating acid-base balance of the body, local variations in the concentration of hydrogen ion are quite likely to impair the effectiveness of some antibiotics [59, 391]. It is of further interest that water diuresis decreases the excretion of hydrogen ion by the kidney [298], and increasing urine pH decreases the sensitivity of the kidney to Pitressin [77]. Obviously, mechanisms of antibacterial action which apply in most tissues of the body may not obtain in the kidney.

Conversely, antibiotics not particularly effective against gram-negative bacteria elsewhere in the body, may, by virtue of excretion, achieve high concentrations in the urine. The best example of this is penicillin [78, 385]. An interesting use of penicillin in the urinary tract is in combination with methicillin for the treatment of pseudomonas infections [346].

Bacteria resistant in vitro to the usual antibiotics present still more difficult problems of therapy. Fortunately, such infections are distinctly unusual in patients without obstruction who have not undergone repeated instrumentation of the urinary tract [249]. Nevertheless, infections with resistant bacteria do occur, and it is sometimes necessary to employ nephrotoxic antibiotics, drugs which should be particularly avoided in this group of patients [230]. Some investigators have infused antibiotics into the renal artery in the hope of achieving high local concentration, but the results do not seem encouraging [185]. Of great interest is the change in antibiotic sensitivities of some urease-producing and citrase-producing bacteria after exposure to organic mercurial enzyme-blocking agents [359]. The change is not uniformly in the direction of increased sensitivity to antibiotics; nevertheless, this approach has been beneficial in selected patients. These studies bear also on the possible nephrotoxicity of bacterial urease [49, 252].

It is important to modify the dosage of various antibiotics in patients with reduced renal function since all these drugs are to some degree excreted in the urine. Some antibiotics are excreted almost exclusively in the urine and, therefore, require small repeat doses at widely spaced intervals to maintain effective tissue concentrations. The decision regarding dosage modification depends on the toxicity of the drug as well as on the extent to which it is normally excreted by the kidney. The details of drug dosage can be obtained by reference to the work of Atuk, Mosca, and Kunin [20] and Kunin [235]. It is sufficient to state here that polymyxin, Colymicin, kanamycin, streptomycin, and vancomycin must be given in reduced dosage to patients with renal insufficiency, and tetracycline and its derivatives and nitrofurantoin should not be used at all under these circumstances. The general subject of infection in renal failure has been reviewed in detail elsewhere [283].

Bacteremia. Urinary tract infection is a common cause of invasion of the bloodstream by gram-negative bacilli. This may follow instrumentation of an infected urinary tract or occur spontaneously. Metastatic infection to distant sites is exceedingly rare [62], but this event serves to deliver bacteria to both kidneys, thereby providing an inoculum for the production of new areas of pyelonephritis. Of greatest clinical significance is the circulatory shock which may be associated with gram-negative bacillary invasion of the bloodstream. It has serious prognostic significance, especially in elderly males with prostatic obstruction, and may not be accompanied by fever or leukocytosis.

Bladder Function and the Indwelling Catheter. Determination of the amount of residual urine in the bladder after micturition is important in evaluating a patient with infection of the urinary tract. The methods employed include catheterization after voiding, radiopaque dye accumulated in the bladder during intravenous pyelography [28], suprapubic scanning after voiding during excretion of ^{131}I-labeled Diodrast (iodopyracet)

[290], and measurement of the amount of PSP excreted in the urine two to four hours after intravenous administration [76, 372]. Whichever method is employed, it must be kept in mind that a patient with urinary tract infection may voluntarily fail to empty his bladder because of discomfort, or may be unable to do so because of partial obstruction of the bladder neck by inflammation and edema.

In the urologic investigation of bladder function of patients with urinary tract infection not responsive to therapy, a diagnosis of contraction of the bladder neck or posterior urethra is frequently encountered. Obstruction to urine flow in these instances is produced by the accumulation of scar tissue showing the changes of chronic inflammation. It is tempting to look to these changes as an explanation for the persistence of infection and treatment failure. Although this may be true in part, the lesions may also be the *result* of persistent infection rather than their cause; furthermore, surgical procedures aimed at removing this inflammatory tissue may fail to alter the course of the infection. This subject will be dealt with in more detail in the next section.

Despite all efforts to avoid placement of an indwelling catheter, there are circumstances when its use is indicated. In these instances, it is important to direct attention to the procedures that will delay the inevitable onset of infection. The methods offering the greatest promise include constant rinsing of the bladder with a dilute neomycin-polymyxin solution [269, 394], careful attention to use of a closed-drainage system [94a, 237, 248a], or perhaps combination of the two [126]. The use of one or the other of these technics seems mandatory to maintain the highest standards of patient care.

The issue is unsettled as to whether systemic prophylactic antibiotics are useful in the prevention of catheter infections. The results have been unsatisfactory in patients requiring in-

dwelling catheters, but kanamycin has been found effective in patients with sterile urine undergoing prostatectomy [318]. Levin [247], after a careful review of this subject, believes that prophylactic antibiotics should also be used in patients with increased risk of infection after a single catheterization and at the time of removal of a catheter in patients with infection, to prevent bacteremia.

URINARY INFECTION IN CHILDREN

The dangers of urinary infection in childhood have been so often emphasized that large numbers of patients are subjected to potentially dangerous procedures, involving instrumentation of the urinary tract and general anesthesia, for inadequate reasons. Diagnoses are employed for which adequate criteria have not been determined, and children are subjected to therapeutic procedures for which benefits have not been established.

It is important to review the data concerned with prognosis of urinary infections in children to try to understand the basis for the attitudes and practices which prevail. Although autopsy and clinical studies are often cited to substantiate the dangers of urinary infections, a clear distinction has generally not been made between subjects with and without gross urinary obstruction [6, 335]. *Review of these data suggests that the overwhelming majority of the serious consequences of urinary infections in children occur in the presence of obvious urinary obstruction.*

A large autopsy study of 1999 children up to 16 years of age dying between 1933 and 1960, excluding cases of sepsis arising outside the urinary tract and gross urinary obstruction, revealed only two examples of chronic pyelonephritis [294]. Even these cases may not have had their renal damage principally as a result of infection since one of these was a 15-year-old girl whose brother had died at age 14 of "nephritis" and renal rickets, and the other was a 10-year-old boy who had chronic glomerulonephritis in addition to chronic pyelonephritis. In another autopsy series comprising 335 children from one day through 10 years of age, eight children were judged to have significant pyelonephritis [223]. Two infants, two and four weeks of age, died of acute pyelonephritis in association with meningitis and bronchopneumonia; two infants aged two months died of diarrhea (water intoxication) and staphylococcal sepsis; and the remaining four included deaths due to infectious stenosis of the larynx, congenital hydronephrosis, astrocytoma, and leukemia. *Thus, it is evident at autopsy that primary pyelonephritis in children in the absence of sepsis, serious disease elsewhere, or gross urinary obstruction is a rarity.*

There have been five major studies of the prognosis of urinary infections in childhood. In the study of Wharton, Gray, and Guild [409] children with the diagnosis of urinary infection were followed for about 10 years. Urine cultures were qualitative and, therefore, inadequate to substantiate the diagnosis of infection at the time of diagnosis or at follow-up examination. Many of the cultures contained staphylococci or streptococci, now known to be mostly a result of contamination. Some of the urine cultures were positive for Salmonella or Shigella, and no pyelographic information was available at the time of original diagnosis to distinguish patients with obvious urinary obstruction from the outset. The same difficulties are encountered in attempting to interpret the data of Woodruff and Everett [417].

In the study of Macauley and Sutton [263], in 1957, 32 children with urinary infections were investigated five years later. Five deaths occurred in children with gross abnormalities of the urinary tract, easily detected by intravenous pyelography. The evidence for nonobstructive pyelonephritis in the remaining children was negligible.

In 1963 DeLuca et al. [80] reported on the follow-up finding in 597 children with non-obstructive urinary infections treated intermittently with antibiotics. It is stated that 210 of these patients eventually developed severe renal damage, but no description is given of the data on which this judgment was made. Of interest is the group of 479 patients given prolonged chemotherapy in whom no mention of the development of renal disease is made.

In the study by Steele et al. [387], although the data are not presented in a way to permit a detailed analysis of the prognosis of obstructive as compared with nonobstructive urinary infection, the following statement is made: "Although patients in the category with no radiographic changes [at the time of detection of infection] had a relatively good prognosis, it is of note that 5 of 23 exhibited recurring urinary tract infection."

Radiologic studies, particularly those of Hodson, have done much to focus attention on the peculiar scarring seen in kidneys of children with urinary infections. There are very few data, however, to document either the development or the course of these scars in relation to the clinical evidence for urinary tract infection. The observations of Persky [313], in particular, support the view that these scars are rarely observed to develop in children with urinary infections, suggesting that they may represent abnormalities which antedate and perhaps evolve independently of the urinary infection.

In summary, review of the studies concerned with urinary infections in children reveals little evidence to suggest that these infections, in the absence of gross urinary obstruction, represent a serious immediate threat to renal function. Considerably more information is necessary, however, to determine the natural history of this disease. There is no doubt that urinary infections may recur or persist over long intervals. The point to be emphasized is that any therapy being consid-

ered for nonobstructive urinary infections in childhood must not introduce risk and operative complications into a disease process which appears generally to follow a benign, or at most, very slowly progressive course.

Diagnosis of infection in children is subject to considerable error, particularly in the newborn period [84a]. Some authors have found the clean-voided sample satisfactory [61, 271], whereas others have emphasized that false-positive clean-voided urine cultures are very common. In the experience of Lincoln and Winberg [248], in the first eight days of life, about 90 per cent of clean-voided cultures were false positives. Braude et al. [50] have had a similar experience. The practice of making the diagnosis of urinary infection and of instituting treatment on the basis of one or two voided cultures in patients who are not seriously ill should be deplored. Lincoln and Winberg [248] have emphasized the need for careful cleansing of the urethral meatus and the importance of repeat cultures before accepting the diagnosis of infection. In doubtful cases subrapubic needle puncture of the bladder seems to be a reasonable undertaking although studies in animals suggest that one should be alert to the possible production of bacteremia when there are large numbers of bacteria in the urine [154, 293]. When urine is obtained directly from the bladder cavity, the detection of any bacteria would be abnormal. However, the presence of low numbers of staphylococci, diphtheroids, or mixed cultures should still raise the strong suspicion of contamination.

Many authors have pointed out the atypical and nonspecific nature of symptoms of urinary infection in children [356a]. It becomes particularly important, therefore, to conduct the bacteriologic studies so as to permit proper interpretation of the results.

In a recent survey of urinary infections diagnosed in a hospital emergency room, two-thirds of the patients who were treated for urinary infections had sterile urine cultures [278]. This gives considerable insight into the extent to which nonspecific complaints may be mislabeled as true urinary infections. Persky [313] has also emphasized the problem of overdiagnosis in children.

If the presence of urinary infection has been established and the child is less than three years of age, it is the current view that an intravenous pyelogram should be performed. Intravenous pyelography should be undertaken when infection is diagnosed in a male of any age. Although some authors believe that all children with urinary infections should have an intravenous pyelogram [158], in females over three or four years of age, in the absence of developmental abnormalities, hypertension, anemia, or other abnormalities, it seems reasonable to treat the infection for 7 to 10 days and consider pyelography if infection should recur. With proper technic, intravenous pyelography is satisfactory for infants, and in most instances in children it should be possible to obtain voiding urethrography during the same procedure [277].

In the presence of a normal intravenous pyelogram the available evidence indicates that the prognosis from the standpoint of renal damage is excellent. If infection recurs after short-term antibiotic therapy, long-term suppression will, in all likelihood, prevent recurrences. It is necessary, of course, to observe these children carefully, and urine cultures should be performed every one or two months.

If it is not possible to achieve sterilization of the urine or if the intravenous pyelogram is abnormal, it is then necessary to consider voiding cystourethography, cystoscopy, and panendoscopy. For obstructive lesions at or above the ureterovesical junction there is little debate as to the need for surgical consultation. Even in these instances, however, it is important to weigh the risks of surgical repair against the results of long-term suppressive therapy. Many obstructive lesions are not progressive, as discussed by Bricker and Klahr in Chapter 27.

In the case of ureteral reflux, the issue as to therapeutic approach is even more controversial. There is evidence, both in man and in animals, that ureteral reflux and damage to ureteral function may result from urinary tract infections, and these effects have been shown in man to disappear with long-term control of infection [228, 280, 355, 392]. Shopfner [366], in a series of patients with urinary infections, found that, after excluding cases with obstructive and neurologic disease, the overwhelming majority (93 out of 120) had "nonobstructive hydronephrosis and hydroureter" [366]. It is important to be certain that control of infection is ineffective before recommending surgical correction of such nonobstructive dilatations [85, 96, 137a].

Lesions such as megacystis, bladder neck obstruction, and meatal stenosis are not easily defined and in the eyes of some authorities are nonexistent [161, 162, 277, 367]. Furthermore, the consequences of surgical correction have not, to my knowledge, been compared with the effects of treatment of infection with antibiotics alone. Despite the inability to arrive at satisfactory definitions and the inadequacy of data evaluating the surgical correction of these lesions, the procedures of meatotomy, transurethral bladder neck resection, or revision of the bladder neck are among the most common procedures applied to children alleged to be suffering from urinary infections [98a, 189a, 405b].

In conclusion, whereas there is no doubt concerning the immediate life-threatening nature of urinary infections in children with gross obstruction to urine flow, the weight of evidence suggests that these infections, in the absence of obstruction, have a natural history similar to that in adults. Furthermore, the primary role of bacterial infection must be given serious consideration in those instances of urinary tract "obstruction" without an obvious mechanical cause. It is frequently possible to relieve such "obstructions" by long-term sterilization of the urine. Finally, diagnoses such as megacystis, bladder neck obstruction, and meatal stenosis are vague and ill defined and should be looked upon with considerable skepticism as justification for surgical procedures whose efficacy has not been demonstrated.

Postscript

Two additional studies, one by Kunin [235a, 235b] and one by Smellie and Normand [370a, 371a], concerned with the prognosis of urinary infections in children have appeared recently. These are important studies of up to 10-year follow-ups of large numbers of children with urinary infections. Both studies emphasize that the prognosis of infections in children with radiologically normal urinary tracts is excellent. Furthermore, *in only rare instances* was it possible to detect the development or progression of renal damage and this occurred in children with vesicoureteral reflux. In the great majority of instances reflux disappeared spontaneously with increasing age and medical therapy. Even when reflux did not disappear, renal disease did not develop in those children in whom antibiotics were successful in controlling urinary infection.

The monograph edited by O'Grady and Brumfitt [299a], in which one of the papers by Smellie appeared, is recommended as an excellent collection of recent clinical studies by British investigators.

Acknowledgments

Supported by U.S. Public Health Service Career Development Award No. 6K3-HD-22, 587, National Institute of Child Health and Human Development, and by Research Grant No. 4767, Institute of Allergy and Infectious Disease.

References

1. Acquatella, H., Little, P. J., de Wardener, H. E., and Coleman, J. C.   The effect of urine osmolality and pH on the bactericidal activity of plasma. *Clin. Sci.* 33:471, 1967.
2. Addis, T.   *Glomerular Nephritis: Diagnosis and Treatment.* New York: Macmillan, 1948. P. 171.
3. Akinkugbe, O. O.   Renal papillary necrosis in sickle-cell haemoglobinopathy. *Brit. Med. J.* 3:283, 1967.
4. Alderman, M. H., and Freedman, L. R.   Experimental pyelonephritis: X. The direct injection of *E. coli* protoplasts into the medulla of the rabbit kidney. *Yale J. Biol. Med.* 36:157, 1963.
5. Allen, A. C.   *The Kidney, Medical and Surgical Diseases.* New York: Grune & Stratton, 1951. P. 336.
6. Allen, T. D.   Pathogenesis of urinary tract infections in children. *New Eng. J. Med.* 273:1421, 1965.
7. Amador, E., Dorfman, L. E., and Wacker, W. E. C.   Urinary alkaline phosphatase and LDH activities in the differential diagnosis of renal disease. *Ann. Intern. Med.* 62:30, 1965.
8. Andersen, B. R., and Jackson, G. G.   Pyelitis, an important factor in the pathogenesis of retrograde pyelonephritis. *J. Exp. Med.* 114:375, 1961.
9. Andersen, H. J.   Clinical studies on the antibody response to *E. coli* O-antigens in infants and children with urinary tract infection, using a passive haemagglutination technique. *Acta Paediat. Scand.* Suppl. 180, 1968.
10. Anderson, L., and McDonald, J. R.   The origin, frequency and significance of microscopic calculi in the kidney. *Surg. Gynec. Obstet.* 82:275, 1946.
11. Andriole, V. T.   Acceleration of the inflammatory response of the renal medulla by water diuresis. *J. Clin. Invest.* 45:847, 1966.
11a. Andriole, V. T.   Effect of water diuresis on chronic pyelonephritis. *J. Lab. Clin. Med.* 72:1, 1968.
11b. Andriole, V. T.   Water, acidosis and experimental pyelonephritis. *J. Clin. Invest.* 49:21, 1970.
12. Andriole, V. T., and Cohn, G. L.   The effect of diethylstilbestrol on the susceptibility of rats to hematogenous pyelonephritis. *J. Clin. Invest.* 43:1136, 1964.
13. Andriole, V. T., and Epstein, F. H.   Prevention of pyelonephritis by water diuresis: Evidence for the role of medullary hypertonicity in promoting renal infection. *J. Clin. Invest.* 44:73, 1965.
14. Andriole, V. T., and Lytton, B.   The effect and critical duration of increased tissue pressure on susceptibility to bacterial infection. *Brit. J. Exp. Path.* 46:308, 1965.
15. Angell, M. E., Relman, A. S., and Robbins, S. L.   "Active" chronic pyelonephritis without evidence of bacterial infection. *New Eng. J. Med.* 278:1303, 1968.
15a. Aoki, S., Imamura, S., Aoki, M., and McCabe, W. R.   "Abacterial" and bacterial pyelonephritis. *New Eng. J. Med.* 281:1376, 1969.
16. Arana, J. A., Kozij, V. M., and Jackson, G. G.   The immunologic status of the host and pyelonephritis: A study of retrograde *Escherichia coli* urinary infection in rats. *J. Immun.* 94:337, 1965.
17. Arean, V. M.   The pathologic anatomy and pathogenesis of fatal human leptospirosis (Weil's disease). *Amer. J. Path.* 40:393, 1962.
17a. Arneil, G. C., McAllister, T. A., and Kay, P.   Detection of bacteria at room-temperature. *Lancet* 1:119, 1970.
18. Ashworth, C. T., and Grollman, A.   Renal lesions in experimental hypertension: Morphological changes in the kidney of rats rendered chronically hypertensive following a period of choline deficiency. *A.M.A. Arch. Path.* 67:375, 1959.
18a. Asscher, A. W.   Screening for urinary tract infection. *J. Roy. Coll. Physicians* (London) 4:219, 1970.
19. Asscher, A. W., Sussman, M., Waters, W. E., and Davis, R. H.   Urine as a medium for bacterial growth. *Lancet* 2:1037, 1966.

19a. Asscher, A. W., Sussman, M., Waters, W. E., Evans, J. A. S., Campbell, H., Evans, K. T., and Williams, J. E. Asymptomatic significant bacteriuria in the non-pregnant woman: II. Response to treatment and follow-up. *Brit. Med. J.* 1:804, 1969.

19b. Asscher, A. W., Sussman, M., and Weiser, R. Bacterial Growth in Human Urine in Urinary Tract Infection. In O'Grady, F., and Brumfitt, W. (Eds.), *Urinary Tract Infection.* (Proceedings of the First National Symposium on Urinary Tract Infection, London, April, 1968.) London: Oxford University Press, 1968. P. 3.

20. Atuk, N. O., Mosca, A., Kunin, C. M. The use of potentially nephrotoxic antibiotics in the treatment of gram-negative infections in uremic patients. *Ann. Intern. Med.* 60:28, 1964.

20a. Bailey, R. R., and Little, P. J. Suprapubic bladder aspiration in diagnosis of urinary tract infection. *Brit. Med. J.* 1:293, 1969.

21. Baker, R., and Connelly, J. P. Bilateral and recurrent renal calculi. *J.A.M.A.* 160:1106, 1956.

22. Bank, N., and Aynedjian, H. S. Individual nephron function in experimental bilateral pyelonephritis: II. Distal tubular sodium and water reabsorption and the concentrating defect. *J. Lab. Clin. Med.* 68:728, 1966.

23. Bank, N., and Bailine, S. H. Urinary beta-glucuronidase activity in patients with urinary tract infection. *New Eng. J. Med.* 272:70, 1965.

23a. Barlow, K. A., and Beilin, L. J. Renal disease in primary gout. *Quart. J. Med.* 37:79, 1968.

24. Bass, H. N. Bubble bath as an irritant to the urinary tract of children. *Clin. Pediat.* 4:174, 1968.

25. Bata, J. E., Gyenes, L., and Sehon, A. H. The effect of urea on antibody-antigen reactions. *Immunochemistry* 1:289, 1964.

26. Beard, R. W., and Roberts, A. P. Asymptomatic bacteriuria during pregnancy. *Brit. Med. Bull.* 24:44, 1968.

27. Beck, D., Freedman, L. R., Levitin, H., Ferris, T., and Epstein, F. H. The effect

of experimental pyelonephritis on renal concentrating ability in the rat. *Yale J. Biol. Med.* 34:52, 1961.

28. Beer, E. Visualization of amount of residual urine. *J.A.M.A.* 107:1886, 2060, 1936.

29. Beeson, P. B. Factors in the pathogenesis of pyelonephritis. *Yale J. Biol. Med.* 28:81, 1955.

30. Beeson, P. B. The case against the catheter. *Amer. J. Med.* 24:1, 1958.

31. Beeson, P. B. Urinary Tract Infection and Pyelonephritis. In Black, D.A.K. (Ed.), *Renal Disease* (2d ed.). Oxford, Eng.: Blackwell, 1964. P. 382.

32. Beeson, P. B. What Is Chronic Pyelonephritis? In Kass, E. H. (Ed.), *Progress in Pyelonephritis.* Philadelphia: Davis, 1965. P. 367.

33. Beeson, P. B., and Rowley, D. The anti-complementary effect of kidney tissue, its association with ammonia production. *J. Exp. Med.* 110:685, 1959.

34. Bell, E. T. *Renal Diseases.* Philadelphia: Lea & Febiger, 1950. Pp. 140–144.

35. Bengtsson, U. A comparative study of chronic non-obstructive pyelonephritis and renal papillary necrosis. *Acta Med. Scand.* 172 (Suppl. 338): 4, 1962.

36. Bengtsson, U. Analgesic nephropathy-chronic pyelonephritis. *Proceedings of the Third International Congress of Nephrology,* Washington, D.C., 1967. Vol. 2, p. 291.

37. Bengtsson, U., Lincoln, K., and Hood, B. Long-term antibacterial treatment of chronic pyelonephritis. *Acta Med. Scand.* 181:641, 1967.

38. Birchall, R. Pyelonephritis — an enigma. *Amer. J. Med.* 28:501, 1960.

39. Blackman, J. E., Gibson, G. R., Lavan, J. N., Learoyd, H. M., and Posen, S. Urinary calculi and the consumption of analgesics. *Brit. Med. J.* 2:800, 1967.

40. Borland, V. G., and Jackson, C. M. Effects of fat-free diet on structure of kidneys of rats. *Arch. Path.* 11:687, 1931.

41. Bowman, R. L., Blume, P., and Vurek, G. G. Capillary-tube scanner for mechanized microbiology. *Science* 158:78, 1967.

42. Braasch, W. F., and Jacobson, C. E.

Chronic bilateral pyelonephritis and hypertension. *J. Urol.* 44:571, 1940.

43. Brainerd, H. D., and Cecil, E. M. Observations on the pathogenesis, course and treatment of non-obstructive pyelonephritis. *Ann. Intern. Med.* 45:232, 1956.

44. Braude, A. I., and Berkowitz, H. Detection of urinary catalase by disc flotation. *J. Lab. Clin. Med.* 57:490, 1961.

45. Braude, A. I., Shapiro, A. P., and Siemienski, J. Hematogenous pyelonephritis in rats: I. Its pathogenesis when produced by a simple new method. *J. Clin. Invest.* 34:1489, 1955.

46. Braude, A. I., Shapiro, A. P., and Siemienski, J. Hematogenous pyelonephritis in rats: III. Relationship of bacterial species to the pathogenesis of acute pyelonephritis. *J. Bact.* 77:270, 1959.

47. Braude, A. I., and Siemienski, J. Production of bladder stones by L-forms. *Trans. Ass. Amer. Physicians* 81:323, 1968.

48. Braude, A. I., Siemienski, J., and Jacobs, I. Protoplast formation in human urine. *Trans. Ass. Amer. Physicians* 74:235, 1961.

49. Braude, A. I., Siemienski, J., and Shapiro, A. P. The Role of Bacterial Urease in the Pathogenesis of Pyelonephritis. In Quinn, E. L., and Kass, E. H. (Eds.), *Biology of Pyelonephritis.* (Henry Ford Hospital International Symposium.) Boston: Little, Brown, 1960. P. 69.

50. Braude, H., Forfar, J. O., and Gould, J. C. Urinary infection in childhood. *Brit. Med. J.* 2:1393, 1964.

51. Brentjens, J. R. H., Vreeken, J., Feltkamp-Vroom, T., and Helder, A. W. Pyelonephritis-like lesions as a late effect of diffuse intravascular coagulation. *Acta Med. Scand.* 183:203, 1968.

52. Breslau, A. M., Gonick, H. C., Sommers, S. C., and Guze, L. B. Pathogenesis of chronic pyelonephritis. *Amer. J. Path.* 44:679, 1964.

53. Brewer, G. E. Present state of our knowledge of acute renal infections; with a report of some animal experiments. *J.A.M.A.* 57:179, 1911.

54. Brewer, T. H. Role of malnutrition, hepatic dysfunction and gastrointestinal bacteria in the pathogenesis of acute toxemia of pregnancy. *Amer. J. Obstet. Gynec.* 84:1253, 1962.

55. Bricker, N. S., Klahr, S., Lubowitz, H., and Rieselbach, R. E. Renal function in chronic renal disease. *Medicine* (Balt.) 44:263, 1965.

56. Brod, J. Chronic pyelonephritis. *Lancet* 1:973, 1956.

56a. Brody, J. I., Oski, F. A., and Wallach, E. E. Neonatal lymphocyte reactivity as an indicator of intrauterine bacterial contact. *Lancet* 1:1396, 1968.

57. Brumfitt, W., and Heptinstall, R. H. Experimental pyelonephritis: The effect of renal vein constriction on bacterial localisation and multiplication in the rat kidney. *Brit. J. Exp. Path.* 40:145, 1959.

58. Brumfitt, W., and Heptinstall, R. H. Experimental pyelonephritis: The relationship of bacterial virulence to the establishment of the renal lesion. *Brit. J. Exp. Path.* 41:552, 1960.

59. Brumfitt, W., and Percival, A. Adjustment of urine pH in the chemotherapy of urinary tract infections. *Lancet* 1:186, 1962.

60. Brumfitt, W., and Percival, A. Serum Antibody Response as an Indication of Renal Involvement in Patients With Significant Bacteriuria. In Kass, E. H. (Ed.), *Progress in Pyelonephritis.* Philadelphia: Davis, 1965. P. 118.

61. Brumfitt, J. R., and Oliver, W. J. The diagnosis of pyelonephritis in childhood: Quantitative culture of non-catheter urine specimens. *Canad. Med. Ass. J.* 86:571, 1962.

62. Bruno, M. S., Silverberg, T. N., and Goldstein, D. H. Embolic osteomyelitis of the spine as a complication of infection of the urinary tract. *Amer. J. Med.* 29:865, 1960.

63. Bryant, R. E., Windom, R. E., Vineyard, J. P., Jr., and Sanford, J. P. Bacteriuria and the course of hypertension. *Clin. Res.* 7:241, 1964.

64. Bulger, R. J. Inhibition of human serum bactericidal action by a chemical environment stimulating the hydropenic renal medulla. *J. Infect. Dis.* 117:429, 1967.

65. Bunts, R. C. Preservation of renal function in the paraplegic. *J. Urol.* 81:720, 1959.

66. Burkland, C. E., and Rosenberg, M. Survey of urolithiasis in the United States. *J. Urol.* 73:198, 1955.

66a. Burry, A. F. The evolution of analgesic nephropathy. *Nephron* 5:185, 1967.

67. Ceremsak, R. J., and Sanderson, D. Perineal prep with pHisoHex: A source of error in urinalysis. *Amer. J. Clin. Path.* 45:225, 1966.

67a. Chadwick, P., and Avila, F. Rapid detection of urinary infections by microscopic observation of growing cultures. *Canad. Med. Ass. J.* 99:892, 1968.

68. Chernew, I., and Braude, A. I. Depression of phagocytosis by solutes in concentrations found in the kidney and urine. *J. Clin. Invest.* 41:1945, 1962.

69. Claireaux, A. E., and Pearson, M. G. Chronic nephritis in a newborn infant. *Arch. Dis. Child.* 30:366, 1955.

70. Clausen, E. Histological changes in rabbit kidneys induced by phenacetin and acetylsalicylic acid. *Lancet* 2:123, 1964.

71. Cobbs, C. G., and Kaye, D. Antibacterial mechanisms in the urinary bladder. *Yale J. Biol. Med.* 40:93, 1967.

72. Cohen, S. N., and Kass, E. H. A simple method for quantitative urine culture. *New Eng. J. Med.* 277:176, 1967.

73. Cohn, Z. A. Determinants of infection in the peritoneal cavity: III. Action of selected inhibitors on the fate of *Staphylococcus aureus* in the mouse. *Yale J. Biol. Med.* 35:48, 1962.

74. Connor, T. B., Berthrong, M., Thomas, W. C., Jr., and Howard, J. E. Hypertension due to unilateral renal disease with a report on a functional test helpful in diagnosis. *Bull. Johns Hopkins Hosp.* 100:241, 1957.

75. Cotran, R. S. Retrograde *Proteus* pyelonephritis in rats: Localization of antigen and antibody in treated sterile pyelonephritic kidneys. *J. Exp. Med.* 117:813, 1963.

76. Cotran, R. S., and Kass, E. H. Determination of the volume of residual urine in the bladder without catheterization. *New Eng. J. Med.* 259:337, 1958.

76a. Cox, C. E., Lacy, S. S., and Hinman, F., Jr. The urethra and its relationship to urinary tract infection: II. The urethral flora of the female with recurrent urinary infection. *J. Urol.* 99:632, 1968.

77. Czaczkes, J. W., Eliakim, M., and Ullmann, T. D. Diminished antidiuretic response to Pitressin in diabetes insipidus during the infusion of sodium bicarbonate solution. *J. Lab. Clin. Med.* 57:938, 1961.

78. Daikos, G. K., and Athanasiadou, M. Penicillin sensitivity of gram-negative enteric bacilli: Successful treatment of urinary tract infections. *A.M.A. Arch. Intern. Med.* 104:378, 1959.

79. Dawborn, J. K., Fairley, K. F., Kincaid-Smith, P., and King, W. E. The association of peptic ulceration, chronic renal disease, and analgesic abuse. *Quart. J. Med.* 25:69, 1966.

80. DeLuca, F. G., Fisher, J. H., and Swenson, O. Review of recurrent urinary tract infections in infancy and early childhood. *New Eng. J. Med.* 268:75, 1963.

81. De Navasquez, S. Further studies in experimental pyelonephritis produced by various bacteria, with special reference to renal scarring as a factor in pathogenesis. *J. Path. Bact.* 71:27, 1956.

82. Dixon, H. G., and Brant, H. A. The significance of bacteriuria of pregnancy. *Lancet* 1:19, 1967.

82a. Dixon, J. M. S., and Clarke, M. A. Experience with agar-filled plastic spoons for the transport of specimens of urine. *Canad. Med. Ass. J.* 99:741, 1968.

82b. Duncanson, R. L., and St. Geme, J. W. Screening for bacteriuria by the miniature culture technique. *Calif. Med.* 109:112, 1968.

83. Durand, A. M. A., Fisher, M., and Adams, M. Histology in rats as influenced by age and diet. 1. Renal and cardiovascular systems. *Arch. Path.* (Chicago) 77:268, 1964.

84. Eastridge, R. R., and Farrar, E., Jr. Effect of water diuresis on an L-form infection in the rat. *Clin. Res.* 16:46, 1968.

84a. Editorial. Bacteriuria in infants. *Brit. Med. J.* 1:185, 1970.

85. Editorial. Defense mechanisms of the bladder. *Lancet* 1:1183, 1968.

85a. Editorial. Hypertension in pyelonephritis. *Lancet* 2:615, 1968.

85b. Editorial. Markers for chronic pyelonephritis. *Lancet* 1:758, 1970.

85c. Editorial. Phenacetin. *Lancet* 2:717, 1968.

86. Editorial. Vesico-ureteral reflux. *Lancet* 1:1072, 1968.

87. Edmondson, H. A., Reynolds, T. B., and Jacobson, A. Renal papillary necrosis with special reference to chronic alcoholism (a report of 20 cases). *Arch. Intern. Med.* (Chicago) 118:255, 1966.

88. Elder, H. A., and Kass, E. H. Renal Function in Bacteriuria of Pregnancy: Its Relationship to Prematurity, Acute Pyelonephritis, and Excessive Weight Gain. In Kass, E. H. (Ed.), *Progress in Pyelonephritis.* Philadelphia: Davis, 1965. P. 81.

89. Emmerson, B. T. Metals and the Kidney. In Black, D. A. K. (Ed.), *Renal Disease* (2d ed.). Oxford: Blackwell, 1964. P. 561.

90. Epstein, F., and Zupa, V. J. Clinical correlates of the Kimmelstiel-Wilson lesion. *New Eng. J. Med.* 254:896, 1956.

91. Erlandson, A. L., Jr., Gagliardi, L. A., and Fisher, M. W. An experimental enterococcal pyelonephritis in mice. *Nature* (London) 184:561, 1959.

92. Fahr, Th. Pathologische Anatomie des Morbus Brightii. In Henke, F., and Lubarsch, O. (Eds.), *Handbuch der speziellen pathologischen Anatomie und Histologie.* Berlin: Julius Springer, 1934. Vol. VI, part 2, p. 809.

92a. Fairley, K. F. Localisation of urinary-tract infection. *Lancet* 1:1212, 1969.

93. Felts, J. H., Mamlin, J. J., and Feezor, C. N. J., Jr. Urinary granulocyte excretion in renal disease. *Arch. Intern. Med.* (Chicago) 113:401, 1964.

94. Finegold, S. M., Miller, L. G., Merrill, S., and Posnick, D. Significance of Anaerobic and Capnophilic Bacteria Isolated from the Urinary Tract. In Kass, E. H. (Ed.), *Progress in Pyelonephritis.* Philadelphia: Davis, 1965. P. 159.

94a. Finkelberg, Z., and Kunin, C. M. Clinical evaluation of closed urinary drainage systems. *J.A.M.A.* 207:1657, 1969.

95. Finnerty, F. A., Jr. Pyelonephritis masquerading as toxemia of pregnancy. *J.A.M.A.* 161:210, 1956.

96. Fisher, J. H., and Darling, D. B. The course of vesicoureteral reflux associated with urinary tract infection in children. *J. Pediat. Surg.* 2:221, 1967.

97. Fitzpatrick, F. K., and Girard, A. E. Pyelonephritis in the mouse: II. Vaccination studies. *Proc. Soc. Exp. Biol. Med.* 127:579, 1968.

98. Fiveash, J. G., Foster, E. A., and Paquin, A. J. Experimental *Escherichia coli* Bacteriuria in the Rabbit. In Kass, E. H. (Ed.), *Progress in Pyelonephritis.* Philadelphia: Davis, 1965. P. 581.

98a. Forbes, P. A., Drummond, K. N., and Nogrady, M. B. Meatotomy in girls with meatal stenosis and urinary tract infections. *J. Pediat.* 75:937, 1969.

99. Fordham, C. C., III, Huffines, W. D., and Welt, L. G. Phenacetin-induced Renal Lesions in the Rat. In Kass, E. H. (Ed.), *Progress in Pyelonephritis.* Philadelphia: Davis, 1965. P. 325.

100. Fox, M. Progressive renal fibrosis following acute tubular necrosis: An experimental study. *J. Urol.* 97:196, 1967.

101. Freedman, L. R. An observation concerning the mechanism of renal cyst formation. *Yale J. Biol. Med.* 33:148, 1960.

102. Freedman, L. R. Discussion. In Quinn, E. L., and Kass, E. H. (Eds.), *Biology of Pyelonephritis.* (Henry Ford Hospital International Symposium.) Boston: Little, Brown, 1960. P. 98.

103. Freedman, L. R. Experimental pyelonephritis: VI. Observations on susceptibility of the rabbit kidney to infection by a virulent strain of *Staphylococcus aureus. Yale J. Biol. Med.* 32:272, 1960.

104. Freedman, L. R. Prolonged Observations on a Group of Patients with Acute Urinary Tract Infections. In Quinn, E. L., and Kass, E. H. (Eds.), *Biology of Pyelonephritis.* (Henry Ford Hospital International Symposium.) Boston: Little, Brown, 1960. P. 345.

105. Freedman, L. R. Pyelonephritis and Urinary Tract Infection. In Strauss, M. B., and

Welt, L. G. (Eds.), *Diseases of the Kidney*. Boston: Little, Brown, 1963. P. 469.

106. Freedman, L. R. Experimental pyelonephritis: XII. Changes mimicking "chronic pyelonephritis" as a consequence of renal vascular occlusion in the rat. *Yale J. Biol. Med.* 39:113, 1966.

107. Freedman, L. R. Chronic pyelonephritis at autopsy. *Ann. Intern. Med.* 66:697, 1967.

108. Freedman, L. R. Experimental pyelonephritis: XIII. On the ability of water diuresis to increase susceptibility to *E. Coli* bacteriuria in the normal rat. *Yale J. Biol. Med.* 39:255, 1967.

108a. Freedman, L. R. The relation of bacteriuria to hypertension. *Milbank Mem. Fund Quart.* 47:33, 1969.

109. Freedman, L. R., and Andrews, E. C. Percutaneous needle biopsy of the kidney. *Conn. Med.* 25:420, 1961.

110. Freedman, L. R., and Beeson, P. B. Experimental pyelonephritis: IV. Observations on infections resulting from direct inoculation of bacteria in different zones of the kidney. *Yale J. Biol. Med.* 30:406, 1958.

111. Freedman, L. R., and Beeson, P. B. Experimental pyelonephritis: VIII. The effect of acidifying agents on susceptibility to infection. *Yale J. Biol. Med.* 33:318, 1961.

112. Freedman, L. R., Kaminskas, E., and Beeson, P. B. Experimental pyelonephritis: VII. Evidence on the mechanisms by which obstruction of urine flow enhances susceptibility to pyelonephritis. *Yale J. Biol. Med.* 33:65, 1960.

113. Freedman, L. R., Phair, J. P., Seki, M., Hamilton, H. B., and Nefzgen, M. D. The epidemiology of urinary tract infections in Hiroshima. *Yale J. Biol. Med.* 37:262, 1965.

114. Freedman, L. R., Seki, M., and Phair, J. P. The natural history and outcome of antibiotic treatment of urinary tract infections in women. *Yale J. Biol. Med.* 37:245, 1965.

115. Freedman, L. R., Seki, M., Phair, J. P., and Nefzger, M. D. Proteinuria in Hiroshima and Nagasaki, Japan. *Yale J. Biol. Med.* 40:109, 1967.

116. Freedman, L. R., Werner, A. S., Beck, D., and Paplanus, S. H. Experimental pyelonephritis: IX. The bacteriologic course and morphologic consequences of staphylococcal pyelonephritis in the rat, with consideration of the specificity of the changes observed. *Yale J. Biol. Med.* 34:40, 1961.

116a. Freeman, R. B., Bromer, L., Brancato, F., Cohen, S. I., Garfield, C. F., Griep, R. J., Hinman, E. J., Richardson, J. A., Thurm, R. H., Winer, C., and Smith, W. M. Prevention of recurrent bacteriuria with continuous chemotherapy. *Ann. Intern. Med.* 69:655, 1968.

117. Friedman-Klien, A., and Freedman, L. R. Unpublished data.

118. Frithz, G. Phenacetin nephropathy in a mother and daughter. *Acta Med. Scand.* 181:529, 1967.

119. Furtado, D., and Garrison, D. The distribution of *Aerobacter aerogenes* in the urinary tract of guinea pigs following ascending routes of inoculation. *J. Urol.* 98:267, 1967.

119a. Gadeholt, H. The cellular content in nontimed specimens of urine. *Acta Med. Scand.* 184:323, 1968.

120. Garrod, L. P. Chemotherapy of infections of the urinary tract. Publication No. 11, Royal College of Physicians of Edinburgh, 1959.

121. Gault, M. H., and Dossetor, J. B. Chronic pyelonephritis: Relative incidence in transplant recipients. *New Eng. J. Med.* 275:813, 1966.

122. Gault, M. H., Rudwal, T. C., Engles, W. D., and Dossetor, J. B. Syndrome associated with the abuse of analgesics. *Ann. Intern. Med.* 68:906, 1968.

123. Gelderman, A. H., Gelboin, H. V., and Peacock, A. C. Lactic dehydrogenase isozymes in urine from patients with malignancies of the urinary bladder. *J. Lab. Clin. Med.* 65:132, 1965.

124. Gilman, A. Analgesic nephrotoxicity: A pharmacological analysis. *Amer. J. Med.* 36:167, 1964.

125. Ginder, D. R. Increased susceptibility of mice infected with mouse adenovirus to *Escherichia coli*-induced pyelonephritis. *J. Exp. Med.* 120:1117, 1964.

126. Gladstone, J. L., and Robinson, C. G. Pre-

vention of bacteriuria resulting from in-dwelling catheters. *J. Urol.* 99:458, 1968.

127. Gloor, F. Die doppelseitige chronische nicht-obstruktive interstitielle Nephritis. *Ergebn. Allg. Path.* 41:63, 1961.

128. Gloor, F. J. Some Morphologic Features of Chronic Interstitial Nephritis (Chronic Pyelonephritis) in Patients with Analgesic Abuse. In Kass, E. H. (Ed.), *Progress in Pyelonephritis*. Philadelphia: Davis, 1965. P. 287.

129. Godley, J. A., and Freedman, L. R. Experimental pyelonephritis: XI. A comparison of temporary occlusion of renal artery and vein on susceptibility of the rat kidney to infection. *Yale J. Biol. Med.* 36:268, 1964.

130. Goldstein, M. The pathogenicity of cocci isolated from the urine. *J. Urol.* 41:237, 1939.

131. Gonick, H. C., Goldberg, G., Rubini, M. E., and Guze, L. B. Functional abnormalities in experimental pyelonephritis: I. Studies of concentrating ability. *Nephron* 2:193, 1965.

132. Gorrill, R. H. Bacterial localization in the kidney with particular reference to *Pseudomonas pyocyanea*. *J. Path. Bact.* 64:857, 1952.

133. Gorrill, R. H. Experimental staphylococcal infections in mice. *Brit. J. Exp. Path.* 32:151, 1956.

134. Gorrill, R. H. The effect of obstruction of the ureter on the renal localization of bacteria. *J. Path. Bact.* 72:59, 1956.

135. Gorrill, R. H. The fate of *Pseudomonas aeroginosa, Proteus mirabilis* and *Escherichia coli* in the mouse kidney. *J. Path. Bact.* 89:81, 1965.

136. Gorrill, R. H., and De Navasquez, S. The pathogenesis and evolution of experimental pyelonephritis in the mouse with special reference to comparable conditions in man. *J. Path. Bact.* 80:239, 1960.

137. Gorrill, R. H., and De Navasquez, S. J. Experimental pyelonephritis in the mouse produced by *Escherichia coli, Pseudomonas aeroginosa* and *Proteus mirabilis*. *J. Path. Bact.* 87:79, 1964.

137a. Govan, D. E., and Palmer, J. M. Urinary tract infection in children — the influence of successful antireflux operations in morbidity from infection. *Pediatrics* 44:677, 1967.

138. Gower, P. E., Haswell, B., Sidaway, M. E., and de Wardener, H. E. Follow-up of 164 patients with bacteriuria of pregnancy. *Lancet* 1:990, 1968.

139. Gray, J. E., Wilkins, J. R., Prestrud, M. C., and Nikitas, C. T. Further characterization of an experimental staphylococcal infection in mice. *J. Infect. Dis.* 101:137, 1957.

140. Greenbaum, D., Ross, J. H., and Steinberg, V. L. Renal biopsy in gout. *Brit. Med. J.* 1:1502, 1961.

141. Grimlund, K. Phenacetin and renal damage at a Swedish factory. *Acta Med. Scand.* 174 (Suppl. 405): 3, 1963.

142. Gullbring, B., Ljungqvist, A., and Richardson, J. Studies on the pathogenesis of serum-induced renal papillary necrosis in the rat. *Lab. Invest.* 15:1486, 1966.

143. Gupta, S. N., Perkash, I., Agarwal, S. C., and Anand, S. S. Antibacterial activity of human prostatic fluid. *Invest. Urol.* 5:219 1967.

144. Gutman, L. T., Schaller, J., and Wedgewood, R. J. Bacterial L-forms in relapsing urinary-tract infection. *Lancet* 1:464, 1967.

145. Gutman, L. T., Turck, M., Petersdorf, R. G., and Wedgewood, R. J. Significance of bacterial variants in urine of patients with chronic bacteriuria. *J. Clin. Invest.* 44:1945, 1965.

146. Guttman, D., and Naylor, G. R. E. Dipslide: An aid to quantitative urine culture in general practice. *Brit. Med. J.* 3:343, 1967.

147. Guze, L. B., and Beeson, P. B. Experimental pyelonephritis: I. Effect of ureteral ligation on the course of bacterial infection in the kidney of the rat. *J. Exp. Med.* 104:803, 1956.

148. Guze, L. B., and Beeson, P. B. Observations on the reliability and safety of bladder catheterization for bacteriologic study of the urine. *New Eng. J. Med.* 255:474, 1956.

149. Guze, L. B., Goldner, B. H., and Kalmanson, G. M. Pyelonephritis: I. Observations on the course of chronic non-obstructed enterococcal infection in the kidney of the rat. *Yale J. Biol. Med.* 33:372, 1961.

150. Guze, L. B., and Haley, L. D. Fungus infections of the urinary tract. *Yale J. Biol. Med.* 30:292, 1958.

151. Guze, L. B., Hubert, E., Kalmanson, G. M. Pyelonephritis: VI. Observations of the effects of congenital partial ureteral obstruction on susceptibility of the rat kidney to infection. *J. Infect. Dis.* 115:500, 1965.

152. Guze, L. B., and Kalmanson, G. M. Persistence of bacteria in "protoplast" form after apparent cure of pyelonephritis in rats. *Science* 143:1340, 1964.

153. Guze, L. B., and Kalmanson, G. M. Action of erythromycin on "protoplast" *in vivo*. *Science* 146:1299, 1964.

154. Guze, L. B., and Kalmanson, G. M. Bacteremia following needle aspiration of the bladder. *J. Urol.* 96:308, 1966.

155. Gwynne, J. F. Chronic pyelonephritis and hypertension. *Aust. Ann. Med.* 9:150, 1960.

155a. Hale, R. W., and McCorriston, C. C. Suprapubic cystostomy with a polyethylene tube. *Amer. J. Obstet. Gynec.* 105:1181, 1969.

156. Haley, L. D. Yeast infections of the lower tract: 1. In vitro studies of the tissue phase of *Candida albicans*. *Sabouraudia* 4:98, 1965.

157. Hamburger, J., Richet, G., Crosnier, J., Funck-Brentano, J. L., Antoine, B., Ducrot, H., Mery, J. P., and deMontera, H. *Nephrology*. (2 vols.) Philadelphia: Saunders, 1968.

158. Haran, P. J., Darling, D. B., and Fisher, J. H. The excretory urogram in children with ureterorenal reflux. *Amer. J. Roentgen.* 99:585, 1967.

159. Harris, R. E., and Dunihoo, D. R. The incidence and significance of urinary calculi in pregnancy. *Amer. J. Obstet. Gynec.* 99:237, 1967.

160. Harrow, B. R. Renal papillary necrosis: A critique of pathogenesis. *J. Urol.* 97:203, 1967.

161. Harrow, B. R. The myth of the megacystis syndrome. *J. Urol.* 98:205, 1967.

162. Harrow, B. R., Sloane, J. A., and Witus, W. S. A critical examination of bladder neck obstruction in children. *J. Urol.* 98:613, 1967.

163. Hart, E. L., and Magee, M. J. Collecting urine specimens: A new method — which does not involve catheterization — for collecting uncontaminated urine specimens for culture. *Amer. J. Nurs.* 57:1323, 1957.

163a. Havgen, J., Strøm, O., and Østervold, B. Bacterial counts in urine: I. The reliability of the loop technique. *Acta Path. Microb. Scand.* 74:391, 1968.

163b. Havgen, J., Strøm, O., and Østervold, B. Bacterial counts in urine: II. A comparison of different methods. *Acta. Path. Microb. Scand.* 77:149, 1969.

164. Headington, J. T., and Bayerlein, B. Anaerobic bacteria in routine urine culture. *J. Clin. Path* .19:573, 1966.

165. Hellström, J. Role of Infection in the Etiology of Renal Lithiasis. In Butt, A. J. (Ed.), *Etiologic Factors in Renal Lithiasis*. Springfield, Ill.: Thomas, 1956. P. 212.

166. Helmholz, H. F., and Field, R. S. Acute changes in rabbit's kidney, particularly pelvis, produced by ligating ureter. *J. Urol.* 15:409, 1926.

167. Henderson, D. A. The aetiology of chronic nephritis in Queensland. *Med. J. Aust.* 1:377, 1958.

168. Heptinstall, R. H. Malignant hypertension: Study of 51 cases. *J. Path. Bact.* 65:423, 1953.

169. Heptinstall, R. H. Renal biopsies in hypertension. *Brit. Heart J.* 16:133, 1954.

170. Heptinstall, R. H. Experimental pyelonephritis, bacteriological and morphological studies on the ascending route of infection in the rat. *Nephron* 1:73, 1964.

171. Heptinstall, R. H. Experimental pyelonephritis: A comparison of blood borne and ascending patterns of infection. *J. Path. Bact.* 89:71, 1965.

172. Heptinstall, R. H. *Pathology of the Kidney*. Boston: Little, Brown, 1966.

173. Heptinstall, R. H. The Limitations of the Pathological Diagnosis of Chronic Pyelonephritis. In Black, D. A. K. (Ed.), *Renal Disease* (2d ed.). Oxford: Blackwell, 1967. P. 350.

174. Heptinstall, R. H., and Gorrill, R. H. Experimental pyelonephritis and its effect on blood pressure. *J. Path. Bact.* 69:191, 1955.

175. Heptinstall, R. H., Michaels, L., and Brum-fitt, W.   Experimental pyelonephritis: The role of arterial narrowing in the production of the kidney of chronic pyelonephritis. *J. Path. Bact.* 80:249, 1960.

176. Heptinstall, R. H., and Stryker, M.   Experimental pyelonephritis: A study of the susceptibility of the hypertensive kidney to infection in the rat. *Bull. Johns Hopkins Hosp.* 111:292, 1962.

177. Hill, G. S.   Experimental pyelonephritis: A microangiographic and histologic study of cortical vascular changes. *Bull. Johns. Hopkins Hosp.* 119:79, 1966.

178. Hill, G. S.   Experimental pyelonephritis: Compensatory vascular alterations and their relation to the development of papillary necrosis. *Bull. Johns Hopkins Hosp.* 119:100, 1966.

179. Hinman, F., Jr.   Mechanisms for the entry of bacteria and the establishment of urinary infection in female children. *J. Urol.* 96:546, 1966.

179a. Hinman, F., Jr.   Bacterial elimination. *J. Urol.* 99:811, 1968.

180. Hobday, J. D.   A simplified culture method for detecting asymptomatic bacteriuria in children. *Pediatrics* 38:903, 1966.

181. Hodson, C. J.   The radiological contribution toward the diagnosis of chronic pyelonephritis. *Radiology* 88:857, 1967.

182. Hodson, C. J., and Wilson, S.   Natural history of pyelonephritic scarring. *Brit. Med. J.* 2:191, 1965.

183. Holle, G.   Significance of renal vessels for natural history of chronic pyelonephritis and calculous pyonephrosis. *Virchow. Arch.* [*Path. Anat.*] 332:494, 1959.

184. Holliday, M. A., Winters, R. W., Welt, L. G., MacDowell, M., and Oliver, J.   The renal lesions of electrolyte imbalance: II. The combined effect on renal architecture of phosphate loading and potassium depletion. *J. Exp. Med.* 110:161, 1959.

184a. Holmgren, J.   On the antibody response to *E. coli* antigens in immunized rabbits and in children with pyelonephritis. Thesis. Orstadius Boktryckeri Aktiebolag. Göteborg, 1969.

185. Hood, B., Bengtsson, U., Isaksson, B., Koll-berg, S., and Rådberg, C.   Intensive treatment of chronic pyelonephritis. *Acta Med. Scand.* 166:205, 1960.

186. Hubert, E. G. Montgomerie, J. Z., Kalmanson, G. M., and Guze, L. B.   Effect of renal physiochemical milieu on serum bactericidal activity. *Antimicrob. Agents Chemother.* P. 29, 1967.

187. Hunter, B. W., Akins, L. L., and Sanford, J. P.   The role of immunity in the pathogenesis of experimental retrograde pyelonephritis. *J. Exp. Med.* 119:869, 1964.

188. Hutt, M. S. R., Chalmers, J. A., MacDonald, J. S., and de Wardener, H. E.   Pyelonephritis. *Lancet* 1:351, 1961.

189. Huvos, A., and Rocha, H.   Frequency of bacteriuria in patients with diabetes mellitus. *New Eng. J. Med.* 261:1213, 1959.

189a. Immergut, M. A., and Wahman, G. E.   The urethral caliber of female children with recurrent urinary tract infections. *J. Urol.* 99:189, 1968.

190. Jackson, G. G., and Grieble, H. G.   Pathogenesis of renal infection. *A.M.A. Arch. Intern. Med.* 100:692, 1957.

191. Jackson, G. G., Kozij, V. M., and Joo, R. L.   Relation of Serogroup Strain Prevalence and *E. coli* Urinary Tract Infections. In Kass, E. H. (Ed.), *Progress in Pyelonephritis.* Philadelphia: Davis, 1965. P. 150.

192. Jaenike, J. R., and Bray, G. A.   Effects of acute transitory urinary obstruction in the dog. *Amer. J. Physiol.* 199:1219, 1960.

193. Järvinen, K. A. J.   Determination of peroxidase in urine. *Brit. Med. J.* 1:379, 1958.

194. Jawetz, E., Hopper, J., Jr., and Smith, D. R.   Nitrofurantoin in chronic urinary tract infection. *A.M.A. Arch. Intern. Med.* 100:549, 1957.

195. Jensen, M. M., and Jackson, N. L.   Influence of urine on viruses. *J. Urol.* 95:87, 1966.

196. Kahler, R. L., and Guze, L. B.   Evaluation of the Griess nitrite test as a method for the recognition of urinary tract infection. *J. Lab. Clin. Med.* 49:934, 1957.

197. Kaitz, A. L.   Urinary concentrating ability in pregnant women with asymptomatic bacteriuria. *J. Clin. Invest.* 40:1331, 1961.

198. Kaitz, A. L., and Hodder, E. W.   Bacteriuria and pyelonephritis of pregnancy. *New Eng. J. Med.* 265:667, 1961.

199. Kallet, H. A., and Lapco, L. Urine beta-glucuronidase activity in urinary tract disease. *J. Urol.* 97:352, 1967.

200. Kalmanson, G. M., Hubert, E. G., and Guze, L. B. Pyelonephritis: IV. Role of serum bactericidal activity and antibody in chronic enterococcal pyelonephritis in the rat. *Proc. Soc. Exp. Biol. Med.* 113:918, 1963.

201. Kalmanson, G. M., Hubert, E. G., and Guze, L. B. Pyelonephritis: V. Role of serum bactericidal activity and antibody in acute pyelonephritis in the rabbit. *Proc. Soc. Exp. Biol. Med.* 113:921, 1963.

201a. Kalmanson, G. M., Montgomerie, J. Z., and Guze, L. B. Influence of the metabolic environment of the kidney on the activity of antibiotics. *Antimicrob. Agents Chemother.* P. 384, 1965.

202. Karabatsos, N., and Herrold, R. D. Some unusual pathogens isolated from the urinary tract. *J. Urol.* 84:187, 1960.

203. Kass, E. H. The role of asymptomatic bacteriuria in the pathogenesis of pyelonephritis. In Quinn, E. L., and Kass, E. H. (Eds.), *Biology of Pyelonephritis* (Henry Ford Hospital International Symposium). Boston: Little, Brown, 1960. P. 399.

203a. Kass, E. H. Bacterial antigen in the kidney. *New Eng. J. Med.* 281:420, 1969.

204. Kass, E. H., Miall, W. E., and Stuart, K. L. Relationship of bacteriuria to hypertension. *J. Clin. Invest.* 40:1053, 1961.

205. Kass, E. H., and Zangwill, D. P. Principles in the Long-term Management of Chronic Infection of the Urinary Tract. In Quinn, E. L., and Kass, E. H. (Eds.), *Biology of Pyelonephritis.* (Henry Ford Hospital International Symposium.) Boston: Little, Brown, 1960. P. 663.

206. Katz, Y. J., Bourdo, S. R., and Moore, R. S. Effect of pyrogen and adrenal steroids in pyelonephritis. *Lancet* 1:1140, 1962.

207. Katz, Y. J., Velasquez, A., and Bourdo, S. R. The prednisolone provocative test for pyelonephritis. *Lancet* 1:1144, 1962.

208. Kay, C. J., Rosenberg, M. A., Fleisher, P., and Small, J. Renal papillary necrosis in hemoglobin SC disease. *Radiology* 90:897, 1968.

209. Kaye, D. Antibacterial activity of human urine. *J. Clin. Invest.* 47:2374, 1968.

210. Kaye, M., de Vries, J., and Mac Farlane, K. T. The initiation of urinary tract infection following a single bladder catheterization. *Canad. Med. Ass. J.* 86:9, 1962.

211. Kaye, M., Pritchard, J. E., Halpenny, G. W., and Light, W. Bone disease in chronic renal failure with particular reference to osteosclerosis. *Medicine* (Balt.) 39:157, 1960.

212. Keane, W. F., and Freedman, L. R. Experimental pyelonephritis: XIV. Pyelonephritis in normal mice produced by inoculation of *E. coli* into the bladder lumen during water diuresis. *Yale J. Biol. Med.* 40:231, 1967.

213. Kellow, W. F., Cotsonas, N. J., Jr., Chomet, B., and Zimmerman, H. Evaluation of the adequacy of needle-biopsy specimens of the kidney. *A.M.A. Arch. Intern. Med.* 104:353, 1959.

214. Kennedy, G. C. Effects of old age and over-nutrition on kidney. *Brit. Med. Bull.* 13:67, 1957.

215. Kennedy, R. P., Plorde, J. J., and Petersdorf, R. G. Studies on the epidemiology of *Escherichia coli* infections: IV. Evidence for a nosocomial flora. *J. Clin. Invest.* 44:193, 1965.

216. Kenny, J. F., Medearis, D. N., Jr., Drachman, R. H., Gibson, L. E., and Klein, S. W. An outbreak of urinary tract infection and septicemia due to *Escherichia coli* in male infants. *Amer. J. Dis. Child.* 104:461, 1962.

217. Keresztury, S., and Megyeri, L. Histology of renal pyramids with special regard to changes due to ageing. *Acta Morph. Acad. Sci. Hung.* 11:205, 1962.

217a. Kerr, Walter S., Jr., Suby, H. I., Vickery, A., and Fraley, E. Idiopathic retroperitoneal fibrosis: Clinical experiences with 15 cases, 1956–1957. *J. Urol.* 99:575, 1968.

218. Kessner, D. M., and Lepper, M. H. Epidemiologic studies of gram-negative bacilli in the hospital and community. *Amer. J. Epidem.* 85:45, 1967.

219. Kimmelstiel, P. Case records of the Massachusetts General Hospital, Case No. 27–1966. *New Eng. J. Med.* 274:1374, 1966.

220. Kimmelstiel, P. Asymptomatic Bacteriuria, a Hypothetical Concept, Should Be

Treated with Caution. In Ingelfinger, F. J., Relman, A. S., and Finland, M. (Eds.), *Controversy in Internal Medicine*. Philadelphia: Saunders, 1966. P. 302.

221. Kimmelstiel, P., Kim, O. J., Beres, J. A., and Wellmann, K. Chronic pyelonephritis. *Amer. J. Med.* 30:589, 1961.

222. Kimmelstiel, P., and Wilson, C. Inflammatory lesions in the glomeruli in pyelonephritis in relation to hypertension and renal insufficiency. *Amer. J. Path.* 12:99, 1936.

223. Kincaid-Smith, P. Vascular obstruction in chronic pyelonephritic kidneys and its relation to hypertension. *Lancet* 269:1263, 1955.

224. Kincaid-Smith, P. Pathogenesis of the renal lesion associated with abuse of analgesics. *Lancet* 1:859, 1967.

224a. Kincaid-Smith, P. Analgesic nephropathy. *Ann. Intern. Med.* 68:949, 1968.

225. Kincaid-Smith, P., and Bullen, M. Bacteriuria in pregnancy. *Lancet* 1:395, 1965.

225a. Kincaid-Smith, P., and Fairley, K. F. Controlled trial comparing effect of two and six weeks treatment in recurrent urinary tract infection. *Brit. Med. J.* 1:145, 1969.

226. Kincaid-Smith, P., McMichael, J., and Murphy, E. A. Clinical course and pathology of hypertension with papilloedema (malignant hypertension). *Quart. J. Med.* 27:117, 1958.

226a. Kincaid-Smith, P., Saker, B. M., McKenzie, I. F. C., and Muriden, K. D. Lesions in the blood supply of the papilla in experimental analgesic nephropathy. *Med. J. Aust.* 1:203, 1968.

227. Kippax, P. W. A study of *Proteus* infections in a male urological ward. *J. Clin. Path.* 10:211, 1957.

228. Kjellberg, S. R., Ericsson, N. O., and Rudhe, U. *The Lower Urinary Tract in Childhood*. Stockholm: Almquist and Wiksell, 1957. Pp. 182–202.

229. Kleeman, C. R., Hewitt, W. L., and Guze, L. B. Pyelonephritis. *Medicine* 39:3, 1960.

230. Kleeman, C. R., and Maxwell, M. H. The Nephrotoxicity of Antibiotics: A Review. In Quinn, E. L., and Kass, E. H. (Eds.), *Biology of Pyelonephritis*. (Henry Ford Hospital International Symposium.) Boston: Little, Brown, 1960. P. 631.

231. Kleeman, S. E. T., and Freedman, L. R. The finding of chronic pyelonephritis in males and females at autopsy. *New Eng. J. Med.* 263:988, 1960.

232. Koletsky, S. Hypertensive vascular disease produced by salt. *Lab. Invest.* 7:377, 1958.

233. Kunin, C. M. The quantitative significance of bacteria visualized in the unstained urinary sediment. *New Eng. J. Med.* 265:589, 1961.

234. Kunin, C. M. Asymptomatic bacteriuria. *Ann. Rev. Med.* 17:383, 1966.

235. Kunin, C. M. A guide to use of antibiotics in patients with renal disease. *Ann. Intern. Med.* 67:151, 1967.

235a. Kunin, C. M. The natural history of recurrent bacteriuria in schoolgirls. *New Eng. J. Med.* 282:1443, 1970.

235b. Kunin, C. M. A ten-year study of bacteriuria in schoolgirls: Final report of bacteriologic, urologic, and epidemiologic findings. *J. Infect. Dis.* 122:382, 1970.

236. Kunin, C. M., Deutscher, R., and Paquin, A., Jr. Urinary tract infection in school children: An epidemiologic, clinical and laboratory study. *Medicine* 43:91, 1964.

237. Kunin, C. M., and McCormack, R. C. Prevention of catheter-induced urinary tract infection by sterile closed drainage. *New Eng. J. Med.* 274:1156, 1966.

238. Kunin, C. M., and McCormack, R. C. An epidemiologic study of bacteriuria and blood pressure among nuns and working women. *New Eng. J. Med.* 278:635, 1968.

239. Lagergren, C., and Ljungqvist, A. The intrarenal arterial pattern in renal papillary necrosis. *Amer. J. Path.* 41:633, 1962.

240. Lagergren, C., and Ljungqvist, A. The intrarenal arterial pattern in chronic pyelonephritis: A micro-angiographic and histologic study. *Virchow. Arch.* [*Path. Anat.*] 335:584, 1962.

241. Lain, L., and Braude, A. I. Diminished pathogenicity of a galactose-deficient mutant of *E. coli* for the kidney. *Clin. Res.* 16:331, 1968.

242. Lancaster, M. G., and Allison, F., Jr. Stud-

ies on the pathogenesis of acute inflammation: VII. The influence of osmolality upon the phagocytic and clumping activity by human leucocytes. *Amer. J. Path.* 49:1185, 1966.

243. Lauler, D. P., Schreiner, G. E., and David, A. Renal medullary necrosis. *Amer. J. Med.* 29:132, 1960.

244. Lefebvre, R., and Genest, J. Study of renal ischaemic tubular atrophy in 79 patients with arterial hypertension. *Canad. Med. Ass. J.* 82:1249, 1960.

245. Lehmann, J. D., Smith, J. W., Miller, T. E., Barnett, J. A., and Sanford, J. P. The immune response of the kidney in experimental pyelonephritis. *J. Clin. Invest.* 47:60a, 1968.

246. Leigh, D. A., Grüneberg, R. H., and Brumfitt, W. Long-term follow-up of bacteriuria in pregnancy. *Lancet* 1:603, 1968.

247. Levin, J. The incidence and prevention of infection after urethral catheterization. *Ann. Intern. Med.* 60:914, 1964.

247a. Liebman, N. C. Renal papillary necrosis and sickle cell disease. *J. Urol.* 102:294, 1969.

248. Lincoln, K., and Winberg, J. Studies of urinary tract infections in infancy and childhood: II. Quantitative estimate of bacteriuria in unselected neonates with special reference to the occurrence of asymptomatic infections. *Acta Paediat.* 53:307, 1964.

248a. Lindan, R. The prevention of ascending, catheter-induced infections of the urinary tract. *J. Chronic Dis.* 22:321, 1969.

249. Lindemeyer, R. I., Turck, M., and Petersdorf, R. G. Factors determining the outcome of chemotherapy in infections of the urinary tract. *Ann. Intern. Med.* 58:201, 1963.

250. Lindholm, T. On renal papillary necrosis with special reference to diagnostic importance of papillary fragments in urine, therapy (artificial kidney) and prognosis: Report of 75 cases, including 12 with papillary fragments in urine. *Acta Med. Scand.* 167:319, 1960.

251. Lipman, R. L., Tyrell, E., Small, J., and Shapiro, A. P. Evaluation of antibiotic therapy in acute pyelonephritis produced by *Escherichia coli* in rats. *J. Lab. Clin. Med.* 67:546, 1966.

252. Lister, A. J. Ph.D. Thesis, University of Cambridge, 1957. Quoted by Gorrill, R. H. Bacteriological conditions leading to destruction of the kidney. *Guy. Hosp. Rep.* 107:405, 1958.

253. Little, P. J. Urinary white-cell excretion. *Lancet* 1:1149, 1962.

254. Little, P. J. The incidence of urinary infection in 5000 pregnant women. *Lancet* 2:925, 1966.

255. Little, P. J., and de Wardener, H. E. The use of prednisolone phosphate in the diagnosis of pyelonephritis in man. *Lancet* 1:1145, 1962.

256. Little, P. J., and de Wardener, H. E. Acute pyelonephritis: Incidence of reinfection in 100 patients. *Lancet* 2:1277, 1966.

257. Little, P. J., McPherson, D. R., and de Wardener, H. E. The appearance of the intravenous pyelogram during and after acute pyelonephritis. *Lancet* 1:1186, 1965.

258. Little, P. J., Sloper, J. S., and de Wardener, H. E. Syndrome of loin pain and hematuria associated with disease of peripheral renal arteries. *Quart. J. Med.* 36:253, 1967.

259. Longacre, A. M., and Popky, G. L. Papillary necrosis in patients with cirrhosis: A study of 102 patients. *J. Urol.* 99:391, 1968.

260. Longcope, W. T., and Winkenwerder, W. L. Clinical features of the contracted kidney due to pyelonephritis. *Bull. Johns Hopkins Hosp.* 53:255, 1933.

260a. Lorrier, J. C., and Valkenburg, H. A. Quantitative urine culture by surface drop method. *Appl. Microbiol.* 18:57, 1969.

261. Lowe, G. K., Henderson, J. L., Park, W. W., and McGreal, D. A. The idiopathic hypercalcemia syndromes of infancy. *Lancet* 2:101, 1954.

262. Lyon, M. L., and Tuttle, E. P., Jr. Differential Effects of Acidifying Agents in Experimental Pyelonephritis. In Kass, E. H. (Ed.), *Progress in Pyelonephritis*. Philadelphia: Davis, 1965. P. 242.

263. Macaulay, D., and Sutton, R. N. P. The prognosis of urinary infections in childhood. *Lancet* 2:1318, 1957.

264. MacDonald, R. A., Levitin, H., Mallory,

G. K., and Kass, E. H.   Relation between pyelonephritis and bacterial counts in the urine. *New Eng. J. Med.* 256:915, 1957.

265. Mahoney, S. A., and Persky, L.   Observations on experimental ascending pyelonephritis in the rat. *J. Urol.* 89:779, 1963.

266. Mallory, G. K., Crane, A. R., and Edwards, J. E.   Pathology of acute and of healed experimental pyelonephritis. *Arch. Path.* 30:330, 1940.

267. Marshall, A. G.   Scars of renal cortex. *J. Path. Bact.* 71:95, 1956.

268. Marshall, S.   Effect of bubble bath on urinary tract. *J. Urol.* 93:112, 1965.

269. Martin, C. M., Vaquer, F., Meyers, M. S., and El-Dadah, A.   Prevention of Gram-Negative Rod Bacteremia Complicating Indwelling Urinary-Tract Catheterization. In Kass, E. H. (Ed.), *Progress in Pyelonephritis*. Philadelphia: Davis, 1965. P. 692.

270. McCabe, W. R., and Jackson, G. G.   Treatment of pyelonephritis: Bacterial, drug and host factors in success and failure among 252 patients. *New Eng. J. Med.* 272:1037, 1965.

271. McCarthy, J. M., and Pryles, C. V.   Clean voided and catheter neonatal urine samples. *Amer. J. Dis. Child.* 106:473, 1963.

271a. McFadyen, I. R., and Eykyn, S. J.   Suprapubic aspiration of urine in pregnancy. *Lancet* 1:1112, 1968.

272. McLeod, J. W.   The hospital urine bottle and bedpan as reservoirs of infection by *Pseudomonas pyocyanea*. *Lancet* 1:394, 1958.

273. Meares, E. M., and Stamey, T. A.   Bacteriologic localization patterns in bacterial prostatitis and urethritis. *Invest. Urol.* 5:492, 1968.

274. Mehnert, B., and Mehnert, H.   Yeasts in urine and saliva of diabetic and non-diabetic patients. *Diabetes* 7:293, 1958.

275. Mehrota, R. M. L.   An experimental study of the vesical circulation during distention and in cystitis. *J. Path. Bact.* 66:79, 1953.

276. Melick, R. A., and Henneman, P. H.   Clinical and laboratory studies of 207 consecutive patients in a kidney-stone clinic. *New Eng. J. Med.* 259:307, 1958.

277. Mellins, H. Z. (Moderator).   A Panel on the Role of Radiology in the Diagnosis of Abnormalities of the Urinary Conduit System. In Glenn, J. F. (Ed.), *Proceedings of a Workshop on Ureteral Reflux in Children*. Washington: National Academy of Sciences–National Research Council, 1967. P. 89.

278. Meyers, A.   Unpublished data, 1968.

279. Miall, W. E., Kass, E. H., Ling, J., and Stuart, K. L.   Factors influencing arterial pressure in the general population in Jamaica. *Brit. Med. J.* 2:497, 1962.

280. Michie, A. J.   Chronic pyelonephritis mimicking ureteral obstructions. *Pediat. Clin. N. Amer.* 6:1117, 1959.

280a. Miller, A. L.   Brown urine — a clue to phenacetin intoxication. *Lancet* 2:1359, 1970.

281. Miller, T. E., and North, J. D. K.   Effect of protein intake on bacterial growth in the kidney. *Brit. J. Exp. Path.* 47:105, 1966.

281a. Mond, N. C., Grüneberg, R. N., and Smellie, J. M.   Study of childhood urinary tract infection in general practice. *Brit. Med. J.* 1:602, 1970.

282. Milne, M. D., and Muehrcke, R. C.   Potassium deficiency and kidney. *Brit. Med. Bull.* 13:15, 1957.

283. Montgomerie, J. Z., Kalmanson, G. M., and Guze, L. B.   Renal failure and infection. *Medicine* (Balt.) 47:1, 1968.

284. Montgomerie, J. Z., and North, J. D. K.   Evaluation of the pyrogen test in chronic pyelonephritis. *Lancet* 1:690, 1963.

285. Monto, A. S., and Rantz, L. A.   The development and character of bacteriuria in pregnancy. *Ann. Intern. Med.* 59:186, 1963.

286. Morgan, J. M., Hartley, M. W., and Miller, R. E.   Nephropathy in chronic lead poisoning. *Arch. Intern. Med.* 118:17, 1966.

287. Mortensen, J. D., Emmett, J. L., and Baggenstoss, A. H.   Clinical aspects of nephrocalcinosis. *Proc. Mayo Clinic* 28:305, 1953.

288. Mostofi, F. K., Verder Brugge, C. F., and Diggs, L. W.   Lesions in kidneys removed for unilateral hematuria in sickle-cell disease. *A.M.A. Arch. Path.* 63:336, 1957.

289. Mou, T. W., and Feldman, H. A.   The enumeration and preservation of bacteria in urine. *Amer. J. Clin. Path.* 35:572, 1961.

289a. Mulholland, S. G., Foster, E. A., Paquin, A. J., Jr., and Gillenwater, J. Y. The effect of rabbit vesical mucosa on bacterial growth. *Invest. Urol.* 6:593, 1969.

289b. Mulholland, S. G., Perez, J. R., and Gillenwater, J. Y. The antibacterial properties of urine. *Invest. Urol.* 6:569, 1969.

290. Mulrow, P. J., Huvos, A., and Buchanan, D. L. Measurement of residual urine with ^{131}I-labeled Diodrast. *J. Lab. Clin. Med.* 57: 109, 1961.

291. Murphy, F. J., Zelman, S., and Man, W. Ascorbic acid as a urinary acidifying agent: 2. Its adjunctive role in chronic urinary infection. *J. Urol.* 94:300, 1965.

292. Murphy, K. J. Bilateral renal calculi and aminoaciduria after excessive intake of Worcestershire sauce. *Lancet* 2:401, 1967.

293. Nelson, J. D., and Peters, P. C. Suprapubic aspiration of urine in premature and term infants. *Pediatrics* 36:132, 1965.

294. Neumann, C. G., and Pryles, C. V. Pyelonephritis in infants and children. *Amer. J. Dis. Child.* 104:215, 1962.

294a. Norden, C. W., Green, G. M., and Kass, E. H. Antibacterial mechanisms of the urinary bladder. *J. Clin. Invest.* 47:2689, 1968.

295. Norden, C. W., and Kass, E. H. Bacteriuria of pregnancy: A critical appraisal. *Ann. Rev. Med.* 19:431, 1968.

295a. Norden, C. W., Levy, P. S., and Kass, E. H. Predictive effect of urinary concentrating ability and hemagglutinating antibody titer upon response to antimicrobial therapy in bacteriuria of pregnancy. *J. Infect. Dis.* 121:588, 1970.

296. Norden, C. W., and Tuttle, E. P., Jr. Impairment of Urinary Concentrating Ability in Pregnant Women with Asymptomatic Bacteriuria. In Kass, E. H. (Ed.), *Progress in Pyelonephritis*. Philadelphia: Davis, 1965. P. 73.

297. Numazaki, Y., Shigeta, S., Kumasaka, T., Miyazawa, T., Yamanaka, M., Yano, N., Takai, S., and Ishida, N. Acute hemorrhagic cystitis in children: Isolation of adenovirus type II. *New Eng. J. Med.* 278:700, 1968.

298. Nutbourne, D. M., and de Wardener, H. E. The effect of a water diuresis on the urinary excretion of hydrogen ions in man. *Clin. Sci.* 20:63, 1961.

298a. Ödegaard, K. Quantitative urine culture. An attempt to preserve the *status quo* of bacterial counts in urine samples by the use of disodium calcium edathamil. *Amer. J. Clin. Path.* 51:409, 1969.

299. O'Dell, R. M., Brazil, W. O., and Schlegel, J. U. Effectiveness of urea in prophylaxis of experimentally induced bacteriuria in rats. *J. Urol.* 97:145, 1967.

299a. O'Grady, F., and Brumfitt, W. (Eds.). *Urinary Tract Infection* (Proceedings of the First National Symposium on Urinary Tract Infection, London, April, 1968). London: Oxford University Press, 1968.

300. O'Grady, F., and Pennington, J. H. Bacterial growth in an *in vitro* system simulating conditions in the urinary bladder. *Brit. J. Exp. Path.* 47:152, 1966.

301. O'Grady, F., and Pennington, J. H. Synchronized micturition and antibiotic administration in treatment of urinary infection in an *in vitro* model. *Brit. Med. J.* 1:403, 1967.

302. Oladsson, O., Gudmundsson, K. R., and Brekkan, A. Migraine, gastritis and renal papillary necrosis: A syndrome in chronic nonobstructive pyelonephritis. *Acta Med. Scand.* 179:121, 1966.

303. Örsten, P. Å. Long term treatment of pyelonephritis. *Acta Med. Scand.* 172:259, 1962.

304. Örsten, P. Å. Asymmetry of renal function with special reference to chronic pyelonephritis. *Acta Med. Scand.* 180 (Suppl. 447): 5, 1966.

305. O'Sullivan, D. J., FitzGerald, M. G., Meynell, M. J., and Malins, J. M. Urinary tract infection, a comparative study in the diabetic and general populations. *Brit. Med. J.* 1:786, 1961.

306. Pandola, G. A., Kreutner, A., Kreutner, K., and Farmer, S. G. Experimental ascending pyelonephritis in rats: Experimental hydronephrosis with sterile pyelonephritis. *Lab. Invest.* 13:1484, 1964.

307. Paplanus, S. H. Bacterial localisation in the kidney. *Yale J. Biol. Med.* 37:145, 1964.

308. Patrick, M. J. Renal infection in preg-

nancy: II. Bacteriuria in pregnancy related to maternal factors. *J. Obstet. Gynaec. Brit. Comm.* 74:17, 1967.

309. Patrick, R. L., Kroe, D. J., and Klavins, J. V. Renal papillary necrosis induced by heterologous serum. *Arch. Path.* (Chicago) 78:108, 1964.

310. Pawlowski, J. M., Bloxdorf, J. W., and Kimmelstiel, P. Chronic pyelonephritis: A morphologic and bacteriologic study. *New Eng. J. Med.* 268:965, 1963.

311. Pears, M. A., and Houghton, B. J. Response of infected urinary tract to bacterial pyrogen. *Lancet* 2:1167, 1959.

312. Perkoff, G. T. Hereditary Chronic Nephritis. In Quinn, E. L., and Kass, E. H. (Eds.), *Biology of Pyelonephritis.* (Henry Ford Hospital International Symposium.) Boston: Little, Brown, 1960. P. 259.

313. Persky, L. Pyelonephritis in children. *J. Urol.* 94:20, 1965.

314. Peters, J. P., Lavietes, P. H., and Zimmerman, H. M. Pyelitis in toxemias of pregnancy. *Amer. J. Obstet. Gynec.* 32:911, 1936.

315. Petersdorf, R. G. Asymptomatic Bacteriuria: A Therapeutic Enigma. In Ingelfinger, F. J., Relman, A. S., and Finland, M. (Eds.), *Controversy in Internal Medicine.* Philadelphia: Saunders, 1966. P. 302.

316. Pfeiffer, E. W. Comparative anatomical observations of the mammalian renal pelvis and medulla. *J. Anat.* 102:321, 1968.

317. Pigeon, G., Saint-Martin, M., and Genest, J. Response to bacterial pyrogen in the differential diagnosis of chronic urinary tract infection. *Canad. Med. Ass. J.* 84:360, 1961.

318. Plorde, J. J., Kennedy, R. P., Bourne, H. H., Ansell, J. S., and Petersdorf, R. G. Course and prognosis of prostatectomy. *New Eng. J. Med.* 272:269, 1965.

319. Politano, V. In Glenn, J. F. (Ed.), *Proceedings of a Workshop on Ureteral Reflux in Children.* Washington: National Academy of Sciences–National Research Council, 1967. P. 132.

320. Pometta, D., Rees, S. B., Younger, D., and Kass, E. H. Asymptomatic bacteriuria in diabetes mellitus. *New Eng. J. Med.* 276:1118, 1967.

320a. Porter, K. A., and Brodie, J. Boric acid

preservation of urine samples. *Brit. Med. J.* 2:353, 1969.

321. Porter, K. A., and Giles, H. McC. A pathological study of 5 cases of pyelonephritis in the newborn. *Arch. Dis. Child.* 31:303, 1956.

322. Prát, V., and Hatala, M. Experimental hematogenous *Escherichia coli* pyelonephritis in the rabbit. *Rozpravy Cesk. Akad. Ved. Rada Mat. Prirod. Ved.* 77:84, 1967.

323. Prát, V., Hatala, M., Benešová, D., and Rossman, P. Pathogenicity of Various Strains of *Escherichia coli* for the Intact Rabbit Kidney and the Effect of Repeated Passage on Renal Tissue. In Kass, E. H. (Ed.), *Progress in Pyelonephritis.* Philadelphia: Davis, 1965. P. 135.

323a. Prát, V., Koníčková, L., Ritzerfeld, W., Losse, H. Experimental infections of the kidneys and urinary tract in pregnant rats *Physiol. Bohemoslov.* 18:243, 1969.

324. Prescott, L. F. Analgesic abuse and renal disease in North-East Scotland. *Lancet* 2:1143, 1966.

325. Prescott, L. F., and Brodie, D. E. A simple differential stain for urinary sediment. *Lancet* 2:940, 1964.

326. Pridgen, W. R., Woodhead, D. M., and Younger, R. K. Alterations in renal function produced by ureteral obstruction. *J.A.M.A.* 178:563, 1961.

327. Prockop, D. J., and Davidson, W. D. A study of urinary and serum lysozyme in patients with renal disease. *New Eng. J. Med.* 270:269, 1964.

328. Raaschou, F. *Studies of Chronic Pyelonephritis.* Copenhagen: Ejnar Munksgaard, 1948.

329. Raaschou, F. Discussion. In Kass, E. H. (Ed.), *Progress in Pyelonephritis.* Philadelphia: Davis, 1965. P. 373.

330. Randall, A. Origin and growth of renal calculi. *Ann. Surg.* 105:1009, 1937.

331. Rantz, L. A. Infections of the urinary tract. *Advances Intern. Med.* 1:137, 1942.

332. Rapoport, M., and Rubin, M. I. Lead poisoning: A clinical and experimental study of factors influencing the seasonal incidence in children. *Amer. J. Dis. Child.* 61:245, 1941.

333. Relman, A. S. Some Clinical Aspects of

Chronic Pyelonephritis. In Quinn, E. L., and Kass, E. H. (Eds.), *Biology of Pyelonephritis*. (Henry Ford Hospital International Symposium.) Boston: Little, Brown, 1960. P. 355.

334. Rengarts, R. T. Asymptomatic bacilluria in sixty-eight diabetic patients. *Amer. J. Med. Sci.* 239:159, 1960.

335. Riley, H. D., Jr. Pyelonephritis. *Advances Pediat.* 15:191, 1968.

336. Riley, H. D., Jr., and Knight, V. Urinary tract infection in paralytic poliomyelitis. *Medicine* (Balt.) 37:281, 1958.

337. Robbins, S. L., and Tucker, A. W. The cause of death in diabetes: A report of 307 autopsied cases. *New Eng. J. Med.* 231:865, 1944.

338. Roberts, A. P., Frampton, J., Karim, S. M. M., and Beard, R. W. Estimation of beta-glucuronidase activity in urinary-tract infection. *New Eng. J. Med.* 276:1468, 1967.

339. Roberts, A. P., Robinson, R. E., and Beard, R. W. Some factors affecting bacterial colony counts in urinary infection. *Brit. Med. J.* 1:400, 1967.

340. Rocha, H., and Almeida, S. S. Experimental pyelonephritis in rats with a glass bead in the bladder. *J. Path. Bact.* 90:668, 1965.

341. Rocha, H., and Almeida, S. S. Experimental pyelonephritis: Observations on mixed infection. *Yale J. Biol. Med.* 37:313, 1965.

342. Rocha, H., and Fekety, F. R., Jr. Acute inflammation in the renal cortex and medulla following thermal injury. *J. Exp. Med.* 119:131, 1964.

343. Rocha, H., Guze, L. B., and Beeson, P. B. Experimental pyelonephritis: V. Susceptibility of rats to hematogenous pyelonephritis following chemical injury of the kidneys. *Yale J. Biol. Med.* 32:120, 1959.

344. Rocha, H., Guze, L. B., Freedman, L. R., and Beeson, P. B. Experimental pyelonephritis: III. The influence of localized injury in different parts of the kidney on susceptibility to bacillary infection. *Yale J. Biol. Med.* 30:341, 1958.

345. Ryan, W. L., Hoody, S., and Luby, R. A

simple quantitative test for bacteriuria. *J. Urol.* 88:838, 1962.

346. Sabath, L. D., Elder, H. A., McCall, C. E., and Finland, M. Synergistic combinations of penicillins in the treatment of bacteriuria. *New Eng. J. Med.* 277:232, 1967.

346a. Saccharaw, L., and Pryles, C. V. Further experience with the use of percutaneous suprapubic aspiration of the urinary bladder: Bacteriologic studies in 654 infants and children. *Pediatrics* 43:1018, 1969.

347. Sanford, J. P., and Barnett, J. A. Immunologic responses in urinary-tract infections. *J.A.M.A.* 192:587, 1965.

348. Sanford, J. P., Hunter, B. W., and Donaldson, P. Localization and fate of *Escherichia coli* in hematogenous pyelonephritis. *J. Exp. Med.* 116:285, 1962.

349. Sanford, J. P., Hunter, B. W., and Souda, L. L. The role of immunity in the pathogenesis of experimental hematogenous pyelonephritis. *J. Exp. Med.* 115:383, 1962.

350. Saphir, O., and Cohen, N. A. Chronic pyelonephritis lenta and the "malignant phase of hypertension." *A.M.A. Arch. Intern. Med.* 104:748, 1959.

351. Sapira, J. D., and Shapiro, A. P. Beta-glucuronidase excretion in hypertensive patients. *Amer. J. Med. Sci.* 253:174, 1967.

352. Savage, W. E., Hajj, S. N., and Kass, E. H. Demographic and prognostic characteristics of bacteriuria in pregnancy. *Medicine* (Balt.) 46:385, 1967.

353. Schainuck, L. I., Striker, G. E., and Cutler, R. E. The functional significance of interstitial pathology in chronic renal disease. *Clin. Res.* 16:168, 1968.

354. Schneierson, S. S. A simplified procedure for performing urinary bacterial counts. *J. Urol.* 88:424, 1962.

355. Schoenberg, H. W., Beisswanger, P., Howard, W. J., Klingenmaier, H., Walter, C. F., and Murphy, J. J. Effect of lower urinary tract infection upon ureteral function. *J. Urol.* 92:107, 1964.

356. Schreiner, G. E. The nephrotoxicity of analgesic abuse. *Ann. Intern. Med.* 57:1047, 1962.

356a. Seeler, R. A., and Hahn, K. Jaundice in

urinary tract infection in infancy. *Amer. J. Dis. Child.* 118:553, 1969.

356b. Seligman, S. J., Deigh, R. A., and Hewitt, W. L. Detection of bacteriuria by a filter paper inoculating strip. *Amer. J. Obstet. Gynec.* 102:890, 1968.

357. Seligman, S. J., and Hewitt, W. L. Urinary Concentrating Tests on Postpartum Bacteriuric Women. In Kass, E. H. (Ed.), *Progress in Pyelonephritis*. Philadelphia: Davis, 1965. P. 558.

358. Selye, H. *The Physiology and Pathology of Exposure to Stress*. Montreal: Acta Endocrinologica, 1950. P. 540.

359. Seneca, H., Lattimer, J. K., and Zinsser, H. H. The chemotherapy of urease- and citrase-producing bacteria of the urinary tract. *Ann. Intern. Med.* 53:468, 1960.

360. Shapiro, A. H. Pumping and Retrograde Diffusion in Peristaltic Waves. In Glenn, J. F. (Ed.), *Proceedings of a Workshop in Ureteral Reflux in Children*. Washington: National Academy of Sciences–National Research Council, 1967. P. 109; discussion, p. 127.

361. Shapiro, A. P. Susceptibility of rats with DCA hypertension to experimental pyelonephritis and aggravation of DCA hypertension by renal infection. *J. Lab. Clin. Med.* 55:715, 1960.

362. Shapiro, A. P. Experimental pyelonephritis and hypertension: Implications for the clinical problem. *Ann. Intern. Med.* 59:37, 1963.

363. Shapiro, A. P., Braude, A. I., and Siemienski, J. Hematogenous pyelonephritis in rats: IV. Relationship of bacterial species to the pathogenesis and sequelae of chronic pyelonephritis. *J. Clin. Invest.* 28:1228, 1959.

364. Sheehan, H. L., and Davis, J. C. Experimental hydronephrosis. *A.M.A. Arch. Path.* 68:185, 1959.

365. Shirai, T., Ellner, P. D., and Sims, E. A. H. Increased Susceptibility to Ascending Pyelonephritis of Rats with Nephrotoxic Antiserum Nephrosis. In Kass, E. H. (Ed.), *Progress in Pyelonephritis*. Philadelphia: Davis, 1965. P. 272.

366. Shopfner, C. E. Nonobstructive hydro-

nephrosis and hydroureter. *Amer. J. Roentgen.* 98:172, 1966.

367. Shopfner, C. E. Roentgen evaluation of distal urethral obstruction. *Radiology* 88:222, 1967.

368. Silk, M. R. Hypertension secondary to hydronephrosis in adult and young animals. *Invest. Urol.* 5:30, 1967.

369. Siller, W. G. Avian nephritis and visceral gout. *Lab. Invest.* 8:1319, 1959.

369a. Simenhoff, M. L., Guild, W. R., and Dammin, G. J. Acute diffuse interstitial nephritis. *Amer. J. Med.* 44:618, 1968.

370. Simonsen, M., Bueman, J., Gammeltoft, A., Jensen, F., and Jorgensen, K. Biological incompatibility in kidney transplantation in dogs: I. Experimental and morphological investigations. *Acta Path. Microbiol. Scand.* 32:1, 1953.

370a. Smellie, J. M. Medical aspects of urinary infection in children. *J. Roy. Coll. Physicians* (London) 1:189, 1967.

371. Smellie, J. M., Hodson, C. J., Edwards, D., and Normand, I. C. S. Clinical and radiological features of urinary infection in childhood. *Brit. Med. J.* 2:1222, 1964.

371a. Smellie, J. M., and Normand, I. C. S. Experience of Follow-up of Children With Urinary Tract Infection. In O'Grady, F., and Brumfitt, W. (Eds.), *Urinary Tract Infection* (Proceedings of the First National Symposium on Urinary Tract Infection, London, April, 1968). London: Oxford University Press, 1968. P. 123.

372. Smith, D. R. Estimation of the amount of residual urine by means of the phenolsulfonphthalein test. *J. Urol.* 83:188, 1960.

373. Smith, H. W. Unilateral nephrectomy in hypertensive disease. *J. Urol.* 76:685, 1956.

374. Smith, J. F. The diagnosis of the scars of chronic pyelonephritis. *J. Clin. Path.* 15:522, 1962.

375. Smith, J. F., and Lee, Y. C. Experimental uric acid nephritis in the rabbit. *J. Exp. Med.* 105:615, 1957.

376. Smith, L. G., Thayer, W. R., Malta, E. M., and Utz, J. P. Relationship of the Griess nitrite test to bacterial culture in the diagnosis of urinary tract infection. *Ann. Intern. Med.* 54:66, 1961.

377. Smythe, C. McC., Rivers, C. F., and Rosemond, R. M. A comparison of the incidence of bacteriuria among hypertensives and matched controls. *Arch. Intern. Med.* (Chicago) 105:899, 1960.

378. Sommers, S. C., Gonick, H. C., Kalmanson, G. M., and Guze, L. B. Pathogenesis of chronic pyelonephritis: II. Effect of repetitive infection. *Amer. J. Path.* 45:729, 1965.

379. Sommers, S. C., Relman, A. S., and Smithwick, R. H. Renal biopsy in hypertension. *Amer. J. Path.* 34:685, 1958.

380. Sowry, G. S. C. Hypertension: The coincidence of conditions. II. *Postgrad. Med. J.* (London) 34:39, 1958.

381. Spark, H., Travis, L. B., Dodge, W. F., Daeschner, C. W., and Hopps, H. C. The prevalence of pyelonephritis in children at autopsy. *Pediatrics* 30:737, 1962.

382. Spühler, O., and Zollinger, H. U. Die chronisch-interstitielle Nephritis. *Z. Klin. Med.* 151:1, 1953.

383. Stamey, T. A. Office bacteriology. *J. Urol.* 97:926, 1967.

384. Stamey, T. A., Fair, W. R., Timothy, M. M., and Chung, H. K. Antibacterial nature of prostatic fluid. *Nature* (London) 218:444, 1968.

385. Stamey, T. A., Govan, D. E., and Palmer, J. M. The localization and treatment of urinary tract infections: The role of bactericidal urine levels as opposed to serum levels. *Medicine* (Balt.) 44:1, 1965.

386. Stamey, T. A., and Pfau, A. Some functional, pathologic, bacteriologic, and chemotherapeutic characteristics of unilateral pyelonephritis in man. *Invest. Urol.* 1:134, 1963.

387. Steele, R. E., Leadbetter, G. W., and Crawford, J. D. Prognosis of childhood urinary-tract infection. *New Eng. J. Med.* 269:883, 1963.

388. Sternheimer, R., and Malbin, B. I. Clinical recognition of pyelonephritis with a new stain for urinary sediments. *Amer. J. Med.* 11:312, 1951.

389. Stuart, K. L., Cummins, G. T. M., and Chin, W. A. Bacteriuria, prematurity and the hypertensive disorders of pregnancy. *Brit. Med. J.* 1:554, 1965.

389a. Sussman, M., Asscher, A. W., Waters, W. E., Evans, J. A. S., Campbell, H., Evans, K. T., and Williams, J. E. Asymptomatic significant bacteriuria in the non-pregnant woman: I. Description of a population. *Brit. Med. J.* 1:799, 1969.

390. Sweet, A. Y., and Wolinsky, E. An outbreak of urinary tract and other infections due to *E. coli. Pediatrics* 33:863, 1964.

391. Tallgren, L. G., and von Bonsdorff, C.-H. The effect of varying the pH level upon the sensitivity of urinary bacteria to antibiotics. *Acta Med. Scand.* 178:543, 1965.

392. Teague, H., and Boyarsky, S. The effect of coliform bacilli upon ureteral peristalsis. *Invest. Urol.* 5:423, 1968.

393. Teplitz, C., Raulston, G. L., Walker, H. L., Mason, A. D., Jr., and Moncrief, J. A. Spontaneous hematogenous pseudomonas pyelonephritis in rats. *J. Infect. Dis.* 114:75, 1964.

394. Thornton, G. F., Lytton, B., and Andriole, V. T. Bacteriuria during indwelling urinary catheter drainage: Effect of constant bladder rinse. *J.A.M.A.* 195:179, 1966.

394a. Tribe, C. R., and Silver, J. R. *Renal Failure in Paraplegia.* London: Pitman Medical Publishing, 1969.

395. Triger, D. R., and Smith, J. W. G. Survival of urinary leucocytes. *J. Clin. Path.* 19:443, 1966.

396. Turck, M., Anderson, K. N., and Petersdorf, R. G. Relapse and reinfection in chronic bacteriuria. *New Eng. J. Med.* 275:70, 1966.

397. Turck, M., Browder, A. A., Lindemeyer, R. I., Brown, N. K., Anderson, K. N., and Petersdorf, R. G. Failure of prolonged treatment of chronic urinary-tract infections with antibiotics. *New Eng. J. Med.* 267:999, 1962.

398. Turck, M., Goffe, B. S., and Petersdorf, R. G. Bacteriuria of pregnancy, relation to socioeconomic factors. *New Eng. J. Med.* 266:857, 1962.

399. Turck, M., and Petersdorf, R. G. The epidemiology of non-enteric *Escherichia coli* infections: Prevalence of serological groups. *J. Clin. Invest.* 41:1760, 1962.

399a. Turck, M., and Petersdorf, R. G. Optimal duration of treatment of chronic urinary tract infection. *Ann. Intern. Med.* 69:837, 1968.

400. Turck, M., Ronald, A. R., and Petersdorf, R. G.   Relapse and reinfection in chronic bacteriuria: II. The correlation between site of infection and pattern of recurrence in chronic bacteriuria. *New Eng. J. Med.* 278: 422, 1968.

400a. Tuttle, E. P., Jr., and Fellner, S. K.   The syndrome of analgesic abuse. *Kidney* 3:1, 1969.

401. Vejlsgaard, R.   Studies on urinary tract infection in diabetes: I. Bacteriuria in patients with diabetes mellitus and in control subjects; II. Significant bacteriuria in relation to long term diabetic management. *Acta Med. Scand.* 179:173, 183, 1966.

402. Vermooten, V.   Geographic, Racial and Climatic Factors in Etiology of Urolithiasis. In Butt, A. J. (Ed.), *Etiologic Factors in Renal Lithiasis.* Springfield, Ill.: Thomas, 1956. P. 238.

403. Vivaldi, E., Cotran, R., Zangwill, D. P., and Kass, E. H.   Ascending infection as a mechanism in pathogenesis of experimental non-obstructive pyelonephritis. *Proc. Soc. Exp. Biol. Med.* 102:242, 1959.

404. Vivaldi, E., Munoz, J., Cotran, R., and Kass, E. H.   Factors Affecting the Clearance of Bacteria Within the Urinary Tract. In Kass, E. H. (Ed.), *Progress in Pyelonephritis.* Philadelphia: Davis, 1965. P. 531.

405. Vosti, K. L., Goldberg, L. M., Monto, A. S., and Rantz, L. A.   Host-parasite interaction in patients with infections due to *Escherichia coli:* I. The serogrouping of *E. coli* from intestinal and extraintestinal sources. *J. Clin. Invest.* 43:2377, 1964.

405a. Waters, W. E., Sussman, M., and Asscher, A. W.   A community study of urinary pH and osmolality. *Brit. J. Prev. Soc. Med.* 21:129, 1967.

405b. Weiss, J. M., Dykhuizen, R. F., Sargent, C. R., and Tandy, R. W., Jr.   Urinary tract infection in girls: I. A computerized analysis of urethral stenosis. *J. Urol.* 100: 513, 1968.

406. Weiss, S., and Parker, F., Jr.   Pyelonephritis: Its relation to vascular lesions and to arterial hypertension. *Medicine* 18:221, 1939.

407. Weyrauch, H. M., and Bassett, J. B.   Ascending infection in an artificial urinary tract: An experimental study. *Stanford Med. Bull.* 9:25, 1951.

408. Whalley, P. J., Martin, F. G., and Pritchard, J. A.   Sickle cell trait and urinary tract infection during pregnancy. *J.A.M.A.* 189: 903, 1964.

409. Wharton, L. R., Gray, L. A., and Guild, H. C.   The late effects of acute pyelitis in girls. *J.A.M.A.* 109:1597, 1937.

410. Williams, J. D.   Some observations on renal biopsy with reference to Bright's disease. *Guy. Hosp. Rep.* 107:373, 1958.

411. Wilson, C., Ledingham, J. M., and Cohen, M.   Hypertension following x-irradiation of the kidneys. *Lancet* 1:9, 1958.

412. Winberg, J.   Renal function in water-losing syndrome due to lower urinary tract obstruction before and after treatment. *Acta Paediat.* 48:149, 1959.

413. Winberg, J.   Renal function studies in infants and children with acute, non-obstructive urinary tract infections. *Acta Paediat.* 48:577, 1959.

414. Winberg, J., Andersen, H. J., Hanson, L. A., and Lincoln, K.   Studies of urinary tract infections in infancy and childhood: I. Antibody response in different types of urinary tract infections caused by coliform bacteria. *Brit. Med. J.* 2:524, 1963.

415. Winterbauer, R. H., Gutman, L. T., Turck, M., Wedgewood, R. J., and Petersdorf, R. G.   The role of penicillin-induced bacterial variants in experimental pyelonephritis. *J. Exp. Med.* 125:607, 1967.

416. Wolstenholme, G. E. W., and Knight, J. (Eds.).   *The Balkan Nephropathy.* Ciba Foundation Study Group No. 30. Boston: Little, Brown, 1967.

417. Woodruff, J. D., and Everett, H. S.   Prognosis in childhood urinary tract infections in girls. *Amer. J. Obstet. Gynec.* 68:798, 1954.

418. Woods, J. W.   Susceptibility of rats with hormonal hypertension to experimental pyelonephritis. *J. Clin. Invest.* 37:1686, 1958.

419. Woods, J. W.   Susceptibility to experimental pyelonephritis when hormonal hypertension is prevented by hypotensive drugs. *J. Clin. Invest.* 39:1813, 1960.

420. Woods, J. W. Non-obstructive *Escherichia coli* pyelonephritis in the rat. *Proc. Soc. Exp. Biol. Med.* 104:116, 1960.

421. Woods, J. W., Welt, L. G., Hollander, W., Jr., and Newton, M. Susceptibility of rats to experimental pyelonephritis following recovery from potassium depletion. *J. Clin. Invest.* 39:28, 1960.

422. Woods, J. W., Welt, L. G., and Hollander, W., Jr. Susceptibility of rats to experimental pyelonephritis during potassium depletion. *J. Clin. Invest.* 40:599, 1961.

423. Yow, E. M. Monzon, O. T., Ory, E. M., and Brennan, J. C. The Microflora of the Urinary Tract. In Quinn, E. L., and Kass, E. H. (Eds.), *Biology of Pyelonephritis.* (Henry Ford Hospital International Symposium.) Boston: Little, Brown, 1960. P. 391.

424. Zikria, B. A., Lasagna, L., and McCann, W. P. The relative importance of blood and urinary concentrations of sulfonamide in the treatment of urinary tract infections. *Bull. Johns Hopkins Hosp.* 103:117, 1958.

425. Zollinger, H. U. Relationship of Renal Toxicity of Drugs to Pyelonephritis. In Quinn, E. L., and Kass, E. H. (Eds.), *Biology of Pyelonephritis.* (Henry Ford Hospital International Symposium.) Boston: Little, Brown, 1960. P. 59.

Index

Index

This Index covers both volumes. Volume I contains pages 1–734; Volume II contains pages 735–1456.

necrosis of
  in malignant nephrosclerosis,
    752–753
  in radiation nephritis, 1059
  in renovascular hypertension,
    770, 771
  in obstructive nephropathy, 1006
Arteriolosclerosis. *See* Nephro-
    sclerosis, arteriolar
Arteriosclerosis of renal arteries.
    See Atheroembolic renal
    disease
Arteriovenous anastomosis
  congenital, 1304
  renovascular hypertension from,
    776
Artery. *See* Arteries, renal
Arthritis
  in dialysis patients, 352
  gouty, and urate nephropathy,
    892, 893
Ascites, in cirrhosis, 1141–1145
Ask-Upmark kidney, 1301
Asparagine excretion
  in Fanconi syndrome, 1095
  in Hartnup disease, 1085
  in Lignac-Fanconi syndrome,
    1092
  in Wilson's disease, 1098
Asterixis
  in acute renal failure, 657
  in uremia, 336–337
Ataxia, in Hartnup disease,
    1084, 1087
Atheroembolic renal disease, 735–
    736, 1039–1046
  angiography in, 178
  from anticoagulants, 1043
  aorta in, 1042
  after aortic surgery, 1043
  after arteriography, 1043
  clinical features of, 736, 1043–
    1045
  and cortical necrosis, 798
  in diabetes, 874
  diagnosis of, 1042, 1045–1046
  erythrocytosis in, 282
  evolution of arterial lesions in,
    1040–1042
  experimental, 1041–1042
  frequency of, 1042
  genesis of vascular lesions in,
    1043
  hypertension in, 736, 777, 787,
    1044–1045
  inciting factors in, 1042–1043

infarction from, 790
morphology of cholesterol crys-
    tals in, 1039–1040
pancreatitis in, 1045
parenchymal changes in, 1042
pathogenesis of, 1042–1043
pathology of, 735–736, 1039–
    1042
renal failure in, 1039, 1043–1044
retinal vessels in, 1045
spontaneous, 1043, 1044
treatment of, 1046
urinary findings in, 1045
Atrophy
  parenchymal, in atheroembolic
    renal disease, 1042
  tubular. *See* Tubules, ischemic
    atrophy of
Auditory loss. *See* Deafness
Autoimmune experimental dis-
    eases
  nephritis, 377, 384–385, 514
  nephrosis, 544–545
Autoregulation of renal function,
    35
Azathioprine
  in glomerulonephritis, 260
  in lupus erythematosus, 849
  in nephrotic syndrome, 588–591
    in childhood, 1379
  in thrombotic thrombocytopenic
    purpura, 861
  in transplantation of kidney,
    1440
Azotemia. *See* Uremia and azote-
    mia

Bacitracin, in renal insufficiency,
    258
Backflow, in radiography, 150–152
Bacteremia
  and focal glomerulonephritis,
    1368
  from infected shunts in hydro-
    cephalus, nephrotic syn-
    drome with, 391
  in urinary tract infections, 709
Bacteria
  in bladder urine, 691, 697
    clearance of, 698, 700
    transport to kidney, 692–693,
      703
    water diuresis affecting, 698,
      699, 700, 708
  cortical necrosis from toxins,
    801, 802–803

urinary tract infections from,
    691
variants in urine after antibi-
    otics, 698–699
Bacteriuria
  asymptomatic, 702
  in children, 1358
  in diabetes, 884
  in polycystic disease, 1230, 1238
  in pregnancy, 694–695, 1188–
    1189
    treatment of, 1189
  and pyelonephritis, 683, 703–704
  treatment of, 260
  in urinary tract infections, 668
BAL. *See* Dimercaprol
Balkan nephropathy, 678–679,
    1265–1266
  clinical findings in, 679
  pathology of, 679
Barbiturate poisoning, dialysis in,
    349
Bartter's syndrome, 225, 1396–1397
  differential diagnosis of, 1397
  prognosis of, 1397
  symptoms of, 1397
  treatment of, 1397
Basal arteries of brain, aneurysms
    of, and polycystic kidneys,
    1228, 1250
Basal cell surface
  of collecting tubules, 26
  of tubules
    distal segment, 23–24
    proximal segment, 17–18
    thin segment, 20
Basal ganglia calcification, in
    hypoparathyroidism, 1111
Basement membrane
  of capillaries in glomerulus, 5–6,
    508
    affecting filtration, 33
    in diabetic glomerulosclerosis,
      876, 882
    in idiopathic glomerulone-
      phritis, 510
  of collecting ducts, in medullary
    cystic disease, 1262
  of filtration membrane, glo-
    merular, 10
  glomerular
    in acute poststreptococcal glo-
      merulonephritis, 435
    in amyloidosis, 835
    antibodies to, 382–387, 514.

Calyx
  hydrocalycosis, 174
  pyelography in caliectasis, 675
Candida, endocarditis from, focal
    glomerulonephritis in,
    466
Cannulation, venous, 785
  complications of, 656
Capillaries
  glomerular, 4–11, 507–508
    in acute poststreptococcal glo-
      merulonephritis, 406, 427,
      435
    in amyloidosis, 835
    basement membrane of, 5–6,
      508. *See also* Basement
      membrane, of capillaries
      in glomerulus
    in diabetic glomerulosclerosis,
      876, 882
    embryology of, 1298
    endothelium of, 5
    epithelium of, 6–7
    filtration membrane of, 10–11
    hydrostatic pressure in, 33, 35
    intercapillary glomeruloscler-
      sis, 497
    intracapillary colliculi, 9
    mesangial cells of, 2, 5, 7–9
    in myelomatosis, 830
    occlusion in hemolytic-uremic
      syndrome, 287
    permeability of, 33, 34
    podocytes of, 7, 508
    in polyarteritis nodosa, 851
    pores of, 33–34
    in radiation nephritis, 1059
    in scleroderma, 858
    slit pores of epithelium, 7, 11
    in thrombotic thrombocytope-
      nic purpura, 860
  peritubular, 12
    removal of substances from,
      43
  venous, 12
Capillaritis, verrucal, in lupus
    erythematosus, 511, 564
Capsule, glomerular. *See* Bow-
    man's capsule
Carbenicillin, in renal insuffi-
    ciency, 257
Carbohydrate. *See also* Glucose
  structural, in glomerular base-
    ment membrane, 879–880

Carbon dioxide, and acid-base
    balance, 67, 69, 73
Carbon tetrachloride
  acute renal failure from, 644,
    650
  tubular disorders from, 1072
Carbonic anhydrase
  and acid-base balance, 73
  deficiency of, renal tubular
    acidosis in, 1119, 1124
  inhibitors of
    in nephrotic syndrome, 600
    in uric acid lithiasis, 895
Carboxylic acids, tubular trans-
    port of, 44
Carbuncle, renal, radiography in,
    176
Carcinoid syndrome, pellagra in,
    1087
Carcinoma of kidney. *See also*
    Tumors
  epidermoid, 1324, 1343
  and nephrotic syndrome, 577–
    578
  radiography in, 162–165
  renal cell, 1321–1323
    chemotherapy in, 1338
    cysts in, 1225
    differential diagnosis of, 1320,
      1321
    erythrocytosis in, 282
    frequency of, 1319
    hereditary aspects of, 1216
    hormonal therapy in, 1338–
      1339
    metastasis of, 1323
      treatment of, 1336–1337
    nephrectomy in, 1335–1336
    radiation therapy, 1337–1338
    symptoms of, 1324–1328
    treatment of, 1335–1339
  squamous cell, 1324, 1343
Cardiac output, and renal func-
    tion, 639
Cardiopulmonary disorders
  in dialysis patients, 352
  in uremia, 239
Cardiovascular system
  in acute poststreptococcal glo-
    merulonephritis, 426–429
  in acute renal failure, 656–657
  in polycystic kidney disease,
    1230, 1236
Caseation, in tuberculosis of kid-
    ney, 1310–1311

Casts
  in tubules
    in amyloidosis, 835
    in calcium nephropathy, 909
    in Lowe's syndrome, 1097
    in myelomatosis, 828–829,
      1099
  in urine, 98–101, 105
    in acute poststreptococcal glo-
      merulonephritis, 432, 433–
      434
    in amyloidosis, 837
    in atheroembolic renal disease,
      1045
    bile-stained, 105–106
    in calcium nephropathy, 914
    in chronic glomerulonephritis,
      492
    in cortical necrosis, 796
    degenerating, 99–100
    diseases with, 105
    epithelial, 99, 106
    erythrocyte, 99, 105
    fatty, 101
    in Goodpasture's syndrome,
      863
    granular, 100
    hemoglobin, 105–106
    hyaline, 101
    in interstitial nephritis, chron-
      ic, 675
    leukocyte, 99, 105
    in Lowe's syndrome, 1097
    in lupus nephritis, 840
    in malignant hypertension,
      757
    in nephrotic syndrome, 549
    normal, 105
    in polyarteritis nodosa, 850,
      851
    in pyelonephritis, chronic, 684
    renal failure casts, 98, 106,
      492
    in thrombotic thrombocyto-
      penic purpura, 860, 861
    waxy, 100
Cataracts, in Lowe's syndrome,
    1391
Catecholamines. *See* Epinephrine;
    Norepinephrine
Catheter, for renal angiography,
    153
Catheterization
  infections from, 691, 697, 784,
    1007

Copper excretion, in Wilson's disease, 1099
Cortex, renal
in infancy, 1351, 1352, 1356
necrosis of, 643–644, 794–806. *See also* Necrosis, cortical
Corticosteroid therapy
in acute poststreptococcal glomerulonephritis, 450
affecting acid-base balance, 74
affecting calcium excretion, 906
affecting calcium levels, 831
affecting localization of immune complexes, 376
affecting Shwartzman reaction, 290
in amyloidosis, 559
azotemia from, 221
in childhood nephrosis, 490
in chronic glomerulonephritis with nephrotic syndrome, 499
complications from, 587–588
in focal glomerulonephritis, 479
in Goodpasture's syndrome, 865
growth retardation from, 605
in hemolytic-uremic syndrome, 291
in hypercalcemic crisis, acute, 917
in lipoid nephrosis, 509
in lupus erythematosus, 848–849
in lupus nephritis, 568
in myelomatosis, 831
in nephrotic syndrome, 584–588, 593
in childhood, 1378–1379
responses to, 1377
in polyarteritis nodosa, 855
potassium depletion from, 934, 943, 958, 959
responses to, in glomerular pathology, 389
in Schönlein-Henoch purpura, 863
in scleroderma, 856, 859
in thrombotic thrombocytopenic purpura, 861
in transplantation of kidney, 1440–1441
withdrawal from, effects of, 1444
Cortisol, plasma levels of, in pregnancy, 1160, 1163
Cortisone, effects in experimental serum sickness, 481

Countercurrent exchanger, 54–55
Countercurrent multiplier, 55–56
in sickle cell disease, 1210
Coxsackie virus, and glomerulonephritis, 440
Cramps, muscular, in uremia, 338
Cranial nerves, in uremia, 337–338
C-reactive protein, in tumors of the kidney, 1330
Creatine
excretion in pregnancy, 1160
tubular reabsorption of, 43
Creatinine
clearance test, 37–38, 108–110
and antibiotic dosage, 259
in children, 1359
in chronic glomerulonephritis, 492
and inulin clearance rate, 109
in obstructive nephropathy, 1025
in pregnancy, 1156, 1158
excretion of
in cystinuria, 1078
and glomerular filtration rate, 222
plasma levels of, 111–114
in acute poststreptococcal glomerulonephritis, 431
in medullary cystic disease, 1260
in pregnancy, 1158
in renal failure with cirrhosis, 1146, 1147
Crescent formation
in chronic glomerulonephritis, 489
in diffuse proliferative glomerulonephritis, 468
in Ellis type 1 glomerulonephritis, 510
in focal glomerulonephritis
embolic, 466
recurrent, 473
in Goodpasture's syndrome, 470, 864
in hereditary nephritis, 472
in nonstreptococcal glomerulonephritis, 414
in polyarteritis nodosa, 851
Crisis
hypercalcemic
in hyperparathyroidism, 315, 916

in sarcoidosis, 916
nephrotic, 548, 603
rejection, in transplantation of kidney, 1441–1442
sickle cell, acute, renal failure in, 651
in urate nephropathy, 899
Crush syndrome. *See* Tubules, necrosis of, acute
Crystalloid composition of kidney stones, 975
Cushing's syndrome
from corticosteroid therapy, 587
malignant hypertension in, 751
Cyclic nephrotic syndrome, 569–570, 606
Cyclophosphamide
in glomerulonephritis, 260
in nephrotic syndrome, 588, 591–593
in childhood, 1379
in renal disease with malignant lymphoma, 578
Cycloserine, in tuberculosis of kidney, 1314
Cylindroids, 101
Cylindruria, 98, 105
from exercise, 447
in hereditary chronic nephritis, 1276
in polycystic kidney disease, 1238
Cyst(s)
abdominal, renovascular hypertension in, 776
of kidney, 1216
angiography in, 166
congenital, 1305–1306
multicystic dysplasia, 1225
multilocular, 1305
polycystic disease, 1225, 1305, 1324
solitary, 1305
medullary cystic disease, 1216, 1259–1266. *See also* Medulla of kidney, cystic disease of
multilocular, 1225
congenital, 1305
percutaneous puncture of, 163
peripelvic, 1225
polycystic disease, 1216, 1223–1253. *See also* Polycystic kidney disease
radiography in, 163, 165–166

Experimental disorders —*Continued*
autoimmune disease, 544–545
from avian antiserum, 541–542
cortical necrosis, 801–805
diabetes, 881
hypercalcemia, 908
hypertension, renovascular, 769–771
infarction, renal, 791–792
nephritis, 373–378, 481, 514, 540–546
nephrocalcinosis, 908
nephrosis, 514
nephrotoxic serum nephritis, 542–543
obstructive nephropathy, 1012–1016
potassium depletion, 935–942, 947–948, 951
preeclampsia, 1166
radiation nephritis, 1064–1065
Extracellular fluid, sodium in, 60–61
Extracts of kidney, hypertension from, 769, 772
Eyes
in acute poststreptococcal glomerulonephritis, 429
in amyloidosis, 558
in atheroembolic renal disease, 1044, 1045
calcific deposits in, 320
in calcium nephropathy, 915
diabetic retinopathy, 882
in glycolipid lipidosis, 1282
in Hartnup disease, 1084
in hereditary chronic nephritis, 1276
in hypertension with polycystic disease, 1239
in Lignac-Fanconi syndrome, 1090
in Lowe's syndrome, 1096, 1097, 1391
in malignant hypertension, 756
in medullary cystic disease, 1264–1265
in renovascular hypertension, 777
retinal disorders. *See* Retinopathy
in uremia, 337–338

Fabry's disease, 1282–1284

Failure of renal function
acute, 637–660. *See also* Acute renal failure
and casts in urine, 98, 106, 492
chronic. *See* Chronic renal disease
functional, 241
postrenal, 641–642
prerenal, 638–641
Familial amyloidosis, primary, 558
Familial nephrosis, 554–555
Fanconi syndrome, 1094–1096
acidosis in, renal tubular, 1119, 1393
biochemical anomalies in, 1095
in cadmium intoxication, 680
in childhood, 1388–1391. *See also* Lignac-Fanconi syndrome
treatment of, 1389
clinical features of, 1388–1389
concentration of urine in, 1095, 1389
with congenital cirrhosis and tyrosinuria, 1391–1392
and cystinosis, 1388, 1389. *See also* Lignac-Fanconi syndrome
etiology of, 1094
hereditary aspects of, 1216
idiopathic, 1390–1391
acidosis in, renal tubular, 1393
incidence of, 1094
and myelomatosis, 827, 1094
phosphate clearance in, 1095, 1389
potassium depletion in, 934
prognosis of, 1095
proteinuria in, 1095, 1389
secondary, 1391–1392
symptoms of, 1095
treatment of, 1095–1096
tubular function in, 1073, 1074, 1095
Fasciculations, in uremia, 335, 338
Fat bodies in urine. *See* Lipiduria
Feet, burning of, in uremia, 339
Fenestrations
in glomerular capillaries, 5
in peritubular capillaries, 12
Ferritin, molecular weight of, 524
Fetal kidney function, 1349–1350
Fever
in acute poststreptococcal glomerulonephritis, 425

in infarction, renal, 790
proteinuria in, 447
in tumors of kidney, 1326–1328
Fibrils
amyloid, 832, 835
collagen, in diabetic glomerulosclerosis, 879
Fibrin deposits, glomerular
in acute poststreptococcal glomerulonephritis, 410
in anaphylactoid nephritis, 393
in chronic renal failure, 284–292
in hemolytic-uremic syndrome, 1373
pathophysiology of, 289–290
in preeclampsia, 1169, 1175
and renal homograft rejection, 284, 292
in Schönlein-Henoch purpura, 862
in toxemia of pregnancy, 393
Fibrinogen levels, in pregnancy, 1169
Fibrinoid material
in amyloidosis, 839
in polyarteritis nodosa, 849, 851
in scleroderma, 856–857
Fibrinolytic agents, in thrombotic thrombocytopenic purpura, 861
Fibroblasts
in glomerular efferent arteriole, 12
in tubules, 14
Fibrocytes, and mesangial cells, 9
Fibrolipomatosis renis, 192
Fibroma of kidney, 1320
Fibromucin fibers, mesangial, in acute poststreptococcal glomerulonephritis, 407
Fibromuscular dysplasia of renal artery, hypertension with, 776, 777–778, 788
Fibrosis
interstitial
in medullary cystic disease, 1262
in radiation nephritis, 1064, 1066
in Lignac-Fanconi syndrome, 1093
perirenal, in radiation nephritis, 1059
retroperitoneal, 1005

focal degeneration in, 409
gastrointestinal symptoms of, 430
genitourinary tract in, 429–430
  treatment of infections, 451
glomeruli in, 406, 409, 435
group A beta-hemolytic streptococci in, 380
hematocrit in, 428, 434
hematuria in, 420, 425, 432
  duration of, 433
hemodynamic changes in, 428–429
and histology of kidney, 435–438
  prognostic significance of, 437–438
hypertension in, 426, 427–428, 442
  in childhood, 1366–1367
  treatment of, 448–449
hypertensive encephalopathy in, treatment of, 448
immunologic mechanisms in, 389, 422–424
  antibiotics affecting, 423
interstitium in, 409, 436
laboratory data in, 432–435
latent period, 411, 424, 442
light microscopy in, 406–409
lipid levels in, 435
macroscopic appearance of, 405
manifestations of, 419–420
mesangial cells in, 406, 407, 410, 489
minimal urinary changes in, 425
mortality in, 440–441
myocarditis in, 428
nephrotic syndrome in, 441, 443, 511
oliguric, 414, 441
  heparin in, 260
  treatment of, 451
pathology of, 405–416
plasma volume in, 428
in pregnancy, 570, 1186
prognosis of, 441–442
progression to latent chronic stage, 411–413
proliferative, 555–556. *See also* Glomerulonephritis,

membranoprolifera-tive
prophylaxis of, 447, 449
proteinuria in, 420, 432, 442
  duration of, 432–433
purpura in, 430
recurrences of, 443
relationship to chronic glomerulonephritis, 487, 489
renal function in, 430–431
resolution of, 410
after respiratory infections, 421
retinopathy in, 429
and rheumatic fever, 430
seasonal factors in incidence of, 422
sedimentation rate in, 434
sex incidence of, 421
silent cases of, 425
and site of preceding infection, 421–422
skin in, 430
after skin infections, 421–422
sodium and water retention in, 428–429, 431
  treatment of, 448
splenomegaly in, 430
systemic symptoms of, 425
tonsillectomy in, 451
treatment of, 447–452
tubules in, 409, 431, 436
type 4 beta-hemolytic streptococci in, 420, 423
type 12 beta-hemolytic streptococci in, 380, 410, 413, 420, 423
type-specific antibodies in, 420, 423, 489
urinary findings in, 430, 432–434
adjuvant-induced, 377, 514
anaphylactoid, 393
  immunologic mechanisms in, 389
and antibodies to glomerular basement membrane, 382–387, 514
  in experimental disease, 382–385
  in man, 385–387
autoimmune mechanisms in, 377
  in experimental disease, 384–385

chronic
  after acute disease, 411, 487, 489
    in childhood, 1368, 1382
  acute exacerbation in, 415–416, 424, 443, 487, 494
    differential diagnosis of, 444
    renal function in, 431
  from antigen-antibody complexes, 846–847
  azotemia in, 493–494
    in childhood, 1382–1383
  in cirrhosis, 1142
  clinical aspects of, 485–500
  definition of, 485–486
  differential diagnosis of, 495–498, 1234
  edema in, 491, 494
  and fat bodies in urine, 552
  fluorescence studies of, 491
  foam cells in, 1277
  hypertension in, 491, 494
  hypocomplementemic, 382, 388–391
  incidence of, 486–487
  laboratory findings in, 491–493
  lobular, 413
  malignant hypertension in, 751
  nephrocalcinosis in, 908
  nephrotic syndrome in, 489, 491, 493, 494
    in childhood, 1382
    treatment of, 499
  pathogenesis of, 487–488
  in pregnancy, 495, 1186–1187
  prognosis and natural history of, 493–495
  proliferative, 413
    heparin in, 595–596
  in Schönlein-Henoch syndrome, 468
  symptoms of, 491
  treatment of, 498–499
  uremic death in, 235
diffuse, 439
  acute, differential diagnosis of, 464
  proliferative
    in Goodpasture's syndrome, 470, 863
    hematuria in, recurrent, 473

experimental, 373–378
localization of, 376
in man, 378–382
subacute, 414, 441
and antibodies to glomerular basement membrane, 514
incidence of, 486
in lupus erythematosus, 841
pathogenesis of, 487
in virus infections, 416, 421, 440
in mice, 378
Glomerulosclerosis, 511
in cirrhosis, 1142
with renal failure, 1147
diabetic, 497, 559–564, 875–884
capillary basement membrane in, 876, 882
clinical features of, 883–884
criteria for diagnosis of, 560
definition of, 875
differential diagnosis of, 497, 1142
diffuse, 875
electron microscopy in, 875–877
and fat bodies in urine, 552
frequency of, 883
genetic theory of, 881–882
hyaline lesions in, 877–878, 882
intercapillary, 511, 875
interstitial lesions in, 668
metabolic theory of, 880–881
nephrotic syndrome, 511, 883
nodular, 875
pathogenesis of, 878–882
in pregnancy, 570
and protein patterns in electrophoresis, 525
intercapillary. *See* Glomerulosclerosis, diabetic, intercapillary
in nondiabetic patients, 564
in sickle cell disease, 1208
tubules in, 563, 877
Glomerulotubular balance
in chronic renal disease, 212
and effective extracellular volume, 215–217
indices of, 215
resetting of, factors in, 215–217
Glomerulus, 1–12
in acute poststreptococcal glomerulonephritis, 406, 409, 435

in acute renal failure, 643
afferent arteriole of, 2–4. *See also* Arterioles
amyloid deposits in, 835
anlage cells of, 9
in arteriolar nephrosclerosis, 737–738
in atheroembolic disease, 1042
basement membrane of. *See* Basement membrane, glomerular
in calcium nephropathy, 910
capillaries of, 4–11, 507–508. *See also* Capillaries, glomerular
in cirrhosis, 1142
in cortical necrosis, 799, 800
in diabetic glomerulosclerosis, 562
efferent arteriole of, 11–12
embryology of, 1298
fibrin deposits in. *See* Fibrin deposits, glomerular
filtration in. *See* Glomerular filtration
foam cells in, 511
in focal glomerulonephritis, 475–476
function in infancy, 1350–1352
in hepatitis, viral, 1140
in hereditary chronic nephritis, 1276
hyalinization of, 511–512
immune injury to, humoral and cellular mediators of, 387
in interstitial nephritis, chronic, 670–671
leukocyte localization in, 387
in Lowe's syndrome, 1097
in lupus nephritis, 840
in medullary cystic disease, 1261
mesangial localization of immune complexes in, 376, 380
in nonstreptococcal glomerulonephritis, 414
in polyarteritis nodosa, 851
in preeclampsia, 1174
in pyelonephritis, chronic, 685
in radiation nephritis, 1059, 1060, 1065
in scleroderma, 857
sclerosis of. *See* Glomerulosclerosis
in sickle cell disease, 1208

streptococcal antigens in, 379–380
in tubular diseases, 1071
and tubules. *See* Glomerulotubular balance
wire-loop lesion in
in lupus erythematosus, 841, 842
in scleroderma, 856, 857
Glucoglycinuria, 1107, 1387
Glucosamine, in calculi, 975
Glucose
in calculi, 975
hyperglycemia in uremia, 237
malabsorption of, and glycosuria, 1107
metabolism in diabetic glomerulosclerosis, 881
plasma levels in glycosuria, renal, 1104
titration curve splay. *See* Titration curve splay
tolerance in uremia, 237
transport maximum in chronic renal disease, 212, 213, 216
tubular reabsorption of, 39–42, 1074
in acute poststreptococcal glomerulonephritis, 431
carrier-mediated transport in, 40
in diabetes insipidus, vasopressin-resistant, 1288
and glomerular filtration rate, 41–42
in glycosuria, renal, 1105
in infancy, 1351
in potassium depletion, 960
in pregnancy, 1161
in urine. *See* Glycosuria
Glucose-6-phosphate dehydrogenase, tubular, in obstructive nephropathy, 1023
Glucuronides, tubular transport of, 44
Glutamic oxalacetic transaminase in serum, in renal infarction, 791, 793
Glutaminase, renal levels in potassium depletion, 959
Glutamine
excretion of, 1075
in Fanconi syndrome, 1095
in galactosemia, 1097

Glutamine, excretion of
  —*Continued*
  in Hartnup disease, 1085
  in Lignac-Fanconi syndrome,
    1092
  metabolism in gout, 894
Glutathione, in erythrocytes, in
    chronic renal disease, 275
Glutethimide poisoning, dialysis
    in, 349
Glycine
  hyperglycinemia, 1103
  and oxalate formation, 1125
  tubular reabsorption of, 43, 1074
Glycinuria, 1075
  in Fanconi syndrome, 1095
  in galactosemia, 1097
  in Hartnup disease, 1085
  hereditary aspects of, 1216, 1386–
    1387
  in Lignac-Fanconi syndrome,
    1092
  in vitamin D resistance, 1110,
    1387
  in Wilson's disease, 1098
Glycogen storage disease
  tubular dysfunction in, 1392
  urate nephropathy in, 892, 900
Glycol, ethylene. *See* Ethylene
    glycol
Glycolate, affecting oxalate excre-
    tion, 982
Glycolic acid excretion, in hyper-
    oxaluria, 983
Glycolipid lipidosis, 1282–1284
Glycosuria, 216, 1104–1107
  in calcium nephropathy, 914
  in childhood, 1385–1386
  diagnosis of, 1104
  in Fanconi syndrome, 1095, 1105
    with myelomatosis, 827
  and glucoglycinuria, 1107
  and glucose-galactose malab-
    sorption by jejunum, 1107
  hereditary aspects of, 1216
  in interstitial nephritis, chronic,
    674
  in Lignac-Fanconi syndrome,
    1090, 1092
  in Lowe's syndrome, 1096, 1105
  in myelomatosis, 1099
    with Fanconi's syndrome, 827
  from nephrotoxic agents, 1100,
    1392

  in pregnancy, 1161–1162
  tubular defect in, 1105–1106
  types of, 1107
  in Wilson's disease, 1098, 1105
Glyoxalate
  activity in hyperoxaluria, 983–
    984
  conversion to oxalate, 1125
Goldblatt hypertension, 769, 770
Goldman equation, 247
Goldstein operation, in polycystic
    kidney disease, 1246
Golgi apparatus
  in glomerular capillary cells
    endothelial, 5
    epithelial, 7
  in tubular cells
    in distal segment, 23
    in proximal segment, 16
    in thin segment, 19
Goodpasture's syndrome, 385–387,
    863–865
  and antibodies to glomerular
    basement membrane, 471,
    480, 514, 864
  in childhood, 1369–1370
  clinical features of, 863
  definition of, 864
  differential diagnosis of, 445
  elution of glomerular antibody
    in, 386
  epithelial crescent formation in,
    470, 864
  fluorescence studies in, 471, 864
  focal glomerulonephritis in, 469–
    471, 479, 863
    transformation to diffuse dis-
    ease, 470
  histology of kidney in, 863
  immunologic mechanisms in,
    389
  nephrotic syndrome in, 579, 863
  pathogenesis of, 471, 480
  and polyarteritis, 865
  proteinuria in, 386, 469, 863
  treatment of, 479, 865
  urinary findings in, 863
Gout
  acidity of urine in, 894
  calculi in, 974, 986
  in lead nephropathy, 670
  primary, 893
  in radiation nephritis, 1053
  and tophaceous renal disease,
    896–897

  uric acid stones in, 891, 893–896
Grafts
  bypass graft in renovascular hy-
    pertension, 789
  of kidney. *See* Transplantation,
    of kidney
  patch graft angioplasty in reno-
    vascular hypertension, 789
Granular casts in urine, 100
Granules in juxtaglomerular cells,
    4
Granulomas
  in lupus erythematosus, 839
  in sarcoidosis, 921
  Wegener. *See* Wegener's gran-
    ulomatosis
Gravity, specific, of urine, 116–117
  in acidosis, renal tubular, 1123
  in infants, 1120
  in acute poststreptococcal glo-
    merulonephritis, 432
  in cortical necrosis, 796
  in hyperparathyroidism, 921
  in polycystic kidney disease,
    1238
Grawitz tumor. *See* Carcinoma of
    kidney, renal cell
Growth hormone, affecting renal
    function, 1159
Growth retardation
  in acidosis, renal tubular, 1394
  in diabetes insipidus, vasopres-
    sin-resistant, 1290
  in Fanconi syndrome, 1388
  in interstitial nephritis, chronic,
    674
  in Lignac-Fanconi syndrome,
    1090
  in nephrotic syndrome, 605,
    1376
Guanethidine, in hypertension in
    chronic renal failure, 254
  in childhood, 1363
Guanidine, uremia from, 236
Guanidinosuccinic acid, in uremic
    urine, 278
Guanidoacetic acid excretion, in
    pregnancy, 1160

Hartnup disease, 1083–1088
  amino acid transport in, 1076
  biochemical abnormalities in,
    1084–1087
  in childhood, 1386
  hereditary aspects of, 1216

jejunal transport defect in, 1085
pellagra in, 1084, 1087
symptoms of, 1084
treatment of, 1087–1088
and tryptophan absorption in jejunum, 1085–1086
tubular transport in, 1073, 1084
Headache, in malignant hypertension, 756
Heart
  in acute poststreptococcal glomerulonephritis, 428
  in acute renal failure, 657
  congestive failure
    in acute poststreptococcal glomerulonephritis, 426
      in childhood, 1367
    in diabetic glomerulosclerosis, 883
    edema in, 250–251
    proteinuria in, 95
    renal function in, 241
  contractility in uremic acidosis, 244
  in dialysis patients, 352
  in polycystic kidney disease, 1228
  in radiation nephritis, 1059
  in scleroderma, 859
  in thrombotic thrombocytopenic purpura, 859–860, 861
  in uremia, 239–240
Heat exposure, proteinuria from, 95
Hemangioma of kidney, 1320
Hematocrit
  in acute poststreptococcal glomerulonephritis, 428, 434
  in acute renal failure, 659
  and blood urea nitrogen, 273
Hematologic studies
  in amyloidosis, 837
  in lupus erythematosus, 838
  in renal failure, 273–292, 658–659
Hematoxylin bodies, in lupus erythematosus, 839, 842
Hematuria, 97
  in acidosis, renal tubular, 1123
  in acute poststreptococcal glomerulonephritis, 420, 425, 432
    duration of, 433
  in acute streptococcal infections, 424, 433

in amyloidosis, 837
in atheroembolic renal disease, 1045
from biopsy procedures, 205
in chronic glomerulonephritis, 492
diseases with, 105
essential, 1211
from exercise, 447
in focal glomerulonephritis, 463, 464, 478
  embolic, 466
in Goodpasture's syndrome, 863
in hepatitis, viral, 1140
in hereditary nephritis, 471, 1275, 1276
in hypocomplementemic glomerulonephritis, 390
in infarction, renal, 790, 791
in malignant hypertension, 757
in nephroblastoma, 1323
in polyarteritis nodosa, 850, 852
in polycystic disease, 1230, 1236
in pyelonephritis
  acute, 701–702
  chronic, 684
in radiation nephritis, acute, 1051
recurrent, 472–474
  in childhood, 1369
  in diffuse proliferative glomerulonephritis, 473
  family history in, 472
  in focal glomerulonephritis, 472–474, 480, 1369
  in hereditary nephritis, 471
  in respiratory infections, 472, 480
in Schönlein-Henoch syndrome, 467, 861
in sickle cell disease, 1208, 1210–1211, 1372
in sponge kidney, 1269
in thrombotic thrombocytopenic purpura, 860
in tuberculosis of kidney, 1312
in tumors of kidney, 1324–1325
Hemodialysis
  in acute renal failure, 653
  anemia in, 253
  in anemia of chronic renal failure, 283
  in childhood, 1364
  folic acid levels in, 276

in Goodpasture's syndrome, 865
historical background of, 343–345
and hyperparathyroidism, secondary, 323
intermittent
  affecting parathyroid glands, 317
  and hyperphosphatemia, 317
neurologic complications of, 340–341
in uremia bleeding tendency, 278
Hemoglobin
  in acute poststreptococcal glomerulonephritis, 434
  in casts in urine, 105–106
  in glomerular filtrate, 34
  in medullary cystic disease, 1260
  molecular weight of, 517, 524
  in polycystic kidney disease, 1238
  in sickle cell anemia, 1207–1208, 1211
Hemoglobinemia, in experimental vascular disease, 290
Hemoglobinuria
  in infarction, renal, 791
  march, 95
Hemolysis
  in chronic renal disease, 253
  in pregnancy, 1191
Hemolytic-uremic syndrome, 285–287, 1373–1374
  in children, 1360
  and chronic glomerulonephritis in childhood, 1382
  corticosteroids in, 291
  heparin in, 260, 291, 1374
  microangiopathy in, 285, 1374
  thrombocytopenia in, 277, 285, 1373
  treatment of, 290–292
Hemopericardium, in uremia, 240
Hemorrhage
  cerebral, in polycystic kidney disease, 1228
  gastrointestinal
    in atheroembolic renal disease, 1045
    in uremia, 238, 254
  pulmonary, and glomerulonephritis. *See* Goodpasture's syndrome
  in renal infarction, 791, 792

in Ellis type 1 glomerulonephritis, 511
in hereditary chronic nephritis, 1276
in medullary cystic disease, 1261
in polyarteritis nodosa, 851
Hyaluronidase excretion, vasopressin affecting, 1289
Hydatid cysts, radiography of, 166
Hydralazine, in hypertension, 255, 449
in childhood, 1363
and prevention of vascular lesions, 771
Hydrarthrosis, in nephrotic syndrome, 546
Hydration. *See* Fluid intake
Hydremia, in chronic renal disease, 275
Hydrocephalus, infected shunts in glomerulonephritis with, 416
nephrotic syndrome with, 391
Hydrochloric acid in gastric juice, in uremia, 238
Hydrochlorothiazide. *See* Thiadiazines
Hydrogen ion excretion, 1117. *See also* Acid-base balance and acidity of urine
Hydronephrosis. *See also* Obstructive nephropathy
angiography in, 164, 165
in childhood, 1003
definition of, 999
and diabetes insipidus
nephrogenic, 223
vasopressin-resistant, 1288, 1290
differential diagnosis of, 1234
erythrocytosis in, 282
in interstitial nephritis, 671
malignant hypertension in, 751
in pregnancy, 695, 1186
in pyelonephritis, chronic, 687
radiography in, 169–174
salt wastage in, 225, 249
unilateral
hereditary aspects of, 1216
in pregnancy, 1186
and ureteral peristaltic waves, 1002
Hydrostatic pressure
in glomerular capillaries, 33, 35
in glomerular capsule, 35
and water movement, 48

β-Hydroxybutyric acid, affecting urate excretion, 892
25-Hydroxycholecalciferol, 310
p-Hydroxyphenylpyruvic acid in urine, in tyrosinemia, 1391
p-Hydroxyphenylpyruvate oxidase, lack of, 1099–1100
Hydroxyproline excretion, in childhood, 1386
Hydroxyproline oxidase deficiency, 1280
Hydroxyprolinemia, 1103
5-Hydroxytryptamine. *See* Serotonin
Hyperaldosteronism. *See* Aldosterone, hyperaldosteronism
Hypercalcemia. *See* Calcium, hypercalcemia
Hyperchloremia, 230
Hyperchloremic acidosis. *See* Acidosis, renal tubular
Hyperemesis gravidarum, 1190
Hyperemia, in renal infarction, 791, 792
Hyperglycemia, in uremia, 237
Hyperkalemia. *See* Potassium, hyperkalemia
Hypermagnesemia, 233–234
Hypernephroma. *See* Carcinoma of kidney, renal cell
Hyperoxaluria. *See* Oxalic acid, hyperoxaluria
Hyperparathyroidism, 921–922. *See also* Parathyroid glands, hyperparathyroidism
Hyperphosphatemia. *See* Phosphate, hyperphosphatemia
Hyperplasia
of juxtaglomerular apparatus, with hyperaldosteronism and hypokalemic alkalosis, 1396–1397
of kidney
compensatory, radiography in, 192–194
congenital, 1301–1302
in potassium depletion, 934, 935
reversibility of, 947
parathyroid. *See* Parathyroid glands, chief cell hyperplasia
Hypersensitivity reactions
angiitis, 854

to antibiotics, 255
Hypertension
in acute poststreptococcal glomerulonephritis, 426, 427–428, 442
in childhood, 1366–1367
treatment of, 448–449
in acute renal failure, 656
in amyloidosis, 557, 833
antihypertensive function of kidney, 774, 775
in atheroembolic renal disease, 1044–1045
in calcium nephropathy, 916
in chronic glomerulonephritis, 491, 494
in chronic renal failure, 254–255
in childhood, 1363
in cortical necrosis, 797
in diabetes, 875, 883
edema from treatment of, 250
and encephalopathy. *See* Encephalopathy, hypertensive
essential
angiotensin infusions in, responses to, 747–748
in arteriolar nephrosclerosis, 736, 739–744
azotemia in, 743–744
blood flow in, renal, 744
diurnal variations in, 747
and chronic renal insufficiency, 254–255, 743, 749
clinical course of, 743–744
concentrating ability in, 747
glomerular filtration rate in, 744
diurnal variations in, 747
in pregnancy, 1171, 1175, 1185
prostaglandin role in, 742
pyelonephritis in, 686–689, 742–743
renal circulatory factors in, 741
renal function in, 740, 743, 744–748
in separate kidneys, 745
renin-angiotensin-aldosterone system in, 741–742
sodium excretion in, 745–746
treatment of, 748–750
vasoexcitor material in, 742

Interstitial nephritis, chronic,
    —*Continued*
    from bacterial infections, 680–
        690. *See also* Pyelone-
        phritis, chronic
    in Balkan nephropathy, 678–
        679
    clinical features of, 674
    colloid cast formation in, 670
    definition of, 668
    glomeruli in, 670–671
    gross appearance of kidney in,
        672–673
    laboratory studies in, 675
    medullary cystic changes in,
        671–672, 674
    papillary damage in, 671
    pathogenesis of, 673–674
    pathology of, 669–673
    pyelography in, 675
    urinary findings in, 675
Interstitium
    in acute poststreptococcal glo-
        merulonephritis, 409, 436
    in amyloidosis, 835
    in diabetic glomerulosclerosis,
        562
    in focal glomerulonephritis,
        476
    in hereditary chronic nephritis,
        1276
    in hyperparathyroidism, 909–
        910
    in medullary cystic disease, 1262
    in nephrocalcinosis, 668–669,
        673
    in nonstreptococcal glomerulo-
        nephritis, 415
    in obstructive uropathy, 669, 673
    in potassium depletion, 936, 946
    in tubular necrosis, acute, 668,
        674
Intestinal conditions. *See* Gastro-
        intestinal tract
Inulin
    clearance test, 36–37, 107–108
    in acute poststreptococcal glo-
        merulonephritis, 431, 436
    in children and infants, 1351,
        1359
    in chronic renal disease, 214
    and creatinine clearance rate,
        109
    in hyperparathyroidism, 921
    in pregnancy, 1156

    in glomerular filtrate, 34
    molecular weight of, 524
Iodinated urographic contrast
        media, tubular transport
        of, 44
Iodopyracet. *See* Diodrast
Iron, serum levels, in chronic
        renal failure, 276
Ischemia
    placental, and preeclampsia,
        1166–1167
    renal
        in cortical necrosis, 799–800,
            802
        mechanisms in, 645–646
Ischemic atrophy of tubules.
        See Tubules, ischemic
        atrophy of
Isoleucine
    excretion in galactosemia, 1097
    tubular reabsorption of, 43
Isoniazid
    pellagra from, 1087
    in renal insufficiency, 257
    in tuberculosis of kidney, 1314
Isothenuria, factors in, 218
Isotonic urine, 57–58
Isotope studies
    in obstructive nephropathy,
        1026
    in polycystic kidney disease,
        1233
    in renovascular hypertension,
        779, 780, 781
    in tumors of kidney, 1333

Jaundice, in renal failure with cir-
        rhosis, 1146
Jejunal dialysis, 346–347
Jejunal transport defect
    in cystinuria, 1073, 1079–1080
    in Hartnup disease, 1085
    from phlorizin, 1106
Joint pains. *See* Bone lesions
Juxtaglomerular apparatus
    in fetus, 1350
    hyperplasia of, with hyperaldo-
        steronism and hypo-
        kalemic alkalosis, 1396–
        1397
    in preeclampsia, 1170, 1174
    in renovascular hypertension,
        779
Juxtaglomerular cells, 4

and erythropoietin production,
        281
    as renin source, 741, 772–773
Juxtamedullary nephrons, 18
    in cortical necrosis, 801

Kanamycin
    deafness from, 1314
    in renal insufficiency, 256
    in tuberculosis of kidney, 1314–
        1315
    in urinary tract infections, 706
Kayexalate. *See also* Resin therapy
    in chronic renal failure, in
        childhood, 1362
    in hyperkalemia, 246
Kayser-Fleischer rings in cornea,
        in Wilson's disease, 1098
Keratopathy, band
    in calcium nephropathy, 915
    in milk-alkali syndrome, 919
    in sarcoidosis, 921
Kernig sign, in uremia, 338
Ketosis, starvation
    from glycosuria, 1106
    in Lignac-Fanconi syndrome,
        1090
Kidney
    anatomy of, 1–28
    antibodies to, 514
    antigenic similarity to lung, 471
    embryology of, 1298–1299
    extract injections, hypertension
        from, 769, 772
    failure of. *See* Failure of renal
        function
    function studies. *See* Function
        studies
    physiology of, 31–77
    transplantation. *See* Transplan-
        tation, of kidney
Kimmelstiel-Wilson disease. *See*
        Glomerulosclerosis, dia-
        betic
Kinin system, activation of, 387
Klebsiella infections of urinary
        tract, 691
Korsakoff's psychosis, in uremia,
        336
Kussmaul respiration, in uremic
        acidosis, 244–245

Laboratory studies, 87–125
Lactescence of serum
    heparin affecting, 530
    in nephrotic syndrome, 529, 548

Obstructive nephropathy
—*Continued*
and exchange between urine and medullary fluids, 1010–1011
experimental, 1012–1016
glomerular filtration rate in, 998, 1013, 1014, 1017, 1025
hydronephrosis in, 999
hypertension in, 1019–1020
idiopathic dilatation in, 1003
incidence of, 1003
from infections, 1003, 1004
intermittent, 1018
lymphatic drainage in, 1011–1012
mechanisms of nephron destruction in, 1007–1008
nephrectomy in, 1028
from neuromuscular defects, 1003, 1005
pain in, 1018
papillary necrosis in, 998, 1006, 1026
pathogenesis of, 1008–1012
pathology of, 1005–1006
pelvic extracellular fluid in, 1010
and physiology of urinary tract, 999–1002
polycythemia with, 1019
polyuria in, 1017, 1018
postoperative treatment, 1031–1032
in pregnancy, 1005, 1186
and pressures in renal pelvis, 998, 1008
pyelography in, 1020–1021, 1026
pyelonephritis in, 998, 1006–1007
pyelovenous outflow in, 1011
reflux of urine in, 1011, 1030
renal function in, 241, 242, 1012–1018, 1025–1027
residual urine in, 1030
sodium excretion in, 1018, 1021–1025, 1032
sustained obstruction in, 1014–1016
tubular reflux in, 1011
from tumors, 1003–1004, 1328
unilateral obstruction in, 1013
renal function in, 1027
uremia in, 1019, 1025
at ureteropelvic junction, 1004
treatment of, 1028
urinary diversion in, 1030–1031

urinary sediment in, 1026
and urinary tract infections, 1003, 1004, 1019
Obstructive uropathy, 641–642, 999
diagnosis of, 642
interstitial changes in, 669, 673
papillary necrosis in, 676
renal function in, 241, 242
in retroperitoneal fibrosis, 1005
ureteral, treatment of, 1028–1029
urinary tract infections in, 695–696, 697–698
in childhood, 710
Occlusive renal vascular disease. *See* Arteries, renal, stenosis of
Ocular signs in uremia, 337–338. *See also* Eyes
Oliguria
in acute poststreptococcal glomerulonephritis, 414, 441
heparin in, 260
treatment of, 451
in childhood, 1361
in cirrhosis, 1140, 1145
in hemolytic-uremic syndrome, 1374
in salt-losing nephritis, 1115
in scleroderma, 856, 857, 859
Ornithine
excretion of
in cystinuria, 1078
in Fanconi syndrome, 1095
in Hartnup disease, 1085
in Lignac-Fanconi syndrome, 1092
in Wilson's disease, 1098
tubular reabsorption of, 1074
Orthophosphate
excretion in hypophosphatasia, 1114
therapy with
affecting calcium excretion, 980, 991
affecting pyrophosphate excretion, 989, 991
Orthostatic proteinuria, 94
in childhood, 1383–1385
Osmol(s), 49
Osmolality of urine, 116–117
affecting bacterial growth, 692, 699, 708
in chronic renal disease, 213
in obstructive nephropathy, 1015, 1017

Osmoreceptors, 50
Osmotic diuresis, 63. *See also* Diuresis, osmotic
Osmotic pressure, 48–49
colloid, and glomerular filtration rate, 35
effective, 50
in Henle loop, 53
and sodium concentration in plasma, 60–61
total, 50
Osteitis fibrosa
with azotemic rickets or osteomalacia, 313, 316
and calcium loss, 306
cystica, in medullary cystic disease, 1264
generalized, 316
parathyroid glands in, 316, 319
vitamin D therapy in, 322
healing of, in dialysis patients, 325
parathyroid enlargement in, 316, 319
Osteodystrophy, renal, 194, 251–252, 1108
alkali therapy in, 311
pathogenesis of, 306
vitamin D therapy in, 313
Osteoid formation, parathyroidectomy affecting, 324, 325
Osteoid seams
mineralization of, 314
uncalcified, in vitamin-D-resistant rickets, 1108
Osteomalacia
in acidosis, renal tubular, 1122–1123
azotemic, 306, 307–308
and osteitis fibrosa, 313, 316
pathogenesis of, 312–313
phosphate-binding agents in, 322
plasma phosphate levels in, 314
radiology in, 314
vitamin D therapy in, 311, 322
radiology after, 314
calcium excretion in, 905
in Fanconi syndrome, 1095
in interstitial nephritis, chronic, 674
in myelomatosis, 1099